KU-543-344

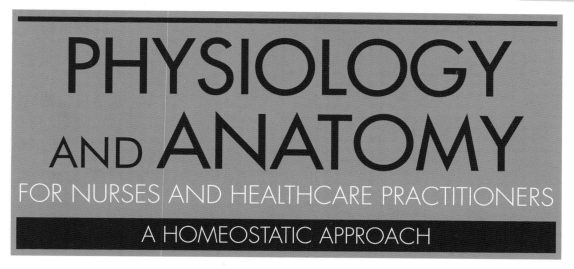

PHYSIOLOGY AND ANATOMY
FOR NURSES AND HEALTHCARE PRACTITIONERS
A HOMEOSTATIC APPROACH

Third edition

John Clancy BSc(Hons), PGCE
Senior Lecturer
Human Applied Sciences
School of Nursing and Midwifery
University of East Anglia
Norwich, UK

Andrew J McVicar BSc(Hons), PhD
Reader
Department of Mental Health and Learning Disabilities
Faculty of Health & Social Care
Anglia Ruskin University
Chelmsford, UK

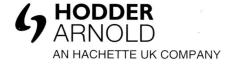
HODDER
ARNOLD
AN HACHETTE UK COMPANY

First published in Great Britain in 1995 by Arnold
Second edition 2002
This third edition published in 2009 by
Hodder Arnold, an imprint of Hodder Education,
an Hachette UK company, 338 Euston Road, London NW1 3BH

http://www.hoddereducation.com

© 2009 John Clancy and Andrew J McVicar

All rights reserved. Apart from any use permitted under UK copyright law, this publication may only be reproduced, stored or transmitted, in any form, or by any means with prior permission in writing of the publishers or in the case of reprographic production in accordance with the terms of licences issued by the Copyright Licensing Agency. In the United Kingdom such licences are issued by the Copyright Licensing Agency: Saffron House, 6–10 Kirby Street, London EC1N 8TS

Hachette UK's policy is to use papers that are natural, renewable and recyclable products and made from wood grown in sustainable forests. The logging and manufacturing processes are expected to conform to the environmental regulations of the country of origin.

Whilst the advice and information in this book are believed to be true and accurate at the date of going to press, neither the authors nor the publisher can accept any legal responsibility or liability for any errors or omissions that may be made. In particular (but without limiting the generality of the preceding disclaimer) every effort has been made to check drug dosages; however it is still possible that errors have been missed. Furthermore, dosage schedules are constantly being revised and new side-effects recognized. For these reasons the reader is strongly urged to consult the drug companies' printed instructions before administering any of the drugs recommended in this book.

British Library Cataloguing in Publication Data
A catalogue record for this book is available from the British Library

Library of Congress Cataloging-in-Publication Data
A catalog record for this book is available from the Library of Congress

ISBN   978 0 340 967591

1 2 3 4 5 6 7 8 9 10

Commissioning Editor: Naomi Wilkinson
Project Editors: Clare Patterson and Joanna Silman
Production Controller: Rachel Manguel
Cover Designer: Laura DeGrasse
Indexer: Dr Laurence Errington

Typeset in 10/12pt Adobe Garamond by Phoenix Photosetting, Chatham, Kent
Printed and bound in Italy

What do you think about this book? Or any other Hodder Arnold title?
Please visit our website: www.hoddereducation.com

PHYSIOLOGY
AND ANATOMY
FOR NURSES AND HEALTHCARE PRACTITIONERS
A HOMEOSTATIC APPROACH

**Books are to be returned on or before
the last date below.**

LIVERPOOL
JOHN MOORES UNIVERSITY
AVRIL ROBARTS LRC
TITHEBARN STREET
LIVERPOOL L2 2ER
TEL. 0151 231 4022

LIBREX-

LIVERPOOL JMU LIBRARY

3 1111 01293 4905

Contents

This book has a companion website available at:
http://www.hodderplus.co.uk/physiologyandanatomy

To access the image library and MCQs included on the website, please register on the website using the following access details:

Serial number: qvhp945bsw32

Preface

The new edition of this popular text continues to present homeostasis as a dynamic concept that provides the basis for understanding health and well-being. It also recognizes how failure to respond to homeostatic disturbances results in homeostatic imbalances responsible for the signs and symptoms of ill health, and how health carers seek to reverse those imbalances by acting as external agents of homeostatic control.

Why *homeostasis*? The concept of homeostasis typically is one of a constant performance or environment, but in physiology such an interpretation is not strictly correct because there must be scope for adaptation to allow people to achieve developmental milestones, or to change performance level according to need – for example, when we perform exercise, when a woman becomes pregnant, when we respond to infection, or when we are recovering from an operation. Homeostasis in the physiological sense therefore represents a dynamism that is central to human functioning. Nevertheless, the concept remains about control; few processes in the body occur by chance, and those that do promote corrective or adaptive responses.

This book is especially concerned with identifying the adaptive responses illustrated in health, the maladaptive processes that are illustrated during ill health, and how the healthcare professional utilises this knowledge in restoring a person's health status or improving the quality of life until death. The intention is to utilize homeostasis as a framework to aid learning and so help the healthcare student to appreciate the physiological rationale of practice.

The education of the healthcare professional places emphasis on producing students and staff knowledgeable about the 'holistic' (physiological, psychological, sociological and spiritual) requirements of health. The integration of physiological functioning into this model has provided difficult in healthcare education, and the need to describe and explain body functioning in the context of an interactive framework prompted the writing of previous editions of this book, as well as many subsequent articles on the theme of homeostasis.

This third edition builds on the successful format, providing nature–nurture interactions as a basis of this interactive framework. The book gives an integrated explanation of body functioning, with descriptions of related anatomy in health, illness and health care. This exciting new edition has been updated and extended to provides the following new material:

- Overview of microbiology and principles of infection management.
- Extended information on pharmacological principles and actions of the major classes of drugs.
- Extended application of physiological functions in relation to specific pathologies, and examples of health care.
- Updates on how the Human Genome Project is beginning to impact on health care.

- More case studies to illustrate the health carer's role as an external agent of homeostatic control.
- New, improved colour design.
- Photographs of common clinical conditions.
- An accompanying website www.hodderplus.co.uk/physiologyandanatomy

The book is divided into six major sections:

- *Section I: An introduction to the human body*. This introductory section considers the construction of the human body and what is meant by cell function. The basic principles of homeostasis are explored in depth. Although each chapter can be read individually, the reader is strongly encouraged to read Chapter 1 first since the principles discussed, and in particular the inclusion of a simple but unique aid to learning – the homeostatic graph – are the foundations for what follows in the other chapters.
- *Section II: The need for regulation*. This second section identifies the fundamentals of human body functioning, including the composition of the body, its chemical reactions (metabolism) and the physiological rationale underlying a healthy diet.
- *Section III: Sensing change and coordinating responses*. This third section explains how the internal (and external) environment is identified by individual or sense organ receptors, and how adaptive responses are enabled and coordinated by the nervous and endocrine systems.
- *Section IV: Effectors of homeostasis*. This section considers further systems of the human body that are themselves capable of bringing about change, and so provide the means of correcting homeostatic disturbances of excess and deficits.
- *Section V: Influences on homeostasis*. The penultimate section considers some of the vital interactive components that promote variation in the human body. It discusses the influence of genes and environmental factors in human development and ageing, and the nature–nurture interactions associated with the perception of pain and distress, and in the control of bodily rhythms over the 24-hour period.
- *Section VI: Healthcare practice: A homeostatic approach*. This final section provides numerous examples of case studies that illustrate homeostatic principles in relation to healthcare problems and how healthcare practitioner may be considered to be an external agent of homeostatic control.

Each chapter provides frequent cross-referencing to other chapters in a manner that can only provide the reader with a greater understanding of the integrated functioning of the human body in health and illness.

Although the book assumes some knowledge of physiology, it identifies and explains the main aspects of function that in turn relate to homeostasis, homeostatic disturbance and homeostatic imbalances. Application Boxes are used throughout to reinforce how healthcare practitioners act as external agents of homeostatic control to minimise, or reverse, functional disturbance in their patients. Activities and reflective questions are included within the text and illustrations of each chapter to test the reader's understanding.

The authors between them have over 50 years' experience of teaching physiology to healthcare practitioners, and they understand what an overwhelming subject the student is faced with when studying physiology and anatomy. Their objective is not for the reader to memorise the contents of each chapter (that would be truly remarkable!), but merely to grasp a general understanding of homeostasis in action, since the book can always be referred to for further reference when needed.

Finally, we hope you enjoy reading the book, and that it will contribute to a better understanding of your role as a healthcare practitioner and of your patients, to the ultimate benefit of both.

John Clancy
Andrew McVicar
October 2008

PS. We would value comments on the value of this book so that the next edition will evolve!

Acknowledgements

For the third edition of *Physiology and Anatomy for Nurses and Healthcare Practitioners: A Homeostatic Approach*, we have enjoyed the opportunity of collaborating with a group of dedicated talented professionals. Accordingly, we would like to take the opportunity to recognize and thank the members of our book team and also the people who have helped and encouraged us along the way.

First, we are extremely grateful to the authors of the case studies, whose contributions to the book have richly enhanced its healthcare application to the principles of homeostasis. Some of these authors are former students who have hopefully been inspired by our teaching since their application of homeostasis to their practice is in turn becoming infectious to the students under their supervision. Please keep spreading the word.

Special mention must be made of one of the authors – Sue Harry – who unfortunately passed away during the writing of this book. This edition is dedicated to the memory of her professionalism, which should be the benchmark to which all healthcare professionals should aspire.

The assistance, support enthusiasm, skill and investment in the text on the part of the editorial and production teams at Hodder Arnold have been equally valuable to make the entire project possible and keep the text, art and production programmes on schedule. Special thanks go to Clare Patterson, Joanna Silman, Naomi Wilkinson, Joanna Koster, Claire Gordon, Andrew Anderson, Carole Goodall and finally, in anticipation of booming sales figures, Max Espley and the sales team.

The clinical photographs have been a signature feature of this third edition, and our particular appreciation goes to Simon Dove and his medical illustrators from the Norfolk and Norwich University Hospital NHS Trust for their help with these valuable resources. Also special thanks go to the patients who have given their permission to use their photographs.

We are grateful too to colleagues for their continued support, for putting up with our enthusiasm when we constantly talked about the third edition, and also for putting up with our mood swings when we were working to deadlines. Our employers, the University of East Anglia and Anglia Ruskin University, in particular our faculties, have given their continued support in this project.

We also appreciate the work of the reviewers of the second edition, whose excellent reviews and evaluative feedback provided the motivation to produce this exciting third edition. We would like to express our sincere gratitude to Nicola Baird, who provided the perioperative expertise throughout the third edition, and Gary Parlett, who reviewed the coronary care input in Chapter 12.

Finally and most importantly, a special thank you to our families: to Rachel, Penny and our beautiful and wonderful children Lauren, Clare and Lisa for their love, smiles, encouragement and support; to our very special parents Ann and Norman Clancy, and James and Mary McVicar; and to our brothers – all these have made this project extremely worthwhile.

John Clancy
Andrew McVicar

Authors of Case Studies

Chapter 2. Breast cancer: Sue Harry and Linda Purdy

Sue Harry RGN, DN, BSc (Hons), CertEd, MA
Former Lecturer in Adult Nursing, University of East Anglia, Faculty of Health, School of Nursing and Midwifery, Norwich

Linda Purdy RGN, RN Child, Dip HE Nursing Practice, Dip HE Children's Nursing, BSc (Hons), Post Grad Diploma (Learning and Teaching)
Sister/Nurse Practitioner in Accident and Emergency, Queen Elizabeth Hospital, Kings Lynn

Chapter 3. Rheumatoid arthritis: Janice Mooney

Janice Mooney RGN, BSc (Hons), PGDHE, DMS, MSc
Lecturer in Primary Care and Director of MSc Advanced Practitioner, University of East Anglia, Faculty of Health, School of Nursing and Midwifery, Norwich

Chapter 4. Diabetes mellitus: Elaine Domek

Elaine Domek RGN, RSCN, ONC, INP, BA, PGCE
Senior Paediatric Nurse Practitioner,
James Paget University Hospitals NHS Foundation Trust
and
Former Lecturer in Children's Nursing, University of East Anglia, Faculty of Health, School of Nursing and Midwifery, Norwich

Chapter 5. Obesity: Penny Goacher

Penny Goacher BSc (Hons), FAETC, MPhil
Lecturer in Human Physiology Applied to Health, University of East Anglia, Faculty of Health, School of Nursing and Midwifery, Norwich

Chapter 6. Hypovolaemia: Judy Barker

Judy Barker RODP, BA (Hons), PGHEP, FETC
Lecturer in Operating Department Practice, University of East Anglia, Faculty of Health, School of Nursing and Midwifery, Norwich

Chapter 7. Cataract: Steve Smith

Steve Smith RGN, BSc (Hons), PGCE, MSc
Lecturer in Adult Nursing, University of East Anglia, Faculty of Health, School of Nursing and Midwifery, Norwich

Chapter 8. Depression: Derek Shirtliffe and Rosie Doy

Derek Shirtliffe DN, Certificate (Child and Adolescent Psychiatry), CertEd, RNLD, BSc (Hons), PhD
Former Lecturer in Learning Disability, Nursing, University of East Anglia, Faculty of Health, School of Nursing and Midwifery, Norwich

Rosie Doy RN (G), RN (MH), NEBSS Cert, CTC, CertEd, MA
Director of Post Registration Studies, and Lecturer in Mental Health, University of East Anglia, Faculty of Health, School of Nursing and Midwifery, Norwich

Chapter 9. Hypothyroidism: John Clancy and Andrew McVicar

John Clancy BSc (Hons), PGCE, CertECBS
Lecturer in Human Physiology Applied to Health, University of East Anglia, Faculty of Health, School of Nursing and Midwifery, Norwich

Andrew McVicar BSc (Hons), PhD
Reader in Physiology Applied to Health Care, Faculty of Health and Social Care, Anglia Ruskin University, Chelmsford

Chapter 10. Pyloric stenosis: Theresa Atherton and Wendy Dubbin

Theresa Atherton RGN, RSCN, DN, BSc (Hons), CertEd, MA
Former Lecturer in Children's Nursing, Nursing, University of East Anglia, Faculty of Health, School of Nursing and Midwifery, Norwich

Wendy Dubbin RGN, RSCN, BSc (Hons), PG Dip, MSc
Course Director/Lecturer – Children's Nursing, University of East Anglia, Faculty of Health, School of Nursing and Midwifery, Norwich

Chapter 11. Deep vein thrombosis: Elizabeth Lorie

Elizabeth Lorie BSc (Hons), RGN
Anticoagulation Nurse Specialist
DVT Clinic, Norfolk and Norwich University Hospital NHS Foundation Trust, Norwich

Chapter 12. Myocardial infarction: Julia Hubbard

Julia Hubbard RN, RNT, DipHE, BSc (Hons), PGDHE, MSc
Director Pre-Registration Nursing and Lecturer in Coronary Care, University of East Anglia, Faculty of Health, School of Nursing and Midwifery, Norwich

SECTION
1

AN INTRODUCTION TO THE HUMAN BODY

Chapter 1

INTRODUCTION TO PHYSIOLOGY AND HOMEOSTASIS

INTRODUCTION TO THE HUMAN BODY, ITS ORGANIZATION, AND THE HOMEOSTATIC BASIS OF BODY FUNCTIONS

You are about to begin the study of the human body. This book will enable you to learn how your body is organized structurally, and how it functions. The study of the human body involves several branches of science: biology, chemistry, physics, mathematics, psychology and sociology. Each contributes an understanding of how the body functions in health, during times of exercise, illness, pain, distress, trauma and surgery. Thus, an understanding of these sciences to varying degrees, and how they link together, is of paramount importance to healthcare professionals, who need to view each patient as an individual. However, it must be stressed at the onset that human beings are biological organisms. We may live in highly sophisticated societies, and have very complex behaviours and different cognitive abilities, but healthcare professionals should not lose sight of the fact that ultimately our 'health' depends upon the functioning of biological structures.

The two branches of science covered in this book that will help you understand the human body are anatomy and physiology. Identifiable within these is the central concept referred to as homeostasis.

Definitions

Human anatomy refers to the study of the structure of the body. Physiology is concerned with the mechanisms of human bodily function. In this book you will see how the structure of the body is custom-built to perform particular functions in health (a sense of well-being). It follows, therefore, that abnormal structure leads to the abnormal functioning associated with ill health. This structural and functional relationship is referred to by biologists as the 'principle of complementarity'.

Homeostasis refers to the automatic, self-regulating processes necessary to maintain the 'normal' state of the body's environment, despite changes in the environment outside that body. Collectively, anatomical structure, physiological function and the maintenance of homeostasis enable the body to attain the basic needs necessary for health and a 'normal' life. This aspect is considered later in this chapter: before contemplating these basic needs, the reader should become familiar with how the body is organized.

Anatomical organization

The outside of the human body has a definite and recognizable shape. The inside has organs, which are located in specific positions relative to one another. The anatomical position of the body provides a reference point when studying or describing the position of body structures. This position is when the person stands erect and faces forward, with arms at his/her side with palms facing forwards. For example, organs such as the heart are drawn according to this convention; features on, say, the left side appear on the right, as though the observer is looking into someone's chest.

A set of standard anatomical terms is used to describe each part of the body, the position of body structures, and their geographical relationships with each other. Many of these regional terms are illustrated in Figure 1.1. The main terms used relate to 'planes of the body', 'relative positioning of organs' and 'body cavity'.

Planes of the body

Body structures can be described in relation to three planes or imaginary lines – median (mid-sagittal), transverse (horizontal) and coronal (frontal) – which run through the body (Figure 1.2). The median plane passes directly along the midline of the body, dividing the body into perfectly symmetrical right and left halves. The transverse plane passes horizontally through the body, dividing it into upper and lower portions. The coronal plane divides the body into front and back portions.

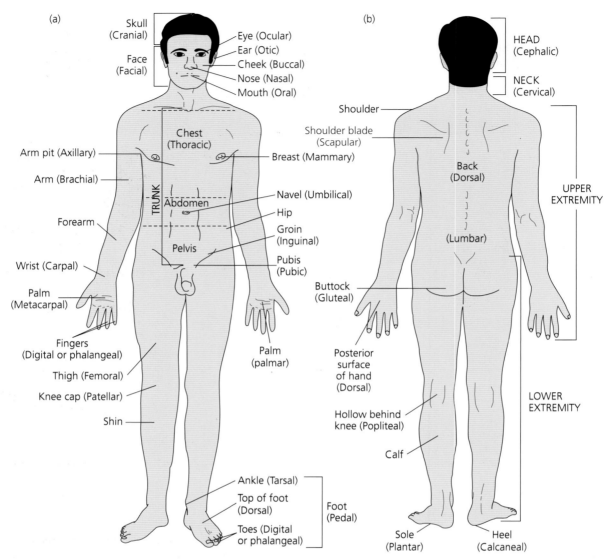

Figure 1.1 Anatomical position. The common names and anatomical terms (in brackets) are indicated for many of the regions of the human body. (a) Anterior view; (b) posterior view

Terms of relative position

Directional terms are also used to describe the position of structures relative to each other (Figure 1.2). For example, 'anterior' and 'ventral' are used interchangeably and refer to the front surface of the body. They also have a broader meaning in the sense of a structure being closer to the front of the body. Examples are 'anterior abdominal wall' or 'the heart is anterior to the spine'. In the same way, 'posterior' may refer to the back surface of the body, or it may mean a structure is nearer to the back of the body. Examples are 'the posterior surface of the arm' or the 'oesophagus (food pipe) is posterior to the heart'. 'Dorsal' is linked similarly to posterior. Similarly, 'medial' indicates that a structure is towards the midline of the body, whereas 'lateral' designates that a structure is away from the midline of the body. 'Proximal' indicates that the structure concerned is nearer the attached end of a limb, and thus the trunk of the body, while a 'distal' structure is further away from the attached end of a limb and/or the trunk. As an example, the shoulder is proximal to the elbow, whereas the elbow is distal to the shoulder.

In the clinical environment, healthcare professionals need to be familiar with these terms so they are all speaking the same language to avoid mistakes being made.

Initially, anatomical terminology may seem unfamiliar and difficult to understand. However, once you have mastered an understanding of basic words, including prefixes (the beginning of a word), roots (the main body of the word) and suffixes

ACTIVITY

Use a biological dictionary to find out what the following terms mean: afferent, efferent, peripheral, deep, superficial, internal, external.

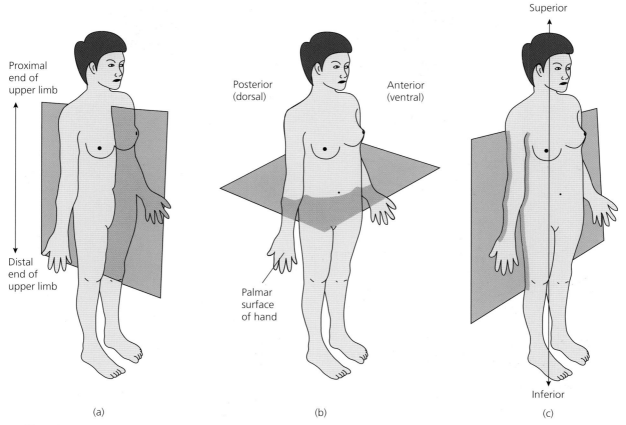

Figure 1.2 Planes through the body. (a) Medial (mid-sagittal) plane; (b) transverse plane; (c) coronal (frontal) plane

Q *Which plane divides the body into (1) anterior and posterior parts, (2) right and left parts that are mirror images of each other, and (3) superior and inferior portions?*

Q *Is the hip proximal or distal to the knee?*

(the end of a word), you will discover the logical and helpful method in which structures are named. For example, once you understand that the prefix 'electro-' means electrical, the root 'cardiac' refers to the heart, and the suffix '-gram' means recording, then the meaning of the term 'electrocardiogram' becomes apparent.

Body cavities

The body can be divided into cavities produced by the bony skeleton (Figure 1.3). These cavities contain the internal organs (viscera). The main body cavities are:

- *The cranial cavity*: the bones of the skull enclose this cavity, which accommodates and protects the brain.

ACTIVITY

Using Appendix C, try to learn 10 common prefixes and suffixes every weekday. When you are satisfied that you know most of the common prefixes and suffixes, learn 20 commonly used roots of the words. This will help you to understand the unfamiliar terminology associated with the clinical area.

- *The spinal cavity*: this is formed by a hole (foramen = 'window') running through the vertebral column. This is called the vertebral canal, and it accommodates and protects the spinal cord.
- *The thoracic cavity*: this is the upper cavity of the trunk of the body. Its confines are the breastbone (sternum), ribs and associated intercostal muscles ('inter-' = between, '-cost' = rib) and cartilage, vertebral column, diaphragm, and the structures below the neck. The cavity contains the windpipe (trachea), two lungs, the heart and its great vessels, the food pipe (oesophagus), and associated nerves and lymphatic supply. The space between the lungs, occupied by the heart, is called the mediastinum.
- *The abdominal cavity*: this is the large lower portion of the trunk. It is confined by the diaphragm, pelvic cavity, spine, abdominal muscles and lower ribs. It accommodates the organs concerned with digestion and absorption of nutrients, and other organs associated with these functions, such as the gall bladder, liver, spleen and pancreas. The kidneys, ureters and adrenal glands are also located in this region.
- *The pelvic cavity*: this is the lowest portion of the trunk, and is a continuation of the abdominal cavity. Its boundaries are

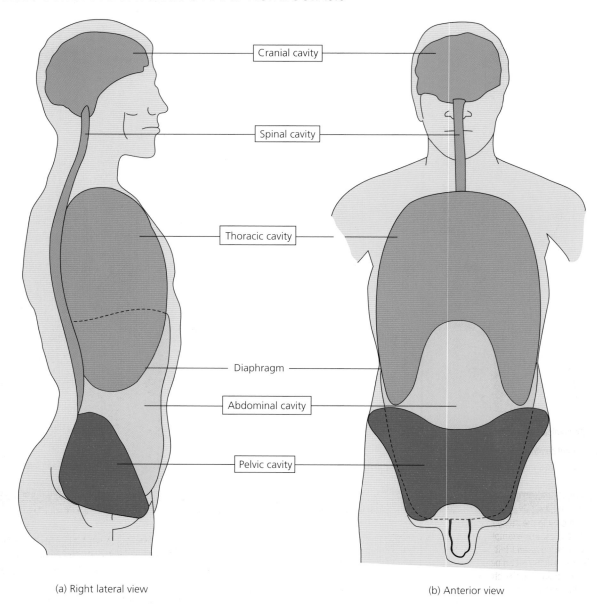

(a) Right lateral view

(b) Anterior view

Figure 1.3 Lateral and anterior views of the human body showing major cavities

Q *What are the confines of (1) the thoracic cavity, (2) the abdominal cavity, and (3) the pelvic cavity?*

the bony pelvis, sacrum and muscles of the pelvic floor. It contains the female reproductive structures, or some of the male reproductive structures (lower ureters, bladder and urethra). Other pelvic organs include the small intestine and the last part of the colon, the rectum and anal canal. It also includes the openings for the urethra, vagina and anus.

Blood vessels, lymphatic nodes and associated nerves are located in all the cavities. Sometimes it is necessary to be much more precise in locating organs of the body. A good example of this is the quadrants and the nine regions associated with the abdomen and pelvic areas (Figure 1.4). A surgeon requires such precision when a surgical incision has to be made.

Using appropriate terminology, describe the anatomical location of the organs of the thoracic and pelvic cavities of the body in relation to each other. Also, look up the prefixes associated with each major organ within the five major cavities of the body.

The basic needs of the human body

The basic needs of the living body identified by biologists as the characteristics of life are:

1 *Feeding or nutrition*: this encompasses the intake of raw materials to maintain life processes such as growth, repair and the maintenance of a normal environment inside the body.

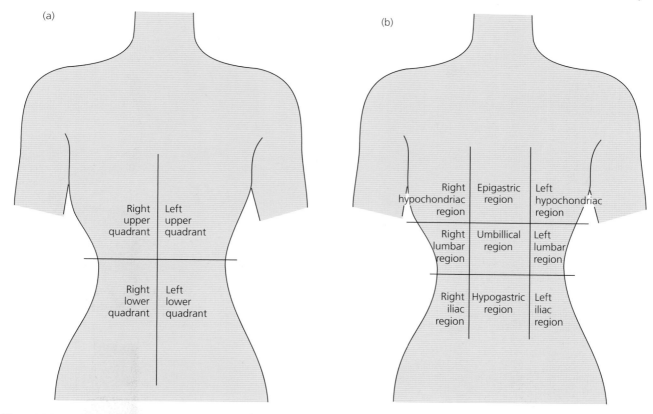

(a)

Right upper quadrant | Left upper quadrant

Right lower quadrant | Left lower quadrant

(b)

Right hypochondriac region | Epigastric region | Left hypochondriac region

Right lumbar region | Umbilical region | Left lumbar region

Right iliac region | Hypogastric region | Left iliac region

Figure 1.4 Anatomical subdivisions: (a) Quadrants of the abdomen; (b) The nine regions of the abdominal and pelvic regions.

Q Which quadrant confines the stomach?

Q Which region confines the appendix?

BOX 1.1 SURFACE ANATOMICAL LANDMARKS AND SOME MEDICAL TERMS

Surface anatomy is the study of external structures and their relation to deeper structures. For example, the breastbone (sternum) and parts of the ribs can be seen and felt (palpated) on the anterior aspects of the chest. These structures can be used as landmarks to identify regions of the heart and points on the chest at which certain heart sounds can be heard using a stethoscope (a process called auscultation). The normal 'lub-dup' sounds of the heart reflect normal structure and functioning of the heart valves. A deviation of this sound to the trained ear reflects abnormal structure and hence functioning.

Anatomical imaging involves the use of X-rays, ultrasound, computed tomography scans, and other technologies to create pictures of internal structures. Both surface anatomy and anatomical imaging provide important information in diagnosing disease. Healthcare professionals will become familiar with such techniques during their training.

The following terms are used to apply anatomy and physiology to some specialties in medical science (you may need to look up the suffix '-ology'):

- *Allergy:* diagnosis and treatment of allergic conditions
- *Cardiology:* the heart and its diseases
- *Endocrinology:* glands that release hormones and hormone disorders
- *Gastroenterology:* the stomach and intestines and their disorders
- *Gynaecology:* disorders of the female urinary tract and female reproductive organs
- *Haematology:* blood and blood disorders
- *Immunology:* mechanisms by which the body resists disease
- *Neurology:* the nervous system and its disorders
- *Obstetrics:* pregnancy and childbirth
- *Oncology:* cancer
- *Ophthalmology:* eye disorders
- *Otorhinolaryngology:* ear, nose and throat
- *Pathology:* diagnosis of disease based on changes in cells and tissues
- *Proctology:* disease of the colon, rectum and anus
- *Toxicology:* poisons
- *Urology:* disorders of the urinary tract and male reproductive organs

2 *Movement*: this is a characteristic in that people, or some parts of them, are capable of changing position.

3 *Respiration*: this refers to the processes concerned with the production of the energy (and related ideal body temperature and pH) necessary to maintain life processes and movement. In humans it involves breathing (external respiration)

and the breakdown of food (internal respiration) inside the cells of the body.

4 *Excretion*: this is the removal from the body of waste products of chemical reactions, and excesses of certain dietary substances (e.g. water).

5 *Sensitivity and responsiveness*: these are the processes

BOX 1.2 ACTIVITIES OF DAILY LIVING

To help nurses direct care to the basic needs of the body, Roper *et al.* in the 1980s devised a nursing model called the Activities of Daily Living (ADL) (Table 1.1).

Table 1.1 Activities of Daily Living (ADLs)

Breathing*
Eating and drinking*
Elimination*
Mobilizing*
Controlling body temperature
Maintaining a safe environment
Sleeping
Personal cleaning and dressing
Working and playing
Communication
Expressing sexuality*
Dying

*Based on basic needs of life. Others relate to further human needs. Table after Roper *et al.* (1990)

There is an underpinning assumption that the foundations of the earlier ADL models postulated by Roper *et al.* were adapted to the characteristics of life identified previously by biologists.

Human beings therefore are self-reproducing systems capable of growing and of maintaining their integrity by the expenditure of energy. They are, however, complex organisms, having cellular, tissue, organ and organ system levels of organization (Figure 1.5).

concerned with monitoring, detecting and responding to changes in the environment inside and outside the human body.

6 *Growth*: this generally implies an increase in size and complexity. It also includes repair of body parts which have undergone damage or need to be replaced.

7 *Reproduction*: this is necessary for the continuation of the species.

LEVELS OF ORGANIZATION

Cellular level

The human body is composed of trillions of microscopic cells. Each cell is regarded as a basic unit of life, since it is the smallest component capable of performing most, if not all, of the characteristics of life (or basic needs). Cells can digest food, generate energy, move, respond to stimuli, grow, excrete and reproduce. To support these activities, cells contain organelles that perform these specific functions (see Figure 2.3, p.24 and Table 2.1 p.25). To facilitate cell function throughout the body, the body contains many distinct kinds of cells, each specialized to perform specific functions. Examples include blood cells, muscle cells and bone cells. Each has a unique structure related to its function (see Figures 1.5 and 2.2, p.24). Receptors on the cell membrane or inside the cell inform genes of the desired function of the cell at any one moment in time. Genes are the controllers of all the cell's chemical reactions (collectively called metabolism), and these act indirectly

through their role in enzyme production. Enzymes are therefore of fundamental importance in the human body since they directly speed up chemical reactions so that they are compatible with a healthy life (Figure 1.6), but optimal enzyme action requires a microenvironment of ideal acidity and temperature. Genes are commonly referred to as the 'code of life' and enzymes as the 'key chemicals of life'. Adenosine triphosphate (abbreviated as ATP) is also another key chemical of life since this chemical is the cell's energy store, which is required to drive metabolic reactions at a rate that is harmonious with health (Figure 1.6). The chemical level of organization regarding cell structure and function is discussed in Chapter 5 under the umbrella term 'chemicals of life'.

Tissue level

A tissue is defined as a collection of similar cells and their component parts that perform specialized functions. There are many different types of tissues, so it follows that there must be different cell types that comprise these tissues. However, the entire body consists of just four primary tissues: epithelial or lining tissues, binding or connective tissues, muscular tissues, and nervous tissues (see Chapter 2, pp.52–8).

Organ and organ system levels

An organ is an orderly grouping of tissues that give it discrete function. Examples of organs are the heart, spleen, ovary and skin. Most organs contain all four primary tissues. In the stomach, for example, the inside epithelial lining performs functions of secretion of gastric juice and absorption of some chemicals such as alcohol. The wall of the stomach, however, also contains muscle tissue (for contraction of the stomach) to help with the breakdown of food, nervous tissue (for regulation), and connective tissue (to bind the other tissues together).

An organ system is a group of organs that act together to perform a specific body function, e.g. the respiratory system maintains the levels of oxygen and carbon dioxide in the blood. These systems work with each other in a coordinated way to maintain the functions of the body. The concepts of tubular (hollow) organs and compact (parenchymal) organs are introduced in Chapter 2, pp.58–9. The details associated with each organ are dealt with in their respective chapters, but the integration of organ function is important to note in this introductory chapter.

Each level of organization is instrumental in sustaining the functions of life for the human body. Table 1.2 illustrates each organ system's involvement in the regulation of the basic needs of the individual.

The basic needs are related to, and interdependent on, each other. For example, we must take in the raw materials of food and oxygen (both metabolites) in order to provide sufficient energy (ATP) to maintain normal body function (Figure 1.6). This energy is needed to support chemical reactions, such as those involved in growth and the muscle contraction necessary for movement. Consequently, these raw materials can be viewed as being the 'chemicals of life' (see Chapter 5).

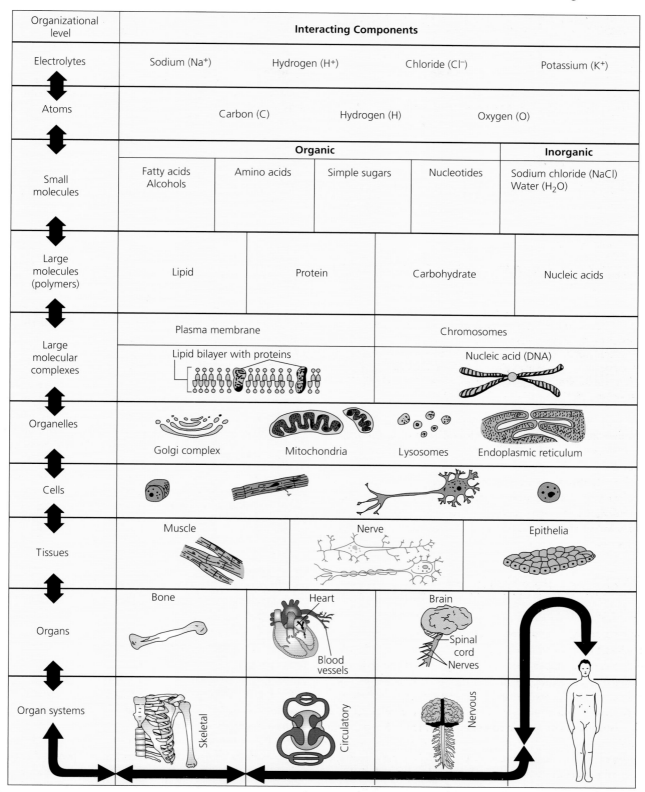

Organizational level	Interacting Components			
Electrolytes	Sodium (Na$^+$)	Hydrogen (H$^+$)	Chloride (Cl$^-$)	Potassium (K$^+$)
Atoms	Carbon (C)	Hydrogen (H)	Oxygen (O)	
Small molecules	**Organic** Fatty acids / Alcohols	Amino acids — Simple sugars — Nucleotides		**Inorganic** Sodium chloride (NaCl) / Water (H$_2$O)
Large molecules (polymers)	Lipid	Protein	Carbohydrate	Nucleic acids
Large molecular complexes	Plasma membrane Lipid bilayer with proteins		Chromosomes Nucleic acid (DNA)	
Organelles	Golgi complex — Mitochondria — Lysosomes — Endoplasmic reticulum			
Cells				
Tissues	Muscle	Nerve	Epithelia	
Organs	Bone	Heart / Blood vessels	Brain / Spinal cord / Nerves	
Organ systems	Skeletal	Circulatory	Nervous	

Figure 1.5 The hierarchy of organizational levels of the human organism indicates that specific interactions at each simpler level produce the more complex level above it.

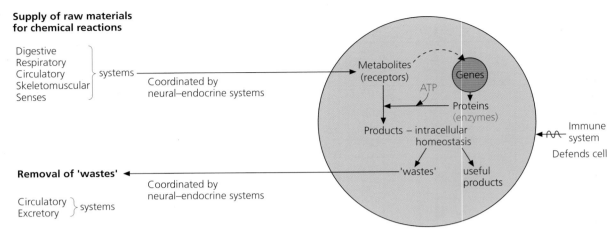

Figure 1.6 Involvement of organ systems in the regulation of intracellular homeostasis

Q Suggest why the following statements are used in physiology: (1) genes, 'the code of life'; (2) enzymes, 'the key chemicals of life'.

Table 1.2 Organ system involvement in maintaining the basic needs of the human body. The table demonstrates that all the organ systems are involved in maintaining the normal environment needed by the cells of the body, to enable them to perform the basic needs of the individual during health

Basic need	Organ systems involved
Intake of raw material	
Food	Digestive
Oxygen	Respiratory
Internal transportation	Circulatory, lymphatic
Excretion	Urinary, respiratory, the skin
Sensitivity and irritability	
Environment outside the body	Special senses, nervous, skeletomuscular
Environment inside the body	Nervous, endocrine
Defence	
Environment outside the body	Skin, special senses
Environment inside the body	Immune, digestive, endocrine
Movement within the environment	Skeletal, muscular, nervous, special senses
Reproduction	Reproductive, endocrine

Chemical reactions also produce waste products; these must be removed from the body to prevent cellular disturbances.

The interdependence of the basic needs means that a failure of one function leads to a deterioration of others (emphasizing further the 'principle of complementary'). For example, malnutrition ('mal-' = bad or poor) results in the retardation of growth and development, lethargy, poor tissue maintenance, a reduced capacity to avoid infection, and a general failure to thrive.

Disorders arise at a cellular level, and, because of the interdependence of the components of the body, this means that a failure of one function leads to a deterioration of others. This is reflected in the diverse signs and symptoms of ill health that require clinical intervention to restore health (or homeostasis). For example, a patient who has had a heart condition may display signs and symptoms that reflect poor functioning of not only the heart, but also lungs and kidneys.

BOX 1.3 ILLNESS – A CELLULAR IMBALANCE

Since health is dependent upon optimal functioning of cellular components – receptors, genes, enzymes – and the cell's microenvironment being ideally suitable for this optimal functioning, it follows that ultimately every illness originates from a functional disturbance arising from the cellular components (i.e. receptors and/or genes and/or enzymes) and/or the microenvironment at the cellular level. Arguably, cellular respiration is the most important chemical reaction in the human body, since its end products (ATP, heat and acidity) are essential in the provision of this ideal environment for optimal cellular metabolism (see Figure 2.11, p.36 and Box 2.1, p.22).

In the context of this introductory chapter, it seems logical to establish the basis for optimum (ideal) biological functioning. The main topic reviewed in the remainder of this chapter is homeostasis.

HOMEOSTASIS: THE LINK WITH HEALTH

An introduction to homeostatic control theory

The word 'homeostasis' literally translates as 'same standing', and is usually taken to indicate constancy or balance. Those students who have entered health care in recent years, having taken courses that have had a significant human biology component, are likely to have come across the term, since it is an important concept, especially in physiological studies.

The idea that a constancy of the internal environment of the human body is essential to life can be traced back to the views of the eminent French physiologist Claude Bernard, in the mid-nineteenth century. The turn of the twentieth century produced many important discoveries of how the body is regulated by hormonal and neural mechanisms.

In order to perform the basic functions of life successfully, there must be a 'consistency' within the body, and in particular in the environment inside cells, called the intracellular fluid ('intra-' = inside). The regulation of the composition and volume of fluids that surround cells, which collectively are called the extracellular fluids, helps to keep this environment constant. The main components of these fluids are discussed in detail in Chapter 6. Briefly, they are:

- *Tissue fluid*: the fluid in which body cells are bathed. It acts as an intermediary between the cells and blood.
- *Plasma*: the cell-free component of blood. Together with blood cells, it circulates through the heart and blood vessels, supplying nutritive materials to cells and removing waste products from them.

Two processes by which the composition of these fluids is kept constant are:

- the intake of raw materials;
- the removal (excretion) of waste products of chemical reactions from the body, or the removal of excess chemicals that cannot be stored, destroyed or transferred to other substances inside the body.

Conventionally, homeostasis is therefore frequently considered to represent a balance or equilibrium between these two processes.

The modern view is that homeostasis is dependent upon an integration of physiological functions, since essentially all the organs of the body perform functions that help to maintain these constant conditions. The authors share the view that all the organ systems are homeostatic controllers that regulate the environment within cells throughout the body (Figure 1.6). This book concentrates on the homeostatic principles of human physiology, emphasizing in particular the role of each system in the maintenance of an optimal cellular environment (i.e. cellular homeostasis). It also discusses the influence of homeostatic control failure in producing some of the more common illnesses (i.e. homeostatic imbalances) that nurses, midwives and other healthcare practitioners are likely to encounter during their careers. In addition, the principles of healthcare intervention are mentioned in relation to the re-establishment of homeostasis and 'health' for the individual.

Principles of homeostasis

Cannon (1932), who introduced the term 'homeostasis', defined homeostasis as 'a condition, which may vary, but remains relatively constant'. It was this definition, together with experience gained working alongside nurses and mid-wives using clinical laboratory values (Table 1.3), that inspired the authors to design the homeostatic graph (Figure 1.7). This is a simplified model to aid the understanding of a patient's physiological and biochemical parameters in health and disease.

Readers of this textbook are strongly recommended to familiarize themselves with this figure before dipping into other chapters, since variants of it are used throughout this book as a model to explain:

- homeostatic principles;
- how components of homeostasis (receptors, genes and enzymes) control cellular and hence body function;
- how the microenvironment (ATP, pH, temperature, composition) of the cell must be tightly controlled to optimize the production of the above homeostatic components and their functioning;
- how failure of the homeostatic components and/or changes to the microenvironment results in illness, and even death;
- an individualized approach to care, in which healthcare interventions are used to re-establish homeostasis for the patient, or to provide palliative care in symptom control to improve the quality of life for the dying patient.

The homeostatic range

The variations in parameter values provide a range within which the parameter can be considered to be regulated. Parameters within the body include: the concentration of chemicals within the body fluids (e.g. blood glucose), an expression of a function of an organ (e.g. heart rate), or the number of a particular cell type (e.g. red blood cell). The fluctuation in parameter values within their normal (or homeostatic) ranges provides the optimal condition in the body (Table 1.3 and Figure 1.7). The range reflects:

- *The precision by which a parameter is regulated*: some parameters, such as body temperature, have a very narrow range (adult values = 36.2–37.7°C), while others, for example blood volume, have a relatively larger range (male adult values = 52–83 mL/kg).

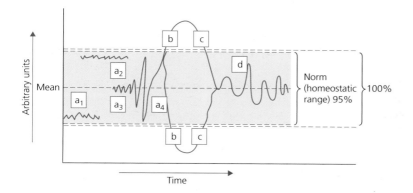

Figure 1.7 Principles of homeostatic control. (a_{1-4}) Homeostatic dynamism: values fluctuating within the homeostatic range, reflecting individual variation within the population (see text for details). (b) Homeostatic disturbance. (c) Homeostatic control mechanisms restore homeostasis. (d) Homeostasis re-established

Q Suggest how the homeostatic range accounts for every individual in the population.

Table 1.3 Normal laboratory blood values*

Clinical chemistry	Normal adult value (homeostatic range)
Sodium	136–148 mmol/L
Potassium	3.8–5.0 mmol/L
Bicarbonate	24–32 mmol/L
Urea	2.6–6.5 mmol/L
Creatinine	60–120 mmol/L
Glucose	Random, 3.0–9.4 mmol/L
CSF glucose	2.5–5.6 mmol/L
Total protein	62–82 g/L
Albumin	36–52 g/L
Globulin	20–37 g/L
Calcium	2.2–2.6 mmol/L
Transaminase	Up to 35 IU/L
pH	7.35–7.45
PCO_2	4.7–6.0 kPa
PO_2	11.3–14.0 kPa

CSF, cerebrospinal fluid; PCO_2, partial pressure of carbon dioxide; PO_2, partial pressure of oxygen.

*Note values are guides for judging health and disease. These ranges have proved to be clinically useful for judging health, disease and recovery in hospital wards and clinics

Q *Describe in scientific terms what is meant by the term 'normal range' when equated with the values expressed in clinical laboratory tables.*

ACTIVITY

Obtain from your clinical directorate a biochemistry ('U&Es') report and note the normal values.

- *Individual variation of values within the population*: one person's normal levels could fluctuate just above the minimum values of the range (Figure 1.7, a_1), while another person's optimal range could fluctuate close to the maximum values (Figure 1.7, a_2). It is also considered normal for some individuals to deviate on either side of the mean (or average) value (Figure 1.7, a_3). To account for all individual variations within the population, it is also possible for some individuals to 'bounce' between the minimum, mean and maximum values (Figure 1.7, a_4).
- *Variation of values within each person according to the changing metabolic demands*: it is quite usual for the maximum and minimum values of some parameters to vary within the individual as the person passes through the different developmental stages of the lifespan (Table 1.3 and Boxes 1.5 and 1.6). The dashed lines associated with the maximum, mean and minimum values in Figure 1.7 indicate the dynamic nature of these values (i.e. for some parameters the maximum value may increase). It is generally well known, for example, that blood pressure increases with the age of an individual, while most other parameter values decrease with adult age (e.g. muscle strength, visual acuity; see Chapter 19, pp.549–33).
- *Variation within each person occurring during times of illness*: (see the case studies in Section VI and the boxes in Chapters

---

BOX 1.4 PREGNANCY AS AN ALTERED STATE OF HEALTH

Midwives often refer to pregnancy as an 'altered state of health'. That is, variations of the homeostatic values of physiological parameters in pregnancy are considered quite normal and necessary for the development of the unborn baby. For example, the hormones oestrogen and progesterone surpass levels experienced in the non-pregnant state. This variation is necessary if implantation and placentation are to ensure structural and functional development of the unborn baby. The new homeostatic range has been adapted to meet the changing anatomical/physiological requirements associated with the developmental stage, pregnancy.

1–18, 21 and 22). Variations also need to account for the changes associated with the individual's sleep–wake activities (circadian patterns, 'circa-' = about, '-dies' = day; see Section VI).

The maintenance of a constant arterial blood pressure is frequently cited in textbooks as an illustration of a homeostatic process at work. However, it is important that this pressure is increased naturally during exercise as it increases blood flow through the exercising muscle, ensuring that the oxygen supply to the muscle supports the increased demand. The elevation of blood pressure in exercise is itself a homeostatic adaptive process. It acts to provide the appropriate environment for the changing chemical needs of muscle, and this highlights the most important feature of homeostasis: physio-

---

BOX 1.5 CLINICAL NORMAL AND ABNORMAL VALUES

In scientific research the term 'normal' means conforming to the usual healthy pattern. The normal (homeostatic) range in statistical terms defines values of parameters expected for 95% of the healthy population (e.g. the normal range of blood pH is 7.35–7.45; Table 1.3). Statistically, this means that 95% of the population (i.e. 95 out of 100 people) has a pH that falls in this range. Thus, the homeostatic range of a parameter is useful in making judgement regarding the health status of an individual. It must, however, be emphasized that each person is unique, and statistically it is expected that 5% of the 'healthy or so-called normal' population (i.e. 5 out of 100 people) naturally fall outside the normal range. These values reflect minor deviations from the homeostatic range, and are considered to be 'normal and acceptable' in clinical practice, and so need no clinical adjustments.

Alternatively, values that reflect large and sudden or long-term deviations from the homeostatic range which cannot be corrected naturally by body mechanisms are termed homeostatic 'imbalance' (i.e. signs and symptoms and/or illness), in which healthcare intervention may be not only desirable but essential to sustain 'normality' for the patient (Box 1.6).

Homeostasis, then, is about the provision of an internal environment that is optimal for cell function at any moment in time, despite the level of activity of the individual. Health occurs when bodily function is able to provide the appropriate environment. This usually entails an integration of the functioning of physiological systems, and its outcome is observed as physical well-being and psychological equilibrium. In order for homeostasis to be maintained, the body must have a means of detecting disturbances (or deviations) to homeostasis; assessing the magnitude of the deviation; and promoting an appropriate response to redress homeostasis (a process known as feedback). Feedback processes also provide the means of assessing the effectiveness of the response.

BOX 1.6 HEALTHCARE PROFESSIONALS – EXTERNAL AGENTS OF HOMEOSTATIC CONTROL

Homeostasis represents the processes necessary for the maintenance of conditions under which cells, and hence the tissues, organ systems and the body, can function optimally. For example, even small changes in a cell's environment, such as fluctuations in temperature, pH, ATP provision or hydration can disrupt the functioning of receptors, genes and enzymes within a cell and may even kill it. The disruptions to homeostasis, if not carefully monitored and controlled by the healthcare professional, could, in the extreme, be lethal for the patient, or at least delay recovery. In summary, health care is aimed at redressing (where possible) homeostasis for the patient. Health promotion and health education in their role of disease prevention are directed at sustaining homeostasis for individuals within the population. Thus healthcare professionals perhaps could be considered as *external agents of homeostatic control* (see 'Health care within a homeostasis framework' p.20 and case studies in Section VI which take this approach).

logical processes provide an *optimal* environment for bodily function which varies from one moment in time to another. While this may involve a near-constancy of some aspects of the environment (e.g. brain temperature), other functions may require a controlled change. The authors share the view that an increase in the white blood cell count, as occurs in response to an infection, and the increase in certain hormones (e.g. adrenaline, noradrenaline, cortisol), as occurs in response to stress, are further examples of homeostatic adaptive process rather than homeostatic imbalances.

Receptors and control centres

The initial disturbance in a physiological parameter is detected by receptors, sometimes referred to as monitors or error detectors. The function of these receptors is to relay information about the deviation to homeostatic control centres (analysers or interpreters). These centres interpret the disturbance as being above or below the homeostatic range, and determine the magnitude of the deviation. As a result, they stimulate appropriate responses via effectors that bring about the correction of the disturbance in order to restore homeostasis. Once the parameter has been normalized, the response will cease (Figure 1.8a, b).

Homeostatic controls

Occasionally, only one homeostatic control mechanism is necessary to redress the balance. For example, when the disturbance of blood glucose concentration exceeds its homeostatic range (hyperglycaemia; 'hyper-' = over or above, 'glyc-' = glucose, '-aemia' = blood) the hormone insulin is released, which promotes glucose removal from blood. More frequently, a number of controls are involved. For example, blood pressure is controlled by a number of neural and hormonal mechanisms

ACTIVITY

Identify the homeostatic controllers and effectors of metabolism within cells.

ACTIVITY

Briefly identify the three homeostatic regulators of acidity in the blood.

(see Figure 12.27, p.346). Another example is when blood acidity exceeds its homeostatic range (a condition referred to as an acidosis), three controls act to reduce the acidity values within the normal range (Clancy and McVicar, 2007a):

- *Buffers*: these chemicals act to neutralize the excess acidity (see Equations 5–9 in Chapter 6, p.130–2).
- *Respiratory mechanisms*: if the buffers are insufficient in removing the acidosis, then the rate and depth of breathing will increase in order to excrete more carbon dioxide, (a potential source of acid in body fluids).
- *Urinary mechanisms*: if the increased rate and depth of breathing are insufficient to remove the acidosis, then the kidneys will produce a more acidic urine and so reduce the acidity of body fluids.

These corrective responses are time dependent; some respond quickly to the disturbance, but if they should fail to re-establish homeostasis this prompts other control mechanisms to correct the deviation. The body therefore has short-term, intermediate and long-term homeostatic control mechanisms. Each controlling mechanism, however, has a limit or capacity on how much they can reverse the disturbance (Figure 1.8c). In the above example, these are the buffers, respiratory and urinary mechanisms, respectively.

Homeostatic feedback mechanisms
Negative feedback

Most homeostatic control mechanisms operate on the principle of negative feedback (i.e. when a homeostatic disturbance occurs, then in-built and self-adjusting mechanisms come into effect, which reverse the deviation). The regulation of blood sugar demonstrates the principle of negative feedback control. An increase in blood glucose concentration above its homeostatic range sets into motion processes that reduce it. Conversely, a blood glucose concentration below its homeostatic range (hypoglycaemia) promotes processes that will increase it. In both situations, the result is that the level of blood sugar is kept relatively constant over periods of time.

Positive feedback

Positive feedback occurs when the disturbance to a parameter results in an enhancement of this disturbance, that is, to promote a value above the homeostatic range rather than returning the value within the homeostatic range (via negative

ACTIVITY

Using the information in this chapter, you should be able to identify the in-built self-adjusting homeostatic mechanisms that are responsible for reversing elevated blood glucose concentration and acidity.

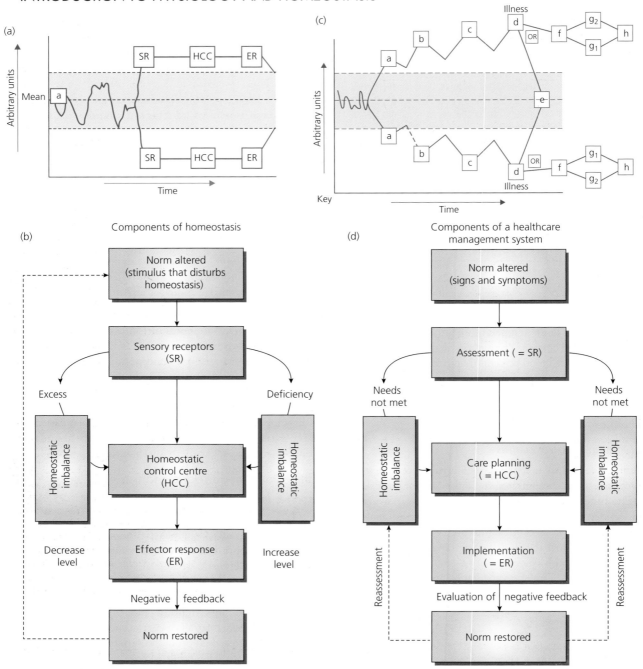

Figure 1.8 Homeostasis. Control, clinical intervention in illness and healthcare management systems. **(a,b)** General schemes demonstrating the roles of receptors, homeostatic control centres, and effectors via negative feedback in a control process. **(a)** Homeostatic dynamism reflecting individual variability. SR, Sensory receptors detect disturbance or deviations from the homeostatic range. HCC, Homeostatic control centres analyse the disturbance and its magnitude of change. ER, Effector response correcting the disturbance, usually by negative feedback. **(c)** Clinical intervention following homeostatic control system failure. a, Failure of receptors and/or short-term homeostatic control system and/or effectors in re-establishing homeostasis (note that there is some reversal of the homeostatic disturbance; however, the limit of these components has been exceeded and the disturbance is enhanced). b, Failure of receptors and/or intermediate homeostatic control system in re-establishing homeostasis (note these mechanisms initially reverse the disturbance; however, the capacity for the reversal is limited hence the disturbance is enhanced). c, Failure of receptors and/or long-term homeostatic control system and/or effectors in re-establishing homeostasis (note these mechanisms demonstrate some reversal of the homeostatic disturbance, but their capacity is exceeded; however, hence the disturbance is still present: i.e. illness arises). d, Healthcare intervention to re-establish patient homeostasis. e, Patient's re-established homeostatic status restored. f, Healthcare intervention is unsuccessful in re-establishing the patient homeostatic status. g_1, Palliative care improves quality of life via symptom control without re-establishing homeostasis. g_2, Health care cannot improve controls symptoms, and the disturbance is enhanced. h, Death occurs as a result of the inability to survive the homeostatic imbalance(s). [a, Represents boxes a_1–a_4 in Figure 1.7, p.11, reflecting the individual variability in the homeostatic range. The blue area represents the norm (homeostatic range) 95%]

Q Describe the function of the components of homeostatic control when there is a deviation in a parameter being monitored.

Q 'Healthcare professionals may be described as external agents of homeostatic control.' Discuss.

ACTIVITY

'Positive feedback is usually regarded as a homeostatic failure.' Discuss this statement.

feedback); positive feedback then results in a further increase, which causes a further increase, and so on. An example is observed during the menstrual cycle just before the release of the 'egg' (ovulation). The high levels of the hormone oestrogen at this part of the cycle reverse its normal inhibition regarding the secretion of luteinizing hormone (LH; release of this hormone is essential for ovulation to take place); the positive feedback now stimulates a surge of LH release, triggering ovulation. Since positive feedback induces change, the effects tend to be transient; most physiological systems utilize negative feedback mechanisms as a means of maintaining stability. An inability to promote change when necessary can, however, cause a change in health. For example, a failure to produce the surge of LH will result in sterility.

HOMEOSTASIS AND ILL HEALTH

If homeostasis and the functioning of homeostatic components provide a basis for health, then ill health will arise when there is a failure of the normal functioning of the components (Figure 1.8c, d). Imprecise functional mechanisms include:

- receptors fail to respond adequately to disturbances in the environment; and/or
- homeostatic control centres fail to analyse sensory receptor information, and/or analyse the information incorrectly, and/or send incorrect information to the effectors; and/or
- effectors fail to respond to corrective directions from the control centres.

All disorders are characterized by a primary disturbance of intracellular homeostasis within tissues somewhere in the body. The disease may be classed according to the primary disorder, such as a respiratory problem, a degenerative disorder, a tumour of a particular tissue, or as being caused by immune system dysfunction or infection. However, all will have consequences for extracellular homeostasis, hence the functioning of cells and tissues other than those involved in the primary disturbance. Thus, health care may be directed at symptoms apparently removed from the primary problem (e.g. relieving constipation in a patient with a breast tumour).

Homeostatic principles in clinical practice

The signs and symptoms of an illness will be related to the cellular homeostatic imbalances induced. For example, people with diabetes are classed as type 1 or insulin-dependent diabetes mellitus (IDDM) or as type 2 or non-insulin-dependent diabetes mellitus (NIDDM). Although not all people can be classified easily, as a general rule IDDM reflects a homeostatic failure of the pancreatic cells to produce the hormone insulin, and NIDDM reflects an imbalance in the target cells that respond to the insulin. The multiple organ system signs and symptoms of diabetes mellitus (see p.635), such as glucose in the urine (glucosuria) and vascular problems caused by fat deposits in the blood vessels (atherosclerosis), reflect a common failure in both types of diabetes in blood sugar management. They, therefore, are the result of a cellular imbalance, as are all illnesses. Furthermore, since cells only produce chemicals then it follows that all illnesses could be referred to as chemical imbalances (Box 1.8).

Clinical intervention in illness and disease is concerned with correcting underlying problems associated with homeostatic

BOX 1.7 HOMEOSTATIC RANGE FLUCTUATIONS

The capacity to modify the homeostatic range is essential in certain circumstances (e.g. pregnancy, see Box 1.4) and is of benefit in other situations (e.g. exercise). Variations in homeostatic ranges and in positive feedback responses provide flexibility to homeostatic processes. As in positive-feedback responses, many of the changes promoted by set-point alteration relate to a specific situation and are short lived. Some resettings are permanent, however, and so promote long-term change. These responses are vital to the process of human development during the individual's lifespan. They allow for growth, functional maturation during fetal development and childhood, puberty changes during adolescence, and changes associated with becoming an adult. However, losing this regulation is associated with old age. Thus, because of the changing or dynamic nature of the parameters in health, the term 'homeostatic' (meaning 'same standing') may now be a little outdated, and in future years it maybe replaced by the more appropriate term 'homeodynamic' (meaning parameter variation). For the purpose of this text the homeostasis term is used.

BOX 1.8 GENERAL PRINCIPLES OF PHARMACOLOGY: ANTAGONISTIC AND AGONISTIC DRUGS

Since all illnesses are homeostatic imbalances of either an excess or deficiency of a product of cellular metabolism, drug companies have been successful in producing drugs that address the excess or deficiency.

Many are broadly classified as antagonistic and agonistic drugs. Generally, antagonistic drugs operate by decreasing the excess product. Conversely, agonists enhance the production of the product that is deficient. How do they do this? Drugs target the specific cellular homeostatic components that are at fault. For example, antagonistic drugs operate by blocking:

- the cellular receptor; and/or
- the gene; and/or
- the enzyme, which is responsible for producing the excess chemical.

Conversely, agonists operate by enhancing receptor activation, and/or the expression of the gene, and/or the enzyme action to increase the cellular product which is deficient.

The drug dosage required for correcting imbalance is dependent on the magnitude of the excess or deficiency (i.e. mild, moderate or severe imbalance) of the chemical products.

Other drugs target the endproducts of cell respiration, i.e. inhibitors or stimulants of ATP, which will slow or increase metabolism, respectively. Drugs may restore normal body temperature (e.g. antipyretics) and pH (e.g. antacids) so as to ensure the microenvironment is ideal for a 'healthy' metabolism via optimizing enzyme action (see Box 2.5, p.32).

The success of the human genomic and proteomics projects will only enhance the number of pharmacological products, which will be tailor-made to the individual's needs; they may also unravel the mysteries of how complementary and alternative therapies work at the cellular level.

imbalances (i.e. managing the symptoms) and enabling the patient to come to terms with the 'disorder'. In other words, clinical practice is concerned with restoring, as effectively as possible, the homeostatic status of the patient at a cellular level (see Figure 1.8 and Box 1.6, p.13; Clancy and McVicar, 1996, 2007a). Using the above example, people with IDDM are treated with insulin injections, whereas diet (and perhaps hypoglycaemic drugs, such as gliclazide, glipizide and metformin) may be sufficient to control the problem in people with NIDDM, since the levels of insulin may be comparable to those of people without diabetes. By promoting normality, healthcare professionals are therefore acting as extrinsic homeostatic mechanisms. Some illnesses, however, such as terminal cancers, are not responsive to therapeutic intervention and, consequently, the imbalance results in long-term malfunction and eventually death. The healthcare professional in these circumstances provides palliative care to improve symptom management and hence the patient's quality of life (Figure 1.8, labels c,f,g and Box 1.6, p.13). There are times, of course, when the healthcare practitioner can do nothing to prevent the death of a patient; for example, patients who suffer a massive blood loss either through trauma following a road traffic accident, or during a major operation, may die from hypovolaemic shock.

Homeostasis is usually considered to pertain to physiological or biochemical processes, and for the bulk of this text we will apply these principles. We also intend to introduce (in this chapter and expand on in later chapters in relation to human development, stress, pain and circadian rhythms), homeostasis pertaining to psychophysiological consistency within the body. Not separating the mind ('psychological') from bodily ('physiological') functions is important because the cells making up the human brain are no different in their basic characteristics from any other cells in the body. Thinking, emotions, behaviour and memories are all subject to the same physical and chemical laws of other functions of the body, and so to understand health fully it is necessary to be familiar with the psychophysiological processes that account for individual differences, as well as with the principles of homeostasis. In summary, individual differences are determined by a person's genes (i.e. nature), which are modified by environmental (i.e. nurture) factors. The person and his/her environment are therefore inseparable. Thus, it is necessary that the nature–nurture implications of a person's health and ill health should be recognized since these interactions provide the foundations of health care. Thus, the authors encourage healthcare professionals to take a transactional (or interactionist) view regarding the patient's condition.

NATURE–NURTURE: AN INDIVIDUALIZED APPROACH TO HEALTH AND HEALTH CARE

Recent approaches to health care:

- recognize that people are individuals. Providing health care that is based solely on common biological change is unlikely to be fully effective for all patients, partly because people

vary biologically, but also because psychological and sociological variations can be profound and so will have an impact on the therapies;
- place an increased emphasis on the psychosocial influences on human behaviour and health. The focus has moved towards understanding how the environment acts on the individual, and hence how this interaction can be manipulated. The biological disturbances produced by such interactions will also be important here.

These are principles embraced by holism. Human beings are complex, so it could be argued that considering aspects of biopsychosocial well-being is itself being divisive, but in practical terms providing effective care requires the healthcare professional to have the appropriate psychological, sociological and biological information necessary to make decisions. Clearly, all three disciplines will underpin the care given (Figure 1.9).

In trying to explain the biological aspects of health, this book will use a systematic format to identify how body systems are constructed and how they function. In doing so, it will identify how changes in one system can induce profound alterations in the functioning of others, and how psychosocial perspectives may also have an impact on biological functioning. This latter interactional approach to health (and health care) is expanded upon here as an introduction and in more detail in the Chapters 20–22, which consider biological functioning in a more holistic framework.

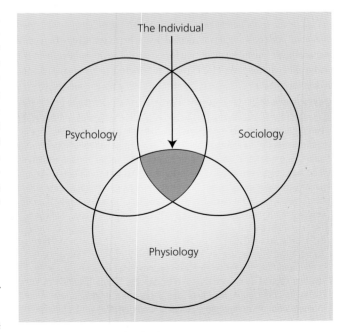

Figure 1.9 A simplistic model of holism

Q What does the term 'holism' mean to you?

BOX 1.9 SMOKING AS AN EXAMPLE OF AN INTERACTIONAL APPROACH TO HEALTH

Smoking frequently commences as a social or psychosocial pastime, but it is a habit that has been known for over 40 years to be associated with long-term health risks. Nicotine in tobacco smoke is a drug that acts as both a stimulant and a sedative. Its stimulant properties arise from the release of adrenaline and through the actions of nicotine on the central nervous system. They include:

- raising heart rate by 10–20 beats/minute;
- raising arterial blood pressure by 5–10 mmHg (07–1.3 kPa);
- raising the concentrations of blood glucose and free fatty acids;
- enhancing memory and alertness;
- improving cognition.

Its sedative properties also relate to its actions on the central nervous system:

- reducing stress perceptions;
- reducing aggressive responses to stressful situations;
- suppressing appetite.

Nicotine is also addictive. Smoking is a widespread behaviour, but it is considered to be the single most important, preventable health risk. Cigarette smoke contains over 2000 chemicals, and the risk to health is multisystemic. Smoking has been shown to substantially raise the risk of developing:

- cancer (lung, laryngeal, oral, oesophageal, bladder, kidney and pancreas): cigarette smoke contains more than 20 known carcinogens, collectively referred to as 'tar';

- chronic lung disease (chronic bronchitis, emphysema): this probably results from adaptive responses to the long-term presence of irritants from the smoke. Responses include increased numbers of goblet cells in the airways, increased mucus secretion (see Figure 2.26c, p.53), and loss of the hair-like processes called cilia that normally produce the 'mucus staircase' that removes mucus from the airways. The mucus provides a medium for bacterial growth;
- coronary heart disease (atherosclerosis): the causative factors are unknown, but there is suggestion that the main cause is the deposition of cholesterol in the walls of blood vessels of the heart (see Box 5.3, p.110 and Figures 12.7c,d, p.313 and 12.13, p.324). The presence of substantial amounts of carbon monoxide in cigarette smoke (and in the blood of frequent smokers) is also thought to have a role through its effect on the carriage of oxygen by blood;
- stroke, possibly linked to long-term cardiovascular adaptations (e.g. high blood pressure or hypertension), but may also be linked to cholesterol deposition in the walls of the blood vessels in the brain.

Smoking by pregnant women increases the risk of underweight babies and premature delivery. In such cases, the placental size is usually smaller than usual. Placental blood flow is likely to be reduced, hence poor fetal growth.

Changes in skin tone are also apparent in frequent smokers, often resulting in excessive facial wrinkling.

INTEGRATED APPROACHES TO HEALTH AND HEALTH CARE

Nature or nurture?

Discussions on the relative importance of biological (i.e. genetic or nature) and environmental (i.e. nurture) aspects have, for many years, provoked heated academic debates, especially in relation to human development. This is particularly the case when considering the factors that influence cognitive and behavioural changes, since both genetic and environmental contributions to psychological development are well recognized. The discussion should also extend to physical factors, since lifestyle interactions undoubtedly induce homeostatic disturbance/imbalance (e.g. see Box 1.9 and Figure 1.10). The exact means by which the environment can influence psychological and physical functions are increasingly the subject of research, and there is now greater emphasis on prevention through health education.

The human genome was published in 2003. One surprise is that there seem to be just 30 000 or so genes in human cells. This is far fewer than the original estimates of 100 000 plus. Early estimates assumed a principle of one gene–one protein; as the number of genes is actually much lower, this suggests

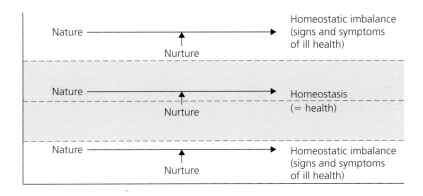

Figure 1.10 Homeostasis and homeostatic disturbance/imbalance/illness: a nature–nurture approach. Homeostasis, hence health, occurs through acquiring healthy nature–nurture interactions. Homeostatic imbalance(s), hence illness, occurs by inheriting the illness gene (nature), which is then exposed to environmental risk factors (nurture). [The blue area represents the norm (homeostatic range) 95%]

ACTIVITY

Various models of care have been developed during the last 40–50 years. Many of these take an 'interactional' stance, and the viewpoints expressed in this chapter are a development of those expressed in the Roy Adaptation Model. Interested readers are directed towards the work of Andrews and Roy (1991).

that there are as yet unrecognized ways by which the genetic blueprint is manipulated in cells to produce the diversity required in the human body. It has also stimulated further debate on the role of environmental interactions, particularly in such complex areas as human behaviour (see p.539 for further information regarding the Human Genome Project).

From the healthcare point of view, it is the interactions with the immediate environment that are of particular relevance, although the influences of the economic and political climates on that environment are also recognized as sources of illness. The application of this model, however, requires a definition of 'environment'. If we take a broad definition, then an individual's environment consists of the physical, chemical, social, emotional and spiritual circumstances in which the individual lives.

Interactions and psychological functions

Childhood and adolescence are viewed as being the main formative periods of our lives, as indicated by the complexity of psychophysiological development during these periods, although behaviour and personality remain labile throughout life.

Our mental faculties have a biological basis, since there are sites within the brain that have roles in, for example, emotion, aggression, sexual behaviour, cognitive functions and memory. The functioning of synapses (i.e. gaps between neurons) requires the activation of appropriate genes within brain neurons, not only for the existence of the neural components of the brain but also to promote neuronal growth and to enable a cell to produce the features necessary for neurochemical transmission at synapses. The observable characteristics produced by the activities of such genes in neural cells might be behavioural or cognitive, so there is a genetic basis to all aspects of psychological function. For example, 'intelligence' is currently considered to be primarily genetic, with 60–80% being accounted for by heredity. The remaining proportion identifies the importance of psychosocial interactions on brain development.

A genetic component helps to explain the apparent familial occurrence of some psychological disorders. By implication, gene mutation should be capable of inducing behavioural disturbance by altering neurological structure and functioning. Putative genes have been identified, but the situation is complicated by the likelihood that behavioural traits are characteristics that involve numerous genes, which increases the complexity of investigation.

Genetic involvement could also help to explain how behav-

ioural disorders are associated with specific neurochemical imbalances, such as an underactivity of neural pathways that utilize the neurotransmitters serotonin and noradrenaline in depressive behaviour (Box 1.10). Pharmacological therapies target this 'nature' component of behavioural disorders, and are an important tool.

Nevertheless, current pharmacological therapies might not reverse a disorder or may only provide a means of managing it. Psychotherapy is an alternative method that uses the lability of neural connections (referred to as 'neuroplasticity') in order to promote appropriate pathways and thus modify behaviour. How such 'environmental' interactions influence the expression of genes and behaviour has not been elucidated. It is clear, however, that to consider only the relative contributions of either genes or environment on psychological function is to take too narrow a perspective. Much of the brain function reflects an interaction of both, and this is reflected in clinical approaches to disorders of mental health (see Box 1.10, and the mental health case studies in Section VI).

BOX 1.10 DEPRESSION AS AN EXAMPLE OF AN INTERACTIONAL APPROACH TO HEALTH CARE

Psychological and sociological studies have made a considerable impact on the understanding of behaviour, yet the continued use of pharmacological therapies, whether as primary or secondary interventions, provides a reminder that the brain is a biological structure. The lack of psychological equilibrium in depression represents a disturbance of the internal environment of the brain, and the promotion of an optimal neural environment has failed. Clinical intervention aims to reverse the disturbance; this is illustrated by the therapeutic approaches used in the treatment of depression.

Depression is characterized in its extreme by a dysphoric mood, or a loss of interest or pleasure. The majority of studies indicate that the activities of monoamine neurotransmitters (noradrenaline and serotonin in particular) are reduced in depressive states, resulting in a functional imbalance between certain neural pathways of the brain. The aim of clinical intervention is to either artificially correct the neurochemical imbalance by using drugs or reverse the neurological change that resulted in the imbalance by using psychotherapy to re-establish neurological balance.

Pharmacological therapies largely involve the administration of drugs that either inhibit the uptake of neurotransmitter from the synapse, and so prolong its action (tricyclic antidepressants and serotonin-reuptake inhibitors), or maintain the presence of neurotransmitter for longer by preventing its breakdown by enzymes (monoamine oxidase inhibitors). The efficacy of these drugs in acute care is well established, but they do not remove the psychosocial cause of the disturbance. Drug companies still invest in producing drugs that activate or inactivate the components of the homeostatic theory (see Figure 1.8, p.14), in an attempt to provide a 'quick fix' to the patient's problems.

Life events and a lack of social support have long been known to act as precipitating factors in the aetiology of depression. Cognitive behavioural therapy has been found to be as effective as pharmacological intervention for acute treatment, and may even be associated with lower rates of relapse.

Both treatments are therefore concerned with re-establishing neurological homeostasis, and an integrated approach should be taken that utilizes the best of each.

BOX 1.11 DYSPNOEA AS AN EXAMPLE OF AN INTERACTIONAL APPROACH TO HEALTH CARE

A balance between lung ventilation and lung perfusion is essential for health (see Box 14.22, p.413). Chronic cardiopulmonary disorders therefore frequently arise from heart disease, such as cardiomyopathies or myocardial infarction, or from lung diseases, such as chronic obstructive airway disease or pneumonia. These might be considered to be the primary problems. A common cause of heart disease is the presence of cholesterol-led atheromatous plaques within the coronary circulation, and that of lung disease is infection or environmental pollutants, such as cigarette smoke. In both cases, there are strong lifestyle or environmental links. Interactional influences on well-being can be framed within systems theory, by placing the individual in the context of component (internal) sub-systems, and wider, external supra-systems (see Figure 1.11). Important features of systems theory is the 'permeability' of boundaries between the various levels indicative of influencing factors between them, and the way in which the different levels are resistant to change in face of those factors – homeostasis could be considered an example of this. Acute pulmonary disorders are also possible, especially with regard to asthma or pneumonia. Once again, both usually have environmental risk factors.

Poor lung ventilation and/or perfusion causes dyspnoea (poor blood oxygenation and difficulties with breathing) and results in difficulty in maintaining the normal gas composition of arterial blood, and hence of the tissues elsewhere in the body. The management of dyspnoea includes some or all of the following:

- *Pharmacological methods*, including the administration of bronchodilators to improve ventilation, steroids to reduce inflammation, mucolytics to loosen mucus secretions, and anti-anxiety drugs to reduce the work of breathing and to reduce the risk of bronchospasm.
- *Physical techniques*, including:
  - positioning of the patient: a semi-prone position uses gravity to reduce pressure from the abdomen on the diaphragm, and hence on the lungs;
  - 'pursed-lip' breathing, to maintain alveolar expansion during breathing out, or 'diaphragmatic breathing' to reduce the work of breathing and to reduce air trapping as a consequence of airway compression during forced exhalation;
  - chest physiotherapy, to remove secretions (and suctioning to facilitate expectoration if necessary);
  - cough control, to facilitate removal of secretions.
- *Psychosocial therapies*, including relaxation and meditation to reduce anxiety and the work of breathing. Reduced anxiety will improve the disposition of the patient, and may also reduce the need for other interventions.
- *Oxygen therapy*, to facilitate oxygenation of alveolar gases; this is a clear example of environmental change that affects physiological parameters.

Thus, the aetiology of disorders that promote dyspnoea often has an environmental component, and the clinical interventions used to alleviate dyspnoea include both biological and environmental factors.

Interactions and physical functions

The success of heath education programmes to reduce physical disorder also indicates that the environment (i.e. lifestyle) has an influence on genetic expression throughout the body. Some of these influences, such as diet, exercise and drug abuse, are well documented. Others are only poorly understood (although the situation is changing rapidly), e.g. the extrinsic factors involved in the development of many cancers. Health education programmes are less apparent in such instances but scientists increasingly recognize causative or modulating agents, and so preventive approaches may eventually be available.

The interactional approach to health and health care in the context of physical functioning is illustrated in Box 1.11.

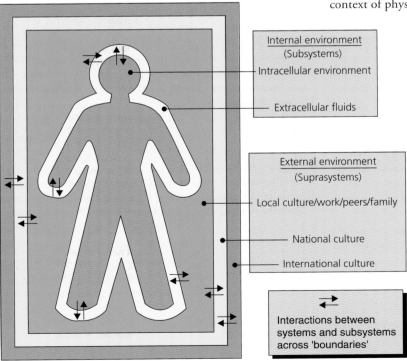

Internal environment
(Subsystems)
Intracellular environment
Extracellular fluids

External environment
(Suprasystems)
Local culture/work/peers/family
National culture
International culture

Interactions between systems and subsystems across 'boundaries'

Figure 1.11 Systems theory and health. The individual represents a system with identifiable subsystems, which relate to intracellular and extracellular environments. The sociocultural environment, in which the individual lives, provides a number of suprasystems. Note the interactions across boundaries between the suprasystems and subsystems. These will influence the health of the individual

Q Which structures within the human body form our link to the environment?

BOX 1.12 HOMEOSTASIS AND THE HEALTHCARE PROCESS

Homeostatic principles are readily discerned within the stages of any healthcare process (compare Figure 1.8b and d, p.14).

- *Assessment and diagnosis.* The assessment of the health deficit and the biological, psychological, social and spiritual needs of the individual correspond to the detection and assessment of change by the receptors of the homeostatic control mechanism.
- *Planning.* The planning of health care, based on the assessment and diagnosis stage, is comparable to the ways by which homeostatic controls analyse and determine the responses needed to correct the disturbance. Furthermore, just as the body has specific homeostatic controls for different parameters, the healthcare practitioner needs to plan care according to the individual's needs. This can be illustrated using the simple example of dietary needs: a small amount of food, presented pleasantly, may be vital to encourage eating in the elderly patient who has a depressed appetite, whereas an energetic young patient will require a bulkier dietary intake, while a patient

with a learning disability may need reminding of what and when to eat.

- *Implementation.* In the healthcare process, implementation refers to putting into action the interventions planned in the previous stage. In a homeostatic perspective, this is analogous to the activation of effectors to produce the appropriate response.
- *Evaluation.* The effectiveness of care is assessed in this stage, much as feedback processes provide a means of evaluating a psychophysiological response. For example, has the injection been given to prevent the patient's pain?
- *Reassessment.* The cyclical nature of the healthcare process is emphasized by this stage, in which the patient is reassessed and new interventions considered if necessary. The dynamism of this process is also observed in homeostatic mechanisms described in this book; parameters fluctuate constantly within their normal ranges, and such changes must, therefore, be constantly reassessed.

HEALTH CARE WITHIN A HOMEOSTASIS FRAMEWORK

Interactions between the individual and the external environment act to change the internal environment of that individual, which is why intrinsic homeostatic processes are so important, since they prevent those changes from becoming destabilizing and causing biochemical change incompatible with well-being. In acting to prevent or reverse the effects of extrinsic influences on the internal environment, healthcare professionals are also demonstrating homeostasis in action (Box 1.12).

Homeostasis therefore provides a working framework for health and health care. Placing holism into a conceptual framework does not mean losing the sense of person, but presents us with the means of viewing the health–ill health continuum.

The impact of extrinsic factors on the internal environment of an individual may be influenced by the degree to which they act upon the individual, and the degree to which the individual is capable of responding to the imposed change. In other words, the impact of extrinsic factors on health will depend partly on the properties of the factors themselves, but also partly on the individual's innate capacity to respond to them. It is therefore also important to note that our ability to maintain psychophysiological equilibrium in the face of environmental stressors will be highly subjective because of genetic variation, the developmental stage of the individual, and individual sociocultural circumstances.

The interactional aspects of health, and the subjectivity that may be observed, are explored further in Chapters 20–22.

CONCLUSION

Homeostasis is a concept used throughout this book to explain how the internal environment is maintained at a level conducive to healthy functioning within the body compartments. Homeostatic control relies mainly upon negative feedback mechanisms that act to reverse disturbances and regulate parameters close to their optimal values. Prevention of parameter variation can be detrimental under some circumstances. The promotion of change via positive feedback mechanisms, or through resetting of homeostatic setpoints, is then of benefit. Failure of negative feedback processes, appropriate positive feedback responses, or setpoint resetting or a reduction in their efficiency, leads to homeostatic imbalance labelled illness.

Homeostasis based on nature–nurture interactions therefore provides a working framework for health and health care whereby the health carer perhaps could be considered as an external agent of homeostatic control. Healthcare processes involving assessment, diagnosis, planning, implementing care and reassessment of care are analogous with the natural components of homeostasis and as such are concerned largely with supplementing normal anatomical, biochemical and hence physiological processes in order to re-establish the homeostatic status (where possible) for the patient. It is with this framework that case studies in Section VI have been written. Chapter 2 emphasises that cells and their chemical products are the basic unit of health, illness and hence healthcare intervention. Most other chapters take a systemic approach to understanding the human body in health and illness emphasizing the homeostatic theme, while, finally, Chapters 19–22 focus more on the nature–nurture interaction in the understanding of human development, pain, stress and circadian rhythms.

SUMMARY

1 Humans are biological beings. The biological construction (anatomy and physiology) of the individual provides the basis for identifying how interactions with the external environment influence the psychophysiological health of the individual.

2 The maintenance of bodily functions regulates appropriate cellular activities, which are determined by enzymes, the products of gene expression, provided that genes receive the appropriate information from receptors.

3 The composition of the intracellular environment will influence the efficiency at which cells operate, and, accordingly, it is regulated so as to be optimal.

4 The concept of homeostasis helps to explain the importance to health of maintaining an optimal environment within which cells must function. 'Optimal' does not necessarily equate with constancy. It also relates to the control of change observed during daily activities of living, times of stress, illness and postoperative recovery, and during the developmental phases of the lifespan.

5 Homeostatic control relies mainly upon negative feedback mechanisms that act to reverse changes and regulate parameters close to the optimal value.

6 Prevention of parameter variation can be detrimental under some circumstances. The promotion of change via positive feedback mechanisms or through a resetting of homeostatic setpoints is then of benefit.

7 Ill health arises when there is a failure to maintain homeostatic functions, either at tissue or organ levels of organization. The interdependency of tissue functions means those homeostatic disturbances and associated signs and symptoms will also arise secondarily to the primary disorder.

8 Healthcare practices are related to homeostasis since they provide the extrinsic effectors that act to restore homeostasis in patient.

9 Homeostasis provides an interactional framework that gives structure to nature–nurture considerations on the basis of well-being and healthcare practices.

ACKNOWLEDGEMENT

An extended version of the material presented in this chapter is available in Clancy and McVicar (1998).

REFERENCES

Andrews, H.A. and Roy, C. (1991) Essentials of the Roy Adaptation Model. In: Roy, C. and Andrews, H.A. (eds) *The Roy Adaptation Model: the Definitive Statement*. Norwalk, CT: Appleton-Lange.

Cannon, W.B. (1932) *The Wisdom of the Body*. New York: Norton.

Clancy, J. and McVicar, A. (1996) Homeostasis. The key concept in physiological control. *British Journal of Theatre Nursing* **6**(2): 17–24.

Clancy, J. and McVicar, A. (1998) Chapter 6. Homeostasis and nature–nurture interactions: a framework for integrating the life sciences. In: Hinchliff, S.M., Norman, S.E. and Schober, J.E. (eds) *Nursing Practice and Health*, 3rd edn. London: Arnold, 122–48.

Clancy, J. and McVicar, A.J. (2007a) Short-term regulation of acid–base homeostasis. *British Journal of Nursing* **16**(16): 604–7.

Clancy, J. and McVicar, A.J. (2007b) Intermediate and long-term regulation of acid–base homeostasis. *British Journal of Nursing* **16**(17): 1016–19.

Roper, N., Logan, W.W. and Tierney, A. (1990) *The Elements of Nursing*, 3rd edn. Edinburgh: Churchill Livingstone.

FURTHER READING

Clancy, J. McVicar, A.J. and Baird, N. (2002) Perioperative practice. *Fundamentals of Homeostasis*. London: Routledge.

Hagedorm, M.I.E. and Gardner, S.L. (1999) Newborn care: hypoglycemia in the newborn. Part I: pathophysiology and nursing management. *Mother Baby Journal* **4**(1): 15–24.

McVicar, A, J. and Clancy, J. (1998) Homeostasis. a framework for integrating the life sciences. *British Journal of Nursing* **7**(10): 601–7.

CELL AND TISSUE FUNCTIONS

The structure of the body can be described on four levels of organization: the chemical level (see Chapter 4), the cellular and tissue levels (both levels described in this chapter), and the organ system levels (see Chapters 7–18).

As discussed in Chapter 1, human physiology is concerned with the 'correct' interdependent functioning of the organ systems, so throughout this book each system is considered as a 'homeostatic control system'. Each has a role to play in maintaining the equilibrium within cells, and hence tissues, organs and organ systems because of the interdependency of these different levels of organizations (see Figure 1.5, p.9). For example, the respiratory system is concerned primarily with maintaining the homeostatic equilibrium of the gases oxygen and carbon dioxide in the blood. This is produced, principally, by way of breathing movements and gaseous exchange between the tiny air sacs in the lungs (called alveoli) and local blood vessels (called pulmonary capillaries). However, the system is ultimately concerned with ensuring that aerobic respiration ('aerobic' = presence of oxygen, 'respiration' = process of producing energy) by cells occurs within its homeostatic range, providing sufficient energy in the form of adenosine triphosphate (ATP) to drive chemical reactions within their normal physiological parameters. In addition to ATP carbon dioxide and water are other products of cellular respiration, and if regulated within their homeostatic range produce the ideal pH for enzymes to function at their optimum. Heat is also another endproduct and if this is within its homeostatic range optimizes enzyme reactions in the cells. The respiratory system is also important in maintaining the acid–base balance of body fluids – it acts as an intermediate homeostatic control of body

pH (Clancy and McVicar 2007a,b, see details in Chapter 6, p.132). The regulation of pH is a necessity since excessive acidity or alkalinity (basicity) threatens cell functions and life. Organ systems cannot operate in isolation. Each works interdependently with others to ensure that the level of chemicals inside cells is maintained, enabling cells to perform the basic characteristics of life. Thus, the respiratory system supports all tissues and organs of the body, primarily by maintaining its component cells.

The focus on cells makes it essential that cell activities are understood by the health care practitioner if the physiological basis of health, the pathophysiological basis of illness and the physiological rationale of health care are to be appreciated. The concept of cells being the 'basic unit of life' was introduced in the first chapter (pp.8–10). In this chapter, the structure and function of the cell will be described in more detail.

ACTIVITY

Before continuing, you should be able to list the basic body needs (characteristics) of life. Refer to Chapter 1 if you are having trouble in remembering.

BOX 2.1 THE IMPORTANCE OF CYTOLOGY IN HEALTH AND ILLNESS

A knowledge of the structure, function and needs of human cells in healthcare curricula is centred on understanding how tissue and organ dysfunction results in ill health, and so provides the rationale for clinical intervention. For example, the condition obstructive respiratory disease induces hypoxaemia (insufficient oxygen in the blood) and hypercapnia (excess carbon dioxide in the blood), and may result in cell death (necrosis) in the patient. The body attempts to correct disturbances through natural homeostatic regulatory components. That is, receptors detect the hypoxaemia and hypercapnia, and send the information to the respiratory homeostatic control centre in the brain. This centre analyses the disturbances and their magnitude before sending information to the effectors (i.e. muscles of respiration), which reverse the disturbance via increasing the rate and depth of breathing. A failure of any of these regulatory devices (i.e. receptors, and/or homeostatic controls, and/or effectors) to re-establish gaseous homeostasis makes healthcare intervention necessary to remove the homeostatic imbalance and restore the 'health' of the individual. That is, the healthcare practitioner is acting as an external agent in homeostatic control when they restore the patient's homeostatic status of blood gases (see Box 1.6, p.13).

CELLULAR LEVEL OF ORGANIZATION

The study of cells is called cytology ('cyt-' = cell, '-logy' = study). This branch of biology investigates how cells are organized in terms of the structure of their component parts, how intracellular homeostasis is maintained, and how they reproduce.

The cells are the basic building blocks, since the body is composed of them and their substances. Just as the body has organs to perform specialized homeostatic functions, cells have component parts called organelles ('little organs') that have specific homeostatic roles within the cell. Their structures are dependent upon the chemical components, such as proteins, lipids and lipoproteins, from which they are made. These

---

BOX 2.2 THE CELL – THE BEGINNINGS OF LIFE

It is usually argued that human life begins as a single cell (zygote) that results from a fusion of the female's egg (ovum) and the male's spermatozoa. The zygote undergoes cell division, producing stem cells, which then give rise ultimately to the trillions of cells that undergo differentiation and specialization into the specific tissues and organ systems of the human body. The potential benefits of stem cell research are explored in Chapter 19.

---

structures in turn are dependent upon their constituent parts: amino acids, fatty acids, and lipids and proteins, respectively (see Figure 1.5, p.9). These substances are thus referred to as being part of the 'chemical basis of life', which are covered in detail in Chapter 3, and ultimately come from the diet, hence the adage, 'We are what we eat.' This, of course, is not strictly correct, since we would be extremely overweight and some dietary components cannot be digested or utilized, and therefore they are removed from the body.

Overview of cellular anatomy and physiology

Cell size, shape and structure

Most cells are microscopic, with the average size ranging from 10 to 30 µm (micrometers, i.e. 10–30 thousandths of a millimetre) in diameter. The largest cell in the body is the female ovum, which is approximately 500 µm in diameter and is just visible to the naked eye (Figure 2.1). The erythrocyte ('erythro-' = red, '-cyte' = cell) of blood is the smallest cell, being about 7.5 µm in diameter. The longest cell, which can measure up to 1 m in length, is the neuron ('neur-' = nerve), but even these are microscopically thin.

Cellular anatomy varies because cells perform different functions to maintain body homeostasis (Figure 2.2). A 'typical' or

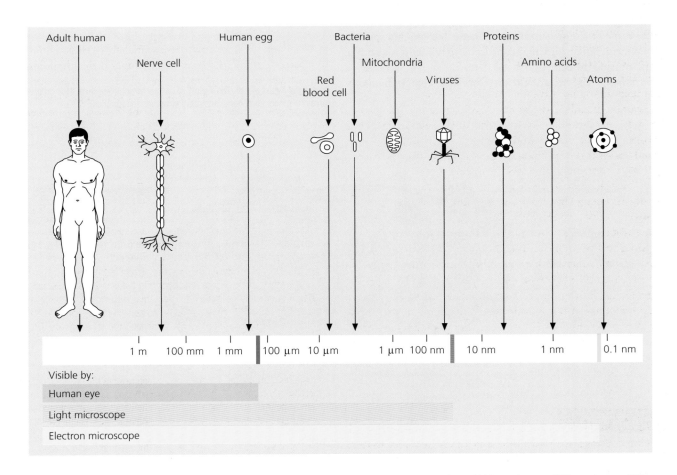

Figure 2.1 Comparison of cell sizes and their components. Note: m, metre; µm, micrometre; nm, nanometre. 1 m = 1000 mm; 1 mm = 1000 µm; 1 µm = 1000 nm

ACTIVITY

Familiarize yourself with the following units. Those units less than 1 mm are not used widely outside science and so may be unfamiliar.

1 m (metre)	= 100 cm (centimetres)	= 1000 mm (millimetres)	= 39.37 inches
1 cm	= 10 mm	= 0.39 inches	
1 mm	= 0.1 cm	= 1000 μm (micrometers)	
1 μm	= 1000 nm (nanometres)		

'generalized' cell is shown in Figure 2.3. This is a composite of many types of cells, and will share features with most cells within the body without being identical to any of them. Generally, cells have five principal parts:

1 *Cell membrane*: this is the outer boundary of the cell. It separates the intracellular ('intra-' = inside) and extracellular ('extra-' = outside) environments.
2 *Cytoplasm*: this is the ground material (or cellular fluid) between the nuclear and the cell membranes that suspends the cell's organelles and inclusions.
3 *Organelles*: these structural components have highly specialized intracellular roles that contribute to homeostasis within and outside the cell.
4 *Inclusions*: these include the secretory and storage chemicals of cells.

Blood cells

Erythrocytes Function: oxygen transport

Leucocytes Function: defence

Neutrophil   Monocyte   Lymphocyte

Muscle cells Function: contraction

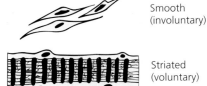

Smooth (involuntary)

Striated (voluntary)

Reproductive cells Function: continuation of species

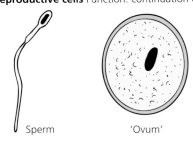

Sperm   'Ovum'

Figure 2.2 Types of cell. The variety of cellular structure reflects their different functions (principle of complementary structure and function)

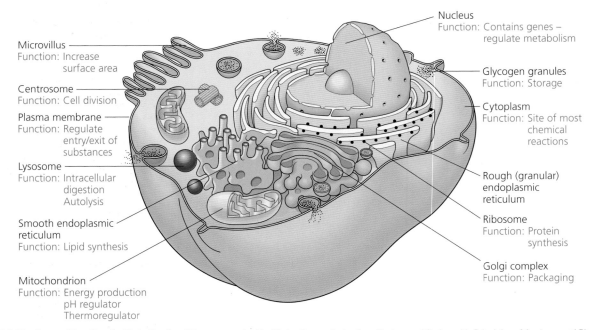

Microvillus
Function: Increase surface area

Centrosome
Function: Cell division

Plasma membrane
Function: Regulate entry/exit of substances

Lysosome
Function: Intracellular digestion Autolysis

Smooth endoplasmic reticulum
Function: Lipid synthesis

Mitochondrion
Function: Energy production pH regulator Thermoregulator

Nucleus
Function: Contains genes – regulate metabolism

Glycogen granules
Function: Storage

Cytoplasm
Function: Site of most chemical reactions

Rough (granular) endoplasmic reticulum

Ribosome
Function: Protein synthesis

Golgi complex
Function: Packaging

Figure 2.3 Structure and function of a 'typical' cell and its components. Modified with permission from Tortora and Grabowski, *Principles of Anatomy and Physiology*, Ninth edition. John Wiley and Sons, Inc, New York. 1999

5 *Nucleus*: this contains the ground material (or nucleoplasm) that suspends the 'vehicles of heredity' (i.e. genes), which are the homeostatic controllers of the cell since they code for all chemical reactions (called metabolism) and are, therefore, responsible for regulating intracellular homeostasis via their role in enzyme production. Genes are composed of deoxyribonucleic acid (DNA).

The homeostatic functions of these cellular components are summarized in Figure 2.3 and Table 2.1, and are considered in detail in the next section.

CELLULAR ANATOMY AND PHYSIOLOGY

Cell membrane

The cell membrane (also known as the plasma membrane) provides a selective barrier between intracellular and extracel-

Table 2.1 Role of cellular components in homeostasis

Component	Appearance	Description	Homeostatic functions
Plasma membrane	Plasma membrane	Outer boundary of the cell. Composed mainly of lipids/proteins as lipoprotein complexes. Also contains carbohydrates as glycoproteins and steroids	Regulates entry/exit of substances. Limits cell size. Important in cell recognition
Cytoplasm	Cytoplasm	Semi-fluid composition enclosed within the plasma membrane	Dissolves reactants necessary for chemical reactions. Houses inclusions (contain storage/secretory products)
Endoplasmic reticulum (ER)	Ribosomes, Rough ER, Smooth ER	A network of membranes throughout the cytoplasm	Rough ER – protein synthesis. Smooth ER – lipid, carbohydrate, and steroid synthesis. ER – segregation of the cytoplasm into different areas of biochemical activity
Golgi body (apparatus)		Flattened stack of disc-like membranes (called cisternae)	Combines large chemicals, e.g. lipoproteins, for organelle synthesis and packaging of materials for export
Lysosome		Membranous sacs of digestive enzymes	Intracellular digestion, autolysis, and destruction of worn-out parts of the cell
Mitochondrion		Large, double-membraned organelle, enclosing important respiratory enzymes	Production of a large proportion of the cell's energy (A TP) requirements. Site for aerobic respiration
Cytoskeleton		Microtubules, Microfilaments	Mechanical support for cellular components (e.g. cilia, centrosomes) maintaining their shape. Aids movement of (i) cellular components (e.g. form spindle for movement of chromosomes during cell division); (ii) substances across the cell's surface (i.e. cilia)
Centrosome (centrioles)		Centralized structure contains centrioles (bundles of microtubules)	Cell division
Nucleus		Enclosed by a nuclear membrane	Maintains intracellular homeostasis via expression and non-expression of genes by enzyme production and inhibition respectively. Contains store of hereditary information (chromosomes)

lular compartments (i.e. it determines what chemicals enter or leave the cell). Both compartments are aqueous (i.e. water based) and so the membrane cannot be composed of water-soluble chemicals, since it would dissolve. It must have structure and composition that does not allow entry and exit of all water-soluble substances, as this would prevent the regulation of their intracellular and extracellular concentrations.

One of the earliest attempts at describing a generalized membrane substructure was by Davson in 1969 (Davson, 1970). Their 'lipid bilayer model' referred to the cell membrane as a 'unit' membrane, since all membrane-bound organelles have the same structure. The main biochemical components are lipids and proteins. Structurally, this model assumed that proteins were associated rigidly with a lipid bilayer. The 'fluid mosaic model' proposed by Singer and Nicolson (1972) suggested a more dynamic structure in which proteins and other molecules could be inserted or removed according to the cells' requirements. The main lipids present are phospholipids and cholesterol. Phospholipids are polarized chemicals, having hydrophilic ('hydro-' = water, '-philic' = liking or attracting) and hydrophobic ('-phobic' = fearing or repellent) ends. Each phospholipid is positioned at right angles to the cell membrane's internal and external surfaces. The hydrophilic heads are exposed to the fluid outside the cell (tissue fluid), and the hydrophobic tails are found inside the membrane; thus water or water-soluble substances (including drugs) cannot enter this region (Figure 2.4).

ACTIVITY

Use a dictionary to define 'lipid', 'protein' and 'carbohydrate'.

According to the fluid mosaic model, the proteins embedded in the cell membrane are like 'icebergs floating in a sea of lipid'. Membrane proteins are broadly classed as integral and peripheral proteins. Integral proteins completely span the membrane and peripheral proteins only partially span it. Membrane proteins have the following specialized functions:

- Some integral proteins have selective transport properties. They form 'pores' or channels extending through the membrane that allow the passage of water, water-soluble substances and specific electrolytes into and out of the cell without having to cross through the lipid layer (Figure 2.4). Other proteins form 'carriers', by which substances can be transported through the membrane (Figure 2.5).
- Some peripheral proteins are 'markers' (called antigens) of specialized cells, hence are important in cell recognition (e.g. ABO blood groupings; see Figure 11.19, p.229) and immunity (e.g. antigens or immunogens; see Figure 13.2a, p.361). The cell membrane also contains carbohydrate chemicals that have been joined (or conjugated) with proteins or lipids, called glycoproteins and glycolipids, respectively (Figure 2.4). These are also important in cell recognition.

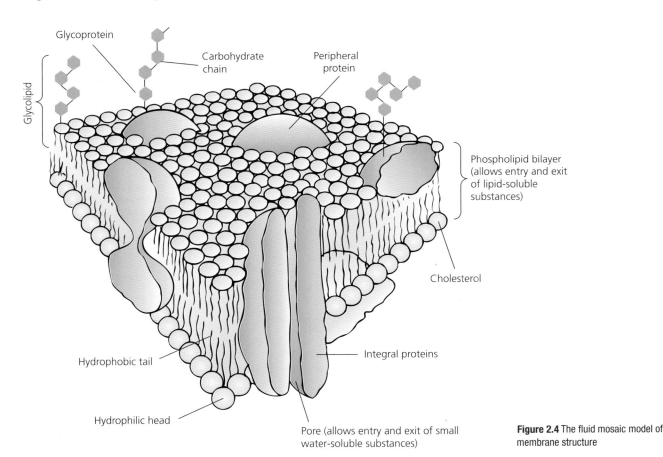

Figure 2.4 The fluid mosaic model of membrane structure

- Some proteins act as receptor sites, or targets, for some hormones (e.g. glucagon, adrenaline and thyroxine; see Figure 9.1, p.208).
- Some proteins are enzymes (e.g. peptidase; see Figure 10.14, p.234) and hence are controllers of chemical (metabolic) reactions within, or associated with, the cell membrane.

The structural components of the cell membrane are thus of fundamental importance in sustaining cellular homeostasis, because of their interaction with chemicals inside and outside the cell, and because they provide the means of controlling entry and exit of substances.

The fluid mosaic model stresses that the cell membrane is constantly changing its shape, since proteins and carbohydrates are mobile within and on the membrane lipids, and because portions of the membrane are continually being removed, recycled and replaced. Membranes also change their shape and surface area when they are taking substances into the cell by enveloping fluid and contents in a process called endocytosis, or secreting substances out of the cell by similar means (exocytosis). The cell must secrete substances that cannot be destroyed, stored or transferred into other substances, since these chemical are surplus to cellular requirements and, as such, are creating a homeostatic disturbance and therefore must be secreted along with 'waste' products of metabolism to sustain intracellular homeostasis. Various factors determine how rapidly such substances are transported, and their mode of transport across the cell membrane.

Factors influencing the transport of substances across the cell membrane

The passage of substances across the cell membrane may be free, restricted or refused. The membrane is, therefore, described as being selectively permeable, and the distribution

Table 2.2 Processes involved in movement of substances in and out of cells

Process	Description	Factors affecting rate	Examples in body
Passive processes	Substances move down their concentration gradients. No cell energy (ATP) required		
Simple diffusion	Net movement of chemicals from regions of a high concentration to regions of a low concentration, until they are distributed evenly	1 Size of chemical 2 Lipid solubility of chemical 3 Charge of chemical 4 Size of gradient 5 Surface area available	Movement of oxygen from lung to blood, from blood to tissue fluid, and from tissue fluid to cells. Vice versa for carbon dioxide
Facilitated diffusion	Plasma membrane integral protein carriers allow passage through protein channels (Figure 2.5)	In addition to the above, availability of carrier	Movement of glucose and amino acids into all cells
Osmosis	Water or solvent chemicals move from regions of a high concentration of water or solvent chemicals through a selectively permeable membrane (Figure 2.6)	1 Concentration gradients (i.e. osmotic pressure gradients) 2 Hydrostatic pressure (can act against osmosis)	Water moves into red blood cells from a hypotonic (weak; high water content) tissue fluid
Filtration	Hydrostatic pressure forces water and small chemicals through selectively permeable membranes from areas of high pressure to areas of low pressure (see Figure 6.2, p.124)	Amount of pressure, size of pores	Capillary exchange when blood pressure is greater than in tissue fluid. Ultrafiltration in the kidney nephron
Active processes	Cell energy (ATP) expenditure allows movement of substances against their concentration gradients		
Active transport	Plasma membrane protein carriers transport ions, chemicals from regions of a low concentration to regions of a high concentration (Figure 2.7)	Availability of carrier chemicals, transported substance, and ATP	Sodium, potassium, magnesium, calcium in all cases
Exocytosis	Cytoplasmic vesicles fuse with the plasma membrane and expel particles from the cell (Figure 2.10)	Availability of ATP	Neurotransmitter release and secretion of mucus
Endocytosis	Membrane-bound vesicles enclose large chemicals, take them into the cytoplasm, and release them		
1 Phagocytosis	'Cell eating'. Ingestion of solid particles. Phagosomes formed (Figure 2.8a)	Availability of ATP	Phagocytes (white blood cells) ingest foreign bodies (e.g. bacteria)
2 Pinocytosis	'Cell drinking'. Ingestion of fluid droplets and their dissolved substances. Pinosomes release contents into cytoplasm (Figure 2.8b)	Availability of ATP	Kidney cells take in nephron fluid containing amino acids
3 Receptor-mediated endocytosis	Specific plasma membrane receptors bind with chemicals, forming ligands, and take them into the cell's cytoplasm via endosomes.	Availability of ATP	Intestinal epithelial cells take up large molecules.

Q List the passive and active homeostatic transport mechanisms of the cell.

of chemicals on either side of the membrane is thus very different. However, the membrane may respond to varying environmental conditions, or intracellular homeostatic requirements, by allowing substances to enter and leave the cell by diffusing through it, or by crossing it by way of pores or carrier mechanisms. Factors affecting the passage of chemicals across the membrane are:

- *Chemical size*: large chemicals enter and leave the cell more slowly than small chemicals.
- *Chemical solubility*: oil or oil-soluble substances pass through the membrane more quickly than water-soluble substances because of the arrangement of the membrane phospholipids. The oils probably dissolve through the lipid layer of the membrane; this property provides a useful means of administering those drugs that can be dissolved in oils, or conjugated with them, and so can be applied to skin as a cream, for example steroids and antihistamine preparations.
- *Chemical charge*: uncharged particles enter more readily than electrically charged ones. Anions (negatively charged particles, e.g. chloride, Cl^-) enter more readily than cations (positively charged particles, e.g. sodium, Na^+). This is because the outer surface of the membrane carries a positive charge, and like charges repel each other and opposite charges attract.
- *Temperature*: an increase in temperature increases the random movement of chemicals and hence promotes the passage of substances across membranes.

The passage of substances across the membrane is a dynamic process, however, and the direction in which they can move across it depends upon their mode of transport. That is, substances move passively by diffusion, or actively by active transport, pinocytosis or phagocytosis. All of these mechanisms play a role in ensuring that biochemical homeostasis in body fluids is maintained. The active and passive mechanisms involved in transporting substances across membranes are summarized in Table 2.2 and are explained further in the next section.

HOMEOSTATIC MECHANISMS BY WHICH SUBSTANCES ARE TRANSPORTED ACROSS THE CELL MEMBRANE

Passive processes

Diffusion

Diffusion is the passage of chemicals from regions of high (strong) concentration to regions of low (weak) concentration of that substance, resulting eventually in its uniform (equal) distribution. Diffusion also acts as a transport mechanism within the cell. For a common domestic example of diffusion, let us consider making a diluted orange drink. If we put water into the tumbler first, and then add the concentrated orange juice, the orange particles diffuse outwards from their point of entry. Initially, the colour is lighter further away from the juice's entry point. Later, the orange solution has a uniform colour because the orange chemicals have moved down their concentration gradient until an even distribution is achieved.

In considering the diffusion of chemicals across a membrane, the process can be subdivided into that of simple diffusion and that of facilitated diffusion because of the restricted nature of the membrane for some substances.

Simple diffusion

Small, uncharged, lipid-soluble substances pass readily across the cell membrane. Diffusion of these chemicals is in both directions, occurring between the intracellular and extracellular compartments. The net passage of the substance depends upon the direction of the concentration gradient. For example, the movement of oxygen from blood to intracellular fluid is necessary to produce energy from the breakdown of food. The movement of carbon dioxide is in the reverse direction to prevent its accumulation inside the cell. Such diffusion movements will be essential since changes in the rate could be disastrous for metabolism and hence for the maintenance of intracellular homeostasis.

Other substances that undergo diffusion include:

- lipid-soluble materials, such as steroid hormones, oestrogens and progesterones;
- small charged particles that are not lipid soluble, such as sodium (Na^+), potassium (K^+) and chloride (Cl^-), but that can diffuse through the membrane through channels provided by integral proteins within it;
- chemicals such as urea, ethanol and water that have a weak charge polarity. Urea and ethanol are fat soluble, and so diffuse through the lipid part of the membrane. Water moves across membranes by osmosis (a special form of diffusion).

Rate of diffusion

Diffusion across the cell membrane is quicker when the following conditions occur:

- A greater surface area is available. In certain areas of the body, the surface area of cells is increased by the presence of finger-like processes called villi and microvilli (see Figure 10.13, p.250). The development of villi and microvilli could be regarded as an evolutionary adaptation by multicellular organisms to ensure a greater rate of absorption of digested foods to maintain their increased metabolic demands.
- There is a greater permeability of the membrane to specific substances. For example, the resting membrane of nerve cells is approximately 20 times more permeable to potassium than to sodium. Consequently, potassium exit from the cell is more rapid than sodium entry. The concentration gradients for potassium and sodium are sustained by an intracellular pump mechanism, called the sodium/potassium ATPase pump (see Figures 8.21, p.188, and 8.22, p.189). Nevertheless, the constant leak of potassium is responsible for the positive electrical charge on the surface of the cell membrane.
- Increased concentration gradients.

Facilitated diffusion

Facilitated diffusion is a quicker mechanism than simple diffusion. The process involves carrier chemicals, usually integral proteins, in the membrane. Carriers transport relatively large

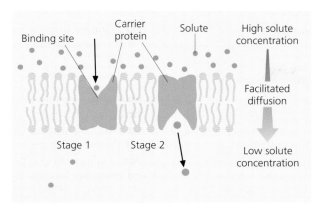

Figure 2.5 Model of facilitated diffusion. A solute chemical (e.g. glucose) is transported across the cell membrane by a carrier protein. Stage 1: carrier chemical binds with the solute, which then changes its shape (stage 2), so that a channel is opened and the solute can pass into the cell's cytoplasm. The process does not use metabolic energy; solute chemicals pass down a concentration gradient

chemicals (e.g. glucose and amino acids) across the membrane, thus releasing these substances into the cytoplasm (Figure 2.5).

Rate of facilitated diffusion

In addition to those factors noted above that increase the rate of simple diffusion, another important factor in controlling the rate of facilitated diffusion is the amount and availability of carrier chemicals. Some carrier-mediated mechanisms are influenced by hormonal actions (see Figure 9.1, p.208). For example, insulin is a hormone (i.e. chemical messenger) that lowers blood glucose concentration and is secreted when the concentration is above its homeostatic range. Insulin enhances the carrier mechanism of glucose, and so facilitates the diffusion of glucose into its target tissues, thereby increasing its utilization inside the cell. The homeostatic regulation of blood glucose concentration is described in detail in Chapter 9, pp.207–8.

Osmosis

Osmosis is the flow of solvent (in most circumstances, water) across a selectively permeable membrane from a dilute to a more concentrated solution. Osmosis is thus a special case of diffusion. Membranes provide little resistance to the movement of water. Therefore, provided that the dissolved substance (called the solute) cannot pass through the cell membrane, then the net effect of osmosis is that more water will move to areas of lower solvent concentrations (= higher solute concentration) than in the opposite direction (Figure 2.6). This continues until the pressure of the increasing vol-

ume of the solution on one side of the membrane counterbalances the movement.

The osmotic pressure of a solution therefore is the force required to stop the net flow of water across a selectively permeable membrane when the membrane separates solutions of different concentrations. The cell membrane maintains different fluid compositions inside the cell relative to outside it. However, there is usually no osmotic pressure difference, as osmosis relates to a difference in the total concentration of **all** solutes, sometimes referred to as the osmotic potential, and this is the same on each side of the membrane. Changes in the total concentration on one side of the membrane can occur. For example, if an individual solute becomes more concentrated, this will subject the membrane to osmotic effects. It is important, therefore, that cells have relatively constant internal and external osmotic pressures to maintain intracellular and extracellular water balance. This principle can be demonstrated by suspending erythrocytes (red blood cells) in a solution, such as 0.9% sodium chloride, which is isotonic ('iso-' =

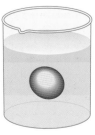

(a) isotonic solution

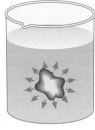

(b) hypertonic solution

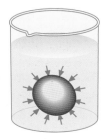

(c) hypotonic solution

Figure 2.6 Osmosis and red blood cells. (a) Isotonic solution; (b) hypertonic solution and crenation; (c) hypotonic solution and potential lysis

Q *Explain why osmosis is referred to as a special case of diffusion.*

BOX 2.3 REHYDRATION THERAPY: A FACILITATED PROCESS

The administration of the solution made up of one tablespoon sugar and one tablespoon salt added to 1 L water (known as rehydration therapy) is an example of facilitated diffusion in action. The sugar facilitates the absorption of salt, hence speeding up diffusion.

BOX 2.4 INTRAVENOUS INFUSION OF NORMAL SALINE

Cells must maintain their isotonic interdependence, otherwise changes in fluid balance, and the resultant effects on solute concentrations, will disturb intracellular homeostasis. Fluids administered intravenously for clinical reasons are normally isotonic to prevent disturbance to intracellular fluid, and hence a potential imbalance. A common fluid used in clinical practice is 'normal' (isotonic) saline (*c.* 0.9%, which means that 0.9 g NaCl is dissolved in every 100 mL of solution) administered as an infusion.

equal, '-tonic' = pressure, strength) to the intracellular fluid. In such an environment there will be random movement of water into and out of cells, but with the absence of an osmotic gradient the volume moved in either direction will be equal. Consequently, there will be no net movement, and the cell volume is unchanged (Figure 2.6a).

When extracellular environments are hypertonic ('hyper-' = strong, above normal), however, water moves out of the cell by osmosis and causes a decrease in cell volume, with the membrane becoming wrinkled or crenated (Figure 2.6b). This process occurs in the homeostatic imbalance of dehydration. Alternatively, when extracellular environments are hypotonic ('hypo-' = weak, below normal), water moves into the cell by osmosis and causes an increase in cell volume. If the extracellular environments are sufficiently hypotonic (i.e. very diluted), water continues to enter until the intracellular pressure exerted on the cell membrane causes the cell to lyse or burst. The lysis of erythrocytes is termed 'haemolysis' (Figure 2.6c).

Filtration

The filtration process forces small chemicals through pores within the membranes of small blood vessels (called capillaries) with the aid of water pressure (referred to as hydrostatic pressure). Movement is from regions of high to low hydrostatic pressures. Chemicals such as proteins in blood are too large to pass through the filter pores and so remain within the vessel. Details of the capillary exchange mechanism, and its modification in the formation of urine by the kidneys, are described in Chapters 6, pp.124–5 and 15, pp.425–8 respectively.

Active processes

Active processes require energy expenditure. The energy is released from an energy storage chemical called ATP produced from the breakdown of food inside the cell (i.e. in the process of cellular respiration; see Figure 2.11). The energy is liberated from ATP breakdown, i.e.

$$ATP \downarrow ADP + P + energy$$

The difference between active and passive processes is that in passive processes, chemicals move down their concentration gradient ('downhill'), and in active processes, chemicals can move from low to high concentration (i.e. against their concentration gradients or 'uphill'). Active processes include:

- active transport
- endocytosis and exocytosis

- phagocytosis
- pinocytosis
- receptor-mediated endocytosis.

Active transport

Active transport involves transporting substances across the cell membrane, usually by integral proteins using the energy released from ATP breakdown as its driving force (Figure 2.7). Active transport carriers are often referred to as 'pumps'. An example is the sodium/potassium ATPase pump; ATPase is an enzyme that releases energy from ATP. This active pump compensates for the diffusion exchange of sodium and potassium. The exchange is a consequence of higher potassium concentration in intracellular fluid and higher sodium concentration in extracellular fluid, and would drastically affect the intracellular environment if the pump was not available to reverse the ion movements. Other examples of pumps are the calcium pumps in muscle cells (see Chapter 17, pp.468–71), and pumps of various cell types that transport amino acids, some simple sugars, iron, hydrogen and iodine.

Endocytosis and exocytosis

These active processes transport large chemicals (collectively called macrochemicals; 'macro-' = large), such as proteins and lipids, that would be difficult to move by diffusion or conventional active transport. The process also moves small amounts of fluid into or out of certain cells. Endocytosis involves enclosing the material to be ingested inside a portion of the cell membrane to form a small vesicle, and then bringing the substance into the cell ('endo-' = inside). The reverse of this process, exocytosis ('exo-' = outside), is an important mechanism by which cells secrete substances. For example, digestive cells secrete enzymes, endocrine cells secrete hormones and nerve cells secrete neurotransmitter secretions using exocytosis.

Exocytosis is an important transport mechanism for all cells. It is necessary for the elimination of waste products of metab-

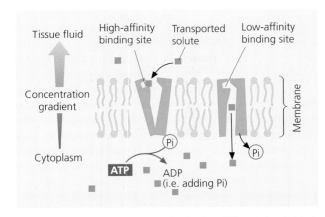

Figure 2.7 Active transport. Phosphorylation (i.e. the addition of phosphate) of carrier chemicals increases their affinity for the specific solute to be transported. Removal of the phosphate from the carrier decreases its affinity for the solute, and it is passed into the cytoplasm. Note use of energy (and phosphate) from ATP, which permits transport of solute against diffusion gradient. ADP, adenosine diphosphate; Pi, inorganic phosphate

olism and for the removal of surplus chemicals that cannot be stored, destroyed or transferred into other materials that the cell can use. The cell organelle known as the Golgi complex is important in exocytosis, and is described later.

Endocytosis and exocytosis are therefore instrumental in maintaining intracellular and extracellular homeostatic ranges of metabolites.

Phagocytosis

This is a form of endocytosis. Phagocytosis literally means 'cell eating', and enables some cells to ingest relatively large particles. An example is the white blood cells, which have a defensive role to ingest foreign particles such as bacteria that have entered the body (see Figure 13.10, p.378). The process begins when the cell membrane encircles the particle by membrane distensions called pseudopodia ('pseudo-' = false, '-podia' = feet). The membrane then folds inwards to form a vesicle called a phagosome, which leaves the cell membrane and enters the cytoplasm. The contents of the phagosome then undergo digestion by enzymes collectively called lysozymes (Figure 2.8a).

Pinocytosis

Another from of endocytosis, pinocytosis literally means 'cell drinking'. In this process, tiny droplets of fluid and their dissolved components stick to the cell membrane, which then invaginates to form a vesicle called a pinosome. This structure separates from the membrane and enters the cytoplasm, and the pinosome contents may then undergo lysozymal digestion (Figure 2.8b).

Receptor-mediated endocytosis

This mechanism involves cell membrane receptors that recognize and bind to specific extracellular chemicals to form chemical–receptor complexes. This area of the cell membrane then invaginates to form a cytoplasmic vesicle called an endosome. The receptors separate and are returned to the cell membrane.

The ingested chemicals may be broken down by lysozymes but may also influence cell functions. For example, the hormone thyroxine enters the cell by this process (see Figure 9.1b, p.208).

Transport across the placenta

Transport across the selectively permeable placenta is via passive and active processes.

Passive transport

Most substances pass through the placenta by passive transport – either by simple or facilitated diffusion. Both types of passive diffusion can only take place 'downhill', i.e. along an electrochemical gradient. Simple diffusion depends on a difference in concentrations of substances, such as oxygen, in the maternal and fetal blood. The speed of transfer varies on the gradient and properties of the substance as well as on the resistance of the membrane.

Facilitated diffusion depends on a concentration difference, but the facilitated diffusion of certain substances, such as glucose, is aided by a carrier protein. These large proteins in the cell membranes speed up the rate of transfer.

Active transport

Active transport (see earlier) takes place against an electrochemical gradient, and energy expenditure is required by the placenta in order for transport to take place 'uphill'. Pinocytosis is used for the transport of even more complex molecules. Material, for example iron, makes contact with the syncytiotrophoblast, which then invaginates to surround it, thus forming a vesicle that discharges its contents onto the fetal side. Iron is found in both the fetal and maternal blood either unbound or bound to transferrin, a protein. Iron concentrations in the fetus are two to three times higher than in the mother. An example of transfer by pinocytosis is of unbound iron through the placenta.

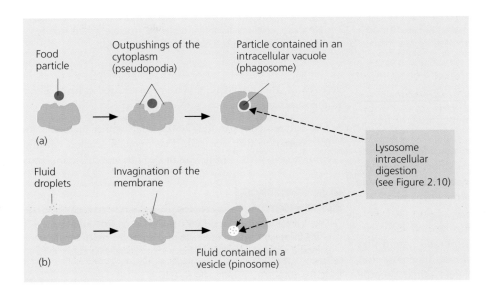

Figure 2.8 (a) Phagocytosis; (b) pinocytosis. SR, sensory receptor; HCC, homeostatic control centre; ER, effector response. (In the graph, box a represents a_1–a_4 in Figure 1.7, p.11, reflecting the individual variability in the homeostatic range)

BOX 2.5 DRUG INTERACTION AT A CELLULAR LEVEL

Since health is dependent upon the correct functioning of the components of homeostasis (i.e. receptors, genes, enzymes, ATP) and the optimal conditions (temperature, pH) for enzymes, then it follows that illnesses are a result of cellular, hence chemical homeostatic imbalances. Therefore, drugs to correct imbalances are aimed at altering alter cellular function by targeting membrane or intracellular receptors, carrier chemicals, chemical pumps, genes, enzymes, product of metabolism, and ATP (Figure 2.9).

It is frequently argued that knowledge regarding drugs is the concern of the medical team. However, the expansion of the role of some health carers (nurses and paramedics) now involves the training that gives them the responsibility to become independent prescribers. The authors would argue that all healthcare practitioners should have a knowledge base, and more so the carer is administering drugs since they must be aware of their site of action in order to state that they are competent for such an administration.

- *Receptors*: some drugs can deceive membrane receptors because they have a shape similar to the natural chemical receptors they usually complex with. For example, diamorphine provides analgesia relief by interacting with the same receptor sites as the body's natural pain killer, the endorphins (see Figure 20.6, p.569 for site of action). Other, lipid-soluble, drugs enter the cell and bind to intracellular receptors, thereby altering cell function by changing gene activity and hence enzyme synthesis. For example, breast cancer is often linked with a homeostatic imbalance of excess of oestrogen, which causes an excess of oestrogen-receptor binding, which is indicated as a factor that causes rapid cell division in breast cancer. Tamoxifen, a drug used in the treatment of breast cancer binds to oestrogen receptors, thus blocking some oestrogen–receptor binding and thereby reducing cell division (see the case study on breast cancer in Section VI, pp.631–2).

Drugs classified as partial agonists operate as agonists or antagonists (see Box 1.8, p.15) depending on the predominant chemical conditions in the body. Clinically, hyaluronidase is used to render the tissues more easily permeable to injected fluids, and is especially useful in some older people since they will have lost receptors as a consequence of the ageing process.

- *Carrier chemicals*: some types of drugs inhibit carrier functioning (e.g. the tricyclic antidepressants such as clomipramine prevent the uptake of certain neurotransmitters associated with depression: see the case study of a woman with depression, Section VI, p.644). Furosemide, a diuretic (used to increase urine production), prevents the movement of ions in the kidney tubule. Alternatively, drugs may also enhance carrier efficiency, e.g. amphetamines (commonly known as 'speed') enter cells to instigate the secretion of noradrenaline in the brain.

Noradrenaline is responsible for the effects (heightened awareness, loss of appetite, etc.) of using these drugs.

- *Pump mechanisms*: local anaesthetics, such as lidocaine and procaine, block the pain impulse by interfering with sodium channels in the membrane, and so prevent nerve cells transmitting the impulse (see 'action potential'; see Chapter 8, p.187). Calcium antagonists, such as nifedipine, are used in the treatment of angina and hypertension, and prevent uptake of calcium ions across the cell membrane of muscle cells of the blood vessels and heart. Calcium is the trigger for muscle contraction, so inhibiting its entry into the muscle cells of the blood vessels causes their relaxation, while heart cells become less contractile, and this decreases blood pressure. See Chapter 17, p.468–71 for details of calcium action in muscle, and the case study of a woman with myocardial infarction, Section VI, p.654. Calcium agonists (such as digitalis) strengthen the heartbeat, and are given to patients with heart failure. Digitalis causes a slight increase in calcium inside the muscle cells of the heart, and so enhances the force of contraction and strengthens the heartbeat (see Box 12.14, p.337).
- *Genes*: the Human Genome Project identified the structure of all the genes within the human being and hence there is now a huge potential for developing drugs for the individual which will cause expression and non-expression of genes to remove homeostatic imbalances of deficiency and excess of chemicals, respectively (see Box 19.8, p.539)
- *Enzymes*: some drugs competitively inhibit normal enzyme action by blocking the active site of the enzyme (see Figure 4.7, p.99). For example, aspirin is given to provide relief from certain types of pain. This drug inhibits the enzyme prostaglandin synthetase, thereby inhibiting the production and secretion of prostaglandin, the most potent pain-producing substance in the body. Other forms of pain relief, such as transcutaneous electrical nerve stimulation, acupuncture, acupressure, touch therapy, Bowen technique, massage, imagery, relaxation and even placebo therapies, also operate at a cellular level. You should be able to understand the site of cellular action of these methods of pain relief after reading Chapter 20 and assimilating Figure 20.6, p.569. Since the completion the Human Genome Project the UK Government have diverted funding to the Proteomics Project, which is basically the identification of enzymes (i.e. the product of gene expression). Once the structure of an enzyme is identified, its active sites can be blocked by drugs designed for the purpose (i.e. in homeostatic imbalances of excess). Alternatively, it may become possible for the enzyme itself to be given as a drug to enhance the production of a chemical (i.e. in homeostatic imbalances of deficiency). Again, this will be very important in developing drugs for the individual.
- *Metabolic inhibitors*: these are drugs that operate by reducing the amount of ATP available in order to reduce metabolism.

CELL ORGANELLES

Organelles have specific roles to play in maintaining the homeostasis of the cell. Their structure helps to maintain the basic needs of the cell. For convenience, they are considered individually in this section, but it should be remembered that they function interdependently, just as organ systems work interdependently to maintain the homeostasis of the body.

Endoplasmic reticulum

The endoplasmic reticulum (ER) is a membrane system that forms an extensive parallel network of cavities called cisternae. Structure and extent vary from cell to cell depending upon the activity of the cell. ER functions associated with cellular homeostasis are:

- The ER provides passageways through which materials are transported within the cell. The organelle makes definite connections with the nuclear and cell membranes, and thus

ACTIVITY

Take a breather from your studies. Then reflect on your understanding of the following transport mechanisms used by the cell to control the entry and exit of chemicals to maintain intracellular homeostasis: diffusion, osmosis, active transport, phagocytosis and pinocytosis.

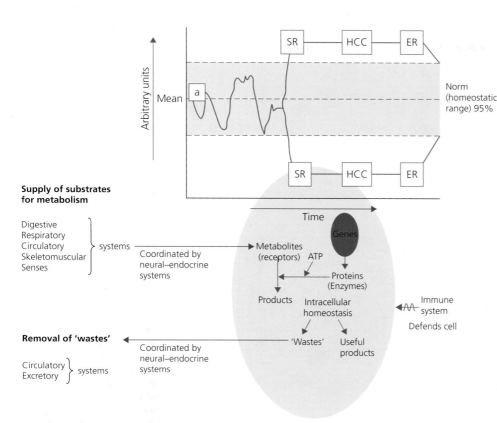

- Activate or deactivate receptors in times and deficiency and or excess imbalances respectively, and/or
- Expression or non-expression of genes in times and deficiency and or excess imbalances respectively, and/or
- *Administer and enzyme agonist-synergists or enzyme antagonist-inhibitors in times and deficiency and or excess imbalances respectively, and/or
- Administer product synergist-synthetic products or anti-products in times and deficiency and or excess imbalances respectively, and/or
- Metabolic enhancers or inhibitors in times and efficiency and or excess imbalances respectively, and/or
- *H^+ ion and body temperature modifiers

Figure 2.9 Clinical cytology provides a rationale for clinical intervention

may be a link between these two structures, and between adjacent cells (Figure 2.10).

- The ER segregates the cytoplasm into areas of different biochemical activity.
- The ER increases the surface area available for a variety of enzymatic reactions.
- The cisternae of the ER act as temporary storage sites for specific chemicals, such as lipids, proteins and glycogen (a carbohydrate storage chemical), which have been produced by the cell.

There are two types of ER, classified according to whether the membrane is associated with ribosomes (small structures concerned with protein synthesis). Both types are often continuous with one another and are interchangeable depending upon the metabolic requirements of the cell.

Rough endoplasmic reticulum

Rough (granular) ER is studded with ribosomes on its outer surface. Ribosomes are involved in protein synthesis; therefore

rough ER is found in all cells since enzymes belong to the protein family of chemicals. Enzymes are necessary to all cells because they catalyse (speed up) chemical reactions, ensuring that the rate of metabolism is compatible with life processes. The rough ER is an extremely important organelle that contributes to maintenance of intracellular homeostasis. It is more abundant in cells that are most actively engaged in protein synthesis (e.g. those that produce hormones and those that produce digestive enzymes).

ACTIVITY

Re-familiarize yourself with the basic needs of the body (see Table 1.2, p.10), because these needs are met by the organelles of the cell.

BOX 2.6 DRUGS AFFECT ENDOPLASMIC RETICULUM FUNCTIONING

Some carcinogens (chemicals that produce cancer) detach ribosomes from the ER, resulting in unusual sites of enzymatic activity, thereby changing the protein synthetic activities of the cell.

Barbiturates (a group of drugs that reduce the activity of the central nervous system) are classified according to their pharmacological actions. Some are general anaesthetics (e.g. thiopentone sodium), and others have hypnotic and sedative actions (e.g. phenobarbitone). Other drugs have tranquillizing properties (e.g. diazepam). All these drugs increase the amount of smooth ER and influence the activity of its enzymes. Some of these enzymes in turn inactivate the effects of barbiturates, which results in barbiturate tolerance and the need for increased dosages of these drugs for them to exert their effects.

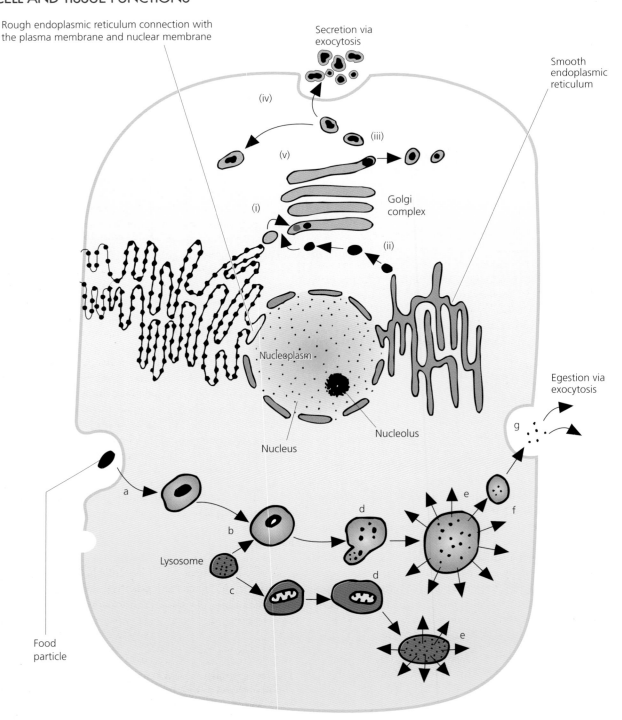

Figure 2.10 The homeostatic roles of the lysosome, Golgi complex and the endoplasmic reticulum. Lysosome: (a) phagosome produced from phagocytosis; (b) lysosome moves toward phagosome; (c) lysosome moves toward 'worn-out' organelle (e.g. mitochondrion); (d) intracellular digestion of particle and organelle; (e) useful products absorbed into the cytoplasm; (f) vacuole contains useless (residual) products; (g) exocytosis (egestion) of the residual products. Golgi complex: (i) protein from rough endoplasmic reticulum; (ii) lipid from smooth endoplasmic reticulum; (iii) conjugated lipoprotein complex in vacuole from the Golgi complex; (iv) conjugated lipoprotein complex secreted from cell; (v) conjugated lipoprotein complex used in cellular metabolism (e.g. production of organelle membrane)

Q Give a reason why the following statements are used in physiology: (1) cell, the 'basic unit of life'; (2) enzymes and ATP, the 'key chemicals of life'; (3) Golgi complex, the 'packaging factory of the cell'; (4) lysosomes, the 'suicide bags of the cell'; (5) genes, the 'vehicles of heredity'.

Smooth endoplasmic reticulum

The smooth (agranular) ER is smooth in appearance because of the absence of ribosomes. The smooth ER is concerned with the synthesis of non-protein substances, which vary from cell to cell. For example, the smooth ER of the adrenal glands and testes produces steroid hormones, while in liver cells cholesterol may be synthesized. The smooth ER of muscle cells is involved in calcium storage (remember calcium is the important trigger for muscle contraction). In addition, the smooth ER of liver cells is important in detoxifying potentially harmful substances, such as drugs and carcinogens.

Golgi complex

The Golgi complex (also known as the Golgi body or Golgi apparatus) is found in all cells except erythrocytes. It is structurally and functionally connected to the ER and consists of four to eight flattened membranous sacs, similar to the smooth ER except that the sacs resemble a stack of dinner plates. The sacs are called cisternae, as they are part of the cavity structures of the ER. The Golgi complex is usually located near the nucleus, facing the cell membrane, from which the contents of the cisternae may be discharged.

Homeostatic roles of the Golgi complex

The principal roles of the complex are to process, sort and deliver chemicals – mainly proteins but also lipids and carbohydrates – to various parts of the cell that need them. In addition, it is responsible for the packaging of secretory products before exocytosis. Thus, secretory cells, such as neurotransmitter-secreting neurons (see Figure 8.23, p.190), cells that produce digestive enzymes (see Table 10.6, p.248), and endocrine cells of the pancreas (see Table 9.2, p.222), have an abundance of Golgi complexes.

Some Golgi complexes remain inside the cytoplasm to perform intracellular roles, such as the regeneration of membranes of organelles and their enzymes so as to replace damaged ones (Figure 2.10).

Lysosomes

These organelles originate from the Golgi complexes. Lysosomes have a thicker membrane than the rest of the organelles because they contain about 40 different 'digestive' enzymes, which must be isolated from the rest of the cell. These are capable of breaking down all the chemical components of the cell, such as the nucleic acids (by enzymes called nucleases), lipids (lipases), proteins (proteases), and carbohydrates (carbohydrases). Collectively, the enzymes are called lysozymes. These enzymes, like most proteins, are synthesized in the rough ER and are transported to the Golgi complex for processing into lysosomal vesicles after leaving the Golgi complex (Figure 2.10). Lysosomes are found in most cells, especially in those tissues that experience rapid changes, such as liver cells (see Figure 10.20, p.261), spleen cells, white blood cells (see Figure 13.10a, p.378), and bone cells.

Homeostatic roles of lysosomes

Lysosome functions include:

- *Intracellular digestion.* Any substance that has been ingested by phagocytosis or pinocytosis is taken into the cytoplasm in a membrane-lined vesicle (phagosome or pinosome). The vesicle coalesces with lysosomes, and lysozymes are released into the sac and break down the substance, mainly into substances that the cell can use. These useful products are absorbed into the cytoplasm and may be: (1) added to the pool of these chemicals in the cell, if required, to maintain their homeostatic ranges; (2) stored in more complex forms; or (3) transferred into other chemicals that can be used. The residue materials that cannot be used are secreted from the cell to prevent a surplus homeostatic disturbance/imbalance occurring (Figure 2.10).
- *Destruction of worn-out parts of the cell.* Defective or damaged organelles are treated in the same manner as above so as not to compromise intracellular homeostasis (Figure 2.10). Sometimes the organelle is referred to as the 'digestive body' or 'dissolving body' of the cell because of these breakdown activities.
- *Autolysis.* For most tissues, cell death during our lifetime is inevitable. Cell death is associated with the release of lysozymes into the cytoplasm, and a process of 'self-destruction' called autolysis. This process accounts for the rapid deterioration of many cells following their death. It also ensures that some material (such as the membrane's lipoproteins, enzymes, etc.) from the dead cells can be reused in the general metabolism. Autolysis therefore has a role in maintaining homeostatic levels of chemicals in the body. Lysosomes are often called the 'suicide bags' of the cell because of this autolytic function.

BOX 2.7 INCREASED LYSOSOMAL ACTION – A CAUSE OF DISEASE

Inappropriate action of lysosomes is problematic. For example, most of us will have experienced the painful effects of sunburn that partly are caused by the effects of ultraviolet light to disrupt lysosomes in skin cells. The consequences are worse in some disease states.

Degenerative diseases (e.g. rheumatoid arthritis) are generally thought to be associated with an increased lysozymal, autolytic activity of specialized white blood cells known as macrophages. Cortisone and hydrocortisone injections are well known for their anti-inflammatory properties. They have a stabilizing effect on lysosomal membranes that reduces this destructive activity of lysosomes. These steroid drugs also suppress the body's immune system. Therefore, they are considered valuable clinical drugs used in the treatment of arthritis, severe allergies, eczema, some cancers and autoimmune diseases, since these conditions become worse if the immune system is activated. However, a low dosage over a short time is advisable since long-term use makes the patient vulnerable to other infections.

Tay–Sachs disease is an inherited condition characterized by protein build-up due to the absence of lysozymes in nerve cells. Children with this condition experience seizures and muscle rigidity because their nerve cells become inefficient.

The lifespan of cells varies enormously. Some cells, such as those of the skin and those lining the gut, have a very quick turnover rate, perhaps just a day or two. Red blood cells live for between 100 and 120 days (see Figure 11.7, p.279), while nerve cells may persist through an individual's life. Some cell materials, such as the protein keratin, found in hair and nails, persist after the death of the cell. Dead cells must be replaced to sustain the structural and functional integrity of the human body.

Mitochondria

The size, shape and number of mitochondria vary from cell to cell depending upon their level and type of activity. Different cell types, however, show the same basic mitochondria structure of a double-membrane organelle (Figure 2.11a). The smooth outer membrane encloses the mitochondria contents, and the inner membrane is arranged in a series of shelf-like projections, almost at right-angles to the longitudinal axis of this comparatively large organelle. The function of these folds (called cristae) is to increase the surface area for the enzymatic reactions involved in cellular respiration (Figure 2.11b).

Homeostatic role of mitochondria

Mitochondria are concerned with aerobic respiration, i.e. the energy-producing process involving the breakdown of fuel (food) chemicals in the presence of oxygen. Some of the energy produced is stored as chemical-bond energy in ATP. This bond energy is simply released as required by the breakdown of ATP (Figure 2.11c). Owing to their energy-producing function, mitochondria are often referred to as the 'power houses of the cell'. They provide about 78% of the cell's energy, the remaining 22% coming from reactions occurring in the cytoplasm; hence, this organelle is of vital importance in prolonging the life of a cell (Box 2.8). Energy from respiration is also liberated as heat (Figure 2.11c). Thus, respiration is an important contributor to the homeostatic regulation of body temperature within the body, and hence optimal enzymatic function. Carbon dioxide and water are also products of respiration, and are important in controlling the acid–base balance of body fluids and also optimal enzymatic function (see Chapter 6, p.128).

Cytoskeleton

Within the cytoplasm of most cells, there are various-sized filaments that form a flexible framework known as the cytoskeleton that provides structural support for the organelles inside a cell. There are four types of filaments: microfilaments (the thinnest), intermediate filaments, thick filaments and microtubules (the thickest).

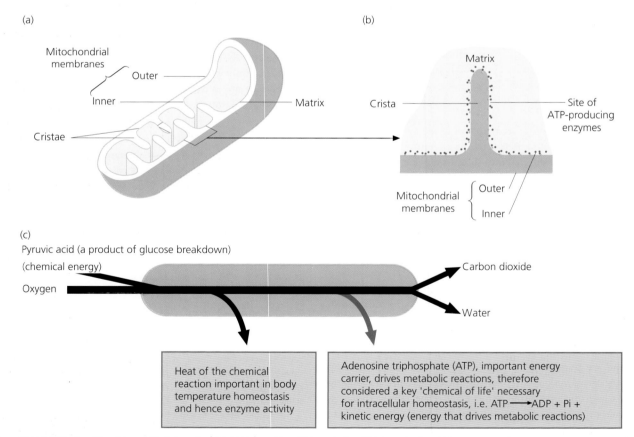

Figure 2.11 (a) Mitochondrion; (b) magnified view of a crista; (c) internal (aerobic) respiration. Pi, inorganic phosphate

Q *Suggest why the mitochondria are referred to as the 'powerhouse of the cell'.*

BOX 2.8 THE PRESENCE OF MITOCHONDRIA INDICATES THE LEVEL OF ACTIVITY OF CELLS

The number of mitochondria present in a cell is determined during the processes of differentiation and specialization of cells that occur during embryological development. Inactive cells can have as few as 100 mitochondria, whereas active cells, such as liver, muscle and kidney tubule cells, can contain thousands of mitochondria. The organelles may be scattered throughout the cytoplasm or located at a specialized site in some cells. For example, thousands of mitochondria are contained in the mid-piece of a sperm cell, and this region acts as the energy generator for the propulsion of the sperm tail (see Figure 18.12, p.502). Many mitochondria are found at the junctions (called synapses) between nerve cells, so chemical messengers (neurotransmitters) can be released actively. There are also numerous mitochondria close to cell membranes involved in active transport (e.g. in the cells of the intestines and kidney).

Mitochondrial enzymes are involved in the respiration process, and a decrease in their production and/or activity has been implicated in causing psychophysiological decline in old people.

Biologists have suggested that it may be that this organelle was once an independent particle, perhaps similar to viruses, which invaded cells and evolved a mutual (or symbiotic) relationship within them.

Mitochondria contain small amounts of DNA and ribosomes, and as a result they can replicate independently and produce their own enzymes. It is thought that the replication process occurs as a homeostatic response to an increased cellular need for ATP, in times of high metabolic demand, e.g. during:

- times of infection and illness, when there is an increased production of white blood cells (leucocytes) to fight off the infection or illness;
- the postoperative period, when the body is in the process of repair and regeneration of body tissues lost or damaged in the surgical procedure;
- times of distress, when there is an increased production of hormones associated with the stress response. Mitochondria play an unexpectedly important role in cell survival in the face of stress, according to a paper in *The Scientist* by Phillips in 2007. The paper suggests that the physiology of the mitochondria is critical for determining whether a cell lives or dies. Several authors have suggested that cells have an extremely neat mechanism to preserve mitochondrial and hence energy levels within the cell in order to prevent cells from undergoing a programmed cell death (called apoptosis; see later).

Homeostatic roles of the cytoskeleton

Microfilaments are composed of a contractile protein called actin. This substance provides mechanical support for various cell structures, and is thought to be responsible for many cell movements.

Intermediate filaments consist of proteins that vary depending upon the cell type, such as keratin found in epithelial cells (i.e. cells that line organs) and neurofilaments found in nerve cells. These filaments help maintain the shape of the cell and the spatial organization of organelles.

Thick fibres are found only in muscle cells. They consist of the contractile protein myosin where it interacts with actin to produce muscle contraction (see Figure 17.6, p.471). Non-filament myosin is found in most cells, however, where its function is to produce local forces and movement.

Microtubules are located in most cells, and are composed of the protein tubulin. These filaments help to support the shape of the cell, and are thought to be an important part of the cell's transporting system, particularly in nerve cells. Microtubules are also components of cilia and flagella, and so are involved in cell movements, and of the centriole, which is involved in the movement of chromosomes during cellular division.

Overall, cytoskeletal structures have important roles in supporting the position of organelles, in cellular movement, and as binding sites for specific enzymes.

Centrosome and centrioles

As its name suggests, the centrosome is an organelle that is located close to the centre of the cell. It is a specialized region of the cytoplasm near to the nucleus, within which are found two small protein structures called the centrioles, positioned at right-angles to each another. Each centriole is composed of a bundle of microtubules (see Figure 2.3, p.24). Each bundle consists of a cluster of microtubules, arranged in a circular pattern, with a central pair isolated from the rest.

Homeostatic role of the centrioles

During cell division, the centrioles move to the opposite sides (poles) of the cell and produce a system of microtubules, called the spindle, which radiates to the equator of the cell (see Figure 2.15c, p.43). Chromosomes become attached to the spindle's equator before migrating to the poles of the cell, seemingly connected to the microtubules (see later). Failure to form a spindle prevents normal cell replication (see Box 2.14, p.44).

Cilia and flagella

These are fundamentally similar structures, differing only in size and their modes of action. The more numerous cilia are generally shorter, often cover the whole surface of the cell and generally are used for moving fluids along channels or ducts. The larger flagella are often found singly, or in small groups, and generally are used to move the whole cell, e.g. sperm cell (Figure 2.12c(ii)).

Both organelles, together with microvilli, are extensions of the cell membrane. They contain microtubules along their length, and in cross-section they show a '9 + 2' pattern (Figure 2.12b(i)). That is, there are nine groups of two tubules arranged in a circle, plus an isolated pair in the centre of the circle. At the base of these organelles is the basal body. This controls the activity of the organelle, and is probably important in their formation. Below the basal body there is a structure similar to that of the centriole; it is thought that the centriole produces the flagella of some cells.

The longitudinal contractile protein filaments that make up these organelles have ATPase activity (i.e. ATP is broken down to provide the energy for the different modes of beating of cilia and flagella).

The beating of cilia is intermittent, not continuous. It has two phases or strokes, called the active (effective) stroke, which produces movement, and the recovery stroke (Figure 2.12c(i)). Ciliary movement is parallel to their surface of attachment.

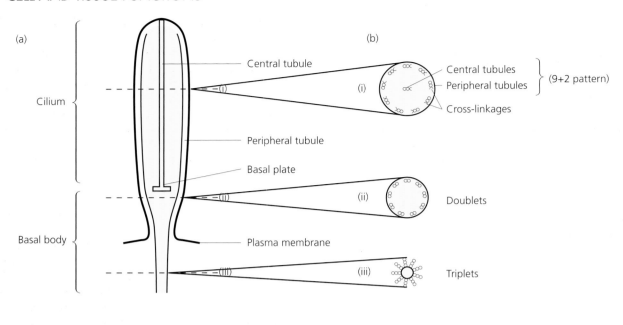

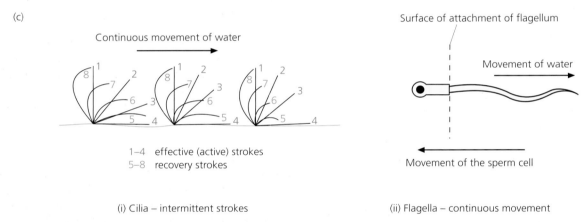

Figure 2.12 (a) Structure of a cilium. (b) Transverse sections of a cilium. (c) Mode of action of cilia and flagella

Q How are cilia, flagella and centrioles related to one another?

Q Give examples of where you would find ciliated cells. Name the male's flagellated cell.

Cilia have a greater density than flagella. This translates the intermittent motion of a single cilium into continuous motion, by ensuring that each cilium begins its cycle of motion slightly before the cilium next to it. Thus, a wave of effective strokes passes across the surface of the cell (like wind over a field of wheat). This movement is referred to as a metachromal rhythm. Flagella are longer, and each can contain several waves of contraction at any one time. They therefore produce continuous effective movement. The movement is at right-angles to the surface of attachment. Flagella are also capable of the active-recovery movements of cilia.

Cytoplasmic inclusions

In addition to organelles, the cytoplasm also contains inclusions. These are a diverse group of chemical substances that are usually food or stored products of metabolism. Thus, inclu-

sions are not permanent cytoplasmic components, as they are continually being destroyed and replaced. Examples of inclusions, and their homeostatic roles, are:

- *melanin*: a pigment present in the outer layer of skin (epidermis). Increasing the deposits of melanin causes tanning of the skin, and occurs as an adaptive protection mechanism against the sun's ultraviolet radiation. The pigment is also found in the hair and the eyes;

- *haemoglobin*: a pigment present in erythrocytes. The principal role of haemoglobin is to transport oxygen in the blood (see Figure 14.12, p.416). It also transports carbon dioxide and so helps regulate the acid–base balance of body fluids (see Chapter 6, p.128);

- *glycogen*: a storage carbohydrate found in liver, fat cells (called adipocytes) and skeletal muscle cells. It is produced

ACTIVITY

You may want to reflect on the reasons why enzymes are referred to as 'biological catalysts' before reading the next section.

from glucose whenever the homeostatic range of blood glucose is superseded;

- *lipids*: stored in adipocytes ('adip-' = fat) whenever the homeostatic ranges of the constituent chemicals, fatty acids and glycerol in blood have been superseded;
- *mucus*: produced in secretory cells that line some organs. Its functions are to lubricate the cells (epithelia) lining these organs, and to contribute to the external defence mechanisms of the body. For example, the mucus produced by the lining of the respiratory system has a protective function against atmospheric microbes that have entered the airways.

Nucleus

Most mature cells possess one nucleus (Box 2.9). The nucleus is the homeostatic control centre for cellular operations. It has two principal roles:

- To store heredity information (genes), and to transfer this information from one generation of cells to the next, and from one family generation to the next.
- To maintain intracellular homeostasis by directing chemical reactions (metabolism). It does this by expressing specific genes in order for the cell to produce appropriate enzymes that ensure that the chemicals inside the cell are within their homeostatic ranges. In addition, since all components outside the cell (i.e. in tissue fluid and blood) are ultimately of cellular origin, genes also regulate these components within their homeostatic ranges.

Mature erythrocytes lack a nucleus and hence genetic material; therefore they cannot duplicate or produce enzymes. They have a low rate of metabolism and so remain functional in blood storage banks.

The shape and location of nuclei can vary, but they are mainly spherical, and are usually positioned near the centre of the cell. A porous double nuclear membrane or envelope encloses the nucleus. Hence the fluid of the nucleus, called nucleoplasm, is in communication with the cytoplasm.

The nuclear membrane is continuous with the ER, which is also attached to the cell membrane. As a result, the nucleus may also be in communication with the tissue fluid (see Figure 2.10, p.34).

Prominent structures enclosed within the nucleus are:

- *nucleoplasm*: a gel-like ground substance that occupies most of the nucleus;
- *nucleolus:* there may be one or two nucleoli present. These membrane-bound organelles consist of protein and nucleic acids (deoxyribonucleic acid, DNA, and ribonucleic acid, RNA). Nucleoli are involved in cell division and are also thought to be involved in the initial metabolic reactions involved in the production of ribosomes. Final stages of ribosomal synthesis occur in the cytoplasm;
- *genetic material*: chromosomes store the heredity information in segments of DNA called genes. Humans have 46 chromosomes in their body (or somatic) cells. Sex cells (or gametes) contain only 23 chromosomes to ensure that at fertilization of the male and female gametes, the first cell associated with life (the zygote) has the full complement of 46 chromosomes.

Genes and protein synthesis

Genes are segments of DNA that contain the instructions for the manufacture of proteins. There are a huge variety of proteins, and it is this diversity that determines the physical and chemical characteristics (phenotype) of cells and, therefore, the human body. Genes control intracellular homeostasis by regulating the production of the enzymes (specialized proteins) necessary for metabolic processes. Since enzymes are the mediators of metabolism, they are often referred to as the 'key chemicals of life'. Human cells contain about 30 000 genes and these are responsible for the correct numbering, sequencing and arranging of the 'building block' molecules of amino acids in the required enzyme.

Most DNA is found in the cell nucleus, but a small amount is located in the mitochondria. The nuclear DNA is too large to pass through the nuclear pores. A gene therefore has to be transcribed, or copied, into a smaller nucleic acid called messenger RNA (mRNA). The mRNA can move freely between the nucleus and the cytoplasm.

Protein (enzyme) synthesis also requires the involvement of another form of RNA, transfer RNA (tRNA). This chemical is responsible for the translation of the original DNA message carried by the mRNA (see below). Actual protein synthesis occurs at the ribosomes, which are mostly attached to ER, although small clusters called polyribosomes ('poly-' = many) are free in the cytoplasm of the cell.

BOX 2.9 GENES – THE LINK WITH METABOLISM AND ILLNESS

The nucleus of each human cell, except gametes, contains the chromosomes that comprise our genetic make-up (genotype) that encodes the observable and measurable characteristics (called phenotypes) that we inherit from our biological parents. These phenotypic characteristics emerge during embryological development as the genes on the chromosomes are expressed to control metabolism of the cell. It is still uncertain how genes are expressed in humans to enable cells to differentiate into a diverse range with specialized functions (skeletal, digestive, renal, etc.) and at a specific time of embryological development (see Figure 19.4, p.526). However, it is generally thought that many environmental factors are the initiators of gene expression. The advances in the human genome and proteonomic projects may unravel these environmental factors (see Chapter 19, pp.554–7).

Chromosomes contain the necessary information to maintain homeostasis of all cells, and hence the functional equilibrium of tissues, organs and organ systems. Interference with this information by cells being infected by viruses, or altered by carcinogens or ultraviolet and ionizing radiation, may lead to homeostatic imbalances, resulting in the malfunctioning of organ systems.

DNA $\longrightarrow$ mRNA $\longrightarrow$ protein
(transcription (translation,
occurs involves tRNA)
within the occurs at
nucleus) ribosomal
level

Structure of DNA

In 1953, Watson and Crick were awarded the Nobel Prize for the discovery that genes were composed of the chemical DNA, which in turn was composed of relatively few types of molecules called nucleotides. DNA consists of two polynucleotide chains (i.e. each consisting of many nucleotides) coiled around each another as a double helix (Figure 2.13a). Each nucleotide consists of (Figure 2.13b):

1 one of the four organic bases: adenine (A), guanine (G), cytosine (C) or thymine (T);
2 sugar (deoxyribose, hence the name deoxyribonucleic acid);
3 phosphate.

The two strands of DNA are arranged so that one is complementary to the other through specific base pairing. Adenine of one strand pairs specifically with thymine in the other strand, and cytosine always pairs with guanine (Figure 2.13b). In discussions of the genetic code the bases are normally referred to by their abbreviations (C, T, A or G).

A sequence of just three of these base pairs provides the code for an amino acid. Since the mRNA that conveys this code to the ribosomes is a copy of only one of the strands of DNA, only the three bases on this strand form that code. This group of three bases is referred to as a triplet (or codon), and the sequencing of triplets along a portion of DNA that code for a particular protein is termed a gene (Figure 2.14a). Smaller genes code for polypeptides, which are the subunits of proteins. A typical gene contains a sequence of approximately 20 000 base pairs, although there is considerable variability between genes. The segment of copied DNA is called the cistron or the sense strand.

Proteins are made up of a large number of amino acids. There are 20 different amino acids available and, since the four

BOX 2.10 EVOLUTION, AND GENE THERAPIES

The genetic 'blueprint' or code in the form of base 'triplets' is used by all organisms and always relates to the same amino acids. It is the metabolism of these amino acids that varies between different organisms, leading to their diversity. This commonality supports the view that all organisms evolved from a common ancestry. This also helps to explain why viruses can replicate in human cells by incorporating their nucleic acid into our own. Similarly, gene therapies under development largely depend upon this process as a mean of inserting genes into defective cells (Munro, 1999) (see Box 19.18, p.556).

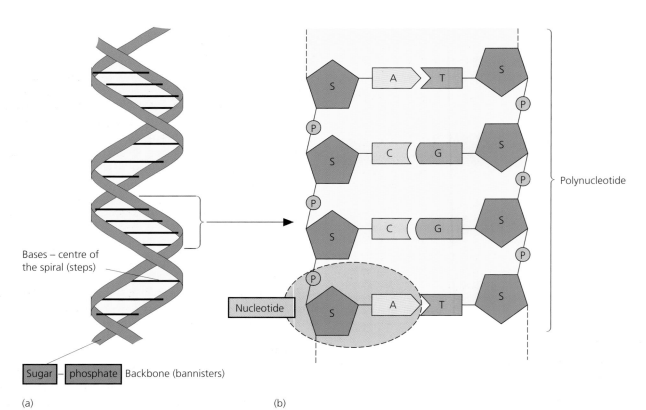

Figure 2.13 (a) The double-helical structure of DNA. (b) Magnified view of DNA components. S, sugar (deoxyribose); P, phosphate; T, thymine; A, adenine; C, cytosine; G, guanine

(a)

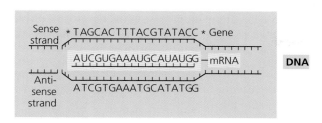

DNA

(b)

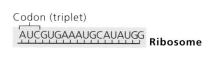

(c)

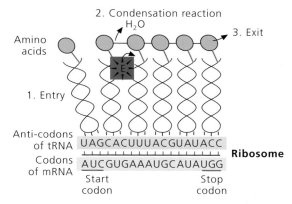

Figure 2.14 Protein synthesis. (a) Transcription: messenger RMA (mRNA) synthesis alongside the DNA strand in the nucleus. Note the gene is composed of the triplets from *to* on the sense strand. (b) mRNA passes out of the nucleus to become attached to ribosomes. (c) Translation: transfer RNA (tRNA) brings the amino acids to the ribosome. E, energy from the breakdown of ATP into ADP + P$_i$ + energy. Note that tRNA anticodons are the original triplets on the sense strand of DNA, which code for the specific amino acids. Pi inorganic phosphate

Q With the aid of this diagram, explain how proteins are synthesized using the following terms: DNA, mRNA, tRNA, codons, sense strand, antisense strand, cistrons, anticodons, transcription, translation, amino acids, proteins, nucleus, ribosomes, polyribosomes, endoplasmic reticulum, cytoplasm, peptide bonds, energy and ATP.

bases can be arranged in 64 different triplet combinations (4 × 4 × 4 = 64), some triplets must code for the same amino acid (Table 2.3). For example, the triplets CCA, CCG and CCC all code for the amino acid glycine.

Structure of RNA

RNA consists of a single polynucleotide strand. Each nucleotide within this strand is composed of:

1 one of the four organic bases: adenine (A), guanine (G), cytosine (C) or uracil (U) (uracil has a similar structure to thymine);

Table 2.3 The mRNA codons for amino acids

UUU } UUC } phe UUA } UUG } leu	UCU } UCC } UCA } ser UCG }	UAU } UAC } tyr UAA } UAG } 'stop'	UGU } UGC } cys UGA 'stop' UGG trp
CUU } CUC } CUA } leu CUG }	CCU } CCC } CCA } pro CCG }	CAU } CAC } his CAA } CAG } gln	CGU } CGC } CGA } arg CGG }
AUU } AUC } AUA } ile AUG met	ACU } ACC } ACA } thr ACG }	AAU } AAC } asn AAA } AAG } lys	AGU } AGC } ser AGA } AGG } arg
GUU } GUC } GUA } val GUG }	GCU } GCC } GCA } ala GCG }	GAU } GAC } asp GAA } GAG } glu	GGU } GGC } GGA } gly GGG }

Key: ala, alanine; arg, arginine; asn, asparagine; asp, aspartic acid; cys, cysteine; gln, glutamine; glu, glutamic acid; gly, glycine; his, histidine; ile, isoleucine; leu, leucine; lys, lysine; met, methionine; phe, phenylalanine; pro, proline; ser, serine; thr, threonine; trp, trytophan; tyr, tyrosine; val, valine.

Q Identify the potential mRNA codons that code for the tripeptide comprised of the following amino acids: alanine, histidine, valine and tyrosine.

Q List the corresponding DNA triplets that code for this codon and tRNA anticodon.

2 sugar (deoxyribose, hence the name 'ribonucleic acid'; see Figure 2.13b);

3 phosphate.

Transcription of the gene code

Transcription is the first stage in protein synthesis; it occurs in the nucleus. The process involves copying the sequence of bases encoded in the DNA chemical into the sequenced nucleotides of mRNA using the enzyme RNA polymerase. The single strand of nucleotides in RNA differs from DNA in that it contains the organic base uracil rather than thymine found in DNA, but the two chemicals are very similar. Consequently, during transcription the adenine of DNA is complementary for uracil.

For example, A DNA template with the base sequence of TAG, CAC, TTT, ACG, TAT, ACC would be transcribed into the complementary strand of RNA as AUC, GUG, AAA, UGC, AUA, UGG (Figure 2.14a). Apart from the insertion of uracil, this sequencing is identical to the complementary strand of DNA (ATC, GTG, etc.).

The template strand of DNA that is copied is called the sense strand, and the one not being transcribed is the antisense stand, since it complements the sense strand.

Translation

Once mRNA has been transcribed from DNA, the DNA reassumes its double-helical structure. The mRNA leaves the nucleus to become attached to the ribosome (Figure 2.14b,c), and its genetic message is translated. Translation occurs in a number of steps:

1 The process begins when the 'front' end of mRNA has attached itself to a ribosome and begins to move across it (Figure 2.14c). In doing so, the ribosome decodes the message by reading the triplets (codons). The first codon acts as a 'start' code; subsequent codons code for specific amino acids. The term 'initiation' refers to the process of positioning the first amino acid at the appropriate mRNA codon site on the ribosome.

2 tRNA chemicals in the cytoplasm are anticodons that are a complementary match for the codons on mRNA. Each tRNA chemical combines with a specific amino acid in the cytoplasm and adds it to the growing chain on the ribosome, according to the sequencing required by the arrangement of codons on the mRNA.

For example, the mRNA codon for the amino acid glycine is GGU, GGC, GGA or GGG, and the respective tRNA anticodons are CCA, CCG, CCU and CCC (Table 2.3). The tRNA that carries glycine from the cytoplasm for incorporation into the growing protein will have one of these anticodons; the tRNA itself will bond only to glycine and to no other amino acid. Note that tRNA anticodons are analogous to the original DNA triplets (except that tRNA has uracil in place of thymine).

3 Following initiation, elongation of the amino acid chain begins with the mRNA moving across the ribosome, one codon at a time. The codon is read by the ribosome, and the corresponding tRNA anticodon brings the specific amino acid and joins it to the previous one. A bond is formed between adjacent amino acids, using energy liberated from ATP catabolism. Further amino acids are added until a terminal 'stop' codon that stops the process is formed (Figure 2.14c). In this way, a polypeptide ('poly-' = many) is produced. Post-translational processing will incorporate this into a final protein molecule.

BOX 2.11 NEONATAL SCREENING IDENTIFIES MUTATIONS

Sickle cell anaemia is a life-threatening condition instigated by a change of just one DNA base pairing. This results in an abnormal gene. The change in base sequencing is called a genetic mutation, and it is responsible for the signs and symptoms of multiple organ system imbalances in the individual. Lees *et al.* (2001) suggested that early treatment (before symptoms develop) could improve both morbidity and mortality. Screening for the condition in the neonatal period would enable early diagnosis and therefore early treatment. Phenylketonuria (PKU) is another disease in which a genetic mutation has occurred. The presence of this abnormal gene means that people with PKU cannot produce an enzyme called phenyl hydroxylase, which is essential for converting the amino acid phenylalanine into tyrosine. Consequently, phenylalanine accumulates in the blood, tissues and central nervous system, resulting in brain damage leading to diminished mental development. Newborns are screened for PKU by the neonatal screening test (previously called the Guthrie heel-prick blood test). Babies identified as having PKU must be given a restricted phenylalanine diet to protect against the effects of the condition (Poustie and Rutler, 2001). Neonatal testing may also screen for hypothyroidism and cystic fibrosis.

GENES AND CELL DIVISION

All cells originate from the division of the zygote. Cell division, an important basic characteristic of life, is necessary to maintain cellular homeostasis. It ensures that:

1 the genetic material (the 'blueprint' for homeostatic function) is transmitted from one cell to another, and from one generation to the next;

2 the development of the organism through cell differentiation and specialization occurs;

3 growth of organisms takes place in specific stages of human development (e.g. neonate to infant to young child);

4 dying, diseased, worn-out and damaged cells are replaced to maintain the structural integrity of the human body, hence ensuring adequate organ system functioning;

5 optimal cell size is not exceeded, since this would lead to intracellular homeostatic imbalances.

Optimal cell size depends on an ideal surface area/volume ratio being achieved, since surface area relates to entry and exit of substances, and volume relates to utilization of the substances. The surface area is the cell's available cell membrane. This regulates the entry and exit of substances and, therefore, accommodates intracellular requirements. As cells grow, the surface area increases at a slower rate when compared with the change in cell volume. This is because the surface area increases with the square of the cell radius, whereas the volume increases with the cube of the radius. If the cell membrane cannot support the increase in volume, then intracellular disturbances and potential imbalances will occur (i.e. there will be insufficient nutrients available and a build-up of waste products of chemical reactions will occur). Cells therefore probably have inbuilt mechanisms that register the point at which cellular function is impaired and cause cell division to preserve the homeostatic status of cells. The components of homeostasis are involved, i.e. intracellular receptors detect the impairment and send the information to the homeostatic control of the cell (gene). The gene produces the enzyme DNA polymerase, which causes cell division to re-establish the surface area/volume ratio compatible for preserving homeostatic function.

There are two types of cell division: somatic (body) cell division (mitosis) and reproductive cell division (meiosis). In each case, the dividing 'parent' cells produce 'daughter' cells.

Mitosis

Mitosis ensures that the daughter cells have the same number of chromosomes (hence genes) as the parent cell, and identical DNA. For this to occur, the DNA of the parent cell must first be duplicated so that one copy can be passed into each daughter cell. Mitosis is therefore sometimes referred to as duplication division. The occurrence of mitosis completes one cell cycle and initiates the next one.

The cell cycle

The cell cycle is the sequence of events by which a cell duplicates its contents and divides into two (Figure 2.15a). The cell

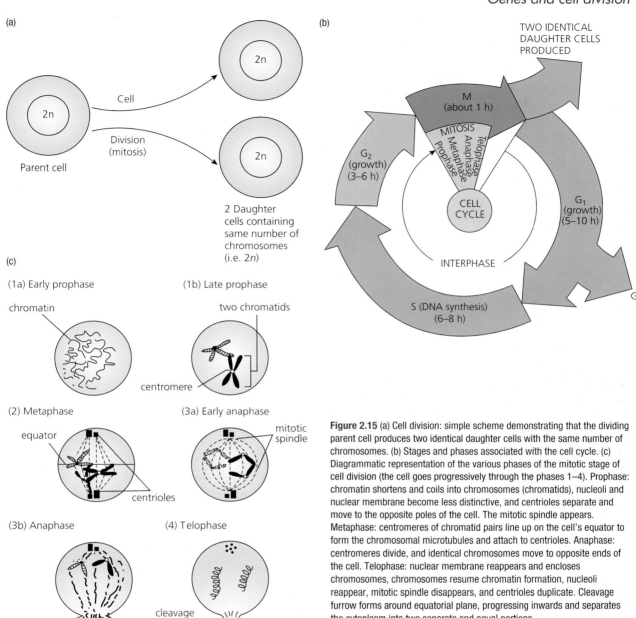

(a)

2n

Cell

2n

Division
(mitosis)

2n

Parent cell

2 Daughter
cells containing
same number of
chromosomes
(i.e. 2*n*)

(b)

TWO IDENTICAL
DAUGHTER CELLS
PRODUCED

M
(about 1 h)

MITOSIS

Telophase
Anaphase
Metaphase
Prophase

G₂
(growth)
(3–6 h)

CELL
CYCLE

G₁
(growth)
(5–10 h)

INTERPHASE

G₀

S (DNA synthesis)
(6–8 h)

(c)

(1a) Early prophase

chromatin

(1b) Late prophase

two chromatids

centromere

(2) Metaphase

equator

centrioles

(3a) Early anaphase

mitotic
spindle

(3b) Anaphase

(4) Telophase

cleavage
furrow

Figure 2.15 (a) Cell division: simple scheme demonstrating that the dividing parent cell produces two identical daughter cells with the same number of chromosomes. (b) Stages and phases associated with the cell cycle. (c) Diagrammatic representation of the various phases of the mitotic stage of cell division (the cell goes progressively through the phases 1–4). Prophase: chromatin shortens and coils into chromosomes (chromatids), nucleoli and nuclear membrane become less distinctive, and centrioles separate and move to the opposite poles of the cell. The mitotic spindle appears. Metaphase: centromeres of chromatid pairs line up on the cell's equator to form the chromosomal microtubules and attach to centrioles. Anaphase: centromeres divide, and identical chromosomes move to opposite ends of the cell. Telophase: nuclear membrane reappears and encloses chromosomes, chromosomes resume chromatin formation, nucleoli reappear, mitotic spindle disappears, and centrioles duplicate. Cleavage furrow forms around equatorial plane, progressing inwards and separates the cytoplasm into two separate and equal portions

cycle consists of two major stages: the interphase, during which a cell is not dividing, and the mitotic stage, during which the cell is dividing (Figure 2.15b).

Interphase

The cell does most of its growing in preparation for cell division during the interphase. It is *not* a 'resting' stage, as described in some textbooks. The interphase has presumably been referred to as the resting stage because a physical charac-

teristic of the phase is the absence of visible chromosomes. DNA appears as a thread-like mass of material within the cell nucleus, and is referred to as chromatin. There are three distinctive phases to the interphase: G_1, S and G_2 (Figure 2.15b); 'S' stands for 'synthesis' of DNA, and 'G' stands for 'gaps' in DNA synthesis.

The G_1 phase occurs immediately following the mitotic phase (i.e. after a new cell has been produced). During G_1, the cell is actively duplicating its organelles and other cellular

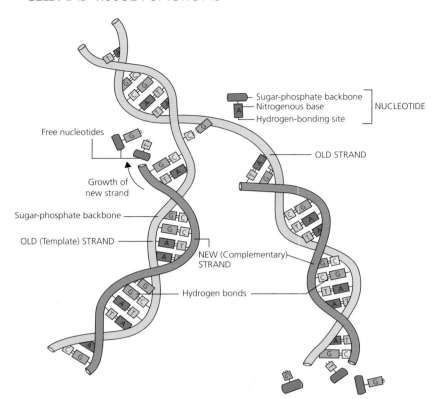

Sugar-phosphate backbone
Nitrogenous base
Hydrogen-bonding site NUCLEOTIDE

Free nucleotides

OLD STRAND

Growth of new strand

Sugar-phosphate backbone

OLD (Template) STRAND

NEW (Complementary) STRAND

Hydrogen bonds

Figure 2.16 Replication of DNA

components, but not its DNA. The centrosome begins to replicate in this phase but does not end until G_2.

The S phase occurs between the G_1 and G_2 phases. During the S phase, the DNA replicates to ensure that the daughter cells formed will have identical genetic material to the parent cell. During DNA replication, its helical structure partly uncoils, and the two strands separate where hydrogen bonds connect the base pairings (Figure 2.16). Each exposed base (known as the template nucleotide) picks up a complementary base nucleotide (with its associated sugar and phosphate).

Uncoiling and complementary base pairing continue until each of the two original DNA strands is joined completely to a newly formed complementary DNA strand. The original DNA has now become two identical DNA molecules.

During the G_2 phase, the cell continues to grow, and enzymes and other proteins are synthesized in preparation for cell division; before mitosis can begin, the cell needs to double its mass and contents. The replication of the centrosome is completed in this stage. Once a cell has completed the G_2 phase, the mitotic stage begins.

BOX 2.14 THE CELL CYCLE AND CHROMOSOMAL DAMAGE

A 'typical' body cell with a cell cycle time of 25 hours has a G_1 phase lasting 5–10 hours, an S phase of 6–8 hours and a G_2 phase of 3–6 hours. The duration of these phases is quite variable according to the ability of the specialized cells to repair, regenerate and divide and so are simply illustrative (see Figure 11.11, p.287). Some specialized cells (e.g. most nerve cells) remain in the G_1 phase for a very long time, and may never divide again. These are said to be in the G_0 state (see Figure 2.15b). However, most cells enter the S phase and thus are committed to cell division. Division is limited in skeletal muscle cells and neurons after specialization because of their complexity.

Although DNA duplication should conserve the genetic make-up of a cell, errors can occur during mitosis, with the consequence that daughter cells may exhibit chromosomal abnormalities such as additional chromosomes. Depending on the extent of the abnormality, such errors during cell division in the adult may not affect bodily function because this reflects the net effect of many thousands of cells. An accumulation of errors with age may, however, contribute to declining function with age, or even to the incidence of certain diseases such as cancers. In the

embryo and fetus, however, when cells are specializing, differentiating and growing, errors in cell division can have a pronounced influence on tissue development and function.

An extra chromosome present in the zygote is called a trisomy ('tri-' = three, '-somy' = bodies). Trisomy may have a devastating effect, since all the cells derived from the zygote will have an extra chromosome (hence extra genes), causing the signs and symptoms that are used to diagnose the syndrome. The best known example is trisomy 21, previously known as Down syndrome, in which the trisomy occurs as an error during meiosis of the female gametes (hence the condition is also known as a maternal syndrome). The range and severity of symptoms in the person with Down syndrome will vary depending upon how many novel detrimental genes associated with their extra inherited genes are expressed. That is, very few signs and symptoms exist if the extra genes inherited only involve the expression of only a small number of novel genes, while signs and symptoms may be severe if the extra genes inherited involve the expression of a large number of novel detrimental genes. (See Figure 19.21, p.543).

BOX 2.15 TUMOURS AND CANCER

All disorders involve a disturbance of cell function somewhere within the body. Many examples are provided throughout this book; this section will concentrate only on disorders of cell division.

A tumour is a swelling produced by an abnormally accelerated period of growth and reproduction of cells (called neoplasm). Tumours are classified as benign or malignant. Benign (non-cancerous) tumour cells are localized and encapsulated. These cells develop singly, or occasionally in small groups, and usually pose no threat to life. They are deemed safe as long as the tumour does not produce symptoms through pressure on vital tissues or become unsightly. Only a small percentage of benign tumours lead to 'secondary' growths (or metastases). These are referred to as 'innocent' tumours and may not necessarily be removed. However, if the size or position of the tumour impairs tissue or organ function, then surgical removal is required. This procedure is straightforward since benign tumours are encapsulated. Post-surgery, there is no danger of secondary tumours and little chance of recurrence.

Malignant (cancerous) tumour cells leave the original tumour site and infiltrate other tissues and organs. This spread (metastasis) is dangerous and difficult to control. This is because at their new sites metastatic cells divide mitotically and produce secondary tumours that will affect the functional capacity of the newly affected tissues or organs (Figure 2.17).

The term 'cancer' refers to a variety of illnesses, many of which are characterized by the appearance of tumours. Cancers are classified according to the type of tissue involved:

* *carcinoma*: malignancy of epithelial cells. Epithelial cells line hollow tubes and organs throughout the body;
* *leukaemia*: malignancy of certain white blood cells;
* *sarcoma*: malignancy of other body cells.

The functions of cancer cells differ from normal cells. The cells are abnormally large or small, and many have chromosomal abnormalities. Cell division is accelerated, and changes in function are largely irreversible. As the number of cancer cells increases, organ function becomes abnormal, and homeostatic imbalances associated with that system and the interdependent organ systems become apparent. Also, cancer cells compete with normal cells for nutrients, thus compromising the function of localized cells.

Aetiology of cancer

Cancer research has yet to demonstrate fully why certain cancer cells behave in the way they do. Nevertheless, much is known about the predisposing factors (Table 2.4). In addition, many environmental carcinogens have been identified, including plant poisons, microbial and animal toxins, tar (benzpyrene) in cigarette smoke, food additives, and deficiencies of vital nutrients such as vitamin A.

Specificity is also observed, since most carcinogens affect only those cells capable of responding to them, and very few carcinogens, such as radiation, affect cells generally throughout the body. In general, cells normally capable of rapid division record a high incidence of cancer, since they are more likely to respond to chemical or radiation carcinogens. Consequently, the incidence of epithelial tissue and stem cell (immature cells prone to rapid division) cancers are very high, while the rates of muscle and nervous tissue cancers are comparatively low.

Principles of correction

Because of the incurable nature of some cancers, prevention is paramount and this obviously involves avoiding exposure to known carcinogens. Should a tumour grow, however, then the odds of survival are markedly increased if the cancer is detected early, especially before it undergoes metastasis. Treatment of malignant tumours must be accomplished by one of the following:

* *Killing the cancer cells*: the treatment for early accessible tumours is surgical removal, accompanied by dissection of the related lymph glands, which may contain some migrating cancer cells. Deep X-ray radiation (radiotherapy), heating and freezing of cells are particularly effective treatments before metastasis. Radiotherapy prevents cell division by using ionizing radiation to break down the chemicals in chromatin and the cytoplasm. Radiation can be directed specifically at the tumour, but other parts of the patient's (and therapist's) body must be protected. The lead aprons worn in X-ray departments protect against these damaging particles.
* *Preventing replication of cancer cells*: cytotoxic drugs (chemotherapy) kill cancerous tissue by preventing mitotic divisions (Moran, 2000). For example, the drugs vinblastine and vincristine prevent mitotic activity of the cancer cells by blocking the assembly of the mitotic spindle. The problem is that these drugs are non-specific in their effects. Consequently, other mitotically active cells, such as those of the gastrointestinal tract, bone marrow and hair, are affected, which explains the side-effects of these drugs, including sore mouth, gastrointestinal tract disturbances, anaemia and hair loss.

The most effective therapies often involve a combination of procedures, such as radiation plus chemotherapy or surgery followed by radiation plus chemotherapy.

At present, tumour cells cannot be poisoned without harming healthy cells. Immunotherapy involves administering substances that enable the immune system to recognize and attack just the cancerous cells, and recent advances in 'designer' drugs also raise the possibility of specific treatments in the future (see Chapter 19, p.556).

Table 2.4 Summary of 'cancer inducers'

Hereditary predisposition Inherited characteristics make the individual more susceptible. Approximately 19 forms of inherited cancers have been identified to date.	**Chronic tissue damage** Injuries, instead of repairing or regenerating the cells affected, can produce cancer cells. For example, skin cancers due to overexposure to ultraviolet radiation (sunlight).
Radiation exposure The governmental health safety standards protect against harmful levels of carcinogenic substances. The problem is that not all the environmental 'pollutants' have been tested for their potential carcinogenicity.	**Age** Gene activity changes throughout life, and thus one's susceptibility to certain cancers changes. For example, colonic cancers are more common in people over 40.
Sex Certain cancers are frequently associated with one particular sex. For example, breast cancer is more common in females.	**Viruses** There are increasing numbers of viruses being linked to certain cancers, e.g. the papillomavirus that is responsible for cervical cancer.
Carcinogen/mutagen factors Many carcinogens are mutagens, since they cause chromosomal changes, e.g. insecticides.	

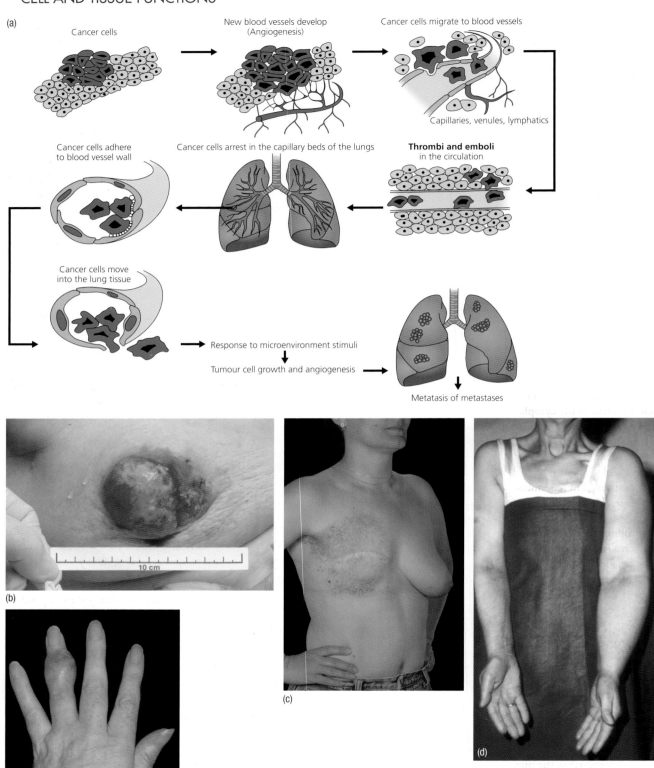

Figure 2.17 (a) The pathogenesis of metastases; (b) patient exhibiting right breast cancer; (c) patient receiving radiotherapy for right breast mastectomy area; (d) patient exhibiting lymphoedema of left arm owing to left breast malignancy; (e) patient exhibiting secondary metastasis in index finger of the left hand, from primary breast cancer site. Figures (b), (c) and (e) reproduced with the kind permission of the Medical Illustration Department, Norfolk and Norwich University Hospital NHS Trust. Figure (d) reproduced with the kind permission of Abrahams *et al.* from *Illustrated Clinical Anatomy*, Hodder, London

Mitotic stage

This stage lasts for about 1 hour. It consists of nuclear division (mitosis; i.e. when the nucleus and its chromosomes divide) and cytoplasmic division (cytogenesis). These events are visible to the microscope.

Biologists divide mitosis into four phases: prophase, metaphase, anaphase and telophase. See Figure 2.15c for a summary of the events associated with each stage.

Meiosis

Meiosis is referred to as 'reduction division', since it ensures that the daughter cells have only half of the chromosome complement, i.e. the cells will have only 23 chromosomes (the haploid number, 'hapl-' = half) in contrast to the 46 chromosomes (the diploid number, 'dipl-' = double) of the parent cell. Reduction division occurs in the male and female sex organs (gonads) during the production of the male and female sex cells (gametes; spermatozoa and ova, respectively) (see Figures 18.11, p.501 and 18.13, p.504). Meiosis is necessary so that the 'normal' chromosomal number is restored in the zygote after fertilization, and if it fails it has major implications for inheritance (see Box 19.10, p.544 and Figure 19.19a, p.543).

The role of genes in cell homeostasis

Many cellular reactions occur in specialized organelles and distinctive areas of the cytoplasm. All metabolic activities directly involve enzymes, and thus are controlled indirectly by the nuclear DNA, since genes are responsible for enzyme production. The availability of enzymes therefore controls biochemical/physiological and psychological activities to ensure homeostasis. The chemical nature of these reactions means, however, that regulating the availability of raw materials (reactants or substrates) and/or products provides another means of controlling metabolic activities. For example, if we restrict the oxygen supply to cells, ATP levels decrease, even though there may be adequate levels of glucose for cell respiration to occur. A decrease in ATP will affect cellular metabolism generally, since it is involved in many chemical reactions. If the levels of oxygen are restored, then (providing glucose levels are adequate) ATP levels will be restored and normal cellular activity will be resumed.

How are genes controlled?

While enzymes provide the link between genes and metabolic activity, the question arises as to how gene activity is expressed at the appropriate time. Various models of control have been proposed. These are based mainly on work with bacteria, and they suggest ways by which genes (DNA) control enzyme synthesis in response to the presence of substrates (reactants), endproducts and/or external regulatory mechanisms. We will discuss only one model here, since it is outside the scope of this book to explore the variety of models that exists.

The operon theory of genetic expression

One way to maintain the intracellular homeostasis is to modulate enzyme production according to the changing microenvironment inside the cell. For example, when the concentration of the endproduct of a reaction is above its homeostatic range, enzymes involved in its production could be inhibited and so prevent further increase (i.e. negative feedback; see Figure 1.8, p.14). The converse is true for an excess of reactants (Figure 2.18), i.e. enzymes are produced to remove the excess, usually by storing, transferring or destroying the chemical in excess. If neither of these mechanisms is possible, then the excess is secreted from the cell to maintain intracellular homeostasis of that chemical (see later). There are many theories of the gene expression to explain the regulation of enzyme synthesis; only one will be discussed – the operon theory – since it is outside the scope of the textbook to discuss other theories.

Jacob and Monod (1961), the proposers of the operon theory, worked with the bacterium *Escherichia coli*. They reported that they could produce two enzymes on demand if the cultured medium of *E. coli* was changed from the monosaccharide glucose to a disaccharide, lactose, made of glucose and galactose. When grown on a glucose medium, *E. coli* was able to use glucose directly in cellular respiration (Figure 2.19a). When grown on a lactose medium, however, the following enzymes were produced:

- *Permease:* produced to make the membrane more permeable (hence the enzyme's name) to lactose, which is a larger chemical than glucose. Remember, large molecules move across the cell membrane at a slower rate than small molecules.
- *Beta-galactosidase:* produced to convert lactose into its constituents, glucose and galactose (Figure 2.19b).

Jacob and Monod explained enzyme production, or induction, by way of the operon theory. They argued that there was a linear segment of DNA called the operon that controlled enzyme (protein) synthesis. In this case, the operon was composed of three genes – two structural and one operator (or promoter):

- *Structural gene:* contains the code necessary for the production of the enzyme. In this case, two structural genes are involved: the permease gene and the beta-galactosidase gene.
- *Operator gene:* controls the transcription of the structural gene necessary for protein synthesis.

Another gene called the regulator (or repressor) gene is involved in operon activity. This gene codes for the production of a regulatory or repressor protein (enzyme) that regulates the activity of other genes within the operon (Figure 2.19c).

The genes and their transcribed proteins therefore interact to provide control over the operon. The overall effects of this interaction are to 'switch on', or express, the structural gene when needed, and to 'switch off', or repress, the structural gene when enzyme production is not needed.

When an enzyme is required, such as when there is an excess of the substrate (reactant), the structural gene is expressed to reduce the substrate level to within its homeostatic range (see

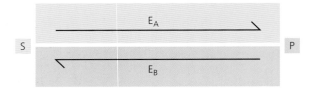

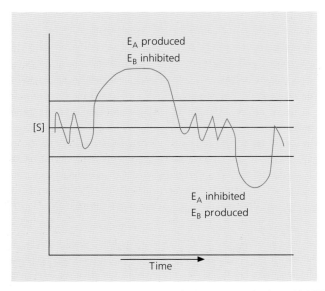 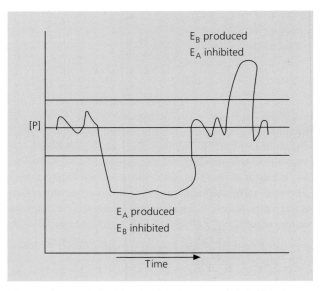

Figure 2.18 Intracellular metabolic homeostasis via enzyme production and inhibition. The reaction goes to the right when there is excess substrate (S) and a deficiency of the product (P). This is controlled by producing enzyme A (E_A), and by stopping the production of enzyme B (E_B). The reaction goes to the left when there is an excess of P and a deficiency of S. This is controlled by producing E_B, and by stopping the production of E_A. The reaction stops when the homeostatic ranges of S and P are achieved

Figure 2.18). Enzyme production may be repressed, for example when there is an excess of the product, or when there is a low level of the substrate specific for that particular enzyme. Using the example above, when *E. coli* is grown on a glucose medium, there is no suitable substrate (i.e. lactose), so there is no need to express the permease or beta-galactosidase structural genes. Consequently, the repressor protein blocks the operator and so represses transcription of the structural gene. This repression prevents the wasteful production of enzymes, a factor that is important in controlling intracellular homeostatic levels of enzymes.

Conversely, when *E. coli* is grown on a lactose medium, permease is produced to allow faster movement of lactose into the cell (a build-up of the substrate thus occurs). It then becomes necessary to express the beta-galactosidase gene to enzymatically convert lactose into its constituent monosaccharides (Figure 2.19b,c).

Gene expression: the link with intracellular homeostasis, health, ill health and development

Enzyme induction and inhibition are directly responsible for maintaining intracellular homeostasis. According to the operon theory, enzyme production involves the activation of the operator gene necessary for synthesis of that enzyme. As

outlined earlier, enzyme synthesis may be promoted by the following situations:

1 The availability of the enzyme is below its homeostatic range (see Figure 1.7, p.11).

BOX 2.16 THE p53 TUMOUR SUPPRESSOR GENE

The gene *p53* (on chromosome 17) regulates mitosis by acting as an inhibitor and as such is a tumour suppressor gene, i.e., its activity stops the formation of tumours. Mutations in *p53* are found in many tumours, and so play a part in the complicated set of connections that lead to the development of many tumours. If a child inherits only one functional copy of the *p53* gene rather that the usual two from their parents, they are more susceptible to developing cancer.

In the cell, *p53* protein binds DNA, which in turn activates another gene to an enzyme, which produces a protein called p21 that interacts with a cell division-stimulating protein (cdk2). In the combined form the cell cannot pass through to the next stage of cell division. Mutant *p53* no longer binds DNA in an effective way and, as a consequence, the p21 protein is not made accessible to perform as the 'stop signal' for mitosis. Thus cells divide non-stop, and form tumours.

While *p53* has an important role in the pathogenesis of human cancers, it is only one factor of a network of events that terminate in tumour formation.

Drug companies are currently trying to develop drugs to modulate such genes or their proteins.

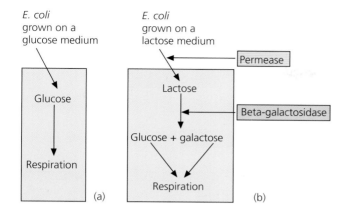

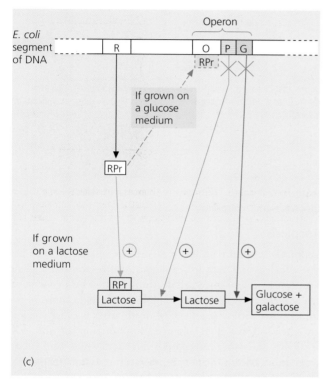

Figure 2.19 The Jacob–Monod operon theory. (a) *Escherichia coli* grown on a glucose medium; (b) *E. coli* grown on a lactose medium; (c) Enzyme induction and inhibition. R, repressor (or regulator gene); O, operator gene; P, permease; G, beta-galactosidase genes (structural genes); RPr, repressor (or regulator) protein; +, enzyme induction; X, enzyme inhibition. Summary: there is enzyme induction when grown on a lactose medium and enzyme inhibition when grown on a glucose medium

Q Using the principles applied to the operon theory, describe how: (1) the levels of intracellular metabolites are controlled; (2) cell specialization occurs; (3) overexposure to ultraviolet light may cause skin cancers; (4) drugs may be used to correct homeostatic imbalances.

BOX 2.17 HYPOTHYROIDISM

A failure to increase enzyme production will result in deficient substrate utilization. For example, in hypothyroidism there is a deficiency of thyroid hormone production. This deficiency means that the synthesis of enzymes involved in the conversion of glucose into energy is compromised, since thyroxine controls the rate of enzyme production. Cell metabolism is therefore depressed, resulting in symptoms such as apathy, slow thought processes, and a slowed pulse rate (for further information see the case study on hypothyroidism in Section VI, p.646).

2 The substrate (metabolite) is beyond its homeostatic range. The excess material must be removed, using further enzymes to remove the homeostatic disturbance hence potential imbalance. For example, in health excesses may be removed in various ways:

(i) The substance may be stored in a related form, e.g. excess intracellular glucose is stored as glycogen by the production of the enzyme glycogen synthetase.

(ii) The substance may be converted into another form; for example some amino acids in excess may be transferred (transaminated) into others if needed (i.e. if their homeostatic levels are compromised). Alternatively, excess of other amino acids may be broken down (deaminated) into energy-producing chemicals (keto acids) and urea. Keto acids are fed into the cellular respiratory pathway; urea is a metabolic waste product that is usually excreted. Transamination and deamination processes are instigated by the synthesis of enzymes known as transaminases and deaminases, respectively.

(iii) Toxic substances (e.g. alcohol), administered substances (e.g. drugs) and circulating substances (e.g. hormones) are converted to less active forms or are destroyed. Failure to produce the enzymes involved will result in prolonged activities of these substances. This is one of the complications of cirrhosis of the liver, in which liver function is severely disrupted. Transamination and deamination occur in the liver. A raised serum transaminase level is indicative of liver disorders.

3 'Old' or defective organelles must be broken down, and new organelles must replace the loss, to ensure intracellular homeostasis. The metabolic reactions involved require enzymatic synthesis and action.

4 Ultimately, a patient's illness (homeostatic imbalance) is a result of an environmentally induced gene expression or repression. Healthcare interventions seek to redress the patient's homeostasis. Interventions operate at a cellular level either blocking or enhancing the gene activating receptors, and/or directly by switching genes on or off, and/or indirectly by modulating gene expression, thus affecting enzyme production or their activities (see Box 2.5, p.32 for further information).

5 The subjective perceptions of pain, stress, and the 'time' inside your body (circadian rhythms) also involves gene–enzyme interactions (these topics are discussed in Chapters 20–22).

BOX 2.20 GENE INVOLVEMENT IN DISEASES THERAPIES

Gene expression is vital to the integrity of metabolic activity in cells. Loss of genes by a mutation (called a deletion) will produce significant alterations to cell metabolism, some of which may be sufficient to induce a disease state (e.g. cri du chat syndrome, p.529). Most disorders that arise from the inheritance of single defective genes have now been identified; most are evident at birth. The most common example in the UK is cystic fibrosis (CF). In up to 90% of patients with CF, pancreatic insufficiency necessitates the use of pancreatic enzyme replacement therapy, but there are concerns about the self-administration of inappropriately high dosages of enzymes (Basketter *et al.*, 2000).

Recent years have also provided increasing evidence for genetic involvement in diseases of adulthood. These disorders seem likely to involve mutations in many genes, or altered gene expression, but the promoting mechanisms are incompletely understood. Some mutations may be inherited, while others are accumulated during life. For example, colorectal cancer tends to occur in middle to late adulthood, and its incidence is greatest in countries with high socio-economic standards. The onset of colorectal cancer is related to prolonged contact between the faecal mass and colon mucosa. A diet low in dietary fibre and high in fats increases the risk of developing the cancer because of the accumulation of substances made by colonic bacteria that mutate DNA. The development of colorectal cancer appears to result from genetic deletions from various chromosomes (Department of Health, 1995). Clearly, an individual who inherits some of these deletions will be at increased risk of accumulating the remaining deletions during life. This helps to explain the occurrence of cancer primarily as a disease of adulthood. Some genes seem to be more crucial in this than others; e.g. people who inherit an altered dominant gene on chromosome 5 exhibit familial adenomatous polyposis coli. These people have a high incidence of polyps (a tumour within the mucous membranes) within the colon, and are more likely to develop colorectal cancer at an earlier age then those people who do not have the gene.

Note the role of diet and lifestyle in this disorder. The aetiology of the cancer is one of gene inheritance (i.e. nature) combined with environmental influences on genes and gene expression (i.e. nurture). The recognition of environmental modification of genes and/or gene expression will result in health education in the not-too-distant future for the prevention of many common disorders, including heart disease and insulin-independent diabetes mellitus. Information obtained from the Human Genome Project has implications for clinical research, and healthcare and nursing practice. The project will revise our understanding of an individual's susceptibility to disease from a nature–nurture perspective. Consequently, innovative clinical tests and gene therapies will evolve to benefit patient care (Munro, 1999).

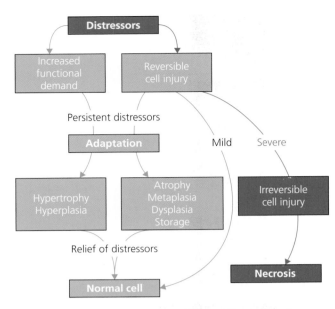

Figure 2.20 Cellular response to stressors. Redrawn with permission from (Rubin, E. *et al. Rubin's Pathology.* Fourth edition (2004) Lippincott, Williams and Wilkins)

Cellular injury and death

Cells adapt to their exposure to 'stressors' via changes in their structure (anatomy) and function (physiology). Cellular adaptation is necessary for the cell to survive. Nevertheless, if the stressors are too powerful, or are long-lasting, the cell's ability to adapt diminishes, resulting in injury and/or death (Figure 2.20). Stressors such as ischaemia can be overcome, as long as it is not too overwhelming and is not long-lasting. Other stressors such as radiation, oxidative stress, chemicals with extreme pH and pathogens can cause injury, followed by cellular death, if the injury is too powerful.

Once the cell has adapted it cannot return to its normal state. Damage to cells beyond the cell's ability of recovery result in cell death. The two main ways in which cells die are apoptosis and necrosis.

Apoptosis

Apoptosis is often referred to as 'cellular suicide'. It may be a physiological and pathophysiological cell response to cell signals. It is a programmed cell death, instigated by a genetic signal, and is an ingenious way to replace cells that cannot restore homeostasis with new cells. Cell death arises because enzyme-led chemical reactions change the function of the cell's organelles and other compounds. Stressors which bring about programmed death include: mutagens (i.e. factors that change genetic material), carcinogens and factors which promote ageing and trauma.

Physiological apoptosis occurs naturally in embryological development, when the cells grow, differentiate and specialize into well-defined tissues, organs and organ systems. For example, embryonic hands begin their developments as outgrowths in the shape of 'buds'; these differentiate into webbed shapes by approximately the fifth week of embryological development. Cartilage and bone development is followed by bone ossification during the seventh week, in association with the transformation of the hand into digits through the process of physiological apoptosis by the eighth week of embryological development. Failure to do this results in a pathological apoptosis, called syndactylism (i.e. the webbing of fingers due to the incomplete separation of soft tissue – see Figure 2.21). It is thought that autoimmune diseases, such as rheumatoid arthritis and diabetes type I, are examples of pathological apoptosis occurring.

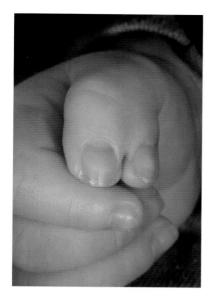

Figure 2.21 Syndactylism of the right thumb (digit 1) and digit 2 finger. Reproduced with kind permission of the Medical Illustration Department, Norfolk and Norwich University Hospital NHS Trust

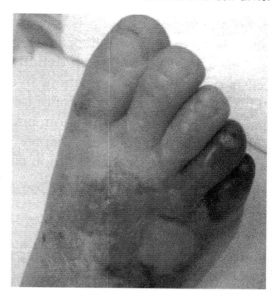

Figure 2.22 Diabetic foot with necrosis of the digits

Necrosis

Cell death by necrosis is a disorderly process related to cellular injury and inflammation. Accompanying cell injury is the depletion of the cell's energy storage component (ATP), and organelles. The cell dies if there is irreparable damage to the mitochondria, since sufficient quantities of ATP cannot be produced to sustain metabolism. Lysozymes are released from lysosomes, resulting in cellular component destruction in a process called autolysis (Figure 2.10). The breakdown of the cell membrane barrier results in the loss of the cell contents. Phagocytes are chemically attracted (via the process of chemotaxis) to the area and these cells digest the cellular debris in the process of phagocytosis (see Figures 2.8a, p.31 and 13.10, p.378). The result is local inflammation and death (necrosis) of cells (Figure 2.22).

Causes of cellular injury and death

Cells can be damaged in many ways that result in injury or death. Physical injury from pathogenic chemicals (e.g. bacterial toxins), mechanical harm (e.g. sports injury) or thermal wounds can cause damage to the cell's anatomy and hence its physiology. A common toxin is alcohol, which can cause injury to the liver if the exposure is prolonged. Cellular damage can result from 'deficit injury', in which cells are deprived of vital metabolites (e.g. oxygen, water, nutrients). This deficit injury is found in conditions of ischaemia, eating disorders such as anorexia nervosa (see the case studies on myocardial infarction, in Section VI, p.654).

Oxidative stress involves exposing cells to active free radicals that are formed by the reaction between oxygen and water during mitochondrial (aerobic) respiration. An example of a free radical is hydrogen peroxide. Damage to cells can occur from

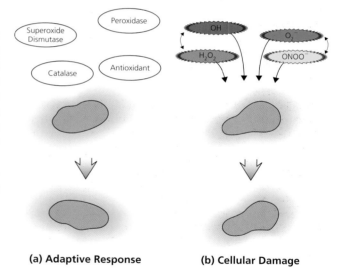

(a) Adaptive Response   **(b) Cellular Damage**

Figure 2.23 Cell response to oxidative stress: (a) cell adapts through appropriate gene expression, i.e. enzymes produced to inhibit free radicals (FR); (b) cell is damaged by inappropriate gene expression i.e. enzymes not produced to inhibit FRs. Redrawn with permission from (Rubin, E. *et al. Rubin's Pathology.* Fourth edition (2004) Lippincott, Williams and Wilkins)

excessive exposure to free radicals (which often cause damage to cells by targeting the genes) *or* an insufficient availability of enzymes, which convert the radical to less harmful substances, hence limiting the cell damage. Free radical injury is implicated in many conditions, for example diabetes, cancer, heart disease, infection, inflammation, through the ageing process and the use of drugs and chemicals (Figure 2.23).

BOX 2.21 EMBRYONIC GERM LAYER DIFFERENTIATION

Each cell type differentiates during embryonic development from the three embryonic germ layers (endoderm, mesoderm and ectoderm; see Table 19.1, p.527). The expression and non-expression of developmental genes (see the earlier discussion on the operon theory) effected by microenvironmental triggers control the process of specialization, e.g. a muscle cell is formed by the expression of genes concerned with the structural and functional development of this cell type, and by the non-expression of other developmental genes such as blood cell genes.

Functional specialization is necessary, as each cell type has an important homeostatic role to play in the person. There is a 'division of labour', so that the individual can carry out the characteristics of life described in Chapter 1, p.68. For example, muscle tissues enable the individual to move, skeletal tissue supports the body, glandular tissues act as secretory cells that release enzymes or hormones, and vascular tissues are involved in the defence of the body. Once they have specialized, some cells lose their ability to perform other functions. For example, the mature red blood cell is concerned with the transport and exchange of respiratory gases, but as a result of this specialization it loses its capacity to divide, since it has no nucleus or nuclear components. Nerve and muscle cells generally also lose this replication function once they become specialized, with the consequence that if such tissues are damaged they are capable of only limited regeneration.

TISSUES AND TISSUE FUNCTION

A tissue is defined as a collection of similar cells and their component parts that perform specialized homeostatic functions. The entire body is composed of only four primary tissue types – epithelial tissues, connective tissues, muscular tissues and nervous tissues – each having many subtypes with different roles.

The study of tissues is called histology ('histo-' = tissue). Histology is concerned with the broader patterns of cellular organization, the structure of tissues, and how this structure is important in determining the tissue's homeostatic functions in the organization of the whole person. Tissues are a good example of the complementary interplay between anatomy and physiology. Biopsy involves using laboratory techniques to examine tissue samples for abnormalities. This is known as histopathology ('patho-' = disease).

The body also contains a number of membranes formed from epithelial cells supported by connective tissue. This chapter is concerned with epithelial and connective tissues, and the types of membrane found in the body. Nervous tissue, skeletal muscle tissue, muscle tissue types, and specialized connective tissues, such as bone and the vascular (blood) tissues, are described in later chapters.

Epithelial tissues

There are three types of epithelia:

- simple epithelia, which are just one cell thick;
- compound epithelia, which are more than one cell thick;
- glandular epithelia, which produce the secretions of the body.

All are derived from the embryonic germ layers, and since they have different structures, they have different functions.

Homeostatic functions of epithelia

- *Protection*: simple (to a limited extent) and compound epithelia protect the underlying tissues from pathogenic invasion, desiccation (drying out) and harmful environmental factors, such as ultraviolet radiation.
- *Transport*: simple epithelia have important roles in controlling the transport of substances across membranous surfaces.
- *Lining*: simple, compound and glandular epithelia line internal cavities and tubes of the body, such as the respiratory and digestive tracts.
- *Secretory*: glandular epithelia are responsible for producing a variety of substances (sebum, sweat, tears, etc.) that have particular homeostatic functions; for example, the production and secretion of sweat are important thermoregulatory mechanisms.

Epithelial tissues consist of flat sheets of cells. All epithelia have a basement membrane, which is a thin layer of 'cementing' material on the underside of the tissue that holds the cells together.

Simple epithelia

Simple (covering and lining) epithelial cells are arranged as a single layer. These tissues are located in areas where they can carry out their roles of absorption or filtration (e.g. the respiratory surfaces of the lung).

Pavement epithelia

The side view in Figure 2.24 demonstrates that this tissue is made up of very thin, flat cells. Squamous epithelia are not found in areas where there is wear and tear, but will be located in areas that are adapted for the homeostatic functions of rapid diffusion, osmosis and filtration, such as in the alveoli of the lungs, the double-membranous Bowman's capsule of the kidney nephrons, the internal lining of the blood vessels and the inner surface of the heart, the lining of lymphatic capillaries, and the serous membranes of the body. These epithelia generally have fluid on one side and blood vessels on the other, so transport can occur between the two. They permit frictionless flow of fluids across their surfaces

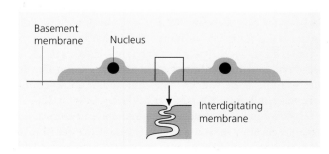

Figure 2.24 Side view of squamous (pavement) epithelium

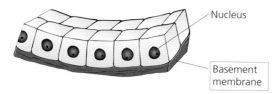

Figure 2.25 Side view of cuboidal epithelium

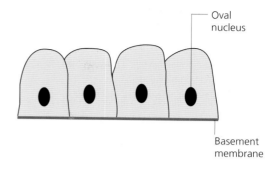

(a)

Cuboidal epithelia

Figure 2.25 is a side view of a cuboidal epithelium; it shows the cubic shape of the cells. These cells are slightly thicker than the pavement tissues, but they are still thin enough for substances to pass through them. This type of tissue is typically concerned with absorption and secretory functions, and is found in, for example, the thyroid gland, sweat glands, germinating layer of the epidermis of the skin, anterior surface of the lens of the eye, surface of the ovaries, and the proximal tubules of the kidneys. In these tubules, the epithelium bears microvilli, which increase the surface area for absorption of water. The nuclei of both squamous and cuboidal epithelia are centralized, and are either round or oval in shape.

Columnar epithelia

Figure 2.26a is a side view of a columnar epithelium; it shows that these cells are taller or thicker than cuboidal cells. The nuclei are oval, and are situated near the base of the cell. Examples of location are the lining of the digestive tract from the small intestine to the anus, and the lining of the gall bladder. The functions of columnar epithelia are varied. They provide a smooth area over which food can pass without friction, protect underlying tissues, and aid food absorption (i.e. the cells in the ileum possess microvilli that increases their surface area; Figure 2.26b). Some intestinal cells are modified columnar cells, called goblet or mucus-secreting cells (Figure 2.26c); their secretions lubricate or moisturize food to aid its passage and the physical and chemical digestive processes.

Some columnar and cuboidal cells have cilia on their free surfaces (Figure 2.26c), which facilitate the movement of materials along the duct. Examples of ciliated epithelia are the linings of the airways, where ciliated cells move inhaled dust particles and microbes from the trachea and areas beyond to the oesophagus, so that they can be swallowed, and the lining of the Fallopian tubes, where the cells move the female gamete to the site of fertilization, and the zygote and developing embryo to the site of implantation.

Compound epithelia

Compound (or stratified) epithelial tissue consists of two or more layers of cells. Only the basal layer lies in contact with a basement membrane. Cells of the other layers are derived from this layer. Compound epithelia are found wherever mechanical stresses are present, such as at the surface of the skin. One of their functions is to protect underlying tissues; others produce secretions, such as those lining the mouth and the anus.

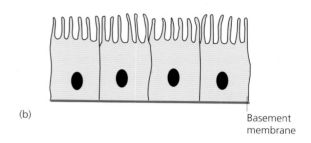

(b)

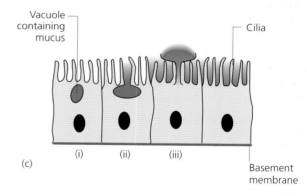

(c)

Figure 2.26 Columnar epithelium. (a) Side view. (b) Bearing microvilli. (c) Containing goblet cells bearing cilia: (i) goblet cell producing vacuole of mucus; (ii) vacuole moves towards the surface of the epithelium, which bears the cilia; (iii) secretion of mucus across the surface of the epithelium

---

ACTIVITY

Identify the type of cell division associated with basal cells.

Stratified epithelia are named according to the shape of the surface cells.

Stratified squamous epithelia

These epithelia are found wherever mechanical stresses are severe. The basal cuboidal, or columnar cells are in contact with the basement membrane, and are actively dividing.

The new daughter cells go through a series of changes before attaining the squamous shape of the most superficial cells. These cells are sloughed off during times of friction. Locations include the lining of the mouth, tongue, oesophagus and vagina (i.e. wet areas that are subjected to wear and tear).

Keratinized stratified squamous epithelia

This is a particular form of squamous epithelium in which the cells contain the waterproofing protein keratin. This enhances the barrier properties of the tissue, making it resistant to friction and aiding the prevention of pathogenic invasion. The epidermis of the skin is an example of this type of epithelium.

Stratified cuboidal epithelium

The role of this tissue is mainly protective. It is located in sweat glands, the pharynx and the epiglottis.

Stratified columnar epithelia

The functions of this tissue are protection and secretion. It is located in the male urethra, and in the lactiferous ducts of the mammary glands.

Transitional epithelia

This is usually made of three or four layers of cells, and is a tissue capable of being stretched. Before stretching, it has a cuboidal shape; when stretched, the cells have a squamous appearance (Figure 2.27). Its expansion properties help prevent rupture of the organ in which it is found (e.g. the lining of the urinary bladder).

Pseudostratified epithelium

This tissue appears to be an epithelium of several layers of columnar or cuboidal cells. It is, in fact, a simple epithelium as all the cells have direct contact with the basement membrane (Figure 2.28). Examples of location are the lining of the larger excretory ducts of many glands, and parts of the auditory (Eustachian) tube, which connects the middle ear with the throat (or pharynx).

Glandular epithelia

This type of epithelium secretes various substances from glandular cells, which either cover a lining epithelium or lie deep in a covering epithelium. The production and secretion of substances requires energy expenditure; therefore the cells have a high mitochondrial content. In addition, they usually have an abundance of ER and Golgi complex, which are responsible for the production and packaging of the secretions.

Glands are classified as either exocrine or endocrine. Their embryological development is summarized in Figure 2.29.

Exocrine glands

Exocrine glands secrete their substances into ducts (either as simple or compound exocrine glands) or directly on to a free surface (Figure 2.30). Secretions from exocrine glands, which are watery, are referred to as serous secretions. In contrast, mucus glands produce viscous (mucous) secretions.

Most glands in the body are exocrine, including:

- *sweat glands*: secrete sweat or perspire to cool the skin. Sweat also contains excretory products such as urea;
- *digestive glands*: the secretions from these glands break down food materials, providing blood and hence body cells with their nutrient requirements;
- *ceruminous glands*: secrete earwax (cerumen), which adheres to atmospheric dust particles and microbes that have entered the outer ear canal, thus preventing their entry into the delicate organs of the inner ear;

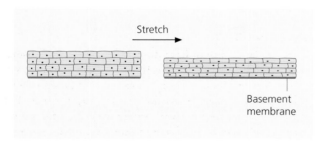

Figure 2.27 Side view of transitional epithelium.

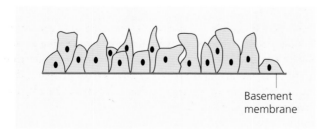

Figure 2.28 Side view of pseudostratified epithelium

Q How are epithelial tissues classified?

Q Where would you expect to find the following tissues: (1) simple cuboidal epithelium with microvilli; (2) simple squamous epithelium; (3) pseudostratified epithelium; (4) transitional epithelium?

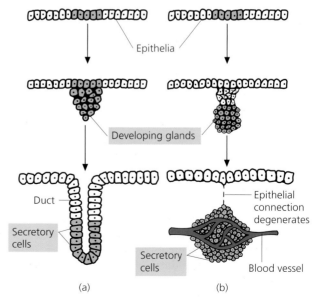

Figure 2.29 Development of (a) exocrine and (b) endocrine glands

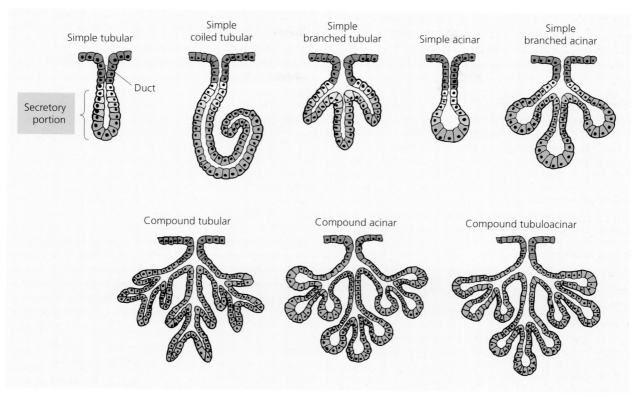

Figure 2.30 Structural types of multicellular exocrine glands. The secretory portions of the glands are indicated in green. The red areas represent the ducts of the glands

- *lachrymal glands*: moisturize and cleanse the surface of the eye by secreting tears. They also contain antibodies, thus act as an external defence mechanism.

Exocrine glands are classified according to the complexity of their ducts, e.g. simple or compound glands, the shape of their secretory structure, e.g. simple or compound tubular (Figure 2.30), or how the gland releases its secretion (Figure 2.31). The mode of secretion is referred to as holocrine, apocrine or merocrine:

- *Holocrine ('holos-' = entire) glands*: secretion from these glands occurs after the entire cell has become packed with secretions causing them finally to lyse or burst, thus releasing these secretions (Figure 2.31a). Future secretions from this tissue depend upon the lysed cell being replaced by the mitotic division of stem cells. An example is the skin's sebaceous (oil) gland cells.
- *Apocrine ('apo-' = off) glands*: the secretory products accumulate at the margin of the cell's membrane (Figure 2.31b). This portion, together with the surrounding cytoplasm, pinches off from the rest of the cell to form the secretion. Further secretions require a period of anabolic reconstruction of the secretory products. An example is the mammary (lactiferous) glands.
- *Merocrine ('meros-' = part) glands*: these cells provide their secretory products in vesicles, which are then exocytosed

(Figure 2.31c). Salivary glands are examples of merocrine tissue.

Endocrine glands

Endocrine glands do not have ducts, and therefore are sometimes referred to as ductless glands. These glands secrete their products (i.e. hormones) directly into the circulatory system, which takes them to a site of action in their target tissues. The endocrine system, together with the nervous system, coordinates all bodily activities in order to provide overall homeostatic functions. The main endocrine glands are illustrated in Figure 9.3, p.212

Mixed glands

Mixed glands contain a mixture of exocrine and endocrine glandular tissue. The pancreas is an example, secreting a variety of hormones (see Table 9.1, p.211) from its endocrine glandular tissue and a host of digestive enzymes (see Table 10.6, p.248) from its exocrine tissue. The male gonads, the testes, are another example.

ACTIVITY

Refer to Chapter 18, p.486–7 to identify the exocrine and endocrine secretions of the testes.

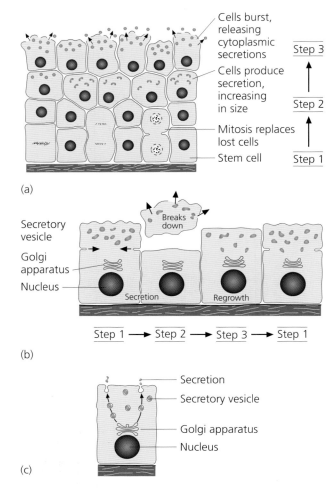

(a)

(b)

(c)

Figure 2.31 Mechanisms of glandular secretion. (a) Holocrine secretion occurs when superficial gland cells break apart. (b) Apocrine secretion involves the loss of cytoplasm. Inclusions, secretory vesicles and other cytoplasmic components may be shed in the process. (c) In merocrine secretion, secretory vesicles are discharged at the surface of the gland cell through exocytosis

Q How do apocrine, merocrine and holocrine glands differ from each another?

Connective tissues

Connective tissues are the most common tissue type in the body. Their general functions are to:

- protect the delicate organs that they surround;
- provide a structural framework for the body;
- support and bind other interconnecting tissue types within organs;
- transport substances from one region to another;
- protect against potential pathogenic invaders;
- store energy reserves.

The binding and supportive connective tissues are highly vascular. An exception is cartilaginous connective tissues, which are avascular ('a-' = absence), and as a consequence repair is not perfect following damage. These various tissues have distinct diverse appearances, but all have three common characteristics: they all possess a fluid, jelly-like or solid ground substance called a matrix, various cell types responsible for secretion of the matrix and various protein fibres.

Connective tissues can be subdivided into the 'true' (proper) connective tissues, and those that are specialized for particular functions (Figure 2.32).

True connective tissues

These contain a viscous matrix and two types of cell:

- *Fixed (immobile) cells*: some of these cells have homeostatic repair functions (e.g. stem cells, fibroblasts or fibrocytes), whereas others have homeostatic defence functions (e.g. phagocytes) or storage functions (e.g. adipocytes, melanocytes).
- *Wandering cells*: these cells have varying properties. Mobile defence phagocytic cells (called macrophages) and mast cells go to sites of injury. The former performs phagocytosis and the latter produce and secrete substances such as histamine and heparin at the site, which have local circulatory effects. T- and B-lymphocytes are wandering cells responsible for the cellular and humoral immune responses (see Chapter 13, p.376–8).

Three different kinds of protein fibres are associated with connective tissues. Collagen fibres are long, straight, stiff and strong, and provide tensile strength. Reticular fibres, made of reticulin, are interwoven between the collagen fibres, adding flexibility to the properties provided by the collagen. Elastic fibres, made of elastin, are branched and stretchable, and give the tissue some elastic properties.

There are four types of true connective tissue: white fibrous tissue, yellow elastic tissue, loose areolar connective tissue, and adipose connective tissue (Figure 2.33).

White fibrous tissue

This tissue may also be termed dense collagen tissue because of the large numbers of these closely packed fibres. There is less matrix associated with this tissue compared with loose connective tissue. The fibres are produced by types of fibrocytes located between the fibres, and are usually arranged in parallel bundles. The tissue appears white or silvery, and is tough but pliable. It is found in tendons, which attach muscles to bone, and in ligaments, which strengthen joints between bones.

Less frequently, the fibres are arranged in an irregular fashion. These tissues form the fascia of muscles, the dermis of the skin, the periosteum (external lining) of bone, and the supportive capsules around organs such as the kidneys and testes.

Yellow elastic tissue

This connective tissue is composed of elastin fibres produced by another type of fibrocyte. These fibres make a loose branching network, and are capable of stretching and returning to their original position. Much more matrix is present than in white fibrous tissue. Examples of location are in those ligaments that must provide more elasticity than collagen ligaments, the trachea, bronchial tubes, true vocal cords, lungs, and the walls of arteries.

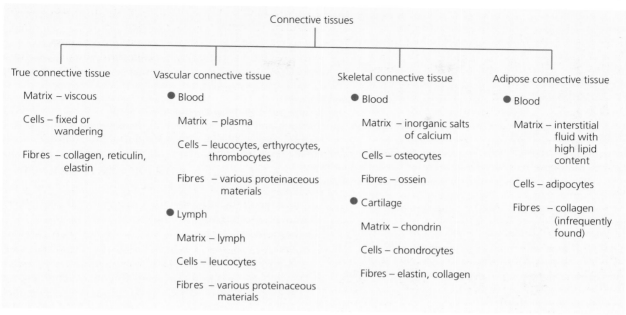

Figure 2.32 Connective tissue classification

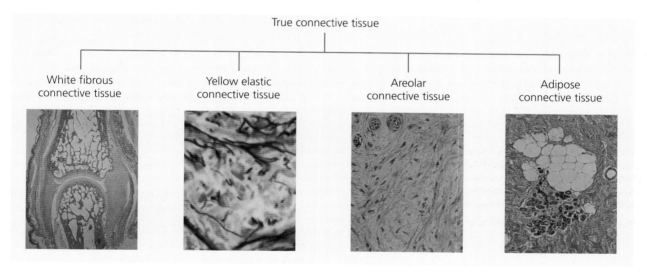

Figure 2.33 True connective tissue classification

Loose areolar connective tissue

This tissue contains the three different types of connective tissue fibres – collagen, elastin and reticulin – and thus has the properties of all three. Cell types present depend upon location, but include macrophages, plasma cells (antibody-producing cells derived from B-lymphocytes), melanocytes (melanin-producing cells) and adipocytes (fat-storing cells). Consequently, this tissue has defence, protective and energy-storage homeostatic functions. Loose connective tissue is found throughout the body. Examples are the mucous membranes, the outer layers of blood vessels and nerves, the choroid layer of the eye, the covering of muscles, the mesenteries of the gut, and the subcutaneous layer of the skin.

The collagen fibres of the subcutaneous layer of the skin firmly fix the skin to the muscle underneath, although the elastin fibres allow some stretching of the skin and allow the skin to recoil immediately, while the reticulin fibres add flexibility. A thick viscous matrix of hyaluronic acid is present, and the enzyme hyaluronidase (which breaks down hyaluronic acid) may be added to hypodermic injections, as this changes the constitution of the matrix into a water consistency and so aids the transportation of drugs, reduces tension and eases the pain of injection. Some bacteria, macrophages and sperm cells also use this enzyme to increase their penetrative capacity.

BOX 2.22 LIPOSUCTION

Suction lipectomy, or liposuction, is the removal of subcutaneous fat ('lipo-' = fat, '-ectomy' = removal of) from certain areas of the body, such as the buttocks, thighs, breast and abdomen. This treatment results in only temporary removal of fat, however, and is not used to treat obesity. It is usually performed for cosmetic reasons.

Adipose connective tissue

This tissue is concerned with the storage of fat. It contains large, fat-containing cells, or adipocytes, but has little matrix and few fibres. It is located subcutaneously (as the fat of the skin) around vital organs, such as the kidneys, at the base and the surface of the heart, and in the marrow of long bones. Its homeostatic functions are the storage and provision of energy (mobilized fatty acids can be utilized by the mitochondria of most cells), insulation to reduce heat loss, and protection of organs against injury.

Other types of connective tissues

These include skeletal connective tissue (see Chapter 3, pp.61–4) and vascular (blood) connective tissue (see Chapter 11, pp.270–1).

Epithelial membranes

Epithelial membranes are not to be confused with epithelial tissue: they are a combination of an epithelium and its underlying connective tissue. They can be subdivided into serous membranes, mucous membranes and cutaneous membranes. Synovial membranes are also found around skeletal joints, but these are not epithelial membranes as they have no epithelia; instead, they are composed of loose connective tissue, elastic fibres, and fat. Synovial joints are considered in detail in Chapter 3, p.84–7.

Serous membranes

Serous membranes (or serosa) cover the surface of organs and consist of a loose connective tissue and a layer of mesothelium, which is an epithelial layer of cells similar to simple squamous epithelium. They are single-membranous structures, but they fold back on themselves, leaving a small space between the 'outer' and 'inner' portions; they therefore appear as a double membrane. The inner, or visceral, membrane covers the surface of the organ and the outer, or parietal, layer attaches it to the wall of the cavity in which the organ lies (e.g. the visceral/parietal pleurae around the lungs and the visceral/parietal pericardia around the heart). The peritoneum, which lines the abdominal and pelvic organs, and body wall, is the largest serous membrane in the body.

Mucous membranes

Unlike serous membranes, mucous membranes (or mucosa) line cavities that open directly to the exterior (i.e. the digestive, respiratory and reproductive tracts). The mucosa has an epithelial layer that secretes mucus. The functions of mucus are to prevent cavities from drying out, to prevent dust and potential pathogenic organisms from passing down the airways, and to lubricate food in the digestive tract so as to ease the passage through the tract and to aid the processes of digestion and absorption.

The structure of the membrane varies according to location and function. For example, in the oesophagus and the anal canal the epithelial layer is stratified, as there is much wear and tear. In the intestine, a simple columnar epithelium aids the absorption of nutrients.

Cutaneous membrane

Finally, the cutaneous membrane (skin) is a complex structure involving a variety of tissues. Its anatomy and function are considered in detail in Chapter 16, p.446–7.

BOX 2.23 WOUND HEALING

Damage to tissue instigates homeostatic adaptive changes (wound healing) to repair and regenerate the tissue's structure and function so as not to compromise the function within the body. For details, see Chapter 11, p.287–96).

ACTIVITY

Distinguish between serous and mucous membranes.

ORGANS

An organ is an orderly grouping of tissues with a discrete function. Organs can be tubular (hollow) or compact (parenchymal).

Tubular organs

During embryological development, the body may be visualized as a large tube containing several inner tubes, such as the respiratory system, cardiovascular system, digestive system, reproductive system and urinary system. Each of these internal tubes has various functions, but structurally they are very similar to each other in that they are all formed of layers of tissues superimposed on one another in a specific way.

Each tubular organ has three basic layers:

- an inner lining tissue, or epithelium, and its underlying binding or connective tissue;
- a middle layer, consisting of alternating layers of muscle and connective tissue;
- an external layer, consisting of connected tissue and an epithelium.

Compact organs

Compact organs may be large (e.g. the liver) or small (e.g. the ovaries). Compact organs also have a common structure. A connective tissue capsule usually encloses the organ. If the organ is suspended in a body cavity, such as the thoracic cavity, it will be surrounded by a serous membrane. One side of the organ has a thicker area of connective tissue that penetrates the organ, forming the hilus. Compact organs have an extensive framework of connected tissue, or stroma. Strands of connected tissue, called septae (or trabeculae), extend into the organ from the capsule and hilus, sometimes dividing the organ into complete sections called lobules. Compact organs consist of functional cells (parenchymal) that predominantly occur in masses, chords, strands or tubules, depending on the specific organ. Parenchyma may be divided into functional distinctive regions, such as an outer cortex and an inner or deeper medulla.

ORGAN SYSTEMS

An organ system is a group of organs that perform a specific body function; for example, the respiratory system maintains the levels of oxygen and carbon dioxide in the blood. The major organ systems of the human body are summarized in Table 1.2, p.10. These systems work in a coordinated way to maintain the homeostatic functions of the body. The details associated with each organ are dealt with in their respective chapters.

SUMMARY

1 Cells vary in size, shape and function. The shape of a cell is related closely to its function, a phenomenon referred to as the principle of complementary structure and function.

2 'Cells: the basic unit of health, illness, healthcare intervention and death'.

3 'Receptors, genes, enzymes and ATP': 'the key to understanding the role of healthcare professionals as external agents of homeostatic control'.

4 Each organ system is an indirect homeostatic regulator of cellular metabolism.

5 'Systemic integration is fundamental in the maintenance of intracellular metabolic homeostasis'.

6 The cell's passive and active transporting mechanisms are homeostatic control processes, since they help to determine the concentration of intracellular metabolites so that the characteristics of life can be performed.

7 Cellular components – organelles – have precise homeostatic functions that are essential in maintaining intracellular homeostasis.

8 The control of organelle function depends on the production of enzymes, the synthesis of which is genetically controlled and environmentally modified, perhaps according to the principles underpinning the operon theory.

9 Homeostatic failures arises through nature–nurture interactions and may result from: inborn or inherited errors of metabolism; inappropriate numbers of chromosomes; the effects of environmental agents (e.g. overexposure to ultraviolet radiation can produce skin cancer) and the ageing process.

10 Clinical intervention is often based upon correcting the functioning of the components of homeostasis, for example genetic failure. This can be direct (e.g. chemotherapy or genetic engineering), or indirect (e.g. through medical or surgical intervention) or by adapting one's lifestyle to avoid harmful environmental agents.

11 Exposure to powerful stressors or prolonged exposure results in adaptation in cell function in order to survive, or cellular injury or cell death.

12 The two main ways in which cells die are apoptosis and necrosis.

13 Tissues perform specialized homeostatic functions essential for the maintenance of overall body homeostasis.

14 There are four principal tissues: epithelial, connective, nervous and muscle tissues. Membranes are composites of epithelial and connective tissue.

15 The principal tissues are classified according to the number of cell layers they possess, their structure and their function.

16 The principle of complementary structure and function predestines the tissue's location. Epithelial tissues, for example, may possess specialized structures such as microvilli, which increase their surface area – these are present in areas concerned with absorption.

17 Glandular epithelia may be simple or multicellular. Their secretions are defined as apocrine, holocrine or merocrine according to how they are released from the cell.

18 Connective tissues possess cells and their products (i.e. fibres and a matrix). They are classified according to the fibre distribution (loose or dense), and usually by the type of fibre they possess (elastin, reticulin and collagen). The exception is adipose connective tissue, which is named after its specialized fat-storage cells, adipocytes.

19 Membranes may be serous, mucous, cutaneous or synovial, the last being the only membrane that does not contain an epithelium and so is not an epithelial membrane.

REFERENCES

Basketter, H.M., Sharples, L. and Bilton, D. (2000) Knowledge of pancreatic enzyme supplementation in adult cystic fibrosis (CF) patients. *Journal of Human Nutrition and Dietetics* **13**(5): 353–61.

Clancy, J. and McVicar, A.J. (2007a) Short-term regulation of acid–base homeostasis. *British Journal of Nursing* **16**(16): 604–7.

Clancy, J. and McVicar, A.J. (2007b) Intermediate and long-term regulation of acid–base homeostasis. *British Journal of Nursing* **16**(17): 1016–19.

Davson, H. (1970) *A Textbook of General Physiology*, 4th edn. Edinburgh: Churchill Livingstone.

Department of Health (1995) *The Genetics of Common Diseases. A Second Report to the NHS Central Research and Development Committee on the New Genetics.* London: Department of Health Publications.

Jacob, F. and Monod, J. (1961) Genetic regulatory mechanisms in the synthesis of proteins. *Journal of Molecular Biology* **3**(5): 318–56.

Lees, C.M., Davies, S. and Dezateux, C. (2001) Neonatal screening for sickle cell disease. *The Cochrane Library*, Issue 1. Oxford: Update Software.

Moran, P. (2000) Cellular effects of cancer chemotherapy administration. *Journal of Intravenous Nursing* **23**(1): 44–51.

Munro, C.L. (1999) Implications for nursing of the Human Genome Project. *Neonatal Network* **18**(3): 7–12.

Phillips, M.L. (2007) Mitochondria regulate cell stress. *The Scientist*, September 2007 **(website)** http://www.the-scientist.com/news/display/53602/

Poustie, V.J. and Rutler, P. (2001) Dietary interventions for phenylketonuria. *The Cochrane Library*, Issue 1. Oxford: Update Software.

Singer, S.J. and Nicolson, G.L. (1972) The fluid mosaic model of the structure of the cell membranes. *Science* **175**(18 Feb): 720–31.

Watson, J.D. and Crick, F.H.C. (1953) Molecular structure of nucleic acids: a structure for deoxypentose nucleic acids. *Nature* **171**: 737. [The original description of the DNA helix.]

FURTHER READING

Cancer Research UK (2008) *Breast Cancer – Key Facts*. London: Cancer Research UK

Cancer Research UK (2008) *Breast Cancer Incidence Statistics*. London: Cancer Research UK.

Denton, S. (2002) *Breast Cancer Nursing*. Cheltenham: Nelson Thornes.

Ogden, J. (2004) *Understanding Breast Cancer, Understanding Illness and Health*. London: Wiley–Blackwell.

Santen, R. (2007) The oestrogen paradox: a hypothesis. *Breast Cancer Research* **9**(Suppl. 2): 1–5.

Smedira, H.J. (2000) Practical issues in counseling healthy women about their breast cancer risk and use of tamoxifen citrate. *Archives of Internal Medicine* **160**(20): 3034–42.

Zack, E. (2001) Mammography and reduced breast cancer mortality rates. *Medical Surgical Nursing* **10**(1): 17–21.

THE SKELETON

INTRODUCTION

A common image from films is that a skeleton is a collection of oddly shaped, dry and dead bones. While there is no doubt that bones are oddly shaped, the reality is that our skeleton is comprised of a dynamic living tissue that is continually remodelled throughout life.

The skeleton and its associated muscles provide support against gravity, and movement, and together comprise a 'skeletomuscular system'. Nevertheless, the skeleton is an organ system in its own right and has the following roles:

- *Body support*: this is essential if we are to maintain a position of our body, and body parts, against gravity: the so-called 'soft' tissues of the body are well named as such as they provide little of such support.
- *Strength and protection*: bone makes the body resilient to impact, while the bony 'box' of the skull and the cage-like structure of the ribs provide protection for vital underlying organs.
- *Calcium phosphate store*: the body contains a relatively large amount of calcium phosphate, the bulk of which is found in bone mineral. The skeleton therefore provides a reservoir of calcium and phosphate ions that can be accessed by the body should blood become deficient in them, or that can be added to if there is excess in blood (see chapter 6, p.127).
- *Synthesis of blood cells*: although not strictly speaking a role of bone, this is a role of the skeleton as bone marrow provides the main site of blood cell production (see Figure 11.3, p.273).

This chapter is concerned with the ways by which bone structure and the skeleton generally provide support and protection for the body. A completely rigid skeleton would provide the best anti-gravity support but movement would be almost impossible. Accordingly, joints between bones are an essential feature of the skeleton, together with associated structures such as joint capsules that encase the joint area. However, their presence provides potential weak points and accordingly reinforcement of the joint by ligaments and muscles are marked features that help to explain some of the irregular shapes that bones must have to accommodate these attachments. Joints are also considered in this chapter, whereas the ways by which skeletal muscles regulate posture and movement are explored in Chapter 17.

This chapter therefore commences by describing the structure of bone, and interactions between the various bone cells in bone growth and shaping. It then continues by providing an overview of the construction of the skeleton and its joints, and also highlights aspects of skeletal structure that facilitate the maintenance of an upright posture, and the absorption of stresses produced during movement.

BONE, BONE CELLS AND BONE HEALING

What is bone?

Bone essentially is composed of a connective tissue; there are various types that provide a degree of support internally (see Figures 2.32, 2.33, p.57 and associated text) but bone is a specific type that it is mineralized by the deposition of mineral salts (a mixture of calcium phosphate and calcium carbonate called hydroxyapatite). A common characteristic of connective tissues is that cells produce around them a matrix of protein. In bone this is largely collagen but there are others including a specific bone protein called ossein, and these are secreted by specialized cells called osteocytes ('osteo-' = bone; '-cyte' = cell). The proteins impart a certain degree of flexibility to bones, which is important as it enables bones to act as a shock absorber during impacts, for example walking. Some proteins, such as osteocalcin, have a role in calcification of the matrix.

Bone tissue has two main forms. The main strength of bone arises from dense mineralized tissue called compact bone, which is relatively heavy, and internally they have reduced density through the presence of 'spongy' bone tissue (called cancellous or trabecular bone), and by cavities. The cavities may be filled with marrow tissue, adipose tissue, or even air in the facial sinuses. Bone, therefore, is lighter than might be anticipated, but it retains its strength through the structure of trabecular bone.

Compact bone

Compact bone is the very hard and dense material that people normally associate with bone. Close examination of a cross-section reveals it to have a complex structure and it actually consists of minute cylindrical structures (< 0.5 mm in diameter) called osteons or Haversian systems (Figure 3.1). Osteons are composed of concentric layers, or lamellae, of bone that enclose a central, or Haversian, canal. This canal runs along the axis of the bone, and conveys blood vessels, lymphatic vessels (see Chapter 13) and neurons (see Chapter 8) into the bone tissue of the osteon. Side canals radiate into the lamellae and so enable blood to perfuse much of the compact bone structure. Other smaller channels, called canaliculi, branch from these side canals and penetrate the compact bone; expansions of the canaliculi (called lacunae) contain the bone cells. The canaliculi are too small to permit the passage of blood vessels and are filled with tissue fluid. Nutrients must diffuse from vessels within the side canals, along the canaliculi to the osteocytes.

The blood vessels in the osteons originate from the outer covering of bone which is a fibrous membrane called the periosteum (see below). The layer of compact bone is usually perforated at points by 'nutrient foramina' (= windows) that permit blood vessels to enter and leave the tissue. These vessels also supply the underlying trabecular bone, and the marrow within the bone cavity.

Trabecular (cancellous, or spongy) bone

Trabeculae are calcified 'beams' that produce a rigid meshwork that give this type of bone the appearance of a sponge, hence the term 'spongy' bone (Figure 3.1). The minute 'archways' and 'beams' provide considerable strength as the meshwork is constructed along the lines of greatest pressure exerted on the bone.

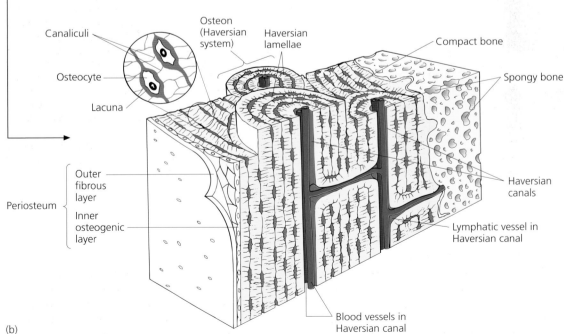

Figure 3.1 Bone tissue: (a) longitudinal section of a long bone; (b) a magnified view of compact bone

Q How does the structure of compact and spongy bone differ?

BOX 3.1 BONE INFECTION AND ABSCESSES

The infection of bone can be blood-borne (see 'Osteomyelitis' in Box 3.8, p.71) but is more likely to arise in open or compound fractures where there is tissue injury. Bone infections may lead to the formation of a fluid-filled area of necrotic tissue called an abscess.

An abscess is a swelling which contains pus, that is detritus from dead cells and perhaps microorganisms. Abscesses are problematic even in soft tissues but at least these tissues provide the possibility of drainage without causing too much structural damage. Those in bone are more difficult to treat:

- They are very painful. Soft tissues expand to accommodate the accumulation of pus but the hard structure of bone prevents this and so pressure builds up.
- Draining an abscess will often necessitate damaging the bone in order to gain access to the area.
- The absence even in healthy tissue of a blood supply through canaliculi means that microorganisms present within the lacuni are not easily accessed by the immune system cells. Similarly, the delivery of blood-borne agents such as antibodies will be less effective. For this reason bone infections will be treated aggressively with quite high doses of antibiotic.

The loss of bone may be extensive leading to a prolonged period of immobility. This also has implications for the individual (see Box 3.5, p.68).

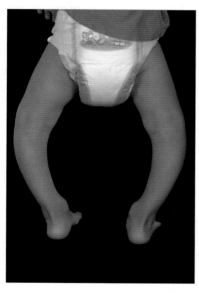

Figure 3.2 Young child with rickets. Reproduced with the kind permission of the Medical Illustration Department, Norfolk and Norwich University Hospital NHS Trust

BOX 3.2 DEMINERALIZATION OF BONE: OSTEOPOROSIS AND OSTEOMALACIA

Osteoporosis

In this condition the bone retains its general structure, but its strength is reduced as a consequence of loss of bone mass (Rosen, 2000). Spongy bone seems to be most affected, but the site of loss can be local or more general.

The loss of bone mineral is normal during the lifespan, commencing when we are in our 40s. As mineral is lost, the anti-gravity support of bone is compromised and this brings with it a substantial increase in the risk of fracture and loss of mobility. Compression fractures of the vertebrae, and fractures of the neck of femur, are frequent consequences of the loss of bone strength (Pountney, 2007; Walker, 2008).

Osteoporosis is a common problem in older people. It occurs in both men and women, though its consequences are most frequently observed in the latter (Gardiner *et al.*, 2007). This is because men on average have stronger (i.e. more calcified) bones than women, and because the hormonal changes that occur around the menopause accelerate mineral loss in women. Sex steroid hormones influence bone mineralization during puberty and this action of the hormones seems to be important in maintaining bone density. The withdrawal of oestrogen after the menopause makes women particularly vulnerable and the incidence of fractures is much higher in elderly women than in age-matched men. There is also evidence for a role of vitamin K in maintaining bone, through its role in promoting the production of bone matrix proteins involved in calcification (Booth *et al.*, 2000). Health education is aimed at encouraging people to maintain as high a bone density as possible in earlier years, through physical activity and adequate diet (Borer, 2005). The former is a direct reference to the effects that physical stress has on the activities of bone cells.

Osteomalacia

This is a rare condition in Western countries. Its cause usually is a deficiency of vitamin D. This vitamin (now viewed as being a hormone) has a vital role in maintaining the calcium ion concentration in blood plasma through its actions to promote calcium uptake from the bowel (see Figure 9.10, p.217 for an explanation of the interplay of hormones involved in calcium balance). Its deficiency means that less calcium is available for bone mineralization. Osteomalacia differs from osteoporosis in that the bone maintains a relatively normal protein matrix and so the ratio of mineral to protein declines, making the bones softer and less supportive. This may not necessarily be caused by inadequate dietary source of the vitamin (or synthesized source: inactive vitamin D is also made in the skin from a precursor) but could also occur as a consequence of malabsorption of the vitamin or through a failure of the liver to activate it. The problem may also be secondary to certain tumours that secrete parathyroid hormone and so promote excessive calcium resorption from bone.

The consequences of having a poorly supportive skeleton is illustrated in children who have the related condition rickets (Figure 3.2), in which the increased pliancy of the bones results in a bowing of the long bones of the legs due to the effects of gravity.

Bone marrow

Bone marrow occupies the spaces within spongy bone and a cavity at the centre of the bone. It too is a connective tissue but is soft unlike the surrounding bone. Protein fibres support adipose (fat) cells and cells involved in blood cell production: all marrow is red at birth because of the synthesis of red blood cells (and white, in lower numbers) that occurs there. By around 2 years of age red marrow becomes restricted to the ends of the long bones, the vertebrae and the flat bones of the skull, pelvis, sternum and clavicle. Elsewhere, adipose tissue dominates, and the marrow becomes 'yellow' and fatty and plays little role in the production of blood.

BOX 3.3 FAT EMBOLISM

The yellow marrow that predominates in many bones can be problematic following bone trauma or surgery. This is because bone damage may result in fat leakage into the circulation. As a consequence, the arrival of fat globules in the coronary, cerebral or pulmonary circulations can act as emboli, and so obstruct the vessels. This is clearly a dangerous occurrence for the person concerned and may even be fatal.

Periosteum

The periosteum is a sleeve of tough, dense connective tissue that covers the surface of bone ('peri-' = surrounding). The outer layer is continuous with tendons (that attach muscle to bone) and ligaments (that reinforce skeletal joints) and so makes a strong junction. Some fibres penetrate into the compact bone, which reinforces the structure and helps to transfer forces from the moving muscles into the bone itself. The inner layer of the periosteum contains osteogenic cells, that is, cells that can be activated to transform into types of bone cells according to need, for example following a bone fracture ('genesis' = creation).

Endosteum ('endo-' = inner)

This is a layer of osteogenic cells that lines all canals within bone, and bone cavities. The transformation of these cells into active bone cells also has an important role in bone repair, including bone remodelling (see next section).

Bone cells

Bone cells are of various types according to their role.

- *Osteocytes*: these are the main cells of fully developed bone. They maintain the protein/mineral matrix.
- *Osteoblasts*: these cells produce new bone, including calcium deposition, and will lay down new bone following injury.
- *Osteoclasts*: these cells are capable of removing mineral from the protein matrix. They are especially responsible for bone resorption during bone remodelling (see below).
- *Osteogenic cells*: these cells are found in the periosteum and endosteum. They are 'stem' cells capable of differentiating into osteoblasts or osteoclasts during times of mechanical stress or injury.

Bone growth

The process of bone growth is illustrated by the changes observed in a long bone such as the femur. At birth, such 'bones' are largely made of cartilage (Figures 3.3 and 3.4). There are, however, two areas in which the process of mineralization (called ossification) is occurring. One of these is within the shaft of the bone, the other within the ends, or epiphyses (singular: epiphysis). The benefit of having a structure that is largely cartilaginous is that it can grow much more rapidly than one that is ossified. The disadvantage is that the 'bone' is poor at weight bearing until much of the shaft has been ossified. Thus, in an older child the 'bone' must be a composite in

BOX 3.4 BONE GROWTH AND GROWTH PATTERNS

Bone growth

The rapid rate of growth observed during childhood occurs largely because of the activity of growth hormone, which stimulates the epiphysial plate to produce more cartilage. During puberty, the growth rate speeds up still further because of the stimulatory action of sex hormones. These hormones, however, are also ultimately responsible for causing bone growth to cease. Thus, not only do they stimulate the epiphysial plate, but they also promote ossification within the shaft and also within the mineralising centre of the epiphysis itself. Eventually the rate of ossification outstrips that of new cartilage growth and the epiphysis becomes ossified and continuous with the shaft. The only remaining sign of the cartilage is a lining of the tip of the bone, as part of the anatomy of the skeletal joint.

Growth hormone is secreted from the pituitary gland and normally is regulated. The hormone especially promotes the growth of long bones; its deficiency in children is not compensated for by the sex hormones, and the individual exhibits dwarfism as growth ceases during puberty. In contrast, excessive secretion of growth hormone in children results in gigantism, in which the long bones are excessively long. If excessive secretion continues into adulthood, the impact of the hormone on other bones becomes apparent, namely the hands, feet and jaws, producing signs of acromegaly (see Figure 9.6, p.215).

Growth pattern

The general pattern of body growth is similar between individuals, although there is variation in the ages at which patterns change. There are slight sex differences in growth rate with girls tending to grow faster during middle childhood years, but boys exceeding girls during later childhood. Both sexes exhibit a pronounced increase in limb length relative to trunk length, and a broadening of the shoulders, chest and trunk.

Growth charts are widely used to document growth rates in children as slow rates have been linked to problems (Wells, 2002). Variation between children is acknowledged but the charts allow for this by providing the expected range for both boys and girls. Where they must be used with caution, however, is in relation to a multi-ethnic population since cultural variations occur that are not allowed for by such standardised charts. The monitoring of growth rates is usually performed within community-based care and in particular is one of the roles of community nurses.

ACTIVITY

Standardized growth charts utilize 'percentiles'. What does this mean?

which the shaft is largely bone, for weight bearing, but the epiphysis continues to be cartilaginous, apart from the centre where mineralization is still occurring, to facilitate continued growth.

Much of the growth takes place between the epiphysis and the bony shaft in an area called the epiphysial plate. Here cartilage-producing cells are arranged in columns that extend from the epiphysis into the shaft. The cells at the epiphysial end of these columns are rapidly reproducing, hence the growth, but those below are maturing, and below them they are becoming encased in mineral by the activity of

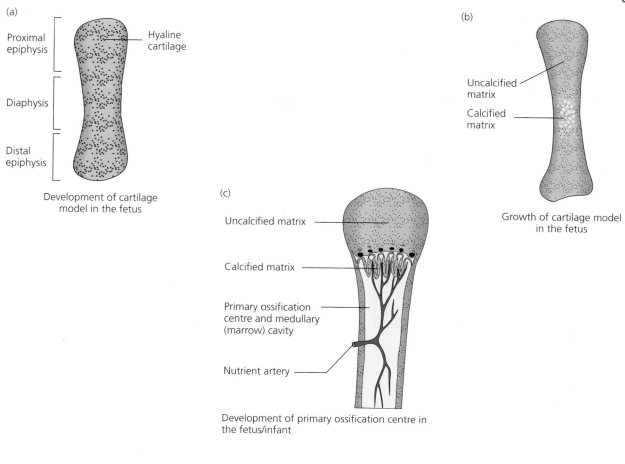

(a)

Proximal epiphysis

Diaphysis

Distal epiphysis

Hyaline cartilage

Development of cartilage model in the fetus

(b)

Uncalcified matrix

Calcified matrix

Growth of cartilage model in the fetus

(c)

Uncalcified matrix

Calcified matrix

Primary ossification centre and medullary (marrow) cavity

Nutrient artery

Development of primary ossification centre in the fetus/infant

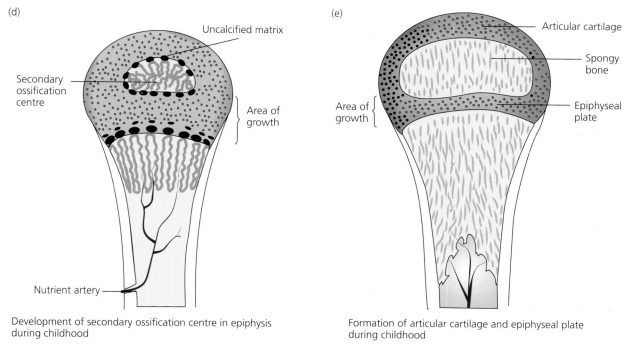

(d)

Secondary ossification centre

Uncalcified matrix

Area of growth

Nutrient artery

Development of secondary ossification centre in epiphysis during childhood

(e)

Articular cartilage

Spongy bone

Epiphyseal plate

Area of growth

Formation of articular cartilage and epiphyseal plate during childhood

Figure 3.3 Bone growth at the epiphysial plate. A change in length is shown. Note how the rate of growth can only be sustained through the growth of cartilage, with ossification occurring behind

LIVERPOOL JOHN MOORES UNIVERSITY
LEARNING SERVICES

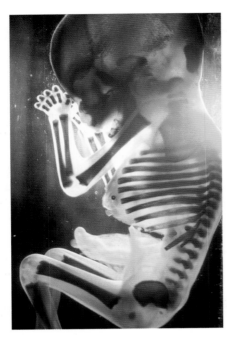

Figure 3.4 Ossification of the long bones and skull of a fetus. The ossification of the shaft of long bones is clear, but the secondary ossification centres in the epiphyses are not. Note that the wrist, elbow, shoulder, knee and hip joints are still cartilaginous. Reproduced with the kind permission of Abrahams *et al.* from *Illustrated Clinical Anatomy*, Hodder, London

osteoblasts. Other cells (osteoclasts) will also be active by removing internal minerals, so helping to extend the marrow cavity as the shaft grows in length. Thus, mineralization of the shaft is in a process of 'catch-up' with the cartilage of the epiphysial plate.

Bone diameter of course also increases as a bone grows in length. This is caused by the activity of osteoblasts, which lay down layers of new bone beneath the periosteum.

Bone remodelling

Bone is a dynamic tissue that continues to be altered throughout life:

- Calcium salts are deposited or removed as required by the body (e.g. in the regulation of plasma calcium ion concentration; see Figure 9.10, p.217).
- There is selective deposition of mineral that results in changes in bone shape that are observed during growth.
- Bone is replaced as 'old' bone is renewed, or the bone has been injured.

The last two processes involve the removal of mineral from one part of the bone and deposition in another. Removal of mineral normally precedes deposition, and so osteoclast cells are active for a period, followed then by osteoblast cell activity.

Physical stress placed on bone is an important stimulus to promote bone remodelling, with calcium deposition in the 'stressed' areas being favoured to increase density. This process ensures maximum strength at the most load-bearing points

within the skeleton, such as the femur head, but the process is more likely to be effective in a young adult than in an older person because the activity of these bone cells is greatest in a younger individual and slows during middle age. Nevertheless, the osteoclasts and osteoblasts continually act to renew bone throughout life.

The control of bone density and shape is little understood. Certainly the hormones parathyroid hormone, calcitonin and vitamin D have an influence on bone mineral (see Chapter 9), but their release and actions primarily relate to the homeostatic control of plasma calcium concentration (Chapter 15) and not to modelling and remodelling of bone. Growth hormone and the sex steroids also have an influence during childhood and puberty but much remains to be discovered.

Bone healing

Fractures or breaks in bone are caused when the forces applied exceed the capacity of the bone to resist them. This may result from accidental application of excessive physical stress on a bone, but can also arise during normal activity if bone density and/or flexibility are severely compromised, for example in osteoporosis. The different types of fracture and examples of healing are shown in Figures 3.5, 3.6 and 3.7.

The main processes involved in wound healing are explained in Chapter 11 (p.287). Healing of bone follows this usual pattern, but there are some subtle differences since body support depends upon a strong skeletal structure. The tissue is actually very good at reorganizing itself, as it simply has to step up the mechanisms involved in remodelling.

The fracture and resultant inflammatory response activate macrophages and other leucocytes, and these instigate debris removal, the activation of fibrocytes and granulation, as part of normal healing processes (see Figure 11.17, p.295). The main difference in bone healing is that the new bone matrix will have to be laid down, mineralized and then the entire structure reorganized so that compact bone and spongy bone is formed. Thus, the activities of the various types of bone cells must follow a pattern so that bone structure is returned to how it was prior to fracture:

- Osteogenic cells in the periosteum/endosteum are converted to osteoblasts.
- The osteoblasts then begin to produce new bone in the fracture area. The activity of these cells is usually to form a hardened mass around the fracture site, called a callus. This provides strength to the fracture area and enables the bone to be brought back into (tentative) use.
- Osteoclast activity then gradually removes the callus, and further osteoblasts will redeposit calcium according to the required bone shape and structure.
- The bone will eventually regain its full structure, though the process may take several months for completion. Once a bone has basically healed after injury, the individual should be encouraged to undertake light exercise, because this stresses the bone slightly and so promotes an increase in bone density.

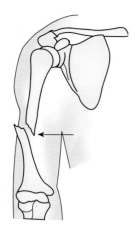

(a) Open fracture/displaced i.e. skin broken and fragments separated.

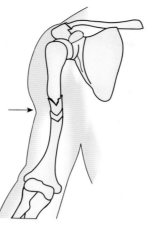

(b) Comminuted fracture i.e. bone broken in 2 or more places. Fragmented.

Direction of fracture		
Type of fracture	*Features*	
Transverse	Across the bone	
Oblique	At an oblique angle to the longitudinal axis of the bone	
Spiral	Fracture forms spiral 'twist' encircling bone; produced by rotatory force	
Linear	Parallel to the longitudinal axis of the bone	

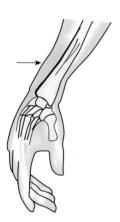

(c) Greenstick fracture i.e. fracture extends only part way through the bone. Usually in children.

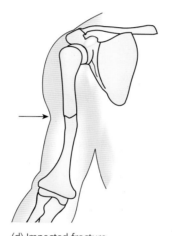

(d) Impacted fracture.

According to deforming force		
Type of fracture	*Features*	
Compression	Adjacent cancellous bones compacted; usually heals rapidly due to minimal soft tissue injury caused by deforming force	
Avulsion	Bone pulled apart; ligaments remain intact	
Stress	Undisplaced microfracture caused by repetitive stress	

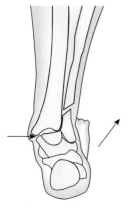

(e) Pott's fracture.

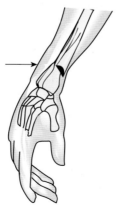

(f) Colles' fracture.

Figure 3.5 Types of bone fracture

Q Name the osteocytes involved in bone healing.

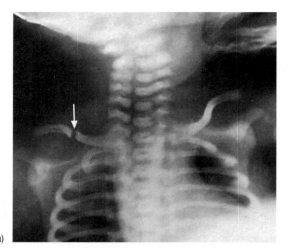

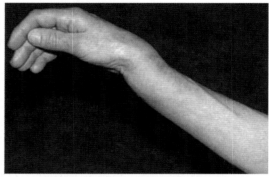

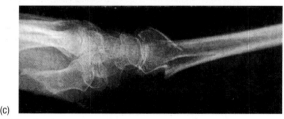

Figure 3.6 Examples of fractures. (a) X-ray of fractured clavicle, (b) photo and X-ray of Colles' fracture. Reproduced with the kind permission of Abrahams *et al.*, *Illustrated Clinical Anatomy*, Hodder, London

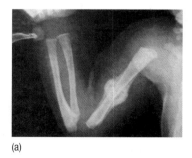

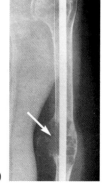

Figure 3.7 Fracture healing. (a) X-ray of a healing fracture of the humerus. Note the callus around the fracture site. (b) Fracture of humerus fixed by an intermedullary nail (arrow indicates bone erosion – this is a pathological fracture through a cancerous process). Reproduced with the kind permission of Abrahams *et al.*, *Illustrated Clinical Anatomy*, Hodder, London

---

BOX 3.5 POSSIBLE CONSEQUENCES OF BONE TRAUMA

The supportive role of bone frequently cannot be utilized following bone trauma, especially of those bones that help to support the body against gravity. Immobility has the following risks:

- *Joint stiffness and contractures*. This could reflect muscle contracture or possible fibrosis of the joint capsule. Physiotherapy and the maintenance of limb movement is essential to prevent this complication and has led to the concept of 'passive exercise'. Although exercise cannot really be considered to be passive, the term reflects the use of extrinsic manipulation of the limb to flex and extend the joint (see Box 17.8, p.474).
- *Deep vein thrombosis* (see Figure 12.18e, p.328). Blood clotting is promoted if blood flow is compromised, either because of localized hypoxia or because trauma has stimulated it. Immobility increases the risk of thrombosis in the legs because the use of muscle to return blood to the heart is compromised and so blood flow is poor. Limb pain, especially during muscle use, may be an indicator of thrombosis, particularly if it is accompanied by tenderness and swelling. Deep breathing and limb exercise will facilitate blood returning to the heart, as will compression stockings (since these reduce the capacity of the limb veins). Early mobilization will also help to reduce the risk.
- *Decubitus ulcers (pressure sores)*. Immobility can restrict blood flow to the skin, and induce hypoxia (= poor tissue oxygenation), since weight compresses the tissue against the bed. Frequent turning, or ripple mattresses, will help to prevent hypoxia. Skin hygiene will help to reduce the incidence of infection, but will also facilitate regular assessment of skin condition.

Other possible complications of bone trauma are:

- *Fat embolism*. The release of fats from adipose tissue within yellow bone marrow may lead to blockage within coronary or pulmonary vessels producing symptoms such as tachycardia or hypoxia.
- *Necrosis of bone*. Bone cells, especially those within compact bone, receive little or no blood even in health. They depend upon diffusion of nutrients from vessels within the vicinity. Bone trauma can remove blood flow completely, leading to cell death. Decisions on mobilizing must consider this possibility since pressure applied to the wound could compromise blood supply still further.
- *Infection*. This is of particular concern if the skin has been broken. Pain, swelling, pus, and pyrexia are indicators. Bone infections are difficult to treat once they become established because of the poor blood supply to bone cells (see Box 3.1, p.63).

Bone shape and external features

Bones are present in various shapes and sizes according to function, but some generalizations can be made:

- *Long bones*: bone length is greater than bone width. Long bones are found in the limbs and provide a wide scope for body movement, but also help to absorb the stresses of body weight.
- *Short bones*: these bones are of nearly equal width and length. They are generally not strong but when collected together produce flexible structures, such as the wrist and ankle.
- *Flat bones*: these are thin, plate-like bones. Their roles are to provide protection (e.g. the skull) and to provide an extensive surface area for the attachment of large muscles (e.g. the shoulder blade or scapula).

BOX 3.6 MANAGEMENT OF FRACTURES

There is no single plan for the management of fractures since the severity of injury, involvement of soft tissue and age of the patient are all variables. The objectives of management are:

- To use manipulation and/or traction to regain the correct position/alignment of the bones and to restore bone fragments to their normal position.
- To immobilize, as necessary (see below).
- To observe for the presence of neuropathy, or of respiratory or mental distress (perhaps indicative of fat emboli; see Box 3.3, p.64), or of shock (due to bleeding).
- To rehabilitate using mobility/load-bearing exercises (see Box 17.1, p.464).

Immobilizing

Immobilizing usually utilizes either plaster casting, fixation of the fracture with a metal pin or plate, or traction. External fixation devices may also be used.

Casting

Casts are made from layers of bandage impregnated with plaster, resin or fibreglass. They are used to immobilize a joint and to hold bone fragments in alignment. The type of cast used depends upon the joint to be fixated. Care includes observing for signs of nerve or circulatory problems such as cool extremity, pain, discoloration, tingling/numbness, weak pulse, paralysis or necrosis. Depending upon the fracture, there may also be risks of fat emboli from the bone marrow, or shock as a consequence of haemorrhage.

Fixation with pins, wires or plates

Where bone fragmentation is extensive the pieces may be held together with internal fixation. The pins, etc. will often be removed as healing progresses but may be left *in situ* either because removal is not feasible or in order to strengthen the resultant new bone.

Traction

Traction (and casting, pins, etc.) aids realignment of broken bones and ensures immobilization of the joint/body part. Traction is used in complex situations. Not only does it immobilize a joint, it also encourages blood supply/healing in the damaged area and helps to prevent contractures from developing.

- *Skin traction*: force (i.e. weights) is applied to the skin, for example via a foam rubber strip.
- *Skeletal traction*: force is applied directly to the skeleton via pins or wires implanted at strategic points.

In each case the amount of force applied will require monitoring and perhaps adjusting, and skin care will be important. With skeletal traction, care must also be taken to prevent infection around the inserted pins (Patterson, 2005).

External fixation devices

These are useful to support a complex fracture where fragment movement is possible even with casting or traction. The devices are especially useful where there is an open wound as they permit wound care. Such devices may also be used to realign bones if there is a congenital abnormality in young children. In this instance the devices encourage appropriate growth.

Note though that immobilization can be counterproductive if a synovial joint is involved. This is because contractures may develop, and shortening of ligaments occur, leaving the individual with a highly restricted movement when the fracture has healed. Sometimes this will respond to physiotherapy, but sometimes movement may not fully return to normality. Accordingly some fractures are not completely immobilized, for example fractures of the shoulder or elbow, but may be held only within a sling. Once pain has subsided the individual will be encouraged to use the limb in a recommended series of exercises, with the aim of reducing any contracture that has already occurred and prevention of further problems.

- *Irregular bones*: these are bones which have complex shapes that are related to their functions, for example the bones of the backbone or vertebral column.
- *Sesamoid bones*: the kneecap, or patella, is the main example of this type of bone. Sesamoid bones strengthen tendons.

Bones also have many irregular external features, arising because of the need for muscle/ligament attachment, for articulating joints between bones, and (sometimes) for the passage of blood vessels, nerves, and lymphatic vessels. These features tend to make the nomenclature of bone anatomy very complex. However, some generalizations can be made:

- Protrusions that serve primarily for muscle attachment are referred to either as processes, tubercles (tuberosities) or trochanters.
- Protrusions that form an articulating surface with other bones, and so have a smooth area lined with joint cartilage, are called condyles.
- Some bones, particularly the flat bones, are strengthened by ridges of bone called crests or spines.
- In some bones the passage of vessels/nerves is facilitated by a notch or groove on the bone.

ANATOMY OF THE SKELETON

The skeleton is comprised of 206 bones, and can be divided into two parts: the axial and appendicular skeletons. The axial skeleton forms the vertical axis of the body, and the appendicular skeleton is so named because these bones are 'appended' onto the axial skeleton (Figure 3.8).

Axial skeleton

The axial skeleton consists of the skull, vertebral column (backbone), ribs and sternum (breastbone) and the hyoid bone (Figures 3.8 and 3.9).

The skull

The skull consists of 8 bones of the cranium and 14 facial bones.

The cranium basically forms a bony 'box' which surrounds and protects the brain. The bones are smooth on the outside but uneven internally as a consequence of brain shape and the presence of blood vessels; brain shape produce three distinct 'bulges', called fossae, on the bones of the cranium. Blood vessels and nerves gain access to the cranial cavity via openings in

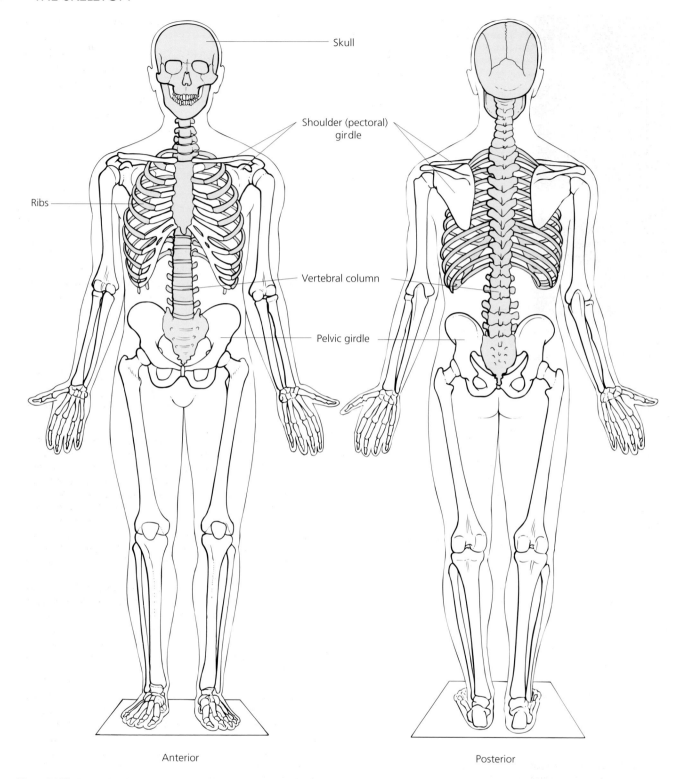

Skull

Shoulder (pectoral)
girdle

Ribs

Vertebral column

Pelvic girdle

Anterior

Posterior

Figure 3.8 The two major divisions of the skeletal system: the axial and appendicular skeletons. The axial skeleton is highlighted

Q List the bones associated with each division of the skeletal system.

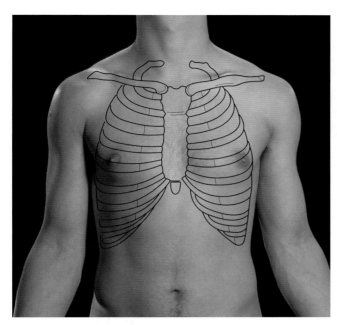

Figure 3.9 Anterior chest wall showing the relative position of the ribs and sternum. Reproduced with the kind permission of Abrahams *et al.* from *Illustrated Clinical Anatomy*, Hodder, London

the skull; for example the spinal cord enters via the foramen magnum at the base of the skull (Figure 3.10).

The facial bones provide attachment for facial muscles, form the mandible (lower jaw), protect cavities such as those of the nose, eyes and sinuses, and form the palate of the mouth. The nomenclature of facial bones is complex, sometimes referring to associated tissues (e.g. the nasolachrymal ducts, which conduct tears from the eye orbit to the nasopharynx, pass through the lachrymal bones of the orbit), but usually referring to the classical names of facial anatomy (e.g. the zygomatic bones form the prominences of the cheeks or zygoma).

The major bones of the skull are identified in Figure 3.10. Most of the joints between them are fixed (i.e. they are held tightly by cartilage and dense connective tissue and do not perform any kind of movement). These are the sutures of the cranium, and the fused joints between many facial bones. Cranial sutures do not fully form until some time after birth.

In contrast to the fixed joints of the skull, the mandibular joint between the mandible and the temporal bone of the

cranium allows a wide range of movement, such as mouth opening, closing, protrusion, retraction and side-to-side movement. The range of articulation is essential because it aids food chewing and communication through facial expression.

The sinuses are air-filled cavities within the frontal, maxillary, ethmoid and sphenoid facial bones (Figure 3.12, p.74). The cavities help to lighten the bone and their association with the nose gives resonance to the voice. Secretions into the sinuses drain into the nasal cavities.

The vertebral column

The vertebral column supports the upright posture of the body, and protects the spinal cord running vertically inside it, but also provides flexibility of movement. Individual vertebral joints between the individual bones provide only limited movement, and are very supportive, but the structure and arrangement of the vertebrae collectively provides the column with a high degree of flexibility in bending forwards – sideways and backward movements remain limited.

BOX 3.7 THE FETAL SKULL

Head size at birth is large relative to that of the trunk (Figure 3.11) and the brain at birth weighs about 25% of its final adult weight. The brain grows rapidly, and this is facilitated by the incomplete jointing of cranial bones, which results in the presence in the infant of membrane-covered spaces called fontanelles. Most fontanelles close during the first few months but the anterior fontanelle is not fully closed for 18–24 months. The actual joints, or sutures, do not form until after 5 years of age, by which time growth of the brain and cranium has slowed considerably.

BOX 3.8 OSTEITIS, OSTEOMYELITIS AND SINUSITIS

Remember that the suffix '-itis' normally infers that inflammation is present. This often results from the presence of infection but there are other factors.

- *Osteitis deformans (Paget disease)*: a condition of unknown cause in which osteoblasts and osteoclasts are excessively active. Bone characteristics change, becoming coarser. The bone increases in size, and any new bone tends to be poorly mineralized. Bones of the axial skeleton are usually involved and the condition results in deformity, extreme pain, fractures and nerve compression. There is normally increased blood flow through the bones as the marrow becomes highly vascular. Treatment is usually by use of drugs such as a biphosphonate like disodium etidronate (Didronel), or perhaps the mineralizing hormone calcitonin (see Chapter 9, p.217) to stabilize the activity of bone cells and so reduce the turnover of mineral.

- *Osteomyelitis*: a condition in which the bone is infected, usually by bacteria. *Staphylococcus aureus* is the most common agent involved and infection is via blood-borne bacteria entering the bone marrow. Children are most susceptible to the condition. The infection is often difficult to eradicate because the lacunae of compact bone are not directly perfused with blood (see text; also Venugopalan *et al.*, 2007) so bacteria that find their way into them are not accessible to the immune system cells, and antibiotics might not access them in a therapeutic concentration. The bone responds to the infection by increased activity of osteoclasts, which resorb bone and increase the size of the lacunae. The consequence is bone weakening in the area of the infection, and the delay in producing new bone can result in abscess formation (see Box 3.1, p.63). Blood vessels in bone also appear to be sensitive to bacterial toxins and there is also risk of bone ischaemia and hence necrosis.

- *Sinusitis*: an infection, usually bacterial, of the air-filled spaces within the facial skeleton. If drainage from the sinuses is disrupted, the build-up of exudate can cause considerable pain. This is exacerbated by the surrounding bone, which being very hard cannot expand to accommodate the volume. As a consequence, the fluid pressure rises within the sinus.

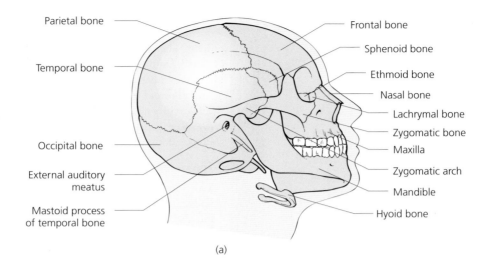

Parietal bone
Temporal bone
Occipital bone
External auditory meatus
Mastoid process of temporal bone

Frontal bone
Sphenoid bone
Ethmoid bone
Nasal bone
Lachrymal bone
Zygomatic bone
Maxilla
Zygomatic arch
Mandible
Hyoid bone

(a)

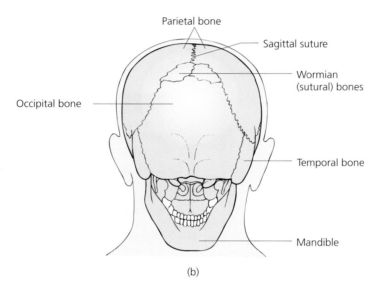

Parietal bone
Sagittal suture
Wormian (sutural) bones
Occipital bone
Temporal bone
Mandible

(b)

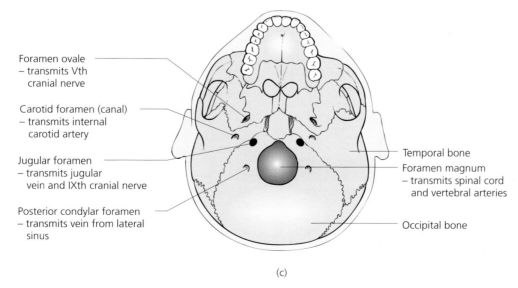

Foramen ovale – transmits Vth cranial nerve
Carotid foramen (canal) – transmits internal carotid artery
Jugular foramen – transmits jugular vein and IXth cranial nerve
Posterior condylar foramen – transmits vein from lateral sinus

Temporal bone
Foramen magnum – transmits spinal cord and vertebral arteries
Occipital bone

(c)

Figure 3.10 The principal bones of the adult skull: (a) lateral view, (b) posterior view and (c) inferior view (this also includes the larger foraminal features)

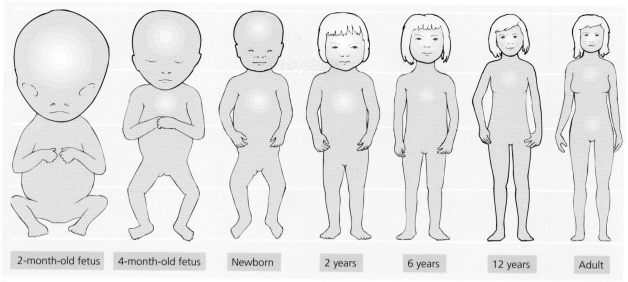

(a)

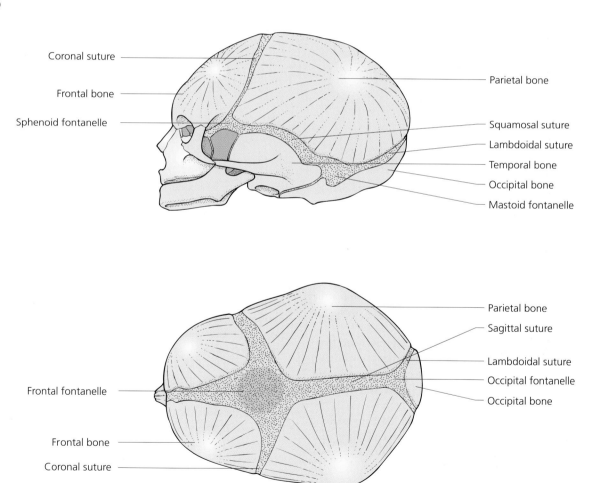

(b)

Figure 3.11 The fetal skull: (a) fetal skull size relative to that of the trunk and (b) the skull of an infant in detail, side view and view from above

Q *How does the fetal skull differ from that of an adult (shown in Figure 3.10)*

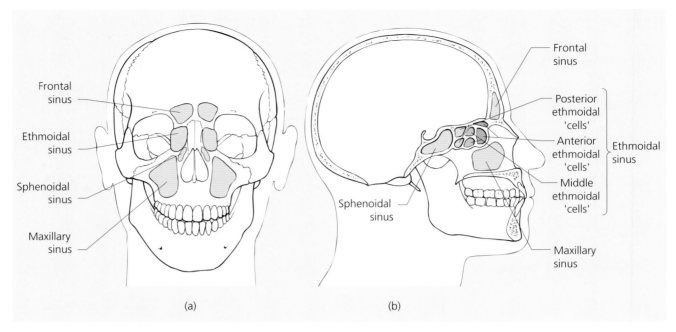

Figure 3.12 The paranasal sinuses, anterior view

Q Are the frontal sinuses medial or lateral to the maxillary sinuses?

The column consists of 33 individual bones (Figure 3.13):

- four cervical (i.e. of the neck);
- twelve thoracic (i.e. of the upper trunk or thorax);
- five lumbar (i.e. of the lower trunk or abdomen);
- five sacral (i.e. of the sacrum, a component of the pelvis);
- four coccygeal (i.e. of the coccyx or 'tail').

The individual bones of the sacrum and coccyx are usually fused together, although the coccyx articulates with the sacrum.

A large central cavity within the cervical, thoracic and lumbar bones, called the vertebral foramen ('foramen' = window), accommodates the spinal cord, while spaces between adjacent bones, called the intervertebral foramina, allow entry/exit for blood vessels and spinal nerves.

The structure of the cervical, thoracic and lumbar vertebrae exhibit differences in size and proportions but generally is similar (Figure 3.13). The main variation is in the first two cervical bones. These (abbreviated C1 and C2) are modified to form a joint with the base of the skull. C1 (also called the atlas) has articulating surfaces on the upper aspect that allow forward and backward movement of the head. C2 (also called the axis) has an upper vertical peg-like feature, the odontoid process, which projects from the body of the bone into the modified vertebral foramen of the atlas, and this allows rotational movement of the head (Figure 3.13). The remaining bones in these

sections of the vertebral column each has a 'body' and three bony processes:

- The *main body, or centrum*, of a vertebral bone provides strength and acts as a shock absorber during postural changes. The size and shape of the centrum varies with position in the vertebral column: the largest centrum is found in the lumbar vertebrae since the lower back is close to the centre of gravity of the body on standing and reinforcement is necessary here. The centrum of a vertebral bone is separated from that of its neighbour by an intervertebral disc, which is comprised of an outer fibrocartilage layer and an inner semi-solid core. The discs contribute to vertebral column flexibility, and also help in absorbing shock during movement. Too severe a shock can, however, cause a herniation of the core through the outer layer, producing a 'slipped disc'.
- Two *lateral processes* articulate with those of their neighbours and provide some muscle and ligament attachment points.
- The *spinous process* on the posterior of the bone also provides attachment for muscles and ligaments. Between them the spinous and lateral processes, and the connecting bars of bone, form a structure called the vertebral arch (as it arches over the spinal cord).

The thoracic vertebrae also have articular surfaces which form joints with the ribs.

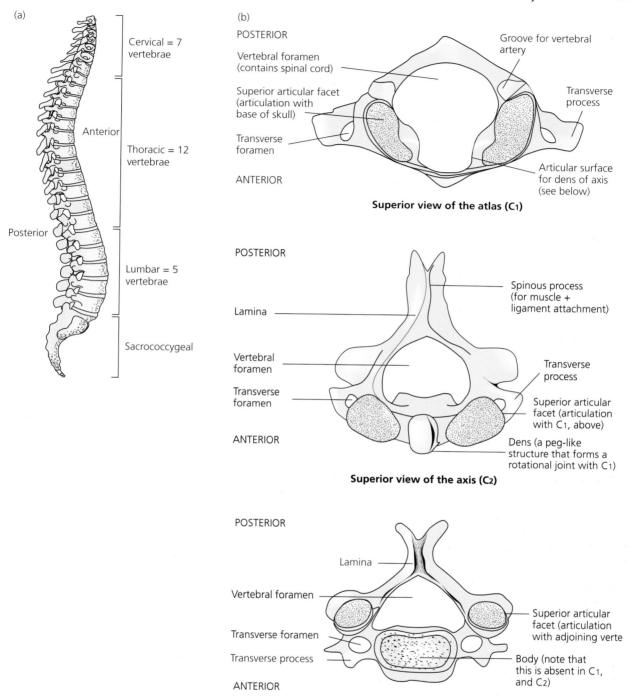

(a)

Cervical = 7 vertebrae

Anterior

Thoracic = 12 vertebrae

Posterior

Lumbar = 5 vertebrae

Sacrococcygeal

(b)

POSTERIOR

Vertebral foramen (contains spinal cord)

Superior articular facet (articulation with base of skull)

Transverse foramen

ANTERIOR

Groove for vertebral artery

Transverse process

Articular surface for dens of axis (see below)

Superior view of the atlas (C1)

POSTERIOR

Lamina

Vertebral foramen

Transverse foramen

ANTERIOR

Spinous process (for muscle + ligament attachment)

Transverse process

Superior articular facet (articulation with C1, above)

Dens (a peg-like structure that forms a rotational joint with C1)

Superior view of the axis (C2)

POSTERIOR

Lamina

Vertebral foramen

Transverse foramen

Transverse process

ANTERIOR

Superior articular facet (articulation with adjoining verte

Body (note that this is absent in C1, and C2)

Superior view of a typical cervical vertebra (C3 – C7)

Figure 3.13 The vertebrae: (a) cervical vertebrae, (b) thoracic vertebrae (*continued overleaf*)

Q *How many vertebrae are there in each region of the vertebral column?*

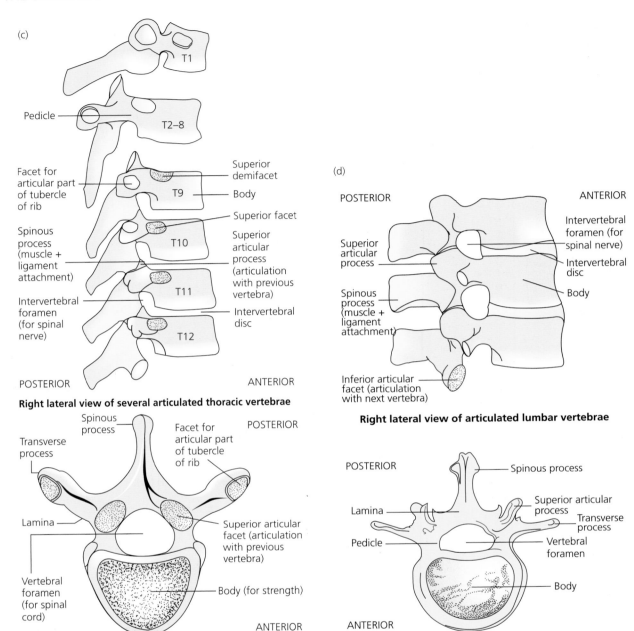

(c)

T1

Pedicle — T2–8

Facet for articular part of tubercle of rib — Superior demifacet
T9 — Body

Spinous process (muscle + ligament attachment) — Superior facet
T10 — Superior articular process (articulation with previous vertebra)

T11

Intervertebral foramen (for spinal nerve) — Intervertebral disc
T12

POSTERIOR — ANTERIOR

Right lateral view of several articulated thoracic vertebrae

(d)

POSTERIOR — ANTERIOR

Superior articular process — Intervertebral foramen (for spinal nerve)

Spinous process (muscle + ligament attachment) — Intervertebral disc — Body

Inferior articular facet (articulation with next vertebra)

Right lateral view of articulated lumbar vertebrae

Spinous process — POSTERIOR
Facet for articular part of tubercle of rib

Transverse process

Lamina — Superior articular facet (articulation with previous vertebra)

Vertebral foramen (for spinal cord) — Body (for strength)

ANTERIOR

Superior view of thoracic vertebra

POSTERIOR — Spinous process

Lamina — Superior articular process
Transverse process

Pedicle — Vertebral foramen

Body

ANTERIOR

Superior view of lumbar vertebra

Figure 3.13 (*continued*) The vertebrae: (c) thoracic vertebrae and (d) lumbar vertebrae

Q How many vertebrae are there in each region of the vertebral column?

BOX 3.9 CURVATURE OF THE VERTEBRAL COLUMN

The vertebral column has a distinct S-shape in side view (Figure 3.14) and the curvatures are referred to as the cervical, thoracic, lumbar and sacrococcygeal curvatures according to the position in the vertebral column. They result from contraction of the muscles of the back and a tightening of ligaments.

Although babies are born with thoracic and sacrococcygeal curvatures, the cervical and lumbar curvatures must develop later. The development of the cervical curvature after about 3 months is necessary if the head is to be held erect, while the development of the lumbar curvature during the latter part of the first year is necessary if the baby is to sit up and eventually stand.

The vertebral curvatures also help ensure that the body's 'centre of gravity' (i.e. the point in the body through which most of the weight acts) lies over the pelvis when we are standing. The lumbar curve is especially important in this respect, and its curvature may increase if weight distribution in the body alters, for example during pregnancy.

The curvatures of the vertebral column also provide a spring-like structure that helps to absorb the forces applied to the skeleton during walking/running. The intervertebral discs also facilitate this role.

Abnormal spinal curvature

The influence of gravity on spinal curvatures is apparent where there is persistent asymmetry of muscle tone and posture:

- *Lordosis*: an exaggerated lumbar curvature. The increased lumbar curvature observed in pregnant women is an example of a temporary lordosis.
- *Kyphosis*: an exaggerated thoracic curvature. It is generally observed in older people, often in association with osteoporosis of the spinal column.
- *Scoliosis*: a lateral curvature (i.e. one that is not usually present). It is most commonly found in the thoracic region of the spinal column, and is frequently seen in young children, and can lead to long-term problems if left untreated. Its presence indicates asymmetric contraction of the lateral muscles of the back often because of unequal skeletal anatomy or muscle physiology.

Physiotherapy can be used to effect in treating abnormal spinal curvatures, especially in children. There are also surgical procedures that can be used to stabilize the spinal column, including fusing vertebrae using bone grafts, or spinal implants such as metallic rods and screws.

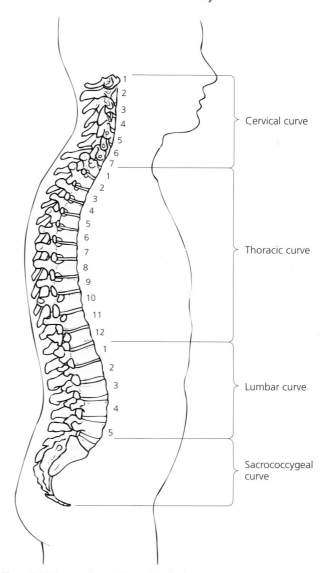

Figure 3.14 The curvatures of the vertebral column

Q How do these curves help to maintain an upright posture?

BOX 3.10 BACK PAIN

Back pain has three general causes: muscle/ligament strain, disc problems and vertebral problems.

- Muscle strains and ligament strains occur when muscles are overstretched or if a joint is forcibly moved against its natural direction of movement. Muscle problems are discussed in Chapter 17 but it is relevant to note here that the increased lumbar curve that is observed in pregnancy places additional stresses on the ligaments of the vertebral column and is largely responsible for the lower back pain that is frequently experienced.
- Should the tough outer layer of a vertebral disc rupture, then the viscous core distends through the fissure and exerts pressure on nearby spinal nerves, or irritates the dura mater, producing pain. This is a 'slipped' or prolapsed disc. Disc degeneration may also be observed, which seems to be age-linked but its cause is poorly understood.
- Vertebral problems include spondylolysis, spondylolisthesis, spinal stenosis and spondylitis. In spondylolysis there is a structural weakening of the vertebral arch of the vertebral bone, leading to increased risk of the facets of vertebrae moving forward through the occurrence of 'microfractures'. The problem is usually hereditary. Spondylolisthesis is a slipping forward of one vertebra over another. If severe then surgery will be required. Spinal stenosis occurs when a nerve root, or several roots, becomes entrapped. It is usually an acquired problem and may require decompression treatment. Inflammation specifically of the vertebral joints is called spondylitis, and ossification of the joint tissue is referred to as ankylosing spondylitis. Both conditions reduce vertebral flexibility and restrict mobility.

People working in environments in which they regularly lift heavy loads are especially at risk of developing chronic back pain. This is an important consideration when using lifting and handling methods in health care (Finucane, 2006).

Ribs and sternum

The sternum is a flat, dagger-shaped bone situated in the anterior midline of the chest (Figures 3.9, p.71 and 3.15). There are three parts to it, called the manubrium, the body and the xiphisternum, and these articulate and facilitate chest expansion during breathing. The manubrium and body have pairs of articular surfaces that form joints with the rib bones, and the manubrium also has surfaces that articulate with the clavicles (or 'collar bones'). The xiphisternum provides attachments for some abdominal muscles and for the diaphragm. It is cartilaginous until well into adulthood, when it ossifies.

The 12 pairs of ribs together form a 'rib cage' that provides protection for the underlying organs of the chest (lungs, heart and associated vessels), provides attachment for postural and respiratory muscles and helps support the shoulder girdle of bones.

Seven pairs of ribs articulate directly with the sternum via cartilages (Figure 3.15); these are referred to as 'true' ribs. Five pairs are not attached directly to the sternum, and so are referred to as 'false' ribs. Of the 'false' ribs, three pairs are attached to the cartilage of the last true rib and two pairs have no individual sternal attachment; these latter are the 'floating' ribs and are attached to the last of the previous 'false' ribs. The 'floating' ribs extend far enough down the back to provide some protection for the kidneys.

Hyoid

The hyoid is a U-shaped bone found at the base of the tongue (see Figure 3.10, p.72). It does not articulate with any other bone or cartilage, but forms an attachment for several muscles involved in chewing and swallowing.

Appendicular skeleton

The appendicular skeleton consists of the limb bones and the bones of the limb girdles.

Shoulder, arm and hand

The shoulder or pectoral girdle consists of the two collar bones and shoulder blades, called clavicles and scapulae, respectively (Figure 3.16). The clavicle is a slender bone that articulates with the sternum at one end and the scapula at the other, provides a site for muscle attachment, and helps to brace the shoulder.

The scapulae are large, flat triangular bones. The blade is strengthened by a ridge or spine on its posterior surface. Although a large bone, the blade articulates at just one end, with the clavicle and humerus of the arm, and much of it is held in place by many muscle attachments and ligaments. Its structure facilitates movement of the shoulder by sliding across the body surface as the shoulder rotates.

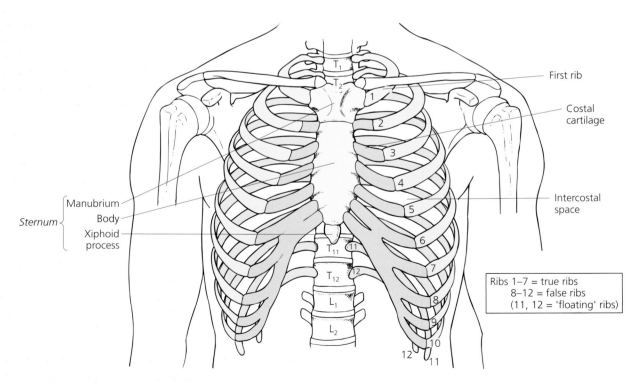

Figure 3.15 The ribs and sternum (anterior view)

Q Why are ribs classified as either true, false or floating ribs?

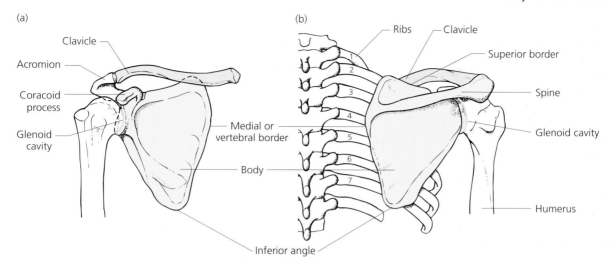

(a)

Clavicle
Acromion
Coracoid process
Glenoid cavity

(b)

Ribs
Clavicle
Superior border
Spine
Glenoid cavity
Humerus
Medial or vertebral border
Body
Inferior angle

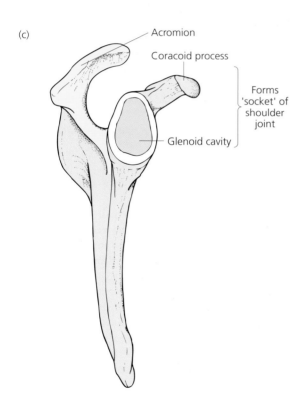

(c)

Acromion
Coracoid process
Glenoid cavity
Forms 'socket' of shoulder joint

Figure 3.16 The pectoral girdle and shoulder joint: (a) anterior view, (b) posterior view and (c) the scapula in lateral view

Q Name the bones of the pectoral girdle.

Q Why is it easier to dislocate the shoulder than the pelvis?

The bones of the arm consist of the humerus of the upper arm, and the ulna and radius of the forearm. The humerus is a long bone that articulates with the scapula at the shoulder and with the radius and ulna at the elbow (Figure 3.17). The joint with the scapula is a 'ball and socket' joint (see p.85) and provides a wide range of movement. At its distal end, at the elbow, the humerus is flattened to form articular surfaces with the ulna and radius. The bone is strengthened at this point by condyles, one of which (the medial epicondyle) is crossed by the ulnar nerve. It is this nerve that is pinched against the humerus (i.e. the 'funny bone') when the elbow is knocked.

The radius bone of the forearm is found on the outer, or lateral, side, while the ulna is found on the inner forearm, or medial side. The radius is the more substantial of the two and the two bones are held together along their length by connective tissue.

The two bones of the forearm produce a complex system of joints that enable the mobility of the forearm:

- The ulna forms a 'hinge' joint (see later) with the humerus and this permits the elbow to be flexed; the end of the ulna is extended as the olecranon process, which forms the 'elbow bone' that fits into a groove at the end of the humerus and helps to prevent overextension of the arm when the elbow is straightened.
- The radius forms a pivotal joint with the humerus and this allows the forearm to rotate. Note however that the radius rotates around the ulna – the hinge joint of the latter cannot rotate.

ACTIVITY

Neither the clavicle nor scapula has a direct connection with the vertebral column. The bones are largely held in place by muscles and ligaments, coupled with the joint between the slender clavicle and the sternum. Such an arrangement gives the shoulder a high mobility – the scapula slides over the posterior surface of the ribs as the joint is rotated – but relatively poor weight bearing. Compare the diagram of the shoulder in Figure 3.16 with that of the pelvis in Figure 3.18. Note how powerful the skeletal structure of the pelvis is compared with that of the shoulder, and the massive muscle attachment areas provided by the pelvis.

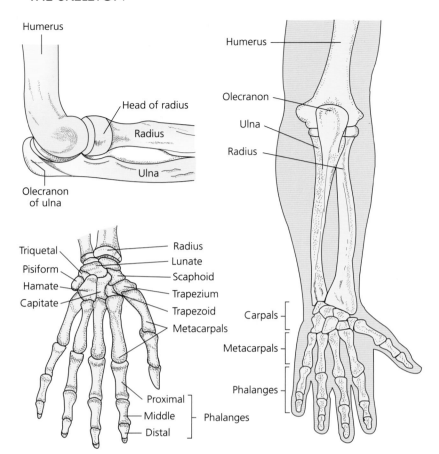

Figure 3.17 Bones of the right forearm (radius and ulna, with detail) and hand

Q Is the radial pulse palpated on the medial or lateral aspect of the wrist?

- Both bones form joints (called ellipsoidal joints – see later) with the bones of the wrist thus allowing a high degree of flexibility of the wrist, but the radius forms a more substantial wrist joint than does the ulna.

The wrist bones are called carpals, of which there are eight in each wrist (Figure 3.17). They are short bones arranged roughly in two rows, and are connected by ligaments. The first row articulates with the radius and ulna, while the other articulates with the five metacarpal bones of the palm. The latter in turn articulate with the finger bones, or phalanges; there are three phalanges in each finger and two in the thumb. The ellipsoidal joints between the phalanges facilitate the hand-grip movement.

Pelvis, leg and foot

The pelvic or hip girdle is the site of the body's centre of gravity and not surprisingly is an extremely robust structure. It is strengthened by fusion of its composite bones and by inflexible joints with the vertebral column (Figure 3.18). The bones also provide large attachment areas for the major postural muscles of the back, buttocks and thigh. Such substantial attachments are essential because the muscles must act to prevent flexing of the hips due to the effects of gravity.

The pelvic girdle consists of a pair of large 'innominate bones' and the sacral bones of the vertebral column. Each 'innominate bone' is actually comprised of three individual bones called the ilium, ischium and pubis, which are fused together to form a strong bowl-shaped structure (Figure 3.18). The junction of the three bones near the lower aspect of the pelvis forms a deep depression called the acetabulum, and this acts as a receptacle for the head of the thigh bone or femur.

The ilium is the larger of the three bones and it is the crest of this bone that can be felt at the hip. It is a large, flattened bone, strengthened by bony ridges or spines, and forms attachments with the large postural muscles of the thigh and buttock. It is joined to the sacrum by ligaments and connective tissue and movement is therefore very restricted. The ischium is also a substantial bone, and supports the weight of the body when sitting. The pubis extends to the front of the lower abdomen; the right and left pubic bones unite at a normally inflexible joint called the symphysis pubis; this joint can become more flexible in women during pregnancy owing to the action of progesterone. The bowl-shaped structure provided by these bones protects the organs of the lower or inferior abdomen, including the reproductive tract.

The femur is a strong, long bone that articulates at the hip and at the knee. The large, rounded head of the femur fits into

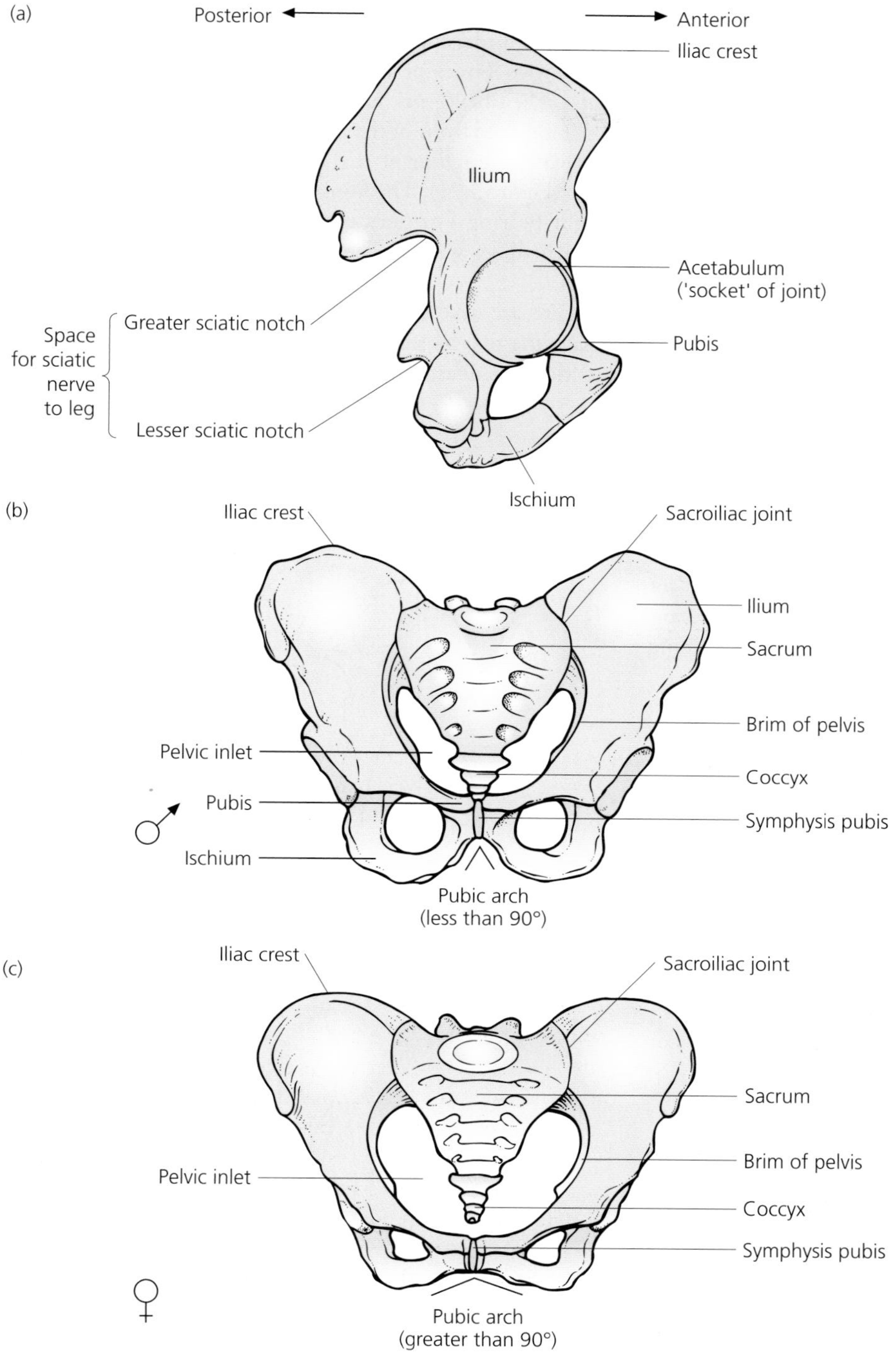

(a)

Posterior ← → Anterior

Iliac crest

Ilium

Greater sciatic notch

Space for sciatic nerve to leg

Lesser sciatic notch

Acetabulum ('socket' of joint)

Pubis

Ischium

Figure 3.18 The pelvic girdle: (a) lateral view of the right side to show the component bones and acetabulum; (b) anterior view of the male pelvis and the female pelvis

Q How does the female pelvic girdle differ from that of the male?

(b)

Iliac crest

Pelvic inlet

Pubis

Ischium

Pubic arch (less than 90°)

Sacroiliac joint

Ilium

Sacrum

Brim of pelvis

Coccyx

Symphysis pubis

(c)

Iliac crest

Pelvic inlet

Pubic arch (greater than 90°)

Sacroiliac joint

Sacrum

Brim of pelvis

Coccyx

Symphysis pubis

BOX 3.11 THE PELVIS IN MEN AND WOMEN

There are noticeable gender differences in the shape of the pelvis. In men the angle subtended by the pubic arch at the point of junction between the two pubic bones is less than 90°, while in the women it is greater than 90°. The reason for this is that the pelvic inlet (the aperture formed by the two halves of the pelvis) must be wider in women to allow passage of a baby, and this widens the pelvis and flattens it slightly (Figure 3.18).

The joint between the pubic bones (symphysis pubis) also exhibits a gender difference in that this joint, which ordinarily has very limited movement, becomes lax in women prior to childbirth as a consequence of the actions of the hormone relaxin. This again is clearly an adaptation that facilitates childbirth.

the acetabulum (socket) of the hip to form a 'ball and socket' joint, and this provides a large degree of rotational and abductional movement. The femur has a distinctive inner curvature (Figure 3.19) that is more pronounced in women because the acetabulum is even further from the body midline than it is in men as a consequence of the wider female pelvis. When standing, the curvature brings the knee joint, shin bones and foot close to the vertical axis of the body and so almost in line with the centre of gravity. This facilitates weight bearing, and means that the centre of gravity is not thrown widely out of position during walking, and so helps maintain balance. The femur curvature also provides a spring-like action and this enables it to absorb some of the forces applied to it during walking. This helps to reduce the 'jarring' effect on the pelvis and vertebral column.

Bony protrusions at the knee end of the femur (called the medial and lateral condyles) provide attachments for the muscles of the lower leg. Processes also articulate with the kneecap, or patella, and with the tibia of the lower leg. The patella is secured in position by extensive cartilages and ligaments (see Figure 3.25, p.86). Such features make the joint very substantial. This is not surprising, as the knee not only has to be strong

to support the weight of the body, but must also receive and withstand forces applied to it in squatting or kneeling.

The two bones of the lower leg are called the tibia and fibula. The tibia forms the shin bone (the prominent crest running along the front of the bone can easily be felt), and articulates with the femur at the knee and with the bones of the ankle (Figure 3.21). The fibula is a more slender bone (it is not weight bearing but does provide some muscle attachments) and articulates with the tibia at the knee end and with ankle bones.

There are seven ankle and heel bones collectively called tarsals, the two largest ones being the talus of the ankle joint and the calcaneus, which forms the heel bone itself (Figures

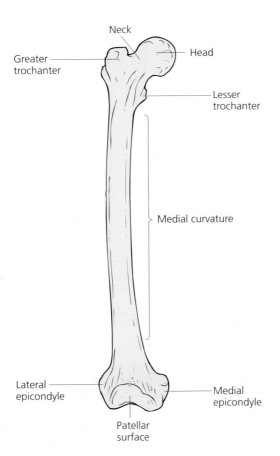

Figure 3.19 The femur

Q How do the ball and socket joints of the pelvis and shoulder compare?

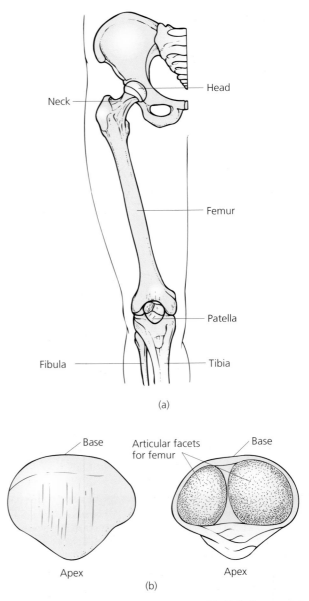

(a)

(b)

Figure 3.20 Bones of the upper leg and kneecap (patella): (a) the femur, anterior view; (b) the right patella: left, anterior view, right, posterior view

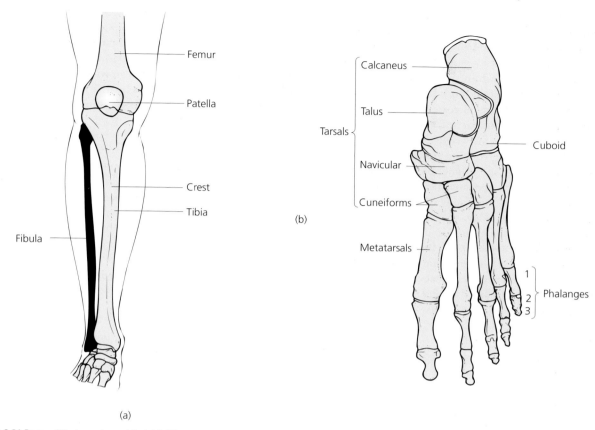

(b)

Figure 3.21 Bones of the lower leg and foot: (a) tibia and fibula, anterior view; (b) the foot

Q Compare the bone structure of the foot with that of the hand (Figure 3.17).

3.21 and 3.22). The instep of the foot is formed from five longer, more slender bones called metatarsals, and these in turn articulate with the proximal bones of the toes (like the fingers, these too are called phalanges). There are three phalanges in each toe, except for the big toe, which has only two.

The metatarsals and associated heel/ankle bones form the foot arches (Figure 3.22). The first three form the high arch, called the medial longitudinal arch, on the inside of the foot, while metatarsals IV and V form the lower arch, called the lateral longitudinal arch, on the outside of the foot. The arched structures are maintained by ligaments and by attached muscles. The main ligament is called the plantar calcaneonavicular ligament (i.e. it is on the underside of the foot, and it attaches to the calcaneus and to the navicular bone of the ankle). A weakening of this ligament causes a failure to maintain the relative positions of these bones and therefore of the high arch, and causes a 'fallen arch' or 'flat foot'.

The foot skeleton during standing and walking

On standing, our body weight is exerted on each ankle, and the weight is then distributed between the heel bone (calcaneus) and the metatarsal bones. The relatively large size of the calcaneus was noted earlier; this is a strong bone, and it also provides a site of attachment for the large calf muscles via the

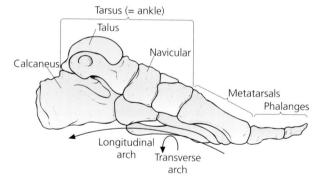

Figure 3.22 The arches of the foot

Q What happens to the foot arches on taking a step?

Achilles tendon running vertically up the back of the ankle. The articulation between the tibia/fibula bones of the lower leg and the main bone of the ankle (the talus) is most stable in the standing position or, especially, when the foot is flexed in the crouching position. Extending the foot, for example if we stand on tip-toe, causes the articulation to occur with the narrower part of the talus; this is a weaker arrangement hence our difficulty in maintaining that stance.

During walking the strength of the calcaneus enables it to withstand the initial impact of the heel with the ground. The body weight is then quickly distributed to the lateral border of the foot along the metatarsals, and eventually across the heads of the metatarsals to that of the first metatarsal bone at the base of the big toe (= the 'ball' of the foot). By this time the heel will have left the ground. Running increases the forces applied during the impact on the ground, and the distal heads of the metatarsals then distribute the weight more evenly. The roles of the toes during walking/running are to provide stability at the point of contact with the ground, but also to impart a forward thrust that facilitates the movement.

The arches also absorb forces applied to the foot, especially during walking/running. Thus they flatten slightly during impact of the foot on the ground and, being highly elastic, release the energy again as they spring back into shape once the foot is lifted. In this way a momentum is imparted onto the movement, raising the energy efficiency of the process. The arches also help to prevent blood vessels and nerves in the foot from being crushed.

Joints

Strictly speaking, a joint is simply the point of contact between bones or between cartilage and bone. Its presence therefore does not always imply movement, though many do. Joints are divided into three categories:

- those between bones which provide little or no movement are called fixed joints;
- those between bone and cartilage are called cartilaginous joints;
- joints that allow movement are called synovial joints and it is the range of types of these joints that enables the body to have a wide diversity of movement.

Fixed and cartilaginous joints

Fixed joints include the sutures of the skull, in which a thin layer of dense fibrous connective tissue unites the bones (during life some sutures become replaced by bone so that there is complete fusion). The joint between the shafts of the ulna and radius of the forearm, and that between the tibia and fibula near the ankle, are other examples of fixed joints, and in these instances provide stability at these points of stress. These latter, however, have more loose and elastic connective tissue than is found in sutures and help the joints to absorb the shock of movement.

Cartilaginous joints include the symphysis pubis between the anterior surfaces of the pubis bones of the pelvic girdle and the discs between the bodies of vertebrae. They differ from fixed joints in that the fibrocartilage present makes the joint slightly more moveable. Such flexibility enables the symphysis to move slightly during birth, and the vertebral column to be flexible and to absorb forces during walking. The joint between the cartilaginous tip of a growing bone, called the epiphysis, and the underlying bone matrix is also a cartilaginous joint, though the presence of bone mineral makes this joint fixed.

Synovial joints

Synovial joints are characterized by the presence of a joint cavity (Figure 3.23). The cavity contains synovial fluid, enclosed within a tough fibrous capsule. The fluid is viscous because of the presence of hyaluronic acid (a normal constituent of cartilage) and is produced as a secretion from the blood plasma. Its role is to provide lubrication, and to provide nutrients for cartilage cells within the joint. An important property of the fluid is that the viscosity reduces as the joint is used, thus increasing the lubricative effects during exercise, much as lubricant oil does in a car engine! Phagocytic cells within the fluid keep the joint free of debris.

The capsule consists of a tough, but flexible, outer layer of dense connective tissue which unites the articulating bones and helps prevent dislocation of the bones. Some of the connective tissue fibres of the capsule are arranged in parallel bundles, which are oriented to provide maximal strength to the joint. Such bundles are called ligaments. The inner layer of the

---

ACTIVITY

Compare the bones of the arm and hand with those of the leg and foot. Note the similarity in terms of bone number and arrangement, but note also how they are adapted to accommodate the respective limb function.

BOX 3.12 DEGENERATIVE CONDITIONS OF SYNOVIAL JOINTS: ARTHRITIS

Inflammatory conditions of synovial joints are referred to collectively as arthritis ('arthro-' = joint).

- *Osteoarthritis*: this is a degenerative (but non-inflammatory in its cause) condition of synovial joints. The causes can be secondary to joint trauma/stresses and congenital factors, or can be idiopathic (i.e. 'primary'). Idiopathic causes are more common and seem to be linked to ageing, perhaps through 'wear and tear' and/or expression of age-related genes. The disorder involves the breakdown of cartilage by enzymes, which results in the flaking and cracking and eventual loss of joint cartilage. As the cartilage thins there is frictional contact between bones, which causes bone erosion, inflammatory responses, and induces pain through the release of pain-producing substances that act on nerve endings (see Figure 20.1, p.562). The problem may be exacerbated over time by calcification of the joint capsule and production of bony outgrowths called osteophytes. Joint flexibility may then be very much reduced.
- *Rheumatoid arthritis (or rheumatoid disease)*: this is an autoimmune disorder of connective tissue and is primarily an inflammatory disease of the joint capsule, articular cartilage and ligaments. There is joint deformity, swelling and pain (Figure 3.24). The cause of the response is obscure, with probably a combination of factors involved, such as genetic susceptibility, hormonal and reproductive factors. (See also the case of a woman with rheumatoid arthritis in Section VI, p.632.)

With extensive damage, correction of a degenerated joint may involve a reconstruction of the joint structure (called arthroplasty) using bone grafts and implants (Gaffo *et al.*, 2006). Total joint replacement with artificial joints may be necessary in advanced inflammatory disease.

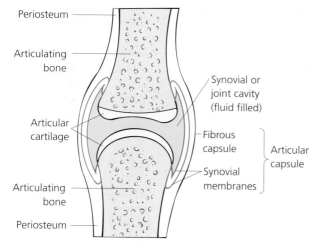

Periosteum

Articulating bone

Articular cartilage

Articulating bone

Periosteum

Synovial or joint cavity (fluid filled)

Fibrous capsule

Synovial membranes

Articular capsule

Figure 3.23 A general synovial joint

Q What other types of skeletal joint are there?

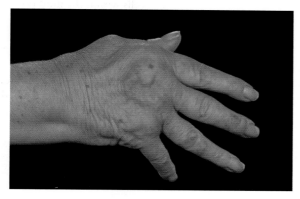

Figure 3.24 Rheumatoid arthritis. Reproduced with the kind permission of the Medical Illustration Department, Norfolk and Norwich University Hospital NHS Trust

capsule consists of loose connective tissue, elastin, and adipose tissue. This is the synovial membrane and it is this that secretes the synovial fluid.

The joint surface of the articulating bones is smoothed by a covering of hyaline cartilage. Additional cartilaginous discs (or menisci) may be present to ensure a tight fit between joint surfaces of very different shapes, for example within the knee (Figure 3.25).

Although the general structure of synovial joints is similar, there are wide variations in the movement they facilitate. Various subtypes of joint are recognized (Figure 3.26) as follows:

- *Ball and socket*: this consists of a ball-shaped surface on one bone fitted into a cup-like socket in another. The advantage of this type of joint is that it permits movement in three planes, including rotation. Examples are the shoulder and hip joints, although the need to maintain posture against gravity means that the hip has less freedom of movement than the shoulder.

BOX 3.13 SPRAINS

Joints subjected to physical stresses must be reinforced if they are not to be dislocated. Those joints which have to support the body weight are reinforced with substantial ligaments and cartilage, and are associated with powerful muscles. For example, the structure of the knee joint (which is actually an aggregate of three joints) is shown in Figure 3.25. Note the presence of extensive ligaments and muscle tendons, and also how the orientation of the fibres of these connective tissues stabilize the joint. Cruciate ligaments ('crux-' = cross) within the joint capsule between the tibia and the femur help to reduce any twisting motion of the knee.

A sprain is an injury to ligaments, produced by a wrenching or twisting movement. There is rapid swelling, worsening with time, and severe pain on movement of the joint. Treatment includes:

- A cold compress applied intermittently for up to 36 hours to suppress pain and swelling.
- Analgesia.
- If necessary, elevate the affected limb to help reduce swelling.
- Mild heat later to improve blood flow and so promote wound healing.
- Immobilization of the joint, usually by splint or elastic dressing.
- Repositioning of the anatomical location of the ligaments, for example through Bowen therapy.
- Teaching the patient to regain use of the joint only gradually, with rest periods.

The joint should also be observed for signs of continuing problems, for example bone necrosis through poor blood supply, or instability that may make repeat dislocation likely.

- *Hinge*: in hinge joints a convex surface of one bone fits into the concave surface of another. This structure provides movement in one plane only. Examples are the elbow, knee and ankle.
- *Pivot joint*: in this joint a protrusion from one bone articulates within a ring (partly of bone, partly ligament) structure on another. The joint provides rotational movement. Examples include the joint between the first two cervical vertebrae (atlas and axis) which allows rotation of the head, and between the proximal ends of the ulna and radius of the forearm, which allows rotation of the forearm and hence of the hands.
- *Ellipsoidal joints*: in these joints an oval-shaped condyle on one bone articulates with an elliptically shaped cavity on another. The structure gives more movement than is possible with a normal hinge joint, by permitting both up/down and back and forth movement. Saddle joints are modified ellipsoidal joints that allow an even greater range of movement in the two planes, though unlike the ball and socket joint do not allow rotation. An example is the joint between the radius and the carpal bones of the wrist.
- *Gliding joint*: in these joints the articulating surfaces are flat and permit movement from side to side and back and forth. Although twisting and rotation might be expected to be possible by this structure, they are normally prevented by ligaments, or by adjacent bones. Examples are those between the carpals of the hand, between the tarsals of the foot, between the sternum and clavicle, and between the scapula and clavicle.

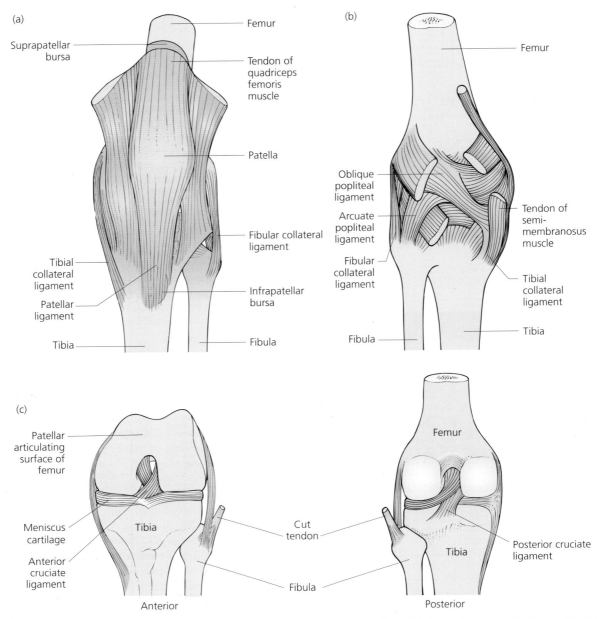

Figure 3.25 The knee joint: (a) anterior view; (b) posterior view. In (c) flexed views are shown to illustrate the cruciate ligaments and menisci cartilages within the joint

Q What is a menisectomy?

Joint dislocation results in joint deformity and loss of normal movement, and pain (Box 3.14). Dislocation also carries with it a risk that blood vessels may also have been damaged. Treatment is to provide analgesia, X-ray to assess the extent of damage, realignment of the joint and immobilization. Surgery may be required if damage is extensive, involving suturing of the torn ligaments and (in the knee) possibly removal of meniscus cartilage. This latter procedure is referred to as a 'menisectomy' and is often performed using an arthroscope to visualize the interior of the joint capsule.

ACTIVITY

Place the tips of your fingers over the joints identified as examples in this section on synovial joints. Can you feel how the skeletal structures are moving according to the differing joint structures?

BOX 3.14 JOINT DISLOCATION

Dislocation is when bones in a joint move from their normal position, with the consequence that the articular surfaces are no longer in contact. The problem may be congenital because a joint has not fully formed or matured, it may be pathological as a result of joint degeneration, or it may be traumatic due to forced movement in an inappropriate plane.

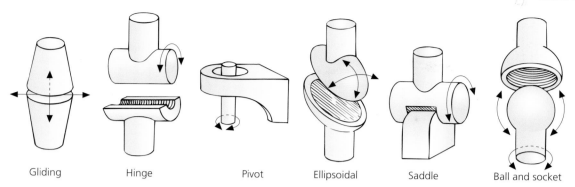

Gliding   Hinge   Pivot   Ellipsoidal   Saddle   Ball and socket

Figure 3.26 Subtypes of synovial joints and their movements

Bursae

Where skin, tendons or muscle rub on the surface of bone as a joint moves, small sacs of fluid called bursae (singular: bursa) prevent friction. These sacs are made of synovial membrane and the fluid is of similar composition to that of synovial fluid.

BOX 3.15 TENDINITIS AND BURSITIS

These are painful inflammatory problems, typically produced by excessive use of a joint, or compression of the joint area. Intervention is to encourage resting the joint until the problem subsides.

SUMMARY

1 Bone tissue is a type of connective tissue, mineralized to give it a supporting role. A bone is composed of two types of bone tissue: compact bone and cancellous (also called spongy or trabecular) bone.

2 Compact bone is a hard and dense tissue composed of tiny cylindrical structures called osteons in which blood vessels and nerves are located within a central canal. Bone cells are found within fluid-filled pockets called lacunae into which nutrients must diffuse from the canals.

3 Cancellous bone consists of little arches of bone that give it a spongy appearance. The structure is still supportive but it also lightens the bone and provides spaces for bone marrow.

4 Bone marrow is red or yellow. Redness is related to blood cell synthesis. Yellow marrow consists mainly of adipose tissue.

5 The shape of bones depends upon their role in the skeleton; for example the major limb bones are long and relatively narrow.

6 The mineral matrix of bone is secreted by specialized cells called osteoblasts. The process continues throughout life as other cells called osteoclasts remove mineral and release it into body fluids. Bone mineral therefore reflects a balance between osteoblast and osteoclast activity.

7 The laying down of new bone mineral is called ossification and is most apparent as cartilage is replaced as bone grows in length.

8 Bone healing also involves ossification but this time not of cartilage. Cells in the connective tissue that covers bone (i.e. the periosteum) transform into osteoblasts and ossify the connective tissue in the area of injury to form a callus. This provides strength to the damaged area but will gradually be replaced as osteoblasts and osteoclasts remodel the tissue.

9 The skeleton consists of axial and appendicular components.

10 The axial component is comprised of the skull, hyoid, sternum, ribs and vertebrae.

11 The appendicular component is comprised of the shoulder and pelvic girdles, the arms and legs, hands and feet.

12 The skeleton provides support for the body but also has features, such as curvatures, that enable it to absorb physical stresses associated with standing and walking.

13 Joints are a feature of the skeleton. Some are immovable but others called synovial joints facilitate movement according to their structure and the activities of associated muscles.

14 Synovial joints are reinforced with ligaments and muscle tendons, especially where they have to support the body against gravity.

15 Synovial joints are found in a variety of forms according to the movement they facilitate.

REFERENCES

Booth, S.L., Tucker, K.L., Chen H., *et al.* (2000) Dietary vitamin K intakes are associated with hip fracture but not with bone mineral density in elderly men and women. *American Journal of Clinical Nutrition* **71**(5): 1201–8.

Borer, K.T. (2005) Physical activity in the prevention and amelioration of osteoporosis in women: interaction of mechanical, hormonal and dietary factors. *Sports Medicine* **35**(9): 779–83.

Finucane, C. (2006) Moving and handling patients safely: a product guide. *International Journal of Therapy and Rehabilitation* **13**(4): 182–6.

Gaffo, A., Saag, K.G. and Curtis, J.R. (2006) Treatment of rheumatoid arthritis. *American Journal of Health-System Pharmacy* **63**(24): 2451–65.

Gardiner, A., El Miedany, Y. and Toth, M. (2007) Osteoporosis: not only in women, but in men too. *British Journal of Nursing* **16**(12): 731–5.

Patterson, M.M. (2005) Multicenter pin care study. *Orthopaedic Nursing* **24**(5): 349–60.

Pountney, D. (2007) Osteoporosis. *Nursing Older People* **19**(3): 19–21.

Rosen, C.J. (2000) Pathophysiology of osteoporosis. *Clinics in Laboratory Medicine* **20**(3): 455–68.

Venugopalan, V., Smith, K.M. and Young, M.H. (2007) Selecting anti-infective agents for the treatment of bone infections. *Orthopedics* **30**(9): 713–17.

Walker, J. (2008) Osteoporosis: pathogenesis, diagnosis and management. *Nursing Standard* **22**(17): 48–60.

Wells, J. (2002) Growth and failure to thrive. *Journal of Paediatric Nursing* **14**(3): 37–43.

THE NEED FOR REGULATION

Chapter 4

CHEMICAL REACTIONS IN CELLS: FUNDAMENTALS OF METABOLISM

INTRODUCTION

'Metabolism' is a generic term that refers to the complex array of chemical reactions that take place during the day-to-day activities of cells. In essence, metabolism is the basis of cell function and understanding the processes involved helps us to understand better the needs of cells, the necessity for the systemic functions of the body to meet those needs, and the foundations of healthcare interventions required to support those systems. Readers may find it useful to refer back to Chapter 1 and remind themselves of the features of integration of cellular homeostasis.

A simple way to consider the basic principles of metabolism is to consider that it encompasses those reactions in which new molecules are produced and used by the body. This entails reactions in which there is a joining together of atoms and molecules, and those in which molecules are broken down into smaller constituent units. 'Anabolism' is a general term for the synthetic processes and 'catabolism' is a term applied to the breaking-down processes. These processes underpin much of the chemistry that is described in this chapter. However, in order to understand this material it is important first to gain an awareness of what atoms and molecules are. Accordingly, the next section provides an explanation of fundamental aspects of chemistry.

OVERVIEW OF BASIC CHEMISTRY

All living and non-living things consist of matter, in gaseous, liquid or solid form, and all matter is made up of a limited number of chemical 'elements' combined together in ways which ultimately produce the huge diversity of substances that make up the natural world. Chemistry is essentially about the properties and behaviours of these elements and their combinations. In biology, the main interest is in the chemistry of living matter, and so is referred to as 'biochemistry'.

Elements

Chemical elements are the basic building units of matter: they are substances that cannot be broken down into simpler substances by ordinary chemical reactions. Ninety-two different elements occur naturally but a dozen or so others too unstable to occur naturally are known to science (for example plutonium). The elements are designated abbreviations, or symbols, mostly based on the first one or two letters of the name of the element although this can appear confusing if it refers to the 'Classical' rather than English, name. For example, symbols of elements abundant in the body are C (carbon), O (oxygen), H (hydrogen), N (nitrogen), Na (= natrium = sodium), K (= kalium = potassium), Ca (calcium), P (phosphorus) and Fe (= ferrum = iron).

The diversity of cell structure and function is made possible because many chemical elements will combine with others to form a myriad of different substances, the properties of which result in the extensive range of chemical reactions that occur from moment to moment within a cell.

Atoms

Each element consists of atoms; needless to say they are minute, of the order of 1/100 millionth of a centimetre in diameter! Some natural substances, such as diamond (a form of carbon) and gold (symbol Au), may be almost entirely comprised of one kind of element. Usually, though, matter consists of two or more different elements combined together in various proportions. An example is the sugar glucose, which is comprised of carbon, oxygen and hydrogen in defined proportions (i.e. $C_6H_{12}O_6$ – see later).

The structure of atoms exhibit two main features: the nucleus and its 'cloud' of surrounding particles called electrons (Figure 4.1a). Physicists have identified a number of different particles and subparticles within the nucleus but the major ones are called neutrons and protons and these are comparatively large and heavy in relation to electrons. Protons and electrons are electrically charged: by convention protons carry a positive charge, electrons a negative one. Atoms have the same number of each and so overall are electrically neutral. Neutrons are uncharged.

The structure of the atoms of one element is different from that of others. All atoms of a given element will have identical numbers of protons (and electrons), and it is differences in the

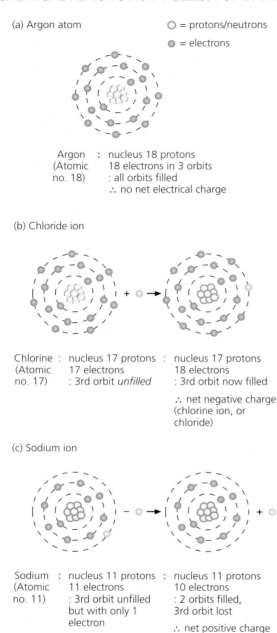

(a) Argon atom

○ = protons/neutrons
● = electrons

Argon : nucleus 18 protons
(Atomic   18 electrons in 3 orbits
no. 18)   : all orbits filled
           ∴ no net electrical charge

(b) Chloride ion

Chlorine : nucleus 17 protons : nucleus 17 protons
(Atomic   17 electrons   18 electrons
no. 17)   : 3rd orbit *unfilled* : 3rd orbit now filled

           ∴ net negative charge
           (chlorine ion, or
           chloride)

(c) Sodium ion

Sodium : nucleus 11 protons : nucleus 11 protons
(Atomic   11 electrons   10 electrons
no. 11)   : 3rd orbit unfilled : 2 orbits filled,
          but with only 1   3rd orbit lost
          electron

          ∴ net positive charge
          (sodium ion)

Figure 4.1 Schematic representation of atoms and ions. In (a), an argon atom is depicted as an example of an inert element. Note how the electron orbits around the nucleus contain a full complement of electrons. In (b), a chlorine atom is shown. In this atom the outer electron orbit is unfilled; in gaining an additional electron the orbit is now filled but the excess electron causes the atom to become negatively charged. This is now a chloride ion. In (c), a sodium atom must lose an electron to ensure that the outer electron orbit is full, thus giving the atom a positive charge; this is a sodium ion

Q Where would the additional electron come from that the chlorine atom requires to form the chloride ion?

numbers present that produce the range of different elements. For example, hydrogen atoms are the smallest atoms and have only one proton and one electron, whereas the biggest naturally occurring atoms, those of uranium, have 92 of each. Despite these differences some elements do have related properties, for example chlorine, bromine and iodine. For convenience chemists arrange elements within these related groups in a 'Periodic Table' (Figure 4.2), in order of the number of protons they have in their atoms; this is called the atomic number, and in Figure 4.2 is depicted above the symbol for each element.

The Periodic Table also shows the atomic mass of an element, as the number below each symbol. The mass (i.e. weight) of an atom reflects the number of protons and neutrons present; electrons are so small that their mass is insignificant in comparison. It is, of course, a miniscule value unless there are trillions and trillions of them, in which case the collective weight can be taken (for example, the weight of a diamond). However, as mass relates to atomic size, it would be erroneous to assume that 1 g of, say, hydrogen will contain the same number of atoms as 1 g of a heavier element such as gold. Hydrogen is the smallest and lightest element and is given a standardized mass of 1. Gold has an atomic mass of 197, that is, its atoms are 197 times heavier than those of hydrogen. Thus, just 1 g of hydrogen will contain the same number of atoms as 197 g of gold. Being aware of these differences in relative mass enables biochemists to compare the number of atoms in substances of different weights, which is important because chemical activity relates to molecule concentration, not weight; it would be erroneous to assume that 250 µg of, say, paracetamol, will contain the same number of active paracetamol drug molecules as 250 µg of a paracetamol/ codeine combination.

Isotopes

Although the nuclei of atoms of one element have a given number of protons, it is possible for them to vary in their number of neutrons. This does not influence the chemical activity of the atom but it does slightly alter its mass. The forms of atoms of a single element with different numbers of neutrons are called isotopes.

In some instances the accumulation of extra neutrons can destabilize an atom, with the result that the nucleus fragments and neutrons are emitted as 'radiation'. Such isotopes are called radioisotopes (Box 14.1). For example, carbon atoms (atomic number = 6) usually have six protons and six neutrons (i.e. the atomic mass is 6 + 6 = 12). Another form of carbon exists which has eight neutrons in its nucleus (i.e. the atomic mass is now 6 + 8 = 14). This form of carbon is referred to as carbon-14 to distinguish it from the usual carbon-12. Both forms are chemically identical but the atomic nuclei of carbon-14 are less stable and emit the excess neutrons as radiation causing them to change to the more stable carbon-12.

I	II											III	IV	V	VI	VII	
								1 H Hydrogen 1									2 He Helium 4
3 Li Lithium 7	4 Be Beryllium 9											5 B Boron 11	6 C Carbon 12	7 N Nitrogen 14	8 O Oxygen 16	9 F Flourine 19	10 Ne Neon 20
11 Na Sodium 23	12 Mg Magnesium 24											13 Al Aluminium 27	14 Si Silicon 28	15 P Phosphorus 31	16 S Sulphur 32	17 Cl Chlorine 35.5	18 Ar Argon 40
19 K Potassium 39	20 Ca Calcium 40	21 Sc Scandium 45	22 Ti Titenium 48	23 V Vanadium 51	24 Cr Chromium 52	25 Mn Manganese 55	26 Fe Iron 56	27 Co Cobalt 59	28 Ni Nickel 59	29 Cu Copper 63.5	30 Zn Zinc 65	31 Ga Gallium 70	32 Ge Germanium 72.5	33 As Arsenic 75	34 Se Selenium 79	35 Br Bromine 80	36 Kr Krypton 84
37 Rb Rubidium 86	38 Sr Strontium 88	39 Y Yttrium 89	40 Zr Zirconium 91	41 Nb Niobium 93	42 Mo Molybdenum 96	43 Tc Techetium (99)*	44 Ru Ruthenium 101	45 Rh Rhodium 103	46 Pd Palladium 106	47 Ag Silver 108	48 Cd Cadmium 112	49 In Indium 115	50 Sn Tin 119	51 Sb Antimony 122	52 Te Tellurium 128	53 I Iodine 127	54 Xe Xenon 131
55 Cs Caesium 133	56 Ba Barium 137	57 La Lanthanum 139	72 Hf Hafnium 178.5	73 Ta Tantalum 184	74 W Tungsten 184	75 Re Rhenium 186	76 Os Osmium 190	77 Ir Iridium 192	78 Pt Platinum 195	79 Au Gold 197	80 Hg Mercury 201	81 Tl Thallium 204	82 Pb Lead 207	83 Bi Bismuth 209	84 Po Polonium (210)	85 At Astatin (210)	86 Rn Radon (222)
87 Fr Fraicium (223)	88 Ra Radium (226)	89 Ac Actinium (226)															

58 Ce Cerium 140	59 Pr Praseodymium 141	60 Nd Neodymium 144	61 Pm Promethium (145)*	62 Sm Samarium 150	63 Eu Europium 152	64 Gd Gadolinium 157	65 Tb Terbium 159	66 Dy Dysprosium 162.5	67 Ho Holmium 165	68 Er Erbium 167	69 Tm Thullium 169	70 Yb Yttterbium 173	71 Lu Lutetium 175
90 Th Thorium 232	91 Pa Protactin 231	92 U Uranium 238	93 Np Neptunium (237)*	94 Pu Plutonium (242)*	95 Am Americium (243)*	96 Cm Curium (247)*	97 Bk Berkalium (249)*	98 Cf Californium (251)*	99 Es Einsteinium (254)*	100 Fe Fermium (253)*	101 Md Mendelevium (256)*	102 No Nobelium (254)*	103 Lw Lawrencium (257)*

*The relative atomic mass of an element whose isotopic composition is variable is shown in parenthesis. Elements marked with * are those which do not occur naturally on earth.*

6 C Carbon 12 — Atomic number — Symbol — Relative atomic mass

Figure 4.2 The Periodic Table of elements. Ninety-nine per cent of the human body is composed of those highlighted

Q *Carbon, hydrogen, oxygen and nitrogen are the most prevalent elements in the body, and hence in our diets. In which dietary constituents would you expect to find these?*

BOX 4.1 RADIOISOTOPES: CLINICAL IMPLICATIONS

Radioisotopes have a number of implications for medicine and health care:

- Iodine is a normal constituent of thyroid hormones and the uptake of a radioisotope of iodine by the gland may be used to assess production of thyroid hormones.
- If the energy of the radiation is large enough then the impact between radiated particles and other atomic nuclei can be used to displace some of the latter's nuclear particles. This is the basis of treating cancer by radiotherapy, the principle of which is to change the chemical structure of the genetic material of tumour cells and so destroy them.
- Conversely, excessive irradiation of normal cells can also make them cancerous, as gene changes cause a loss of control of cell division. Chapter 2 identified how the rate of cell division is regulated through the activities of certain genes: the proto-oncogenes are those that are potentially capable of causing a cell to divide out of control should they be expressed uncontrollably, whereas tumour suppressor genes are those that place a brake on the process. Mutation of the latter in particular is linked to cancer.
- In more recent developments, imaging the activity of parts of the brain has become possible by administering the sugar glucose that has been produced so that it contains a radioisotope of carbon.

Electrolytes (ions)

While atoms are electrically neutral, some can lose or gain electrons and so disturb the balance between positive and negative charges. The atom is then called an ion. The loss of electrons gives the ion a net positive charge since the protons will now be in excess of the electrons, while a gain of electrons gives it a net negative charge, as the number of electrons will now exceed the number of protons. The charge means that a solution of ions will now carry an electric current and so another term for them is electrolytes: this is the term most widely used in clinical practice.

Electrolytes arise for those elements that have electrons unevenly distributed around the nucleus. Electrons spin in a series of orbits around the nucleus that for convenience can be visualized as a series of concentric circles (see Figure 4.1a); the orbits actually equate to energy levels or 'shells' around the nucleus. The number of orbits depends upon the number of electrons that the atom has, and hence may vary between elements. Each orbit has a maximum number of electrons that it can contain: the first orbit at most holds only 2, the second orbit 8, and the third 8 (in smaller atoms) or up to 18 (in large atoms). Whichever is the outermost orbit of the atom, its stability is determined according to whether or not the orbit has its maximum quota of electrons.

If the number is submaximal this confers the atom with its chemical property, as the atom will tend to interact with others to fill that outermost orbit. This is the basis of atoms combining to form molecules; for example oxygen gas is a molecule of two oxygen atoms (see below). An alternative is for the atom to fill the outer orbit by gaining electrons from another atom, but without combining with it. Another possibility is to lose electrons and remove that orbit entirely, thus making the (full) preceding one the new outer orbit. In gaining or losing electrons the electrical balance between protons and electrons will then have changed leading to an overall electrical charge; the atom will have become an ion. For example:

- Chlorine (symbol Cl) atoms have the atomic number 17 (Figure 4.2) and so normally have 17 protons and 17 electrons. This means that their will be three electron orbits, but the outermost one will only contain seven electrons (2 + 8 + 7; see Figure 4.1b). For maximum stability the orbit must be filled by accepting one more electron (note: the alternative of losing as many as seven electrons is not feasible). The 'atom' will now have 17 protons and 18 electrons, giving it a net negative charge: this is the chlorine (or chloride as it is usually called) ion; it is given the symbol Cl^-. The extra electron is taken from another atom, for example sodium, which would then also become an ion.
- Sodium (atomic number 11) normally would have 11 protons and 11 electrons, with just one of the latter in an outer orbit (2 + 8 +1; see Figure 4.1c). To achieve maximum stability the atom would have to lose that electron and so lose that orbit (note: the alternative of acquiring another seven electrons to fill the outer orbit is not feasible). This leaves the 'atom' with 11 protons and 10 electrons, and hence a net positive charge; this is the sodium ion; it is given the symbol Na^+. The lost electron could contribute to another ion, for example the chloride ion mentioned above.

If an electric current is passed through a solution containing chloride ions, the ions move towards the positive electrode, called the anode; negative charged ions are often referred to as 'anions' for this reason. Similarly, an electric current passed through a solution of positive ions causes the ions to move towards the negative electrode (the cathode), and so these ions are often referred to as 'cations'. This principle is used in, for example, electro-plating base metal with silver.

In combination, a cation and an anion make a 'salt'; for example sodium chloride (NaCl = common or table salt) is a combination of sodium and chloride ions. This salt is a solid white crystal and must be dissolved in water for the ions to be separated:

Salts and ions are readily available from our diets, and our body fluids contain a considerable number of types of ion in a range of concentrations (see Chapter 6). The presence of an electrical charge makes ions chemically active and most have important physiological actions, and so the concentrations of

ACTIVITY

Refer to the discussion to explain why sodium ions have one electrical charge, zinc ions two, and aluminium ions three. Why are these ions positively charged rather than negative?

ions dissolved in our body fluids must be closely controlled. Much is now understood of those processes but little is known about the regulation of some, such as zinc (Zn^{2+}) and aluminium (Al^{3+}), which are found in such low concentrations that they are referred to as 'trace' elements.

In contrast, the atoms of some elements, such as helium (symbol He), have just the right number of electrons to fill their orbits and therefore do not have to lose or gain electrons for stability. These are called 'inert' elements as that stability means that they do not readily take part in chemical reactions. This makes helium (a gas) useful in clinical evaluations of lung function as it can be breathed in without physiological consequence (see Chapter14, p.409).

Combining atoms to produce molecules

When two or more atoms combine in a chemical reaction the resultant substance is considered to be a 'molecule'. If the molecule contains atoms of different elements it may be referred to as a 'compound', although the term 'molecule' tends to be used generically.

Various forms of chemical bonds are recognized.

Ionic bonds

Salts (see previous section) are molecules in which the attraction of opposing electrical charges produces an 'ionic' bond that holds the ions together.

Covalent bonds

Other bonds are more common in biological systems, especially those called covalent bonds in which atoms are bonded together through the sharing of electrons.

For example, an atom of oxygen (atomic number 8) has eight electrons and so has only six in its outer orbit (2 + 6; see Figure 4.3a). For maximum stability an oxygen atom therefore must gain two electrons in order to fill the outer orbit. In this instance the atom does not usually become an ion but instead it shares electrons with another atom, such as another oxygen atom. Between them they will still only have 12 electrons in their outer orbits (6 + 6) but by sharing there will be brief moments when each atom will have a full complement of electrons (eight) in its orbit. The time spent without a full complement becomes negligible and so in effect the two atoms have attained stability.

The oxygen atom could, of course, share electrons with atoms of other elements, and this is illustrated in Figure 4.3b in which an oxygen atom is sharing electrons with two hydrogen atoms. Hydrogen (atomic number 1) has only one electron in its outer orbit (remember that this is the first orbit and can maximally hold two electrons) and by sharing electrons

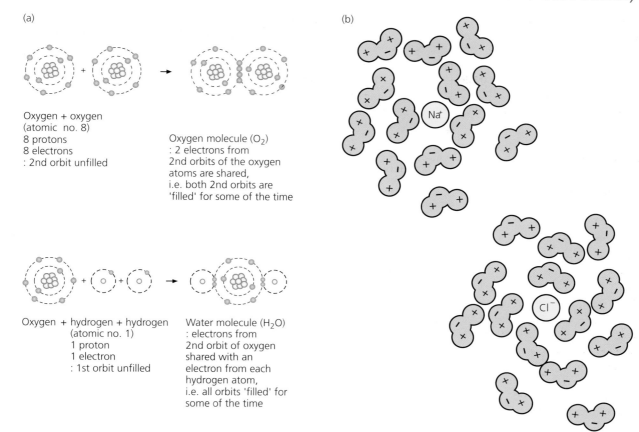

(a)

Oxygen + oxygen
(atomic no. 8)
8 protons
8 electrons
: 2nd orbit unfilled

Oxygen molecule (O_2)
: 2 electrons from
2nd orbits of the oxygen
atoms are shared,
i.e. both 2nd orbits are
'filled' for some of the time

Oxygen + hydrogen + hydrogen
(atomic no. 1)
1 proton
1 electron
: 1st orbit unfilled

Water molecule (H_2O)
: electrons from
2nd orbit of oxygen
shared with an
electron from each
hydrogen atom,
i.e. all orbits 'filled' for
some of the time

(b)

Figure 4.3 Bonding between atoms. In (a) oxygen atoms have formed covalent bonds with another oxygen atom to form an oxygen molecule (i.e. O_2) or with two hydrogen atoms to form a molecule of water (H_2O). In (b), the uneven distribution of electrical charge within a water molecule means that the molecule can act as a solvent of atoms/molecules that also have a charge. This is how, for example, table salt (sodium chloride) dissolves in water (see text)

with oxygen the hydrogen atoms will also each 'gain' for periods the extra electron they need for stability. Such covalent bonds are essential to life; they are relatively easy to form, but are stable and are not expensive in terms of the energy required.

In these examples the molecule consisting of two oxygen atoms is given the symbol O_2 (the subscript number denotes the presence of two atoms) and is the form in which oxygen is found in the atmosphere. The molecule or compound consisting of an oxygen atom and two hydrogen atoms is given the symbol H_2O (i.e. water). Note how the change in constituents alters the properties of the substance. Oxygen and water molecules are relatively simple as they involve just a few atoms. Some atoms have a capacity to share many more electrons and so more complex molecules are possible. For example, a carbon atom (atomic number 6) has four electrons in its outer orbit (2 + 4; see Figure 4.4). To 'gain' the four electrons it requires to fill the outer orbit a carbon atom may, perhaps, share electrons with four hydrogen atoms to produce the molecule CH_4 (called methane, a gas), or perhaps with atoms that include another carbon atom. This latter carbon atom may, of course, combine with yet more atoms to gain the additional three electrons it now requires for stability, and so the process may con-

tinue. Potentially such molecules may involve hundreds of atoms and are said to be 'macromolecules' ('macro-' = large) and there are many examples of these in cells, for example carbohydrates, proteins and fats.

The capacity of carbon atoms to combine with so many others makes it a particularly versatile element. It is perhaps not surprising, therefore, to find that carbon-based compounds form the chemical basis of all living organisms. The chemistry of carbon and its compounds is referred to as 'organic' chemistry to distinguish it from the chemistry of other elements (called 'inorganic' chemistry).

Hydrogen bonds

A further type of bond is that referred to as a 'hydrogen bond'. This again entails attraction between opposite electrical charges but is different from an ionic bond because there is no donation or loss of any electrons. The charge on a hydrogen atom comes about because of disproportionate sizes of atoms within the structure of a molecule. Remember that atom size is especially related to the number of positively charged protons in its nucleus. Hydrogen is the smallest of atoms, with just one proton, so any other elements it is joined to within a molecule will have bigger atoms. Thus, if hydrogen forms a covalent

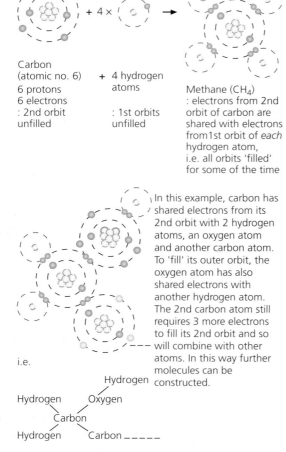

Carbon
(atomic no. 6)
6 protons
6 electrons
: 2nd orbit
unfilled

+ 4 hydrogen
atoms

: 1st orbits
unfilled

Methane (CH$_4$)
: electrons from 2nd
orbit of carbon are
shared with electrons
from 1st orbit of *each*
hydrogen atom,
i.e. all orbits 'filled'
for some of the time

In this example, carbon has
shared electrons from its
2nd orbit with 2 hydrogen
atoms, an oxygen atom
and another carbon atom.
To 'fill' its outer orbit, the
oxygen atom has also
shared electrons with
another hydrogen atom.
The 2nd carbon atom still
requires 3 more electrons
to fill its 2nd orbit and so
will combine with other
atoms. In this way further
molecules can be
constructed.

i.e.

Hydrogen
Hydrogen   Oxygen
        Carbon
Hydrogen   Carbon _____

Figure 4.4 The versatility of carbon: the building of simple or complex organic molecules

Q Look closely at the diagram of the carbon atom. How many electrons does it have in its outer orbit? How many can it contain when full? How many electrons could it share with other atoms?

bond, the sharing of electrons tends to be unequal; the shared electrons will spend most of their time around the bigger nucleus, leaving the hydrogen atom deficient for much of the time and the other atom in surplus (for example the oxygen within a water molecule). This disproportionate sharing causes the hydrogen atom to have a weak positive charge and the associated atom a slight negative charge. A hydrogen bond forms when the molecule is electrically attracted to other charged molecules. These bonds take little energy to form and require little to break them, and are widespread in the body. For example:

- The charged hydrogen atoms in amino acids cause different ones in a protein molecule to interact with each other, thus producing the three-dimensional shape vital to its role.
- Hydrogen bonds between the constituent molecules of DNA help to hold the two chains of the DNA molecule

together. The two chains must be separated during the processes of DNA replication or RNA transcription (see Chapter 2, p.41), and the presence of hydrogen bonds means that this is done easily and efficiently.

- Hydrogen bonds between water molecules and electrolytes in solution help to keep the electrolytes apart and prevent them recombining with each other through ionic bonding (see Figure 4.3b). This property helps to explain why water is such a good solvent and hence why body fluids can contain so many different ions (see Chapter 6). In contrast, those substances such as lipids that do not carry a charge are poorly soluble in water. This too is important for us because it makes the (uncharged) lipid-based cell membrane insoluble in body fluids, and so it can form an effective barrier between the aqueous environments inside and outside cells. This enables cells to maintain a composition of fluid inside them that is quite different from that of the fluids outside.

Isomers

Isomers are molecules that have the same chemical formula but the constituent atoms are arranged slightly differently, giving the molecules different properties. Examples of important biochemical isomers are the sugars glucose, fructose and galactose. These are the major 'simple' sugars that we obtain from our diets (see Chapter 5, p.107) but all have the formula $C_6H_{12}O_6$. Their molecule shape is essentially a ring made from the six carbon atoms, with oxygen and/or hydrogen attached to each of these. However, the arrangement of the hydrogen and oxygen atoms is slightly different in the three sugars and this is sufficient to change their properties (e.g. fructose tastes much sweeter than the others). The differences also mean that biochemical pathways that utilize glucose to yield energy cannot do the same with fructose and galactose, much of which has to first be converted to glucose in the liver (though some cells can utilize them directly using different pathways, for example spermatozoa).

Even just one type of sugar can exist in slightly different form. For example, glucose can have a sequence of oxygen and hydrogen atoms that are designated a 'right-handed' formation, or a sequence that is a mirror-image ('left-handed' configuration). The 'right-handed' form is referred to as D-glucose (as opposed to L-glucose) and, in clinical terminology, as dextrose.

OVERVIEW OF METABOLISM

It was noted at the start of this chapter how the term metabolism relates to all chemical interactions in the body. Indeed, much of the discipline of biochemistry is concerned with this, so this book can at best provide only an insight into those processes that are especially important to understanding physiological functioning.

The formation of chemical bonds (i.e. anabolic reactions) between atoms or molecules clearly requires the constituent atoms or molecules (called the reaction substrates) to be present in adequate amounts, together with the input of sufficient energy for the bonds to be made (Figure 4.5). The substrates generally are provided by three possible sources:

- *Digestion of food*: taking glucose as an example, this is released by the breakdown of complex dietary carbohydrates.
- *Breakdown of substances and mobilization of stores*: this is illustrated by the release from the liver of glucose from the breakdown of the storage carbohydrate glycogen (a process called glycogenolysis).
- *Conversion from other substances*: for example, glucose can be generated by conversion of other non-carbohydrate sources, such as amino acids and fatty acids, in a process called gluconeogenesis.

The energy required to form chemical bonds is provided by its release from bonds between atoms in other molecules. This process of breakdown of molecules is generally referred to as catabolism. Thus, catabolism and anabolism are closely interrelated in cell functions (Figure 4.5). The first critical stage in providing cells with adequate energy is to break down 'fuels' (i.e. mainly glucose but also amino acids and fatty acids – see Chapter 5) in those specific catabolic processes called respiration, which are explained in more detail in a later section. Within cells, most respiration takes place within the mitochondria. This basically presents the cell with two problems:

- How to harness the energy so that it is not lost as heat.
- How to transfer the energy to other parts of the cell.

The solution is to incorporate the energy into further chemical bonds in a small molecule that is much more readily available to cell processes. That molecule is adenosine triphosphate (or ATP), and is discussed in Chapter 2 (p.30; see also Box 4.4). Thus, at points within a cell the ATP is broken down again to its constituents (adenosine diphosphate and

phosphate; ADP + P) to release the bond energy once more. The ADP and P are recycled in forming more ATP.

Less than 50% of the energy released by cellular respiration is actually harnessed. Similarly, energy is also lost as heat when it is released from ATP. Overall, the efficiency is normally only of the order of 20–25%, and even athletic training will not raise this by more than just a few per cent. In other words, some 70–80% of the energy released is lost as heat. Much of this must be dissipated from cells because excess heat breaks the weak hydrogen bonds that act to hold together many molecules. However, not all heat is immediately lost from the body since maintaining a core temperature of about 37°C is also necessary (see Chapter 16, p.454). Some of the heat produced by metabolism is therefore conserved to maintain the core temperature.

Substrate and energy provision therefore facilitates cell functioning, but within cells the appropriate catabolic and anabolic reactions must also proceed in an appropriate way, and at a rate conducive to the demands placed on the cell. This is largely ensured by the presence of chemicals called enzymes that act as catalysts: they accelerate a specific chemical reaction but do not actually take part in it themselves and so are not changed by it. These chemicals were also identified in Chapter 2 (p.47) as they are key chemicals in the regulation of cell chemistry, and hence cell structure and function. They are discussed in more detail in the following section.

Enzymes

By promoting a specific reaction, perhaps just one of thousands of reactions occurring within a cell, enzymes increase the rate at which that reaction proceeds. This will be vital if that biochemical process is to be compatible with life.

In chemical terms, enzymes are polypeptides or proteins (proteins are made of polypeptides combined together), that is to say, they are large molecules composed of lots of amino acids. Cells produce a huge variety of enzymes and the nomenclature for them used by biochemists and clinicians can be bewildering:

- Some enzymes have generic names according to the chemical group on which they act. For example, a 'protease' is an enzyme that breaks down proteins; the digestive enzyme, pepsin, is one of these.
- The name of an enzyme can be more specific. For example, 'sucrase' is a digestive enzyme that breaks down dietary sucrose into its constituent simple sugar units of glucose and fructose.
- Sometimes an enzyme is named after its chemical action, for example a 'dehydrogenase' enzyme is one which dehydrogenates (i.e. removes a hydrogen atom from) a molecule, a 'hydroxylase' enzyme adds a hydroxyl group (-OH) to the molecule, and a 'transaminase' is involved in the conversion of one amino acid into another type. Box 4.2 provides examples.

Note that enzyme names usually end in the suffix '-ase'. Enzymes may also contain a non-protein cofactor without

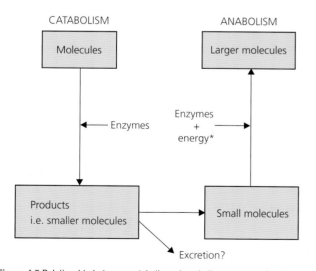

Figure 4.5 Relationship between catabolic and anabolic processes. Some products of catabolism (and perhaps anabolism) may not be useful to cells and so will be removed from the cell and excreted. *Note that the energy required for anabolism will be provided by the catabolism of fuels (e.g. glucose molecules)

BOX 4.2 ENZYME SPECIFICITY: CARDIAC AND LIVER ENZYMES

Enzymes produced by a cell are normally for its own use, and in addition to those enzymes common to processes in all cells, such as those involved in respiration, they will also include enzymes that relate to the role of that particular cell type. These enzymes may become detectable in blood if the cells are damaged and so may be isolated and used for diagnostic purposes. For example, the appearance in blood of the enzymes LDH (lactic dehydrogenase), HBD (hydroxybutyrate dehydrogenase), GOT (glutamate oxaloacetate transaminase) and GPT (glutamate pyruvate transaminase) is used as an indicator of myocardial infarction or liver damage (see also Box 10.28, p.264, and Box 10.29, p.266).

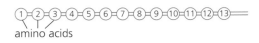

(a)

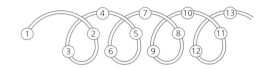

(b)

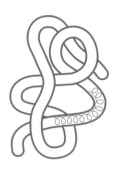

(c)

Figure 4.6 Primary, secondary and tertiary structure of enzymes. (a) Primary structure: an amino acid chain determined by the genetic code of the cell. (b) Secondary structure produced by folding and coiling of the amino acid chain. (c) Tertiary structure: a three-dimensional structure produced by further coiling and folding. Note that (b) and (c) arise from interactions between certain amino acids in the primary structure, producing a final structure that is characteristic and specific to that enzyme

Q *Why is the three-dimensional structure of an enzyme important?*

which it will not function. These cofactors may be ions, such as calcium and magnesium, or complex molecules called coenzymes, such as some B-group vitamins.

It is the structure of the enzyme that enables it to have a specific role as a catalyst. Like all proteins, the enzyme molecule is mainly composed of a large number of smaller constituent molecules called amino acids, of which there are only 20 different types. The synthesis of an enzyme within a cell commences with various amino acids being joined together in a sequence that ultimately is determined by the 'genetic code' provided by DNA (see Figure 2.14, p.41); this is referred to as its 'primary structure' (Figure 4.6). The actual sequencing is important because some amino acids then interact with others along the chain, by forming hydrogen bonds, (see earlier) that cause the structure to coil (= secondary structure) and bend (= tertiary structure) (Figure 4.6) eventually producing a complex three-dimensional shape. Bearing in mind that the molecule might be up to several hundred amino acids in length, the number of possible combinations and permutations of 20 different types of amino acid is colossal, and so there is tremendous scope for variety in protein size and shape. The shape produced is of particular significance for enzymes and for proteins that contribute to cell structures.

The significance of shape to enzyme action can be illustrated by applying a 'lock and key' model (Figure 4.7). This model suggests that the enzyme (= the 'lock'; see 'E' in Figure 4.7) accepts a molecule which has a complementary shape (= the 'key'; see 'A' in the diagram) to form *an enzyme–substrate complex*. The three-dimensional structure of the enzyme molecule means that only substance A will fit into it. In this example, the enzyme's action promotes the separation of the compound into two of its constituent compounds; let us call these 'B' and 'C'. However, it is also clear from Figure 4.7 that substances B and C could also individually fit into the enzyme shape, and so the enzyme might also promote bonding between them, and hence the reforming of substance A. This is an important feature of a catalyst: reactions that involve enzymes are reversible. The question therefore arises as to which substance(s) a cell would produce using this enzyme: A or (B + C). Generally this is determined by the relative amount of either A or (B + C) present since the predominant substrate is more likely to gain access to the enzyme's active site. Thus if A is in excess of (B +

C) then this is more likely to attach to the enzyme, generating further B and C; if (B + C) is in excess then the reaction is likely to generate A. This is referred to as competitive binding, and has a number of applications (Box 4.3).

Following on from this example, if B and C are used in some capacity within the cell, or they are secreted from it, then there will be fewer to compete with A for the binding sites on the enzyme. Thus, provided that there is an adequate amount of A around then production of (B + C) will increase. In this way, increased utilization of B and/or C is matched by increased production and so cell homeostasis is maintained.

From this discussion it should be obvious that a lack of a particular enzyme will prevent a certain reaction from occurring, while a surfeit of the enzyme could cause the reaction to proceed too quickly. The control of the enzyme is achieved by regulating its synthesis or by interfering with its availability (see Figure 2.18, p.48). Other enzymes will also be involved in these processes: this is a classic example of the inter-relationships that operate in living organisms and contribute to homeostasis.

(a)

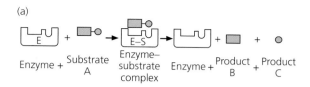

(b)

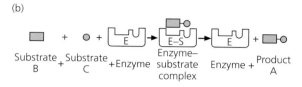

Figure 4.7 Enzyme–substrate reactions. Note how a single enzyme can promote the production of products from a certain substrate, but can also promote reformation of the substrate from those same products

Q Refer to the text. What determines whether the enzyme will form products or substrate?

DETAILS OF CELLULAR RESPIRATION

Energy production by cells 1: cellular respiration and the generation of ATP

As noted earlier, cellular respiration (sometimes referred to as internal respiration) is the process of breaking chemical bonds to release energy essential for cell activities. Oxygen must be available for it to be efficient: this, and the production of carbon dioxide as a waste product, means that the term 'respiration' is also applied to lung function where the gases are exchanged (sometimes referred to as external respiration), and the lungs comprise the respiratory system (see Chapter 14).

Cellular respiration is a very complex process, involving glucose, fatty acids or amino acids as fuels. Mostly, it entails the release of energy from chemical bonds within glucose molecules. It commences with the uptake of glucose by a cell which then enters a sequence of conversions, catalysed by a battery of enzymes, that ultimately generates a net 38 molecules of ATP from a single molecule of glucose:

The first eight molecules of ATP are produced in the cell cytoplasm by reactions that do not use oxygen; this is referred to as anaerobic respiration ('an-' = without, 'aer-' = air).

The remaining 30 are produced using oxygen in a process referred to as aerobic respiration, which takes place within the mitochondria of the cell.

The next sections consider the aerobic and anaerobic processes in more detail.

Energy production by cells 2: aerobic respiration
Aerobic respiration of glucose

You should read this section in conjunction with Figure 4.8.

Glucose is a relatively large molecule ($C_6H_{12}O_6$), insoluble in lipid and unable to diffuse directly into the cell. It therefore

BOX 4.3 COMPETITIVE BINDING

Competitive binding will apply wherever substances have to compete for a spot on a protein.

An example is the action of the enzyme carbonic anhydrase that is found in red blood cells. In the tissues this enzyme promotes the formation of bicarbonate ions from carbon dioxide (see Chapter 6, p.130), which is present in relatively high concentrations. Within the lungs the carbon dioxide concentration falls as the gas is excreted. Competitive binding then favours the conversion of bicarbonate ions to more of the gas which can then also be excreted.

In another example, phenylketonuria (PKU) is an inherited condition in which the amino acid phenylalanine is not fully utilized. As a consequence, its concentration in the blood rises and it begins to compete more effectively for the protein-carrier process that transports amino acids into the brain. Thus, the developing brain of a child, which has a large demand for all types of amino acid, can become deprived as uptake is dominated by phenylalanine transport. Intervention is aimed at reducing the phenylalanine concentration by restricting its presence in the diet. Control has to be instigated early – PKU is normally tested for by midwives within 7–10 days of birth.

Some drugs also use competitive binding; they compete for binding sites of hormones or other biological messengers such as neurotransmitters. In doing so they prevent the actions of that chemical (i.e. they are antagonistic drugs); for example, salbutamol (Ventolin) is an antagonist of adrenaline and is used to reduce the actions of adrenaline on lung airways during an asthma episode.

BOX 4.4 METABOLIC RATE

The text identifies how cellular respiration is the initial, critical step in the provision of energy required for other chemical processes within cells. Cellular respiration therefore is equated to the 'metabolic rate' of the cell. As most of the ATP (3038 molecules per molecule of glucose) produced by respiration involves utilizing oxygen, measuring how much oxygen someone uses per minute provides a useful means of measuring the metabolic rate of the entire body.

In considering an individual's metabolic rate it is necessary to consider two aspects: the basal metabolic rate (BMR) and the increment caused by activity.

The BMR relates to the basic processes that keep us alive, including cell division during tissue repair (or growth in children or in the pregnant woman). It will vary between individuals primarily because of differences in gender, age and body size, and so is normally expressed as a value that has been standardized. The BMR of an individual normally varies only slightly (until age-related factors come into play). Clinically, however, it is elevated:

- in metabolic disorders such as hyperthyroidism ('hyper-' = greater than normal) in which an excessive production of thyroid hormones raises the rate above the normal range;
- in a fever (pyrexia) when substances (pyrogens) released from infectious organisms, or white blood cells produced in response to their presence, act to reset the homeostatic set point for body temperature;
- after surgery or trauma through the activities of the stress hormone, cortisol.

The increment in metabolic rate that is observed from activity relates to:

- physical activities;
- mental activities;
- digestion and assimilatory activities after eating a meal.

Physical activity level makes the most important contribution and so is a factor in dietary recommendations (see Chapter 5, p.112).

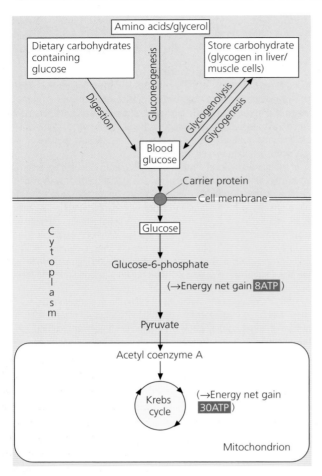

Figure 4.8 Glucose metabolism (or cellular respiration). Note that this is a very simplified diagram of the processes involved. Once glucose has entered a cell, it undergoes many conversions, promoted by numerous enzymes. The ATP that is produced in the cytoplasm does not require oxygen (i.e. this is anaerobic respiration). That produced in the mitochondria occurs in a process that utilizes oxygen (i.e. this is aerobic respiration). Each molecule of glucose generates a net 38 molecules of ATP. Overall the equation for the reaction is: $C_6H_{12}O_6 + 6O_2 \rightarrow 6CO_2 + 6H_2O$

Q *How many molecules of ATP are gained from a molecule of glucose by anaerobic and aerobic respiration? Which process is the more efficient of the two?*

enters cells through facilitated diffusion, via carrier proteins that 'flip' the sugar across the cell membrane. The molecule is then converted within the cytoplasm, via a series of enzymatically driven reactions that do not utilize oxygen, to a substance called pyruvate. By not involving oxygen this is actually an anaerobic stage (see below), referred to as glycolysis, but is integral to the whole process of aerobic respiration of glucose. As already noted, above, it generates eight molecules of ATP from one molecule of glucose. The pyruvate then enters the cell's mitochondria where it is converted using another enzyme into a substance called acetyl coenzyme A, the significance of which is explained later. Acetyl coenzyme A enters yet another complex series of enzymatically controlled reactions called the

tricarboxylic acid (TCA, or Krebs) cycle. This cycle of reactions is important because the stepwise reactions release energy in a slow, controlled fashion that makes the harnessing of the energy as ATP much more efficient, hence the 30 molecules of ATP produced per molecule of glucose that enters the original process. The TCA cycle involves the use of oxygen, and so is the actual aerobic stage.

One feature of the aerobic stage is that electrons are released from atoms during the reactions and these are then transferred along a series of further chemicals found in the membranes of mitochondria. This is the actual process that requires oxygen and is the main source of energy release and ATP generation. The chemicals concerned are called cytochromes (otherwise referred to as the electron transport chain). One important cytochrome is derived from the B vitamin niacin and so this must be present in our diet. Some substances, such as cyanide, are highly toxic to this stage of respiration, effectively preventing generation of adequate ATP and hence are potentially lethal.

The aerobic metabolism of glucose via the TCA cycle produces 'waste' products in the form of carbon dioxide and water, the excesses of which are removed from the body via the lungs/kidneys (see acid–base homeostasis in Chapter 6). Homeostatic regulation of the functioning of these organs ensures that the removal is sufficient to prevent a build-up of these wastes.

BOX 4.5 ORAL GLUCOSE/ELECTROLYTE THERAPY

The means by which glucose enters into cells is an example of facilitated diffusion, which was described in Chapter 2. The process is made more efficient by utilizing the concentration gradient for sodium, which is greater than that of glucose, to drive the carriage. To do this, sodium ions must also combine with the carrier protein. Glucose uptake by cells of the small intestine operates in the same way, and this is one reason why electrolytes are incorporated into oral rehydration solutions used to counteract the consequences of diarrhoea.

Aerobic metabolism of fatty acids and amino acids

You should read this section in conjunction with Figure 4.9.

Cells also have the enzymes necessary for the respiration of fatty acids (from fat) and certain amino acids (from protein). While glucose ordinarily is the main 'fuel' for respiration, some fatty acid metabolism occurs continuously alongside that of glucose and normally accounts for about a third of energy production. Amino acids normally contribute some 15% to the basal metabolic rate.

Within cells, the fatty acids or amino acids are converted into the intermediary substance acetyl coenzyme A identified earlier in the metabolism of glucose. In so doing they can now enter the same TCA cycle (Figure 4.9) and generate ATP. Some amino acids, and the glycerol released from the breakdown of stored fats, can also be converted to pyruvate and enter the TCA cycle, or alternatively the pyruvate may be converted to glucose for use elsewhere in the body.

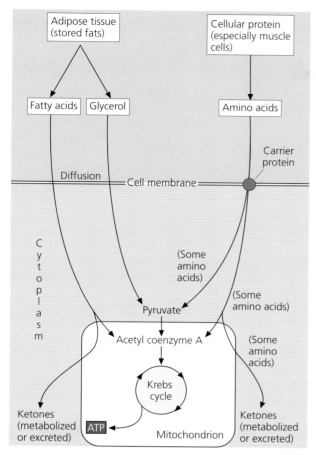

Figure 4.9 Aerobic metabolism of fats and proteins. Note that certain amino acids, and glycerol from fats, may be converted to pyruvate and so may be used to generate new glucose molecules (gluconeogenesis). Note also that the metabolism also produces ketones as byproducts, unlike the carbon dioxide and water produced by glucose metabolism (see Figure 4.8)

Q Undernourishment, or altered metabolism in diabetes mellitus, tends to favour the metabolism of fats and proteins. The excessive amount of ketones produced may then become a problem. Why?

This complex interplay is useful for two main reasons:

1 Glucose, fatty acids, glycerol and some amino acids can all be converted to acetyl coenzyme A and so all are sources of energy via the TCA cycle in mitochondria. Under normal circumstances, therefore, it is highly unlikely that cells will be starved of metabolic fuels.

2 The capacity of cells to convert glycerol or some amino acids to glucose means that the availability of glucose can be increased to support tissue repair in damaged tissues, or to support muscles during exercise. The process of producing glucose from non-carbohydrate sources is referred to as gluconeogenesis (which translates as the 'creation of new glucose') and is stimulated by the hormones cortisol (in wound healing) and adrenaline (in exercise).

Upon entering the TCA cycle, the metabolism of acetyl coenzyme A will lead to the production of carbon dioxide and water, as noted in the metabolism of glucose. However, converting fatty acids and amino acids to acetyl coenzyme A in the first instance also produces substances called ketones. These may be excreted in urine or reused by some tissues for energy, for example cardiac muscle, but there is a limit to the effectiveness of such processes. For example, the extent of the increased fatty acid and amino acid metabolism that is observed in the disorder diabetes mellitus, when it is poorly controlled, means that ketone production is excessive. Ketones:

- Are detectable as a pear-drop smell on the individual's breath, a situation referred to as ketosis.
- May appear in blood as ketoacids, and if in excess of what can be excreted in urine will induce an acidosis (i.e. excessive acidity; see Chapter 6, p.132).

Energy production by cells 3: anaerobic metabolism

Although most energy (and hence ATP) that is produced by cells involves the use of oxygen, the sections above also noted that an anaerobic stage is integral to the overall process of respiration involving glucose. It was also noted that the anaerobic process is considerably less productive of ATP than is the aerobic stage. Nevertheless, that ATP production makes an important contribution, though it is insufficient on its own to sustain cell functioning for very long. In addition, the process produces lactic acid. This is highly toxic to cells and so has to be removed or at least deactivated; lactic acid is taken up from blood by the liver where it is detoxified.

During sharp bursts of exercise, or during prolonged and severe exercise, the oxygen supply to muscles may not be sufficient to maintain the aerobic stage. Some muscle cells do have an interim oxygen store, the pigment myoglobin (similar to the blood pigment haemoglobin), but this source is soon depleted and so anaerobic metabolism must play a more significant role. The reduced production of ATP and increased generation of lactic acid can limit exercise capacity (for example in producing a 'stitch'), and the consequential build-up of lactic acid after exercise has finished must be metabolized. The deoxygenated myoglobin must also be replenished with oxygen. The metabolism of lactic acid by the liver after exercise involves oxygen and, together with the reloading of myoglobin, means that oxygen consumption will have to be greater than is usual at rest; this extra is called the 'oxygen debt' and explains why people breathe heavily after exercise even though they have stopped the activity.

Clinically, circulatory disorders such as coronary arterial disease may also compromise the blood supply, and hence delivery of oxygen, to tissues, causing them to become hypoxic. Anaerobic respiration then becomes a more important contributor to cell function; the effects of hypoxia can range from fatigue/reduced tissue functioning to cell death.

BOX 4.6 APPLICATION: HYPOXIA

If oxygen supply to a tissue cannot match cellular requirements then aerobic metabolism declines and the production of lactic acid increases as anaerobic metabolism begins to dominate. The tissue is said to be hypoxic ('hypo' = less than normal; 'oxia' = oxygenation). The inefficient production of ATP by anaerobic metabolism means that ATP production will soon become inadequate, while the excessive production of lactic acid may also disrupt cell structures and their functions.

Hypoxia has three main causes:

1 Inadequate oxygenation of blood by the lungs. This is referred to as 'hypoxic hypoxia' since it arises from hypoxic lungs. This could occur because of:
 (i)   reduced atmospheric oxygen pressure at high altitude;
 (ii) poor lung ventilation because of lung disorder;
 (iii) poor distribution of air breathed into the lungs because of lung disorder.
 For the last two causes, therapy includes supporting lung function, perhaps even by using ventilation procedures (see Chapter 14).
2 Inadequate capacity of blood to transport oxygen. This may be caused by anaemia arising from insufficient amounts of haemoglobin in blood, or from the effects of toxic chemicals such as carbon monoxide pre-

venting normal oxygenation. Therapy aimed at improving lung ventilation will have little effect in these circumstances since the haemoglobin available in the blood will already be saturated with oxygen (see Chapter 14).

3 Inadequate perfusion of tissues with blood. This is referred to as 'stagnant hypoxia' as the blood present in the tissue becomes depleted of oxygen. This could be local as blood supply to an area is compromised or widespread as in circulatory shock. The aim of therapy is to restore blood perfusion as soon as possible.

In severe hypoxia (for example in shock) or in anoxia (i.e. when no oxygen is present) it is important to note that there is a point at which the effects of oxygen lack are irreversible; from then on the cells will die even if oxygenation is restored. For an active tissue like the brain this is of the order of 3–4 minutes, but for a less active tissue such as the hand this might be 30–40 minutes. Cooling the tissue reduces its metabolic rate and this explains why individuals who are hypothermic (i.e. too low a body temperature) can sometimes survive lengthy periods in cold seas or cold air temperatures. It is also a principle that is widely used in the transportation of transplant tissue.

REGULATION OF METABOLISM

This chapter has described how metabolism is determined by a number of factors, not least the supply of substrates to cells, the entry of substrates into cell structures, and the production/activities of appropriate enzymes that will catalyse reactions. The means of control are therefore going to be varied; much of it is controlled by hormones, but any physiological disorder could be expected to disrupt metabolism somewhere in the body. Some hormones are considered specifically as mediators of metabolism because they directly influence the concentrations of fuel molecules in blood, or their utilization by cells. This section focuses on the actions of these particular hormones, the disorders related to which are classed in clinical circles as 'disorders of metabolism'.

Various hormones are instrumental in regulating the glucose content of blood and its utilization by cells (see also Chapter 9, p.222):

• Insulin promotes glucose uptake by cells when blood glucose concentration is increased following absorption of a meal that contains carbohydrate. Cellular respiration will therefore increase (which is why we feel warm after a large meal) but the uptake of glucose by the liver will also will lead to the production of a glucose store (glycogen), or even to its conversion to fatty acids and perhaps amino acids. Insulin is the only hormone that acts to reduce blood glucose concentration and a failure to produce insulin, or a failure of cells to respond to it, results in the condition diabetes mellitus, which is characterized by a persistent increase in blood glucose concentration (= hyperglycaemia; Box 4.7).

• Glucagon acts in an opposite fashion to insulin, and elevates blood glucose concentration when it falls below the homeo-

static range (for example, between meals or during stressful episodes such as serious illness or major surgery). It does so by mobilizing glucose from glycogen stores, and by promoting gluconeogenesis from fatty acids and amino acids.

• Adrenaline and cortisol also promote gluconeogenesis in times of stress and provide additional metabolic support by mobilizing glucose, fatty acids and amino acids, and so increase their input into cell respiration. Examples of this are seen in the stress response (see Chapter 21, p.598).

• Growth hormone modulates the mobilization of metabolic fuels, primarily amino acids and fatty acids essential in sustaining childhood growth. Its normal activities also include a 'diabetogenic' action in that it acts to cause insulin resistance in some tissues, thus raising blood glucose concentration and potentially making glucose more available to others. Chronically high levels of the hormone exacerbate this action and will eventually cause insulin production to decrease.

• Thyroid hormones act as regulators of the basal metabolic rate, rather than as mediators of fuel availability. A deficiency in their production or actions can have profound effects on child development, especially mental development. In adults a deficiency of thyroid hormones (hypothyroidism) leads to a depressed basal metabolic rate, with symptoms of lethargy, fatigue, feeling cold and lowered pulse rate (see Box 9.7, p.217). Hyperthyroidism, when excess thyroid hormones are produced, causes the opposite – increased basal metabolic rate, hyperactivity, feeling hot and a rapid pulse rate.

• Leptins are produced by adipose tissue and are thought to act within the hypothalamus to promote a reduction in food intake, and feeling of satiety (see Box 4.8 and Chapter 5, p.119).

BOX 4.7 METABOLISM IN DIABETES MELLITUS

Normal ranges for 'fasting' glucose concentration in blood plasma:

Newborn = 2.2–3.3 mmol/L (at 1 day)
Child = 3.3–5.5 mmol/L
Adult = 3.9–5.8 mmol/L

Diabetes mellitus produces medium and long-term symptoms related to an increased blood glucose concentration arising from inadequate production of, or responses to, the hormone insulin. The medium term relates to the increased production of urine and the risk of urinary tract infections as a consequence of the presence of glucose in the urine (glycosuria). The presence of ketosis is also likely to occur at or around this time, that is the concentration of ketones in blood will increase and the 'pear-drop' odour of a type of ketone, called acetone, will be noticeable on the person's breath. In addition, there is a continual risk that inadequate dietary and insulin control may result in episodes when blood glucose concentration is too low (referred to as hypoglycaemia: 'hypo' = less than normal; 'glyc-' = glucose; '-aemia' = of the blood). Brain cells in particular are sensitive to this and behavioural changes including aggression may be observed, and the problem may even progress to coma and perhaps death.

In addition, hyperglycaemia ('hyper-' = greater than normal; 'glyc-' = glucose; '-aemia' = of the blood) in diabetes also influences cell function, particularly of sensory nerve cells and cells in the walls of small blood vessels. Long-term control is aimed at facilitating glucose utilization by cells, thus reducing the occurrence hyperglycaemia, and the production of ketoacids from ketones. Long-term problems are largely related to the slow deterioration of nerve cell function and the microcirculation, particularly in the feet, kidneys and eyes, arising from the actions of glucose on these tissues. The rise in fatty acid concentrations in blood also increases the risk of heart disease.

The risks of coma and damage to tissues have resulted in aggressive therapeutic approaches to control the individual's blood glucose concentration. Much of this, however, involves a self-care regime and patient education is therefore essential. One of the difficulties associated with diabetes care is that people will often report feeling well – the damage arising from the increased glucose is insidious – and lapses in control may occur as a consequence. In addition, imposing rigorous control may also be perceived by the individual as being too demanding, and of placing unacceptable restrictions on their lifestyle.

See the case study of a child with insulin-dependent diabetes Section VI, p.634.

BOX 4.8 METABOLISM AND OBESITY

Fatty acids make a substantial contribution to cellular respiration, and it is noted in Chapter 5 just how useful fat stores are to us. Obesity represents excessive fat storage and is a health risk for the following reasons:

- The emphasis on fat means that there is usually hyperlipidaemia ('hyper-' = excess; '-aemia' = in blood). This raises the risk of lipid deposits, or atheroma, in blood vessels and hence of coronary heart disease, hypertension and stroke.
- The excessive body weight makes it harder for muscles to move the body, raising the effort required. The stress placed on the heart to maintain circulation even under normal circumstances is therefore increased.
- Obesity is often associated with a resistance to the actions of the hormone insulin, raising blood glucose concentrations. It is thought that this effect predisposes the individual to insulin-independent diabetes mellitus.

Obesity represents an imbalance in which either the individual is predisposed to storing (and synthesizing) fat, or there is a level of energy utilization (i.e. activity) that is inadequate for the level of fat intake. In the latter, this illustrates the biological importance of energy stores: the body does not excrete excess metabolic fuels but stores them, presumably in case of lack of food. Sedentary lifestyles are of concern in the developed world and are thought to be an important factor in the increasing incidence of obesity in the UK.

Predisposition to obesity is also likely in some individuals. Recent interest has focused on the genes involved in the production and actions of adipose hormones called leptins. Their elevation in blood with obesity has led to suggestions that they may be involved in the genesis of this condition. A strain of obese mouse that has a defect in leptin function is known, and these mice respond well to injections of the hormone. However, most common forms of human obesity are not related to the specific gene defect that is observed in this mouse and so the role of leptins in obesity, though likely, remains unclear.

BOX 4.9 APPLICATION: METABOLIC RESPONSES TO SURGERY

Surgery promotes metabolic responses that represent a resetting of homeostatic means as a consequence of the release of metabolic hormones in response to the surgical trauma (including pain). Their actions to promote metabolism, are those associated with a 'stress' response. As such they should be viewed as an adaptive process to the situation that helps to promote survival. Readers should refer to Chapter 21 and to Clancy *et al.* (2002) since these explain the stages of their release in relation to stress theory.

The hormones adrenaline, cortisol and growth hormone are involved, and promote the breakdown of glycogen and fat stores and so mobilize glucose and fatty acids. A raised blood glucose concentration (or hyper-glycaemia) is observed that favours the functioning of tissues, especially the brain. Many tissues will also generate energy from the released fatty acids. The significance of increased mobilization of metabolic fuels is that cell division and tissue growth and repair are facilitated.

The availability of metabolic fuel is also facilitated by glucose synthesis prompted by the actions of cortisol to induce protein breakdown and the conversion of the amino acids to glucose by the liver. Protein synthesis is also decreased, exacerbating the reduction in protein, and muscle loss may be observed. The persistence of protein depletion may hinder long-term wound healing and have implications for the general welfare of patients.

SUMMARY

1 Metabolism encompasses those chemical reactions that lead to synthesis (i.e. anabolism) or breakdown (i.e. catabolism) of substances by cells.

2 Atoms of elements provide the basic units of which chemical molecules are comprised.

3 Ions, or electrolytes, are formed when certain atoms lose or gain electrons in order to improve the stability of their atomic structure. These are positively or negatively charged according to whether they lose or gain electrons. The presence of an electrical charge makes ions chemically and physiologically active. Ions are constituents of body fluids.

4 Molecules are formed when two or more atoms bond together. This may entail electrical attraction (e.g. hydrogen bonds) or a sharing of electrons (i.e. covalent bonds). Both types of bond are relatively easy to form. Covalent bonds in particular are involved in anabolism and catabolism. Forming bonds in anabolic processes requires an input of energy and so metabolic rate equates with the energy production by cells to facilitate this.

5 Enzymes are proteins that act as catalysts and so promote anabolism or catabolism according to the relative availability of substrates (this is referred to as 'competitive binding'). Their role depends upon their precise three-dimensional structure arising from the sequence of amino acids of which they are composed. This sequence is determined by DNA and hence explains how genes determine cell structure and functions.

6 Cellular respiration describes the processes by which enzymes cause the release of energy by breaking molecular bonds. Respiration provides an intermediary chemical, ATP, and this transfers energy from these energy-producing processes to all areas of the cell for utilization.

7 Glucose is the main substrate for respiration. One molecule of glucose generates 38 molecules of ATP. Eight of these molecules are produced in the cytoplasm by processes that do not require oxygen; this is referred to as anaerobic respiration. The remaining 30 molecules of ATP are produced within mitochondria by aerobic respiration, that is, using oxygen.

8 Aerobic respiration of glucose entails a gradual change to the glucose molecule and the harnessing of energy as it is released. One of the substances produced during this process is called pyruvate and this can also be produced by cells using fatty acids and some amino acids. In this way cells can utilize these fuels in addition to glucose.

9 Aerobic respiration of glucose generates carbon dioxide and water as waste substances. Carbon dioxide is a source of acid and so must be excreted via the lungs.

10 Aerobic metabolism of fatty acids and amino acids generates ketones, a source of ketoacids. These must also be removed, this time by the kidneys and liver.

11 Anaerobic processes generate lactic acid; this too is removed by the liver and kidneys.

FURTHER READING

Texts on metabolism and biochemistry abound. Readers might find the following useful in relation to some of the specific points raised in this chapter regarding metabolism in surgery, diabetes mellitus and obesity.

Clancy, J., McVicar, A. and Baird, N. (2002) Chapter 7: Anaesthesia, stress and surgery. In: *Fundamentals of Physiology for Perioperative Practitioners*. London: Routledge, pp.212–36.

Dominiczak, M.H. (2007) *Flesh and Bones of Metabolism*. Edinburgh: Mosby.

Williams, G. and Pickup, J.C. (2004) *Handbook of Diabetes*, 3rd edn. Oxford: Blackwell Science.

NUTRIENTS AND NUTRITION

INTRODUCTION

The biology of nutrition pays scant regard to how good food tastes but is concerned with what nutrients it supplies. Our diet has to provide all of the chemicals that are necessary for cell metabolism, for the production of cell structures, and for the body fluids within and outside cells. In recognition of this a German philosopher, Ludwig Feuerbach (1804–1872), once quipped

> *'Man ist was man isst'* ('one is what one eats').

Although not technically correct, the quip is not far from the truth. For example, plant proteins are very different from those in the human body, but they provide the building blocks for our cells to make proteins that are essential for us.

However, eating is not simply a biological function; it is also a psychosocial phenomenon. Some issues to be considered by practitioners include:

- The individual's need for independence, if possible.
- Privacy while eating may be desirable, or social communication may also be preferred.
- Ward routines may disturb eating behaviours.
- Individuals have distinct dietary habits.
- Specific groups have specific dietary needs (e.g. cultural aspects or developmental stage).
- Age and gender influence the preferred diet.
- Positioning and use of utensils may be influencing factors for patients requiring help with eating.
- Sick people may have poor appetites: observe the amounts eaten and observe for signs of under-nutrition.
- Poor mouth care may affect eating behaviours.
- Financial constraints may prevent the eating of an ideal diet and so dietary recommendations must be flexible enough to be cost-effective for the individual.
- A working knowledge of the functioning of the gastrointestinal tract should improve the understanding of dietary factors in individuals with disordered functions.

All of these can affect an individual who requires the support of health and social care services. Additional practices

BOX 5.1 ENTERAL AND PARENTERAL NUTRITION

The normal means of feeding is not always possible in various disorders and so food must be delivered directly into the digestive system (enteral nutrition) or into the circulatory system (parenteral nutrition).

- Enteral feeding entails the delivery of foodstuffs in a semi-liquid state into the stomach, or possibly even the intestine, using a tube that has been inserted via the oesophagus (Bourgault *et al.*, 2007). This is clearly an unpleasant procedure for a patient, and may not always be effective if bowel dysfunction prevents digestion and/or absorption of nutrients.
- In parenteral feeding, sterile food solutions are administered intravenously via a catheter placed in a convenient vein. Parenteral nutrition supplies the range of constituents of a normal diet, other than nucleic acids and fibre. Feeds are available in a range of compositions or formulae, and if necessary can be made up in pharmacy according to dietetic advice. The intention is to maintain organ function and fluid/electrolyte balance until enteral or oral feeding becomes possible.

relate to the care of people for whom eating independently is not possible and so alternative modes of delivery of nutrients have to be applied (Box 5.1). For this text, however, the focus is the nutrition requirements of a healthy diet, and some of the health issues related to these.

NUTRIENTS AND THEIR DIETARY SOURCES

Introduction: a balanced diet

Approximately 95% of the mass of the human body is comprised of the elements carbon, hydrogen, oxygen and nitrogen in various combinations to form carbohydrates, proteins, lipids and water. Another 4% (mainly bone) is made up of phosphorus and calcium, while the remaining 1% consists of about 18 other elements, such as potassium and sodium. Our diets should therefore contain the same elements but will also have to contain 'fibre' (not really a nutrient) to aid the function of the bowel in digesting food; digestion is essential because many of the foods we eat contain the elements in complex molecules and these must be reduced to simpler ones if they are to be absorbed into the body. Dietary composition also has to be considered in relation to its energy content (also considered a 'nutrient'), since the diet must meet the energy requirements of cells. It is important that all individuals have the appropriate amount of each type of nutrient; this is then referred to as a balanced diet. A person's illness, or surgery, or life stage may result in recommended changes to their diet, but this is usually related to palatability of the food, or to alterations to the food composition, in order to meet any specific needs.

This section identifies the constituents that should be present in a normal diet in health, and how this is influenced by life stage. To obtain the necessary range of nutrients, the Government (Food Standards Agency 2007 see http://www.food.gov.uk/healthiereating) recommends that a balanced diet contains:

- plenty of starch-containing foods;
- at least five portions of a variety of fruits and vegetables per day;
- some protein-rich foods (plant and/or animal);
- dairy products, but choosing reduced-fat versions (or small amounts of full-fat versions);
- small amounts of saturated fat, salt (sodium chloride) and sugar.

There are recommendations regarding the intake of almost all nutrients. Recommended intakes of nutrients are calculated from their rates of utilization, storage or excretion and are continually under review. The aim of such recommendations is to ensure that everyone receives sufficient amounts of each nutrient, although there are difficulties in establishing a standard for all as the needs of the body change according to the individual's age and stage of development, and there are individual differences in the rates at which nutrients are absorbed from the bowel: as an illustration, someone who absorbs a nutrient at half the rate of another individual must eat twice as much to obtain the same amount. A number of indices (collectively called Dietary Reference Values; Department of Health, 1991; see also the British Nutrition Foundation for additional reference values: http://www.nutrition.org.uk) have been developed that meet the needs of almost everyone. Readers may also be aware of data provided on food packaging which relates to the recommended daily allowance (RDA), based on estimated average requirements.

The principal nutrients within a healthy diet are:

1 carbohydrates (other than 'fibre')
2 proteins
3 lipids (including fats)
4 energy (not a chemical but considered a dietary constituent)
5 fibre (mainly forms of carbohydrate)
6 vitamins
7 minerals
8 nucleic acids
9 water.

Carbohydrates, proteins and fat comprise the bulk of our food but all of the above constituents are necessary for the maintenance of growth and health.

BOX 5.2 ANOREXIA NERVOSA, BULIMIA AND OBESITY

Anorexia is a condition that is characterized by a body weight that is at least 15% below the minimum standard for age, gender and stature. Anorexia nervosa is an emaciated state arising from psychological cause that produces complex symptoms related to general nutrient deficiency. It is a complex disorder, found most commonly in adolescent women, and appears to arise from concern over changes in body weight during puberty. Hunger and appetite are suppressed, although individuals may also resort to laxative abuse, enemas and self-induced vomiting.

Bulimia and obesity are conditions in which food volume in excess of body requirements is eaten. This usually arises from socio-psychological disturbances, although there is also some evidence for an inherited propensity to obesity.

- Bulimia is a condition whereby an individual impulsively consumes a large amount of food in a short space of time. Self-induced vomiting, or even laxative abuse, is then used in an attempt to prevent weight gain or perhaps promote weight loss. Many people with bulimia have a normal body weight or are only slightly overweight.
- Obesity (Figure 5.1) is a condition in which body weight is at least 20% above the 'ideal'. Excess weight is a consequence of excessive fat deposits and results from a prolonged intake of energy in excess of body requirements. The most widely applied index to evaluate excess weight is the body mass index or BMI, and is calculated as weight/height^2. A BMI of 20–25 is considered healthy, and 30+ indicates obesity. However, BMI is influenced by muscle bulk too, and body build in general, and so its use has been criticized. Intra-abdominal fat has been known for some time to present the greatest health risk (Donahue and Abbott, 1987) and consequently new measures for monitoring obesity have been proposed, notably waist circumference and sagittal (i.e. cross-sectional) abdominal diameter. (See the case of an obese boy, Section VI, p.636.)

Correction of anorexia, bulimia and obesity generally requires an understanding of the psychological cause of the disturbed physiological homeostasis (Wiedeman and Pryor, 2000).

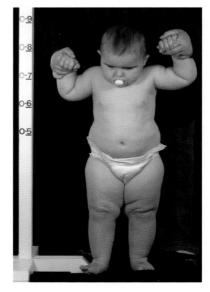

Figure 5.1 Obesity in a child of 18 months. Reproduced with the kind permission of the Medical Illustration Department, Norfolk and Norwich University Hospital NHS Trust

Carbohydrates

Carbohydrates are widespread in nature, being important energy stores in plants and animals. Their chemical molecules contain atoms of carbon ('carbo-'), hydrogen ('hydr-') and oxygen (indicated by '-ate'), and have various functions in cells:

- they are the primary energy source;
- they may act as energy reserves;
- they may be incorporated into, or combined with, other molecules;
- they may have roles in membrane functions or are structural components of those membranes;
- some may be converted into other substances, such as the constituents of proteins and lipids, and so supplement these.

Carbohydrates, then, are very versatile. There are a number that we obtain from our diets, and they can be divided into three main subgroups: monosaccharides, disaccharides and polysaccharides.

Monosaccharides ('mono-' = single; 'saccharide' = sugar) are 'simple sugars' that contain from three to seven carbon atoms in their molecules and are highly soluble in water. Important dietary examples are:

- *Pentoses* ('penta-' = five; they have five carbon atoms in their molecule): for example, ribose is a constituent of nucleic acids (hence deoxyribonucleic acid; DNA).
- *Hexoses* ('hexa-' = six; they have six carbon atoms in the molecule): for example, glucose is the most important source of energy in cells. Other examples are galactose and fructose.

Disaccharides ('di-' = two) consist of two monosaccharide molecules joined together. Important ones in our diets are:

- *Sucrose* (cane, beet or table sugar): a common example of a disaccharide, and is formed by combination of the monosaccharides glucose and fructose.
- *Lactose* (milk sugar): a combination of glucose and galactose.
- *Maltose* (malt sugar): a combination of two glucose molecules (Figure 5.2a); maltose in our diet is mostly commercially produced.

Polysaccharides ('poly-' = many) consist of numerous monosaccharide molecules joined together, and may be very large molecules. Unlike monosaccharides and disaccharides they are usually poorly soluble in water, and so form important components of cell membranes, and the means of storing carbohydrates within cells. Dietary important ones include the following:

- Starch is found in plants, is made from numerous glucose molecules, and is an important dietary source of that sugar. On average, starch comprises 60% or more of the carbohydrate in our diet, and large quantities are stored in the stems, roots, tubers and seeds of food plants.
- Glycogen is the animal equivalent of starch, and also is composed of glucose molecules. It forms a convenient means of storing that sugar in cells, primarily in the liver and in skeletal muscle, but the glycogen content of animal tissues generally is low and so it is not a significant dietary source of glucose.
- Cellulose, dextrin and lignin are found in plants and are composed of glucose molecules, but they are constructed differently from starch and cannot be broken down by our digestive system to release the constituent sugars. However, they are important in our diets because they provide fibre.

Simple (monosaccharide) sugars can be absorbed directly from the bowel, but polysaccharides (other than fibre) and disaccharides must be digested to yield their 'simple' sugar constituents (Table 5.1). From the above it is clear that glucose molecules are the predominant simple sugars within the composition of dietary carbohydrates – this is our most important 'fuel' and even other hexose sugars from our diets, such as fructose and galactose, are largely converted to glucose in the liver. Eating carbohydrates therefore causes the concentration of glucose in blood to rise. The rate of change has implications for the release of the hormone insulin, which acts to enhance utilization of the glucose (see Chapter 9, p.222) and consequently blood glucose homeostasis. A diet that regularly induces rapid increases in blood glucose after a meal is currently thought to be a risk for the eventual development of insulin insensitivity (perhaps leading to diabetes mellitus) and other long-term meta-

Table 5.1 Common carbohydrate constituents (excluding fibre) of a Western diet

Carbohydrate class	Examples	Source	Products
Polysaccharides	Starch	Plant tissues	Digested to glucose
	Glycogen	Animal tissues, especially liver	Digested to glucose
Disaccharides	Sucrose	Sugar cane/beet	Digested to glucose and fructose
	Maltose	'Malted' foods (from starch)	Digested to glucose
	Lactose	Milk	Digested to glucose and galactose
Monosaccharides	Glucose	Fruits, honey, vegetables	Absorbed and utilized as glucose
	Fructose	Fruits, honey, vegetables	Absorbed and utilized as fructose or converted to glucose
	Galactose	Digestion product of lactose	Converted to glucose in liver
Sugar alcohols	Sorbitol	Fruits, and manufactured from glucose	Converted to fructose in liver
	Inositol	Cereal brans, and manufactured from glucose	Inositol is inert

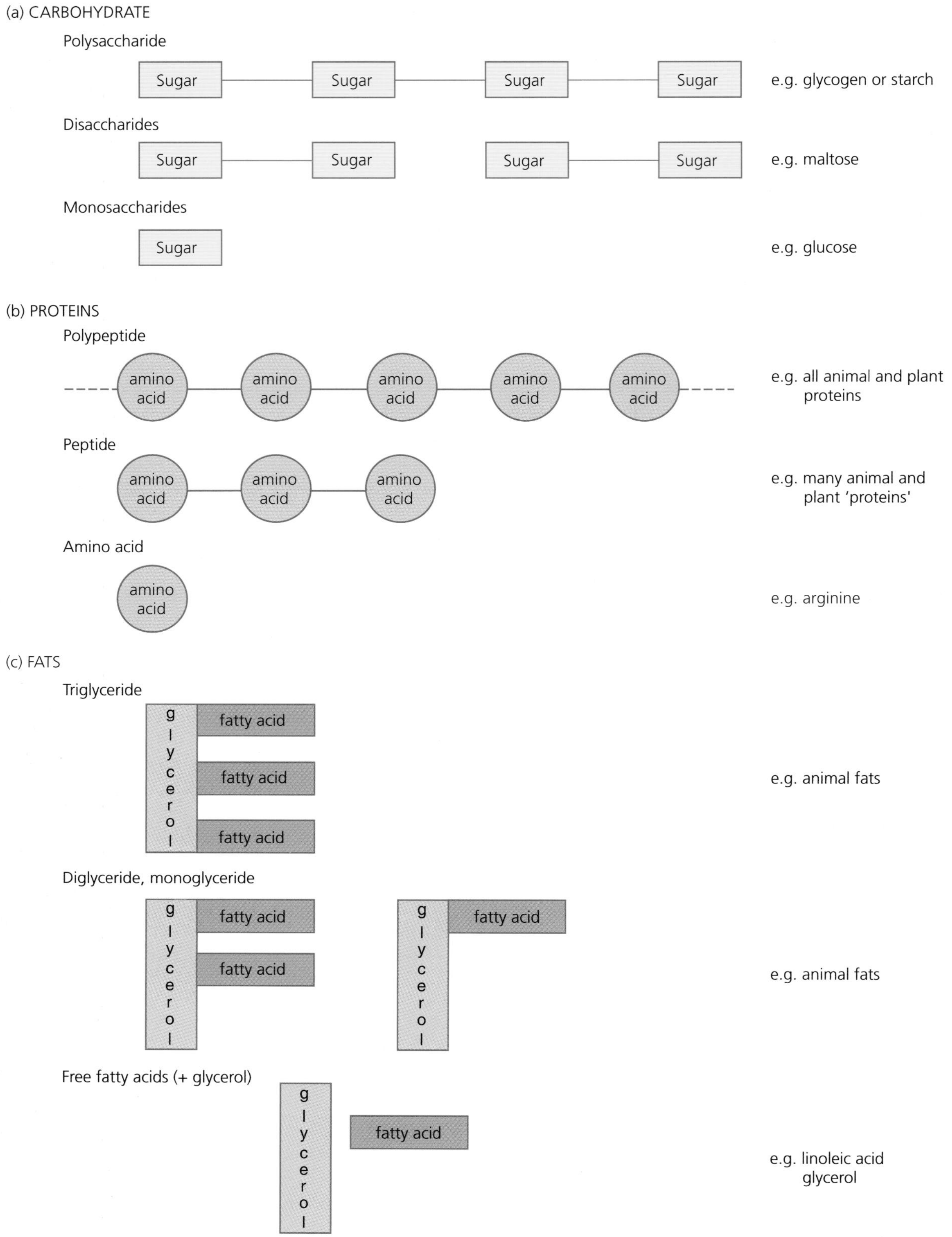

(a) CARBOHYDRATE

Polysaccharide

| Sugar | — | Sugar | — | Sugar | — | Sugar |

e.g. glycogen or starch

Disaccharides

| Sugar | — | Sugar | | Sugar | — | Sugar |

e.g. maltose

Monosaccharides

| Sugar |

e.g. glucose

(b) PROTEINS

Polypeptide

- - - amino acid — amino acid — amino acid — amino acid — amino acid - - -

e.g. all animal and plant proteins

Peptide

amino acid — amino acid — amino acid

e.g. many animal and plant 'proteins'

Amino acid

amino acid

e.g. arginine

(c) FATS

Triglyceride

glycerol — fatty acid
glycerol — fatty acid
glycerol — fatty acid

e.g. animal fats

Diglyceride, monoglyceride

glycerol — fatty acid
glycerol — fatty acid

glycerol — fatty acid

e.g. animal fats

Free fatty acids (+ glycerol)

glycerol   fatty acid

e.g. linoleic acid glycerol

Figure 5.2 Outline of the structure of the main food groups: (a) polysaccharides, (b) polypeptide (protein) and (c) triglyceride (fat; a form of lipid). Note how each is an example of a macromolecule ('macro-' = large) but each has distinctive molecular subunits (simple sugars, amino acids and fatty acids, respectively) that form the 'building blocks' of the macromolecule

bolic consequences such as coronary heart disease. Carbohydrates that promote a rapid change in blood glucose are accorded a 'high glycaemic index (GI)' score (70+), while those that produce a moderate rate of change are accorded a 'low GI' score (55 or less). Low GI foods are therefore considered better for us and include sources low in glucose or those with very complex carbohydrates that are digested slowly, such as most fruits and vegetables, wholegrains, beans and lentils. High GI foods include sources in which the carbohydrates are less complex, or in which glucose is present, such as processed foods and beer. However, the GI score can be surprisingly high in some fruits (e.g. watermelon) and vegetables (e.g. potatoes): there are databases of GI ratings for readers interested in this topic, for example http://www.glycaemicindex.com.

Carbohydrates are so widely available in our foods, for example in potatoes, pasta and rice, that in the UK dietary excess is a greater problem than deficiency. Excessive carbohydrate intake contributes to obesity through the conversion of glucose to glycerol, a constituent of fats. Deficiency results in weight loss but the widespread availability of carbohydrate means that it usually arises through conscious abstention, for example in weight-reducing diets or in the condition anorexia nervosa (Box 5.2). Metabolic deficiency, as distinct from dietary deficiency, arises when there may be adequate simple sugars in body fluids but they cannot enter cells in sufficient amounts to maintain metabolism. For example, in diabetes mellitus cells literally are 'starved' of glucose and in galactosaemia the liver is unable to take up galactose from blood. The deficiency affects normal metabolism, but the resultant excess in blood also has a consequence for health, for example in promoting neuropathy and renal failure (in diabetes) and neurological problems (in galactosaemia; especially in infants).

Lipids (including fats)

The group of substances collectively referred to as lipids are present in various forms within the body. A normal diet will contain a range of lipids, but most will be animal fats and vegetable oils since they provide animals and plants with important energy stores. Like carbohydrates, lipids are composed of the elements carbon, hydrogen and oxygen but they have a very different molecular structure, which makes them poorly soluble in water. The basic constituents of lipids are small molecules called fatty acids, which collectively may be part of large, complex molecules (fats and oils), or may occur individually, though modified:

- *Fats (and oils)*: consist of molecules in which fatty acids combined with a molecule of glycerol (Figure 5.2c); they are sometimes referred to as triglycerides, diglycerides or monoglycerides because respectively the fat molecule contains three, two or just one fatty acid.
- *Cholesterol*: a modified fatty acid that is biologically important because it is used to make cell membranes (see Chapter 2 and Box 5.3).
- *Phospholipids* (e.g. steroid hormones and prostaglandins; see

Chapter 9, p.206): these are modified fatty acids that contain an atom of phosphorus in their molecule.
- *Glycolipids*: modified fatty acids in that they have been combined with a carbohydrate molecule. They are found on the surface of cell membranes where they provide marker sites, for example the antigens responsible for blood groups (see Chapter 11, p.296).
- *Lipoproteins*: lipids that have been combined with protein molecules. Important examples are high-density lipoprotein (HDL) and low-density lipoprotein (LDL), two means by which cholesterol is carried in blood (Box 5.3). The combination of protein with cholesterol makes the molecule soluble in water. Other important lipoproteins are found in the bowel where they aid the solubility of lipids for digestion (see Chapter 10, p.254).

Dietary lipid provides us with about 40 different naturally occurring fatty acids. These differ in two main ways. First, they differ in the number of carbon atoms that form the chemical 'backbone' of the molecule; for example long-chain fatty acids have 14–25 carbon atoms. Second, they differ in the 'saturation' of the constituent carbon atoms with hydrogen atoms; in this context, fatty acids (or the fat molecule containing them) are themselves frequently referred to as saturated or unsaturated.

A carbon atom has the capacity to form four individual chemical bonds through the sharing of four of its electrons (see Chapter 4 for atom structures). In a fatty acid, two of those bonds are taken up by one atom bonding with two other carbon atoms – this is the basis of forming the chain of carbon atoms typically found in the molecular structure of a fatty acid. If the two remaining bonds are taken up by two hydrogen atoms, then the carbon atom is now bound to a total of four other atoms: the two carbons and the two hydrogens. It cannot form further bonds unless one or more of the adjacent atoms are replaced; the carbon atom therefore is said to be 'saturated'. In a saturated fatty acid (or fat) all of the carbon atoms are in this state. Alternatively, the carbon atom might share all four of its electrons with the two adjacent carbon atoms, in other words it is now only bound to two molecules: the two carbons. Such bonds are referred to as a 'double' bond, in recognition that each takes up two potential bonding sites. Its significance is that a carbon atom may free up a site to bond with a further atom, yet still remain bound to its adjacent carbon atom, in much the same way as saturated carbon atoms have. In a monounsaturated fatty acid there is just one double bond within its molecule, whilst in a polyunsaturated fatty acid there may be several.

All of this seems somewhat esoteric for healthcare practices but the distinction is important. Saturated fatty acids can be converted by the liver into cholesterol, and while cholesterol is crucial to us in making cells, its excess poses significant health risks (Box 5.3). Unsaturated, especially polyunsaturated, fatty acids are of less risk and so the dietary recommendation is that most fat intake is unsaturated (see the section on 'Energy' below).

The overall fat content of food, and its saturated/unsaturated composition, varies depending upon the source:

- Beef, lamb, and pork are rich sources of fats, even when visible fat is removed. 'White' meat of poultry is low in fat but duck and goose may contain as much fat as beef. Animal fats may be saturated or unsaturated and the cholesterol content varies; for example, egg yolk and dairy fats are high in cholesterol.
- Fat in fresh fish varies according to species. Thus, cod and haddock have low fat contents while that of mackerel is quite high. The fat in fish is usually unsaturated, and the cholesterol content is normally low.
- Most vegetable fats are polyunsaturated, with the exception of olive oil (which is monounsaturated) and palm and coconut oils (which are saturated). Plants do not synthesize cholesterol.

A deficiency of fatty acids is rare as our metabolism can utilize a wide range, non-specifically. However, some individual polyunsaturated fatty acids are considered essential for life. These are commonly referred to as omega-3 and omega-6 fatty acids; they all have a number of unsaturated carbon atoms in their molecules but there is commonality at the third or sixth position in the two groups respectively.

Omega-3 fatty acids are important for normal growth, and have been implicated in the maintenance of cell membranes; for example, they have been linked to neurological improvements in children with learning problems, and to coronary blood vessel health, though some of the evidence for these actions remains speculative at this time. Fish oil is a good source of omega-3 fatty acids, but some vegetable oils may contain them.

Omega-6 fatty acids are also involved in growth, and are also associated with healthy tissue integrity for example of the skin and kidneys. In addition, one (arachidonic acid) is the precursor for the synthesis of eicosanoid hormones, that is prostaglandins, thromboxanes and leukotrienes (see Chapter 9). Vegetable oils are the main dietary source of omega-6 fatty acids, especially from nuts.

A degree of interconversions between fatty acids is possible, and there are just three 'essential' fatty acids that should be present in our diet: one omega-3 (alpha-linolenic acid) and two omega-6 (linoleic and arachidonic acids). For this reason, synthetic fatty or oily foods, for example margarine, often contain added essential fatty acids.

Proteins

Protein is available as animal or vegetable protein. In an average Western diet about one-third of dietary protein comes from plant sources and two-thirds from animal sources. Animal sources are meat and fish (i.e. primarily from muscle) and dairy products. The main plant sources are seeds including cereals, peas, beans and nuts. Root vegetables and green vegetables generally are poor sources, although potatoes contain significant amounts.

Protein molecules are largely composed of carbon, hydrogen and oxygen, but also contain nitrogen, while sulphur and phosphorus are also frequently present. The basic building units of proteins are called amino acids (see Figure 5.2b). Digestion of food in the bowel (see Chapter 10) releases the

---

BOX 5.3 CHOLESTEROL

Normal ranges for (total) cholesterol concentration in blood:

Child = 3.11–5.18 mmol/L
Adult = 3.63–8.03 mmol/L
(note: this range exceeds the recommended upper limit; see below)

Cholesterol is the basic ingredient of cell membranes, and a precursor for the synthesis of steroid hormones. Although it is essential to health, plasma concentrations of cholesterol above 5.0 mmol/L are associated with an increased risk of cardiovascular disease; there are suggestions that the target should be even less than this (Pottle, 2007). Some authorities suggest that it is important to also consider which form the cholesterol is in. To be transported in blood lipids are normally combined with another molecule (usually a protein to make a lipoprotein), in order to make them soluble. A high concentration of cholesterol as low-density lipoprotein (LDL; see text) is thought to predispose to the formation of fatty plaques within blood vessels because it is in this form that the lipid is deposited in the tissues. Excess lipid is then removed from the tissues as high-density lipoprotein (HDL) and this returns to the liver where the excess is broken down or passed into bile.

An ideal ratio of HDL:LDL in blood is 2:1, that is, it favours removal of excess cholesterol from tissues. Factors have been recognized that reduce LDL, though it is also suggested that the means of raising HDL should also be explored (Safeer and Cornell, 2000). Factors that promote a favourable ratio are:

- *Oestrogens*: women have an advantage up to the menopause, but

the incidence of heart disease rises rapidly after menopause at least partly because of increased formation of atheroma.
- *Exercise*: active people have a better lipid profile.

Negative factors are:

- *Lack of exercise*: causes a fall in HDL and hence a fall in the HDL:LDL ratio.
- *Smoking*: also causes a decrease in HDL.
- *Excessive cholesterol in the diet*: increases LDL concentrations.
- *Excessive saturated fat in the diet*: this is converted in the liver to cholesterol, promoting high concentrations of LDL.
- *Familial hypercholesterolaemia*: this is an inherited condition in which a gene mutation prevents uptake of excess cholesterol by the liver, and hence prevents metabolism of excess lipid.

Dietary cholesterol is not necessarily an indicator of the likely level in blood, because our liver can convert saturated fatty acids to cholesterol. This is the reason why dietary recommendations are that both cholesterol and saturated fat content of the diet should be limited. Soluble fibre in the diet reduces the uptake of cholesterol from the bowel and so helps to reduce blood cholesterol (see 'Fibre' section). Cholesterol levels in blood may also be reduced using cholesterol-lowering drugs, particularly if the hypercholesterolaemia is resistant to dietary control. For example, the most effective drugs that lower LDL-cholesterol in blood are those classed as statins, which inhibit cholesterol synthesis by the liver.

constituent amino acids from protein, which are then absorbed and utilized, primarily in the process of protein synthesis within our cells, thus converting food protein to our (human) protein. There are 20 naturally occurring amino acids and our cells require the whole range to be available. Although our diets should provide the complete range some amino acids can be synthesized from others by the liver in a process called transamination, and this can compensate for any shortfall, at least transiently. However, there are 10 amino acids (12 in infants) that cannot be synthesized in this way. These are called the 'essential' amino acids, and must be provided in our diets. They are: arginine, histidine, isoleucine, leucine, lysine, methionine, phenylalanine, threonine, tryptophan and valine.

Animal and plant proteins differ in their essential amino acid content: most animal proteins have the full range of amino acids and so are 'complete' proteins, but vegetable proteins may not always contain adequate amounts of all essential amino acids. Thus, wheat protein is deficient in lysine, but some bean proteins are rich in this. In contrast, wheat protein is a rich source of cysteine, which is lacking in bean protein. Wheat and beans therefore contain 'complementary proteins' in that, if eaten together, they will provide the range of amino acids necessary for a balanced diet.

Protein is widely available in our foods, but tends to represent a more expensive component than other nutrients. Consequently, protein excess is rare, and deficiency is more common, either through malnutrition or because of metabolic changes (Box 5.4). Kwashiorkor is an example of protein deficiency arising from malnutrition. It is very rare in the UK, but more common in the tropical regions. When it is observed it is more likely to involve a child since children need relatively large protein intakes to maintain normal growth. Kwashiorkor has a complex array of symptoms, some of which have also been related to inadequate vitamin and mineral intake. Muscle wasting, growth failure and a general 'failure to thrive' are characteristic. A deficiency in plasma protein concentration (referred to as hypoproteinaemia) is also observed, contributing to the development of oedema, as the forces that regulate the exchange of fluid within the extracellular body fluid compartments (see Chapter 6) become unbalanced. Hypoproteinaemia is also observed secondary to the loss of protein in urine in some renal conditions (e.g. nephrotic syndrome), or in liver failure (e.g. cirrhosis); oedema is also a complication of those disorders.

Energy

Although not exactly a nutrient, energy is required by the body to maintain the basal activities of cells and to sustain an increase in those activities when required, and so it is considered to be an integral part of our diet. Energy is derived from metabolizing carbohydrate, lipid and proteins and so dietary provision is usually expressed in relation to the intake of these 'fuels'. Carbohydrates form the main source of energy but the ideal proportion of carbohydrate, relative to fats and protein remains the subject of debate. It is currently considered that:

- Carbohydrates should comprise about 50% of energy intake. In view of the association of certain sugars, such as sucrose, with dental caries, it is considered that only 10% of energy requirements (i.e. only about one-fifth of total carbohydrate intake) should come from this source (referred to as extrinsic sugars).
- Dietary fats should contribute about 35% of our energy needs, but the type of fatty acid present must also be taken into account. Only 10% of energy should be supplied by saturated fatty acids, because of their association with cholesterol deposition in blood vessels.
- Dietary protein provides about 15% of energy needs.

Food packaging usually identifies the total energy content of the food, and still frequently gives it in (kilo)calories, which represents the energy released when chemical bonds are broken during metabolism, Thus, 1 g of carbohydrate (or protein) produces approximately 4 kcal of energy during metabolism, while 1 g of fat produces around 9 kcal. Clearly, fats are a much richer source of energy, weight for weight, than carbohydrate. However, although we have the capacity to metabolize fatty acids, most cellular energy is derived from carbohydrate metabolism (indeed, we can also convert some fatty acids to

---

BOX 5.4 EXCESSIVE PROTEIN CATABOLISM

Protein normally forms only a relatively small resource for energy production, and most energy is derived from the metabolism of carbohydrate and fat. Consequently, it is not surprising to find that the body does not store protein in the same sense, but rather resorts to breaking down muscle protein, or perhaps depleting plasma proteins, to supply amino acids as necessary. Protein utilization is increased when there is a deficit of carbohydrate and fatty acids for metabolism, for example:

- *In starvation.* Even when fully replenished the glycogen stores of the body can only support a supply of carbohydrate for 12 hours or so, and so starvation quickly begins to promote the mobilization of fatty acids from fat stores, both as fuel and for their conversion to glucose via a process referred to as gluconeogenesis (see Chapter 10, p.263). As fat stores deplete then protein is increasingly broken down to provide amino acids for the same purposes.
- *In uncontrolled diabetes mellitus.* In this condition glucose cannot enter cells in sufficient quantities to maintain normal energy metabolism. As in starvation, fats and proteins are mobilized to provide alternative fuels.

- *After major surgery.* Several hours after surgery the individual enters a 'flow' phase characterized by the mobilization of metabolic fuel (see Box 21.7, p.601, also Clancy *et al.*, 2002), which supports cell division, tissue growth and repair. Glucose and fatty acids are released, and gluconeogenesis takes place. If nutrition does not meet these extra demands, there is a risk that muscle breakdown will then occur to provide amino acids for energy, which in extreme circumstances may lead to muscle wasting. Protein depletion appears to slow a patient's recovery from surgery and so is best avoided.

Protein metabolism can be monitored through the urinary excretion of the waste products urea and 3-methylhistidine, a substance strongly indicative of muscle protein loss.

carbohydrate), and this explains the greater dietary requirement for carbohydrate than fats. In contrast, storing energy as fat makes much more sense; being overweight by, say, 8 kg owing to excess fat stores would be equivalent to an excess 18 kg if the same energy had been stored as carbohydrate!

By definition a calorie is the amount of heat required to raise the temperature of 1 g of water (i.e. 1 mL) by 1°C; it is not an empirical unit (there are other forms of energy). The calorie has now largely been superseded by the joule and one calorie is equivalent to 4.2 joules (i.e. 1 kcal = 4.2 kJ). Foods may show energy content in both units but the calorie value is likely to disappear eventually.

The amount of energy required by an individual is dependent upon two factors: the basal metabolic rate (BMR) which cells exhibit in terms of basic functioning, cell division etc. and the individual's physical activity level (PAL) (see Box 4.4, p.99). As the name implies, BMR is the overall energy utilization when the body is totally at rest and no additional influences such as a recent meal or recent exercise are imposed. Its value in adults is around 7000 kJ/day (approximately 1700 kcal/day). The physical activity level is a factor used to convert the BMR to an energy intake recommendation. For little or moderate activity, the PAL value is around 1.3 in women and 1.4 in men and so the daily energy required would be approximately:

In women: 7000 × 1.3 = 9100 kJ (2167 kcal) per day.

In men: 7000 × 1.4 = 9800 kJ (2333 kcal) per day.

With very heavy exercise, the respective PAL values are about 1.8 and 1.9, and the energy requirement per day therefore will alter accordingly to over 13 000 kJ (3000+ kcal) per day.

An energy intake that exceeds our energy requirement will mean that the excess is stored: our body conserves rather than excretes excess fuels, presumably as a measure to ensure a supply should food supplies dwindle. Being overweight, or obese, therefore is more common in Western countries than is undernutrition, and is an increasing health problem: for example, in England the proportion of men who were overweight or obese increased from 6% to 66% between 1982 and 2002, while in women there has been a corresponding increase from 8% to 57% (Health Survey for England 2002). Reducing the incidence of obesity is now a priority for the National Health Service in the UK. To lose weight it is essential to reduce energy intake so that energy consumption is now in excess of energy intake. Most authorities advocate moderate control of dietary energy intake, but an increase in physical activity as well. 'Reducing diets' mainly seek to reduce energy intake, sometimes very rapidly, but this usually leaves the individual feeling very hungry and so compliance with the diet becomes burdensome and more likely to fail. Some diets aim to resolve this by including soluble fibre (see below) to absorb water and hence 'bulk up' the food, increasing the sense of being full. Others have sought to change the way in which energy metabolism occurs. A good example of this is the 'Atkins diet', which is carefully constructed with the intention of favouring fat metabolism, while supporting it with some carbohydrate metabolism as well. New pharmaceutical preparations are also likely to appear – a drug that will promote rapid weight loss for minimal effort will be very popular!

Fibre

Dietary fibre is mainly the carbohydrate component of ingested plant material that cannot be fully digested. Strictly speaking, fibre is not a nutrient because it does not contribute to body chemistry, but it is nevertheless an important dietary constituent that appears to have a number of beneficial effects (Blackwood *et al.*, 2000; Aman, 2006). Fibre is classed according to whether or not it is soluble. Cereal bran is an important source of insoluble fibre, and beans, oat bran and cabbage-type vegetables are rich sources of soluble fibre.

Insoluble fibre (e.g. uncooked cellulose):

- absorbs water, rather than dissolving in it. This helps to increase the water content of faecal stools, thus making them easier to pass, and so helping to prevent constipation and complications such as haemorrhoids ('piles');
- promotes muscle movements of the bowel (called peristalsis; see Chapter 10, p.239). This reduces the transit time required for faecal matter to pass through it, and so reduces the time available for microorganisms present to produce a substance called deoxycholate, a known carcinogen, from bile salts secreted into the bowel from the gall bladder. Dietary fibre therefore may help to reduce the risk of bowel cancer.

Soluble fibre (e.g. hemicellulose, pectin, gum) interferes with the absorption of fatty acids and of bile salts, which are produced from cholesterol, leading to further cholesterol and fatty acid utilization in the body, so helping to reduce blood lipid concentrations and helping to reduce the risk of atheroma plaques forming within blood vessels.

Excess fibre in itself is not harmful as it is not digested within the bowel or absorbed into the body tissues. However, its effect on transit time, which might be heightened because of the irritation it might cause of the walls of the bowel, greatly increases faecal frequency, may cause soreness in the anal area as a consequence, and may produce general feelings of bloating and bowel discomfort.

Deficiency of fibre is associated with constipation as the stools become hardened and less easily passed.

Vitamins

Vitamins are a diverse group of substances, the majority of which cannot be synthesized by our cells and so must be present in the diet, although in only small quantities, to sustain growth and metabolism. Some act as coenzymes: that is, they work in conjunction with certain proteins within cell biochemistry.

Thirteen vitamins are currently known to be essential for life (Tables 5.2 and 5.3). Historically, their nomenclature is largely based on letters of the alphabet, though revisions have over time produced a confusing, seemingly incomplete list.

Table 5.2 Fat-soluble vitamins

Vitamin	Source	Storage in body	Homeostatic functions	Effects of deficiency	Effects of excess
A	Liver, green leafy vegetables. Synthesized in gut from betacarotene	In liver	Maintains epithelia	Atrophy of epithelia, e.g. dry skin and cornea, increased susceptibility to respiratory/urinary/digestive tract infection, skin sores	Anorexia, dry skin, sparse hair, raised intracranial pressure in children; blurred vision, enlarged liver in adults
			Provides visual pigment Bone/tooth growth	'Night blindness' Slow bone/tooth growth	
D	Synthesized as provitamin D_3 in skin using ultraviolet light. Also in fish liver, fish oils, egg yolk, milk	Slight at most	Absorption of calcium and phosphate from gut	Demineralization of bone (rickets in children, osteomalacia in adults)	Excess calcium absorption from gut Calcium deposition in soft tissues
E	Nuts, wheatgerm, seed oils, green leafy vegetables	In liver, adipose tissue and muscle	Inhibits catabolism of membrane lipids Promotes wound healing and neural function	Abnormal organelle/plasma membranes. Oxidation of polyunsaturated fatty acids	Toxic build-up unlikely
K	Produced by intestinal bacteria. Also in spinach, cauliflower, cabbage and liver	In liver and spleen	Synthesis of blood clotting factors	Delayed blood clotting	Haemolysis and increased bilirubin in blood in children; otherwise toxic build-up unlikely

Thus, the one identified as vitamin 'B' was found to consist of a group of substances each with individual actions, and so numbers (e.g. B_1, B_2) were introduced, while others were eventually found not to be true vitamins at all and so were deleted from the series (e.g. there is no vitamin B_4 or vitamin G). Matters were also complicated when some were found to have existing names, for example vitamin B_3 was found to be nicotinic acid that had already been identified as being vital to health.

Vitamins are also classified according to whether they are soluble in water or fat. Thus, vitamins A, D, E and K are classed as fat-soluble vitamins, while vitamins of the 'B' complex and vitamin C are classed as water-soluble vitamins:

- Fat-soluble vitamins (Table 5.2) require the presence of fatty acids in the bowel for their absorption, and also may be stored in fat (adipose) tissue and in the liver to a limited degree.
- Water-soluble vitamins (Table 5.3) are excreted rapidly and so little is stored. The exception is vitamin B_{12}; the liver contains sufficient vitamin B_{12} for a 2–3 year supply.

As the body has limited stores of vitamins, deficiencies rather than excesses are more likely to occur. Deficiency is avoidable with a balanced diet and large build-ups of vitamins are unlikely from normal dietary intakes, though they are possible if vitamin preparations, currently popular, are taken. Recommended doses from supplements should be adhered to since vitamin excess, especially of fat-soluble vitamins, can raise stores to toxic levels. Thus, excess vitamin D promotes excessive uptake of calcium from the bowel with the consequence that the mineral begins to be deposited in soft tissues, while an accumulation of vitamin A within the liver can cause liver damage.

Vitamins have a wide range of functions, and are found in a variety of foodstuffs that are only summarized in Tables 5.2 and 5.3, since it is outside the scope of this textbook to discuss their value in detail. However, such information does not emphasize the criticality of vitamin actions and the reader is introduced here to the functions of vitamin K, as an example of the importance of vitamins in a healthy metabolism.

The main role ascribed to vitamin K is as a coenzyme essential for the production of various blood clotting factors (II, VII, IX and X; see Chapter 11) but recent research indicates that it also has a role in the normal calcification of bone. Vitamin K is produced by bacteria living in the intestines and so deficiency is extremely rare, though immature intestinal function and flora make infants more susceptible. In adults, deficiency may occur if the intestines are badly damaged, or if there is a problem in the absorption processes: this is a fat-soluble vitamin so people with impaired lipid absorption (e.g. coliac disease, Crohn's disease, ulcerative colitis and chronic pancreatitis) may become deficient in vitamin K. In such malabsorption syndromes an oral preparation (menadiol sodium phosphate) is administered which facilitates absorption of the vitamin. Dietary deficiency may also occur in malnourished patients (e.g. alcoholic disorders and patients undergoing long-term parenteral nutrition that is deficient in the vitamin). Miscellaneous causes include patients who have received massive blood transfusion, disseminated intravascular coagulation nephrotic syndrome, cystic fibrosis and leukaemia.

Vitamin K deficiency causes:

- Bleeding, especially in response to minor or trivial trauma, as a consequence of reduced synthesis of clotting proteins. Clinical manifestations in adults are only evident if serum thrombin concentration is severely reduced (hypoprothrombinaemia). In

Table 5.3 Water-soluble vitamins

Vitamin	Source	Storage in body	Homeostatic functions	Effects of deficiency	Effects of excess
B₁ (thiamin)	Whole grain, eggs, pork, liver, yeast	Not stored	Coenzyme in carbohydrate metabolism. Essential for acetylcholine (neurotransmitter) synthesis	Build-up of pyruvic/lactic acids. Energy deficient. Partial paralysis of digestive tract/skeletal muscle (i.e. beri-beri). Degeneration of myelin sheath (polyneuritis)	Toxic build-up unlikely
B₂ (riboflavin)	Small quantities produced by gut bacteria. Also in yeast, liver, beef, lamb, eggs, whole grain, peas, peanuts	Not stored	Component of coenzymes in carbohydrate and protein metabolism, especially in eye, blood, skin, intestinal mucosa	Blurred vision, cataracts. Lesions of intestinal mucosa. Dermatitis. Anaemia	Toxic build-up unlikely
B₃ (niacin or nicotinamide)	Yeast, meats, liver, fish, whole grain, peas, beans. Also synthesized from amino acid tryptophan	Not stored	Component of coenzyme NAD in intracellular respiration. Assists breakdown of cholesterol	Hard, rough, blackish skin. Dermatitis, diarrhoea (pellagra). Psychological disturbance	Burning sensation in hands/face, cardiac arrhythmias, increased glycogen utilization
B₆ (pyridoxine)	Salmon, yeast, tomatoes, maize, spinach, whole grain, liver, yoghurt. Some synthesized by gut bacteria	In liver and muscle	Coenzyme in fat and amino acid metabolism	Dermatosis of eye, nose, mouth. Nausea. Retarded growth	Toxic build-up unlikely
B₁₂ (cyano-cobalamin)	Liver, kidney, milk, eggs, cheese, meats. Not found in vegetables. Requires intrinsic factor from stomach for absorption	In liver	Coenzyme for haemoglobin synthesis and amino acid metabolism	Pernicious anaemia. Nerve axon degeneration	Toxic build-up unlikely
Folate (folic acid, folacin)	Synthesized by gut bacteria. Also in green leafy vegetables and liver	Not stored	Synthesis of nucleotides. Red/white blood cell production	Macrocytic anaemia due to abnormally large red blood cells	Toxic build-up unlikely
Pantothenic acid	Liver, kidney, yeast, cereals, green vegetables	In liver and kidney	Constituent of coenzyme A in carbohydrate metabolism, gluconeogenesis and steroid synthesis	Fatigue. Muscle spasms. Lack of some steroid hormones	Toxic build-up unlikely
Biotin	Synthesized by gut bacteria. Also yeast, liver, egg, yolk, kidney	Not stored	Component of coenzymes for pyruvic acid utilization in cellular respiration	Mental depression. Muscular pain. Dermatitis. Fatigue. Nausea	Toxic build-up unlikely
C (ascorbic acid)	Citrus fruits, tomatoes, green vegetables	A little in plasma	Promotes protein metabolism. Promotes formation of connective tissue. Detoxifier. Promotes wound healing	Retardation of growth. Poor connective tissue repair/growth (scurvy), including swollen gums, tooth loosening, fragile blood vessels. Poor wound healing	Not toxic. Note: no evidence for effect to prevent infection

infants the bleeding may be especially serious, including intracranial and retroperitoneal bleeding, and can present as early as 1–7 days, and as late as 3 months, postpartum. It is clinically recommended, with the consent of the mother, that all newborn babies should be given vitamin K (as phytomenadione) to prevent vitamin K deficiency bleeding (called haemorrhagic disease of the newborn). For breast-fed babies, further doses may be administered at 1 week and again at 4–6 weeks of age.

• Altered calcium metabolism. Calcification of arteries and other soft tissue may occur with, for example, damage to the cardiovascular system leading to cardiac valve replacement or coronary arterial bypass surgery. Deficiency of vitamin K may also result in abnormal accumulation of calcium in the brain, with potential impact on cognition. The kidneys and pineal gland are also vulnerable to excess calcium infiltration. In contrast the skeleton is a compromised by a deficiency in calcium (thus promoting osteoporosis; see Chapter 3).

In infants, birth defects may be observed, such as underdevelopment of the nose, face, bones and fingers, linked to vitamin K deficiency.

- Symptoms similar to Type 2 diabetes mellitus. Vitamin K levels are abundant in the pancreas and may be important in the production of insulin.

Other risk factors associated with in vitamin K deficiency include:

- Over-anticoagulation with oral coumarin drugs, e.g. warfarin, which act by interfering with vitamin K metabolism in the liver cells and so are used to reduce the synthesis of clotting proteins. Their effects can be antagonized by giving vitamin K.
- Exacerbation of diseases involving endogenously produced coagulation inhibitors (e.g. lupus).
- Biliary tract disease, e.g. common duct destruction, primary biliary cirrhosis, leading to decreased fat absorption, and hence deficiency of fat-soluble vitamins.
- Exacerbation of some drug actions, for example of salicylates and barbiturates.

Minerals

Minerals and mineral salts such as sodium chloride (table salt) and sodium bicarbonate (baking powder) have the property that they dissociate into their constituent ions when dissolved in water. Body fluids contain a variety of ions, and changes in this ionic environment through dietary intake could potentially have adverse effects on cell function (Table 5.4). The concentrations of most ions in body fluids therefore must be regulated if homeostasis is to be maintained (see Chapters 6: Body fluids, and 15: The kidneys and urinary tract).

Minerals are also important structural constituents (but not in a storage capacity, except calcium and iron). For example, sulphur is an essential constituent of many proteins (it is found in certain amino acids such as cysteine), iron is a constituent of the blood pigment haemoglobin and calcium and phosphorus are constituents of bone. Some minerals, for example copper, selenium, zinc, aluminium, iodide and fluoride, are required in such small amounts that they are considered 'trace' elements, but they have important roles. For example, iodine is a constituent of thyroid hormone, fluoride is a component of bone

Table 5.4 Dietary sources and functions of selected minerals

Mineral	Source	Function	Effects of deficiency
Calcium	Milk, egg yolk, shellfish, green leafy vegetables	Formation of bones/teeth Blood clotting, muscle contraction Muscle/nerve action potentials Endo- and exocytosis Cell division	Loss of bone density, e.g. osteomalacia/ rickets
Phosphorus	Milk, meat, fish, poultry, nuts	Formation of bones/teeth Buffer chemical Muscle contraction/nerve activity Component of ATP, DNA, RNA and many enzymes	Deficiency rare
Potassium	Widespread; 'Lo-salt'	Action potential of muscle/nerve cells	Neuromuscular depression
Sodium	Widespread; table salt	Major osmotic solute of extracellular fluids Action potential of muscle/nerve cells	Hypovolaemia
Chlorine (chloride)	Non-processed foods; usually found with sodium, e.g. table salt	Involved in acid–base balance Major osmotic solute of extracellular fluids Formation of gastric acid	Deficiency usually occurs with sodium
Magnesium	Beans, peanuts, bananas	Constituent of many coenzymes Role in bone formation and muscle/nerve cell functions	Muscle weakness Convulsions Hypertension
Trace minerals Iron	Widespread but especially meats, liver, beans, fruits, nuts, legumes	Component of haemoglobin Component of chemicals involved in cell respiration	Anaemia
Iodine (iodide)	Seafood, cod-liver oil, iodized table salt	Component of thyroid hormones	Thyroid hormone deficiency (induces thyroid goitre)
Fluorine (fluoride)	Tea, coffee, fluoridated water	Component of bones/teeth	Decreased bone/teeth density
Zinc	Widespread, but especially meats	Component of some enzymes Promotes normal growth, spermatogenesis Involved in taste and appetite	Dermatitis Growth retardation Diarrhoea
Copper	Eggs, wholewheat flour, liver, fish, spinach	Haemoglobin synthesis Component of some enzymes, or acts as cofactor	Retarded growth Cerebral degeneration
Chromium	Yeast, beer, beef	Involved in insulin synthesis Maintains HDL concentrations in plasma	Rare – may be involved with diabetes mellitus

HDL, high-density lipotrotein.

and tooth mineral, and zinc and selenium are important enzyme cofactors.

Minerals generally are found dissolved in body fluids and so are not stored to any degree (calcium and phosphorus are significant exceptions as most of the body content of these minerals occurs in bone). Since most minerals are not stored, deficiency may arise if dietary intake does not match mineral excretion. Most minerals are abundant in foodstuffs but deficiencies of trace minerals may arise as their sources are more restricted. Dietary supplements are widely available but excessive intake of some trace minerals can be detrimental if the minerals are actually stored. For example, excessive iodine has toxic effects on the thyroid gland (causing *thyrotoxicosis*) while excessive iron is a cause of poisoning in young children. Excessive fluoride causes mottled teeth and porous, brittle bones.

Nucleic acids

Nucleic acids form the genetic material of cells. There are two types of nucleic acid (see Chapter 2): DNA and ribonucleic acid (RNA). Both are very large molecules, comprising a 'backbone' of molecules of the sugar ribose and of phosphate molecules, to which are attached sequences of molecules called purines and pyrimidines, often referred to as 'bases' (but not to be confused with 'bases' involved in acid–base regulation in the body).

As cells die some of their nucleic acid constituents will be reused, but some is broken down to uric acid and excreted in urine. The constituents required by cells to synthesize nucleic acids must therefore be obtained in part from the nucleic acids ingested in our diets, following their digestion and absorption in the gut. The structure of nucleic acids is similar in all organisms and so they are readily available in natural foods. However, processed foods tend to be low in nucleic acids.

Water

Water is familiar to us in our everyday life, and makes up a substantial proportion of our body volume: 50–70% depending upon the proportion of fat, which is relatively deficient in water. However, it would be wrong to regard it as being a simple space-filler in our tissues. It was noted in Chapter 4 that the distribution of electrical charges in water molecules (viz. hydrogen bonds; see p.95) make it an excellent solvent for other charged particles, for example ions, collectively referred to as 'solutes'. The presence of an electrical charge also means that water molecules may take part in some metabolic reactions, or are themselves produced by chemical reactions.

An excess of water can be viewed in two different ways. First, over-hydration from over-drinking is a rare phenomenon as the body regulates body water content very efficiently, and these processes are unlikely to be overwhelmed by excessive ingestion of water over a very short time because there are conscious 'brakes' on our desire to do so. However, the latter may be overcome if that desire is reduced, for example through cognitive depression induced by drugs, or through excessive anxiety. Second, water in the body is compartmentalized into body fluids of particular volume and composition (see Chapter 6). Redistribution of water can result in relative excess within the compartments, even when total body content is normal, for example oedema occurring as a consequence of excessive extracellular fluid.

We must excrete water, either as sweat or urine, or in faeces, and so it has to be replenished from our diets, mainly as the fluids we drink but note that even the driest of foods contain a significant amount of water; for example, breakfast cereals contain about 10% water by weight. Dehydration is not unusual, although the kidneys are normally so good at conserving water that we can manage by drinking around a litre per day, but urine concentration will be strong and there may be urinary tract irritation, and possibly even deposition of salts (e.g. calcium as renal stones) in the long term. There are suggestions that adults should drink 2–2.5 L/day to maintain a good state of hydration.

LIFESPAN INFLUENCES ON RECOMMENDED DAILY INTAKES OF NUTRIENTS

Notions of a balanced diet must also take into account the differing needs of the body at different stages of human development. This section provides only an overview of additional dietary considerations; further details are available from guidelines published by the UK Department of Health (1991, 1997 and 1998) and available from the British Nutrition Foundation (http://www.nutrition.org.uk).

Newborn to infant

There are two nutritional considerations during this period of life: the requirements of the nursing mother and those of the baby, who is entirely dependent at this time.

Human milk is highly varied in composition, and changes even between feeds. In general, 100 g of breast milk provides about 290 kJ (70 kcal) of energy and the energy cost to the mother during lactation will be of the order of 2000 kJ (or 500 kcal) per day. Some of this energy is supplied from fat deposits stored by the mother during pregnancy but much must be supplied by the mother's diet. The energy costs will also increase with time as the growth of the baby accelerates. In proportionate terms the energy needs of the baby during the first 6 months of life are higher than at any other time of life (Figure 5.3).

The birth weight of the infant will double during the first year of life and nutritional requirements will change periodically. Provision of all nutrients remains important but particularly important nutrients during this time are protein (for growth), iron (for blood), vitamin D (to promote calcium uptake by the bowel), calcium and fluoride (for bone and teeth development, even before teeth have erupted). If breast-feeding, the nursing mother must increase her intake of these nutrients. The dietary needs for iron usually increase only after the first 5–6 months as the baby's stores are normally quite high at birth.

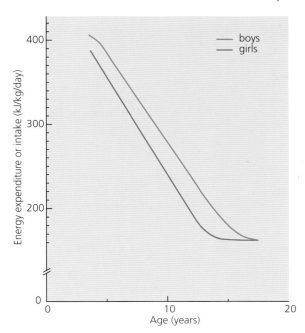

Figure 5.3 Energy requirements standardized for body weight in boys and girls up to the age of 18 years

Not all infants are breast-fed initially and infant formulas are commercially treated to modify their composition. Although nutritionally adequate, these formulas will be deficient in other constituents of breast milk, especially antibodies. Cow's milk is an unsuitable alternative (Box 5.5).

Babies are developmentally unready for solid food until about 4 months of age, although cultural practices may result in weaning babies before or after this. In particular, they have difficulty in moving food to the back of the mouth for swallowing and they have difficulty digesting cereals. Delay in weaning runs the risk of inducing protein deficiency as the

---

BOX 5.5 BREAST MILK VERSUS COW'S MILK

Substituting cows' milk for breast milk is not recommended:

- there is less lactose in cows' milk;
- the protein of cows' milk, mainly casein, is harder to digest (although human milk also contains a little casein);
- the absorption of iron from breast milk is also considerably more efficient than from cow's milk;
- cow's milk contains more sodium, which places a greater demand on the infants' kidneys to excrete the load;
- the range of free amino acids contained in breast milk is beneficial as there are more 'essential' dietary amino acids for infants than adults (12 rather than 10);
- the vitamin content of cow's milk is very different from that of breast milk;
- the baby may also respond to allergens present in cow's milk.

Infant formulas are used widely as substitutes for breast milk. The UK Department of Health (1996, 2008) has published guidelines on these, and issues on infant feeding generally.

---

growth of the baby accelerates. It is also important to note that infants are less able to synthesize amino acids in their livers as older children and adults are, and there are 12 essential amino acids, not 10, in this age group.

Growing child and adolescent

Growth during childhood accelerates as the child enters puberty. This is therefore a critical period for nutrition and recommended intakes of all nutrients increase sharply. For example, protein intake might increase almost threefold between the ages of 3 and 14 years. Energy requirements relative to body size are much higher in children and adolescents than in adults in order to support the rate of growth and the high levels of physical activity exhibited by this group. The energy intake might almost double between 3 and 14 years of age.

Adults: 18–50 years

Growth effectively ends between the ages of 19 and 22 years and nutrition then largely becomes a case of maintenance. Energy requirements of this age group are particularly influenced by levels of physical activity, but on average are about 8.5 MJ/day (2000 kcal/day) in women and 10.5 MJ/day (2500 kcal/day) in men. Dietary considerations of a balanced diet should apply to this age group, as outlined throughout much of this chapter.

Pregnancy

The diet of a pregnant woman must support the increased tissue mass produced by an increased uterus size, the fetus and placenta, an expanded blood volume and extra fat deposits, and maintain the increased metabolic activity related to that increased mass (Box 5.6). The third trimester is particularly important in this respect and this suggests that additional energy intake (of about 800 kJ/day or 200 kcal/day) is most important during that period.

Many women report a change in their sense of smell and taste during pregnancy, and develop food cravings for a while. Some surveys indicate that craving salty and/or sweet foods is most common, leading to a view that cravings possibly represent an underlying desire to obtain specific nutrients, for example sodium chloride or energy. Sometimes the craving may be for inorganic material; one theory is that this represents a desire for minerals. However, the evidence for a craving linked to actual need is weak. In most instances the craving arises even though there is not an actual deficiency. It remains a poorly understood phenomenon.

Adults: 50–75 years

The ageing process is most noticeable after about the age of 50 years when physical activity may decline, basal metabolism diminishes, digestive activity is reduced, secretions (e.g. of saliva) are less pronounced, perceptions of taste and smell change and lifestyles alter. However, nutrient requirements are generally the same as at 30 years old, except that less energy is needed.

BOX 5.6 NUTRITIONAL REQUIREMENTS IN PREGNANCY

Most nutritional requirements are increased during pregnancy but these often can be obtained through a well-balanced diet. The following are considered to require specific attention:

- *Carbohydrates*: in line with fetal growth, carbohydrate requirement increases during pregnancy but to reduce the risk of maternal tooth decay it is better to obtain this from polysaccharides, i.e. from bread, potatoes, rice rather than from 'extrinsic' sugars in sweets, cakes etc.
- *Proteins*: similarly, requirement for protein increases during pregnancy and lactation. About 39 g/day is required during pregnancy (compared with about 36 g/day in a non-pregnant adult woman), and 46 g/day during lactation. However, excessive intake may impair fetal growth, and dietary intake in the UK is usually sufficient.
- *Lipids*: lipid requirement also increases slightly during pregnancy but dietary intake in the UK is usually sufficient.
- *Fibre*: the requirement for fibre increases during pregnancy in order to aid maternal bowel functions. The recommended daily amount (RDA) is 30 g but it should be noted that too much can inhibit absorption of iron from food.
- *Vitamins*:
  - Vitamin A. Recommended daily amount in pregnancy rises from about 2000 to 2500 IU (i.e. International Units; see Appendix A: Units of measurement) but the use of vitamin supplements should

be avoided as high levels have been found to influence birth defects.
  - Folic acid. Deficiency of folic acid (a B vitamin) is associated with neural tube defects (NTDs) in embryos (see Box 19.3, p.529). A supplement (0.4 mg/day) is therefore recommended before and during the first trimester of pregnancy. If there is a previous history of NTD then daily supplementation of 5 mg is recommended.
  - Vitamin E. The requirement increases in pregnancy and helps to prevent premature delivery, spontaneous abortion and stillbirth. However, dietary intake in the UK is usually sufficient and supplements are recommended only for those at high risk.
- *Minerals*:
  - Iron. The requirement for iron increases during pregnancy but routine supplements are no longer recommended in the UK since dietary intake (and maternal storage) is usually sufficient.
  - Calcium. The requirement for calcium increases in pregnancy and is thought to help prevent premature labour. However, dietary intake in the UK is usually sufficient and supplements are recommended only for those at high risk.
  - Zinc. This is the most important mineral for successful pregnancy outcome. Requirements increase by 30% in pregnancy and 40% during lactation. The RDA is 20 mg but in the UK this is usually met by dietary intake.

Adults: 75+ years

Most people over 75 years of age show a decrease in activity levels compared with a 50–60-year-old, although there is a wide variation. BMR is appreciably decreased above 75 years of age. Appetite therefore diminishes and this can have an implication for nutritional homeostasis (see next section).

Food requirements, and hence appetite, generally diminish over the age of 75 years as metabolism slows, but there is a risk that the low food intakes observed in inactive elderly people may not provide adequate amounts of other nutrients for health. It is therefore especially important that food is presented in a palatable and appetizing way, and that the food eaten is of adequate quality. Sadly, caring institutions sometimes fail to meet these criteria and carers should be aware of what food, if any, is eaten by elderly people, either at home, in the community or in hospital.

REGULATION OF NUTRITION

The obesity 'epidemic' in Western countries, noted earlier, provides evidence that body weight is at best only poorly regulated by physiological mechanisms; nutrition on the whole is poorly regulated, and controlling the intake of most individual nutrients is coarse and imprecise. Nevertheless, some physiological 'drives' have been identified and are referred to here.

Of course, people also eat for pleasure and for social purposes, and this is a powerful influence on what they eat, how much they eat, and even how often they eat. Accordingly, health promotion and education measures in this context are strong, and the UK Government has established a Scientific Committee to advise on this issue (Department of Health, 1999).

Energy (carbohydrate, lipids and proteins)

We have a drive to obtain high-energy foods, storing those 'fuels' that are in excess of body needs at the time. They therefore tend to be very popular with people, but not for their specific nutrient content, or even for the source of energy. Thus, while carbohydrates, lipids and proteins form the bulk of our diets, their general intake is non-specifically related to the drive for energy, and there are public health concerns that (in the UK) average diets contain energy in excess of requirement, and in the form of excessive saturated fat and carbohydrate. Nevertheless, there are physiological processes that have an identifiable role in regulating food intake. In that context, two aspects must be considered (Woods, 2005):

What determines the interval before the drive to eat reappears? Brain nuclei within the hypothalamus have been implicated in providing the drive to eat. Increased local concentrations of metabolic fuels, that is, glucose and fatty acids, within the hypothalamus, seem to be influences, but more important signals come from the secretion of the hormones insulin (from the pancreas) and leptin (from adipose tissue, especially in the abdomen). Both are secreted into blood in proportion to the amount of fat that is stored in the body, and act on the hypothalamus to influence food intake. Thus, increased adiposity raises the level of secretion of leptin, which then acts to reduce food intake, while weight loss increases its secretion and so stimulates food intake. Administering these hormones directly into the brain has also been shown to reduce food intake and body weight.

What determines how much we eat during a meal (satiety)? There is evidence that various substances/hormones, secreted from the gastrointestinal tract in response to the presence of food and/or digested food products, may act as controllers. For example, the secretion of the hormone cholecystokinin (CCK; released from the ileum and pancreas) is low before food is consumed, but increases when fat products are present in the small intestine (see Chapter 10, p.250), and its actions are rapid enough to have an impact during the timeframe of a meal. Experimentally, the administration of CCK has also been found to decrease meal size, while providing an antagonist of its actions increases meal size. Conversely, the secretion of ghrelin, a hormone secreted from the wall of the stomach, increases between meals but decreases when food is consumed, and experimental administration of ghrelin increases the size of meal consumed.

There is evidence that obesity may arise when there is resistance to many of these various factors, especially to leptin. The implication is that hormones and secretions, together with sensory nerve activity from the gastrointestinal tract, act together to regulate hunger perception, and meal size. The picture is very complex, however, as there is a range of different secretions from the bowel that may influence food intake, including by altering the sensitivity to others. Nevertheless, the evidence sheds some light on the mechanisms for regulating food intake, and hence of body weight. One difficulty we have, though, is that eating is not simply related to biological need: in Western countries it is rare for the desire to eat to arise from biological deficit or need, and psychosocial factors are significant. The current obesity 'epidemic' in the UK indicates that the biological control of energy intake, and body weight, can readily be overcome.

Water balance

Provided that drinking water is available, the water content of our body does not normally deviate more than ± 2% from normal. Regulation is via the monitoring of the total concentration of solutes in blood plasma; if we begin to dehydrate this rises and draws water out of cells by the process of osmosis, in turn raising solute concentration within the cells, and reducing cell volume. Specialized nerve cells within the hypothalamus act as receptors of this change, giving us a perception of thirst and promoting water conservation by the kidneys. Overhydration promotes opposite changes and responses. Details can be found in Chapter 6.

Minerals and vitamins

Eating a range of natural foods will normally ensure the provision of adequate amounts of these nutrients. Perhaps as a consequence of this, we do not have a 'drive' to seek them out. The exception is sodium chloride. This salt is the main contributor to the solute concentration that determines water balance (above) and so the two processes are inextricably linked. Thus, a deficit of sodium chloride will be interpreted by the body as over-hydration (viz. the salt appears to have become diluted) and so water is excreted. Most sodium chloride is found in the extracellular fluids, including blood plasma, and a decreased blood volume raises our preference for salty foods and promotes sodium chloride conservation by the kidneys (see Chapter 6).

Fibre

Many natural foods provide a rich source of fibre, but processed foods are often deficient. Modern diets therefore may cause constipation as the stimulation of peristaltic movements of the bowel are reduced. The discomfort of this can act to promote greater intake of fibre-containing foods. While this should not be viewed as a biological regulator, the mechanism can be related to homeostatic theory!

SUMMARY

1 Nutrients provide the substrates for all body structures, and the constituents of body fluids.

2 A balanced diet contains adequate daily amounts of all nutrients.

3 Carbohydrates include complex polysaccharides, smaller disaccharides and simple sugars, or monosaccharides. Dietary carbohydrates are digested to their monosaccharide components, of which glucose is the most prevalent.

4 Proteins are composed of amino acids. Some amino acids, having been ingested with proteins, may be converted to different ones within the liver but 10 (12 in infants) cannot: these are 'essential' amino acids and must be present in the diet.

5 Lipids are composed of fatty acids, perhaps modified or combined with glycerol to form glycerides or fats. Fatty acids are saturated or have degrees of unsaturation; that is, their chemical structure has bonds that can be opened to accept other atoms or molecules.

6 Saturated fatty acids may be converted within the liver to cholesterol, an example of a modified lipid. This is an important lipid in the body, but potentially can have detrimental effects on blood vessels.

7 'Energy' is considered to be a nutrient: on average, 50% of energy intake should be as carbohydrates, 35% as lipids and 15% as protein. Energy requirements relate to the BMR and to physical activity levels.

8 Fibre is not digested in the conventional way, if at all, but has beneficial effects on the bowel.

9 Vitamins are a complex group of chemicals that have a range of functions. Small quantities of each are required but they are central to living processes. Some are fat-soluble, others water-soluble. Fat-soluble vitamins may be stored to a limited degree but this makes toxic levels a possibility, although an unlikely one, on normal diets. Vitamin deficiency is more likely to be a problem.

10 Minerals range from some that are very abundant to those that are trace elements. Most are not stored to any degree and so a regular intake is necessary. This means that trace element deficiency is possible.

11 Nucleic acids, that is DNA and RNA, must also be synthesized by dividing cells. While components are reusable some are metabolized and so nucleic acids must be present in the diet. Growth requires additional nucleic acid.

12 Water is often taken for granted but is a vital component of body chemistry, as a solvent and as a determinant of volume.

12 Nutrient requirements change during life, primarily as a consequence of growth during childhood, and declining metabolic rates in later adulthood. Pregnancy and lactation have further implications for maternal dietary requirements.

REFERENCES

Aman, P. (2006) Cholesterol-lowering effects of barley dietary fibre in humans: scientific support for a generic health claim. *Scandinavian Journal of Food and Nutrition* **50**(4): 173–6.

Blackwood, A.D., Salter, J., Dettmar, P.W. and Chaplin, M.F. (2000) Dietary fibre, physicochemical properties and their relationship to health. *Journal of the Royal Society of Health* **120**(4): 242–7.

Bourgault, A.M., Ipe, L., Weaver, J., Swartz, S. and O'Dea, P.J. (2007) Development of evidence-based guidelines and critical care nurses 'knowledge of enteral feeding. *Critical Care Nurse* **27**(4): 17–22.

Clancy, J., McVicar, A. and Baird, N. (2002) *Perioperative Practice. Fundamentals of Homeostasis*. London: Routledge.

Department of Health (1991) *Dietary Reference Values for Food Energy and Nutrients for the UK*. London: HMSO.

Department of Health (1996) *Guidelines on the Nutritional Assessment of Infant Formulas*. London: HMSO.

Department of Health (1997) *Healthy Diets for Infants and Young Children. A Guide for Health Professionals*. London: HMSO.

Department of Health (1998) *National Diet and Nutrition Survey: People Aged 65 Years and Over*. London: HMSO.

Department of Health (1999) New Scientific Advisory Committee On Nutrition. Press Release. Food Standards Agency. www.food.gov.uk

Department of Health. Health Survey for England 2002. http://www.dh.gov.uk/en/Publicationsstatistics/PublishedSurvey/Health SurveyforEngland

Department of Health (2008) *Pregnancy, Childbirth and Infant Care*. London: HMSO.

Donahue, R.P. and Abbott, R.D. (1987) Central obesity and coronary heart disease in men. *Lancet* **ii**: 1215.

Pottle, A. (2007) Measuring cholesterol levels. Clinical skills: 9. *Nursing Standard* **21**(46): 42–7.

Safeer, R.S. and Cornell, M.O. (2000) The emerging role of HDL cholesterol. Is it time to focus more energy on raising high density lipoprotein levels? *Postgraduate Medicine* **108**(7): 87–90.

Wiedeman, M.W. and Pryor, T.L. (2000) Body dissatisfaction, bulimia, and depression among women: the mediating role of drive for thinness. *International Journal of Eating Disorders* **27**(1): 90–5.

Woods, S.C. (2005) Signals that influence food intake and body weight. *Physiology and Behaviour* **5**: 709–16.

FURTHER READING

British Nutrition Foundation: http://www.nutrition.org.uk

Guenter, P., Jones, S. and Ericson, M. (1997) Enteral nutrition therapy. *Nursing Clinics of North America* **32**(4): 651–68.

Jebb, S.A. and Moore, M.S. (1999) Contribution of a sedentary lifestyle and inactivity to the etiology of overweight and obesity. Current evidence and research issues. *Medical Science, Sports and Exercise* **31**(11 Suppl.): S534–41.

BODY FLUIDS

INTRODUCTION

Fluids within the body provide the environment in which biochemical reactions take place, and contain an extensive range of substances, a reflection of the range of metabolic processes that take place. However, when considering the physiology of body fluids it is usual to focus on water and also electrolytes (ions) since minerals are among the most abundant constituents. Minerals were introduced in Chapter 5 within the context of nutrition, and this chapter describes their role in cell function. It also provides an overview of body fluid homeostasis, though most details on this are provided in a later chapter in relation to kidney functioning (see Chapter 15). Before reading this chapter, readers may find it helpful to first revisit the sections on atoms, electrolytes and water in Chapter 4.

BODY FLUID COMPARTMENTS

Essentially our body fluids are composed of water with substances dissolved within it. Some of that water is found within cells, while the rest occupies the various spaces and cavities, for example within blood vessels, the abdomen and around the brain. That within cells is referred to as the intracellular fluid compartment, that outside as the extracellular fluid compartment. The adult body contains some 40–45 L of water (Figure 6.1), equivalent to about two-thirds of our body weight. Approximately 25 L of this is intracellular fluid, and 18 L or so comprises the extracellular fluid.

All body fluids contain minerals of various types; these are electrically charged and, consequently, they are often referred to as electrolytes, or ions. The presence of the electrical charge makes them chemically active and their physiological activities are discussed in the next sections.

Extracellular fluids

The fluid that bathes cells is not a continuous, single compartment but is subdivided into:

- *interstitial or tissue fluid*: this is the component that bathes most of our cells; approximately 12 L in volume in adults;

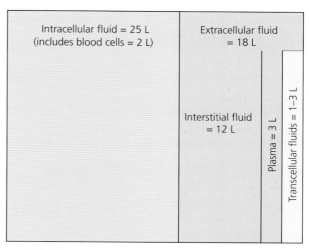

Figure 6.1 Body fluid compartments. Strictly speaking, transcellular fluids are part of the extracellular compartment but they have compositions very different from that of plasma and interstitial fluid, and so are usually considered separately (Tables 6.1 and 6.2)

Q Give four examples of a transcellular fluid.

BOX 6.1 FLUID COMPARTMENTS IN INFANTS

Infants have a higher percentage of total body water compared with older children and adults. In addition, the daily exchange of extracellular fluid through secretion and reabsorption occurring within the gastrointestinal tract is relatively much higher, and may be equivalent to as much as 45% of total body weight per day. Such differences in infants are attributed to relative differences in body and organ sizes, and the immaturity of physiological processes concerned with fluid balance. As a consequence impairment of fluid intake can rapidly alter the level of hydration, for example in persistent vomiting.

- *blood plasma*: this is approximately 3 L in adults; note that the blood cells come under the intracellular compartment;
- *transcellular fluids*: ('trans-' = across) these specialized fluids occupy distinct, specific spaces, and are secreted into them by the epithelial cells that line them. An example is the

BOX 6.2 'THIRD COMPARTMENT' SYNDROME

The body has two major fluid compartments: the extracellular and intracellular fluids. 'Third compartment' syndrome occurs if the volume of fluid in a location suddenly becomes excessive. The additional fluid derives from the blood plasma and tissue fluids and so promotes a redistribution of these fluids, leading potentially to circulatory collapse.

The commonest causes of 'third compartment' syndrome are surgery and peritonitis:

- Surgery can cause a cessation of gastrointestinal activity, including peristaltic contractions. Fluid secretion in the stomach and duodenum (which is normally quite high but much is reabsorbed again later in the intestines) continues but without peristalsis does not pass along the bowel to the absorptive sites. Consequently, the fluid content of the bowel may become excessive.
- Peritonitis can cause 'third compartment' syndrome because the peritoneum membrane that lines the abdomen becomes much more permeable to fluids and proteins, leading to an accumulation of fluid within the abdomen, referred to as peritoneal oedema, or ascites. As with the bowel fluids, the accumulation of peritoneal fluid can occur quite quickly, hence the (apparent) occurrence of a significant 'third compartment'.

cerebrospinal fluid around the brain and spinal cord. Because they are secreted, each has its own particular composition that may be very different from the rest of the extracellular fluids. Collectively the volume is about 1–3 L in adults.

Interstitial (tissue) fluid and blood plasma

Cellular function requires substances to be transported to and from the cells but, close though the microscopic blood vessels or capillaries may be, they remain separated from the cells by the interstitial fluid that bathes them. Substances could, and do, simply diffuse across between the two types of fluid, but this is very slow and inefficient, and a better system is used in which the substances are actually 'carried' by fluid movement to and from the cells.

Fluid movement entails the passage of water, with its dissolved solutes, out of the plasma through microscopic pores in the blood vessel walls into the interstitial fluid, and thence back into the plasma again. Thus the two fluids are continuous and so the electrolyte compositions of blood plasma and interstitial fluid are almost identical (Table 6.1). One requirement for the movement of fluid in this way is that the pores in the blood vessel walls must be highly permeable to water and solutes. However, pore size is not large enough to permit a significant passage of large molecules, such as proteins, and so the plasma has a considerably higher protein concentration than does the interstitial fluid. The protein concentration gradient between plasma and interstitial fluid is one of the main factors in causing the exchange of fluid, which is explained in a later section.

The main electrolytes present are sodium, potassium, chloride, calcium, bicarbonate and phosphate. Of these, sodium and chloride are by far the most abundant (Table 6.1), while potassium, calcium and phosphate ions are present in relatively low concentrations. In considering electrolyte composition of plasma it is also important to be aware that 'free' calcium and 'total' calcium concentrations will be different. This is because only about half of plasma calcium content is in the free, chemically active form; the remainder is chemically bound to plasma proteins and so will not directly influence cell function. However, the 'free' concentration will change rapidly should the bound calcium be released. Binding is influenced by the acidity of the blood, and the release of bound calcium does not normally occur because the plasma is kept slightly alkaline. Hydrogen ions (i.e. acid) produced by metabolism are held at a low concentration (i.e. they have been 'buffered') by also being bound to other substances, primarily bicarbonate ions in blood plasma (see later). Reference to Table 6.1 shows that the concentration of bicarbonate ions is relatively high in both plasma and interstitial fluid, though nowhere near that of sodium or chloride. Phosphate ions present can also act to 'buffer' hydrogen but the concentration of phosphate must be kept very low (Box 6.3) and so that action is less important.

Table 6.1 Concentrations of main ionic constituents of intracellular and extracellular fluids

Constituent	Extracellular fluid Blood plasma (mmol/L)	Interstitial fluid (mmol/L)	Intracellular fluid Skeletal muscle cell (mmol/L)
Cations			
Sodium (Na^+)	142	145*	12
Potassium (K^+)	4.3	4.4	150
Calcium (Ca^{2+})	1.2**	1.2**	4
Anions			
Chloride (Cl^-)	104	117*	4
Bicarbonate (HCO_3^-)	24	27*	12
Phosphate (HPO_4^{2-}, $H_2PO_3^-$)	2	2	40
Proteins (g)	70	Approximately 0	25
pH	7.4	7.4	7.0

*Slight differences in plasma result from negative charge on plasma proteins.
**Ionized calcium. Total calcium concentration in plasma is about twice this.

BOX 6.3 CALCIUM AND ARTERIOSCLEROSIS

Calcium salts, such as calcium phosphate, have a relatively low solubility in water, evidenced by deposits found in kettles and central heating systems in 'hard' water areas. In the body, this can be useful because it aids the deposition of calcium and phosphate in bone. Elsewhere in the body the calcification of tissues is normally detrimental, for example the calcification of brain tissue in some neurological disorders. Arteriosclerosis is a 'hardening' of the arteries as a consequence of calcification of the blood vessel walls, often secondary to scarring. It is irreversible and is a causative factor in high blood pressure (hypertension) and in thrombosis (the occlusion or partial occlusion of a blood vessel by a blood clot). Many factors might contribute to the problem but one risk factor is the local concentration of calcium and phosphate ions. In plasma and interstitial fluid the concentration of calcium and phosphate ions, and associated ions such as those of hydrogen phosphate ($HPO_4{}^{2-}$), is close to that at which the salts will start to precipitate out of solution. Arteriosclerosis is normally avoided because the low concentrations of these ions is closely regulated.

Transcellular fluids

The transcellular fluids are separated from blood plasma by a continuous layer of cells (i.e. by an epithelium) and are produced as secretions of those cells. They include

- cerebrospinal fluid around the brain and spinal cord;
- gastric fluid in our stomachs;
- intestinal fluid;
- intraocular fluid in our eyes;
- synovial fluid within (synovial) skeletal joints;
- secretions such as saliva, semen, cervical fluid and sweat.

The total volume of transcellular fluid is variable, particularly because of changes in the secretion of gastric and intestinal fluids after a meal, but in general amounts to some 1–3 litres. Their composition may be kept near constant, as in the cerebrospinal fluid, or may vary according to the circumstances at the time, as in gastric fluid. The solutes found in these fluids are of the same types as found in other extracellular fluid but their respective concentrations are different from that of the blood plasma and the interstitial fluid (compare Tables 6.1 and 6.2). This is because the cells that secrete them exert some control on the composition of the resultant fluid.

Intracellular fluids

Tissues have widely differing functions so it is not surprising to find that there is variation in the composition of intracellular fluid, depending upon which tissue is studied. Some generalizations can be made, however, and the composition of fluid from muscle cells, as shown in Table 6.1, gives a general impression.

The fluids inside and outside a cell are of course separated by the cell membrane, which is largely lipid and not very permeable to solutes unless there are pores. There are indeed pores but they are 'selective' and consequently intracellular fluids have a very different composition from that of the interstitial fluid that bathes the cells. The situation is complicated by the presence in cell membranes of ion-transporting processes such as the sodium/potassium exchange pump (see Chapter 2) which actively transports sodium ions from the intracellular fluid and releases them into the extracellular fluid while potassium is transported in the opposite direction. Thus, intracellular fluids contain high concentrations of potassium but relatively low concentrations of sodium (see Table 6.1); in general terms this is the opposite situation to that found in the extracellular fluids.

Calcium ions take part in many reactions within the cell, for example by acting as cofactors that aid the actions of certain enzymes. It may seem surprising therefore that the intracellular concentrations of calcium ions are similar or even lower than they are outside the cell (see Table 6.1). However, the availability of calcium ions is a factor in the control of many biochemical reactions, for example in muscle contraction (see Chapter 17, p.468). To control availability, a large proportion of the calcium content of a cell will be bound to proteins and released from them as required. The total calcium content (ionized + bound) of cells, therefore, will be more than the ionized component indicates.

Phosphate is abundant within cells, while bicarbonate ion concentration is considerably lower than that found in extracellular fluids. These ions act as buffers, an important role considering the continual production of hydrogen ions by metabolism (see 'Acid–base homeostasis', later). Phosphate ions are also an integral part of cellular metabolic processes. For example, phosphate-based compounds such as ATP act as energy transporters within the cell (see Chapters 2 and 4).

Table 6.2 Mean ionic concentrations of some transcellular fluids

Fluid	Na+ (mmol/L)	K+ (mmol/L)	Cl− (mmol/L)	HCO3− (mmol/L)	pH
Saliva	33	20	34	0	6.6
Gastric juice	60	9	84	0	3.0
Bile	149	5	101	45	8.0
Pancreatic juice	141	5	77	92	7.7
Cerebrospinal fluid	141	3	127	23	7.5
Sweat	45	5	58	0	5.2

Movement of water and solutes within and between compartments

Within compartments

Fluid compartments are not static since water, with its constituents, is constantly on the move:

- Within the intracellular compartment, fluid movement occurs as cytoplasmic streaming.
- Within the extracellular compartment, fluid movement is a process of bulk flow and also an exchange between the blood plasma and the interstitial fluid.
- There is exchange between the interstitial fluid and intracellular fluid.

Cytoplasmic streaming

This circulation of fluid within a cell occurs as a consequence of a combination of random motion of molecules, small diffusional gradients and small thermal gradients operating across the cell. This flowing of the fluid helps to move substances around the cell, a process that is more efficient than if diffusion alone was the only mechanism.

Bulk flow

Bulk flow provides the means of transporting substances on a large scale and in the shortest possible time. Examples are the propulsion of foodstuff and fluid through the digestive tract, and the flow of blood through the cardiovascular system.

Exchange between the plasma and interstitium

An exchange of fluid and solutes between the plasma and the interstitial fluid is essential in order to transfer substances from the plasma through the interstitial fluid to the cells at a rate that is conducive to normal cell function. The exchange of fluid occurs in tissues, where capillary blood vessels come into the proximity of cells. Capillary exchange occurs as a result of:

- having the wall of the capillary fully permeable to water and most solutes, although not to most large molecules such as proteins; and
- the interplay of physical forces that promote such movements.

The forces involved in capillary exchange are illustrated in Figure 6.2. Basically, the relatively high hydrostatic or fluid

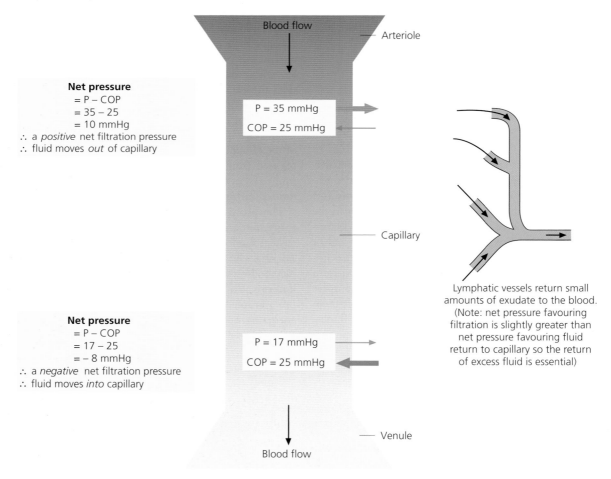

Net pressure
= P − COP
= 35 − 25
= 10 mmHg
∴ a *positive* net filtration pressure
∴ fluid moves *out* of capillary

Net pressure
= P − COP
= 17 − 25
= − 8 mmHg
∴ a *negative* net filtration pressure
∴ fluid moves *into* capillary

Blood flow
Arteriole
P = 35 mmHg
COP = 25 mmHg
Capillary
P = 17 mmHg
COP = 25 mmHg
Venule
Blood flow

Lymphatic vessels return small amounts of exudate to the blood. (Note: net pressure favouring filtration is slightly greater than net pressure favouring fluid return to capillary so the return of excess fluid is essential)

Figure 6.2 Fluid exchange between plasma and interstitial fluid across the capillary wall. The net movement of fluid into or out of the capillary will largely depend upon the difference between the pressure favouring outward movement (the hydrostatic or blood pressure in the capillary, P) and that favouring inward movement (the osmotic pressure caused by plasma proteins, called the colloid osmotic pressure, COP)

Q Why don't the electrolytes in plasma contribute to the osmotic pressure component of capillary exchange?

BOX 6.4 OEDEMA

This box should be read in association with Figure 6.2.

Oedema is an accumulation of fluid in the interstitial compartment as the consequence of a disturbance in the capillary exchange of fluids. It may have a number of causes:

- Elevated capillary hydrostatic pressure as a consequence of:
  - dilation of blood vessels entering the tissue, as occurs in inflammation or during hot weather; or
  - increased backpressure from veins as occurs in congestive heart failure; or
  - (in legs) as a consequence of gravity following standing for a long while, especially if the valves of leg veins are ineffectual.
- Decreased colloid osmotic pressure (caused by hypoproteinaemia; 'hypo-' = lower than normal; '-aemia' = blood) as a consequence of loss of plasma proteins via the urine, or reduced synthesis of plasma proteins, as occurs in various liver conditions or in malnutrition, or of plasma dilution resulting from fluid overload.
- Blocked drainage of interstitial fluid by lymphatic vessels, perhaps caused by a tumour, parasitic organisms or by tissue damage.

Oedema may form:

- peripherally, either locally or generalized. Local oedema might be gravitational (e.g. of the ankle) or perhaps might be caused by obstruction of tissue drainage during surgery or because of positioning of an immobile patient. Generalized oedema is more likely to involve an elevated central venous pressure (e.g. in congestive heart failure) or hypoproteinaemia (e.g. owing to urinary loss of protein in nephrotic syndrome);
- in the abdomen (peritoneal oedema, or ascites) as a consequence of increased fluid secretion across the peritoneum (e.g. in liver failure where the reduced circulation of blood through the liver raises the pressure in the hepatic portal vein);
- in the lungs (pulmonary oedema) as a consequence of increased secretion of fluid out of the pulmonary capillaries (e.g. elevated pulmonary capillary pressure as a consequence of left-sided heart failure).

Although treatment must aim to correct the underlying cause, sometimes a degree of relief may be provided simply by using gravity to reduce the capillary hydrostatic pressure. This may simply involve sitting the individual up to help relieve pulmonary oedema, but could also require tilting the bed or suspending limbs, depending upon the site of the oedema.

Drugs (diuretics, for example furosemide) may be also be used to promote urinary sodium and water excretion and so reduce extracellular fluid volume and oedema. Alternatively, treatment may be aimed at reversing a reduced plasma protein concentration by the infusion of plasma extracts or synthetic protein.

---

pressure within the capillary tends to force fluid out from blood plasma and into the interstitial fluid, but this force is opposed by osmosis induced by the plasma proteins that are retained in the capillary: specifically referred to as the colloid osmotic pressure, or oncotic pressure. Where blood enters a tissue, the net pressure favours movement of fluid out of the blood vessel. However, this loss of fluid means that the hydrostatic pressure diminishes along the capillary. Thus, towards the other end of the capillary a point will be reached when the colloid osmotic pressure now exceeds the hydrostatic pressure, and so fluid will then be drawn back into the vessel. As a result, there is virtually no difference in the volume of blood that enters a tissue in an artery and leaves it in a vein.

The prevention of protein leaking into the interstitial fluid is essential to this process, otherwise the colloid osmotic pressure would also decrease along the capillary. In reality, small quantities of protein do penetrate the interstitium and this slight alteration in the balance of forces acting across the capillary wall results in a small net loss of fluid from the plasma. The leaked proteins, and the accumulated interstitial fluid, are returned to the circulatory system via the lymphatic system (see Chapter 13).

Exchange between interstitial and intracellular fluids

In Chapter 2 it was described how water may pass through a selectively permeable membrane, such as the cell membrane, by a process of osmosis. Thus, movement of water across the cell membrane will occur if the solution on one side of the membrane has a higher solute concentration than the solution on the other side. There are a number of solutes present in body fluids, including various ions and substances such as glucose, proteins and urea, and so the potential osmotic effects of these fluids is determined by the net effect of the concentration gradients of these individual solutes. The term normally used to denote the osmotic potential of a solution is the 'osmolality' and is measured by the effect that solutes have to depress the freezing point of water (Box 6.5). Note that the osmolality gives no information as to the variety or types of solute present or of their individual concentrations, only their net effect.

BOX 6.5 OSMOTIC PRESSURE, OSMOTIC POTENTIAL AND OSMOLALITY

Osmosis is referred to in various ways, depending upon its context:

- 'Osmotic pressure' relates to the notion that water movement across a selectively permeable membrane could be prevented if a pressure is applied to the opposite side of the membrane. The amount of pressure to be applied will be directly related to the extent of osmosis, and so enables scientists to quantify the osmosis. The concept of osmotic pressure is most important in relation to fluid exchange across a blood capillary (Figure 6.2) since here blood pressure is counteracted by the osmotic pressure exerted by the plasma proteins.
- 'Osmotic potential' is a qualitative term that is usually used when solutions are compared; for example 'normal' saline (see later) is considered as having the same osmotic potential as body fluids even though their compositions are different.
- 'Osmolality' converts osmotic potential (and osmotic pressure) into a value that is based on the effects of solutes to lower the freezing point of water. Normal body fluids have an osmolality of about 285 milliosmoles (mOsm)/L. The measurement enables comparisons to be made more readily than by using osmotic pressure, and is the way osmotic content of blood and urine are recorded.

Since water moves so easily across cell membranes it is unlikely that a difference of osmotic potential between intracellular and extracellular fluids will last for long because equilibration will soon occur and make the total osmotic potential of the two compartments very similar. One consequence of this is that:

- Should the individual become dehydrated, water is first lost from the extracellular fluid, which increases the solute concentration. This will osmotically remove water from cells and so also result in cellular dehydration.
- Over-hydration through excessive water intake produces opposite events, leading to over-hydration of cells and dilution of solutes. Over-hydration should not be confused with oedema (see Box 6.4), since it results in an increase in cell volume and a dilution of body fluids, whereas oedema is an accumulation of extracellular fluid only, without dilution.

Obvious external signs of dehydration are a dry oral mucosa and 'hollowing' of tissue around the eyes, and a loss of skin turgor. However, both dehydration and over-hydration usually affects the whole body, and hence the function of all cells, since a near-constant intracellular environment is necessary for optimal functioning. Symptoms of neurological dysfunction are initially the most noticeable if the change in water balance becomes moderate to severe, with individuals experiencing headaches or, if the imbalance is even more severe, lethargy, personality changes, mental confusion, or even coma and death.

ACTIONS OF WATER AND ELECTROLYTES AND PRINCIPLES OF BODY FLUID HOMEOSTASIS

Water and ions are continually added to our body fluids through our diets; most ions ingested in our foods are absorbed from the bowel and this is the case whether we are deficient in them or not. Our diets normally contain more than adequate amounts of the major ions and the ionic constitution of our body fluids is mainly determined by the rate at which they are excreted, especially in the urine. In order to regulate the ionic contents of our body fluids the rate of addition and the rate of excretion must be kept equal (i.e. we must remain in a state of ionic balance, a classic example of homeostasis).

If normal regulatory processes are operating, then fluctuations in the electrolyte content of body fluids occur when there is a mismatch between intake and excretion, and are most likely to occur in those fluids that exchange substances with our external environment, in other words in the extracellular fluid (Figure 6.3). The homeostatic mechanisms that regulate body fluid composition are stimulated by such changes. The detection of change in the extracellular fluid involves specialized receptor cells. Body fluid homeostasis is enlarged upon in Chapter 15, when kidney function is described in detail, but to put much of the present chapter into a healthcare perspective, it is useful at this point to consider the actions of the constituents of body fluids and how they relate to those processes.

Water

As noted previously, water is the solvent in which most of the chemical reactions that comprise metabolism take place. Clearly, the concentrations of solutes dissolved in that water will change according to the rate of addition and removal of those solutes, but they can also be altered by adding or removing water since this will dilute or concentrate the fluids (and will also alter their volume). Thus changes in water balance could be expected to alter cell functions and so water homeostasis is essential.

The body is normally able to regulate water balance very effectively. For example, as already noted, dehydration will cause the movement of water out of cells by osmosis, thereby concentrating the intracellular fluid. This causes the receptor cells (called 'osmoreceptors' – see Chapter 15) to initiate changes in water intake and excretion, by influencing our perception of thirst and promoting a reduction in urine volume. Over-hydration will have opposite effects on the osmotic pres-

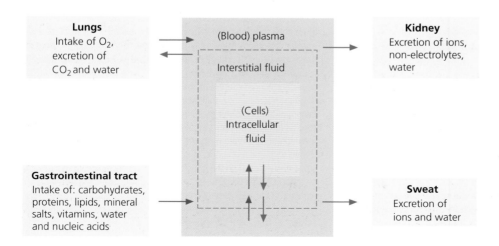

Lungs Intake of O$_2$, excretion of CO$_2$ and water

(Blood) plasma

Interstitial fluid

(Cells) Intracellular fluid

Kidney Excretion of ions, non-electrolytes, water

Gastrointestinal tract Intake of: carbohydrates, proteins, lipids, mineral salts, vitamins, water and nucleic acids

Sweat Excretion of ions and water

Figure 6.3 Schematic diagram of the exchanges of water and solutes between fluid compartments and the external environment. Note that it is the composition of blood plasma that is most susceptible to rapid change, and that interstitial fluid and hence intracellular fluid will be indirectly influenced by those changes

sure of plasma, and will suppress thirst and promote the production of a large volume of dilute urine. The intention is to remove excess water and so restore the balance state.

Sodium and chloride (Na⁺; Cl⁻)

Sodium and chloride ions are the most abundant electrolytes in extracellular fluid, and are usually considered together. They have two areas of activity:

- The ions influence cell membrane processes:
  - Sodium ions aid the carriage of large molecules, such as glucose and amino acids, into cells by combining with their protein carrier molecule in the cell membrane; the concentration gradient for sodium causes diffusion into the cell.
  - Chloride ions, being negatively charged, may interfere with the movement of positive ions. For example in parts of the central nervous system chloride ions suppress the electrical changes that occur when the nerve cells are stimulated by interfering with the diffusion of sodium or potassium ions, and so provides a physiological means of inhibiting nerve transmission (see Chapter 8, p.188).
- Being so abundant, these ions are the main contributors to the osmotic potential of extracellular fluid, and so have a role in the distribution by osmosis of water between the extra- and intracellular compartments.

The means of controlling sodium chloride balance relates to the osmotic activities of the ions. An increased sodium chloride intake (e.g. in salty food) will raise the sodium chloride concentration of extracellular fluid, promote osmosis from cells, and cause thirst and renal water retention; in other words, the responses that are normally associated with dehydration (above). However, unlike the control of water balance alone, the changes here are induced by the intake of the salt – the person may already have been in a state of water balance and so the volume change induced by the responses would be in excess of normal. The excretion of sodium (and the excess water) by the kidneys is stimulated by the resultant increase in blood volume, detected by stretch receptors located within the circulatory system.

Potassium (K⁺)

The concentration gradient for potassium across cell membranes is mainly responsible for the electrical status of the cell membrane (remember that the concentration of potassium

BOX 6.6 HYPERNATRAEMIA AND HYPONATRAEMIA

Hypernatraemia ('hyper' = greater than normal, 'natrium-' = sodium, '-aemia' = of blood) occurs when blood sodium concentration is persistently greater than normal values. It usually results from an inability to regulate sodium concentration, for example in renal failure, or from dehydration. Hyponatraemia ('hypo' = less than normal) often reflects excessive hydration of the extracellular fluids but can arise if there is excessive loss of the ion, for example with vomiting.

Therapy must relate to the underlying cause, depending upon whether or not there is a change in water balance. This will usually entail assessment of how salt and water input and output compares.

BOX 6.7 HYPERKALAEMIA AND HYPOKALAEMIA

When blood potassium concentration is increased to above the normal range this is referred to as hyperkalaemia ('hyper-' = greater than normal, 'kalium' = potassium, '-aemia' = of the blood). Although some adaptation by cells is possible, the elevated potassium may cause nerves and muscles to become overexcited, most noticeable as an increased heart rate. Hyperkalaemia may be caused by an inability to excrete potassium adequately, as in renal failure or a dysfunctional adrenal gland. Excessive hyperkalaemia can cause death, and clearly this has to be considered if potassium infusions are administered.

Hypokalaemia ('hypo-' = less than normal) will have the opposite effect making heart cells more difficult to excite, leading to a decreased pulse rate. Hypokalaemia can be induced by excessive use of those diuretic drugs that promote potassium excretion, or again by a dysfunctional adrenal gland. Regular observations of pulse rates are important in these settings.

Therapy for hyperkalaemia includes treating underlying factors, such as acidosis in which hydrogen ions enter cells and are exchanged for potassium ions, and improving excretion of the ion (e.g. by use of oral or rectal ion exchange resins). Treatment for hypokalaemia will usually entail oral potassium supplements; potassium infusions are normally only used when considered necessary because of the potential for over-infusion leading to hyperkalaemia.

inside the cell is much greater than that outside). This is referred to as the 'resting membrane potential' and variations in the potassium gradient will change it slightly, making it approach or deviate further from the threshold value at which nerve and muscle cells becomes activated (for details, see Chapter 8, p.187). Thus, an increase in extracellular potassium concentration makes the membrane easier to stimulate, and a decrease in makes the cell more difficult, perhaps even impossible, to stimulate using physiological stimuli.

Since the plasma potassium ion concentration can have such a profound effect on excitable cells it is not surprising that the plasma concentration is monitored directly, and an increase in concentration alters the excretion of potassium in urine.

Calcium (Ca²⁺)

Calcium has two major areas of activity:

- Intracellular actions. Many hormones act by stimulating the release of calcium ions from stores within target cells, and these promote the actions of certain enzymes in the cell. In muscle cells the ions are necessary for the contractile process (see Chapter 17), though smooth and cardiac muscle cells have little calcium storage and so it is necessary for these cells to take up calcium ions from the extracellular fluid; following contraction these cells then pump the ions back out again. Drugs classed as 'calcium antagonists' interfere with this process and help to prolong muscle contraction in the heart.
- The threshold membrane potential at which excitable cells are stimulated is influenced by the calcium ion concentration of extracellular fluids. For example, a reduction in calcium ion concentration reduces the threshold with the result that the cell is more easily stimulated.

BOX 6.8 HYPERCALCAEMIA AND HYPOCALCAEMIA

Hypercalcaemia ('hyper-' = greater than normal, '-aemia' = of blood) is a persistent elevation of blood calcium ion concentration above the normal range. It occurs usually either as a consequence of a failure of regulating the transfer of the ion into and out of bone (usually because of a hormone imbalance, especially of parathyroid hormone), or because of excessive acidity in blood (which releases calcium from that bound to plasma protein). The short-term consequence is a reduction in the activity of nerve and muscle cells; for example constipation arising from diminished bowel movements may be observed.

Hypocalcaemia ('hypo-' = less than normal) may arise because of inadequate uptake from the gut, excessive transfer to bone or excessive renal losses. The problem is frequently caused by hormone deficiency but may also be induced by alkalosis due to sudden depletion of hydrogen ion concentration in blood, for example in excessive breathing during anxiety (which removes too much carbon dioxide, a source of acidity). Muscle spasms may be observed as nerve and muscle cells become over-excitable: carpopedal spasm (of the hand) is an observation frequently seen in anxiety-induced hypocalcaemia.

Therapy for hypercalcaemia involves treating the underlying cause but may also entail promoting the loss of calcium in urine by enhancing renal losses (e.g. using saline infusion to promote urine production and electrolyte loss). Treatment for hypocalcaemia may be by oral supplement but calcium gluconate infusion may be used if severe.

The pronounced effects that calcium ions exert on excitable cells means that the calcium ion concentration of extracellular fluid must be closely monitored. However, responses to a change in plasma calcium ion concentration are complex as calcium balance involves the level of transfer between plasma and bone, the rate of uptake from the bowel and the rate of excretion in the urine (see Figure 9.10, p.217).

Bicarbonate and phosphate (HCO_3^-; HPO_4^{2-})

Bicarbonate and phosphate ions are the main ions that buffer acidity produced by hydrogen ions generated through metabolic processes. An excess or deficiency of buffers alters the concentration of hydrogen ions present, thus compromising the regulation of acidity (see next section).

The concentration of bicarbonate ions in blood plasma is therefore regulated by responses to acidity changes (see the following section) through alterations in its production (from carbon dioxide) and excretion (as carbon dioxide in the lungs, as bicarbonate in urine). Phosphate excretion in urine is also affected by the regulation of acidity, but it is also linked to that of calcium. When combined with calcium, phosphate ions contribute to the main mineral component of bone. Bone is continuously resorbed and reformed, and so there is a continual release and uptake, respectively, of phosphate to and from the extracellular fluid. It is therefore not surprising to find that regulation of the concentration of phosphate ions in blood plasma is linked to the control of calcium.

Hydrogen

Although these ions are present in only very small concentrations, the importance of hydrogen ions in pathology makes it worthy of mention here, but is explored in more detail in the next section. Hydrogen ions have a potent damaging effect on protein structure and function and so their concentration must be regulated very closely; it is directly monitored. Increased acidity stimulates the removal of carbon dioxide, a source of acidity, via the lungs. Alternatively, an increased acidity of blood passing through the kidneys promotes the urinary excretion of hydrogen ions. By a related mechanism the kidney may also alter the buffering (neutralizing) capacity of plasma by changing the excretion bicarbonate ions.

ACID–BASE HOMEOSTASIS

The preceding discussion on bicarbonate and hydrogen ions identifies their links to the regulation of body fluid acidity. The regulation of this is complex, not least because hydrogen ions are generated from metabolic sources and not simply obtained from diet. The term 'acid–base homeostasis' refers to those processes that act together to regulate the hydrogen ion concentration of body fluids. Hydrogen ions are highly reactive, and readily influence the weak bonds that are responsible for the three-dimensional shape of protein molecules. Those proteins that are enzymes are catalysts that accelerate chemical reactions within the body so that they are compatible with life, and loss of their structural integrity will compromise that function and may even become life threatening. The following describes the background chemistry to acids and alkalis, the sources of hydrogen ions and the regulation of hydrogen ion concentration in fluids. This discussion is available in extended form in Clancy and McVicar (2007a,b).

Acids and alkalis

In body fluids, those chemical molecules called acids separate into positively charged hydrogen ions (H^+) and the negative ions that they had been associated with. 'Strong' acids ionize completely and so release **all** their hydrogen ions (see Equation 1a), but weak acids do not ionise completely and so do not release all their hydrogen ions (see Equation 1b).

Equation 1a: strong acid, e.g.

$$HCl \Leftrightarrow H^+ + Cl^-$$

Hydrochloric acid   Hydrogen ion   Chloride ion

Equation 1b: weak acid, e.g.

$$H_2CO_3 \Leftrightarrow H^+ + HCO_3^-$$

Carbonic acid   Hydrogen ions   Bicarbonate ions

Note: The symbol $\Leftrightarrow$ signifies that the reaction is reversible. In these equations, the acid separates (dissociates) when the reaction moves to the **right**. For strong acids, any tendency for the reaction to move towards the left, and hence reform acid, is ineffective because the reformed acid molecule will reionize immediately (i.e. the reaction to the right is always favoured so that at any one time there will be more ions than acid). For a weak acid, the acid reforms when the reaction moves to the **left** but the tendency for the acid to dissociate is weak, and so at any one time the reaction will provide more acid molecules than ions.

In these examples, the negatively charged ions are either chloride or bicarbonate. In Equation 1b, the latter recombines with H^+ to form undissociated acid molecules, and so they are given a distinct collective term, 'bases'. There are other chemicals that produce negatively charged ions that also may act as bases if hydrogen ions are present from another source, yet do not produce hydrogen ions when they dissociate. For example:

Equation 2:

$$NaOH \rightarrow Na^+ + OH^-$$

Sodium hydroxide → Sodium ions + Hydroxyl ions

Potentially:

$$H^+ + OH^- \rightarrow H_2O$$

Hydrogen ion + Hydroxyl ion → Water

In doing so, they are in effect neutralizing the acidity produced by the source of H^+. The sodium hydroxide in this example is referred to as an 'alkali'.

To summarize:

- An acid produces hydrogen ions when it breaks down (dissociates) making a solution acidic. Some acids dissociate very readily and are therefore referred to as 'strong' acids. Others do so less readily and so are 'weak' acids.
- A base is a negative ion that is also produced by the breakdown of a weak acid and may recombine with hydrogen ions to reform the acid molecule. The breakdown of strong acids does not produce effective bases because any tendency for the acid to reform is counteracted by the stronger tendency for the acid to immediately break down again.
- An alkali does not produce hydrogen ions when it dissociates, but it does produce negative ions that are capable of combining with hydrogen ions should they be present from another source; this may be a weak or a strong acid, thus neutralizing the acidity and making a solution alkaline.
- Note that because bases also remove hydrogen ions, effectively neutralizing the acidity, they too can make a solution alkaline if they are in excess.

BOX 6.9 GASTRIC ACID: A SOURCE OF HYDROCHLORIC ACID IN THE BODY

Although acids have a variety of uses in the body, the reactivity of strong acids is such that roles for this type of acid are very limited. For example, you are probably aware that fluid in the stomach is acidic, sometimes highly so. The acid present is hydrochloric acid and has important roles in destroying microorganisms in food we eat, and in providing the environment necessary to activate the digestive enzyme pepsin. The corrosive nature of this strong acid is immediately apparent by the burning sensation produced if some is refluxed into the oesophagus, or during a bout of indigestion. The need for a thick protective mucus lining in the stomach is clear, yet cells of the stomach wall still may only survive for a day or two even in health. Excessive erosion of the stomach lining produces a gastric ulcer.

The pH scale and pH of body fluids

pH values, measured using a pH meter, relate to the concentration of hydrogen ions in a solution. The unit of measurement for the concentration of ions in is the 'mole' where 1 mole represents the number of ions that would weigh 1 g. The concentration of ions in body fluids is normally in a range indicated in millimoles per litre (mmol/L) where 1 mmol is 1/1000 of a mole (see Table 6.1). However, the hydrogen ion concentration in body fluids is much less than even this, and is converted into a micro-unit of measurement (called nanomoles per litre, nmol/L, where 1 mmol = 1 000 000 nmol). The pH (= '**p**otential of **H**ydrogen') provides a more convenient means of expressing such low concentrations.

Solutions have a pH of 1–14, in which a value of 7 is neutral and equates to that of pure water in which hydrogen (H^+) ions and alkali ions (OH^-) are present in very small quantities but are equal e.g.:

Equation 3:

$$H_2O \Leftrightarrow H^+ + OH^-$$

Water ⇔ Hydrogen ion + Hydroxyl ion

This therefore provides a reference point for the acidity/alkalinity of solutions. Acidic solutions have a pH value of less than 7; the greater the excess of hydrogen ions, the more acidic the solution becomes, and hence the lower the pH value. Alkaline solutions have pH values of above 7; the more alkali/base ions there are relative to hydrogen ions, the higher the pH values. pH therefore is a reflection of the balance between the presence of acids, and of alkalis/bases. One important aspect to note, however, is that pH is not a linear scale, and a change in just one pH unit corresponds to a 10-fold change in hydrogen ion concentration (Box 6.10).

BOX 6.10 pH AND HYDROGEN ION CONCENTRATION

The pH of blood averages 7.4 in health though a value between 7.35 and 7.45 is considered normal. A pH of 7.4 actually represents a concentration of hydrogen ions of 40 nmol/L, which is slightly less than that of 'neutral' water in which the hydrogen ion concentration is 100 nmol/L. Thus, blood is slightly alkaline.

Decreased pH values reflect an increased hydrogen ion concentration, and increased pH represents a decreased hydrogen ion concentration. The pH scale is an example of a logarithmic scale: this means that a change in a single pH unit represents a 10-fold change in hydrogen ion concentration. Thus, a pH of 8 represents a hydrogen ion concentration only one-tenth of that at neutral pH 7, while a pH of 6 represents a 10-fold increase. When acidity in the stomach is about pH 3 during digestion this represents a concentration of hydrogen ions of 1 million nanomoles per litre (i.e. 1 mmol/L). To put this into context, pH 3 represents a 25 000-fold greater increase in hydrogen ion concentration than is present in blood at pH 7.4, yet the pH has changed by only 4.4 units. This relationship between pH and hydrogen ion concentration must be borne in mind when interpreting blood analysis data, and some clinicians even advocate using hydrogen ion concentration data rather than pH.

Intracellular fluids

Arguably, the most important chemical reaction in the body is intracellular respiration, since its endproducts include the energy required for life processes. Food (usually glucose) is broken down initially without oxygen in the cytoplasm of cells, and finally with oxygen within the mitochondria. These processes were described in Chapter 4 but in the context of this section, it is useful to summarize:

Equation 4 – a summary of cellular respiration:

$$C_6H_{12}O_6 \;+\; 6O_2 \;\rightarrow\; 6CO_2 \;+\; 6H_2O \;+\; \text{Energy}$$

Glucose   Oxygen   Carbon dioxide   Water   (as ATP and heat)

Note: The single arrow to the right indicates that this reaction is unidirectional (i.e. glucose molecules cannot reform in this reaction so carbon dioxide is a 'waste' product to be excreted).

The carbon dioxide generated may combine chemically with water to form carbonic acid, the weak acid identified in Equation 1b earlier. If this acid ionizes it will produce H^+ ions and bicarbonate ions (HCO_3^-) also noted in Equation 1b. Together the reactions can be represented as:

Equation 5:

$$CO_2 \;+\; H_2O \;\Leftrightarrow\; H_2CO_3 \;\Leftrightarrow\; H^+ \;+\; HCO_3^-$$

Carbon dioxide   Water   Carbonic acid   Hydrogen ion   Bicarbonate ion

Thus, an increased generation of carbon dioxide when metabolism is increased could be anticipated to generate more hydrogen ions, and hence promote an increase in acidity (decreased pH), for example accompanying:

- the stress response since there is an increased production of stress hormones in an attempt to adapt to stress;
- an infection because there is an increased number of white blood cells in an attempt to fight off pathogens;
- trauma since there is an increased cellular division as part of the repair and regeneration process;
- strenuous exercise as there is an increased frequency and prolongation of muscle contraction.

Other acids also generate hydrogen ions, for example sulphuric acid from the metabolism of amino acids, and ketoacids from the metabolism of amino acids and fatty acids. If pH homeostasis within the cell fails then the resultant increased acidity (referred to as 'acidosis'; see Box 6.12) will affect health by impairing enzyme activity, if it is prolonged. Excess hydrogen ions must be secreted from cells into extracellular fluid, raising the potential that the pH of those fluids (viz. of blood) will change as a consequence.

Extracellular fluids: pH of arterial blood

The normal range for pH of arterial blood is 7.35–7.45; the range indicates close regulation – if it was not then it would impact on the release of excess hydrogen ions from within cells, and influence protein function in blood itself. It becomes impossible to sustain life when arterial pH is below 6.8 or above 7.8 (Lynes, 2003), though the individual will be seriously ill even before pH has changed to those extreme values. Blood contains a number of sources of acidity but as with intracellular fluids the main one is from carbon dioxide (namely, carbonic acid).

pH regulation

The control of pH is concerned with ensuring an adequate balance of hydrogen ions and bases. It is achieved through three mechanisms:

1. Through the action of bases to 'buffer' body fluids, that is, acting to prevent an increase in acidity when hydrogen ion generation is increased.
2. Through excretion of carbon dioxide, the source of carbonic acid. This is achieved through gas exchange by the lungs.
3. Through excretion of hydrogen ions in urine.

Buffer mechanisms

Buffer mechanisms are chemical reactions that occur moment-by-moment and so provide us with a rapid, short-term regulation of pH. Two types of buffers exist:

- *Acid buffers*: these chemicals are bases that act like sponges to 'mop up' H^+ ions if the body fluid has H^+ ions that exceed the homeostatic requirements. In Equation 6, Buffer X (= B^-) is an 'acid buffer' since it will promote combination with H^+ producing, in this illustration, 'HB'.
- *Alkaline buffers*: these chemicals are acids that donate (or release) H^+ ions if the body fluid is deficient in them. In Equation 6, Buffer Y (= HB) is an alkaline buffer since a rise in its concentration will promote its break down to H^+ and B^- ions.

Equation 6:

$$H^+ \;+\; B^- \;\Leftrightarrow\; HB$$

Buffer X   Buffer Y

The activities of these two types of buffer are illustrated by considering the carbonic acid–bicarbonate system, the principal buffer system of the extracellular body fluids, including arterial blood. If there is an excess of hydrogen ions then this will tend to drive the reactions shown in Equation 1b towards the left, thus generating carbonic acid molecules from H^+ and HCO_3^-. Carbonic acid (H_2CO_3) is a weak acid and much of this newly generated carbonic acid will not instantly dissociate again – in effect, free hydrogen ions have been removed, and so the pH value is maintained. Thus, the bicarbonate ions have acted as an acid buffer.

There is a risk that this action of bicarbonate ions may become excessive and take the buffering too far, leading to a rise in pH as the blood becomes more alkaline. However, as bicarbonate ions are used up, a shift in the equilibrium of Equation 1b occurs so that the reaction to the right is favoured. Carbonic acid breakdown begins to increase, releasing hydrogen ions as it does so. Again, the pH value is maintained. Thus, the carbonic acid has acted as an alkaline buffer.

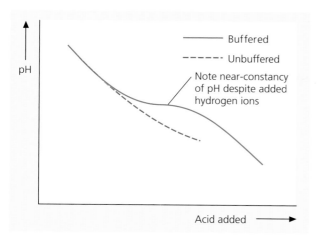

Figure 6.4 Influence on pH of adding acid (i.e. hydrogen ions) to either a solution that is unbuffered (dotted line) or one that contains a buffer chemical (solid line). Note the plateau region where pH is held almost constant by the buffer

Q The near-constancy of pH in the plateau region indicates that the added hydrogen ions have not affected the acidity of the solution. What has happened to them?

Note how a strong acid cannot operate in this fashion; in the example in Equation 1a, any tendency for chloride ions to 'mop up' hydrogen ions must fail as the hydrochloric acid molecules (HCl) that would form will immediately dissociate and so hydrogen ions will, almost instantly, become 'free' once more. Only weak acids can provide buffers, and they effectively maintain the pH of fluids within a relatively narrow range – see Figure 6.4. The effectiveness can be overwhelmed, however, if hydrogen ion production exceeds the capacity of the fluid to buffer it (Box 6.10).

Buffer systems also operate within cells. Here the carbonic acid–bicarbonate system operates but it is of lesser importance relative to the situation in blood, as bicarbonate ions generally are in much lower concentration. Other bases are present, especially phosphates and proteins (e.g. haemoglobin). Phosphate in cells is found in two forms: hydrogen phosphate (HPO_4^{2-}) and dihydrogen phosphate ($H_2PO_4^{-}$). Note the difference in the number of negative charges: hydrogen phosphate has two and so can combine with H^+ to form dihydrogen phosphate ions, which now will only have one charge:

Equation 7:

$$HPO_4^{2-} \quad + \quad H^+ \quad \Leftrightarrow \quad H_2PO_4^{-}$$

Hydrogen phosphate ion   Excess hydrogen ion   Dihydrogen phosphate ion

Thus, hydrogen phosphate acts as an acid buffer, mopping up excess hydrogen ions.

Dihydrogen phosphate is also sometimes referred to as 'acid phosphate' because like bicarbonate ions, above, hydrogen ions may be released (producing hydrogen phosphate once

BOX 6.11 SHORT-TERM REGULATION OF ACID–BASE HOMEOSTASIS: BUFFERING CAPACITY

Buffers operate constantly as the equilibrium of chemical reactions, such as those in Equation 5, shift towards one side or the other, promoting the breakdown of a weak acid, or the reformation of that acid.

Nevertheless, the effectiveness of the system can only be maintained according to the amount of buffer present (referred to as the 'buffering capacity'). For example, imagine a situation where the base concentration is far in excess of H^+:

$$10H^+ \quad + \quad 20B^- \quad \rightarrow \quad 10BH \quad + \quad 10B^-$$

In this example, 10 excess hydrogen ions produced by metabolism are removed by 10 of the 20 available acid buffers (B^-), leaving a lot of buffer still available. Fluid pH has been buffered.

Now consider a further increase in the generation of H^+:

$$20H^+ \quad + \quad 20B^- \quad \rightarrow \quad 20BH$$

In this example, 20 excess hydrogen ions have now been removed by the base. pH continues to be controlled but at the expense of reaching the maximum buffering capacity.

Now consider even further addition of H^+:

$$30H^+ \quad + \quad 20B^- \quad \rightarrow \quad 20BH \quad + \quad 10H^+$$

Metabolism has produced an excess of 30 hydrogen ions of which 20 are removed by the individual's buffering capacity. However 10 free hydrogen ions are still present, and hence the pH will not be fully restored to normal; the buffering capacity has been exceeded.

Raising the buffering capacity of body fluids
Patients in critical care often suffer from disease, the shock of trauma, or metabolic responses that have arisen through surgery, and this places them at risk of developing an acid–base imbalance, usually an acidosis, because the buffering capacity of blood is inadequate for the level of acid production (Coombs, 2001). Historically, bicarbonate ions were administered to patients with signs of acidosis in order to increase the buffering capacity of body fluids. For infusions, however, bicarbonate is not now normally present as a constituent of an infusate as it carries a risk of converting the acidosis into an alkalosis if excessive. An alternative source may be provided through incorporating lactate into the infusate; this is converted only gradually to bicarbonate by the liver.

more) if pH has to be lowered. Thus it may also act as an alkaline buffer.

For proteins, each constituent amino acid molecule has the following basic formula:

$$NH_2 - \underset{\underset{R}{|}}{\overset{\overset{H}{|}}{C}} - COOH$$

where R simply represents atoms that vary according to the amino acid in question. As amino acids are joined together in a protein the presence of the NH_2^- (called an amine group) at one end of the growing molecule, and the COOH (called a carboxyl group) at the other is retained. In the slightly alkaline conditions that normally occur, the carboxyl end loses its hydrogen atom thus becoming a negative ion (referred to as proteinate anion). This allows proteins to behave as acid buffers, since they can 'mop up' hydrogen ions, if they are in excess:

Equation 8:

$$\underset{\substack{\text{Proteinate} \\ \text{anion}}}{NH_2\text{-Protein-COO}^-} + \underset{\substack{\text{Excess} \\ \text{hydrogen ion}}}{H^+} \Leftrightarrow \underset{\substack{\text{Uncharged} \\ \text{protein}}}{NH_2\text{-Protein-COOH}}$$

The protein molecule is now uncharged but if further H^+ ions are present the amine group may now also pick up a hydrogen ion; thus the protein becomes overall positively charged (called a proteinate cation):

Equation 9:

$$\underset{\substack{\text{Uncharged} \\ \text{protein}}}{NH_2\text{-Protein-COOH}} + \underset{\substack{\text{Excess} \\ \text{hydrogen ion}}}{H^+} \Leftrightarrow \underset{\substack{\text{Proteinate} \\ \text{cation}}}{NH_3^+\text{-Protein-COOH}}$$

Each protein molecule therefore potentially can pick up two excess hydrogen ions, making it an important acid buffer. The chemical reactions are reversible and so the hydrogen ions can be released once more should hydrogen ions begin to be deficient and so proteins can also act as alkaline buffers.

Respiratory mechanisms

Referring back to Equation 5, it was noted how there is a complex relationship between carbon dioxide, carbonic acid and hydrogen/bicarbonate ions. The direction in which the reaction is likely to proceed is influenced by the relative concentrations of the different components. An increase in carbon dioxide concentration in body fluids therefore tends to increase hydrogen ion concentration and lower the pH value. Conversely, if hydrogen/bicarbonate ions are increased the buffering and reformation of carbonic acid increases, and the reaction may be driven towards the dissociation of the acid to carbon dioxide and water. That part of the equation depends upon the presence of an enzyme, carbonic anhydrase, to catalyse it. In cells and tissues, conditions and the enzyme favour the incorporation of carbon dioxide into carbonic acid, and hence towards the generation of hydrogen ions and bicarbonate ions. In the lungs the opposite is promoted – the carbonic acid forms carbon dioxide, which is then eliminated via expiration from the lungs. Note how bicarbonate ions in extracellular fluid also provide the means of conveying carbon dioxide from the tissues to the lungs; no wonder there is so much bicarbonate in plasma.

The change in excretion of carbon dioxide can be rapid as acidity of blood is one of the ways by which the body indirectly monitors carbon dioxide concentration. However, such responses tend to be short-lived as detection of the subsequently reduced carbon dioxide content of blood acts to reverse the response. In established acid–base disturbances, for example ketoacidosis in uncontrolled diabetes mellitus, it is not unusual to observe this increased lung ventilation because a tolerance to the reduction in carbon dioxide content has taken place through the resetting of homeostatic set points (see Chapter 14, p.419), a process that takes several days to occur. This is referred to as 'respiratory compensation' (Box 6.11).

Renal mechanisms

Our kidneys play an essential role in acid–base homeostasis, since many buffer ions and hydrogen ions can be directly removed from the body in urine (Woodrow, 2004). The kidneys may increase the excretion of hydrogen ions by replacing other positive ions in urine, such as sodium (Na^+), thus making the urine more acidic. The excess hydrogen ions may also be excreted in combination with other molecules, for example dihydrogen phosphate (see earlier). In excreting more hydrogen ions, the kidneys also absorb more bicarbonate ions, thus recycling this important acid buffer (Woodrow, 2004). The processes are described in more detail in Chapter 15. The increased excretion of hydrogen ions in urine is an adaptation that takes several hours or more to become effective, and so 'renal compensation' mechanisms are intermediate or longer-term regulators of acid–base balance.

Acidosis and alkalosis

The normal pH values of body fluids reflect the integrated activities of the three regulatory mechanisms (above). One simple way to view the process is that the continual production of acids, and hence hydrogen ions, by metabolism is prevented from disturbing pH values by buffering, but the acids or hydrogen ions must at some point be excreted otherwise that mechanism will become overwhelmed. A failure of one or more of these regulatory mechanisms will produce a disorder:

- If there is excess acidity, this is referred to as an 'acidosis' (Box 6.12). Acidosis is a set of signs and symptoms including headache, blurred vision, fatigue, weakness, possibly tremors and delirium.
- If there is an acid deficiency then this is referred to as an 'alkalosis' (Box 6.13). Symptoms include irritability, weakness, muscle cramps, dizziness, carpopedal spasm and paraesthesia. The promotion of neuromuscular symptoms relates to the influence that the pH change has on the concentration of free calcium concentration (see earlier), which in alkalosis lowers the threshold sensitivity for activation of nerves and muscles.

Boxes 6.12 and 6.13 identify that acid–base disturbances can have a metabolic or respiratory cause. Diagnosis includes analysis of arterial blood gas composition and associated electrolytes particularly bicarbonate (and chloride, which changes if bicarbonate ions are in excess or deficient), which informs of a patient's oxygenation, ventilation and acid–base homeostasis, and the possible causes of respiratory or metabolic dysfunction. Practitioners should be fully aware of the principles of acid–base homeostasis since they are frequently members of the clinical team to receive the arterial blood gas measurements. The reader is directed to an article by Allen (2004), which identifies a simple four-step approach that enables arterial blood gas interpretation even when all the complexities

BOX 6.12 ACIDOSIS

Understanding a patient's blood pH aids the assessment, diagnostics, planning and implementation of health care, and in re-evaluating a healthcare intervention.

Acidosis is observed when there is an excessive acidity of body fluids, producing an arterial blood pH of < 7.35. There are two origins of this condition (Figure 6.5):

- *Metabolic acidosis*: in metabolic acidosis, hydrogen ions are usually produced somewhere in the body in excess of the normal regulatory processes, for example ketoacidosis in a patient with diabetes mellitus, or lactic acidosis in a person performing strenuous exercise. Alternatively a metabolic acidosis arises through excessive hydrogen ion retention, for example in a patient experiencing kidney failure, or through excessive loss of bicarbonate from the body, for example in diarrhoea.
- *Respiratory acidosis*: this arises because the respiratory mechanisms are not excreting enough carbon dioxide, for example in patients who have obstructive and/or restrictive airway diseases.

Compensatory processes occur. In chronic metabolic acidosis, the respiratory rate and depth of respiration both increase and this response increases CO_2 excretion, and hence reduces this source of acidity.

Unless it is the cause of the disturbance, then the renal system excretes more hydrogen ions, thus lowering the pH of urine, and retains more bicarbonate ions, thus increasing the buffering capacity of the blood.

Base excess

It is not unusual for bicarbonate ion concentration to be higher than normal in a respiratory acidosis because carbon dioxide generates bicarbonate as well as hydrogen ions (see Equation 5); consequently carbon dioxide retention appears to paradoxically elevate plasma bicarbonate concentration in addition to promoting an acidosis. However, the increment can be estimated and the actual concentration compared with this to give an indication of any further bicarbonate retention as a result of renal compensation. 'Base excess' is a term used by doctors to estimate the extent of the compensatory response to an acidosis. This value is important because raising the buffering capacity of blood may be part of the therapy to reduce an acidosis, and the base excess makes it more likely that over-correction may occur.

However, whatever the cause, if the acidosis is chronic in nature then these intermediate and long-term homeostatic pH regulators can only be considered to be partly effective and a degree of acidosis will persist.

BOX 6.13 ALKALOSIS

Alkalosis indicates a deficiency of hydrogen ions in body fluids, indicated by an arterial blood pH of > 7.45. Again there are two origins of this condition (Figure 6.5):

- *Metabolic alkalosis*. This is observed when there is bicarbonate ion retention, for example because drugs have promoted renal reabsorption of the ion, or because over-secretion of steroid hormones (e.g. Cushing's disease) has done the same. The buffering of hydrogen ions in blood is then excessive.
- *Respiratory alkalosis*. This is caused by an over-excretion of carbon dioxide through hyperventilation, for example that experienced in extreme anxiety states. In that example the state is normally only transient (i.e. acute respiratory alkalosis). Chronic respiratory alkalosis is extremely rare.

It is unlikely that compensatory mechanisms will be alerted in acute respiratory alkalosis, as these are slow to be established. In order to readdress acid–base homeostasis quickly the patient who is hyperventilating can breathe in and out of a paper bag, therefore breathing in 'exhaled carbon dioxide' (an indirect source of hydrogen ions) that would then reverse the respiratory alkalosis.

In chronic alkalosis, the compensatory responses will be the opposite to the mechanisms that operates in chronic respiratory and metabolic acidosis, in that they act either to retain carbon dioxide, thus increasing this source of acidity, or to increase bicarbonate excretion in urine, thus decreasing the bicarbonate concentration of the blood, thereby reducing its buffering capacity.

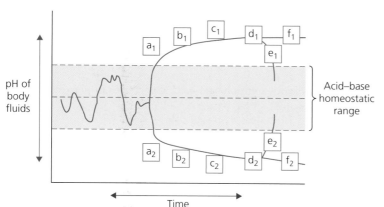

Key:

a_1 = Alkaline buffers attempt to donate hydrogen ions in order to decrease the pH, in an attempt to re-establish pH homeostasis

a_2 = Acid buffers attempt to 'mop up' hydrogen ions to increase pH, in an attempt to re-establish pH homeostasis. (Note: Both buffers are short-term regulators of body fluid pH and the graph demonstrates that the buffering capacity is being exceeded, since homeostatic disturbances of body fluid pH are still evident [b_1/b_2])

b_1/b_2 = The intermediate regulators of breathing are alerted in an attempt to re-establish pH homeostasis. See text for details. For example, in the case of b2 (a potential acidosis), both the rate and depth of breathing are increased to remove more carbon dioxide (a source of acid) from the body to correct the potential acidosis. (Note: The graph demonstrates that the re-establishment of body fluid pH is beyond the capabilities of the intermediate regulators, since homeostatic disturbances of body fluid pH are still evident [c_1/c_2])

c_1/c_2 = The long-term regulators of the renal system are alerted in an attempt to re-establish pH homeostasis. See text for details. For example, in the case of b_2 (a potential acidosis) the rate of excretion of hydrogen ions by the kidneys is increased in an attempt to re-establish pH homeostasis. [Note: The graph demonstrates that the re-establishment of body fluid pH is beyond the capabilities of the renal regulators, since homeostatic imbalances of body fluid pH are still evident (d_1/d_2)]

d_1 = Alkalosis

d_2 = Acidosis

e_1/e_2 = Clinical intervention to re-establish the patient's pH homeostasis of body fluids

f_1/f_2 = Death due to uncontrolled extreme alkalosis and acidosis

Figure 6.5 Summary of the regulators of acid-base homeostasis. Note that acid–base homeostatic range corresponds to the normal variation in hydrogen ion concentration that reflects the pH range necessary for optimal enzyme activity in a healthy individual. Reproduced, with permission, from J. Clancy and A.J. McVicar (2007), Intermediate and long term regulation of acid–base homeostasis, *British Journal of Nursing* **16**(17): 1076–9

discussed in this article are not fully understood. The following key points are an extraction from that paper:

- Large increase in PCO_2 (partial pressure, approximately 4.5–6 kPa) makes the patient acidotic through the generation of carbonic acid.
- Insufficient PCO_2 makes the patient alkalotic through a deficiency of carbonic acid.
- Large increase in HCO_3^- (normally approximately 22–26 mmol/L) makes the patient alkalotic through an excess of buffer.
- Insufficient HCO_3^- makes the patient acidotic through a deficiency of buffer.
- If the level of PCO_2 is causing the problem, it is respiratory in nature.
- If the level of HCO_3^- is causing the problem, it is metabolic in nature.

USE OF INFUSATES IN PRACTICE TO SUPPORT BODY FLUID COMPARTMENTS

The infusates used to support body fluids can be divided into those that are colloids, those that are crystalloids, and those that are blood cell preparations. Blood cell preparations are not considered here; their uses are self-explanatory and are noted in Chapter 11. This section only provides an overview of the common colloidal and crystalloid infusates, primarily to relate their use to the discussion in this Chapter.

See the case study of a 25-year-old man undergoing emergency surgery, Section VI, p.639.

Colloidal infusates: plasma expanders

A colloid is a substance that forms a viscous consistency with water. Colloidal infusates may be of protein (e.g. Gelofusine) or carbohydrate (e.g. dextran). Both types can be used to replace plasma protein when it is very deficient and this will restore to normal the osmotic pressure owing to colloids in plasma. This helps to restore fluid exchange in the tissues while the production of plasma proteins recovers, and the use of colloid infusions, therefore, is to support the plasma subcompartment of the extracellular fluids. Protein infusions are more effective than dextrans but carry a higher risk of inducing an immune response.

Crystalloid infusates

These infusates dissolve in water and are used to support the extracellular and/or intracellular fluids, according to need, including the level of osmotic potential required:

- *Isotonic infusates*: remember that osmosis relates to a concentration gradient and not upon individual types of solute: solutions may have the same overall solute concentration and so have the same osmotic properties. The osmotic potential of these solutions is the same as that of the body fluids themselves. Cells suspended in any of them will not show a change in their state of hydration, at least not initially (dextrose is the exception as cell hydration will gradually increase when the glucose is utilized – see below). Thus, the solutions noted are

---

BOX 6.14 INTRAVENOUS THERAPY

Access to the vascular compartment must be made aseptically to prevent the introduction of infectious agents. The access is normally through:

- Peripheral venepuncture in which a needle is inserted through the skin into a superficial vein, often in the hand or arm, and connected to a catheter tubing. A 'butterfly' needle is often used because the flanges can be taped to the skin and so keep the needle *in situ*. The purpose of the catheter is to facilitate regular blood sampling, to infuse a medication, to commence fluid therapy or to administer radio-opaque/radioactive material.
- Insertion of a large-bore catheter into a major vein, normally a subclavian vein, internal jugular vein or femoral vein. Such catheters enable the measurement of central venous pressure or to deliver large volumes of fluids or viscous fluids as are used in total parenteral nutrition.

Infusates may be administered using a bag/drip feed method in which gravity and blood flow at the needle tip encourage the addition of fluid to blood at the needle tip, or via a pump (syringe driver).
Complications (see Biswas, 2007) may arise from:

- Phlebitis, which is a redness and swelling of skin at the site of venepuncture. Irritation or pain is usually present. The inflammation represents a defence response to infection, the chemicals being delivered into the vein or to the needle/catheter material. Apart from being unpleasant for the patient, phlebitis also raises the risk of blood clotting (thrombophlebitis) at the needle tip sufficient to cause an embolus.
- Extravasation because the needle tip has exited through the wall of the vein, leading to infusate delivery into the surrounding tissue, resulting in swelling (i.e. oedema) and pallor as blood flow to the area is compromised.
- Blockage, either at the tip of the needle (protein deposition, blood clot or compression of tissue against it) or through a kink in the catheter tubing.

---

said to be isotonic ('iso-' = same) to body fluids.

- *Hypertonic infusates*: these solutions have an osmotic potential that is greater than that of body fluids. Thus, cells suspended in them will shrink as water is lost by osmosis. Such infusates are not as widely used as isotonic ones but do have a value in practice where there is excessive intracellular hydration, or to promote water movement from a transcellular fluid.
- *Hypotonic infusates*: hypotonic infusates are rarely used because these infusates have an osmotic potential less than that of body fluids and so cells will take in water rapidly by osmosis, resulting in cell swelling, and even lysis. A 5% dextrose solution provides a means of slowly improving cell hydration and so reduces the risks of cell swelling, and is a preferred means of promoting cell hydration (see below).

Various solutions are used as infusates in practice (see also Table 6.3).

Saline (sodium chloride solution)

Sodium chloride is found predominantly within the extracellular fluid, and so this infusate largely supports that compartment. The most widely used saline is 'normal' or 'isotonic' saline (0.85% sodium chloride solution; i.e. 0.85 g per 100 mL). This has an osmotic pressure similar to that of body fluids and so water in the infusion will not move into cells in any quantity. In some circumstances 'hypertonic' saline

Table 6.3 Composition of crystalloid infusates (in mmol/L)

	Na$^+$	Cl$^-$	K$^+$	Ca^{2+}	Lactate
5% dextrose	0	0	0	0	0
0.9% saline	153	153	0	0	0
Hartmann's (lactated Ringer's) solution	131	111	5	2	29

may be used (e.g. 2.5% sodium chloride solution) to raise the osmotic pressure of extracellular fluids and so cause the withdrawal of water out of cells by osmosis.

Dextrose

This is a solution of glucose. It is usually administered as an isotonic solution (5%; i.e. 5 g per 100 mL) and so might not be expected to promote water movement in or out of cells. However, unlike saline, the glucose will gradually be taken up by cells and utilized, effectively leaving water behind. The loss of solute means that water can now pass into cells by osmosis, thus helping to hydrate the intracellular fluid. Nevertheless, 5% dextrose should be viewed essentially as an isotonic infusate.

Dextrose/saline

This isotonic infusate combines the advantages of both saline and dextrose in that cell hydration is slowly promoted (by the dextrose component) but the saline component also helps to ensure that some of the infusion remains within the extracellular compartment.

Hartmann's solution

Hartmann's solution provides a more comprehensive support for extracellular fluid than just saline alone. It is sometimes referred to as a 'lactated Ringer's' solution. A Ringer's solution is one that is isotonic and has an electrolyte composition that closely matches extracellular fluid: Hartmann's solution approximates to human extracellular fluid except that it contains lactate rather than bicarbonate ions. The lactate ions are converted to bicarbonate by the liver and so bicarbonate is added to blood, but it is added at a much slower rate than if it was in the infusate. This helps to reduce the likelihood of bicarbonate overload.

Potassium

Potassium chloride solution may occasionally be infused to quickly increase the potassium concentration in blood plasma. However, infusion runs the risk of inducing potassium overload if it is administered quickly, and so this infusate is not widely used in general settings. If it is required, potassium support is usually provided by the potassium in Hartmann's solution, or by potassium in combination with saline or glucose, in which the potassium concentration is close to the normal values for extracellular fluid and onset of hyperkalaemia therefore unlikely. Injections of a bolus of solution that has a high concentration of potassium chloride may be used in cardiac units in order to stimulate the heart.

SUMMARY

1 Body fluids are subdivided into the extracellular and intracellular compartments.

2 The extracellular fluid is composed of blood plasma, the interstitial fluid and transcellular fluids. Transcellular fluids are secreted by specialized epithelia and therefore have a different ionic composition from that of the rest of the extracellular fluid.

3 Blood plasma and interstitial fluid have very similar compositions because interstitial fluid is continually being formed from plasma, and returned to it, in the capillary beds of tissues. Pores in the blood vessels are sufficiently large to allow passage of water and the majority of solutes, except plasma proteins.

4 Normal cell function, appropriate for the tissue in which it is found, requires the rigorous regulation of all the processes that take place. Ions play a central role in determining cell function and part of homeostatic regulation requires a control of the intracellular ionic environment.

5 Intracellular fluids and the interstitial fluid are separated by the cell membrane. The properties of this lipid membrane enable cells to have different ionic compositions from the surrounding fluid.

6 Although the maintenance of cell membrane functions helps to regulate intracellular fluid composition, the intracellular environment, and cellular volume are also influenced by the extracellular fluid composition. The regulation of extracellular fluid composition and volume helps to stabilize cell membrane activities, and is also necessary to ensure that chemical processes occurring in this fluid progress efficiently.

7 An important aspect of water and ionic regulation is that a balance between input and output (excretion) is maintained. Much of the regulatory process involves the control of urinary excretion of ions and water. Detection of an imbalance involves specialized receptors that respond to aspects specific to the actions of the electrolyte concerned.

8 The input–output equation becomes more complex when the substance concerned is produced by the body itself. The regulation of body fluid acidity and alkalinity (pH) is a complicated interaction between the production of hydrogen ions by metabolism, the removal of these ions out of solution by 'buffer' chemicals' and ultimately the excretion of the hydrogen ions by the kidneys, or excretion of a major source of hydrogen ions, carbon dioxide, by the lungs.

9 Disturbances in fluid and electrolyte balance are commonplace, both in day-to-day living (relatively minor since diets and homeostatic changes in renal function rapidly correct the imbalance) and clinically (potentially severe).

10 Clinical therapies frequently entail the infusion of fluids to support body fluid volume and composition.

11 Infusates include blood cells, plasma, crystalloids (e.g. saline or glucose) and colloids (to support plasma volume). There is a variety of crystalloid infusates, and the choice is determined by the disturbance and, in particular, to the fluid compartment that requires most support.

REFERENCES

Allen, K. (2004) Four step method of interpreting arterial blood gas analysis. *Nursing Times* **101**(1): 42–5.

Biswas, J. (2007) Clinical audit documenting insertion date of peripheral intravenous cannulae. *British Journal of Nursing* **16**(5): 281–2.

Clancy, J. and McVicar, A. (2007a) Short-term regulation of acid-base homeostasis of body fluids. *British Journal of Nursing* **16**(16): 1016–21.

Clancy, J. and McVicar, A. (2007b) Intermediate and long-term regulation of acid–base homeostasis. *British Journal of Nursing* **16**(17): 1076–9.

Coombs, M. (2001) Making sense of arterial blood gases. *Nursing Times* **97**(27): 36–9.

Lynes, D. (2003) An introduction to blood gases. *Nursing Times* **99**(11): 54–5.

Woodrow, P. (2004) Arterial blood gas analysis. *Nursing Standard* **18**(21): 45–52.

SECTION III

SENSING CHANGE AND COORDINATING RESPONSES

THE SENSES

INTRODUCTION

Chapter 1 identified that homeostasis is a concept that was derived in relation to the maintenance of the internal environment of the body, and how that is important to health and well-being, but also acknowledged the dynamic nature of the processes involved because that environment is under continuous challenge from the external environment. For homeostasis to be effective, therefore, the body must be able to detect internal and external changes if there is to be a corrective or adaptive response. In other words there must be a 'sensory system' that is able to detect the diverse range of stimuli that have an impact on the body, and 'control' and 'effector systems' that can produce a breadth of responses necessary to ensure that the internal environment remains optimal.

Sense or perception?

Strictly speaking, the body receives information regarding its internal and external environments via our 'senses'. This term is often equated with 'sensation' or 'perception', for example that of sound or touch, but it is important to note that these terms refer to our capacity to be consciously aware of a change to some aspect of our environment whereas this is not the case for all of our senses. While a sense such as pain must be perceived to provide us with the information that tissues have been damaged or are threatened, being continually aware of what is happening to body fluid composition, blood pressure or body temperature would not be practical in normal life, except when the changes are extreme and require conscious action.

Our senses require the presence of receptors. These are found throughout the body, and range in structure from complex cells, such as those of the retina of the eye, to 'simple' surface molecules such as are found on the cell membrane within synapses at nerve cell junctions, or on cells that are the targets for hormones. Synapses, and hormone actions, are described in Chapters 8 and 9. Similarly, receptors that support many of the self-regulating processes involved in homeostasis are also considered elsewhere; for example the role of receptors in maintaining water homeostasis is recognized in Chapters 6 and 15. Consequently, this chapter only explains some of the general principles involved, and the classification used, but does

---

BOX 7.1 CONSCIOUSNESS

Arousal, say from sleep, commences when neural activity from the brainstem 'wakes up' the rest of the brain, especially the cerebral cortex (see Chapter 8, p.194). Consciousness, however, implies something beyond this: a capacity of the brain to make us 'aware'. The fundamental need for neurological interpretation of sensory information if an individual is to be 'conscious' has implications during surgery when consciousness and arousal are inhibited by general anaesthesia or brain injury.

From a sensory viewpoint, 'consciousness' means that we can consciously perceive our environment and interpret it in a meaningful way. How this interpretation of sensory information occurs continues to elude science, and provides a distinction between physiology and psychology. The use of radioactively labelled markers, such as glucose, is now providing insight into the neurological changes that accompany 'thinking', but how a pattern of neural activity is translated into a mental image remains unknown.

Coma appears to represent a failure of consciousness; comatose individuals show no apparent recognition of sensory input (although input from, say, the lungs that does not entail 'awareness' may still be operative). Interestingly, triggering memory through the use of familiar sounds or voices has sometimes been successful in reversing the coma.

BOX 7.2 THE SENSES IN HOLISTIC PRINCIPLES OF HEALTH

The task of incorporating physiological processes into a framework based on holistic principles of health can at times present a challenge (see Chapter 1, p.10). This is especially the case when attempting to place systemic functioning into the context of psychosocial interaction. Understanding the senses can provide insights into the holistic nature of health (and health care) since it is our senses that provide us with the image of our world. This image is constructed by the brain according to the information it receives, but if we consider those senses that are 'translated' into a mental, conscious perception then the image will also be influenced by the context in which it was received. Our senses provide the links with our environment, especially the social environment, and so the contextualization of stimuli, based on experiences, is an important aspect of subjectivity and individuality. Recognizing this provides the means by which the psychosocial and physical aspects of health can be integrated and applied to individualized care (see Chapter 20 onwards).

ACTIVITY

The individuality of perceptions is sometimes difficult to comprehend; for example, we all 'know' what colour is. However, as a simple exercise, try explaining to a friend what the colour red is. In doing so note how often you need to resort to the use of examples, rather than identifying exactly what the colour is. How can you be sure that your image of a red bus is exactly the same as that of your friend? How might you explain to someone who has never seen the colour red before just what it is (this is a hypothetical situation but an interesting exercise nonetheless!)?

not explore the physiology of these senses any further. Much of the chapter encompasses those senses referred to as the 'special senses', the functions of which mainly relate to the monitoring of the external environment.

RECEPTORS AND THEIR ROLES

Sense receptors and sensory modalities

The sensing of environmental change normally requires the presence of specialized receptor cells sensitive to a specific stimulus. For example, dehydration causes a rise in the osmotic pressure of plasma and this is detected by cells that are sensitive to the resultant change in volume of fluid within them. Dehydration is unlikely to be a localized occurrence – in this example the detected change would be indicative of an alteration in osmotic pressure throughout the body. The receptors therefore need only be located in an appropriate position; osmotic receptors are located within the hypothalamus, close to the pituitary gland that secretes the hormone responsible for altering kidney function when we are dehydrated. In contrast, sensing touch at the fingertips conveys absolutely no information of, for example, what is happening to our feet! Touch receptors therefore must be distributed about the body.

The specific type of stimulus detected by a receptor is called its modality (= mode or kind), for example touch, pressure or temperature. Many of our receptors are unimodal ('uni-' = one), that is, they are so specific that they are able to detect an individual modality, such as osmotic pressure, and their responses, therefore, only relate to the intensity of stimulation. Some receptors are bimodal; for example the joint receptors involved in movement control can detect the degree of movement of the joint (an intensity mode) and the rate of change of that movement (i.e. its acceleration). Other receptors are referred to as being polymodal ('poly-' = many) and can detect very complex stimuli. For example:

- vision involves the detection of the intensity of light (brightness) and also its wavelength (colour vision);
- hearing involves the detection of sound intensity (loudness) and also frequency (tones);
- both smell and taste involve the detection of chemical intensity (concentration) and also type (for example, pungent, floral or acrid smells, and sweet, sour or salty tastes).

These senses are accorded the term 'special' senses. Their complexity is such that their receptors are organized into anatomical features recognizable as sense organs: the eye, ear, nose and tongue. Pain, too, is polymodal in that it has qualities of both intensity and type (throbbing, aching or stabbing, sharp), and some texts include this as a 'special' sense, although there are no specific sense 'organs' as such for pain. In recognition of the particular relevance of pain to healthcare professions, this 'sense' has been placed into a separate chapter (Chapter 20) and only brief mention of it will be made in this one.

The special senses provide another contrast to other senses in that most receptors can only provide information of the occurrence of an event (a change to the body) while the special senses provide a predictive capability. For example, touch indicates contact, while the stimulation of osmotic receptors mentioned earlier indicates that a change in water balance has already occurred. However, receptors for vision, hearing and smell all provide information on circumstances or changes that may be operative some distance from the body, and so enable a cognitive assessment as to their likely impact on the body before the event. Similarly, perceiving an unpleasant taste allows us to reject a substance from our mouth that could perhaps be injurious to the body, and pain provides us with a warning that further tissue damage will ensue unless we respond to its cause. Thus, the information provided by our special senses enable us to take measures if necessary and so either prevent a disturbance in homeostasis, or at least minimize it – or perhaps even to encourage it if it is likely to be desirable!

General characteristics of receptors

Transduction

Receptors associated with the sensory nervous system are transducers: they convert the stimulus into an alternative form by altering the electrical properties of the cell membrane of the receptor. This is achieved by an alteration in the distribution of electrolytes between the intracellular and extracellular fluids. The distribution of some types of ions across cell membranes is not equal and, consequently, there is ordinarily a slight difference in the number of negative and positive charges on each side of cell membranes causing them to exhibit a voltage difference (called a resting electrical potential), with the inside of the cell being negative with respect to the outside (see Chapter 8, p.186 for more details). Receptor cells and other excitable cells, such as nerve and muscle cells, have the capacity to change the permeability of their membranes to certain ions (usually sodium or potassium), leading to their movement into or out of the cell, and a subsequent change in the voltage. Such changes are called generator potentials and their rate of production relates to the degree of stimulation.

Generator potentials occur extremely rapidly and, when added together (called 'summation'), may meet or exceed a 'threshold' level and trigger events within the receptor cell. Depending upon the type of receptor, these may, for example,

BOX 7.3 FACTORS THAT INFLUENCE RECEPTOR SENSITIVITY

The threshold of stimulation that is required to stimulate receptors, and hence determines their sensitivity to stimuli, alters with age and some conditions that affect peripheral nerve cells, such as diabetes mellitus. In these instances the sensory nervous system is less efficient at detecting change in the internal or external environment, leading to increased homeostatic disturbance. For example, diminished receptor sensitivity (and receptor number) probably has a role in the reduced efficiency of the regulation of blood pressure in elderly people, and in the reduced tactile senses in people with diabetes.

promote the release of a hormone by a gland cell, or perhaps generate further electrical changes (called action potentials) in sensory nerve cells associated with the receptor, for example a touch receptor in the skin. The threshold level for a specific stimulus determines the sensitivity of the receptor and so is a factor in the efficiency of homeostatic control. Thus, receptors will have a low threshold in the homeostatic regulation of those parameters that have narrow homeostatic ranges.

Receptor fields

Sensory receptors may be discrete cells (e.g. in the retina of the eye) or nerve endings (e.g. touch receptors in the skin). Those that are nerve endings may be extensively branched and extend over an area called a receptor field. Some receptor fields are large, others small: the smaller the field the greater our ability to 'place' the stimulus (Figure 7.1). For example, the points of a pair of compasses applied to the fingertips can be discerned as two distinct points even when they are only about 1.5 mm apart. This is because the fingertips have a high receptor density with small receptor fields in which the stimulus is detected by more than one receptor even when the points are close together. On the back, however, the two points are only separately discerned when some 35–40 mm apart. This is because the receptor density is less and the field for each receptor is large, and so when the two points are close together they actually stimulate nerve endings from the same nerve cell (i.e. just the one receptor) and so cannot be discerned as two stimuli.

Adaptation

Receptors of many senses exhibit a decreasing sensitivity in response to continued stimulation, even though the stimulus is still present. Touch is a typical example: life would be very unpleasant if we were to be constantly distracted by being aware of contact with our clothes, with chairs, with the ground, or with spectacles, etc. In these instances, once the stimulus has been received, and perhaps acted upon, it becomes more important to detect a new change rather than to remain aware of the 'safe' old one. Thus, these types of receptors adapt to the new stimulus and so can respond again if the stimulus changes.

Receptors may be 'slow-adapting' (referred to as tonic) or 'rapid-adapting' (or phasic). The former tend to be those receptors that provide information regarding relatively steady

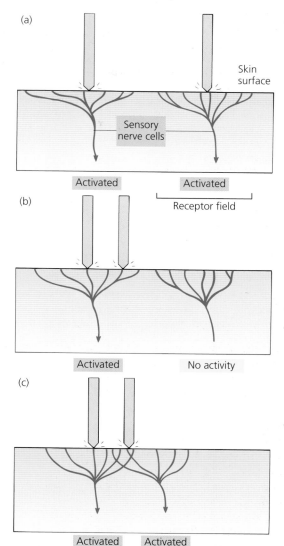

Figure 7.1 Two-point discrimination. In (a) the two points are in contact with two receptor fields and so will be detected by each of the two neurons. In (b) the points are too close together to be discriminated as both are in contact with the same receptor field, and hence neuron. In (c) the overlapping receptor fields helps to discriminate two points even when the contacts are close together as both neurons are activated but one possibly more than the other

Q Give an example where two-point discrimination is (1) excellent; (2) poor.

states of the body, such as blood composition and body position, which change relatively slowly. Rapidly adapting receptors are important if states can change rapidly since they may convey moment-to-moment information regarding changes in the stimulus. For example, receptors in our skeletal joints not only provide information that the joint has been flexed but also how rapidly it was flexed (i.e. its velocity). This is essential if movement is to be controlled (see Chapter 17).

Overview of the types of receptor in the body

Receptors are sometimes referred to according to their location. This is usually a collective term, however, and does not distinguish receptor type. For example 'cutaneous' receptors are those found in the skin, while 'visceroreceptors' are those found in the viscera or internal organs of the body. A more usual means of classification relates to the kind of stimulus the receptors detect.

Mechanoreceptors

Mechanoreceptors are sensitive to mechanical deformation and include receptors of touch, pressure, vibration and stretch. They are relatively simple in structure consisting of the terminals of sensory nerve cells, which are either 'free' or are encapsulated. These receptors include touch receptors, proprioreceptors and auditory receptors.

Touch receptors

- *Merkel's discs*: disc-like arrangements of 'free' nerve terminals in contact with epidermal cells in the skin, that respond to touch.
- *Meissner's capsules* are egg-shaped structures in the dermis of the skin (i.e. deeper than Merkel's discs) containing nerve terminals that also respond to touch.
- *Pacinian corpuscles* are oval structures distinguished by their concentric onion-like layers of connective tissue. Nerve terminals are found within the layers. They are pressure receptors (from sustained touch) and are located in deep subcutaneous tissues, in submucosa tissue, in tissue around joints and in mammary glands.
- *Root hair plexus*: 'free' nerve endings are wrapped around the base of a hair root and respond to deformation induced by movement of the hair shaft when it is touched or if there is a breeze.

Proprioreceptors

Proprioreceptors are a group of various receptors involved in the control of posture and movement ('proprio-' = position).

- *Muscle spindles*: stretch receptors that contain nerve endings in contact with modified skeletal muscle fibres. They respond to changes in muscle length and have a crucial role in the control of muscle contraction (see Chapter 17, p.476).
- *Golgi tendon organs*: also stretch receptors within the tendons and monitor the tension induced when the attached muscle contracts. They seem to have a protective role and cause muscle contraction to suddenly cease (i.e. 'give way') if the tension threatens injury.
- *Joint receptors*: provide information about the position of the joint and also about how rapidly the position is changing during movement. They consist of nerve endings associated with connective tissue within the joint.
- *The vestibular apparatus of the inner ear*: includes three semicircular canals attached to a distended structure called the vestibule (Figure 7.2). The base of each canal connects with the vestibule via a distended region called an ampulla within which are found the receptor cells, the hair-like cilia of which are embedded in a gel projection called the cupula.

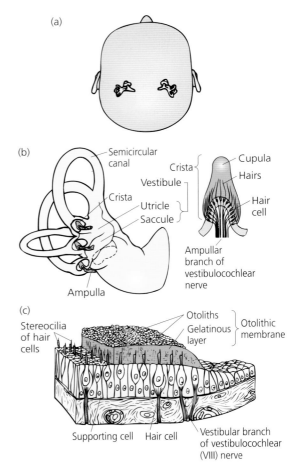

Figure 7.2 The vestibular apparatus of the inner ear. (a) Relative position within the head. (b) The vestibular structures – utricle, saccule and semicircular canals; an enlarged crista is shown. Details of the utricle and saccule are shown in (c). See text for explanation

Q The receptor cells are often referred to as hair cells. Why?

Movement of the head causes fluid to flow within the canals, and this deflects the cupulae and so stimulates the receptor cells, thus providing information that the head has moved. The vestibule itself contains two sac-like areas called the utricle and saccule (Figure 7.2), both of which also contain receptor cells. These also have hair-like cilia projecting into a membrane; on the surface of this gel-like membrane lie small crystals of calcium carbonate called otoliths ('oto-' = ear, '-liths' = stones) which slide over the surface of the membrane when the head is moved. This distorts the projections of the receptor cells and stimulates them.

Auditory receptors

These are described later, but basically respond to a distortion produced by pressure waves in the fluid of the inner ear.

Thermoreceptors

Thermoreceptors are 'free' nerve endings that have properties that enable them to respond to fluctuations in temperature. There are 'hot' and 'cold' receptors that respond to different temperature ranges, although the ranges overlap. Together they provide information over a range of skin temperatures.

Chemoreceptors

Chemoreceptors are sensitive to changes in the concentration of chemicals within the body fluids. This is a diverse range of receptors, where the cells have surface chemicals that specifically interact with the substance to be monitored. When activated these sensory cells may:

- be sensory nerve cells, that are stimulated directly by the substance(s) concerned – taste and smell (described later) are examples;
- promote electrical activity in sensory nerve cells that are associated with the receptor cell, as in the detection of increased blood acidity by the carotid bodies;
- promote the release of a hormone from the receptor cell itself, which therefore is a gland cell, as in the release of aldosterone from the adrenal cortex when blood potassium is elevated, or the release of insulin from pancreatic beta-cells when blood glucose concentration is elevated.

Nocireceptors

Nocireceptors (or nociceptors) are responsive to noxious stimuli. Nociceptors are usually referred to in relation to pain, and are still not fully understood. They seem to be free nerve endings, some of which at least are sensitive to chemicals released from damaged cells in the vicinity. However, others appear to be those of other senses, such as touch or temperature, which convey an unpleasant sensation when stimulated excessively.

Photoreceptors

Photoreceptors are sensitive to light. These are cells of the retina of the eye and their details are provided in a later section.

Interpretation of receptor activity

Overview

Electrical activity generated by receptors associated with sensory nerves is conducted to the central nervous system (i.e. spinal cord and brain). Within the brain, it is integrated, coordinated and, if appropriate, interpreted as a conscious perception of the stimulus. The pathway along which sensory information travels is generally:

Receptor ⟶ Transmission ⟶ Interpretation
(sensory nerve/ (cerebral cortex
thalamus of brain) of brain)

This plan is very simplistic, however, and other pathways involve other parts of the brain before activity enters the thalamus. Similarly, information may be transmitted to parts of the brain other than the cerebral cortex, such as the cerebellum (involved in movement control; see Chapter 17), and may not always involve transmission through the thalamus, although this usually is the case. Even processing may not involve the brain, with the information being integrated by the spinal cord. Details of some of the major sensory pathways are pro-vided in the next subsection. The reader may find it useful to cross-reference with anatomical details of the central nervous system provided in Chapter 8, especially of the thalamus, cerebral cortex and cerebellum.

Sensory pathways

Sensory activity from peripheral receptors enters the grey matter within the spinal cord via the 'dorsal roots' of the spinal nerves (Figure 7.3). There some of the nerve cells synapse (interact) with others that ascend the cord to the brain. Some of these ascending nerve cells are found in the lateral (side) and anterior (front) aspects of the spinal cord and pass directly to the thalamus within the brain. Accordingly these pathways are called the lateral and anterior spinothalamic tracts, respectively. The tracts carry discrete sensory information: in general the lateral tract conveys information from nociceptors and thermoreceptors, while the anterior tracts carry information from touch and pressure receptors in the skin. One feature of these tracts is that the neurons within the cord that are stimulated by incoming sensory nerve cells actually cross over to the other side of the cord before passing to the thalamus. In this way, information from receptors on one side of the body passes to the opposite side of the brain.

In contrast, those sensory nerve cells that carry activity from touch receptors in deeper tissues, and from proprioreceptors (especially those in joints), do not synapse immediately within the cord. Rather they turn and ascend the spinal cord themselves, passing up the posterior (rear) aspects of the cord (Figure 7.3; note that a sensory nerve cell passing from our toes to the brain must therefore have a length of about 1.5–2 m). Accordingly, these pathways involve posterior spinothalamic tracts; these are actually observable as surface features on the cord and are called dorsal columns. The nerve cells eventually interact with clusters of nerve cells within the brainstem, called the dorsal column nuclei, the fibres of which then cross over to the other side and then pass to the thalamus, and thence to other brain areas, particularly the cerebral cortex. As with the other spinothalamic tracts, the crossing over of neurons within the brainstem means that the left side of the brain receives information from the right side of the body and vice versa.

Proprioreceptor activity from muscles may also ascend via the posterior spinocerebellar tract (which therefore lies in a posterior aspect and passes to the cerebellum at the back of the brain) of the spinal cord. The role of these receptors and the cerebellum in relation to the control of posture and movement are discussed in Chapter 17.

BOX 7.4 SPINAL CORD NERVE BLOCKS

The ascending sensory nerve tracts in the spinal cord are relatively superficial, and the sensory nerve cells within them clustered together. For nociceptors (pain) this arrangement is very useful because epidural or intraspinal analgesic drugs can be administered very close to their position in the lateral spinothalamic tracts of the spinal cord, producing effective nerve block and hence preventing onward transmission of pain signals to the brain (see Figure 20.1, p.562).

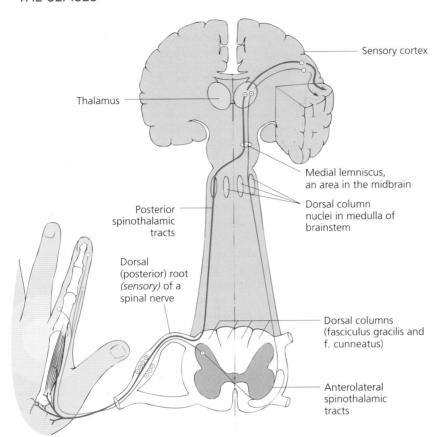

Figure 7.3 Routes of transmission from sensory receptors to the sensory cortex: the spinothalamic tracts

Labels in figure:
- Sensory cortex
- Thalamus
- Medial lemniscus, an area in the midbrain
- Dorsal column nuclei in medulla of brainstem
- Posterior spinothalamic tracts
- Dorsal (posterior) root *(sensory)* of a spinal nerve
- Dorsal columns (fasciculus gracilis and f. cunneatus)
- Anterolateral spinothalamic tracts

BOX 7.5 CROSSOVER OF NERVE TRACTS

The text identifies the major sensory tracts of nerve cells within the spinal cord: the lateral and anterior spinothalamic tracts and the posterior spinothalamic tracts, or dorsal columns. A feature of these is that all are paired tracts, with one passing up one side of the cord, one the other. Another feature is that all 'cross over' at some stage to the opposite side of the brain. Similarly, 'motor' nerve cells (that activate tissues such as muscles and glandular tissues) also pass down the cord in tracts, again crossing over. Thus, one side of the brain receives information from the opposite side of the body, and sends nerve activity to that side. This is the reason why a severe stroke localized to one side of the brain can produce profound effects on muscle activity on one side of the body, whilst the other is little affected.

The special senses of vision, hearing, smell and taste are in the head and so electrical activity does not pass via the spinal cord but goes direct into brain tissue via cranial nerves. The activity either passes directly to the thalamus, and thence to the cerebral cortex, or passes via other parts of the brain particularly within the brainstem and hypothalamus, and so may miss out the thalamus entirely.

THE SPECIAL SENSES

This section considers in detail the anatomy and physiology of the 'special' senses of vision, hearing, taste and smell. The pre-

dictive element of the special senses was described earlier and has obvious advantages in the course and planning of actions, the consequences of which are that the internal environment is more likely to be optimal if challenging or threatening situations can be avoided. The special senses facilitate our capacity to operate in the range of environments with which we come into contact each day, and help us to maintain independence of our actions. In so doing it could also be said that these senses play a role in our social and psychological well-being, in addition to the maintenance of physiological homeostasis.

Vision

Overview

Vision requires the detection of light; the receptor cells of the eye contain chemicals – referred to as visual pigments – which absorb light and consequently break down into component molecules that activate the cell membrane of the receptor, and in turn stimulates action potentials in associated sensory nerve cells. The pigment chemical then reforms. In intense light the pigment quickly breaks down again, repeating the process.

The ratio of undissociated to dissociated pigment provides a means of monitoring light intensity (brightness), while having different pigments that respond optimally to certain wavelengths provide a means of detecting colour. Light receptors therefore respond to light within the relatively narrow range of wavelengths determined by the pigments present. This is why we cannot see light at the extreme ends of the spectrum (infrared or ultraviolet light) without the use of aids to convert it into the visible range (e.g. night-vision monitors).

The process of vision is summarized thus:

Light → Receptor → Associated → Transmission → Interpretation
　　　　(retina)　　 nerve cell 　(optic nerve/　 (cerebral
　　　　　　　　　　　　　　　　　 thalamus 　　　 cortex
　　　　　　　　　　　　　　　　　 of brain)　　　 of brain)

General anatomy and of the eye

The eye is basically a sense organ that focuses light waves onto the receptor cells, but with the capacity to adjust the amount of light incident on the receptor region. Its anatomy is related to these functions.

The eye is approximately spherical, with a white-coloured, fibrous, protective and supportive layer called the sclera. At the front of the eye the sclera is considerably thinner and becomes the delicate and transparent cornea. A thin layer of modified skin, the conjunctiva, extends from the eyelids to the sclera surrounding the cornea (Figure 7.4a) and this helps to protect the lining within the socket. Laterally the sclera is attached to the bone of the orbit of the skull by six extrinsic muscles that produce lateral and vertical movement of the eye upon their contraction or relaxation. The muscles are controlled by the oculomotor and trochlear nerves (cranial nerves III and IV: see Figure 8.5, p.167). The optic nerve carries sensory activity from the retina, and exits the rear of the eye where the nerve sheath fuses with the sclera.

Lubrication of the sclera and, in particular, the cornea is provided by secretions from the lachrymal or tear gland found at the top outer area of each eye. Secretions drain into the nasal cavity via the lachrymal duct that originates at the inner corner of each eye, and explains why our noses seem to fill when we are tearful. Tears also provide a means of irrigating the eye when an irritant is present.

Below the sclera lies a vascular layer called the choroid, which provides it with nutrients. The choroid extends from

BOX 7.6 STRABISMUS AND NYSTAGMUS

Strabismus is a condition in which an eye drifts from position when the gaze is focused on an object. Often referred to as 'lazy eye' it arises because of an imbalance in control of the ocular muscles. The eye must be trained by covering the normal eye at times, making the other eye dominate the vision.

Nystagmus is a rhythmic movement of the eyes, producing a flickering effect. Nystagmus may be caused by an incorrect conditioning of this reflex, in which case it is usually present from childhood. However, nystagmus can also suggest the occurrence of neurological disturbance or drug abuse.

A flicking movement can also be stimulated by a sudden change in the stimulation of the vestibular or balance apparatus of the ear (called a vestibular–ocular reflex). This is thought normally to operate when the head is turned suddenly, thus keeping the eyes facing forward. However, excessive stimulation, such as that produced by a revolving chair or a fairground ride, may cause a rhythmic flickering to occur. This can look alarming but is not harmful and lasts for only a few seconds.

BOX 7.7. CONJUNCTIVITIS

Conjunctivitis is an inflammation of the conjunctiva caused by an infection or by the presence of irritants (Mead, 2000). Antibiotic creams may be administered. Eyewashes might also be used, although the possibility of cross-infection to other individuals, or to the other eye, means that they must be used with caution.

the rear of the eye to the ciliary body, which in turn forms the iris (Figure 7.4b). The lens is suspended from the ciliary body by the suspensory ligaments, and the ciliary body also contains smooth muscle cells capable of altering the shape of the lens. Lying within the choroid are nerves of the parasympathetic and sympathetic branches of the nervous system that control lens shape (for focusing) and enter the iris to alter the aperture (to increase or decrease the amount of light entering the eye).

The inner coat of much of the eye consists of the light-sensitive retina. This extends from the ciliary body around the inner surface of the rear of the eye and it is in this layer that the light receptor cells – the rods and cones – are found. The retina also has its own nerve cells associated with the receptor cells, and aid in processing of the information before it is passed on into the optic nerve. The receptors are considered in more detail below. Two features worth mentioning here are that the inner surface of the retina contains the blood vessels that maintain the layer, and that the exit point of the optic nerve (called the optic disc) is devoid of receptors, and so is called the blind spot. The presence of blood vessels on the retina surface clearly does not affect our capacity to see, but is useful clinically as it allows the vessels to be observed (Box 7.8) for signs of disorder. Ideally, light must not be focused on the optic disc as the lack of receptors there will impair vision. Not surprisingly the 'blind spot' is off-centre and incident light largely avoids it. In addition, the light from an object that does fall onto the blind spot in one eye will fall elsewhere on the retina of the other eye.

BOX 7.8 OBSERVING THE RETINA

Observing the retinal blood vessels, using an ophthalmoscope, is an important clinical aid in the diagnosis of, for example, cerebral hypertension. This is because any distension of a blood vessel produced by a higher than normal blood pressure within the eye will compress any vessels passing immediately below it. Such compressions can be observed. Diabetes mellitus also has an adverse effect on retinal blood vessels (Watkinson and Seewoodhary, 2008). Early signs of deterioration can be detected by observing the vessels.

Use of the ophthalmoscope entails shining a thin beam of light into the eye and peering through a lens arrangement that allows an image of the retina to be seen (Figure 7.5). This normally means that the practitioner must hold the ophthalmoscope very close to the eye, which can be a somewhat disconcerting experience for some people.

The pupillary constriction that would be anticipated by use of the light, and which would prevent observation of the retina, is prevented by the use of a drug that blocks the parasympathetic nerve endings responsible for causing the contraction of the pupil. Thus, a drug such as atropine is administered in eye-drops a short time before the investigation. Unfortunately, the effect lasts for a few hours and so patients should avoid bright lights and ideally be escorted home.

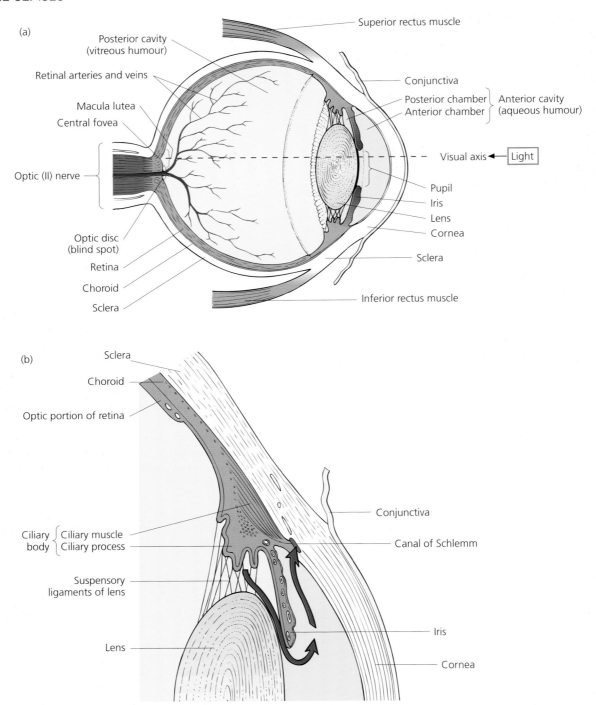

Figure 7.4 (a) General features and visual axis of the eye. (b) Enlargement to show detail of the iris, ciliary body, and the circulation of the aqueous humour

Q What is glaucoma?

In this way the brain can also compare the images from both eyes and remove any perception of a blind spot.

The lens of the eye divides the eyeball into two fluid-filled compartments (Figure 7.4a). The anterior compartment contains aqueous humour, which is a thin, watery fluid that is constantly being formed by the ciliary body and then reabsorbed by the canal of Schlemm at the base of the ciliary body. This circulation of fluid is important because the cornea and iris are devoid of blood vessels and so rely on the fluid for nutrients. The compartment behind the lens is filled with vitreous humour (literally 'glass-like'), a colourless fluid made jelly-like by the presence of small amounts of mucoprotein. This is the

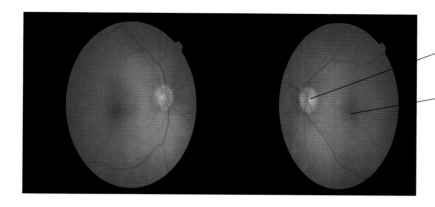

Forea ('yellow spot')

Exit of optic nerve (optic disc or 'blind spot')

Figure 7.5 The normal retina as viewed using an ophthalmoscope. Reproduced with the kind permission of the Medical Illustration Department, Norfolk and Norwich University Hospital NHS Trust. See also Figure 7.9, p.151

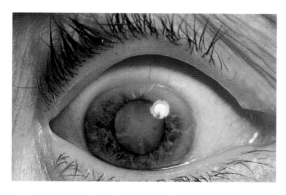

Figure 7.6 Cataract; note the milky opacity of the lens behind the pupil. Reproduced with the kind permission of Abrahams *et al.*, from *Illustrated Clinical Anatomy*, Hodder, London.

largest compartment and the fluid, once formed, cannot be replaced even if lost by injury. It facilitates light transmission without diffracting ('bending') it excessively, or diffusing it, and provides pressure within the eye that helps maintain its shape.

Light enters the eye through the cornea, passes through the lens and ultimately arrives at the receptor cells of the retina. Although widespread in the retina, the receptor cells are particularly dense at the 'yellow spot' or fovea, an area lying in line behind the lens that is devoid of blood vessels. The fovea is packed with cone receptors, which convey colour vision, although small numbers of these will also be found in other areas of the retina. Some rods will also be present in the fovea but they are mainly found outside it. Thus, the image of whatever is the centre of our attention is focused onto the fovea for high definition, colour analysis and clarity, but peripheral images can still be discerned though not in such detail.

BOX 7.9 EYE SURGERY

Techniques for eye surgery have advanced considerably in recent years especially with the advent of laser treatments.

Corneal transplantation.

The cornea does not have blood vessels and this is very useful from the point of view of corneal transplants since immune cells do not gain access and so tissue rejection presents less of a problem than elsewhere in the body. The surgery does result in the loss of some aqueous humour but this will be replaced as more is secreted from the canal of Schlemm.

Glaucoma

If the rate of secretion of aqueous humour exceeds that of its resorption then an increased humour pressure will result, called glaucoma. The presence of the lens at the rear of the cavity prevents the pressure being dissipated throughout the vitreous humour. Consequently, the cornea bulges resulting in greater diffraction ('bending') of light and hence blurred vision, especially around the edges of the image. As pressure increases it is then transmitted to the vitreous humour, which consequently crushes the retinal blood vessels. Retinal damage and blindness may result if it is untreated. Treatment is aimed at preventing the pressure developing in the aqueous humour by improving fluid drainage through the canal of Schlemm, either by surgery or by the pharmacological contraction of iris sphincter muscles to release the occluded duct. Alternatively, a trabeculectomy operation may be performed in which a

valve is placed within the sclera behind the upper eyelid, and this allows drainage of excess fluid.

Cataracts

A cataract (Figure 7.6) is a lens that has lost its transparency because of biochemical changes to the proteins within it. This will prevent the transmission of light, resulting in blindness. Correction is often by removal of the lens, while leaving the membrane at the back of the lens intact so that the vitreous humour is preserved, followed by implantation of an artificial lens. The preferred method of removing the lens is 'phacoemulsification' in which a small diamond-tipped blade is inserted through the edge of the cornea to allow access of other micro-equipment. The anterior capsule of the lens is removed and the lens itself disintegrated using ultrasound or laser ablation. A flexible lens is then inserted and secured. This method enables insertion of an artificial lens without the need for an extensive incision (and sutures) to the cornea. It is a rapid technique and usually does not entail a stay in hospital.

See also the case of a woman with cataracts, Section VI, p.641.

Detached retina

This is a separation of part of the retina, often as a result of eye trauma that has caused a deformation of the eyeball, such as a blow to the orbit. Laser therapy is used to reattach the separated tissue. Scarring may cause loss of some retinal cells but, as with the blind spot (see text), the brain can use vision from the other eye to compensate for this.

The foveal cones are minute, only 2–3 μm in diameter. If we imagine two very fine beams of light incident on the fovea, the difference in the angle as the beams hit the fovea can be as small as one-hundredth of a degree yet still stimulate adjacent receptor cells. In this way, light from very small variations in appearance of an object will still fall on different receptor cells and so enable us to distinguish the detail. The ability to discern detail is called visual acuity (Box 7.10).

The iris aperture, the lens and the cornea provide a breadth of vision that is referred to as the visual field. Amazingly, the curvature of the cornea enables us to see beyond 180°; with two eyes looking directly ahead the visual field is of the order of 210°, that is we can see forwards, sideways and a little back too. Objects at the perimeter of such a wide field of view may not be observed in detail, but any movement is easily detected. In fact, movement within the visual field is an extremely potent stimulus that causes a reflex movement of the eyes so that the moving object can be scrutinized to determine if we should be interested in it. Note that, however deep a conversation you might be having, a bird, car, other person, etc., moving unexpectedly within your field of view causes an unconscious, albeit usually momentary, glance at it. The control of eye movement is described later.

Physiology of vision

If we are to observe something in full detail, the light rays coming from whatever has attracted our attention must be focused if its image is to be formed at the fovea. In other words light rays are bent or refracted on entering the eye so that they fall onto that particular part of the retina. The retina must then be able to convert those rays into nerve cell activity, for interpretation. Vision, therefore, can be considered to involve four stages:

1 The refraction of light waves onto the receptor cells of the retina, especially the fovea.
2 The transformation of light into electrical activity.
3 The interpretation of electrical signals generated in the eye.
4 The control of the amount, or intensity, of the light so that this is appropriate and does not under- or over-stimulate the receptor cells.

Light refraction

Light rays are refracted (bent) when they pass from one medium into another, for example note how the image of an object is distorted when it is submerged in water. Most of the refractive power of the eye is actually in the cornea as light passes through its cells, and little further refraction occurs through the humours. The lens therefore provides the all-important final focusing of light onto the retina. The lens is basically a concentric series of transparent layers of lens fibre (i.e. proteins) enclosed within a transparent capsule. The curvature of the lens capsule is flexible and may be distorted by contraction or relaxation of the muscle cells of the ciliary bodies to which the lens is attached. A very rounded lens refracts light more effectively than one that is slightly curved, thus distortion of the lens alters its 'focal length'. If we are looking at a near object, light from it must be greatly refracted to bring it into focus on the retina (Figure 7.7). In contrast, light from a distant object requires less refraction: the lens is said to 'accommodate'. It is usually the case that after about 40–45 years of age the close focusing or accommodating ability of the lens begins to decline as its structure and biochemistry changes, and a need to wear spectacles becomes more likely.

Activation of the retinal receptor cells

A section through the retina is illustrated in Figure 7.9 (p.151). It appears to be inverted in that the receptor cells lie below the associated nerve cells and, for much of the retina below, the blood vessels. Such barriers are of little consequence because light is a powerful energy source, although acuity is aided by the lack of vessels in the fovea.

The receptor cells can be subdivided into those that are sensitive to wavelengths of light within the visible colour range (the cones) and those that are most sensitive to low light intensities and do not convey colour (the rods). A typical rod cell is shown diagrammatically in Figure 7.10. It contains the usual

---

BOX 7.10 MEASURING VISUAL ACUITY

In practice, acuity is readily measured by the reading of letters of different sizes (called Snellen tests). These include rows of letters that should be visible to an observer at certain distances away. The letters are designed so that their height will subtend an angle of one-twelfth of a degree if it is read at the appropriate distance. Thus a person standing 6 m (20 feet) away should be able to read the appropriate row of letters and this is called 6/6 (or 20/20) vision. In contrast, if a person standing 6 m distant can only accurately read larger letters that should normally be readable from further distances (e.g. 18 metres, called 6/18 vision) then they have an acuity defect.

BOX 7.11 BLURRED VISION

Blurred or distorted vision results from a failure of the refraction of light rays to focus an image on the retina:

- A thickened lens or elongated eyeball will cause the image to be focused at a point in front of the retina (a condition called myopia or near-sightedness; Figure 7.8a).
- A long, slimmer lens or a shortened eyeball may cause the focal point to fall behind the retina (a condition called hypermetropia or long-sightedness; Figure 7.8b).
- An irregular curvature of the lens or cornea will disturb the focusing of central and peripheral aspects of an image and this is called astigmatism (Figure 7.8c).
- The capacity for a lens to accommodate to near objects diminishes with age, producing an inability to focus on near objects, or presbyopia.

All of these disorders are correctable with appropriate spectacle lenses. For example, a convex spectacle lens will cause convergence of light rays before they are incident on the cornea and this will correct a refractory deficiency as in long-sightedness (Figure 7.8b). Similarly a concave lens will cause divergence of light rays and correct excessive refraction produced by the eye, as in short-sightedness.

Blurred vision can also arise if there is a loss of lens transparency through a change in its structure (a cataract; see Box 7.9)

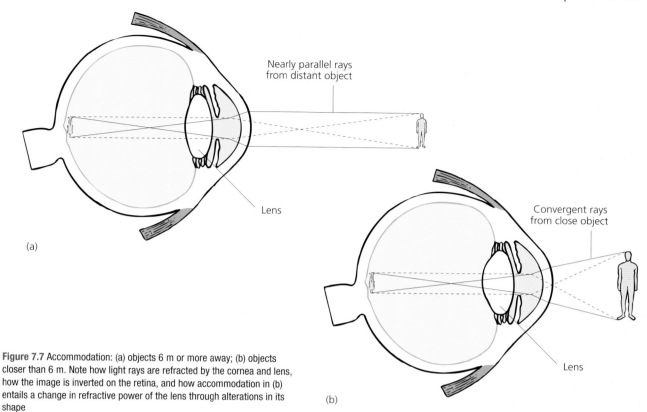

Figure 7.7 Accommodation: (a) objects 6 m or more away; (b) objects closer than 6 m. Note how light rays are refracted by the cornea and lens, how the image is inverted on the retina, and how accommodation in (b) entails a change in refractive power of the lens through alterations in its shape

cell organelles but also contains light-sensitive pigment. This pigment, called rhodopsin, is composed of two molecules, retinene (a derivative of vitamin A) and opsin. Light promotes the breakdown of rhodopsin into its constituents and, when this occurs, the membrane potential of the receptor cell alters and action potentials are produced. The two substances then recombine to reform the pigment, which is then available to respond once more to light.

The sensitivity of rod cells to light is determined by the amount of undissociated rhodopsin relative to dissociated pigment:

- In bright light, at any given time most of the pigment is dissociated because it breaks down immediately upon reforming, and this reduces its sensitivity.
- In contrast, much of the pigment is undissociated in poor light; the availability of the pigment makes the eye most sensitive in dim light.

Thus, if a person enters a dark room from a bright one sensitivity increases substantially during the first few minutes as pigment re-forms. Sensitivity increases still further during the next 20 minutes or so, but monochromatic (black and white) vision will dominate since the cones require much greater light intensities to function. This increased sensitivity when light is poor is called visual adaptation and allows us to gain some vision even when there is very little light available. Of course, if that person then re-entered a brightly lit room the effect

would be dazzling, as rhodopsin would dissociate in large quantities, producing an overwhelming stimulation of the retina. Eventually, adaptation would again occur as a new balance of dissociated to undissociated pigment became established and vision restored.

Cones behave in a similar fashion to rods but they contain slightly different pigments called visual purples. These exhibit peak sensitivity to light wavelengths corresponding to violet–blue, bluish green–yellow and orange–red (Figure 7.11) and are therefore referred to as 'blue', 'green', or 'red' cones. On average, they are most sensitive to the wavelengths necessary to make up 'white' light, which is a combination of blue, green and red light (as shown by the spectrum of colour when the wavelengths are separated in a rainbow). The human eye cannot discern infrared and ultraviolet light unless aids are used.

Evidence suggests that 'colour vision' depends upon what proportions of blue, green and red cones are stimulated. This 'trichromatic' theory does not explain why we are able to distinguish metallic colours, or 'brown', but to see the full range of visible colours does require the correct proportions of the three types of cone to be present. It is also clear that people who are deficient in particular cones have a colour 'blindness' appropriate to the deficit (Figure 7.12). In principle, the deficiency could be in any of the primary colours, but most combinations are only rarely affected and red–green deficiency is most common. Colour-deficiency is a sex-linked occurrence

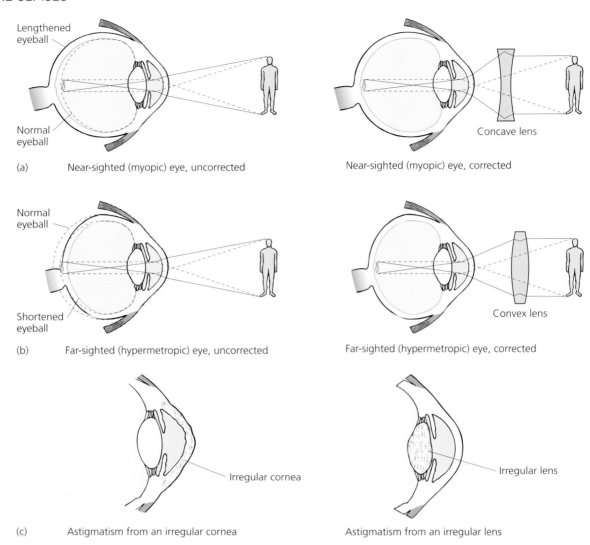

Figure 7.8 (a) Near-sighted vision and its correction. (b) Far-sighted vision and its correction. (c) Astigmatism, in which the sharp focusing of an image is compromised by a scattering of light rays by an irregular cornea or lens

Q When is a spectacle lens said to be (1) convex; (2) concave? Which type of lens is used in short-sightedness?

(genes on the X chromosome are responsible), being found in about 8% of men but less than 1% of women.

Electrical activity of rods and cones at threshold or above will promote a change in the membrane potential of the sensory nerve cells that they synapse with. The retina contains a complex arrangement of interacting nerve cells (Figure 7.9) that provide initial sensory processing before action potentials are conducted into the optic nerve and thence to the brain. Thus, some processing of the information occurs before the nerve activity even leaves the eye.

Interpretation of the visual signals

Electrical activity passes from the retinal cells to the optic nerve (cranial nerve II; see Figure 8.5, p.167) and thence to the brain. Activity from the left side of the retina of each eye passes to the right side of the brain and vice versa (Figure 7.13). The crossover of neural pathways from the left and right sides of the retina occurs at the optic chiasma, a structure that lies just anterior to the pituitary gland at the base of the brain. The significance of crossover is that it enables a comparison of the data from each eye, and it is this that helps us to perceive depth in the visual world, and hence three-dimensional images. After crossing over, the bundles of nerve cells pass to a part of the thalamus called the dorsal lateral geniculate body but in doing so they remain tightly packed into discrete nerves. Lesions of these parts of the pathway cause a profound loss of vision (Figure 7.13). After the thalamus, however, the neural pathways diverge and become more dispersed, and so electrical activity from the retina eventually arrives at various parts of the brain for processing. The dispersion means that a lesion in these brain areas can have unusual consequences for vision.

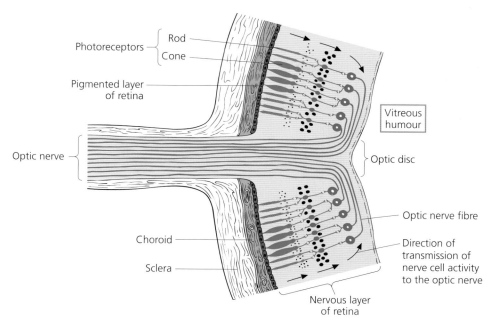

Figure 7.9 The retina. Blood vessels have been omitted for clarity

Q Why is the retina sometimes said to be 'upside down' in terms of its structure?

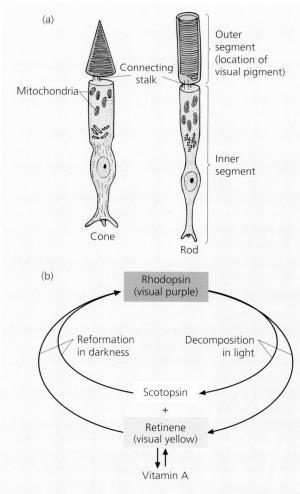

Figure 7.10 Rods, cones and visual pigment. (a) Receptor cell types of the retina. (b) The behaviour of visual pigment (rhodopsin) in light and dark

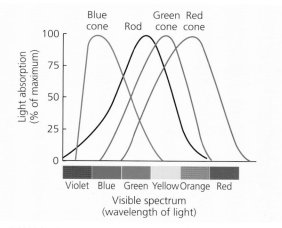

Figure 7.11 Light absorption by rods and cones

Q How might the cones enable us to see yellow?

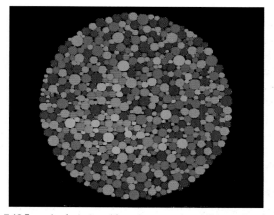

Figure 7.12 Example of a test card for red–green colour deficiency. People with red–green deficiency should read the number 4; those without red–green deficiency should read the number 42. Copyright Isshinkai Foundation, Tokyo, Japan. Reproduced with permission

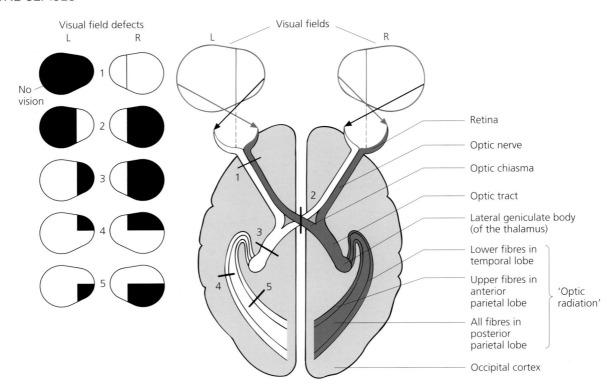

Figure 7.13 Visual pathways and the effects of lesions at various points to produce visual field defects. Note that information from the right side of each retina passes to the right side of the brain, that from the left to the left side of the brain

The visual perceptional areas of the brain comprise virtually all of the occipital lobe of the cerebrum, parts of the frontal/parietal motor cortex, and parts of the brainstem (see Chapter 8). Recognition of an object probably involves the cognitive analysis of the topographical features of the object, for example its edges, based at least partly on memory but also involving degrees of reasoning that involve memory circuits within the brain. The mechanism of the latter is still unclear.

Other parts of the brain that receive sensory input from the eye provide additional information and/or influence behaviour. They include:

- The suprachiasmatic nucleus (i.e. it lies above the optic chiasma) of the hypothalamus. This is thought to control the sleep–wake circadian rhythmicity in response to light cues (see Chapter 22, p.614).
- The accessory optic nuclei and superior colliculi of the brainstem. These are involved in controlling eye movement, and so must be linked to vision.
- The pretectum areas of the brainstem (see Chapter 8, p.175). These are involved in controlling pupil diameter, and hence reactions to light intensity.

Control of the intensity of light entering the eye

It was described earlier how retinal receptor cells are able to adapt to differences in light intensity and how this is an important homeostatic response that enables us to maintain vision in both poor light and bright light. The efficiency of the process is influenced by the amount of light entering the eye: in poor light the adaptation will be restricted by very low light levels; in bright light the process will be limited by excessive light. Adaptation, therefore, is facilitated by admitting as much light as possible under poorly illuminated conditions, and by restricting the entry of light under bright conditions.

Upon entering the eye light must pass through the pupil of the iris. This contains pigmented cells but also contains antagonistic smooth muscle cells arranged in a radial and circular fashion. As their names suggest, the radial cells extend from the centrally located pupil to the periphery of the iris, and the

---

BOX 7.12 HALLUCINATIONS AND DREAMS

If the visual cortex is stimulated without the use of the eyes then light or even images can be discerned. For example a blow to the back of the head causes us to perceive 'stars' as nerve cells in the visual areas of the brain are activated by the mechanical stimulus. Even more interestingly, electrical stimulation of certain areas of the cerebrum may produce an image constructed from the impulses produced in the nerve cells. Dreams too are constructed from electrical impulses in these areas. Such effects serve to emphasize that the integration of electrical impulses in cognitive processing is responsible for the 'construction' of mental images.

Similarly, inappropriate stimulation of the auditory cortex produces auditory hallucination (i.e. the hearing of sounds that are not actually present).

BOX 7.13 PUPIL DIAMETER AS A MEANS OF ASSESSMENT

It is important in health care to understand how pupil diameter is controlled because pupil dilation will occur in response to sympathetic activity during times of heightened excitement and agitation, but will also be observed:

- if a patient is in danger of entering circulatory shock as sympathetic stimulation is then enhanced;
- in states of depressed mental function, especially a drug overdose, when the reflex response to light is sluggish or even absent (stimulation of the retina with a light pen will then not produce a normal reflex constriction of the pupil);
- in a patient with a brainstem trauma who may also not respond normally to the light pen (the autonomic reflex involves neurological structures within the brainstem for its coordination; for this reason, pupil response to light stimulation is a part of the assessment of 'brain death').

circularly arranged cells extend circumferentially around the pupil. In bright light parasympathetic nerve activity stimulates contraction of the circular muscle cells, and relaxes the radial ones, resulting in a constriction of the pupil. In dim light, sympathetic nerve activity contracts the radial cells and relaxes the circular ones, resulting in pupil dilation. The aperture of the pupil can therefore be altered according to light conditions. The process works as a reflex and so occurs automatically and very rapidly. The reflexes operate via parts of the brainstem.

The influence of sympathetic activity to dilate the pupil may also play a role in the all-out activity called the 'fight, flight and fright' response in the alarm stage of the general adaptation syndrome (see Chapter 21, p.596). This is because pupil dilation increases the illumination of peripheral areas of the retina and may even expand the visual field. Visual perception will therefore be heightened under threatening circumstances, although during times of excitement, pupil dilation may even be a sexual attractant in the appropriate setting!

Control of eye movement

The physiology of vision also includes the control of eye position in relation to focusing on near or distant objects, and in relation to following a moving object. Thus, if the attention is switched from a distant to a near object, the eyes must converge so that the image of the object still lands on the fovea of each eye (Figure 7.14a). Continual assessment of the position of the image ensures that it is kept on the fovea; as the object moves toward the eyes then the image is returned to the fovea by further convergence, even to the extent of causing the eyes to be 'crossed' when the object is very close! The neurological processing that is necessary to control these movements takes about one-fifth of a second and this limits the accuracy of the convergence: to put this into context, it means that the last visual fixation that a batsman, for example, has on a cricket ball travelling at 160 km/hour will be when the ball is still more than 10 m away from him. Anticipation is then essential. The delay has implications when we are following a rapidly moving object, for example when driving a car.

At other times we may wish to focus on an object that is moving laterally across the visual field. Movement within the visual field is a potent stimulus to attract attention and the eyes will usually reflexly focus on an unexpected moving object (Figure 7.14b), and perhaps track it as it moves across the visual field should we be interested in it. This 'visual pursuit' of a moving object is a complicated process and involves a 'programming' by the brain of the direction and speed of movement. Provided that the movement is not too rapid, tracking is very smooth (Figure 7.14c). If the movement is rapid, however, the eyes must carry out extremely quick catching-up movements and this means that, for a fraction of a second, the brain is programming itself to work out where the object will be. These rapid eye movements are called saccades (Figure 7.14d) and similar movements, without the 'programming', are also performed in, for example, scanning a piece of text or a painting. They are among the fastest movements that the body is capable of producing, but may be problematic if the programming is delayed (Box 7.14).

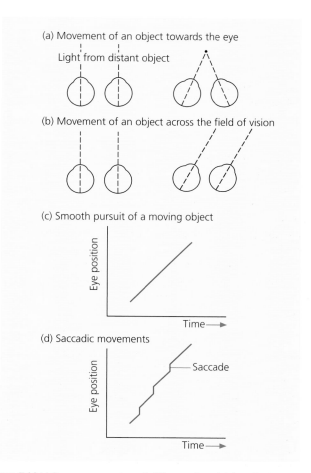

Figure 7.14 (a) Convergence movement of the eyes to maintain an image on both retinas when an object moves towards the eyes. (b) Pursuit movement of the eyes to maintain images on both retinas when an object moves across the visual field. (c) Tracking diagram for pursuit movement. The straight line indicates 'smooth' pursuit. (d) Tracking diagram for pursuit movement when an object is moving quickly. Saccadic ('jumping') movements must be used to enable the eyes to catch up with the position of the object

BOX 7.14 ALCOHOL AND VISION

Excessive alcohol slows down the integration involved in the processing of movement of an object in the visual field:

- Convergence movements are slowed, making it difficult to judge distance and so making stopping distance much longer when following a car.
- If following an object across the visual field the individual typically will have to perform saccades to keep up (Figure 7.14d), even at relatively slow rates of movement. However, saccades are only effective if the brain can register the new position. The delay introduced by alcohol means that by the time the saccade is accomplished, the object has moved on again. In other words, the object is not exactly where the brain thinks it is, leading to poor judgement!

Hearing

Overview

'Sound' is the perception of small pressure waves generated in air or water by a moving or vibrating object (e.g. the vocal cords of the larynx). The vibrations set up alternate compressions and decompressions of the air and convey different features of sound:

- The number of compressions per second (or cycles per second; 1 cycle/second = 1 Hertz or Hz) gives the sound its frequency, which is perceived as 'pitch' or tone.
- The amplitude of the compressions gives sound its 'intensity' or loudness. Sound intensity is measured in decibels: rustling leaves have a decibel rating of 15, that of conversation 45. The ear is very sensitive and can normally detect intensities almost as low as 0 decibels and frequencies over a range of 20–20 000 Hz. A sound intensity of 115–120 decibels produces pain within the ear and persistent exposure to 90–100 decibels can cause permanent hearing damage.

Sound intensity and frequency are complex modalities but some generalizations can be made regarding the basis of their detection:

Pressure → Outer ear → Middle ear → Inner ear → Neural
waves   (tympanic   (ossicles: (receptor   pathways
(in air/water) membrane)   transmission) cells: neural (processing/
                                          stimulation) interpretation)

There is therefore a complex means of transmission of pressure waves to the receptor cells, but it is the pattern of distortion of receptor cells within the inner ear that seems to be important in conveying information regarding sound intensity and frequency.

General anatomy of the ear and physiology of hearing

The ear is divided into three component parts: the external, middle and inner ear (Figure 7.15).

The visible external ear, or pinna, is deeply folded and this introduces minor perturbations in the sound pressure waves incident on the pinna, which helps in locating its source. Comparison of signals from both ears also facilitates the location of sound, for example an ear will receive sound from that side of the head just moments before the opposite ear does (i.e. there is a very slight time delay).

The aperture of the external ear penetrates the skull via the auditory meatus, or external auditory canal, which terminates at the eardrum, or tympanic membrane. This membrane is under a degree of tension and vibrates at the same frequencies as those of pressure waves incident upon it. Earwax (cerumen) helps to maintain the health of the skin within the external auditory canal and also helps to collect particles from the air, thus protecting the eardrum. Hairs within the meatus also help to filter particles. Excessive production of wax can impair hearing, especially if it becomes impacted on the eardrum (see Chapter 16, p.454).

Vibrations of the tympanic membrane are transferred to the bones that provide a transmission system in the middle ear. These small bones, or ossicles, are called the malleus, incus and stapes, and are suspended within an air-filled chamber (Figure 7.16a). They provide a link between the tympanic membrane and the inner ear (cochlea). Having a 'middle ear' conveys four major advantages:

- The force of vibration is amplified by the ossicles. This is essential as the aperture to the inner ear is relatively small and, in addition, the inner ear is fluid-filled and so requires more energy to produce pressure waves within it.
- The middle ear chamber connects directly with the nasopharynx (the cavity at the back of the nose) via the Eustachian or auditory tube. Thus, any major change in external air pressure can quickly be applied to the middle ear by opening the aperture of the auditory tubes in the nasopharynx through swallowing. In this way the pressure on either side of the tympanic membrane is equilibrated, and any 'ballooning' of the eardrum as a consequence of a pressure gradient across it is therefore prevented. This protects the membrane from damage, but is only effective if air pressure changes are slow, or not too excessive. It will not protect against very sudden, large changes in air pressure such as occur in explosions, when the membrane may then perforate.
- Pressure waves established in the inner ear pass through the spiral-shaped cochlea and exit into the middle ear (see later). The air within the middle ear chamber provides the means of dissipating these pressure waves, thus making the receptor cells in the cochlea receptive once more to further stimulation.
- If our external environment is extremely noisy, the inner ear can be protected from excessive vibration of the tympanic membrane by altering its contact with the ossicles, and hence reducing their transmission. This is achieved by the contraction of small muscles that pull the malleus bone away from the tympanic membrane (a muscle called tensor tympani), and the stapes bone away from the aperture to the inner ear (a muscle called stapedius). This mechanism is a reflex, analogous to the reduction of pupil diameter that is observed when the eye is exposed to bright light, that prevents excessive stimulation of the receptor area – another

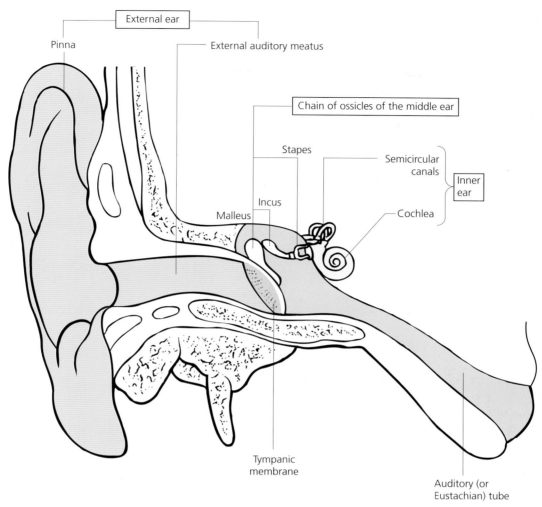

Figure 7.15 General anatomy of the ear.

example of homeostatic adaptation. There is a slight delay in the adaptation occurring, so entering a noisy room can seem almost deafening at first, while exiting a noisy room into a quiet one initially makes hearing difficult.

The stapes bone, the final link in the chain of ossicles, has a flattened surface that makes contact with the membrane that occludes the aperture to the inner ear. This aperture, called the 'oval window' or fenestra ovalis, is the route of transmission into the inner ear, which contains:

- the cochlea involved in hearing;
- the components of the vestibular apparatus involved in balance.

BOX 7.15 OTITIS MEDIA, AND OTITIS MEDIA WITH EFFUSION

The auditory tube may allow bacteria from the nasopharynx to enter the middle ear, causing inflammation, a condition called otitis media (Berry, 2000). Young children are especially at risk because of the relatively short length of the tube. Antimicrobial drugs may prevent further progress of infection.

If there is pus and inflammatory effusion this will interfere with the functioning of the ossicles in the middle ear, reducing clarity of hearing, while the pressure exerted on the inner ear produces continuous low-level stimulation of the receptor cells, perceived as a ringing or hissing sound, called tinnitus (see Box 7.17, p.158). The condition is referred to as otitis media with effusion, commonly referred to as 'glue ear'.

Antimicrobial drugs may be prescribed (see Mandel and Casselbrant, 2006) but the presence of effusion also means that there is a risk of the middle ear pressure rupturing the tympanic membrane, and a risk of a spread of infection to the inner ear. Because of this, clinicians may recommend the insertion of a small tube, or grommet, through the tympanic membrane to relieve the pressure produced by the build-up, although the value of grommets has been questioned and they are less popular today than they were in the past (Thompson, 2000). The grommet is removed once the infection has been cleared using antibiotics, and the middle ear has cleared of pus. The point of insertion of the grommet then heals.

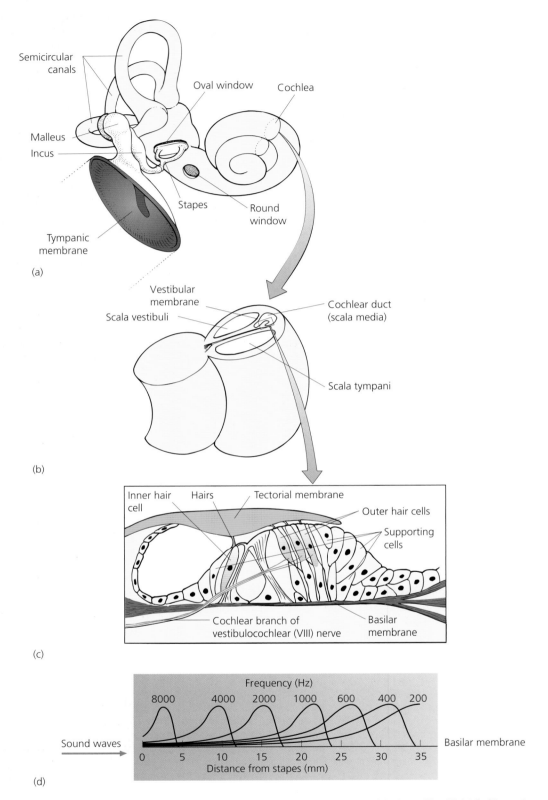

(a)

(b)

(c)

(d)

Figure 7.16 Structures involved in hearing: (a) anatomy of the middle and inner ear; (b) general structure of the the cochlea; (c) detail of the anatomy of the cochlea to show the hearing receptors and associated structures (called the 'organ of Corti'); (c) cross-section through the scala media; (d) the role of vibrations of the basilar membrane in the cochlea to provide initial frequency discrimination of sound waves. Low-frequency sounds are most effective at a distance from where sound enters the cochlea at the stapes, while high-frequency sounds are most effective close to the stapes

Q How do sound waves pass from the air to the basilar membrane?

The vestibular apparatus is described elsewhere, in its role to monitor balance and the position of the head (see Chapter 17, p.475). It is the transference of vibration from the ossicles to the cochlear fluid that activates the receptor cells involved in hearing.

The cochlea is shaped like a snail shell. The coils increase the surface area of the receptor membrane within them, and a cross-section through the cochlea is shown in Figure 7.16b. The figure shows how the cochlea is divided into three fluid-filled compartments called the scala media, scala vestibuli and scala tympani. The fluid inside the scala media is referred to as endolymph ('endo-' = inner) and bathes the receptors and associated structures (below). The fluid in the scala vestibuli and scala tympani is referred to as perilymph ('peri-' = surrounding). The fluid names help to reinforce how the cochlea operates:

- First, sound waves are transmitted from the 'oval window' into the endolymph of the scala media where they stimulate the receptor cells.
- The pressure then has to be dissipated, achieved by the passage of the pressure waves into the perilymph of the scala vestibuli, and then into the other chamber, the scala tympani, via a small hole at the tip of the cochlea.
- The pressure waves are then transmitted from this compartment into the middle ear via the 'round window' or fenestra rotunda.

Figure 7.16c illustrates a cross-section through the scala medial chamber. The structure shown is clearly very complex but it can generally be described as one in which the receptor cells 'sit' on a membrane, called the basilar membrane, with their hair-like cilia projecting into a gel-like matrix, the tectorial membrane. Sound vibrations in the endolymph cause the basilar membrane to be deflected and a wave of oscillations to pass along it. The hair projections of the receptor cells are distorted and it is this that results in the generation of action potentials in the sensory nerve endings.

The conduction of sound waves through the water-based endolymph is highly efficient. Low-frequency sounds travel easier than high-frequency ones and evidence suggests that low-frequency components of sounds produce the greatest oscillation of the basilar membrane towards the apex of the cochlea, while high-frequency sounds stimulate the earlier sections. This is illustrated in Figure 7.16d. In this way the basilar membrane provides the first stage in enabling the ear to differentiate sound frequency. The amplitude of vibration of the membrane seems to provide information about the intensity of the sound waves. Thus, as with vision, some processing of the stimulus is provided by the sensory organ itself. The full process is extremely complex, however, and beyond the bounds of this book.

The sensitivity of the cochlea depends upon the frequency of the sound waves. Although the ear can detect frequencies of 20–20 000 Hz, it is most sensitive to the range of frequencies associated with human speech (i.e. 1000–4000 Hz) (Figure 7.17).

BOX 7.16 AUDIOGRAM

Clinically, an initial hearing test involves assessment of the intensity 'threshold' of sounds across a range of frequencies. An audiogram can then be produced which, when compared with norms, indicates any loss of hearing at given wavelengths (Figure 7.17). Tones generated via headphones are conducted to the inner ear by the usual route, but tones can also be conducted via bones of the skull. Conduction of sound through bone (by applying the tone to the mastoid process of the skull, behind the ear) bypasses the middle ear and any hearing defect can then be narrowed down to an inner ear or middle ear deficit. Hearing difficulties may also arise through errors in the interpretation by the brain of signals arriving from the ear.

Disruption of the conduction pathway of the middle ear is called conduction deafness.

Inner ear problems include the effects of excessive endolymph pressing down on the basilar membrane, impairing the receptor cells. Recent developments in microtechnology have seen the testing of cochlear implants – electrodes connected to a transducer behind the ear that stimulate the cochlear nerve directly. Impairment of cochlear nerve function causes nerve deafness.

Impairment of cochlear nerve function causes nerve deafness. Nerve deafness frequently disturbs the vestibular apparatus of the inner ear, producing further symptoms of vertigo and nausea. Collectively, this is called labyrinthine disease. More commonly this results from infection of the inner ear, trauma, local arteriosclerosis, allergies or ageing.

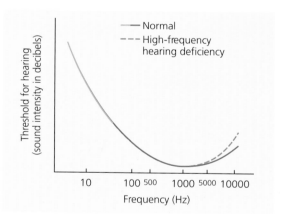

Figure 7.17 An audiogram to detect the range of frequencies that may be heard, and the sensitivity of hearing

Q Where do you think the range of frequencies for the human voice might lie on this graph?

Interpretation of auditory signals

Sensory nerve fibres from the receptors in the cochlea pass via the cochlear fibre bundles of the vestibulocochlear nerve (cranial nerve VIII, sometimes called the auditory or acoustic nerve; see Figure 8.5, p.167) to the cochlear nuclei of the brainstem (Figure 7.18). Here they connect with other nerve cells which subsequently connect with other nerve cells within various 'nuclei' of the brainstem, including the inferior colliculi, before passing to a part of the thalamus called the medial geniculate body (see Chapter 8 for the location of these brain

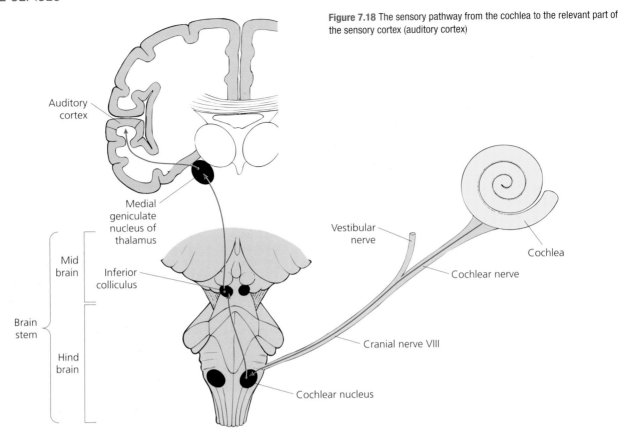

Figure 7.18 The sensory pathway from the cochlea to the relevant part of the sensory cortex (auditory cortex)

BOX 7.17 TINNITUS

Tinnitus is a term given to a persistent ringing sound in the ears. It is therefore a symptom, rather than an actual condition. It seems to be present when the production of excessive endolymph depresses the basilar membrane. Meniere's syndrome and inner ear infection both promote tinnitus, but it is observed in a number of disorders, and is often poorly understood. Treatment depends upon cause (Kaltenbach, 2000) and may include destruction of tissue using ultrasound, a reduction in endolymph secretion through the use of diuretics, local vasodilation using an elevated blood CO_2 content or, in extreme cases, surgical intervention.

ACTIVITY

Put on a blindfold and place a nose-clip over your nostrils. Ask a friend to place a piece of apple or onion in your mouth without telling you what it actually is. Can you tell what the piece is, and the difference between the two? Repeat the test but this time ask your friend to inform you what the piece is of. Can you now tell the difference between them? Explain your findings.

---

structures). Neurons then carry the signal to the auditory area of the cerebral cortex (of the temporal lobes). Sensory nerve cells from each ear interact within the brain and each temporal lobe actually receives input from both ears; damage to one temporal lobe therefore normally has minimal effects on hearing. A further pathway within the brainstem also carries information to the reticular formation, a structure which, among various functions, is involved in the sleep–wake cycle. Thus, sound is an effective waking stimulus even from deep sleep.

Taste and smell
Overview

Taste and smell receptors are highly specialized chemoreceptors and are stimulated when molecules interact with comple-

mentary molecules on the surface of the receptor cells. Unlike other chemoreceptors, however, these receptor cells respond to an enormous range of molecules. Before detection the molecules must first be dissolved in water, which is provided by saliva and nasal secretions. The two senses are not mutually exclusive and stimulation of the olfactory receptors of the nose is an important aspect of taste, even though taste is looked upon as being a feature of the oral cavity. This is readily demonstrated in the activity above.

The tongue and physiology of taste (= gustation)

Taste is sensed by receptor cells that are present in 'buds' on the surface of the tongue, and on the epiglottis, pharynx and palate. Each 'bud' consists of four types of cell, some of which are chemoreceptors, while others are responsible for nutritive support (Figure 7.19a). There are some 10 000 taste 'buds' on

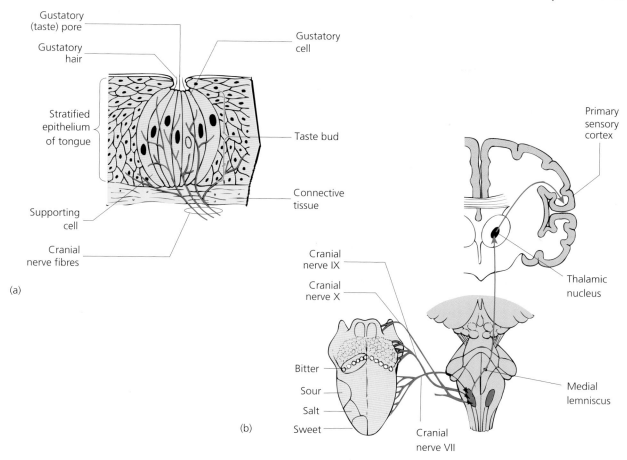

Figure 7.19 Taste (gustation): (a) receptor cells; (b) the sensory pathway from the tongue to the relevant part of the sensory cortex

the tongue alone and these are clustered together in structures called 'papillae':

- fungiform papillae contain up to five taste 'buds';
- vallate papillae contain up to 100 buds;
- filiform papillae are smaller than the other types and contain few if any taste buds.

Between them, the buds provide four basic tastes: sweet, sour, bitter and salt. The taste buds responsible for these modalities are arranged in particular areas of the tongue (Figure 7.19b), but all four are 'tasted' to various degrees by the receptors of the palate, epiglottis and pharynx:

- 'Sweet' tastes are desirable as they imply a rich caloric value of the food present in the mouth.
- 'Bitter' and 'sour' tastes may be offensive; if extreme the food may be rejected as potentially toxic.
- 'Salt' and 'acidic foods' may or may not be considered desirable. For example, salt depletion of the body fluids stimulates a 'salt' appetite and salty foods may then be chosen in preference to others.

The four kinds of taste buds do not appear to differ in terms of their cell structures and the ways in which the molecules

generate nerve activity in associated sensory nerve cells is still debatable. Thus, lysyl-taurine (a kind of peptide) tastes 'salty' yet clearly does not contain sodium chloride, lead salts taste 'sweet' yet do not contain sugars, and a protein modifier (called miraculin) makes 'acidic' substances taste sweet. Genotypes may be involved in taste discrimination; for example genetic variation means that only a proportion of people can taste the substance phenylthiocarbamide (PTC).

The sensory pathway for taste can be illustrated as:

Chemical → Taste → Associated → Transmission → Interpretation
receptor (tongue) nerve cell (cranial nerve/ (cerebral
(tongue) brainstem/ cortex)
thalamus)

Interpretation of taste

Activity from the anterior two-thirds of the tongue pass via the facial nerve (cranial nerve VII) to the brainstem (Figure 7.19b). The glossopharyngeal nerve (cranial nerve IX) conveys activity from the posterior third. Fibres from the pharynx, epiglottis and palate pass to the brainstem via the vagus nerve (cranial nerve X; see Figure 8.5, p.167). Within the brainstem, all inputs pass to a collection of nerve cells within the medulla oblongata (the nucleus of the tractus solitarius) from which fibres pass to specific areas of the thalamus. They then synapse with other neurons, which pass to the cortex of the parietal lobe.

The nose and physiology of smell (olfaction)

The sense of smell depends upon chemoreceptors present within the mucous membrane of the nasal epithelium, an area measuring around 5 cm^2 in the roof of the nasal cavity. The presence of two nostrils helps in the determination of the direction from which a smell originates because they introduce a slight delay in the stimulation of one part of the olfactory epithelium relative to the other. There are some 10–20 million receptor cells in the nose (with other supportive or secretory cells) and these are in fact modified nerve cells. The nerve endings are expanded into olfactory 'rods' from which cilia project into the bathing fluid layer; molecules dissolved within mucus interact with surface molecules in the cilia membrane (Figure 7.20). Proteins present within the fluid are thought to facilitate the presentation of odour molecules to the receptors.

Like taste, the sense of smell appears to involve more than simply an interaction between a chemical molecule and a complementary molecule on the surface of the receptor. Odour-producing molecules are generally small but odour is more dependent upon molecular configuration than on size. For example, the chemicals camphor and hexachlorethane smell identical but are very different molecules with different chemical properties. The olfactory cells are particularly sensitive at detecting characteristic odours, and humans can distinguish up to 4000 different odours! However, the detection of intensity of particular odours is not so well developed.

How such a diverse range of odours can be detected is unknown. Attempts to classify smell modalities have suggested that odours can be separated into seven types: putrid, musky, floral, pungent, peppermint, ethereal and camphoraceous. A combination of these is suggested to produce the range of odour perceptions of which we are capable. The diversity of odours goes beyond the limits of these modalities, however, and to call these 'primary' odours would be misleading. Pain fibres also originate in the olfactory epithelium and are stimulated by irritative characteristics of odours, for example peppermint and chlorine. Sneezing and tear secretion are reflexly induced after stimulation of these fibres, and these are clearly defensive mechanisms against a perceived noxious vapour.

Adaptation to a stimulus is also noticeable with smell, and may only apply to a single odour within a collection of odours; the 'thresholds' for other odours are unchanged. Adaptation allows us to remain within a particular environment without constantly perceiving a particular dominant odour, unless it is noxious. The mechanism is unknown but probably involves modulation of receptor function and of central processing.

The sense of taste can be summarized as:

Chemical receptor (nerve ending) → Associated nerve cells → Transmission (cranial nerve/ brain nuclei) → Interpretation (cerebral cortex)

Interpretation of olfactory signals

Sensory nerve cells extending from olfactory receptors terminate in the olfactory bulb, a distended terminal of the olfactory nerve (cranial nerve I; see Figure 8.5, p.167), where they connect with other nerve cells in what are called the 'olfactory glomeruli' (Figure 7.20). These connect with further nerve cells within the vicinity, before neural activity passes via the olfactory nerve to various structures within the limbic system of

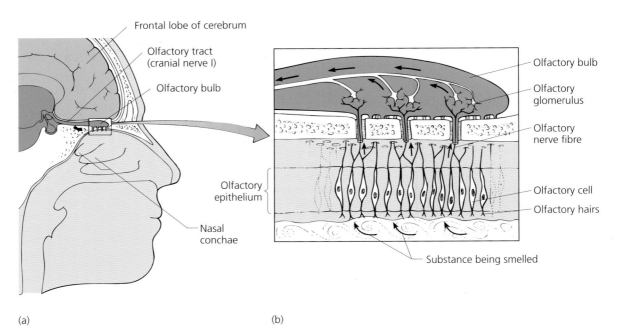

(a) (b)

Figure 7.20 Smell (olfaction): (a) location of receptors; (b) detail of the olfactory bulb

the brain (see Chapter 8), including an area of the cerebral cortex. Smell appears to be unique among the senses in that sensory neural activity does not relay via the thalamus in the brain.

Initial processing of the activity probably occurs in the olfactory glomeruli but final processing occurs in the primary olfactory cortex located in the temporal lobe of the cerebrum. Pathways linking the limbic system with the hypothalamus provide the input to hypothalamic 'drive' centres associated with odours, for example autonomic arousal and sexual arousal.

SUMMARY

1. The homeostatic control of physiological systems and cellular function is dependent upon the facility to 'sense' changes in all aspects of the internal environment, and of many elements of the external environment.

2. Senses depend upon receptor cells that have specializations, usually of the cell membrane, that enable them to respond to specific parameters. Some senses are polymodal in that they can detect more than one quality of a stimulus. These are the special senses of vision, hearing, taste, smell (and pain).

3. Receptors are transducers. That is, they can take a particular stimulus (light, sound, etc.) and convert this into electrochemical nerve impulses.

4. The generation of nerve impulses increases with intensity of stimulation, but a threshold must be exceeded before a nerve impulse is transmitted from the receptor.

5. Information from peripheral senses passes to the brain via tracts within the spinal cord. Numerous relays may be involved but almost all pass through the thalamus of the brain on the way to the sensory areas of the cerebral cortex.

6. The eye is a sense organ which causes light rays to be focused onto receptors of the retina. Biochemical features of the receptors allow us to perceive light of different wavelengths (colour) as well as intensity.

7. Information from the retinal receptors passes via the thalamus to various components of the brain, particularly the visual cortex of the occipital cerebral lobe. Processing produces 'vision' and is also important in controlling eye movement.

8. The ear consists of external, middle and inner structures; the inner structures include the organs of hearing and of balance. Transmission of sound to the fluid-filled inner ear occurs via small ossicles within the air-filled middle ear.

9. Pressure waves induced in the cochlea of the inner ear are converted into electrochemical signals which provide both intensity and frequency information. Electrochemical activity passes to various parts of the brain, but especially to the auditory cortex of the temporal lobes.

10. Taste and smell result from stimulation of chemoreceptors of the tongue and nasal cavities. Although involving an interaction between receptor molecules present on the receptor cell membranes and food or odour molecules, the process is more complex than a simple 'lock and key' mechanism. The actual mechanism is not understood, but it enables us to detect a wide variety of different molecules.

11. Information from the nose and tongue passes to various structures within the brain. Apart from the cerebral cortex, other important olfactory processing areas include structures of the limbic system.

REFERENCES

Berry, P. (2000) Otitis media in children: diagnosis, treatment and prevention. *Postgraduate Medicine* **107**(3): 239–41.

Kaltenbach, J.A. (2000) Neurophysiologic mechanisms of tinnitus. *Journal of the American Academy of Audiology* **11**(3): 125–37.

Mandel, E.M. and Casselbrant, M.L. (2006) Recent developments in the treatment of otitis media with effusion. *Drugs* **66**(12): 1565–76.

Mead, M. (2000) Procedures for practice nurses. The illness conjunctivitis. *Practice Nurse* **19**(5): 215–16.

Thompson, J. (2000) Clinical update. Otitis media with effusion. *Community Practitioner* **73**(8): 728–9.

Watkinson, S. and Seewoodhary, R. (2008) Ocular complications associated with diabetes mellitus. *Nursing Standard* **22**(27): 51–60.

THE NERVOUS SYSTEM

INTRODUCTION

A capacity to sense change, and to promote an appropriate effector response, are fundamental features of a homeostatic process. Many of our senses involve the nervous system, at least in part (see Chapter 7), and many effectors are also mediated by nerves. Consequently, the network of nerves throughout the body is extensive and complex. Of even more complex anatomy are the brain and spinal cord as these must interpret incoming sensory data, and produce the appropriate neural output to tissues. The different elements that comprise the anatomy of the nervous system, and their physiology, are described in this chapter. This is a difficult topic and readers should explore the 'Overview' section before the later sections, since this highlights some general features of the nervous system.

As an introduction, it is important first to make a distinction between 'nerves' and 'nerve cells'.

Nerves

What is a nerve?

Nerves form an extensive network of conducting pathways, which spread throughout the body and provide a means of rapid communication between parts of the body. A cross-section through a nerve shows that it consists of a tough protective covering of connective tissue, called the epineurium ('epi-' = upon, 'neurium' = neural matter) in the form of a tube, and numerous bundles of sectioned nerve cells within the tube (Figure 8.1). The bundles of nerve cells, or fasicles, are separated from others by more connective tissue, called the perineurium ('peri-' = surrounding), and by blood vessels. Each nerve cell is surrounded by a further, delicate, connective tissue layer called the endoneurium ('endo-' = inner).

Nerves, then, are conduits for collections of nerve cells, or to be more precise, the long processes that are a feature of many nerve cells. The structure of nerve cells is described below but the elongated processes are often simply referred to as nerve fibres. Thus, a nerve might be viewed as nerve fibres bundled together rather like wires in an electrical cable:

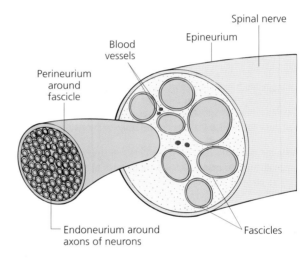

Figure 8.1 Section through a peripheral nerve

Q The epineurium, perineurium and endoneurium are examples of types of connective tissue. What are the characteristics of this kind of tissue?

- There are fibres that are processes from nerve cells that convey activity from the brain and/or spinal cord to the tissues of the body; these will mediate effector responses in a homeostatic process.
- Other fibres convey activity from the tissues to the brain/spinal cord; these will mediate sensory input from receptors in a homeostatic process.
- The diameter of the nerve is determined by how many nerve fibres are present within it, and so changes along its length as nerve fibres enter or exit. This usually means that a nerve is at its thickest close to its connection with the brain or spinal cord.

Nerve nomenclature

Nerves are frequently named according to their origin and/or to where their activity passes. For example, pelvic nerves

BOX 8.1 LOSS OF NERVE SUPPLY TO A TISSUE

A single nerve may contain thousands of nerve fibres (i.e. nerve cells or neurons) that connect more than one tissue with the brain/spinal cord. For example, the femoral nerve (found in the thigh; the name relates to the bone of the thigh, called the femur) will contain nerve cells that connect with the muscles of the leg, the bone and joints of the limb, and the blood and lymphatic vessels, and skin of the limb. Nerve trauma, therefore, will influence all of the tissues innervated by that nerve.

Some regeneration of nerve connections is possible after trauma but success depends upon two factors:

- Are the severed ends of nerve cells able to remake contact? The partial restoration of senses observed in the skin of reconnected hands or feet suggest that this can occur.
- Can surviving nerve fibres (assuming that the nerve trauma has left some of the nerve intact) branch to connect with cells that have lost their nerve connections? There is evidence that this may occur, with nerve cells sending out connections to cells, for example muscle cells, in the vicinity.

Reforming connections probably involves the local secretion of chemical nerve growth factors, in conjunction with chemical attractants. Some of these chemicals have been identified and may also be involved in the outgrowth of nerves toward their target tissues in the embryo/fetus. These substances have potentially important clinical applications, for example in stimulating the regeneration of spinal cord after spinal trauma.

rons will ultimately change tissue functions and so may also be referred to as motor neurons:

- The cell body of such efferent cells is located at one end of the neuron, either within the spinal cord itself or within intermediate neural structures called ganglia (singular, ganglion) that may be some distance from the spinal cord but which will themselves connect with the cord (e.g. see later section on the autonomic nervous system).
- The elongated section of the nerve cell that makes up the nerve fibre of an efferent neuron is termed an axon (Figure 8.2).
- One feature that is observed in efferent neurons is that their cell bodies have extremely fine branching processes, called dendrites (dendron = Greek for 'tree'). These are important because it is via these processes that the nerve cell is able to receive electrical inputs from other nerve cells in the vicinity.
- The end of the axon within the target tissue will also normally terminate in fine branching processes, referred to simply as axon terminals, and they will conduct impulses from the axon towards cells within the vicinity.

Afferent (or sensory) neurons

Those nerve cells that carry impulses from sensory receptors within the tissues to the brain/spinal cord are collectively called afferent ('affere-' = to carry towards) neurons. Afferent neurons may be called sensory neurons, because the information they convey usually originates at sensory receptors:

- In these neurons the cell body is found as an 'off-shoot' from the fibre. For most of these cells this is usually close to where they enter the spinal cord (Figure 8.2) and the large number of cell bodies present produces a distension of the nerve at this point. This is called a spinal ganglion; another name is dorsal root ganglion because these afferent cells enter the posterior or dorsal aspect of the spinal cord.

contain nerve cells that pass to/from the pelvic region, while the optic nerve originates in the eye. Unfortunately, the nomenclature is not always so obvious. The names of many nerves derive from Latin or Greek and may refer to features other than sources or targets. For example, the name of the nerve called the vagus is Latin for 'wandering' and refers to the extent to which this nerve extends throughout the thorax and abdomen of the body. Branches from the vagus innervate a variety of organs, and so naming the nerve according to source or target is not feasible. Nerve nomenclature is therefore complex. Specific nerves are mentioned elsewhere in this book where relevant but will only be named in this chapter if appropriate to the discussion, or as examples.

Nerve cells (neurons)
Structure of nerve cells

Nerve cells are commonly referred to as neurons, and their elongated processes (fibres) may be very long, up to 1.5 m or more for a sensory nerve cell passing from a toe to the brain. In contrast, the processing of information within the brain or spinal cord usually involves neurons that are short and which interact with many neighbouring nerve cells. All neurons contain cell organelles such as a nucleus and mitochondria, but these are largely localized to a distended portion called the cell body.

Efferent (or motor) neurons

Those nerve cells that extend from the brain or spinal cord and pass to tissues elsewhere in the body are collectively said to be efferent ('effere-' = to carry away from) neurons. These neu-

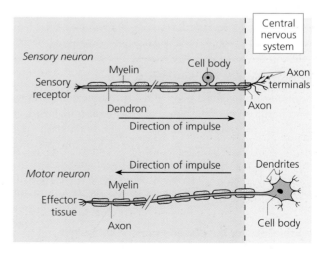

Figure 8.2 Sensory and motor neurons within the nervous system. Note that a single peripheral nerve contains both sensory (afferent) and motor (efferent) neurons (i.e. they are mixed nerves)

- The elongated fibre of the cell that extends from the sensory receptor to the cell body is called the dendron, and that from the cell body to the spinal cord the axon.
- The axon terminals of a sensory nerve cell will form junctions with dendrites of other neurons within the spinal cord.

Thus, the dendron conducts nerve impulses towards the cell body, the axon away from it. In efferent cells described above, the cell body is situated at one end of the cell so there is no dendron, only an axon. However, it was noted that efferents cell have 'dendrites', that is, small branching features that conduct impulses towards the cell body.

Myelin: Schwann cells

Nerve cells must conduct electrical impulses and their dendrons/axons are frequently (but not always) covered with an insulating fatty material called myelin that helps to increase the rate of conduction (Figure 8.2). Myelin is secreted by non-neural cells, called Schwann cells, that are closely associated with the neurons and which lie down the myelin in concentric layers around the nerve fibre. Nerve conduction is considered in a later section but it is important to note here that myelin never forms a complete sheath along a nerve cell. Gaps, called nodes of Ranvier, are essential because myelin is not a complete insulator and electrical current must be regenerated from time to time, and this requires access to tissue fluid by the cell membrane.

The synapse: a junction between nerve cells

Actual physical contact between cells is not usually present although the 'gap' is minute, only of the order of 20 nm (i.e. 20 millionths of a millimetre) wide. The whole structure at the end of the dendrite or axon terminal, including the 'gap', is called a synapse and plays a central role in whether or not nerve impulses are transmitted from one neuron to another. The process is mediated by a chemical released from the terminals, referred to as a neurotransmitter. Synaptic function, with examples of how it can influence nerve transmission, is described in a later section.

OVERVIEW OF THE NERVOUS SYSTEM

Organization of the nervous system

The discussion so far has highlighted that some nerve cells pass to and from tissues of the body, and the brain/spinal cord, and that neural processing takes place in the brain/spinal cord. Accordingly, the nervous system can be divided into two broad anatomical components: (a) the peripheral nervous system of nerves which conduct impulses to and from tissues, and (b) the central nervous system in which processing of information occurs (Figure 8.3).

Organization of the peripheral nervous system

The organization of peripheral nerves can be subdivided according to the functional aspects and the tissues served (Figure 8.3):

- *Autonomic nerves* mediate those changes in tissue functions that are generally involuntary, and coordinate the functions of most organs in the body, though in certain cases, autonomic function may be voluntarily overridden. For example, the ability to empty an unfilled urinary bladder voluntarily is achieved by the exercising of voluntary control of those autonomic nerves involved. Similarly, stress relaxation techniques also demonstrate limited conscious control of the resting heart rate, which is a parameter under the involuntary control of the autonomic nervous system.
- *Somatic nerves* are those nerves that promote the contraction of voluntary muscles, and in particular mediate the control of posture and movement.

The role of autonomic nerves in controlling organ functioning, and hence homeostasis, is considered in more detail in a later section. The role of somatic nerves in mediating muscle contraction is considered in Chapter 17 in relation to the skeletomuscular system and posture maintenance. For now, note that the distinction is not always clear-cut, as the roles of the autonomic and somatic branches sometimes overlap in the control of the body. For example, breathing involves contraction of the diaphragm and of intercostal muscles and this is mediated by somatic nerves, but autonomic nerves influence airway resistance. Similarly, the contraction or relaxation of the urinary bladder is an autonomic function, but bladder emptying also requires voluntary relaxation of the external

---

ACTIVITY

Terminology used in neurophysiology

If you have been following the text you should by now be appreciating just how confusing the terminology related to the nervous system can be! It might be worth reviewing this by considering the following summary:

Central nervous system: this comprises the brain and spinal cord, which coordinate sensory information transmitted from the tissues of the body and promote an appropriate nerve activity to the tissues.

Peripheral nervous system: this is a collective term for the system of nerves, and associated structures called ganglia, that transmit impulses either to the central nervous system, or from it to the tissues.

Somatic nerves: this branch of the peripheral nervous system comprises those nerves that convey impulses to and from skeletal muscle.

Autonomic nerves: this branch of the peripheral nervous system is composed of those nerves that convey impulses to and from the organs of the body.

Afferent neurons: a general term used for those nerve cells within peripheral nerves that convey impulses to the central nervous system. These will normally have receptors at their peripheral terminal and so may also be referred to as sensory neurons.

Efferent neurons: a general term for those nerve cells within peripheral nerves that convey impulses from the central nervous system to tissues (skeletal muscle or other tissues of the body; i.e. distinction between somatic and autonomic nerves may not be made). Because these neurons act to change tissue functions they are often referred to as motor neurons.

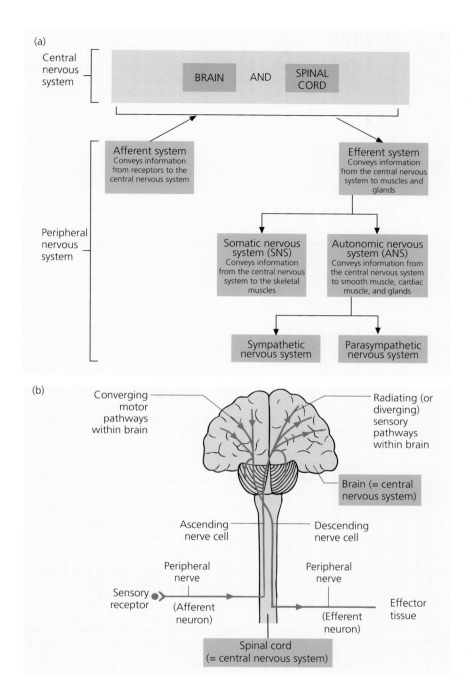

Figure 8.3 (a) General layout of the nervous system. (b) Afferent and efferent pathways. Note how afferent pathways are said to 'ascend' and efferent pathways 'descend'

sphincter muscles of the pelvic floor, unless bladder distension is excessive in which case relaxation becomes involuntary!

Spinal nerves

Most peripheral nerves, whether autonomic or somatic, enter or exit the central nervous system via the spinal cord, at which point they are generally called spinal nerves, of which there are 31 pairs (Figure 8.4). Each spinal nerve contains afferent and efferent neurons of both the autonomic and somatic nervous systems, and it is only at some distance from the cord that the two branches can be distinguished. Spinal nerves enter/exit the spinal cord between the vertebrae and so are at a distance from the brain; clearly, the spinal cord must also contain neural pathways of both the somatic and autonomic systems, and these will conduct neural activity to and from appropriate parts of the brain.

Spinal nerves do not have names attached to them and are normally referred to by the position of the vertebrae from between which they extend (e.g. 'thoracic 2' emerges via the second thoracic vertebrae). Once the somatic and autonomic branches have separated, however, then names will be applied. For example, the intercostal muscles of the chest wall are innervated by the intercostal nerves that branch from the thoracic spinal nerves.

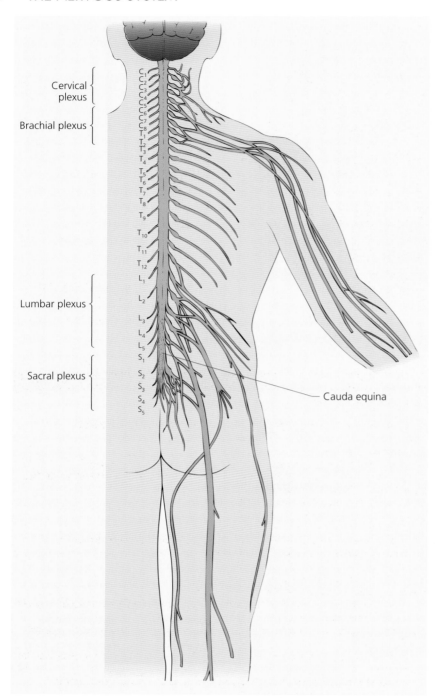

Cervical plexus

Brachial plexus

Lumbar plexus

Sacral plexus

Cauda equina

Figure 8.4 General organization of spinal nerves, and the somatic nervous sytem (plexus = aggregation of nerves or neurons). C, cervical; T, thoracic; L, lumbar; S, sacral. Numbers refer to vertebrae within the respective parts of the vertebral column/spinal cord

Q How many thoracic spinal nerves are there?

Cranial nerves

The remaining peripheral nerves are notable because they do not pass via the spinal cord but instead connect directly with the brain. They are usually considered separately from the spinal nerves, and collectively are called the cranial nerves of which there are 12 pairs (Figure 8.5 and Table 8.1). Cranial nerves are named according to appearance or function, but there is also a conventional method of numbering them using roman numerals (Figure 8.5 and Table 8.1). They innervate tissues of the head and neck, with the exception of the vagus (i.e. pair X); this

is an extremely long nerve that passes through the thorax and abdomen and innervates the organs of these areas.

It was noted above how spinal nerves include afferent and efferent nerve cells of both the autonomic and somatic nervous systems, as they are the common conduits into the cord itself. The cranial nerves are more variable in this respect:

• Cranial nerves may contain afferent neurons, mainly originating from the eyes, ears, nose, mouth, facial tissues and arteries of the neck, or efferent neurons, which supply various muscles, salivary glands, etc., or they may contain both

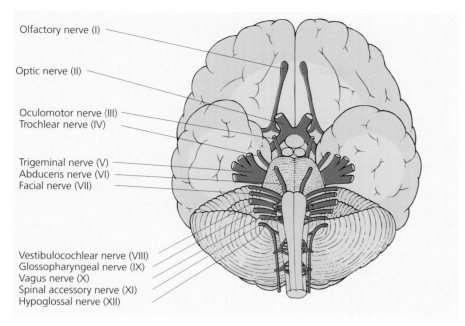

Olfactory nerve (I)

Optic nerve (II)

Oculomotor nerve (III)
Trochlear nerve (IV)

Trigeminal nerve (V)
Abducens nerve (VI)
Facial nerve (VII)

Vestibulocochlear nerve (VIII)
Glossopharyngeal nerve (IX)
Vagus nerve (X)
Spinal accessory nerve (XI)
Hypoglossal nerve (XII)

Figure 8.5 The cranial nerves and their origin in the brain (see also Table 8.1)

Q How many cranial nerves are there?

Table 8.1 Functions of the cranial nerves

Cranial nerve	Homeostatic function	Tissues innervated
Olfactory (I)	Sensory	From olfactory epithelium of the nose
Optic (II)	Sensory	From retinal cells of the eye
Oculomotor (III)	Motor	To the rectus muscles (inferior, superior, medial) and inferior oblique muscles that move the eyes
		To the upper lip area
Trochlear (IV)	Motor	To the superior oblique muscle of the eye
Trigeminal (V)	Ophthalmic sensory	From areas around the orbits of the eyes, nasal cavity, forehead, upper eyelids and eyebrows
Maxillary	Sensory	From the lower eyelids, upper lip, upper gums and teeth, mucous lining of the palate, and the skin of the face
Mandibular	Mixed	Sensory from the skin of the jaw, lower gums and teeth, and lower lip
		Motor to the muscles of mastication, and the floor of the mouth
Abducens (VI)	Motor	To the rectus muscles (lateral) that move the eyes
Facial (VII)	Mixed	Sensory from taste receptors (anterior two-thirds of tongue)
		Motor to muscles of facial expression; includes visceral efferents (autonomic nervous system) to the submandibular and sublingual salivary glands, and tear glands
Vestibulocochlear (VIII)		
Vestibular	Sensory	From the vestibular apparatus (balance organs) of the inner ear
Cochlear	Sensory	From hearing receptors of the cochlea of the inner ear
Glossopharyngeal (IX)	Mixed	Sensory from the pharynx, tonsils, and posterior third of tongue; includes visceral afferents (autonomic nervous system) from carotid arteries and aortic arch
		Motor to pharynx (i.e. swallowing movements), and visceral efferents (autonomic nervous system) to parotid salivary glands
Vagus (X)	Mixed	Sensory from the pharynx, larynx and oesophagus, and visceral afferents (autonomic nervous system) from the thorax and abdomen
		Motor to the larynx, pharynx and soft palate (swallowing movements), and visceral efferents (autonomic nervous system) to viscera of the thorax and abdomen
Accessory (XI)		
Cranial	Motor	To the pharynx, larynx and soft palate (swallowing movements)
Spinal	Motor	To the sternocleidomastoid and trapezius muscles of the neck
Hypoglossal (XII)	Motor	To the musculature of the tongue

(Table 8.1). For some of these nerves the efferent neurons are solely autonomic or somatic. For example, movement of the eyeballs requires stimulation of the ocular muscles of the orbit of the eye via the oculomotor nerve (i.e. a somatic function; 'oculo-' = of the eye), while basal control of the heart involves the vagus nerve (i.e. an autonomic function).

- Some cranial nerves contain neurons of both branches. For example, the glossopharyngeal nerve mediates contraction of the muscles of the pharynx for swallowing (a somatic function; 'glossus' = tongue) and saliva production from certain salivary glands (an autonomic function).

Organization of the central nervous system

The general anatomy of neurons of the brain and spinal cord is similar to that of peripheral neurons in that they consist of a cell body with fibre-like structures (dendron and axon), and branching terminals (dendrites and axon terminals). Similarly, synapses permit interactions to occur between cells. Estimates of the number of cells that each brain cell interacts with suggest that a single neuron may be directly associated with ten thousand others! The brain contains some 100 000 million (i.e. 100 billion) neurons and the potential 'circuitry' is therefore unimaginably extensive.

The central nervous system also contains non-neural cells. These are called neuroglial cells and estimates suggest that they outnumber neurons by as much as 10:1 and so comprise much of the brain mass. They can be subdivided according to their position and function, as outlined in Table 8.2. Note also that the Schwann cells mentioned earlier in relation to the production of a myelin sheath around nerve cell axons are also a type of neuroglial cell.

Neural organization of the spinal cord

In general the neurons of the cord may be considered under three categories:

1. Those with fibres that pass up the cord to the brain, and so form part of the afferent pathways, now referred to as 'ascending'.
2. Those with fibres that pass down the cord from the brain, and so form part of the efferent pathways, now referred to as 'descending'.
3. Neurons that provide connections between various ascending and descending neurons, called interneurons ('inter-' = between).

BOX 8.2 THE BRAIN AS A 'STABLE' TISSUE

We are probably born with most if not all of the central nervous system neurons that we will have in life. Brain growth and development during childhood therefore involves neuronal growth, the forming of connections, or synapses, between neurons with appropriate others, and the growth of neuroglial tissue (i.e. non-neural support cells).

The complexity of neural connections within the brain makes cell division unlikely since it would disrupt the brain 'circuitry'. It appears that neurons remain with us for the duration of our lives. Some may die, although current thinking is that ageing does not have a pronounced effect on neuronal numbers but can have a profound effect on the maintenance of synapses. The lack of cell division activity means that this 'stable' tissue does not readily form tumours; most brain tumours arise from the more reproductively active glial cells, hence the term 'glioma' used for this kind of tumour.

The axons of ascending and descending neurons pass along the periphery of the cord, and so in cross-section the insulating layer of myelin on many of these neurons makes these areas appears white in colour; hence this area is referred to as the 'white matter' of the spinal cord. The cell bodies of these neurons, however, are found more centrally in the cord and the absence of myelin around the cell bodies makes this area appear darker (hence 'grey matter' – an inaccurate term because although the tissue appears grey post-mortem, in life it is pink).

Neural organization of the brain

Superficially the brain can be observed to consist of a number of structures relating to the forebrain and hindbrain; the midbrain is not visible (see Box 8.3 for explanation of these terms).

Table 8.2 Neuroglial cells; support cells for neurons

Type of cells	Description	Homeostatic function
Central nervous system		
Astrocytes ('astro-' = star, '-cyte' = cell)	Star-shaped cells with numerous processes. Protoplasmic astrocytes found in grey matter of the CNS; fibrous astrocytes found in white matter	Twine around nerve cells to form supporting network in brain and spinal cord; attach neurons to their blood vessels
Oligodendrocytes ('oligo-' = few, 'dendro-' = tree)	Resemble astrocytes in some ways, but processes are fewer and shorter	Give support by forming semi-rigid connective tissue rows between neurons in brain and spinal cord. Produce myelin sheath around neurons of the CNS
Microglia ('micro-' = small, '-glia' = glue)	Small cells with few processes derived from monocytes. Normally stationary, but may migrate to site of injury. Also called brain macrophages	Engulf and destroy microbes and cellular debris
Ependyma (= upper garment)	Epithelial cells arranged in a single layer. Range in shape from squamous to columnar. Many are ciliated	Form a continuous epithelial lining for the ventricles of the brain (spaces that form and circulate cerebrospinal fluid) and the central canal of the spinal cord
Peripheral nervous system		
Neurolemmocytes (Schwann cells)	Flattened cells located along the nerve fibres. Cells encircle the axon many times to form a series of concentric rings. Inner layers contain myelin	Produce insulating sheath of myelin around nerve fibres, to enhance conduction velocity of impulses along the axon

CNS, central nervous system.

BOX 8.3 THE EMBRYOLOGICAL BRAIN

The positions of structures within the brain are determined during embryonic development and reference to those positions usually relates to the terms given to embryonic features. The developing brain is first distinguishable as three enlargements called the forebrain, the midbrain and the hindbrain (Figure 8.6).

- The forebrain later subdivides into two further structures: the cerebrum and the thalamus and hypothalamus.
- The midbrain develops as groups of nuclei of grey matter lying quite deep within the brain, and tracts of nerve axons conducting information into and out from higher structures.
- The hindbrain subdivides into the cerebellum, and the pons varolii and medulla oblongata.

ing area and so the convolutions enable more of this processing tissue to be contained within the skull.
- A striking feature of the external appearance of the cerebrum is the occurrence of lobes (paired; one on each side of the brain), and these are named after the bones of the skull that overlie them: frontal lobes, parietal lobes, occipital lobes and temporal lobes.
- The frontal lobes are separated from the parietal lobes that lie behind by a large involution called the 'central sulcus', while the temporal lobes are delineated on each side by an indentation called the 'lateral fissure'.

Hindbrain structures that are visible externally include the cerebellum (a two-halved structure lying at the base of the brain; Figures 8.6 and 8.7a) and the pons varolii and medulla oblongata (distended areas of the part of the brain that lie at the top of the spinal cord).

Internally, sections through the brain reveal:

- 'white matter' which is composed of myelinated nerve fibres that connect different parts of the brain;
- clusters of processing neurons (i.e. grey matter) called nuclei within the white matter; Figure 8.9, p.173 illustrates why they are sometimes likened to 'islands' within the white matter. Note the distinction between brain nuclei and the nuclei of cells);
- fluid-filled spaces called ventricles (not to be confused with the ventricles of the heart). The fluid is a special form of tissue fluid called cerebrospinal fluid (CSF) and this circulates around the brain and the spinal cord and helps to maintain a precise cellular environment (see Figure 8.16, p.181).

Much of the external features of the brain are dominated by the highly convoluted cerebrum of the forebrain (Figure 8.7a):

- The two halves of the cerebrum are referred to as cerebral hemispheres and their separation is clearly indicated by a deep cleft, called the 'longitudinal fissure'.
- The outer surface of the cerebral hemispheres is referred to as the cerebral cortex (cortex = bark, as in tree bark), which is largely composed of 'grey matter' because of the presence of huge numbers of nerve cell bodies that are not myelinated.
- The ridges of the convolutions are called gyri (singular, gyrus) while the indentations between the ridges are called sulci (singular, sulcus). The convolutions increase the surface area of the cerebrum (to about 0.2 m² in an adult) and this is of note because the cerebral cortex is an important process-

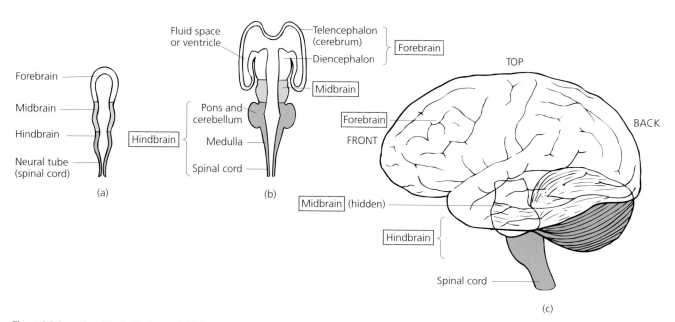

Figure 8.6 An outline of brain development. (a) Commencement of development of the head-end of the neural tube in the embryo. (b) Further development of the three main components of brain structure. Note that the forebrain and hindbrain in particular have enlarged in relative terms. (c) Side view of the final brain. Note how the orientation of the forebrain has changed relative to the mid- and hindbrain, and much of these latter are now enclosed by the forebrain

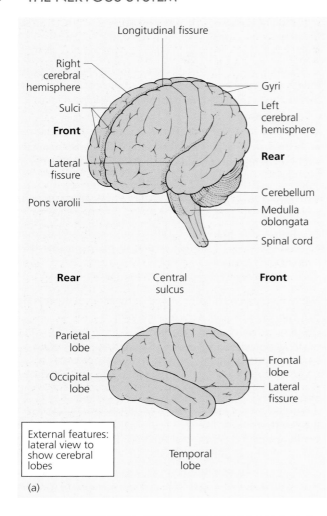

External features: lateral view to show cerebral lobes

(a)

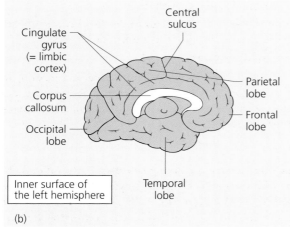

Inner surface of the left hemisphere

(b)

Figure 8.7 (a) External features of the brain. (b) The cerebral hemispheres

Q What is the corpus callosum?

BOX 8.4 STEREOTAXIS

The anatomy of the brain has been extensively recorded and functions ascribed to various features. Surgical techniques have developed over the decades such that neurosurgeons are able to use catheters or electrodes to manipulate or ablate areas of the brain. The features are common to everyone and placement of these implants is facilitated by the use of stereotaxic equipment in which a frame is used to direct them to specific 'coordinates' within the brain, based upon stereotaxic atlases. The method has been considerably improved by the development of imaging techniques such as computed tomography (or CT scans) that enable the surgeon to visualize the positioning of the electrodes.

The effectiveness of the method has been demonstrated in some patients with Parkinson's disease, a condition in which dysfunction of cerebral ganglia produces disorder of movement control. Placement of electrodes and their stimulation reduces or even removes the tremor associated with the condition. Longer-term movement control has also been demonstrated.

BOX 8.5 LOSS OF NEURONS WITHIN THE CENTRAL NERVOUS SYSTEM

A loss of neurons, for whatever reason, will obviously prevent transmission of neural activity along the usual routes. Neurons may be damaged by various means including:

- Direct physical trauma resulting from head injury, or crush effects of a tumour or (in the spinal cord) prolapsed intervertebral discs.
- Indirect physical trauma as in cerebral ischaemia, for example as a consequence of cerebral haemorrhage, and raised intracerebral pressure, owing to excess cerebrovascular fluid, as in hydrocephalus and meningitis, or presence of a haematoma.
- Toxin damage, for example the effects of ions of 'heavy' metals on brain development.
- Some disorders in which (central nervous system) neurons degenerate are of unknown aetiology, although autoimmune responses or inherited causes have been implicated (e.g. motor neuron disease or Alzheimer disease).

Whereas peripheral damage may induce localized loss of function (see Box 8.1, p.163), loss of neurons in the central nervous system can cause disorders that are extensive and devastating. These include cognitive disorders (e.g. cerebral palsy; Alzheimer disease, Creuzfeldt–Jakob disease), motor disorders (e.g. cerebral palsy, epilepsy, motor neuron disease, Creuzfeldt–Jakob disease), autonomic disorders (e.g. respiratory dysrhythmias) and endocrine disorders (e.g. pituitary hyposecretion).

Correction may be aimed at preserving remaining function by removing the underlying cause, such as relieving raised intracranial pressure, or treating an infection. Drug treatments may be used to suppress any inflammation, and tumours may be surgically removed, although additional damage may be incurred in the process. Generally, though, the correction of trauma is limited, and care is often directed at alleviating symptoms, providing therapies that reinforce remnant functions, and providing support.

In certain circumstances, non-progressive brain damage may be improved, though not reversed, by reinforcement of behavioural or social patterns (e.g. 'conductive therapy' in children with cerebral palsy). This probably promotes the development of new neural synapses within the affected areas.

DETAILS OF THE ANATOMY OF THE BRAIN

This section considers in more detail the neural organization of the central nervous system and also identifies some of the roles ascribed to parts of the brain. The major features discussed here are: the forebrain, the midbrain, the hindbrain, the meningeal membranes, the fluid ventricles and CSF and the vasculature of the brain.

The forebrain

As noted previously, the forebrain consists of the most obvious external feature of the brain, namely the highly convoluted cerebrum. There also are some deeper structures, the thalamus and hypothalamus, which develop embryologically from forebrain tissue that together comprise the 'diencephalon' ('between brain') (Figure 8.6b).

The cerebrum

The cerebrum is divided into two hemispheres, connected by a large bundle of myelinated axons called the corpus callosum (Figure 8.7b). This allows communication between the hemispheres and links geographically similar positions. Each hemisphere consists of outer areas that comprise the cerebral cortex, and deeper cerebral nuclei, which may interact with each other, with the cerebral cortex, or with midbrain and hindbrain structures.

Cerebral cortex: (i) the hemispheres

The cortex is comprised of 'grey' matter and represents a collection of major processing areas. The hemispheres have various functions but some generalizations regarding perceptual functioning can be made (Box 8.6).

Cerebral cortex: (ii) the frontal lobes

The frontal lobes are involved in the planning, execution, and evaluation of actions, and their advanced development is considered to reflect the acquisition of intelligence. The cortex includes an area called the motor association area (Figure 8.8) in which information concerning planned actions is collated and passed to the primary motor cortex area, located just forward of the central sulcus that separates the frontal and parietal lobes. This area determines most of the final efferent output to muscles, including those of voluntary eye movements and speech (this latter especially involves the frontal lobe of the left hemisphere; see p.196).

Cerebral cortex: (iii) the parietal lobes

The parietal lobes are especially involved in sensory reception and perception. An area just behind the frontal lobe, directly behind the motor cortex, is called the primary somatosensory cortex (Figure 8.8) and receives information from the 'somatosenses', that is the 'body' senses of touch, pressure, temperature and pain. Information from this area passes to various parts of the brain, including the sensory association area of the parietal lobes. This is a large area that extends into the occipital and temporal lobes (and so receives input from

those lobes also), and is involved in the perception of a stimulus, the integration of various stimuli and in memory.

Cerebral cortex: (iv) the occipital lobes

The occipital lobe consists mainly of the visual cortex (Figure 8.8) and so receives most of its input from the eyes.

Cerebral cortex: (v) the temporal lobes

The temporal lobe has already been mentioned as consisting of part of the wider sensory association area. It also receives sensory information from the ears and consists mainly of the auditory cortex (Figure 8.8).

Cerebral nuclei

Although the cerebral cortex is 'grey matter', below it lies substantial 'white matter', indicative of myelinated axons of nerve cells which convey information through the brain from one area to another. However, set within the white matter are clusters of grey matter, or nuclei, which collectively comprise processing areas called the basal ganglia and the limbic system.

The basal ganglia are a collection of interconnected structures within both hemispheres (Figure 8.9) involved in the control of movement. They interact with the motor cortex and are described in more detail in Chapter 17 in relation to the control of muscle contraction and posture.

The limbic system, shown in Figure 8.10, is another collection of interconnected structures that surround the centre of

---

BOX 8.6 HEMISPHERE DOMINANCE

Curiously, the cortex of the right hemisphere receives most of its sensory information from the left side of the body, and the left hemisphere receives it from the right side. Similarly, the hemisphere controls the contraction of muscles on the opposite side of the body. In this way, being left- or right-handed indicates that one hemisphere is dominant. People who are right-handed will have a dominant left hemisphere, while left-handed people will have a dominant right hemisphere. The left hemisphere seems to be more effective at analysing information presented to it in changing sequences, and is considered important in logic and mathematical analysis (that is, 'scientific' functions). The right hemisphere appears more effective in the analysis of shape, form and space ('artistic' functions) and studies have suggested that left-handedness gives a propensity to artistic abilities. This separation of functioning must be treated with caution, however, since both hemispheres will be involved in functions and the effect is not powerful: there is no conclusive evidence that right-handed people are always better mathematicians!

Transmission of information between the hemispheres must take place and, as noted, this is via the corpus callosum that connects the two. Failure to transmit this information because of trauma to the corpus callosum means that communication between the hemispheres will be incomplete. For example, the language centres on the left side of the brain might not communicate with the right side of the brain. Thus, a request for the individual to raise their left hand will not produce a response because muscle contraction on the left side of the body depends upon nerve activity from motor areas on the right side of the brain. Similarly, sensory stimuli applied to the left side of the body cannot be described, since sensory information from that side will pass to the right side of the brain but cannot be relayed to the language centres on the left side.

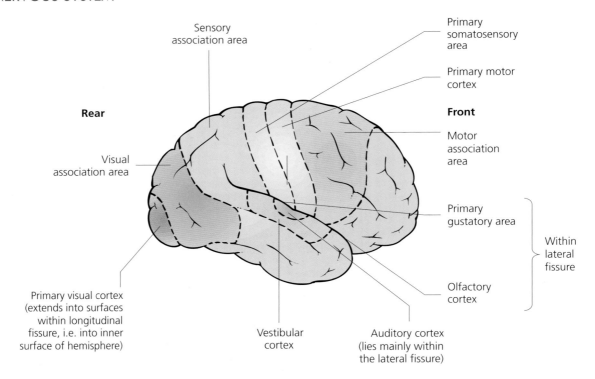

Figure 8.8 The cerebral cortex: general functional anatomy

Q How do these functional areas relate to the cerebral lobes shown in Figure 8.7?

the forebrain, for example the hippocampus (named because of its passing resemblance to the shape of a seahorse) and the amygdala (= almond). Some of the cerebral cortex is also part of the limbic system, especially that along the lower edge (limbus = border) of the cerebral hemispheres, within the fissure between them. Much of that area is readily distinguishable from the rest of the cortex, and is called the cingulate gyrus (though it is frequently referred to simply as the limbic cortex). The limbic system has a role in memory, behaviour and emotions, and has featured widely in popular literature in recent years, especially in connection with aromatherapy since activity in the olfactory nerve (cranial nerve I) passes directly to limbic structures. Smell can be highly evocative of memories of past events, and can also be mood-enhancing.

The diencephalon (thalamus and hypothalamus)

The 'diencephalon' consists of cerebral nuclei deep within the cerebrum that separate it from the midbrain. They are distinguished from the cerebrum through embryological development and there are two major components: the thalamus and the hypothalamus (see Figure 8.9b).

The thalamus is a large, two-lobed structure, which acts as a relay centre for neural information (mainly from sensory receptors) on its way to the cerebral cortex. It is composed of several smaller functional nuclei (Figure 8.11) from which axons pass to specific areas of cortex. For example, the lateral (i.e. at the sides) geniculate nuclei receive input from the eyes and relay it to the visual cortex, and the medial (i.e. at the middle) geniculate nuclei receive input from the cochlea of the ear and relay it to the auditory cortex. Not all thalamic nuclei receive information directly from senses, however. For example, the ventral (i.e. at the bottom) geniculate nuclei receive input from the cerebellum (part of the hindbrain) and relay it to the motor cortex in its role in mediating conscious movement.

The hypothalamus is a relatively small centre at the base of the brain, located under the thalamus ('hypo-' = below) (Figures 8.9b and 8.12). It contains several nuclei, and tracts of axons. The nuclei modulate the autonomic nervous system and, via the pituitary gland, the release of several major hormones; the hypothalamus provides an important link between the brain (especially parts of the limbic system) and the functioning of other physiological systems, and its role in this respect is described in the relevant chapters. In addition, the hypothalamus is involved in behavioural organization since it contains the centres of human 'drives', that is, eating, drinking and sexual behaviours. The hypothalamus also contains the centre for temperature regulation.

(a)

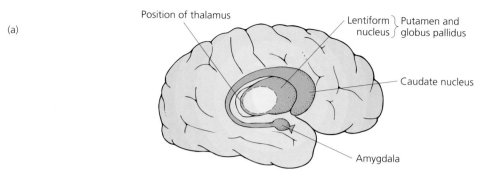

Position of thalamus

Lentiform nucleus } Putamen and globus pallidus

Caudate nucleus

Amygdala

(b)

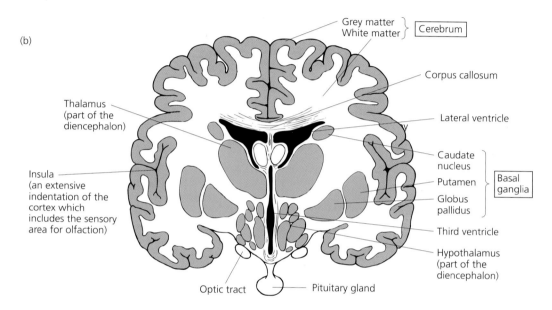

Grey matter } Cerebrum
White matter }

Corpus callosum

Thalamus (part of the diencephalon)

Lateral ventricle

Caudate nucleus } Basal ganglia
Putamen }
Globus pallidus }

Insula (an extensive indentation of the cortex which includes the sensory area for olfaction)

Third ventricle

Hypothalamus (part of the diencephalon)

Optic tract

Pituitary gland

Figure 8.9 The basal ganglia of the forebrain: (a) longitudinal section to show the positions of the main nuclei; (b) cross-section to show the main ganglia relative to other brain structures

Q *What are the ventricles?*

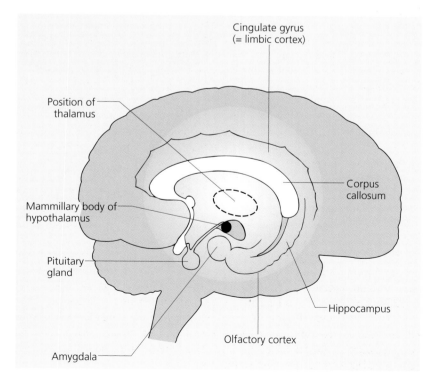

Cingulate gyrus (= limbic cortex)

Position of thalamus

Corpus callosum

Mammillary body of hypothalamus

Pituitary gland

Hippocampus

Amygdala

Olfactory cortex

Figure 8.10 The relative positions of major components of the limbic system

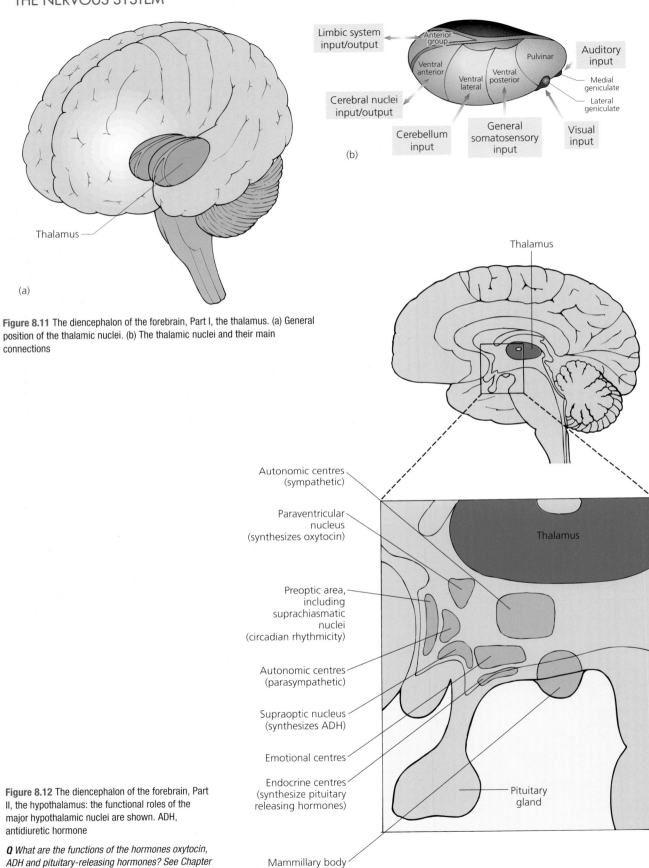

Figure 8.11 The diencephalon of the forebrain, Part I, the thalamus. (a) General position of the thalamic nuclei. (b) The thalamic nuclei and their main connections

Figure 8.12 The diencephalon of the forebrain, Part II, the hypothalamus: the functional roles of the major hypothalamic nuclei are shown. ADH, antidiuretic hormone

Q What are the functions of the hormones oxytocin, ADH and pituitary-releasing hormones? See Chapter 9 for details.

BOX 8.8 NEURODEGENERATIVE DISORDERS

Some neurological disorders can be pinpointed to quite precise parts of brain anatomy. For example, Parkinson's disease is promoted by a decline in activity within neural pathways associated with a midbrain nucleus called the substantia nigra. In contrast some disorders produce profound changes that are much more widespread, for example, Alzheimer disease and Creuzfeldt–Jakob disease (CJD), and so the damage that arises is much less focused, although some of the consequences of the damage might relate to particular areas of the brain. Both diseases are progressive and disabling.

Alzheimer disease

Alzheimer disease still prompts debate as to whether it represents accelerated ageing or a specific disease state. This is because the extent to which aging processes contribute to disorders of late adulthood is not always clear. Alzheimer disease produces a loss of reasoning, abstraction, language and memory, and the failure of such cognitive functions through this disease, and other causes, is frequently referred to as 'dementia'. First described by Alois Alzheimer in 1907, the most obvious changes in brain anatomy are the formation of plaques and neurofibrillary tangles. The former are extracellular deposits of amyloid beta-protein, while the latter are dense tangles of proteinaceous fibres present within the cytoplasm of certain neurons. The plaques and tangles are not unique to the disease, however, as both occur to a lesser degree in the brains of elderly people. An understanding of the aetiology of Alzheimer disease could therefore give information as to how plaques develop in ageing brains.

Much is now known about the genetics and molecular biology of Alzheimer disease (Drouet *et al.*, 2000), and plaque development is thought to result from a defective enzymatic processing of the precursor of amyloid beta-protein, a 'normal' protein found on cell membranes. In some people, there is a familial link with the disease (involving alleles on chromosome 21), while people with Down syndrome (i.e. trisomy 21) also exhibit a propensity to develop the condition. There is some evidence, therefore, that a propensity to the condition can be inherited. However, the familial link is not especially strong and this suggests that Alzheimer disease largely arises because the molecular changes that promote plaque formation are also influenced by environmental risk factors (Brown *et al.*, 2005). This is an area of debate but some studies have implicated smoking, alcohol and metal poisoning (e.g. aluminium) as risk factors.

Creuzfeldt–Jakob disease (see Barnett, 2002)

CJD is a 'prion' disease – it is caused by infection of the nervous system with a type of protein that seems to be capable of causing normal cell surface proteins to transform, and so become dysfunctional. Prions are resistant to the action of protease enzymes and so are not digested when taken in from a dietary source. With new-variant CJD (nv-CJD) the protein originates in cows, where it causes bovine spongiform encephalitis (BSE), and transfers to humans in food products that contain neural tissue from infected cows. The protein appears to make its way to the central nervous system, possibly via peripheral nerve cells. Within the brain its resistance to proteases enables it to interact with cell surface proteins, seemingly causing them to change molecular shape, leading to widespread vacuolation, a degeneration of neural tissue that produces sponge-like features. Very little is understood about prion diseases generally but there is also suggestion that perhaps some people have surface proteins that are more susceptible to change than those of other people, and therefore perhaps there is a genetic susceptibility. The evidence is speculative at present, and in relation to nv-CJD is complicated by an incubation period that seemingly is of several years.

The midbrain

The midbrain is a relatively small region of the brain, lying deep within the brain, and consists of two major component parts called the tectum and the tegmentum (Figure 8.13a,b). The midbrain also contains the cerebral aqueduct, the centrally placed channel that connects the third and fourth fluid-filled ventricles of the brain.

The tectum (= roof)

The tectum forms the dorsal, or posterior, part of the midbrain. It consists of a number of nuclei, the most prominent ones appearing as four external bumps on the brainstem (Figure 8.13a), being:

- the pair of superior (i.e. upper) colliculi which receive sensory input from the eyes, via the thalamus, and are involved in the control of eye movement;
- the pair of inferior (i.e. lower) colliculi which receive input from the ears as part of the auditory pathway.

The tegmentum (= covering)

The tegmentum lies anterior to the tectum and contains several nuclei (Figure 8.13c). Prominent ones include:

- The substantia nigra (= black substance; these neurons contain melanin) connect with certain basal ganglia of the forebrain and contribute to the modulation of impulses that will eventually exit the cerebral cortex and evoke muscle contraction. Parkinson's disease and Huntington's disease are both consequences of failure in some respect of these nuclei.
- The red nucleus projects to the spinal cord and is part of those pathways (referred to as the extrapyramidal tracts; see Chapter 17, p.481) which convey the information out of the brain to the muscles.
- Part of the reticular (= net) formation, a diffuse area that extends back into the hindbrain. It is a relay centre of some sensory information to the thalamus, but has also been found to have a role in determining the sleep–wake cycle, and in movement control.

The hindbrain

The structures of the hindbrain visible as external features are the cerebellum, pons varolii and medulla oblongata (Figure 8.14a).

The cerebellum

The cerebellum (= little brain) is a large structure located behind and below the rest of the brain. In general structure it resembles that of the cerebrum: it has a cortex of 'grey matter' which connects with a set of subcortical structures called the

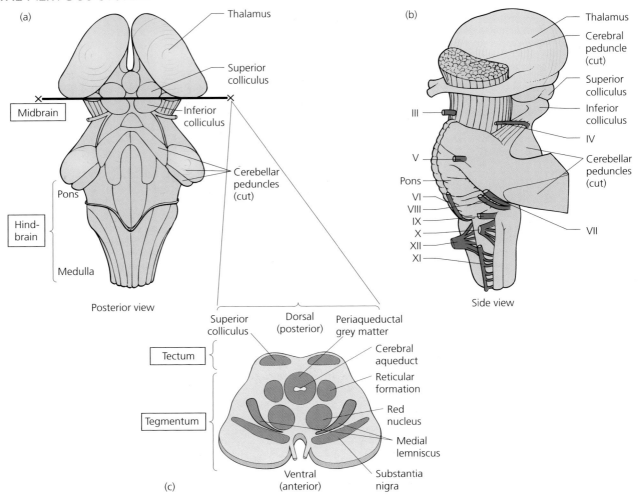

Figure 8.13 (a) Midbrain features, and the brainstem, posterior view. (b) Side view to show exit of cranial nerves. (c) Section through the midbrain at X–X in (a) to show the main nuclei of the midbrain.

Q Which parts of the hindbrain are included as components of the 'brainstem'? (See Figure 8.14.)

Q What is the cerebral aqueduct? (See Figure 8.16.)

cerebellar nuclei. Three pairs of large tracts of nerve cells are associated with the cerebellum:

- The inferior and middle cerebellar peduncles, that connect with the medulla oblongata and the pons varolii of the hindbrain, respectively. The cerebellum receives sensory inputs via these tracts from the eyes, vestibular apparatus of the ears and from sensory receptors around the body.
- The superior cerebellar peduncles that communicate with the midbrain, providing an output that enables a 'fine tune' modulation of activity that eventually evokes muscle contraction during movements (see Chapter 17). The cerebellum, therefore, helps to coordinate movement, particularly the production of smooth movement, and of fine movements such as are involved in writing, playing sport, etc.

The pons variolii

The pons is visible externally as a large bulge at the front of the brainstem (Figure 8.14a). There are numerous nuclei of cells within the pons, such as:

- the reticular formation (this continues into the tegmentum mentioned above);
- part of the respiratory centres (the 'apneustic' centre) that coordinate this system (others are in the medulla; see later);
- nuclei of various cranial nerves, providing connecting relays for sensory or motor activity related to the head and neck;
- those that are part of the pathways by which sensory information passes from the spinal cord to appropriate parts of the brain, or form part of the pathways by which efferent activity from motor areas of the brain converge before leaving the brain, for example the lemnisci (singular, lemniscus), that traverse both the medulla and pons, from which activity passes to the thalamus and from there to the cerebral cortex (Figure 8.14b).

Another large tract of fibres worth mentioning here are those that form the cerebellar peduncles (see above), which carry sensory information arriving in the pons and pass it on to the cerebellum, and also relay information coming out of the cerebellum to the midbrain and cerebral cortex.

(a) External features and position of the cardiovascular centres and respiratory centres

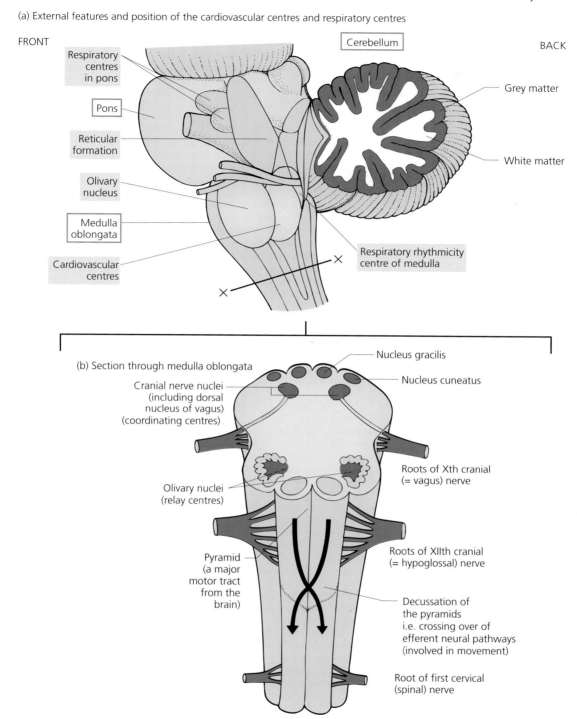

Figure 8.14 The hindbrain: (a) external features and internal position of the cardiovascular and respiratory centres, and of the reticular formation; (b) spinothalamic sensory tracts of the medulla, section and anterior aspect

The medulla oblongata

The medulla is the section of hindbrain that links the brain with the spinal cord and much of its anatomy therefore involves tracts of axons of nerve cells that carry information into and out of the brain:

- The gracile and cuneate fasciculi (there are two of each) are noticeable externally on the posterior aspect of the medulla. These tracts carry sensory input into the brainstem from the spinal cord (Figure 8.14b).
- The pyramids pass through the anterior aspects of the medulla and carry efferent activity to the muscles. It is in the

medulla that the tract from the one side of the brain crosses over (called 'decussation') to the opposite side of the spinal cord (Figure 8.14b). In this way, one side of the brain mediates contraction of muscles on the opposite side of the body (remember that sensory information passing into the brain eventually passes to the hemisphere opposite to the side of the body from which it originated).

Internally the medulla also contains nuclei, for example:

- the gracile and cuneate fasciculi terminate at the gracile and cuneate nuclei respectively, from which axons project toward the thalamus (Figure 8.14);
- diffuse areas of neurons, and various nuclei, comprise the respiratory 'inspiratory' and 'expiratory' centres and the cardiovascular 'accelerator' and 'depressor' areas (Figure 8.14a) that modulate these systems;
- the olivary bodies, which are two oval-shaped protrusions noticeable on the anterior surface of the medulla (Figure 8.14b) inside which are found the inferior olivary nuclei (these sac-like structures, together with accessory nuclei, act as relay centres for transmission of activity from various parts of the brain and spinal cord to the cerebellum).

In addition to receiving afferent information from peripheral autonomic neurons, the areas of the medulla that are involved in promoting respiratory and cardiovascular responses also receive inputs from areas of the hypothalamus. These are responsible for the mediation of psychological influences on autonomic responses, for example in the stress response.

The meningeal membranes

The brain and spinal cord are covered by three epithelial membranes, collectively called the meninges (Figure 8.15):

- an outermost layer called the dura mater;
- a middle layer called the arachnoid mater;
- an innermost layer called the pia mater.

Dura mater

The dura mater is a thick, tough protective/ supportive layer comprised mainly of the protein collagen. There are two components:

- An inner layer (sometimes confusingly referred to as the 'meningeal' layer) which is continuous between the brain and spinal cord, and forms inwardly folding membranes, or septa, that project into the major indentations of the brain and so help to support it. The most prominent of these septa is called the falx cerebri and extends down into the longitudinal fissure between the two hemispheres. The layer also extends out along the 'roots' of the cranial and spinal nerves, and forms a protective sheath until they exit the skull and vertebrae respectively.
- An outer layer which is really the periosteum lining of the bones of the cranium.

Venous sinuses, which eventually return blood flowing out of the brain to the jugular veins, may be found between these two layers.

BOX 8.9 THE BRAINSTEM AND 'BRAINSTEM DEATH'

Parts of the hindbrain (the pons varolii and medulla oblongata), the midbrain, and parts of the thalamus of the forebrain are sometimes referred to as the brainstem. This is because they provide the 'stem' to which the cerebellum of the hindbrain and the cerebrum of the forebrain appear to be attached, and through which all activity into and out of these structures therefore arises or passes. Brainstem structures:

- act as a conduit for neural impulses passing into and out of the brain (this will apply to sensory/motor impulses from and to the rest of the body, but also includes impulses from the balance organs of the ear and also to and from muscles of the eye);
- contain brain centres (nuclei) that are especially involved in the control of vital body functions, for example breathing and blood pressure.

The brainstem introduces important considerations in clinical practice. For example, the pons and medulla contain the reticular formation that is involved in arousal, and which is inhibited by general anaesthetics. The brainstem also contains the autonomic nuclei that are responsible for coordinating breathing, heart rate and blood vessel constriction/dilation, and acts as a conduit for other features of the autonomic nervous system. The brainstem also contains the main sites of action of morphine and so has a role to play in analgesia.

Accordingly, 'brainstem death' is considered to represent a condition that represents the death of the individual (Edwards and Forbes, 2003) and this is an important factor in determining if an individual on life support equipment is likely to recover. Tests include:

- An electroencephalogram (EEG) to monitor brain activity, especially in relation to sensory activity.
- The presence or absence of a pupil light response. The pupil of the eye is controlled by the nerve activity produced in response to the level of light stimulation of the retina (see Chapter 7, pp.152–3). The nerve pathway involved includes brain centres within the hindbrain. 'Brainstem death' will mean that the reflex does not occur.
- The presence or absence of a vestibular–ocular reflex. Sudden movement of fluid within the vestibular apparatus of the inner ear (see Chapter 7) produces a reflex horizontal movement of the eye. The nerve pathway that stimulates this passes through the brain stem, and so the reflex will be absent in 'brainstem death'.
- The presence or absence of a corneal touch reflex. Blinking in response to contact with the cornea of the eye is a defence response and operates via a reflex passing through the brainstem. This reflex too will be absent if there is 'brainstem death'.

Arachnoid mater

The arachnoid mater is a delicate membrane of loose connective tissue that lies between the dura mater and the pia mater. A narrow space separates the arachnoid mater from the overlying dura mater, referred to as the subdural space. In places the arachnoid mater penetrates the dura mater to project into the blood of the superior sagittal sinus; these projections are the arachnoid villi (villus = finger-like projection) that reabsorb CSF back into the blood. Trauma may cause bleeding into the subdural space (called a subdural haemorrhage) and produces a clot (a subdural haematoma). If acute, the haematoma may form within hours after the trauma, if subacute perhaps in one or more weeks. The bleeding may also be chronic over weeks or even months. The mass of the haematoma compresses underlying brain tissue, commonly causing raised intracranial

(a) Around the brain

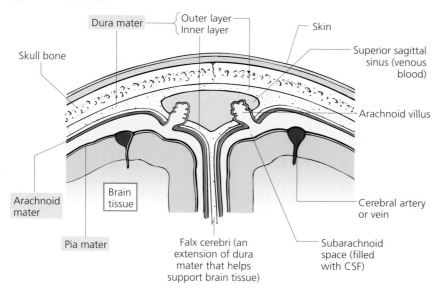

Note: Arachnoid and pia mater are connected by a network of bridging strands (called trabeculae) that help to maintain the patency of the subarachnoid space

(b) Around the spinal cord

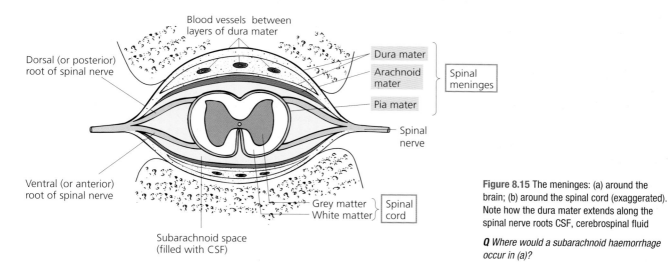

Figure 8.15 The meninges: (a) around the brain; (b) around the spinal cord (exaggerated). Note how the dura mater extends along the spinal nerve roots CSF, cerebrospinal fluid

Q Where would a subarachnoid haemorrhage occur in (a)?

BOX 8.10 MENINGITIS

This is an inflammation of the meningeal membranes induced by an infectious agent. Pain receptors are found in the meninges (but not in the brain tissue) and severe headache is observed. Apart from any localized effects of the inflammation on adjacent brain/spinal tissue, the meningeal vessels also become more permeable, and secrete too much fluid and, therefore, raise intracranial pressure. This has generalized cerebral effects, and the condition is life threatening. Irritation of cranial and spinal nerves could explain the associated symptoms, such as neck stiffness, tinnitus and head retraction.

Meningitis may be caused by infection with bacteria, viruses, fungi, parasites or by the actions of toxins. Bacterial meningitis usually involves

Neisseria meningitidis and is often referred to as 'meningococcal meningitis'. Children and adolescents are particularly at risk. Other agents are *Streptococcus pneumoniae* and *Haemophilus influenzae*. The bacteria are common agents found within the nasopharynx and so the mode of entry to the meninges remains unclear, though it is normally blood borne. Viral meningitis normally produces milder symptoms.

Diagnosis usually entails the sampling of cerebrospinal fluid. This is usually clear and colourless but becomes turbid if there is meningeal infection because of the occurrence of large numbers of leucocytes. Differential white cell count is used to distinguish the occurrence of bacterial or viral meningitis.

pressure (i.e. an elevated pressure of CSF around and within the brain; see below).

A much larger space, referred to as the subarachnoid space, separates the arachnoid mater from the underlying pia mater, and contains the CSF (see below) that bathes the brain and spinal cord. Enlargements of this space in certain parts of the brain, and at the base of the spinal cord, are used clinically to obtain samples of CSF. The patency of the space is maintained by a meshwork of bridging strands called trabeculae between the arachnoid mater and pia mater. Head trauma may cause bleeding into the subarachnoid space. There is often an inflammatory reaction in these membranes, and the clot (or subarachnoid haemorrhage) impairs circulation of CSF and its reabsorption. Again, brain tissue is compressed and displaced by the blood mass. There is commonly a rapidly developing headache, visual and motor impairment and loss of consciousness. Mortality rates are relatively high and the risk of rebleeding and mortality is a major risk, especially in the first 24 hours. For this reason it is important to monitor for vital signs and general state of consciousness.

Pia mater

The pia mater covers the actual surface of the brain and spinal cord, and forms a sheath around cranial nerves and spinal nerve roots as they traverse the subarachnoid space. The pia mater is composed of loose connective tissue and so resembles the arachnoid mater in structure, but it is also rich in blood vessels that supply the underlying neural tissue. The pia mater also lines the cerebral ventricles and forms the choroid plexus, the membrane that secretes the CSF.

BOX 8.11 THE BLOOD–BRAIN BARRIER AND DRUGS

The secretory epithelium that produces cerebrospinal fluid (CSF) forms a 'blood–brain barrier' as only lipid-soluble substances, or those with transport facilities within the epithelial cell membranes, can cross into the CSF. This barrier is clinically important, as psychometric drugs must be capable of crossing it if brain function is to be affected.

For example, in people with Parkinson's disease there are certain neural pathways that utilize dopamine as a neurotransmitter but are deficient in the chemical. However, dopamine itself cannot be administered because it does not cross the barrier. Levodopa is a drug that is commonly prescribed, which crosses the blood–brain barrier into the brain and is then converted into dopamine within the brain.

General anaesthetics and alcohol are lipid-soluble and are not influenced by the barrier. The rapid onset of action of these drugs is an indication of their rapid transit into the brain.

Cerebrospinal fluid

As noted previously, the brain and spinal cord do not consist entirely of tissue; spaces filled with CSF are evident. The CSF provides the brain with:

- a protected environment;
- hydraulic suspension of the brain matter;
- protection against mechanical damage to blood vessels and the membranous linings of the brain by preventing friction with the skull.

By their nature, neurons are particularly susceptible to changes in their intracellular/extracellular environment, and even the normal fluctuations of blood glucose concentration

---

BOX 8.12 EXCESS OR DEFICIENT CEREBROSPINAL FLUID (CSF) VOLUME

Excess CSF: Raised intracranial pressure
At any given time there is approximately 120–150 mL of CSF circulating around the adult brain. The fluid is continuously being secreted from, and reabsorbed into, the blood plasma and so the volume present represents a homeostatic balance between the rate of secretion and rate of reabsorption (note: about 600 mL of fluid is produced/reabsorbed each day). This normally is not problematic but an increase in the volume present may be caused by:

- inflammatory conditions, such as meningitis, that disrupt the reabsorptive areas;
- brain trauma, for example stroke, in which tissue damage or bleeding disrupts the circulation of the fluid and so prevents it from reaching the reabsorptive areas – consequently, the continued secretion causes the CSF volume to rise;
- a blockage of the routes of fluid circulation, for example the cerebral aqueduct between the third and fourth fluid ventricles, by a brain tumour;
- a congenital failure in the formation of the cerebral aqueduct during brain development.

Raised intracranial fluid volume, and pressure, is therefore a form of (cerebral) oedema and is called hydrocephalus (literally 'water on the brain'). Consequently, tissue is forced outward but unlike other oedematous states, there is no room for brain tissue to expand with the fluid volume since it is enclosed within the bony box of the skull. Its impact with the skull disturbs neural functioning and may even cause neural loss if the

compression is severe. Severe headaches and cognitive disturbances are common but the compression can be fatal, especially if the fluid accumulation is rapid. In benign intracranial hydrocephalus, the onset is relatively slow. The causes are largely unknown, although previous history of head injury might be a factor. The slow accumulation of CSF produces a gradual onset of symptoms that may delay diagnosis. The outcome again could be fatal. In congenital hydrocephalus, the incomplete formation of a bony skull for a period after birth makes the bones of the skull more movable, and the raised intracranial pressure typically produces a 'high dome' head. The onset of raised intracranial pressure is usually gradual.

Treatment is aimed at removing any cause of the accumulation of CSF. This might entail removing the source of inflammation, removing a blood clot, removing excess fluid until recovery from trauma occurs or surgical implantation of a catheter into the subarachnoid space or ventricles to enable drainage of CSF back into the venous system. The latter often fails as the catheter tip blocks, and patients may require repeat placement. This can have consequences for the patient's quality of life (Gelling et al., 2004).

Deficiency of CSF
Loss of CSF might be observed in people who have undergone epidural anaesthesia in which a catheter is inserted between the vertebrae into the spinal cavity (epidural = upon the dura. This describes the placing of the anaesthetic). In this procedure, fluid may leak from the insertion point. The fluid loss influences neural functioning; headaches again are characteristic.

that arise through eating patterns would be disturbing for them (neurons do require glucose but operate most effectively if the CSF concentration is held almost constant). To ensure an even tighter homeostatic control of the extracellular environment than is normally observed in blood, the central nervous system must largely be physically isolated from the blood.

The CSF remains isolated from blood by being secreted by cells of the pia mater that line the larger fluid spaces; in other words the CSF is one of the 'transcellular' fluids of the body. Utilizing a secretory process means that the fluid composition can be very closely regulated; this helps to protect the neurons from the short-term, moment-to-moment fluctuations observed in composition of blood plasma.

There are four main fluid spaces, or ventricles (Figure 8.16a). Three (i.e. two large lateral ventricles, and the third ventricle) lie deep within the forebrain, whilst the fourth is in the hindbrain. Most CSF is secreted into the lateral ventricles, which connect with the third ventricle via the interventricular foramina ('inter-' = between; 'foramina' = windows). The third ventricle is connected to the fourth ventricle by the cerebral aqueduct within the midbrain.

The CSF flows from the ventricles into the subarachnoid space (see 'The meningeal membranes', above) and from there around the brain (Figure 8.16b). Some CSF passes into the subarachnoid space of the spinal cord and so circulates around the cord neurons. Fluid flow is promoted by the action of cilia, although head and vertebral movements help. The fluid is eventually reabsorbed back into the blood via the arachnoid

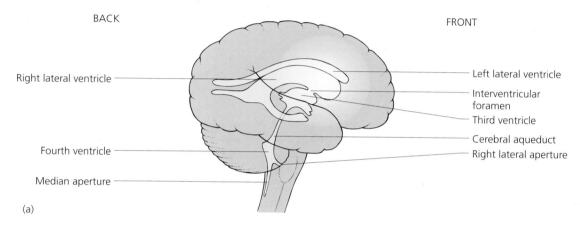

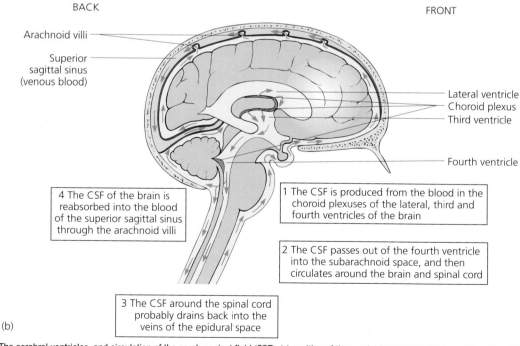

Figure 8.16 The cerebral ventricles, and circulation of the cerebrospinal fluid (CSF): (a) position of the cerebral ventricles; (b) circulation of the CSF. The choroid plexus is the tissue that secretes the CSF; 1–4 are key points within the CSF circulation

Q What is the role of the arachnoid villi?

villi (see above). Clearly, the rate of reabsorption must balance the rate of secretion, if CSF volume is to be maintained. The means of regulation of the process is unclear.

Vasculature of the brain: the cerebral circulation

The brain is supplied with blood by four arteries (Figure 8.17a):

- Two internal carotid arteries that branch from the two 'common' carotid arteries within the neck. The internal carotids penetrate the base of the skull and run along the base of the brain (the other branches, the external carotid arteries, supply the face and neck). Upon entering the skull, each internal carotid artery divides to form an anterior and a middle cerebral artery, and these supply blood to the anterior half to two thirds of the brain.

- Two vertebral arteries that ascend the vertebral column, and penetrate the skull via the foramen magnum, through which the spinal cord passes. The vertebral arteries combine to form a single basilar artery, which runs along the anterior (or ventral) aspect of the hindbrain and sends branches into the hindbrain and midbrain. It eventually divides to form a pair of posterior cerebral arteries that supply structures at the rear of the cerebrum.

Although the carotids and vertebral arteries would appear to be responsible for supplying blood to different parts of the brain, the internal carotids and the basilar artery are interconnected at the base of the brain. Communicating arteries

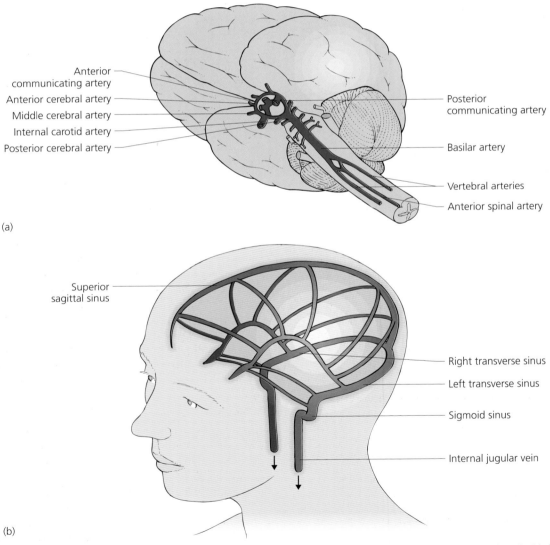

(a)

Anterior communicating artery
Anterior cerebral artery
Middle cerebral artery
Internal carotid artery
Posterior cerebral artery

Posterior communicating artery
Basilar artery
Vertebral arteries
Anterior spinal artery

(b)

Superior sagittal sinus

Right transverse sinus
Left transverse sinus
Sigmoid sinus
Internal jugular vein

Figure 8.17 The cerebral vasculature. (a) Cerebral arteries; the anterior and posterior communicating arteries join the cerebral arteries to form the 'circle of Willis'. (b) Venous drainage

Q What is the advantage of having a circle of Willis?

Q To where do the jugular veins pass?

branch from the sites of origin of the anterior cerebral and posterior cerebral arteries to form the 'circle of Willis' (Figure 8.17a). Blood can, therefore, pass from the carotid arteries to the posterior cerebral arteries, or from the basilar artery to the anterior and middle cerebral arteries. Having four arteries supplying the brain, and vessels that connect anterior and posterior vessels, are adaptations that help to prevent blood flow to the brain being compromised, a feature that probably reflects the high metabolic activity of the brain and the sensitivity of brain cells to disturbances in their immediate environment.

Blood drains from the brain via small veins that empty into blood sinuses (i.e. spaces) within the dura mater (a meningeal membrane – see above). The largest of these is called the superior sagittal sinus (Figure 8.17b) and lies within the fold of membrane called the falx cerebri. Most venous blood eventually drains into a pair of transverse sinuses, which run forward inside and along the base of the skull and empty into the internal jugular veins. These eventually join in the neck with the external jugular veins, which drain other parts of the head and neck, to form the 'common' jugular veins.

BOX 8.13 CEREBROVASCULAR ACCIDENTS (CVAs, STROKES)

A CVA occurs when a portion of the brain is deprived of blood, and hence of oxygen and glucose. Cerebral thrombosis caused by clot formation at the site of an atherosclerotic plaque, cerebral embolism caused by drifting clots, fatty masses or air bubbles and cerebral haemorrhages are all common causes of CVA, and may cause loss of neurons, or an increase in fluid pressure on underlying nerve cells.

Symptoms of CVA depend upon which part of the brain is damaged, and therefore which cerebral artery (see text) is affected:

- a CVA involving the anterior cerebral artery particularly affects the motor and sensory cortex;
- a CVA involving the middle cerebral artery will have similar effects but may also include speech and auditory defects;
- a CVA in the posterior cerebral artery will affect the visual cortex, and the limbic system;
- loss of blood supply via the basilar artery may partly be compensated for by blood passing through the circle of Willis. Nevertheless, damage to the cerebellum and brainstem can be severe. Loss of brainstem functions will also affect autonomic control.

Blockages to cerebral arteries can be temporary, and symptoms short-lived. These are called transient ischaemic episodes (or attacks; often abbreviated as TIAs) and can precede more serious attacks. They are most frequently observed in older people as a consequence of age-related changes to blood supply.

Initial symptoms of a stroke may also be exaggerated by the swelling of surrounding tissues, and so neural function may improve with time as the swelling subsides. Care is particularly directed at facilitating neurological improvement (Cross, 2008). Anticoagulant therapy can help to reduce the likelihood of further clotting and so prevent exacerbation of the problem. Surgical intervention to remove a blood clot may also be necessary to relieve raised intracranial pressure or to improve circulation. Preventive surgery, for example on aneurysms, is also possible in some cases. The reduction of risk factors, such as high blood pressure (hypertension), is an important part of health promotion strategies.

See the case of a person with impaired mobility following a stroke, Section VI, p.666.

DETAILS OF THE ANATOMY OF THE SPINAL CORD

Nerve cells and tracts

The spinal cord lies within the vertebral bones, passing through the spinal foramen of each bone, and is covered by the three meningeal layers, noted earlier. The main functions of the spinal cord are to provide a means of transmitting motor activity from the brain to the tissues via peripheral nerves, and to carry sensory activity from around the body to the brain. On descending the vertebral column therefore, diameter decreases as spinal nerves exit. On reaching the level of the second lumbar vertebra (towards the lower back) the cord divides into a mass of neural structures which are the roots of various nerves that enter or exit the vertebral column below this point. The structure is reminiscent of a horse's tail and so is called the cauda equina ('cauda' = tail; 'equina' = horse; Figure 8.4).

Nerve 'roots' leave the cord, and cauda equina, at intervals to form the spinal nerves; the 'roots' fuse after leaving the cord within spaces between the vertebrae (the vertebral foramina), to form the nerves themselves. Thus, at each vertebral joint there is a pair of posterior (or dorsal) and anterior (or ventral) nerve roots (Figure 8.18). There are 31 pairs of spinal nerves, the subdivisions of which relate to the skeletal subdivisions of the vertebral column (see p.165):

- eight pairs arise from the cervical vertebrae;
- twelve pairs arise from the thoracic vertebrae;
- five pairs arise from the lumbar vertebrae;
- five pairs arise from the sacral vertebrae;
- one pair arises from the coccygeal vertebrae.

Sensory neurons within the spinal nerves form the dorsal nerve root, while the motor neurons form the ventral root. In other words, sensory information passing along the nerves to the cord enter the posterior aspect of the cord, while motor information passing from the cord into the nerves exits from the anterior aspect of the cord. The cell bodies of the sensory neurons are found in the same area of the dorsal root and produce the distension called a dorsal root ganglion (Figure 8.18). The cell bodies of motor neurons lie within the cord itself so there is no comparable structure in the ventral root.

The arrangement of paired spinal nerves produces what appears to be a 'segmental' arrangement, with a specific spinal nerve perhaps supplying a very localized segment of the body. To a large extent this is in fact the case and clinically has significance when considering sensory nerves. Thus, the epidural administration of an analgesic agent into the vicinity of the spinal cord could block pain transmission from a number of tissues but they will be located in a similar part of the body. The further the nerve is away from the spinal cord, the more dispersed the nerve endings tend to be but even in the skin there are sensory areas that map to a particular spinal nerve. These areas are called dermatomes (Figure 8.19).

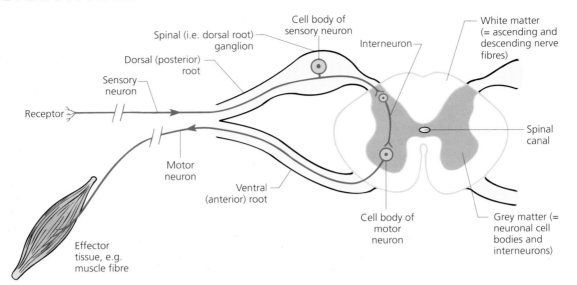

Figure 8.18 Spinal nerve roots and the general appearance of the cord

Q What do the terms 'ventral' and 'dorsal' mean?

White matter

The white matter of the cord is found at its periphery, and consists of myelinated nerve fibres that descend or ascend the cord, and is highly organized with the neurons forming 'columns' of tissue within the cord periphery. Within the columns, the neurons are arranged into distinct 'tracts' (Figure 8.20a):

- The dorsal columns consist of axons of sensory neurons which, on entering the cord, turn to ascend it and terminate by synapsing with other nerve cells within the medulla of the hindbrain, from which neurons cross over to the opposite side before ascending further. Functionally these neurons carry sensory information from mechanoreceptors, particularly those associated with the skin (see Chapter 7, p.142).
- The lateral and ventral columns contain nerve fibres in tracts that ascend (i.e. are sensory) or descend (i.e. are motor) the cord.
- Ascending tracts consist of nerve cell fibres which convey information from
  - temperature and pain receptors, as well as pressure receptors of the skin and proprioreceptors of the muscles and joints. Unlike those of the dorsal columns, the nerve cells entering the cord immediately synapse with others, the

Figure 8.19 Distribution of dermatomes. The diagram provides a sensory 'map' of the body surface. Each dermatome is an area of skin that is served by a pair of spinal nerves, or by cranial nerve V (trigeminal nerve). The letters and numbers refer to the origin of the nerve

Q Where would nerve activity stimulated by injury to the left little finger pass into the spinal cord?

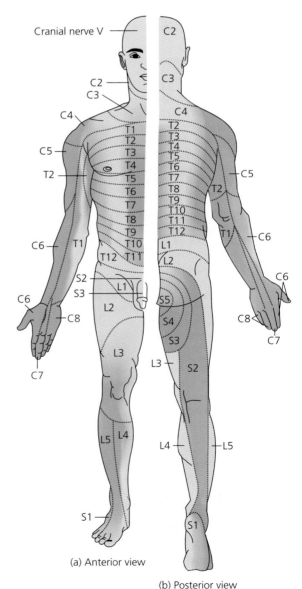

(a) Anterior view

(b) Posterior view

axons of which then ascend in the tracts. Some of these neurons ascend on the same side as the afferent neuron enters the cord; others cross over to the opposite side before ascending the cord. The destination in the brain of the ascending tracts of these columns was considered in Chapter 7. Most eventually pass to the thalamus within the forebrain, from whence information passes out to other brain areas. Accordingly, they are collectively referred to as spinothalamic tracts (perhaps preceded by anterior, lateral, etc.).

- There are various descending tracts (Figure 8.20a), and these are referred to according to where they originate within the brain, for example corticospinal tracts originate within the cerebral cortex. Each tract consists of motor neurons that eventually synapse with other efferent neurons, which pass via spinal nerves to the tissues of the body.

Grey matter

In cross-section, the central portion of the cord appears as a somewhat H-shaped, or butterfly-shaped, area (Figures 8.18 and 8.20b). This is the grey matter of the cord and consists of unmyelinated nerve cell bodies, axons and glial cells.

Sensory neurons entering the cord pass into the grey matter. At this point, the grey matter is called the dorsal horn since it is the 'arm' of the H-shape closest to the dorsal (i.e. posterior) surface of the cord. Depending upon their role (see white matter, above) they then either turn to enter the ascending columns, or they form synapses with other cells in the grey matter may relay with small interneurons (i.e. neurons between other ones; sometimes called relay neurons) which may be entirely confined within the grey matter or project to other parts of grey or white matter. These cells, therefore, provide communication channels in the cord. Other parts of the grey matter comprise the cell bodies of motor neurons, the

(a) White matter

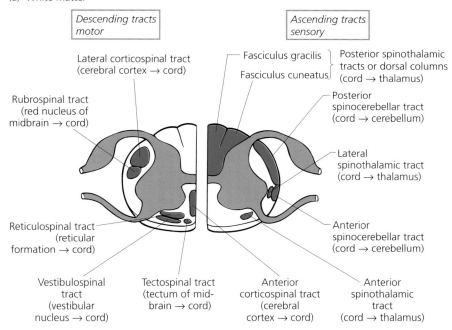

(b) Grey matter

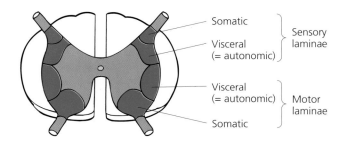

Note: Various laminae are present within each group, e.g. substantia gelatinosa within sensory groups

Figure 8.20 Structural organization of the white and grey matter of the spinal cord: (a) white matter; (b) grey matter

Q What is it that makes white matter 'white'?

axons of which project into the ventral root of a spinal nerve via the ventral or anterior horn (i.e. the 'arm' of the H-shape closest to the ventral surface of the cord). The cell bodies of these cells will receive information from descending neurons from the brain, or from interneurons within the grey matter.

The arrangement of cell bodies within the 'horns' of grey matter conveys an image of layers of cell bodies and interneurons. Cells within the grey matter are said to have a laminar arrangement, not columnar as in white matter, and laminae have been identified in which cell bodies/interneurons are found that are part of specific neural pathways. For example, the laminae referred to the substantia gelatinosa have a particular role in modulating the transmission of pain impulses (see Chapter 20, p.563) and neurons of the lateral areas of the grey matter are particularly involved with the autonomic branch of the peripheral nervous system. In other words there is once again a high degree of neural organization (Figure 8.20b). The types of cell present, and communication, reflect the three main functions of the grey matter, which are:

- initial processing and/or relay of incoming sensory information;
- relay and/or final processing of outgoing motor activity;
- an integrative role modulating motor output in direct response to sensory input without involving the brain (i.e. reflex responses).

Spinal canal

The spinal canal runs along the centre of the cord and extends into the medulla of the hindbrain where it communicates with the fourth ventricle, or fluid space, of the brain. The canal is filled with CSF, which circulates down the cord and back to the brain by the action of the ciliated epithelium that lines the canal. As within the brain, the fluid provides a protected environment, a hydraulic support for the delicate tissue and shock absorbance.

Vasculature of the spinal cord

The spinal cord has a complex arterial blood supply:

- Anterior and posterior spinal arteries descend the surface of the cord, and are derived from the vertebral arteries and from cerebellar arteries (branches of the basilar artery which supply the cerebellum of the hindbrain). Branches penetrate into the neural matter of the cord.
- In addition, this blood is joined by arterial blood supplied by small vessels which branch from intercostal, cervical and lumbar arteries and penetrate the cord via spaces between the vertebrae.

DETAILS OF NEURAL PHYSIOLOGY

There are three broad aspects to the basic functioning of the nervous system.

- First, if electrodes are placed close to a nerve then electrical activity can be detected whenever neurons within it are active. Thus, the activity of neurons involves change to their electrical properties in order to generate an 'impulse' (i.e. a change in voltage), and to conduct the impulse to other areas.
- Second, in conducting impulses neurons must have properties to ensure that they are conducted in the appropriate direction, and are transmitted from one cell to another. This latter process involves special junctions called synapses.
- Third, the brain has areas of distinctive, often specific, processing (e.g. the 'motor cortex'). The passage of impulses to and from the brain, and within it, therefore is by discrete pathways. The processing of information by the central nervous system is essentially one of an integration of these neural pathways, and frequently involves various parts of the brain. Such integration is necessary for all the diverse properties associated with brain function, ranging from the somatic control of posture (see Chapter 17), to the autonomic regulation of blood pressure (see Chapter 12), to cognitive functions such as memory (this chapter).

This section considers these three aspects in detail.

Membrane potentials: generating the nerve impulse
The 'resting membrane potential'

The 'resting membrane potential' is the voltage difference that is present across a cell membrane when it is at rest. It is present in most, if not all, cells but has particular significance in nerve and muscle cells, and in some secretory cells, because these cells have the capacity to alter that voltage and generate an electric current. This is the basis of the nerve impulse.

The membrane potential arises because of the way in which electrolytes are distributed across the cell membrane. In Chapters 2 and 6 it was emphasized how the phospholipid cell membrane has selective permeability properties. Although it is permeable to small, uncharged molecules such as urea and carbon dioxide, the permeability to electrically charged substances such as electrolytes is very low, and this enables the maintenance of a different electrolyte composition of intracellular and extracellular fluids. Thus, sodium provides the highest concentration of positively charged ions in the extracellular fluids – about 10-fold higher than inside cells – while that of potassium is about 30-fold more concentrated within the cells. Similarly, the main negatively charged ion outside cells is chloride (about 10 times more concentrated than in intracellular fluid) while proteins, amino acids and phosphates are the main negatively charged electrolytes inside cells (fluid composition is discussed further in Chapter 6).

In practice there is a 'leak', albeit slow, of positive charge from the cell, mainly because of the diffusion of potassium (K^+) ions outwards. Although the long-term effects of this leak of charge is compensated for by the sodium/potassium exchange pump of the cell membrane (Chapter 2, p.30), it is sufficient so that at any given time there is a net positive charge on the external surface of the membrane, and hence a relative excess of negative charge on the inside. In other words, the membrane is polarized. The polarization is therefore rather like that of a battery, and placement of microscopic electrodes across the cell membrane will detect a voltage. The value is minute, of the order of 70 millivolts (usually written as –70 mV, i.e. negative inside with respect to outside the cell), though the actual value varies slightly between cells.

The action potential

Nerve and muscle cells are considered to be 'excitable' cells because their cell membranes have the capacity to alter their ionic permeabilities in response to a stimulus. They can do this because their membranes contain specific ion 'channels', which are proteins through which ions may diffuse. In order to control that diffusion, however, molecular structures must provide 'gating' mechanisms. Regulating the opening or closing of these 'gates' determines which ions are most free to diffuse across it. Consider the following hypothetical situation where numbers represent the electrical charges (positive) of ions of sodium entering a cell, or potassium leaving it:

Equation 1a:

$$5 - 10 = -5$$

| +ve charges entering the cell (sodium ions) | +ve charges leaving the cell (potassium ions) | i.e. net *negative* charge inside the cell |

Thus, more positive charge (as potassium ions) is leaving than is entering, and so the inside of the cell becomes electrically negative relative to the outside. This might represent a 'resting' situation (i.e. the membrane potential when the cell has not been stimulated).

Now consider if the membrane is stimulated and the permeability to sodium is increased. More positive charge enter as sodium ions diffuse in:

Equation 1b:

$$10 - 10 = 0$$

| +ve charge entering the cell (sodium ions) | +ve charge leaving the cell (potassium ions) | i.e. no net charge inside the cell (electrically neutral) |

At this point the number of positive electrical charges entering and leaving the cell are the same and so there is no electrical difference across the membrane. If the sodium permeability continues to increase, as it does when the nerve cell is stimulated, then more positive charge moves in as sodium diffusion increases:

Equation 1c:

$$15 - 10 = +5$$

| +ve charge entering the cell (sodium ions) | +ve charge leaving the cell (potassium ions) | i.e. net +ve charge inside the cell |

Thus, more positive charge is now entering the cell than is leaving it. Note how the polarity of the membrane changes compared with the resting state in Equation 1a. The reversal of electrical charge (from negative to positive) is referred to as depolarization and is the critical event in the generation of a nerve impulse.

Now consider what happens if the sodium permeability is reduced once again, to its resting value, but the potassium permeability is increased:

Equation 1d:

$$5 - 15 = -10$$

| +ve charge entering the cell (sodium ions) | +ve charge leaving the cell (potassium ions) | i.e. net *negative* charge inside the cell |

In this situation more potassium ions are now diffusing out of the cell and so the polarity has now returned to the state seen at rest (negative) but it has increased in strength. In this example, the membrane is said to be hyperpolarized compared with at rest (i.e. it will take a bigger stimulus to make it depolarize as above). This is what happens during the recovery phase following the stimulation of a nerve cell.

What makes the nerve cells change their membrane potential is the stimulation provided either by activity at a sensory receptor, or at a synapse with another nerve cell; the same effect can be produced artificially by application of an electric current, hence the devastating effects of electrocution. Putting the above equations more closely into the context of nerve cell stimulation:

- Once stimulated the cell membrane begins to depolarize as sodium channels begin to open and sodium ions (i.e. positive charge) begin to diffuse into the cell, mainly promoted by the concentration gradient for sodium between the extracellular and intracellular fluids. The value of the membrane potential will therefore begin to move towards electrical neutrality (Equation 1b).
- At a certain threshold value the sodium channels open fully dramatically raising the permeability, and sodium ions then move rapidly into the cell (Equation 1c). The movement is so rapid that the membrane potential assumes a positive value (in reality bigger than indicated above, about +30 mV; positive inside the cell with respect to outside) because of this influx of positive ions. The depolarization produces an 'action potential' (as distinct from the 'resting' potential), in other words a nerve impulse. The response is 'all or none'. Graded responses are not possible so an action potential is either produced or not. Thus, the level of nerve activity is determined by the number action potentials being generated per second, and conducted along the nerve cell. The process can be considered a 'positive' feedback mechanism in which the slight potential change prior to threshold promotes further change, leading to the full response.
- Once an action potential has been generated, the cell membrane cannot be restimulated. If a new impulse is required, for example because a train of action potentials is passing along the nerve cell, then the membrane must be restored to, or close to, its original resting membrane potential. This repolarization is achieved by a rapid diffusion of positive charge out of the cell. Those sodium ions that had entered the cell when it was stimulated will be pumped out eventually but not quickly enough for the membrane to be reset

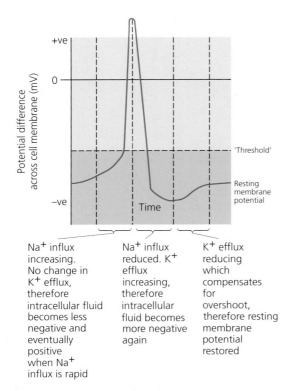

Na⁺ influx increasing. No change in K⁺ efflux, therefore intracellular fluid becomes less negative and eventually positive when Na⁺ influx is rapid

Na⁺ influx reduced. K⁺ efflux increasing, therefore intracellular fluid becomes more negative again

K⁺ efflux reducing which compensates for overshoot, therefore resting membrane potential restored

Figure 8.21 The action potential and changes in Na⁺ and K⁺ movement across the cell membrane. See text Equations for explanation

Q How does the inside of the cell membrane become positively charged during an action potential?

quickly. The outward movement of positive charge is promoted by the opening of potassium channels, which now allow the diffusion of potassium ions (i.e. positive charge) out of the cell down their concentration gradient (Equation 1d).

- The net loss of positive charge is, in fact, transiently excessive and the membrane is hyperpolarized (see Equation 1d). This is actually advantageous as it does not immediately restore the sensitivity for restimulation, and so once the nerve impulse has moved along a stage in the nerve fibre, retrograde stimulation is unlikely to occur and the impulse therefore moves in just one direction. Repolarization is actually very quick and the whole action potential from depolarization to full repolarization takes place in a millisecond (1/1000 second) or so.

The various voltage changes observed during an action potential are depicted in Figure 8.21. The ease at which the cell can be stimulated is a measure of its excitability, and depends upon how close the resting membrane potential is to the threshold potential. Excitability is another example of homeostatic principle in action: the effects of altering parameters which influence either the membrane potential or the threshold potential enables a change in excitability when necessary. Thus the presence of the hormone adrenalin during exercise, or in the stress response, moves the resting potential towards threshold and so increases excitability (which

BOX 8.14 HOMEOSTATIC IMBALANCES IN THE GENERATION OF ACTION POTENTIALS

The capacity to generate action potentials is central to nerve cell functioning, and depends upon a number of factors:

- The distribution of electrolytes across the cell membrane. The main ionic influences on neural function are the effects of altering potassium and calcium concentrations within the extracellular fluid. Such imbalances frequently arise because of disorders of fluid homeostasis induced by endocrine defect, renal failure or dietary deficiency. The effect of potassium changes is to alter the resting membrane potential, either depolarizing it toward threshold (in hyperkalaemia; neurons become more excitable) or hyperpolarizing it away from threshold (in hypokalaemia; neurons become less excitable). Calcium ion disturbances influence the 'gating' mechanisms and therefore alter the threshold at which an action potential is generated. Thus, hypocalcaemia induces a lowering of the threshold (membrane more excitable) and hypercalcaemia raises it (membrane less excitable).
- The presence of ion 'channels' within the membrane. Nerve cells will ordinarily possess such channels. In myelinated axons, however, the channels are concentrated at the nodes of Ranvier (Figure 8.22b). Should the insulative layer of myelin be lost, then current decrement from the membrane may be so extensive that subsequent nodes are not stimulated. This is one of the problems associated with multiple sclerosis.
- The capacity to open and close the ion channels at appropriate times. If membrane potentials, and the threshold potential, are normal then this should not be a problem. Some drugs, however, interfere with the 'gating' mechanisms. This can be of clinical advantage since drugs with this effect include some anaesthetics.
- Temperature. Physiologically, body temperature will be controlled within tight limits, but hypothermia is a common occurrence, particularly in elderly people, and this will reduce neural function throughout the body. The principle is also often used in surgery, and in the use of 'freeze' sprays to treat sport injuries.

improves the speed of a reflex action), and the sinoatrial node of the heart undergoes faster cyclical depolarizations that generate the heart beat (see Chapter 12, p.316; see also box 8.14).

Conduction of nerve impulses
Conduction along the nerve fibre (dendron/axon)

The generation of an action potential by a nerve cell is only one part of nerve cell function: the electrical activity must also be conducted to appropriate tissues. The basic process in propagating a nerve impulse along a nerve fibre is the destabilization of sodium channels in adjacent parts of cell membrane by the electric current generated by an action potential. This causes an influx of positive charge and a shift in membrane potential towards threshold; once this is reached another action potential is generated at this new point in the cell membrane (Figure 8.22a). In this way, an action potential is regenerated along successive parts of the membrane, i.e. along the axon, dendron or dendrite of the cell. How the nature of the action potential ensures unidirectional movement of the impulse was described in the previous section.

The ease of conduction through a cell membrane of electric current generated by an action potential will be related to the electrical resistance of the membrane. Large-diameter axons

(a) Unmyelinated neuron

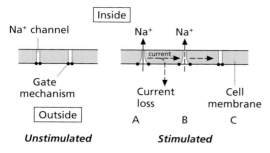

(b) Myelinated neuron

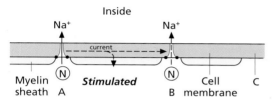

Figure 8.22 Sodium channels, membrane currents and conduction in (a) unmyelinated and (b) myelinated neurons. In each case the sodium channels are fully open at A and so the membrane is fully permeable to Na⁺ and an action potential is generated. At B the channels are beginning to open in response to the electrical current that was generated at A and so the membrane begins to approach threshold. At C the channels are still closed but will subsequently respond to current produced at B. In this way the impulse is said to 'propagate' along the nerve cell. Note that the presence of myelin in (b) reduces loss of current out of the cell and so increases the distance between the sodium channels. Ⓝ, node of Ranvier

BOX 8.15 MEASURING NERVE CONDUCTION

Placing electrodes at a strategic point along a nerve pathway can detect stimulation applied to it physiologically, or electrically. Allowing for the distance between the point of stimulation and detection of the impulses, and the time taken for the impulses to arrive at the electrodes, enables the calculation of the nerve conduction velocity. Doing this evaluation can be useful in assessing a reflex action (see Chapter 17 for description of these). Muscles too require electrical stimulation from an associated nerve cell and similar techniques can be used to evaluate transmission of activity into the muscle.

Myelin is secreted by certain neuroglial cells (called Schwann cells in the peripheral nervous system, and oligodendrocytes in the central nervous system; see earlier section). The process of myelination results in the enveloping of the nerve axon by concentric layers of this insulative lipid. However, despite its insulative properties, the current generated by the neuron still leaks slowly through the myelin. Therefore, there must be gaps at intervals within the myelin sheath at which the cell membrane can be depolarized again in order to regenerate the current. Such gaps are called the nodes of Ranvier (see p.164) and current can be envisaged as 'jumping' from node to node (ion channels concentrated at the nodes are responsible for producing action potentials; Figure 8.22b). This process is called saltatory conduction in contrast to the continual conduction observed in unmyelinated neurons. There is still an influence of axon diameter, however, as this will be a determinant of the required distance between nodes, and therefore the number of times an action potential has to be regenerated along the neuron.

The presence of myelinated and unmyelinated neurons, and neurons of different diameters, means that a range of conduction velocities can be observed within the nervous system, and one of the main classifications of fibre type relates to conduction velocities and the presence or absence of myelin (Table 8.3). An application of this is provided in Chapter 20 in relation to pain physiology.

Conduction between cells: the synapse

At some point within a neural pathway the activity generated by action potentials in a nerve cell must be transmitted to another cell: either another neuron, or a muscle cell, or a glandular cell. If there were actual physical contact between cells

have a lower resistance than small-diameter ones, and so conduct electric current more rapidly (and are also easier to stimulate). The rate at which an axon conducts impulses is called its conduction velocity and for axons without an insulative layer of myelin ranges from 2 to 30 m/second, depending upon axon diameter. In context, 30 m/second will convey a nerve impulse along a single fibre from a toe to the brain in less than 1/15 second. In general though, only the smallest diameter axons are unmyelinated. The presence of myelin on axons of other neurons reduces current loss to the tissue fluids bathing the cell and so increases the conduction velocity. Conduction velocities can be achieved that would otherwise require fibres of extremely large diameter if they lacked myelin. Thus, myelinated nerve fibres conduct impulses at velocities of up to 120 m/second (over 400 km/hour), and a nerve impulse from toe to brain would now take around 1/60 second.

Table 8.3 Nerve fibre classification and properties

Class	Conduction velocity (m/s)	Myelination	Nerve fibre diameter (μm)
A			
Alpha (α)	50–120	Myelinated	8–20
Beta (β)	30–70	Myelinated	5–12
Gamma (γ)	10–50	Myelinated	2–8
Delta (δ)	3–30	Myelinated	1–5
C	0.5–2	Unmyelinated	< 1

C fibres normally comprise almost half the nerve fibres in a peripheral nerve, and all the postganglionic neurons of the autonomic system. An additional sensory nerve fibre classification is sometimes used, in which class I and II fibres correspond to Aα, Aβ and Aγ fibres, class III correspond to Aδ fibres, and class IV fibres correspond to C fibres.

then this would present little difficulty, as the impulse would be conducted as before. Such connections seem to be present in some parts of the brain, and between cells of cardiac muscle (which must also conduct electrical activity). The limitations of such connections, however, are:

- Direct connections make unidirectionality of the conduction of impulses between cells difficult to sustain. This means that in complex processing areas a 'short-circuiting' might be possible when spurious nerve activity could eventually end up going back along the nerve cell from which it originated.
- They do not permit any kind of modulation. Thus, any activity in one nerve cell will immediately trigger activation of the next one. As already noted, some brain pathways do appear to act in this way, but for most it is important that sometimes the onward transmission can be delayed or even prevented (for example, if we were to block the transmission of pain).

These difficulties are resolved since most junctions do not involve physical contact. Such junctions are called synapses.

A synapse is shown diagrammatically in Figure 8.23 from which it can be seen that a small fluid-filled space exists between the neurons. This is called the synaptic cleft and is filled with interstitial fluid; although it is microscopically small (of the order of just 20 nm across; 20 millionths of a millimeter), the electric current generated by nerve cells is so small that it represents a significant barrier to the direct conduction of the neural impulse. The neuron that is conducting an impulse terminates at the synapse as a distended bulb-like structure called a synaptic end-bulb (sometimes referred to as a bouton; = terminal button). When reference is made to synaptic function, this neuron is called the presynaptic neuron. The postsynaptic neuron is the next in the pathway.

Microscopically it can be seen that the synaptic end-bulb contains thousands of minute sacs, called synaptic vesicles. Each vesicle contains a small amount of chemical synthesized in the cell body of the neuron that has been transported to the end-bulb via the cytoplasm. When an action potential arrives at an end-bulb a few of the vesicles move to the membrane and quickly release their contents into the synaptic cleft (Figure 8.23). Molecules of the chemical then rapidly diffuse across the narrow cleft and interact with receptor molecules on the surface of the (postsynaptic) membrane of the next cell. This interaction between chemical and receptor induces changes in the ionic permeability of the postsynaptic membrane, and hence in its membrane potential, which if sufficient to meet the threshold will trigger the generation of a new action potential in this cell thus ensuring onward transmission of the 'impulse'. Collectively, these chemicals are therefore called neurotransmitters.

Having interacted with postsynaptic receptors, the neurotransmitter is removed from them by the actions of enzymes, and this leaves the receptors free to interact with further chemical should it be released from the presynaptic membrane. Excess neurotransmitter within the cleft either diffuses out of the synapse into the interstitial fluid, or is actively transported back into the presynaptic neuron. Only the presynaptic cell

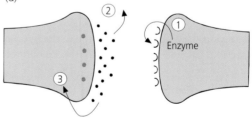

Figure 8.23 The synapse and mode of activation: (a) resting synapse; (b) arrival of action potentials at the (presynaptic) membrane; (c) activation of the postsynaptic membrane; (d) restoration of the resting state

Q What is the role of the neurotransmitter chemical?

can release neurotransmitter, and it does not have the receptors for this neurotransmitter and so cannot be self-activated. This explains the unidirectionality of neural pathways but it does not explain how the transmission can be modulated. To understand how this occurs it is necessary to consider the distinction between those synapses that are 'excitatory' and those that are 'inhibitory'.

Excitatory and inhibitory synapses

The release of only small amounts of a neurotransmitter from a single presynaptic end-bulb will not necessarily be sufficient to produce an action potential in the postsynaptic neuron. It does cause a slight change in the resting membrane potential, however, as sodium channels begin to open; this slight depolarization is called an excitatory postsynaptic potential (EPSP) and brings the membrane potential closer to that of threshold. The EPSP therefore makes the membrane more easily stimulated so that, should further neurotransmitter release occur, following the rapid arrival of another action potential, then the additive effect of individual EPSPs that are generated may reach threshold and trigger an action potential. This action potential will be propagated along the postsynaptic cell as described earlier.

In practice, EPSPs last for only a few milliseconds, and so summation will only occur if several adjacent end-bulbs are activated more or less simultaneously or if the same synapse is activated a few times in quick succession by the arrival of a train of impulses. The whole process is highly complex but has a big advantage since nerve cells are rarely 'quiet'. They sporadically produce action potentials, perhaps because the local environment has been temporarily disturbed or because mechanical movement of the cell membrane has activated it, and the consequences would be potentially disastrous if they activated the pathways. Fortunately, these sporadic potentials are not sufficient to induce threshold depolarization of the next cell and so tissues do not receive what would otherwise be confusing messages.

The picture presented so far is one of excitation: the neurotransmitter excites the postsynaptic cell membrane and if the EPSPs are of sufficient magnitude this triggers another nerve impulse. The problem with this is that it means that pathways will always be excited when a nerve cell is adequately stimulated. Flexibility to enable the nervous system to allow a pathway to be active or inactive is facilitated by the involvement of synapses that are inhibitory.

In these synapses, the release of small amounts of a neurotransmitter from a single synaptic end-bulb causes changes to the permeabilities of the membrane such that a slight hyperpolarization of the postsynaptic membrane, not depolarization, occurs. The slight hyperpolarization produced is called an inhibitory postsynaptic potential (IPSP) and which can be additive to enhance the hyperpolarization. By causing the membrane potential to move further away from its threshold value, IPSPs make the membrane less responsive to those excitatory potentials from other interacting nerve cells; in other words, the synapse has been 'switched off'. This concept of synapses being 'switched on' (excited) or 'switched off' (inhibited) is explored further in Chapter 20 where the 'gate' theory for pain transmission is discussed.

Neurotransmitters that cause excitation, and hence promote the forward continuation of the nerve impulse, are referred to as excitatory neurotransmitters. Those that induce hyperpolarization are called inhibitory neurotransmitters. Inhibitory synapses generally act in one of the following ways:

- by preventing the actions of the neurotransmitter from the end-bulb of an excitatory neuron so that an action potential is not produced in the postsynaptic cell. This is a stabilizing effect on the postsynaptic membrane and is therefore called postsynaptic inhibition (Figure 8.24a);
- by preventing depolarization of the end-bulb of an excitatory presynaptic neuron, effectively preventing the release of the excitatory neurotransmitter itself. This is called presynaptic inhibition. It seems to be the most common process (Figure 8.24b).

Table 8.4 Examples of neurotransmitters and neuropeptides

Substance	Homeostatic actions
Neurotransmitters	
Acetylcholine (ACh)	Released by some neuromuscular and neuroglandular synapses, and at neuronal synapses in the central nervous system
	Acts mainly as an excitatory neurotransmitter, but also has inhibitory functions
Serotonin (5-HT)	Concentrated in certain neurons in the brainstem
	Acts as an excitatory neurotransmitter
	May induce sleep
	Also involved in sensory perception, temperature regulation, and control of mood
Noradrenaline (NA)	Released at some neuromuscular and neuroglandular synapses
	Also found in neural synapses of the brainstem: mainly excitatory
	May be involved in arousal, dreaming, and regulation of mood
Gamma-aminobutyric acid (GABA)	Concentrated in the thalamus, hypothalamus, and occipital lobes of cerebrum; mainly inhibitory
Dopamine (DA)	Inhibitory in substantia nigra of midbrain
	Involved in emotional responses and subconscious movements of skeletal muscles
Neuropeptides*	
Substance P	Excitatory in pain pathways within central nervous system (see Chapter 20)
Enkephalins	Inhibitory in pain pathways within the thalamus and spinal cord
Endorphins	Inhibitory (see Enkephalins) especially within the midbrain
	May have a role in memory and learning
Dynorphin	Inhibitory (see Enkephalins); 50 times more powerful than beta-endorphin

*Neuropeptides are neurotransmitters, but some are also neuromodulators that are produced elsewhere but will interact with the synapse where they are also found.

A variety of excitatory and inhibitory neurotransmitters have been identified in the nervous system (Table 8.4). Importantly, any given presynaptic neuron can only produce one type of transmitter substance, and so determines the nomenclature used to describe a neuron. For example, adrenergic neurons

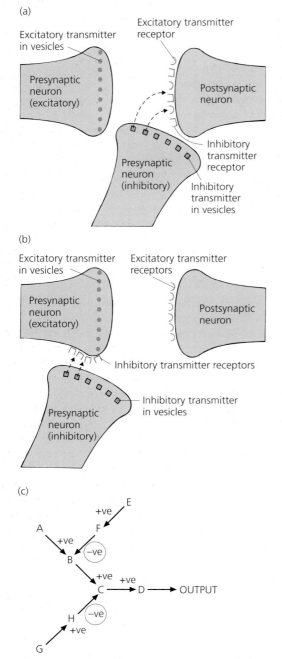

Figure 8.24 Inhibition of synapses, and its role in integrative responses. (a) Postsynaptic inhibition, in which the membrane is stabilized by the inhibitory neurotransmitter and so prevents generation of an action potential. (b) Presynaptic inhibition in which the inhibitory neurotransmitter stabilizes the presynaptic neuron and prevents it from releasing its neurotransmitter. (c) Schematic integration. A–H are neurons: note how activity from D will depend upon the presence or absence of inhibitory influences from neurons F and H. In this way, output from D may be modulated according to the balance between the activation of neurons A, E and G

Q What is the role of inhibitory neurons?

release noradrenaline at their synapses, and cholinergic neurons produce acetylcholine. Similarly, drugs that mimic these chemicals are referred to as adrenergic or cholinergic drugs. It was noted early in this chapter that a single brain cell might interact with perhaps 10 000 other nerve cells. Some of those synapses may be excitatory and some inhibitory, utilizing different neurotransmitters accordingly. Thus, according to the situation, the nerve cell might be activated (excited) or deactivated (inhibited), 'switching on or off' the pathway in which it is involved. This is illustrated simplistically in Figure 8.24c. An example noted in earlier sections on the brain identified that while most neural output to muscles derives from the motor cortex, there are other structures (various brain nuclei) that act to modulate that output; this latter capability reflects the integration if inhibitory pathways within the excitatory one (see Chapter 17). Pharmacological interventions are aimed at interfering with any imbalance in the excitatory and inhibitory pathways (for example see Boxes 8.16 and 8.17). Other examples of synaptic integration are considered in the next subsection.

BOX 8.16 IMPORTANCE OF MAINTAINING A BALANCE BETWEEN INHIBITORY AND EXCITATORY NEUROTRANSMITTERS

Since the output from neurons within processing areas of the brain is determined by the net effects of excitatory and inhibitory inputs during the integration of nerve cell activities, a disturbance in one or other can have drastic effects on brain function. For example, the movement problems of Parkinson's disease (see Box 17.13, p.482) at least partly result from the lack of the inhibitory transmitter dopamine, leading to excessive expression of excitatory pathways (producing the characteristic tremor). Correction is aimed at restoring the balance. Thus, levodopa (a precursor to dopamine) may be administered to people with Parkinson's disease to replace the missing dopamine, or an antimuscarinic (anticholinergic) drug may be used to reduce the activity of acetylcholine in the excitatory pathway.

Another example, which in some people cannot at present be corrected in this way (Mann and Pons, 2007) is epilepsy. Here neural activity normally modulated within the cerebral cortex seems to radiate out from a point to produce foci of intense activity that produce loss of consciousness and muscle contractions typical of fitting. Support and help with prevention of episodes are the main aims of care (Splevings, 2000).

BOX 8.17 MOOD STATES: DEPRESSION

Clinical depression is a mood disorder (or group of disorders) that seems to involve an imbalance of excitatory and inhibitory neurotransmission in certain parts of the brain (frontal lobe, limbic system, hypothalamus). Various neural pathways are involved, as indicated by the range of drugs available:

- *Serotonin (or 5-HT) agonists* (e.g. fluoxetine or Prozac): stimulate the receptors to this excitatory neurotransmitter in serotinergic synapses.
- *Tricyclic antidepressants*: promote release of the excitatory neurotransmitter noradrenaline in adrenergic synapses.
- *Monoamine oxidase inhibitors*: inhibit the breakdown of noradrenaline and therefore prolong its concentration in the synaptic cleft, in adrenergic synapses.
- *Lithium*: enhances the release of serotonin (excitatory) in serotinergic synapses.

However, drug therapy is not curative and cognitive approaches to restore neurological homeostasis can prove more therapeutic.

See the case of a woman with depression, Section VI, p.643.

BOX 8.18 HOMEOSTATIC IMBALANCES IN CONDUCTION VELOCITY OF NEURONS

Reflex responses to stimuli will be depressed if conduction in those spinal neurons involved is reduced, but a slowing of conduction velocity within the brain will also have severe effects on integrated neural circuitry. Reductions in conduction velocity, or in the extreme a failure for action potentials to be conducted at all, arise either because of neuronal problems or because of synaptic dysfunctioning.

Neuronal problems
Some causes of a reduced conduction velocity are:

* When the myelin sheath of axons deteriorates, as in multiple sclerosis. This condition is still poorly understood. The rate of deterioration of myelin seems to be slowed by the use of anti-inflammatory drugs, which slow the development of sclerotic (scar) tissue in demyelinated areas. Corrective treatment is not yet possible and care is generally aimed at facilitating maximal possible function (Barnes, 2007).
* When hypothermia also reduces conduction velocity via its slowing effect on the generation of action potentials.
* Peripherally, when inflammatory demyelinating disease (such as the cause of Guillain–Barré syndrome) will also slow conduction. Motor dysfunction causes muscle weakness. Conversely, sensory activity may actually be enhanced in Guillain–Barré syndrome, presumably because of altered receptor sensitivity, with the individual experiencing heightened cutaneous sensation of pain, temperature and touch. This condition usually reverses and care is directed at supporting the patient, with life support if necessary, until recovery occurs. Extensive rehabilitation is usually necessary (Worsham, 2000).

Synaptic dysfunction
Synaptic function involves the synthesis and secretion of neurotransmitters and its interaction with receptors on the postsynaptic membrane, removal of excess transmitter chemical and degradation of the chemical/receptor ligand so that the receptor is free to interact with more chemical when released. Errors can occur at all stages of the process:

* Myasthenia gravis is a condition in which muscle weakness occurs because of a defect at the neuromuscular synapse, probably because of a shortage of available postsynaptic receptors to the neurotransmitter acetylcholine, or of an excess of acetylcholinesterase, the enzyme that removes acetylcholine from the postsynaptic receptors.
* Parkinson's disease and Huntington's disease are disorders characterized (at least in early stages) by disorders of movement control, and are primarily caused by a deficiency in the neurotransmitters dopamine and gamma-aminobutyric acid (GABA), respectively, from certain neurons of the brain (see also Box 17.13, p.482).

Correction of synaptic dysfunction is aimed at restoring the missing transmitter (see Box 8.16) or by prolonging the actions of the transmitter that is released, as in the administration of acetylcholinesterase inhibitors to myasthenia gravis patients.

BOX 8.19 NEURAL INTEGRATION AND SENSORIMOTOR DEVELOPMENT

It is considered that most neurons that the brain will have are present at birth. Thus, brain growth during childhood results from a proliferation of non-neuronal cells (the neuroglial cells) and the growth of processes from the neurons themselves. The latter establish communication links with neurons in the vicinity or at a distance. Much of the gross plan of the brain is established during fetal development, when axon growth is directed to appropriate areas by a 'scaffolding' of glial cells and by chemical attractants. Such connections are essential to the development of the circuitry of the brain, and it is their integrative functions that determine brain activities. Thyroid hormones are essential for this functional development of the brain in the fetus and in early childhood, particularly in relation to cognitive functions.

Motor and sensory functions mature faster than cognitive functions such as those of memory and reasoning. Early sensorimotor development is essential if the child is to be able to assume an upright posture, to walk, to acquire speech, and to gain voluntary control of urinary and anal sphincters. Autonomic efficiency will also increase, leading to better homeostatic regulation and improved physical performance. Fine motor skills therefore take time to become established.

The formation of synaptic connections between neurons is facilitated by 'reinforcement' of their activities. Accordingly, physical activity, play and other primary and secondary socialization processes promote both sensorimotor and cognitive development. This increases the complexity of activities performed, which in turn facilitate further neural development.

Integrated functions

Integrated neural circuitry commences before birth and is introduced here by Box 8.19 which considers the need for integration in early sensorimotor developments.

Spinal reflexes as an example of integration

Reflexes are responses that do not involve extensive integration of activity by the brain for their initiation. The main advantage of having reflex neural pathways is that responses to sensory stimulation can occur much more rapidly than they would if processing by the brain was involved. This is illustrated by the withdrawal reflex of a limb in response to pain, which requires contraction of muscles that, when stimulated, will move the limb away from the stimulus. For example, standing on a tack stimulates pain receptors at the puncture site, and the afferent sensory activity passes to the spinal cord. Here the afferent neuron synapses directly within the anterior horn of grey matter with the appropriate motor neuron which, when activated, causes the appropriate muscle to contract (Figure 8.25). This is a simple example of what is called a monosynaptic reflex arc (i.e. the whole neural pathway has only one synapse, thus only two neurons – one sensory and one motor – are involved. The neurotransmitter that is released in the synapse will be an excitatory one.

However, withdrawing the limb acts to unbalance the body, and so other muscles in the opposite limb and in the back will therefore also contract, while others will relax, so that some semblance of balance is maintained. Such responses will involve interneurons within the grey matter of the cord that also synapse with the (pain) sensory neuron as it enters the cord. These in turn will synapse with motor neurons to those other muscles. The interneurons that initiate muscle contraction elsewhere will utilize excitatory synapses, but those that cause muscle relaxation will 'switch off' basal activity in the relevant motor neurons by utilizing inhibitory synapses. In this way, an integrated pattern of muscle contraction/relaxation is produced.

Note that the initial response, the withdrawal of the limb, has been entirely processed by the spinal cord, although information regarding the stimulus and the change in position of the limb will be transmitted to the brain. The role of the withdrawal reflex in homeostasis is evident in this example, since failure to withdraw the limb could potentially result in more damage to the tissues of the foot.

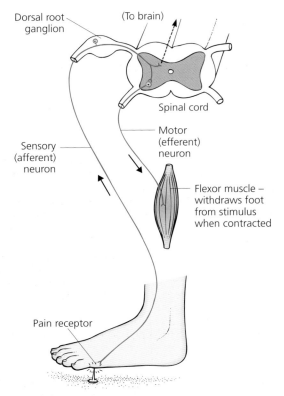

Figure 8.25 A simple monosynaptic reflex arc in response to a painful stimulus. Note that the brain is not involved, although neural information will be transmitted to the brain to keep it 'informed' of the new limb positioning. The full response will be more complex since other muscles will also be affected by the movement

Examples of cerebral neural integration

The brain has an extensive role in the control of tissue and organ functions within the body, via the autonomic nervous system, the hypothalamic–pituitary gland hormonal axis and the mediation of skeletal muscle contraction. These functions are largely dealt with later or in Chapters 9 and 17, and this section will only concentrate on some of the brain's cognitive functions. The aim is to present, albeit simplistically, an overview of such functions, the intention being to emphasize the necessity of integrating the activity from various areas of the brain. Much of the physiology of cognitive function is still unknown, and in some instances, insight has only been gained in recent years. What constitutes 'consciousness', however, remains an enigma: a physiological basis has not been ascertained as yet. This is a complicated topic area and readers interested in this area are recommended to read the works of Susan Greenfield (especially Greenfield, 2004).

Example 1: sleep

Arousal is associated with increased activity in areas of the reticular formation within the upper pons and midbrain regions (see Figures 8.13, p.176 and 8.14, p.177). The pathways use noradrenaline as an excitatory neurotransmitter and the activity radiates to the thalamus, hypothalamus, cerebral cortex and other parts of the hindbrain (Figure 8.26). Sleep arises when activity from the reticular formation is inhibited. Evidence suggests that sleep is a period during which information is sifted and its emotional impact assessed. Memory is updated accordingly. The sleep–wake cycle is an important biological rhythm which appears to be associated with the suprachiasmatic nuclei of the hypothalamus (i.e. nuclei located above the chiasma, the 'crossover' of optic nerve pathways; see Chapter 23, p.614). Neurons from this area pass to the brainstem and cerebral cortex. Sleep and wakefulness are deter-

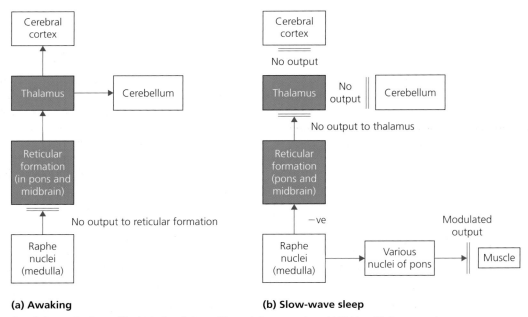

(a) Awaking

(b) Slow-wave sleep

Figure 8.26 Interactions between structures of the brainstem during waking and slow-wave sleep. (a) Waking; (b) slow-wave sleep

Table 8.5 Electroencephalogram (EEG) patterns in (a) levels of consciousness and (b) stages of sleep

(a) Levels of consciousness

Wave	Frequency (cycles/second) of EEG waves	State of consciousness
Alpha (α)	8–23	Awake but quiet
Beta (β)	14–25	Awake but tense (note waves are asynchronous during normal increase in mental activity)
Theta (θ)	4–7	Emotional stress
Delta (δ)	< 3.5	Deep sleep, or anaesthesia (slow wave)

(b) Sleep stages

Sleep stage	Observed EEG
1	Low-voltage wave interrupted periodically by bursts of α-waves
2/3	Progressive decline to 2–3 cycles/second, i.e. δ-waves
4 (REM)	Bursts of desynchronized β-waves similar to those in wakefulness; lasts for 5–30 minutes, recurring approximately every 90 minutes

REM, rapid eye movement sleep, or paradoxical sleep.

mined by balancing the activities of the various brainstem nuclei, and hence their impact on the cortex.

The electrical activity of the cortex undergoes four distinct phases during sleep, as shown in Table 8.5:

- The first two stages are characterized by irregular waveforms associated with consciousness or shallow sleep.
- The 'deep' sleep of stage 3 is characterized by the occurrence of synchronized patterns of activity with a slow frequency, and so is called 'slow-wave' sleep. Slow-wave sleep seems to involve an inhibitory action of nuclei within the medulla oblongata, particularly those called the raphe nuclei, via neurons that utilize the inhibitory transmitter serotonin (Figure 8.26).
- The fourth stage is characterized by alternation between slow waves and patterns of activity reminiscent of stages 1 and 2. Such patterns produce changes in heart and breathing rates, and rapid eye movements are observed (and so stage 4 is called rapid eye movement, or REM, sleep), while generally there is a pronounced muscular paralysis. Dreaming occurs in this stage and it seems to relate to bursts of electrical activity passing from the pons (of the brainstem) to the visual cortex of the occipital lobe. REM (stage 4) sleep, which includes a degree of cortical excitation, seems to involve noradrenergic neurons from the reticular formation, and excitatory cholinergic neurons from various other nuclei within the pons. The latter are probably inhibited during slow-wave sleep but the inhibition is modulated during REM sleep. The nuclei of the pons also seem to be responsible for the inhibition of spinal cord motor neurons (causing the paralysis) during REM sleep (note that acetylcholine is excitatory, therefore the neurons in the pons nuclei must synapse with other inhibitory ones for this effect).

Although these nuclei can be said to induce sleep or wakefulness through inhibitory or excitatory actions, what actually regulates sleep is less clear. The presence of sleep-inducing substances, released into the CSF, has been implicated (see Chapter 22) but their role remains debatable. Pharmacological interventions utilize some of those known to be involved in induction of sleep (Box 8.20). What is clear is that the pattern of sleep changes through adulthood, and time spent in slow-wave sleep decreases (van Cauter *et al.*, 2000).

BOX 8.20 SLEEP-PROMOTING DRUGS

Benzodiazepines are the main class of drug used to promote sleep. These drugs act agonistically on some receptor subtypes of gamma-aminobutyric acid (GABA), an inhibitory neurotransmitter. Anticholinergic drugs may also be used which block acetylcholine receptors in the arousal pathway.

Melatonin, produced by the pineal gland and implicated in regulating the sleep–wake cycle (possibly via actions on the suprachiasmatic nucleus of the hypothalamus), is also under investigation as a sleep-promoting drug (Pandi-Perumal *et al.*, 2007). It is not registered as such in the UK at the time of writing.

Many general anaesthetics and sedative drugs also act to inhibit the output from the reticular formation, resulting in lowered states of arousal and even unconsciousness.

Arousal

The release of the neurotransmitter noradrenaline is stimulated, and its reuptake reduced, by amphetamine drugs. Dopamine release may also be promoted within the limbic system. The excitatory role of noradrenaline and dopamine in synapses associated with the neurology of arousal means that these drugs could maintain an artificially high level of arousal, and is the reason for amphetamine abuse.

Example 2: memory

Memory is considered to have two components: short- and long-term. Short-term memory has a duration of several seconds or a few minutes at most, and has limited volume. It seems to be associated with the persistent excitability of neurons within the cerebral cortex that appear to reverberate within neuronal circuits, the oscillation of activity remaining for perhaps several minutes before declining. Such memories can be converted into long-term ones by consolidation of the information.

Long-term memory is not associated with persistent neural activity. Experimental evidence suggests that the numbers of synaptic connections are increased and that individual synapses are sensitized or primed so that they are more likely to be stimulated should similar sensory information arrive later.

The learning that underpins memories can be:

- *Perceptual (visual)*: perceptual learning utilizes the visual association area of the temporal lobe of the cortex.

- *Stimulus–response conditioning (an association between two stimuli)*: involves the amygdala nuclei of the limbic system, which seems to act as a mediator between sensory inputs and behavioural responses. The amygdala, however, has a complex circuitry and receives inputs from various parts of the brain, while neurons pass from it to the autonomic nuclei of the brainstem, and to the hypothalamus. Some areas of the cerebellum also appear to be involved in conditional learning.
- *Relational (an association between two events) learning*: involves the hippocampus (of the limbic system) which consolidates short-term memories. Various nuclei of the thalamus are also involved in the process, and in the recall of information from long-term stores. Memory also involves the area of cerebral cortex called the limbic cortex.

Acetylcholine is an important excitatory neurotransmitter of memory circuits within the hippocampus and the limbic cortex. Dopamine is also involved (probably as an inhibitory transmitter) in areas of the limbic cortex, while endogenous inhibitory or excitatory opiates are important in the amygdala. The complexity of memory is such, however, that various other neurotransmitters have also been implicated, and this is evidence of complex, multiple neuronal circuits.

Example 3: speech and language

Areas of the left hemisphere dominate in the comprehension of language and in the production of speech (Kent, 2000). This seems to be most appropriate considering the general 'analytical' properties of that hemisphere. The right hemisphere includes cortical areas involved in the understanding of the meaning of words, and applies emotional overtones to the voice.

Comprehension of speech begins within the auditory pathways, particularly in Wernicke's area of the auditory cortex in the superior aspect of the left temporal lobe (Figure 8.27). In contrast, speech is synthesized in a cortical area of the left frontal lobe, called Broca's area. This area lies adjacent to the motor cortex responsible for producing movement of the tongue, lips and larynx in the enunciation of speech. It is thought that Wernicke's area in some way contains memories of the features of auditory sounds, turning them into words, while Broca's area contains memories of the motor output required to verbalize words. Neurons from Wernicke's area project to Broca's area via a tract of nerve fibres called the arcuate fasciculus.

The 'meaning' of words is stored within parts of the sensory association cortex, and the motivation to speak is supplied by areas of the motor cortex.

Example 4: emotional behaviours

'Behaviours' are diverse functions of the brain, but some generalizations can be made regarding the role of the limbic system and hypothalamus (see Figures 8.10, p.173 and 8.12, p174):

- The amygdala nuclei convey a behavioural awareness and ensure that patterns of response are appropriate to an individual's situation.

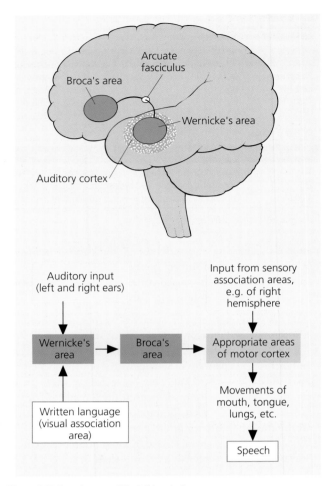

Figure 8.27 Speech areas of the left hemisphere

Q What might be the consequences of trauma to Broca's area?

- Different areas of the hippocampus are involved in different emotions, such as rage and passivity.
- The limbic cortex appears to provide the association required between activity passing to and from various areas of cerebral cortex and the rest of the limbic system.
- Aggressive behaviours especially involve medial (offensive behaviour) and dorsal (defensive behaviour) areas of the hypothalamus. Both project to nuclei of the midbrain for expression. The amygdala is also involved and neurons pass from here to the hypothalamus and midbrain. Interestingly, the amygdala responds to the presence of sex steroids, suggesting a role in sexual aggression.
- Sexual behaviour involves various areas. The area of the basal forebrain lying anterior to the chiasma of the optic nerves determines copulatory behaviour and territorial aggression in men, and maternal behaviour in women. The ventromedial nuclei of the hypothalamus determine copulatory behaviour in women. Sexual behaviours are modulated by areas of the limbic cortex.

ACTIVITY

Readers should review the earlier section ('Overview of the nervous system') on the general organization of the nervous system before commencing this section.

THE AUTONOMIC NERVOUS SYTEM

The autonomic nervous system is that part of the nervous system that mediates the functioning of most organs of the body. It therefore has a dominant role in the homeostatic control of the internal environment. For this reason it is included here as a separate major subsection.

Anatomical organization of the autonomic nervous system

The autonomic nervous system comprises both central and peripheral elements. It is especially involved in the involuntary control of organs and tissues. Like other peripheral nerves, the nerves of this system will comprise both afferent (sensory) and efferent (motor) nerve cells. Earlier in this chapter, it was noted that the term 'motor' is used to convey an impression of promoting activity, especially in muscle cells (i.e. motor). The term has to be used more broadly for the autonomic nerves because some will stimulate the target tissue when they are activated, but others will inhibit it. For example, autonomic nerves to the heart may increase heart rate, while others decrease it, and some nerves increase gut motility while others

decrease it. In this way, tissue functioning can be enhanced or reduced by autonomic motor nerves according to the situation, and this provides the level of flexibility that is required to maintain homeostasis.

An individual autonomic nerve/nerve cell will either increase or decrease the activity of tissue cells; it does not do both. If tissues are to be activated or deactivated according to circumstances then different nerves/nerve cells must be present. Accordingly, the autonomic nervous system can be subdivided into two subdivisions called the sympathetic and parasympathetic divisions (Figure 8.28), that usually act in a complementary way in various homeostatic control processes (Figure 8.29). There is no hard and fast rule as to which subdivision does what, but generally sympathetic nerves act to stimulate a tissue, and parasympathetic nerves inhibit it; in other instances the reverse is true.

Parasympathetic division

The general layout of the nerves of this division is relatively straightforward, and basically consists of the vagus nerve (cranial nerve X), certain neurons of various other cranial nerves, and nerves which originate from the sacral (i.e. lower back) region of the spinal cord (Figure 8.28). This is why this division is sometimes termed the craniosacral division.

As mentioned earlier, the vagus nerve passes from the brainstem, down through the thorax and abdomen, sending branches to various viscera as it goes along (vagus = wandering). The parasympathetic functions of the vagus and other cranial nerves are summarized in Table 8.1. The sacral nerves

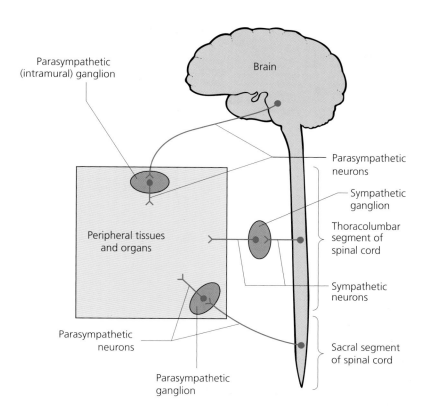

Figure 8.28 General organization of the autonomic nervous system

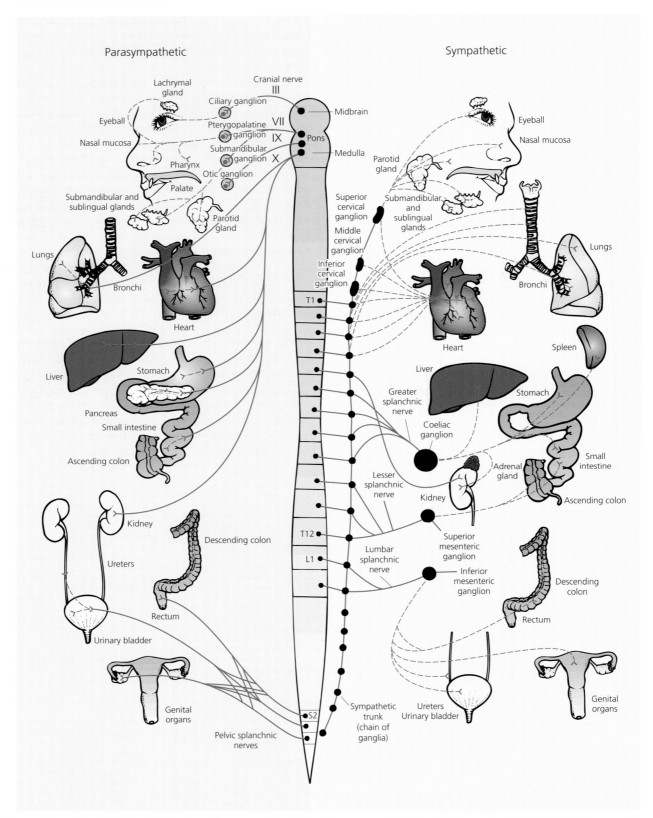

Figure 8.29 Innervation of the viscera by the autonomic nervous system. Although the parasympathetic division is shown only on the left side of the figure, and the sympathetic on the right, keep in mind that each division is found on both sides of the body. Solid lines, preganglionic neurons from the spinal cord to the peripheral ganglia; dotted lines, postganglionic neurons from the ganglia to the tissue cells

Q What is the advantage of having organs supplied with both parasympathetic and sympathetic nerves?

help to control lower abdominal functions such as micturition and defecation.

The layout of the parasympathetic division is, in fact, slightly more complicated than this because the nerves first synapse with shorter efferent nerves, which then interact with the target tissue. The aggregated cell bodies of these latter nerves form the intramural ganglia (Figure 8.28) and are usually found very close to (or even within) the tissues served by the nerves. The nerve cell axons leading from the cord to these ganglia are therefore usually referred to as preganglionic fibres, ('pre-' = before) while the shorter ones from the ganglia to the target cells are postganglionic ('post-' = after). These terms are especially used in pharmacology texts in relation to actions of the neurotransmitters (see Box 8.21, Figure 8.31 and related text).

Within the central nervous system, parasympathetic neurons synapse with cell neurons in various nuclei, which are also in communication with sensory areas of the cortex, the thalamus and hypothalamus, and other nuclei of the brainstem. The sacral nerves must also have projections along the spinal cord to and from the brain.

Sympathetic division

The anatomy of the sympathetic division can appear to be much more complex than that of the parasympathetic division (Figure 8.29). Sympathetic nerves leave the spinal cord (via the usual spinal nerve roots) at regular intervals between the 6th cervical and 2nd lumbar vertebrae, hence a term sometimes used is the cervicolumbar division. The sympathetic nerves soon dissociate from the spinal nerves, however, and short nerves (containing preganglionic fibres) run to the sympathetic ganglia, which form a chain alongside the vertebral column (Figures 8.29 and 8.30). The postganglionic neurons are generally much longer and extend from synapses within these ganglia to the target tissues. Modifications of this layout of sympathetic ganglia occur, however. For example, the coeliac ganglion lies some distance from the cord (Figure 8.29). This ganglion actually involves synapses from a number of sympathetic nerves from the cord, and is commonly called the solar plexus.

Within the central nervous system the sympathetic division involves nerve cells that ascend or descend the spinal cord, and includes various nuclei within the brain. As with the parasympathetic system, connections within the hypothalamus and brainstem are particularly important in sympathetic functions.

Summary of the physiology of the autonomic nervous system

The details of the functions of the sympathetic and parasympathetic divisions are outlined in Table 8.6, while the specific

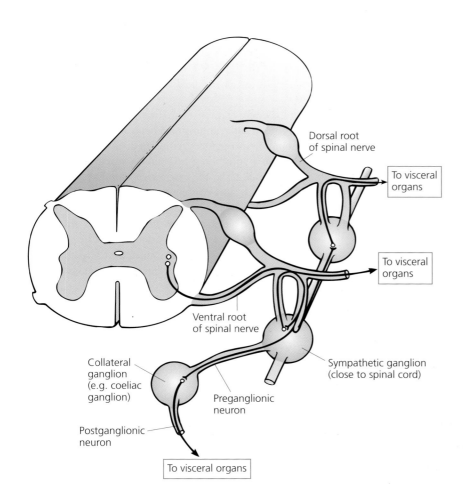

Figure 8.30 Efferent neurons of the sympathetic nervous system. Note the 'relay' function of the sympathetic ganglia

Table 8.6 Comparison of the sympathetic and parasympathetic nervous systems

Structure	Sympathetic innervation	Parasympathetic innervation
Eye	Dilates pupil; accommodation for distance vision	Constricts pupil; accommodation for near vision
Salivary glands	Concentrated secretion stimulated	Watery secretion stimulated
Sweat glands	Increased secretion	Not innervated
Cardiovascular system		
Blood vessels		Not innervated, except in penis and clitoris: dilation
To skin	Vasoconstriction	
To skeletal muscles	Vasodilation	
To digestive viscera	Vasoconstriction	
Heart, rate and force of contraction	Increases	Decreases rate
Blood pressure	Increases	Decreases*
Adrenal gland	Medulla secretes adrenaline + noradrenaline	Not innervated
Respiratory system		
Diameter of airways	Increases	Decreases
Respiratory rate	Increases	Decreases
Digestive system		
Sphincter muscles	Contract	Relax
General level of activity	Decreases	Increases
Secretory glands	Inhibited	Stimulated
Urinary system		
Kidneys	Decreases urine production	Not innervated
Bladder	Relaxes muscle of bladder, contracts internal sphincter	Contracts bladder muscle, relaxes internal sphincter
Male reproductive system	Increases glandular secretion; ejaculation	Erection through action on blood vessel

*Indirect effect as consequence of actions on heart rate.

roles of autonomic nerves in regulating the functions of organs and organ systems are highlighted in the relevant chapters. The question as to which division is responsible for exciting a tissue is very much related to the situation under which they are activated. For example, exercise has a marked stimulatory effect on the sympathetic division (producing the 'fight, flight and fright' responses), and so is responsible for promoting responses that facilitate physical activity. Thus, changes in sympathetic nerve activity promote the following excitatory responses:

- cardiac output is raised by increasing the heart rate and force of contraction;
- an initial vasodilation of muscles is induced to raise blood flow through them (although metabolic factors then become more important in this respect);
- arterial blood pressure is maintained despite pronounced muscle vasodilation, by inducing vasoconstriction in various other tissues;
- peripheral vision is enhanced by inducing dilation of the pupils;
- excess heat produced by the raised metabolic rate is removed by stimulating sweat secretion;
- glycogen stores in the liver and muscle are broken down to provide more glucose as fuel;
- somatic nerve excitability is enhanced, thus speeding up reflexes and promoting more rapid movements.

In contrast, exercise is also facilitated through the actions of sympathetic nerves to inhibit:

- the motility and secretory activity of the gut (which is appropriate in view of the concurrent vasoconstriction in the gut);
- smooth muscle tone in the airways (bronchodilation then occurs which facilitates lung ventilation).

The net effect of the responses of various systems is to maintain cellular homeostasis, particularly within the active muscles.

The parasympathetic division tends to be activated in response to emotional experiences. For example:

- contemplating the eating of food raises activity in the vagus nerve and induces gastric acid secretion and increases gut motility;
- relaxation therapy causes heart rate to decrease, partly through stimulation of appropriate neurons within the vagus nerve (though it also reduces sympathetic activity);
- emotional shock promotes bronchoconstriction and may even inhibit the heart to the extent that blood pressure falls, and fainting occurs, as a consequence of cerebral ischaemia;
- sexual stimulation induces vasodilation in the penis (male) or clitoris (female) and these actions represent the main example of a direct effect of the parasympathetic nervous system on specific blood vessels (in contrast to sympathetic nerves, which have a pronounced effect on blood vessels within many tissues).

ACTIVITY

Refer to the actions of adrenaline identified in Chapter 9 (p.220), and in Chapter 20 (p.598) and compare these with the actions noted here of the sympathetic nervous system. Note the similarity. Why is this? You might refer to Table 8.6 for further help. How quickly would the sympathetic nervous system change tissue functions? How long would adrenaline take to do likewise? Refer to the 'Introduction' in Chapter 9 where there is a comparison of nervous and hormonal properties.

Neurotransmitters of the autonomic system

The principle of a single nerve cell being capable of producing only one particular transmitter is applicable also to the autonomic nervous system. The examples of autonomic actions described in the previous section indicate that the neurotransmitters can have either excitatory or inhibitory effects on tissues, depending upon the tissue.

The nerve endings of postganglionic neurons of the sympathetic nervous system release noradrenaline which interacts with receptors on the membrane of cells within the target tissue (the hormone adrenaline, released when sympathetic nerves to the adrenal gland are stimulated, may also act on these receptors; Figure 8.31). Whether the response that ensues is stimulatory or inhibitory is determined by the type of receptor that is present. Receptor subtypes, classified as alpha- and beta-receptors, will be present in appropriate tissues (Box 8.21). In addition, some sympathetic nerve cells release other transmitter chemicals that are related to noradrenaline, called dopamine and serotonin, and these interact with their own receptors (of which there are further subtypes, e.g. dopamine receptors are referred to as D_1, D_2 or D_3 receptors).[1] Although there are receptors to these other substances within various tissues, for example the kidneys, the major clinical interest is in their roles as neurotransmitters within the central nervous system.

---

[1]The interest in dopamine is more focused on its actions as a central neurotransmitter, rather than its actions peripherally in the autonomic nervous system. Thus, D_1 and D_2 receptors are found in nerve terminals of the striatum, a collection of neural tissue that includes the cerebral nuclei called the caudate nucleus and the putamen. The terminals originate in the brainstem nucleus called the substantia nigra and comprise what is referred to as the nigrostriatal pathway. The terminals secrete dopamine and disorders here, primarily of the D_1 receptor to the neurotransmitter, are implicated in Parkinson's disease. D_3 is of interest in relation to the actions of dopamine within the limbic system, especially in connection with schizophrenia, although this is a hotly debated topic.

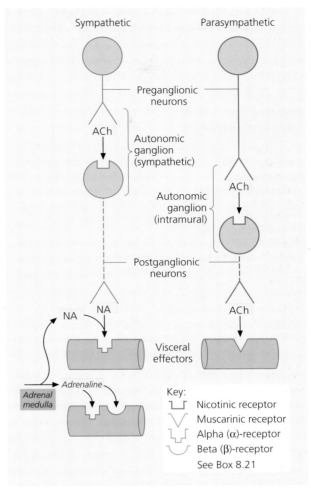

Figure 8.31 Neurotransmitters of the sympathetic and parasympathetic branches of the autonomic nervous system. NA, noradrenaline; ACh, acetylcholine

Q *Which neurotransmitter is produced by the preganglionic neurons?*

Q *Which neurotransmitters are produced by the postganglionic neurons?*

BOX 8.21 AUTONOMIC NERVOUS SYSTEM: RECEPTORS AND DRUGS

Drugs acting on the autonomic nervous system are classed as adrenergic or cholinergic drugs according to the receptors that are activated or inhibited; these receptors are for the catecholamines (adrenaline, noradrenaline) and acetylcholine, respectively. Similar receptors are also found within the central nervous system since both groups of chemicals also act as neurotransmitters there. Each category includes receptor subtypes according to subtle variations in the molecular structure of the receptor. Drugs have been developed that interact predominantly with one or other subtype, acting as agonists (i.e. activate the receptor) or as antagonists (i.e. no activation of the receptor, and receptor blockade against the intrinsic substance). They provide a means for therapeutic interventions on tissues and organs in which these subtypes are located.

1. *Adrenergic receptors:* those for adrenaline and noradrenaline are classed as:
   - Alpha-1 – found especially in arterial muscle.
   - Alpha-2 – found mainly on platelets, postsynaptically on blood vessels, in the pancreas and in brain synapses.
   - Beta-1 – found on cardiac muscle cells.
   - Beta-2 – found on smooth muscle in the bronchioles of lungs.

Other subtypes of both alpha- and beta-receptors have been identified and seem likely to result in new pharmaceuticals.

2. *Cholinergic receptors:* these only relate to acetylcholine but there are subtypes.
   - Muscarinic receptors mediate most of the parasympathetic actions in peripheral organs. There are three main subtype of receptor, although no selective drugs are yet available:
     (i) M1 receptors are found in synapses in the central nervous system and in sympathetic ganglia (with nicotinic receptors, see below).
     (ii) M2 receptors are found on cardiac cells.
     (iii) M3 receptors are found on gland cells, and smooth muscle cells of viscera.
   - Nicotinic receptors, of which there are two main subtypes here: ganglionic and muscle receptors.
     (i) Ganglionic receptors are found in synapses in parasympathetic and sympathetic ganglia. Similar receptors are also found within the brain and it is these that promote the alertness associated with cigarette smoking.
     (ii) Muscle receptors are found in neuromuscular junctions with skeletal muscle.

Postganglionic nerve cells within the parasympathetic division release acetylcholine, and receptor subtypes to this neurotransmitter, called muscarinic and nicotinic receptors, also exist for this substance. Just to confuse matters, acetylcholine is also the neurotransmitter released by preganglionic nerve cells within the sympathetic ganglia (Figure 8.31). Here the acetylcholine and drugs (e.g. nicotine) that act on nicotinic receptors for acetylcholine may provoke some sympathetic activities such as a faster heartbeat.

SUMMARY

1 Nerves, or more precisely nerve cells (neurons), provide the means of rapid communication necessary for the regulation of many homeostatic processes.

2 The nervous system has two main anatomical divisions: the peripheral nervous system, which conducts neural activity to and from tissues, and the central nervous system, which analyses information before promoting a response.

3 The peripheral system is subdivided into that branch that controls skeletal muscle in the regulation of body posture and movement (called the somatic system), and that which is involved in the regulation of visceral functions (called the autonomic system). In general, we can exert considerable conscious control over the former, but the latter is under involuntary control.

4 Peripheral nerves enter/exit the spinal cord as spinal nerves, between the vertebrae. Sensory neurons enter the dorsal (or posterior) aspect of the cord, while effector (or motor) neurons exit via the ventral (or anterior) aspect.

5 The central nervous system consists of the brain and spinal cord.

6 The brain develops embryologically as three distinct components which increase in complexity during development. These are the forebrain, midbrain and hindbrain.

7 The forebrain consists of the cerebral hemispheres (with both cortical and subcortical processing areas) and deeper structures called the thalamus and hypothalamus. The cortex and subcortical areas have particular roles in cognitive processes, in the control of movement and in the receipt and interpretation of sensory information. The hypothalamus is especially involved in the 'drives' of the body and in stress responses and also in coordinating circadian rhythms. The thalamus is predominantly a relay centre for information passing into and out of the forebrain.

8 The midbrain contains many brain 'nuclei' and nerve tracts, and forms the area between the forebrain and the hindbrain. It provides aspects of movement control but is also a route of information passage into and out of the brain.

9 The hindbrain consists of structures at the top of the spinal cord, but also includes the cerebellum, which have integrative functions particularly in relation to arousal, the control of movement and the control of the autonomic system. Some of these structures (the pons varolii and medulla oblongata) form the brainstem with the midbrain.

10 The CSF provides the environment that bathes cells of the brain and spinal cord. The fluid is secreted into fluid ventricles and circulates around the central nervous system. It is eventually reabsorbed into the venous blood across special areas of the meningeal membranes that surround the brain and cord.

11 The spinal cord has a precise organization, consisting of tracts of nerve cell fibres that ascend or descend the cord within the 'white' matter, and layers of cells that integrate activity or act as relays within central 'grey' areas. Integrative functions of the cord include the production of reflexes.

12 Nerve cell activity is generated by the movement of electrical charge across the cell membrane, as an action potential. The membrane can be stabilized, however (i.e. the action potential inhibited), by the antagonistic movement of other ions, which prevent the action potential being generated. This forms the basis of neural integration (a switching mechanism within the nervous system) and takes place at junctions called synapses between nerve cells.

13 Synaptic function involves the release of neurotransmitters which modulate ionic movements across the membrane of the next cell in the pathway. Some chemicals are excitatory, others inhibitory. Within the central nervous system the ionic environment surrounding the cells is tightly controlled (to enable membrane events to be regulated) by regulating the composition of the bathing fluid, the CSF.

14 Many cognitive functions of the brain have now been attributed to various brain structures, and involve a variety of neurotransmitters. The balance between excitatory and inhibitory pathways is essential for 'normal' functions.

15 The autonomic nervous system also operates via neurotransmitters and numerous receptor subtypes to these chemicals have been identified and enable the system to exert complex control of visceral functioning. The system is subdivided into the sympathetic and parasympathetic branches that, in general, exert opposing actions on tissues in response to visceral afferent input.

REFERENCES

Barnes, F. (2007) Care of people with multiple sclerosis in the community setting. *British Journal of Community Nursing* **12**(12): 552–7.

Barnett, F. (2002) Nursing patients with variant Creutzfeldt–Jakob disease at home. *British Journal of Community Nursing* **7**(9): 445–50.

Brown, R.C., Lockwood, A.H. and Sonawane, B.R. (2005) Neurodegenerative diseases: an overview of environmental risk factors. *Environmental Health Perspectives* **113**(9): 1250–6.

Cross, S. (2008) Stroke care: a nursing perspective. *Nursing Standard* **22**(23): 47–60.

Drouet, B., Pincon-Raymond, M., Chambaz, J. and Pillot, T. (2000) Molecular basis of Alzheimer disease. *Cellular and Molecular Life Sciences* **57**(5): 705–15.

Edwards, S.D. and Forbes, K. (2003) Nursing practice and the definition of human death. *Nursing Inquiry* **10**(4): 229–35.

Gelling, L., Iddon, J., McVicar, A. and Pickard, J. (2004) Measuring progress in patients with CSF circulation disorders: quality of life and hope. *Journal of Clinical Nursing* **13**: 589–600.

Greenfield, S. (2004) *The Private Life of the Brain*. London: Penguin.

Kent, R.D. (2000) Research on speech motor control and its disorders: a review and prospective. *Journal of Communication Disorders* **33**(5): 391–428.

Mann, M.W. and Pons, G. (2007) Various pharmacogenetic aspects of antiepileptic drug therapy: a review. *CNS Drugs* **21**(2): 143–64.

Pandi-Perumal, S.R., Srinivasan, V., Spence, D.W. and Cardinali, D.P. (2007) Role of the melatonin system in the control of sleep: therapeutic implications. (includes abstract) *CNS Drugs* **21**(12): 995–1018.

Splevings, D. (2000) The nurse's role in achieving optimal epilepsy management. *Community Nurse* **6**(8): 34–5.

van Cauter, E., Leproult, R. and Platt, L. (2000) Age-related changes in slow wave sleep and REM sleep and relationship with growth hormone and cortisol levels in healthy men. *Journal of the American Medical Association* **284**(7): 861–8.

Worsham, T.L. (2000) Easing the course of Guillain Barre syndrome. *RN* **63**(3): 46–50.

INTRODUCTION

Cells and tissues require an appropriate rate of delivery of specific nutrients and metabolites if they are to maintain intracellular homeostasis. This is achievable only by the homeostatic regulation of the functions of other tissues and organs because of the 'division of labour' and the interdependency of chemical–cell–tissue–organ systems that is observed in the body (see Chapter 1, pp.8–10). Physiological function therefore cannot be static, since systemic function must be responsive according to the needs of the individual at any given time (see Figure 1.7, p.11). Although some tissues are able to exert limited intrinsic control on some of their activities, the overall homeostatic regulation of cells, tissues and the integration of organ functions are provided by the coordinating systems of the body: the nervous and hormonal systems (see Figure 1.6, p.10).

Nerve cells and hormones provide a means of communication between different parts of the body. The principles of nervous function were described in Chapter 8, but it is worth considering here the advantages and disadvantages of the two coordinating systems in order to place hormones in the context of homeostatic regulation.

General comparison of neural and hormonal systems

Hormones are produced in specific secretory or gland cells in one part of the body, then secreted and transported in extracellular fluid (usually blood plasma) to their receptor sites on target cells elsewhere in the body. In contrast, nerve cells extend from one tissue to another, and so provide a direct anatomical communication link. However, they also depend upon the production and secretion of neurotransmitters into extracellular fluid (usually tissue fluid) at synapses; these neurotransmitters then interact with receptors on the target cells.

- Both hormones and neurotransmitters combine with cellular receptors in order to activate or deactivate genes/gene products to regulate target cell metabolism, to maintain intracellular homeostasis. In summary, hormones and neurotransmitters activate or inhibit chemical reactions involved in the storage, transference, destruction and/or secretion of cellular chemicals which are in excess and/or production of chemicals that are deficient (see Figure 2.9, p.33).

- The distances travelled by neurotransmitters to the target cell are microscopic, and nerve cells have the advantage that they can convey 'messages' (i.e. impulses) very rapidly to the target cells. The disadvantages are that this direct link must be established with every target cell within a tissue; that anatomical link must be maintained, since neural damage may irreversibly prevent communication.

- The rapidity with which neural impulses are conducted means that target cells can be induced to alter their activities within fractions of seconds. In contrast, the time taken to induce the secretion of hormones from stores within secretory cells (or to produce them first in some cases), and to conduct them to targets, means that responses are much slower (of the order of several minutes to 1–2 hours, depending on the hormone). Hormones, therefore, are important in regulating medium- or long-term homeostatic functions of tissues, such as controlling body fluid composition or growth. Hormone operation would clearly be unsuitable, for example, in the rapid change in cardiovascular function that is necessary to control blood pressure at the moment when we stand up (see Figures 12.22, p.340 and 12.27, p.346).

- Both systems can act concurrently in the regulation of an organ. For example, the rapidity of neural responses is advantageous in the moment-to-moment coordination of gut motility, but the slower response to hormones is more appropriate in the control of gut secretions (although neural activity can also alter these).

- Some nerve cells in the hypothalamus of the brain also produce hormones and therefore represent an overlap between the systems. It is partly through such secretions that the brain can alter body function.

- Nervous activity modulates the release of certain hormones, and some hormones influence neural activity. The two systems, therefore, may not always act in isolation.

- From a clinical viewpoint, the fact that both systems utilize the release of a chemical, and its interaction with target receptors, means that many drugs used to modulate these processes have similar modes of action, either as receptor

BOX 9.1 ANTAGONISTIC AND AGONISTIC DRUGS

The role of hormones clearly depend upon their interaction with receptor molecules, which are located on the target cell's membrane or within its cytoplasm or nucleoplasm. Neurotransmitters released at nerve endings are similarly dependent upon receptor interaction. Drugs that influence receptors are used widely in medicine (see Box 1.8, p.15). An antagonistic drug is one that will combine with the receptor chemical but not activate the resultant cell response. In doing so, it prevents the hormone gaining access to the receptor; these types of drugs are often referred to as 'blockers' (e.g. a beta-blocker interferes with a beta-receptor for adrenaline). In contrast, agonistic drugs interact with, and activate, the receptor in the same way as the hormone would do (e.g. salbutamol mimics the actions of adrenaline on the airways, and so aids breathing in conditions such as asthma; see the case study of a boy with asthma, Section VI p.659).

Antagonistic drugs, therefore, are useful when hormone or neural responses must be reduced, and agonistic drugs are used when there is a hormone deficiency or when it would be useful to promote the actions of a hormone or nerve in their absence.

antagonists or agonists (Box 9.1), or as agents that interfere with chemical synthesis, storage or release.

- The overlap in actions of nerves and hormones in determining biological functioning is illustrated by the stress response and by sexual behaviour.
- Part of the stress response is referred to as the 'alarm' stage (see Figure 21.6, p.598). In this stage, an individual's physiology is altered first by activation of the sympathetic nervous system, which produces an immediate response, and then by the hormone adrenaline, which provides a back-up to the neural actions. Both act to increase the output of blood from the heart, and to alter blood flow to the tissues, in preparation for physical activity. The response is very similar to that promoted by adrenaline alone (indeed, a similar chemical, noradrenaline, is produced at the endings of the sympathetic nerves), and sympathetic activation causes this hormone to be released; its actions support those of the nerves.
- Sexual behaviour is complex. Basically, behaviour results from neurological functioning in the brain. Nerve cells within certain parts of the brain that are involved in such behaviours also act as target cells for the (gonadal) sex hormones, which modulate the functions of these cells, producing some of the features associated with female and male behaviours. Not all such behaviours can, of course, be attributed simply to hormone actions, but there is often a hormonal influence.

Hormones, therefore, may act independently of nerves, or in association with them. Functions of nerves are the focus of Chapters 8 and 17, and other actions are noted at specific points throughout this book. This chapter describes the main hormonal (or endocrine) glands of the body, and the actions and roles of their secretions.

OVERVIEW OF THE ANATOMY, PHYSIOLOGY AND CHEMISTRY OF THE HORMONAL SYSTEM

In order to have breadth of understanding as to how the hormonal system functions, it is necessary to consider:

- the nature of hormonal secretions;
- the chemistry of hormonal secretions;
- how secretory tissue is organized;
- how hormones induce a change in target cell activity;
- the general principles of how hormone release is regulated.

What is a hormone?

The term 'hormone' was coined around 100 years ago. Translated, the term means 'I excite', which reflects the role of hormones as chemical messengers that alter the activities of cells. The actual definition is much more involved, however. By definition, a hormone is a 'substance produced by cells in one part of the body that is secreted into the blood in response to a specific stimulus and in amounts that vary with the strength of the stimulus, and has its actions in the body some distance from the site of secretion'.

This definition may be applied to the major hormones of the body, but various other chemical messengers are now recognized that do not fit it:

- *Autocrine secretions*: released into the tissue (interstitial) fluid but influence the activities of the cell that secreted them. An example is the way in which oestrogen hormones secreted by ovarian follicle cells during the menstrual cycle stimulate the same cells to secrete further oestrogen (a temporary positive feedback mechanism; see Chapter 1, pp.13–14).
- *Paracrine secretions*: released into tissue fluid and influence the activities of other cells but again within the immediate vicinity. Delivery of the secretion to the target cells is by diffusion through the fluid; the secretion is not blood-borne. Prostaglandins (see later) are examples of paracrine secretions; these are produced by most tissues and provide an intrinsic modulation of cellular functions.
- *Pheromones*: released out of the body (i.e. secreted and excreted) and change the behaviour of other organisms. There is considerable evidence for their presence in a variety of species, and it is thought that humans also produce pheromones as sexual attractants, probably via apocrine sweat.

The breadth of these secretions highlights the difficulty in defining precisely the term 'hormone'. This chapter uses the term in its broadest sense, as defined above, while recognizing that this still omits autocrine secretions.

Names of hormones

Hormones are often named after their actions or the processes involved in those actions. For example:

- *Testosterone*: from the testes (the suffix '-sterone' indicates that this is a steroid hormone).

- *Oestrogen*: promotes oestrus (female fertility; menstrual cycle).
- *Antidiuretic hormone*: prevents diuresis (the production of copious volumes of urine).

Some hormones are frequently referred to by a collective name. An example is the tropins, a term used to indicate that the hormone's action is to promote the release of another hormone. For example, gonadotropins are those hormones that act on the gonads to stimulate the release of testosterone (in men) or oestrogens (in women). You will become more familiar with the names of hormones as you read this and other chapters of the book.

Hormone chemistry

Hormones are a diverse range of substances. Basically, they can be divided into four types: peptides, catecholamines, steroids and eicosanoids. Examples are given later, but some general features of their functional chemistry are noted here.

Peptides

Peptides are small molecules composed of amino acids (Figure 5.2b, p.108). These are soluble in water, but are only poorly soluble in lipid, so after production they can be stored in membrane-bound vesicles within the secretory cells. Secretion, therefore, can be almost immediate, and occurs by exocytosis of the vesicles following their fusion with the plasma membrane of the cell (see Figure 2.10, p.34). The interaction of peptides with target cells requires the presence of specific membrane receptors on the surface of those cells (Figure 9.1). Examples of peptide hormones include insulin, glucagon, vasopressin and oxytocin.

Catecholamines and thyroxine

Catecholamine hormones are derivatives of the amino acid tyrosine; therefore, they all share a similar chemical structure. They are only slightly soluble in lipid, so they can be stored in intracellular vesicles hence released quickly. They also require the presence of surface membrane receptors on target cells for their actions (Figure 9.1). The similarity of their chemical structure may cause an overlap in those actions, although membrane receptor subtypes are found in certain tissues that enable each hormone to have specific actions in those tissues. Adrenaline and noradrenaline are examples of catecholamines.

The hormone thyroxine produced by the thyroid gland is also synthesized from tyrosine, and is stored within the thyroid gland. Although not strictly considered to be a catecholamine, its basic structure is very similar (but also has important differences; see later). It also requires the presence of surface membrane receptors on target cells (Figure 9.1). However, in this instance the hormone–receptor complex is passed internally into the cell where it acts directly on genes to produce the proteins that mediate its action; other hormones act on gene products already in place. This means that responses that are dependent upon thyroxine release are relatively slow in onset,

perhaps of the order of 1–2 hours (rather than minutes or tens of minutes, as for many other hormones).

Steroids

Steroid hormones are all are derivatives of the lipid cholesterol. Examples include testosterone, oestrogens, cortisol and aldosterone. Their mode of action is quite different from that of other hormone groups. Because they are highly lipid soluble, they diffuse easily through cell membranes; therefore they cannot be stored, and must be produced as required. Steroid hormones pass into their target cells, where they interact with intracellular receptors. Once inside the cell, steroids act directly to change gene activities (similar in principle to the mode of action of thyroxine, above), so they are relatively slow in onset of actions.

Steroids have very similar molecular structures and so some overlap in their actions can occur. For example, the influence of oestrogens on fluid balance during the menstrual cycle arises partly through a stimulation of aldosterone receptors in the kidney.

Eicosanoids

Eicosanoids are derivatives of arachidonic acid (an omega-6 fatty acid; see Chapter 5, p.110), which itself may be derived from other essential dietary fatty acids, such as linoleic acid. They are, therefore, lipid soluble, and so must be produced as required. Eicosanoids act intracellularly in target cells.

Eicosanoids include the prostaglandins, thromboxanes and leukotrienes. The hormones are produced following the secretion of arachidonic acid from within the cell membrane, and their target cells are usually local to the site of production. These hormones seem primarily to be intrinsic regulators of the tissue that produces them. Examples include prostaglandin E_2, prostaglandin $F_{2\alpha}$, prostaglandin I_2 (also called prostacyclin) and thromboxane A2.

ACTIVITY

If you are unsure what an essential fatty acid is, look it up in a dictionary

---

BOX 9.2 UK AND US NOMENCLATURE

Many clinical texts originate from the USA and so include reference to American terms. The names, and the spelling of those names, of many drugs have recently been standardized. One of the commonest aspects that confuses is the terminology in relation to catecholamines. In the UK, the names 'adrenaline' and 'noradrenaline' are still frequently used, which reflect the origin of the hormones in the adrenal glands ('ad-' = beside, 'renal' = of the kidneys). In the USA, these hormones are called epinephrine and norepinephrine, respectively, because they originate from the epinephric glands ('epi-' = upon, 'nephro' = the kidneys).

Organization of secretory tissues: exocrine and endocrine glands

Cells that secrete chemicals are frequently collected into discrete areas of tissue or glands. Some glands release their secretions onto the outer surface of the body; these are called exocrine glands. Their secretions include mucus, saliva, digestive enzymes, tears, earwax, sebum and sweat. Many exocrine glands (e.g. salivary glands) require ducts to transport their secretions. Not all exocrine glands are ducted, however; some cells that secrete digestive enzymes, and those that produce mucus, release their secretions directly. But how is this outside the body? Chapter 10 notes how the gut is basically a tubular structure passing from the mouth to the anus. Despite various modifications along the way (e.g. the stomach and intestines) the tube-like structure remains apparent. It is, in theory, possible to pass a thread from mouth to anus (we do not recommend that you try this!), so the lumen of the gut can actually be considered to be continuous with the outer surface of the body. This is why digestive secretions are considered to be exocrine in nature.

Hormones are not produced as exocrine secretions (although pheromones are, which again highlights the difficulties of establishing a simple definition for hormones). Those glands that secrete the major hormones of the body are referred to as endocrine glands, which is why the study of hormones is called endocrinology. This process does not require the presence of ducts to transport the secretions, as they can be secreted directly into the extracellular fluid. Hence, these glands are sometimes referred to as ductless glands (this is a bad choice of term, since we noted above that some exocrine glands also do not have ducts).

In a few instances, a glandular tissue has both exocrine and endocrine functions. For example, the pancreas is partly an exocrine gland that releases digestive juices into the duodenum via the pancreatic duct, but it also has 'islets' of endocrine tissue that secrete hormones such as insulin directly into the circulatory system. The pancreas, therefore, is a mixed gland. The testes are also mixed glands (see Chapter 18).

Inducing a change in target cell activity: second messenger chemicals

The amount of hormone that is released from a gland is considerably diluted in extracellular fluid, and so interactions with target cell receptors are of a relatively low key, perhaps involving only one or two molecules of hormone. This makes them very potent, but also means that, once a hormone has interacted with the target cell receptor, the responses of the target

cell must involve an amplification of the signal until it is sufficient to produce an effective change in target cell activities. The amplification is provided by the generation of other messenger chemicals within the cytoplasm of the cell following the combination between the hormone molecule and cell receptor. In this way, the hormone is viewed as being the 'first messenger' and the chemicals produced within the target cell are 'second messengers'.

Second messengers to peptide, catecholamine and eicosanoid hormones

For these particular hormones, second messengers are produced when the hormone interacts with a surface membrane receptor. There are a number of examples of second messengers, the most important one is cyclic adenosine monophosphate (abbreviated as cyclic AMP, or cAMP). Calcium ions and certain modified membrane lipids (e.g. inositol triphosphate) are also second messengers. It is the deactivation of the second messenger process, together with the enzymatic separation of the hormone molecule from its receptor that results in cessation of the target cell response to a hormone.

The discovery of second messengers, and recent advances in understanding their actions, have opened up new avenues for pharmacological research. Some drugs that modulate their actions are available (e.g. phosphodiesterase inhibitors act on the enzyme phosphodiesterase to prevent the breakdown of cAMP and so prolong its actions); additional drugs and refinements can be expected in the future.

Second messengers promote the activation of a group of enzymes called protein kinases that activate certain proteins within the cell. These in turn activate further enzymes called phosphorylases (phosphorylate is a term used to indicate the chemical combination of a substance with a phosphate molecule) that then activate other proteins. While this is clearly a very complex process it is necessary because numerous stages of chemical activation produce a 'cascade' (see also Figure 11.15, p.291) that is responsible for the amplification of the signal. Thus, for example, just one molecule of the hormone glucagon, which promotes the breakdown of glycogen to glucose in liver cells, induces the generation of more than one million molecules of glucose. This is how hormones are such potent substances.

Having a second messenger system also has other advantages in that by having more than one second messenger system operating a single cell may act as a target for more than one hormone, and may be induced to respond identically or differently to the different hormones. For example:

- the hormones glucagon (a peptide) and adrenaline (a catecholamine) promote the same second messenger within liver cells, skeletal muscle cells and fat cells and so both cause the release of glucose from glycogen stores in these cells. In this way, glucose can be mobilized under different circumstances: glucagon helps to prevent basal blood glucose concentration from decreasing too far, and adrenaline raises blood glucose concentration during times of physical activity or in the alarm stage of the stress response (Figure 9.1a);

ACTIVITY

Refer to Chapter 18, pp.486–7 and identify the endocrine and exocrine secretions of the testes.

'Hormones are endocrine secretions.' Refer back to the earlier definition of a hormone and explain what this means.

- insulin promotes a different second messenger that causes liver cells, skeletal muscle cells and fat cells to produce glycogen from glucose. In this way, the same cell that responds to glucagon by breaking down glycogen into glucose can be made to act oppositely by storing glucose as glycogen. These target cells can therefore respond to a situation when blood glucose concentration must be reduced (i.e. the insulin action) or when it has to be increased (i.e. the glucagon action), thus helping to maintain blood glucose homeostasis.

Second messengers for thyroid hormones and steroids

For thyroid hormones (thyroxine), the entire membrane receptor/hormone combination is internalized by the cell, and cell activation then results from a very different sequence of events from that observed during activation by peptides and catecholamines. Thus, thyroxine triggers gene transcription and so will promote enzyme production; it is these enzymes that then alter cell activity (Figure 9.1b). The principle of amplification and second messengers still applies, but as already noted this mode of action is generally slower than that of peptide hormones and catecholamines. It is perhaps of significance that thyroxine controls basal metabolic processes, so a rapid mode of action is not necessary.

The mode of cell activation by steroids is generally similar to that of thyroid hormones, except that steroids are lipid soluble and receptors to them are found within the cytoplasm of target cells, rather than on the cell membrane. Like thyroxine, steroids also promote gene transcription and enzyme production. Similarly, steroid hormones are essentially concerned with processes (such as blood volume regulation and reproductive functions) that do not require an instant response.

BOX 9.3 LACK OF HORMONE RECEPTORS IN TARGET TISSUES

Inadequate target tissue response results if there is a lack of receptors to a hormone, as this prevents the tissue from 'recognizing' the hormone when it is present. An example is the disturbance of glucose metabolism in a form of non-insulin-dependent diabetes mellitus, in which tissues do not respond to the hormone insulin even though it is released from the pancreas.

Clinical intervention in such cases is directed at using alternative means to control the parameter that the hormone regulates. For example, in the case of non-insulin-dependent diabetes mellitus, the patient will be advised on dietary control of carbohydrate and fat consumption, but may also receive a metabolism-promoting drug, such as metformin, to facilitate cell functions in the absence of insulin. It is also possible that target cells may fail to respond to a hormone because of an underlying disorder of the cells or the tissue itself. However, the problems arising from the lack of response to the hormone are then considered to be secondary to the cause of disorder, although improving hormonal actions might still be part of the treatment.

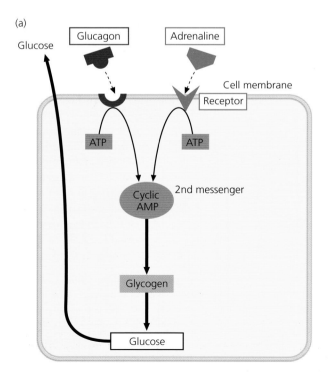

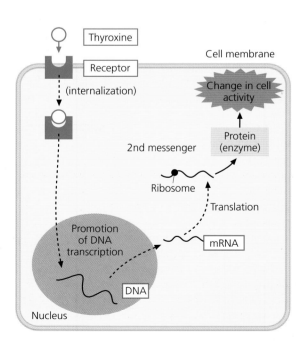

Figure 9.1 Second messenger chemicals. (a) The second messenger chemicals are activated by peptide and catecholamine hormones after their interaction with receptors in the cell membrane. (b) The interaction between steroids and thyroxine with their respective receptors trigger events directly within the cell. mRNA, messenger RNA

Regulation of hormone release: general principles

Details of stimuli for the release of individual hormones, and the control of that release, are given in the next section. As an introduction, it is worth considering here general aspects of the stimulus required, and the regulation of secretion.

The stimulus

Many hormones have essential roles in the homeostatic regulation of psychological function and physiological systemic functions. The stimuli for hormonal secretion therefore relate to a diverse range of parameters, such as mood-changing stimuli (e.g. time of the year), composition of body fluids, blood pressure, blood volume, body temperature or nutrient content of digestive chyme. For example, the hormone vasopressin (also known as antidiuretic hormone or ADH) plays a vital role in the maintenance of body water content (see Chapter 15, p.433. It is therefore appropriate that the release of this hormone is in direct response to the increased osmotic pressure of body fluids that occurs when we are dehydrated. As the osmotic pressure is corrected, the stimulus declines and hormone secretion is reduced accordingly. The amount of vasopressin released, and hence the extent of the kidney response, is related directly to the magnitude of the change in osmotic pressure. From a homeostatic perspective, this type of relationship helps to prevent fluctuations in the parameter concerned by reversing any changes that have occurred.

In contrast, some hormones are released in order to induce change; this shift in homeostatic set points promotes optimal conditions according to the needs of the body at that particular time. Thus, adrenaline has an important role in the heightening of cardiovascular responses during exercise, and the stress response; once the exercise has finished, or the stressors are removed, the release of the hormone declines again. Adrenaline also induces metabolic change and will have widespread effects throughout the body. Under such circumstances, adrenaline is released through nerve activity to the adrenal gland from the brain. Note the transience of this relationship; prolongation of the change eventually produces homeostatic imbalance as the homeostatic set points do not return to their usual setting, and in this instance there will be increased blood pressure even at rest.

Other hormones promote permanent change because this is developmental; for example, sex hormones from the gonads control fertility in adulthood, but during puberty they are also responsible for instigating sexual maturity and the development of secondary sexual characteristics. This promotion of permanent change requires a resetting of homeostatic parameters (see Figure 1.7, p.11 and associated text), much as responses to exercise and stress did in the previous examples, but this time the resets are permanent. Stimuli operating within this changed state then provide the control of hormone release necessary to maintain fertility. For sex steroids, this is usually via other hormones.

Principles of control

In the examples given above of the actions of vasopressin during dehydration, and of adrenaline in exercise and stress, the

ACTIVITY

Concepts of negative and positive feedback are prominent in this section, and in this chapter generally. You are advised to review Chapter 1 before proceeding further.

removal of the stimulus directly reverses the change in hormone release. This is a simple negative feedback 'loop'; it involves a 'short loop', since there is only one stage to the process as it comes from the action of the hormone itself (Figure 9.2a).

The number of stages involved in the eventual secretion of some hormones utilizes a 'long-loop' feedback system. This is frequently observed when the initial stimulus for the release of a hormone entails other intermediary hormones (Figure 9.2b). Cortisol is one such hormone (see later; Figure 9.12, p.219) that is released from the adrenal gland in response to the intermediary, adrenocorticotropic hormone (ACTH). The names of intermediary hormones normally have the suffix '-tropic'

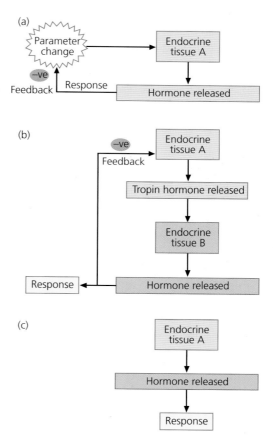

Figure 9.2 Feedback loops in the homeostatic control of the release and/or actions of hormones. (a) The feedback to hormone release operates as a 'short loop' and comes from the action of the hormone itself. (b) The feedback is 'long looped' and entails other hormones. (c) The loop is 'open' since there is apparently no feedback

Q *Which of these feedback loops is likely to promote the most closely regulated control of hormone release?*

(e.g. another is gonadotropic hormone); a 'tropin' is a hormone that stimulates the release of another. Indeed, a more modern name for ACTH is corticotropin. The presence of cortisol in blood acts as a negative feedback signal to switch off the secretion of corticotropin, leading to a decline in cortisol release and hence the eventual switching on of the release of corticotrophin so that cortisol is secreted once again. Long-loop feedback systems tend to be found when very close control of hormone secretion is necessary, or when cognitive processes must connect in some way with a gland; for cortisol, the intermediary corticotropin is secreted from the pituitary gland (see below) at the base of the brain during stress.

In contrast, there are occasions when certain hormones are released that do not appear to have a negative feedback mechanism to control their secretion. For example, growth hormone promotes a variety of metabolic actions, none of which could be envisaged as providing a stimulus to decrease its secretion. This is called an 'open-loop' system (Figure 9.2c), although it might just be the case that the feedback mechanism remains to be discovered. For example, the secretion of insulin-like growth factor 1 (IGF-1; in older texts referred to as somatomedin) from the liver is promoted by growth hormone and this does have a negative feedback effect on growth hormone secretion, but is not responsible for all of the actions of growth hormone: IGF-1 stimulates cell division in various tissues.

Finally, there are a small number of instances when positive feedback operates. In positive feedback, the response to the hormone is to increase the stimulus, leading to yet greater hormone secretion. The cycle, therefore, is one of rapidly increasing hormone activity, rather than maintenance. An example is the effect of uterus tension during labour to stimulate the release of the hormone oxytocin, which then causes the development of further tension, and hence further hormone release.

Examples of feedback loops in the regulation of the secretory activities of individual endocrine glands are described in detail in the next section.

HOMEOSTATIC FUNCTIONS OF THE HORMONES

Hormones have essential roles in psychological and physiological homeostasis. Although hormonal actions are diverse, there is a degree of overlap, and examples have been given throughout this book in which interactions between secretions are important for the overall control of some parameters. For example, blood pressure regulation involves a number of vasoconstrictor hormones of different chemistries and origins. For clarity, however, this section will take a systematic approach, and describe the secretions of individual endocrine tissues, the locations of which are shown in Figure 9.3. A summary table of the secretions of these glands, and their regulation, is also provided (Table 9.1).

BOX 9.4 HYPOSECRETION AND HYPERSECRETION OF HORMONES

Gland dysfunctioning is generally classed as causing either hyposecretion or hypersecretion. Specific examples are given later, but we will introduce the general principles here (see Figure 9.4).

Hyposecretion
Inadequate secretion of hormone can have a number of causes:

- the endocrine cells may lack receptors to the activating stimulus (e.g. through the production of autoantibodies, as in the underactive thyroid disorder called Hashimoto's disease; see Section VI, p.646 for the case of a patient with hypothyroidism). Ageing will also reduce hormonal secretion, partly because of receptor deficiencies as rate of receptor production and maintenance declines as a consequence of the ageing process;
- hyposecretion might reflect an inability of glands to produce the hormone, as in insulin-dependent diabetes mellitus. Lack of synthesis usually results from genetic mutation, and may be inherited, congenital or acquired (e.g. from the effect of ageing);
- a deficiency, usually dietary, of the precursor molecule may lead to inadequate synthesis (e.g. a lack of iodine in the diet may cause thyroxine deficiency). Overgrowth or hypertrophy of the gland as a consequence is a homeostatic maladapted response in an attempt to raise hormone secretion. Dietary deficiencies as causes of hormonal disorder are rare in Western societies.

Hyposecretion can sometimes be improved with drugs that stimulate production and/or secretion of the hormone from the gland. Often, however, correction requires hormone replacement therapy. This term is frequently applied to the administration of oestrogens in postmenopausal women, but it can be used to mean any circumstance in which an individual is administered hormone therapy. The hormone is normally a synthetic form of the natural chemical.

In the near future it is almost certainly going to be possible to insert endocrine 'stem' cells, which can produce the hormone that is deficient or absent in hyposecretory imbalances. The introduction of pancreatic islet cells is likely to be the first success with stem cell transplantation, since the British government has invested substantial amounts of money in developing this therapy. The identification of hormone genes will also undoubtedly be developed as further avenues to treat hormonal deficiency diseases.

Hypersecretion
Hypersecretion commonly results from a failure of the negative feedback mechanism that controls hormone release:

- The feedback failure usually results from a lack of receptors to the feedback signal to the gland cells, but what makes these receptors decline is unclear. Autoimmune responses are thought to be a frequent cause.
- Gland hypertrophy, and overactivity of its cells, is also seen when there is a tumour present, since tumour cells may 'escape' negative feedback processes. Alternatively, elevated plasma concentrations of a hormone might reflect non-glandular secretion of the hormone. Thus, the actual gland might continue to be regulated closely via a negative feedback, but tumours elsewhere, which do not have the appropriate receptors and are unresponsive to feedback control, could produce the hormone even when this is inappropriate. The secretion of a hormone by a site other than that of the gland is referred to as ectopic.

Principles of correction might involve using a drug to suppress hormone production or to antagonize its actions. Availability of such drugs is limited at the present time. Surgery (partial or total gland removal) to reduce the gland is another option. Again further treatment will be developed following the successful discoveries of the human genomic and proteomic projects.

Table 9.1 Summary of the secretions, actions and regulation of some of the major endocrine glands

Gland	Hormone	Target	Action	Homeostatic regulation
Hypothalamus	*Releasing hormones	Anterior pituitary	Release of various hormones (see text)	Negative feedback from target endocrine secretions Neural input to hypothalamus
	*Inhibitory hormones	Anterior pituitary	Inhibit release of various hormones (see text)	Unclear Neural input to hypothalamus
Anterior pituitary	Corticotropin (ACTH)	Adrenal cortex	Release of glucocorticoid hormones	Negative feedback from glucocorticoid Hypothalamic regulatory hormones
	Thyrotropin (TSH)	Thyroid follicles	Release of thyroxine	Negative feedback from thyroxine Hypothalamic regulatory hormones
	Gonadotropins, i.e. luteinizing hormone (LH), follicle-stimulating hormone (FSH)	Gonads	Oestrogens and progestins (female), testosterone (male)	Negative feedback from gonadal hormones
	Growth hormone (GH, somatotropin)	Various tissues	Metabolic (see text)	Unclear Hypothalamic regulatory hormones
	Prolactin	Breast (female) Unclear in male	Lactation (role in male unclear)	Unclear Hypothalamic regulatory hormones
	Melanocyte-stimulating hormone (MSH)	Melanocytes in skin	Promotes melanin synthesis	Unclear Hypothalamic regulatory hormones
Posterior pituitary	Vasopressin (antidiuretic hormone, ADH)	Kidney, arterioles	Water retention Vasoconstriction (blood pressure regulation)	Negative feedback from plasma osmotic pressure, and arterial blood pressure
	Oxytocin	Breast and uterus (unclear in male)	Lactation, labour Role in male unclear	Negative feedback from suckling Positive feedback from uterus during labour
Thyroid	Thyroxine (T3, T4)	Various tissues	Metabolic, especially role in basal metabolic rate	Thyrotropin from anterior pituitary gland
	Calcitonin	Bone	Promotes calcium deposition	Negative feedback from plasma calcium ion concentration
Parathyroid	Parathyroid hormone (PTH)	Bone, kidney	Promotes calcium resorption from bone Activates vitamin D in kidney (i.e. promotes calcium uptake from bowel)	Negative feedback from plasma calcium ion concentration
Adrenal cortex	Glucocorticoids, e.g. cortisol	Various tissues	Metabolic, permissive influence on other hormones	Corticotropin from anterior pituitary
	Mineralocorticoids, e.g. aldosterone	Kidney	Promote sodium reabsorption from renal tubule, promote potassium secretion (i.e. excretion)	Negative feedback from effects on blood volume (via changes in renin production), or plasma potassium concentration
	Gonadal steroids	Gonads	Influence on reproductive tract, but not regulatory	Unclear
Adrenal medulla	Catecholamines (adrenaline, noradrenaline)	Heart and circulation, also various other tissues (see text)	Promote cardiac function Promote vasoconstriction (blood pressure regulation)	Sympathetic nervous system activity
Duodenum	Secretin and CCK–PZ	Digestive glands, gall bladder, pancreas, stomach	Promote secretion of pancreatic fluid and enzymes, bile secretion, regulate gastric emptying	Presence of food products in duodenum
Pancreas	Insulin	Liver, skeletal muscle	Promotes glucose utilization	Negative feedback from blood glucose concentration
	Glucagon	Liver, skeletal muscle	Promotes glucose mobilization from stores	Negative feedback from blood glucose concentration
	Somatostatin	Insulin- and glucagon-secreting cells of pancreas	Modulates release of insulin and glucagon	Presence of insulin or glucagon
Gonads: ovaries (female)	Oestrogens (e.g. oestriol), progestins (e.g. progesterone)	Reproductive tract, breast and secondary sexual characteristics	Regulation of menstrual cycle. Behavioural effects	Gonadotropins (LH and FSH) from anterior pituitary
Gonads: testes (male)	Androgens (e.g. testosterone)	Reproductive tract and secondary sexual characteristics	Regulation of spermatogenesis, and accessory glands of reproductive tract Behavioural effects	Gonadotropins (especially LH) from anterior pituitary

*Hypothalamic regulatory hormones include specific releasing and inhibitory hormones that act on the secretion of individual hormones from the anterior pituitary gland.
CCK–PZ, cholecystokinin–pancreozymin

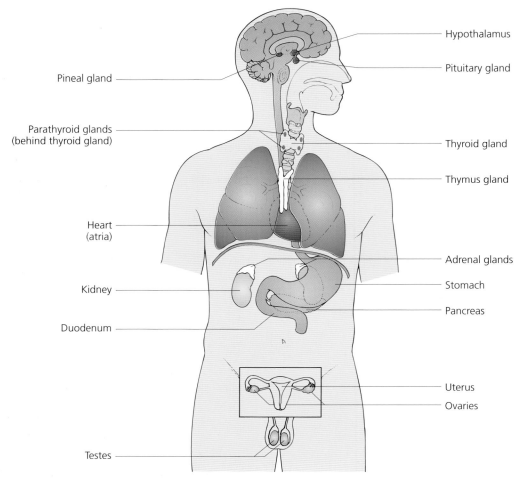

Figure 9.3 Location of the major endocrine glands

The hypothalamus and the pituitary gland

The hypothalamus lies at the base of the brain, and the pituitary gland is located just below it, attached to it by a 'stalk'. Together they form a functional unit often referred to as the hypothalamic–pituitary axis because the hypothalamus mediates the secretion of hormones by the pituitary gland; however, it is convenient to consider the two separately.

The hypothalamus

The hypothalamus is a part of the forebrain (see Chapter 8, p.172). It has a diverse range of functions, including the control of 'drives' of human nature (feeding, drinking, sexual behaviour), the control of body temperature and the establishment of a daily metabolic rhythm (circadian rhythm; see Chapter 22, p.610). It shares some functions with other parts of the brain, particularly with areas of the limbic system that are responsible for emotion, anxiety and aggression.

Being a part of the brain, the hypothalamus contains nerve cells. Some of these have a glandular role; cells that produce and secrete the hormones are referred to as neuroendocrine cells, because they are both nerve cells (i.e. neurons) and gland cells. The glandular cells of the hypothalamus will secrete their hormones when stimulated, but being neurological tissue, that secretion may also be influenced by higher brain centres. Thus, many of the psychological influences on physical function, such as stress and circadian rhythm changes, occur through the activities of the hypothalamus.

Most of the hormones produced by the hypothalamus are released into small blood vessels that form a direct link between the hypothalamus and pituitary (Figure 9.5). These hormones are conveyed to cells within the anterior lobe of the pituitary gland, which themselves produce further hor-

ACTIVITY

The blood vessels that pass from the hypothalamus to the anterior pituitary gland are examples of portal vessels (i.e. they carry blood directly from one capillary bed to another without passing through a vein or artery). Establishing this portal circulation from the hypothalamus is thought to determine the onset of puberty. The largest portal vessel in the body is the hepatic portal vein. Refer to Figure 10.18 (p.225) and associated text and identify why this is also a portal vessel.

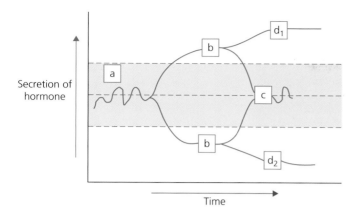

Figure 9.4 General scheme for the regulation of hormone secretion. a, Secretion operating within homeostatic norms; b, disturbance of secretion; c, restoration of normal secretion by negative feedback responses to the hormone actions or other hormones (see Figure 9.2, p.209); d_1, imbalance from continued hypersecretion owing to failure of negative feedback; d_2, imbalance from continued hyposecretion owing to failure of stimulation of the gland or failure of the gland to produce hormone. [a, Represents boxes a_1–a_4 in Figure 1.7, p.11, reflecting the individual variability in the homeostatic range. The blue area represents the norm (homeostatic range) 95%]

mones, so the hypothalamic hormones involved are referred to as either releasing or inhibiting hormones (or factors), according to their actions on the pituitary gland, and are usually named after the pituitary hormone that they influence (Table 9.1).

Other hypothalamic hormones are secreted directly from nerve endings within the posterior lobe of the pituitary. The hormone, having been produced in the cell body of the neuron located within the hypothalamus, is transported along the axon of the nerve cell to the terminals, where it is stored in vesicles ready for secretion. It is conventional, however, to consider these particular secretions as being pituitary rather than hypothalamic hormones.

The roles of hypothalamic secretions, and the control of their release, are considered below.

The pituitary gland

The pituitary gland (or hypophysis) is of mixed embryological origin: the anterior part is formed from an upgrowth of the oral cavity of the embryo, while the posterior part is a down-growth from the overlying brain. This helps to explain how the anterior lobe is comprised of non-neural cells, while the posterior lobe is comprised of neural tissue.

The anterior lobe

The anterior lobe (or adenohypophysis) comprises some 75% of the pituitary by weight. It consists of two parts:

- the *pars distalis*: secretes most hormones of the anterior lobe;
- the *pars intermedia*: a small piece of glandular tissue that lies between the pars distalis and the posterior lobe of the pituitary gland (Figure 9.5). It is occasionally referred to as the intermediate or middle lobe of the pituitary gland, but it is functionally linked to the pars distalis.

The hormones produced by the anterior lobe are identified, together with their main actions, in Table 9.1. All are peptides. Most are tropins that act on other endocrine tissues in the body, and therefore regulate the production of their secretions; for this reason, the anterior lobe has been called the 'master gland'.

BOX 9.5 DYSFUNCTIONING OF THE ANTERIOR PITUITARY GLAND

Strictly speaking, such disorders include those arising from problems in the secretion of anterior lobe tropins, such as gonadotropin and thyrotropin, but these are considered in relation to the target glands (see Boxes 9.7, p.217 and 9.11, p.221). This box considers only disorders of growth hormone and prolactin, hormones that have direct effects.

Hyposecretion of growth hormone retards childhood growth, resulting in small stature but normal body proportions (a condition known as pituitary dwarfism). It is important that any growth deficiencies are identified during childhood, since the calcification of growth plates in the long bones at puberty will prevent further growth. Slowed growth is normally detected by regular attention to growth assessments. Synthetic growth hormone can be administered during childhood, if tests identify a deficiency, in order to improve growth rate. The hormone also has metabolic effects in the adult, and is released primarily during sleep in order to repair and regenerate body tissues. Hyposecretion will therefore have metabolic consequences relating to slowed tissue maintenance and poor wound healing.

Hypersecretion of growth hormone promotes excessive growth in children, leading to pituitary giantism. In adults, when the growth plates of longer bones have been calcified, excessive secretion promotes growth of the skeleton, especially in the extremities, leading to exaggerated features (known as acromegaly – see Figure 9.6), such as the frontal bone of the skull, mandibular bones, hands and feet. Hypersecretion may also occur from ectopic sites, such as tumours. Antagonistic drugs may be given (e.g. to counteract secretion from tumours) or alternatively destruction of part of the pituitary gland may be required. However, acromegalic changes are irreversible once they are established.

Hypersecretion of prolactin may be seen after birth when the hormone is released in increasing quantities to promote lactation. Drugs that promote the release from the hypothalamus of prolactin inhibitory hormone may be used to reduce the hypersecretion.

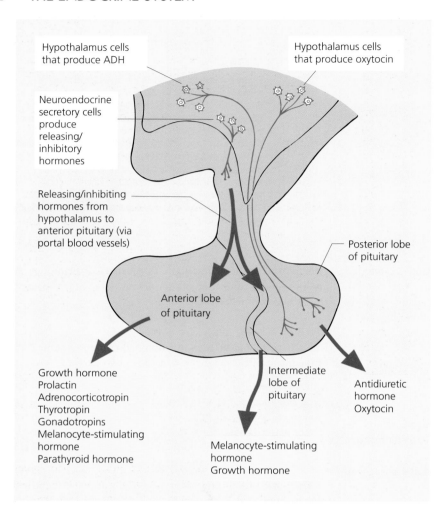

Hypothalamus cells that produce ADH

Hypothalamus cells that produce oxytocin

Neuroendocrine secretory cells produce releasing/ inhibitory hormones

Releasing/inhibiting hormones from hypothalamus to anterior pituitary (via portal blood vessels)

Posterior lobe of pituitary

Anterior lobe of pituitary

Growth hormone
Prolactin
Adrenocorticotropin
Thyrotropin
Gonadotropins
Melanocyte-stimulating hormone
Parathyroid hormone

Intermediate lobe of pituitary

Antidiuretic hormone
Oxytocin

Melanocyte-stimulating hormone
Growth hormone

Figure 9.5 The hypothalamus–pituitary gland axis and the main hormones secreted. ADH, antidiuretic hormone

Most of the secretory cells of the anterior lobe are subject to a long-loop negative feedback inhibition from the secretions of their target endocrine tissues (further details are given when the individual target glands are discussed). A schema was given in Figure 9.2b, and negative feedback was identified in Chapter 1, p.13 as the main means by which body functions, and hence homeostasis, can be regulated. The process places a high degree of control on the pituitary gland, and this need for precise control reflects the potency of its hormones.

Most hormones of the anterior lobe are released in response to the presence of hypothalamic releasing hormones. Some, namely growth hormone, melanocyte-stimulating hormone (MSH) and prolactin, are controlled primarily by hypothalamic inhibitory hormones, although the situation is complicated by the presence of releasing hormones. It is unclear why the control should be different from that of other anterior lobe secretions, but it may relate to their actions since they are not tropins and so have direct effects on non-glandular tissues: growth hormone has widespread metabolic effects (another name for growth hormone is somatotrophin; 'soma' = body, 'troph' = nutrition); MSH (which is the main secretion of the

pars intermedia) promotes pigmentation of skin melanocytes, and prolactin promotes milk production during lactation. Growth hormone is also secreted from the middle lobe.

The posterior lobe

We noted earlier that the posterior lobe (or neurohypophysis) is composed of neural tissue. Thus, the lobe is sometimes referred to as the pars nervosa (nervous part). The gland consists of axon terminals that contain vesicles of hormone produced by the cell bodies of the nerve cells within the hypothalamus. The posterior lobe secretes two hormones: vasopressin and oxytocin.

Vasopressin (or ADH) is produced by cell bodies within a part of the hypothalamus called the supraoptic nucleus (i.e. they lie above the optic nerves close to where they cross over). Vasopressin is involved in the control of water balance via its retentive actions in the kidney (hence its alternative name), and the control of blood pressure via its vasoconstrictor actions. The hormone is released following the stimulation of osmoreceptors in the hypothalamus (responding to the effects of dehydration) or arterial baroreceptors (responding to

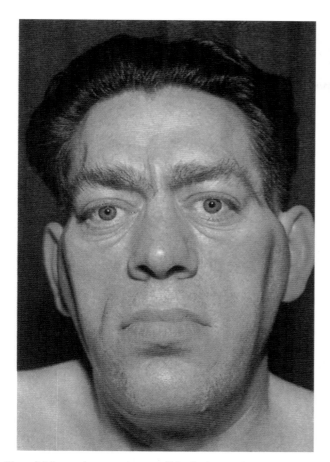

Figure 9.6 A case of acromegaly, exemplifying the heavy enlargement of the front of the lower jaw. Reproduced with permission from Boucher I, Ellis H and Fleming P, *French's Index of Differential Diagnosis*, 13th edition. London: Hodder Arnold

BOX 9.6 DYSFUNCTIONING OF THE POSTERIOR PITUITARY GLAND

Hyposecretion of vasopressin (or renal resistance to its actions) is known as diabetes insipidus (not to be confused with diabetes mellitus), and means that the kidneys are unable to conserve water efficiently. Copious volumes of dilute urine are produced because the urinary concentration mechanism is compromised (see Chapter 15, p.433), leading to persistent dehydration. Synthetic vasopressin is administered when the disorder is caused by hyposecretion. Diabetes insipidus may be inherited or acquired, for example as a consequence of brain surgery in the area of the hypothalamus.

Hypersecretion of vasopressin is known as syndrome of inappropriate antidiuretic hormone secretion (SIADH). Water conservation is constantly promoted, even if the patient is well hydrated, and overhydration and body fluid dilution (called hypo-osmolality), and an expansion of body fluid volume (hypervolaemia), occur.

The main documented action of oxytocin is during birth. Hypersecretion of oxytocin is extremely rare, but its concentration in blood at stages of labour may be increased above that achieved by normal secretion by administration of synthetic hormone in order to progress labour.

The thyroid gland

The thyroid gland is a gland in the neck with a butterfly shape (Figure 9.7a). It has four lobes that straddle the lower end of the trachea. It secretes tri-iodothyronine (T3), tetra-iodothyronine (T4) and calcitonin.

T3 and T4

These are derived from the amino acid tyrosine. Their names simply reflect the number of iodine atoms that are incorporated into each hormone molecule. They are released together and have similar actions, although T4 (commonly called thyroxine) is the main secretion.

The need for iodine to be incorporated into the molecules of thyroid hormones is one of the main reasons why iodine must be included in our diet. The iodide ion is actively taken up by the gland and initially incorporated into tyrosine molecules attached to a protein called thyroglobulin that is stored in extracellular spaces within the lobules of the gland (Figure 9.7b,c). The gland therefore is able to concentrate iodine within it, and the uptake of administered radioisotopic iodine is a clinically useful means of monitoring thyroid function.

When required, T3 and T4 are generated quickly from thyroglobulin and released into the blood. Release is promoted by thyroid-stimulating hormone (TSH; increasingly known as thyrotropin) from the anterior pituitary gland, which in turn is released in response to TSH-releasing hormone from the hypothalamus (see Figure 9.8 for details of thyroxine control). Both thyroxine and TSH have negative feedback actions on the hypothalamus and anterior pituitary cells, and there is, therefore, a tight control on thyroid hormone release. The need for this is clear when one considers that the main function of thyroxine is to determine basal metabolic rate.

hypotension). Correction of water balance or blood pressure removes the stimulus and provides the negative feedback that causes hormone secretion to decline.

Oxytocin is synthesized by cell bodies within the parts of the hypothalamus called the paraventricular nuclei (i.e. they lie alongside the cerebral ventricles). Oxytocin is involved in labour, and is released as a reflex response to increasing tension of the uterus wall. The hormone causes the uterus to contract, and a positive feedback operates that makes hormone secretion, and hence uterine tension, increase further. Delivery of the baby, and resultant loss of uterine tension, causes the hormone secretion to decline again. Oxytocin is also released during suckling, when it promotes the release of breast milk (see Figure 18.10c, p.499). Its release declines when the baby stops feeding – another negative feedback response. Men also produce oxytocin but its actions are unclear. There is some evidence that the hormone is released during orgasm and aids the transportation of semen by contracting the vas deferens (and also of the oocyte in women by contracting the oviducts), and there is also some support for its involvement in regulating fluid balance, but these findings remain speculative at the present.

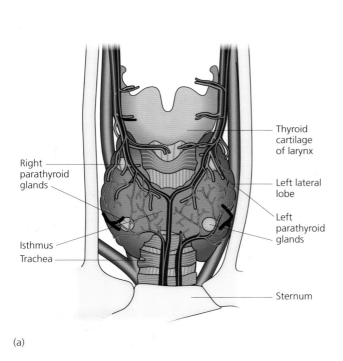

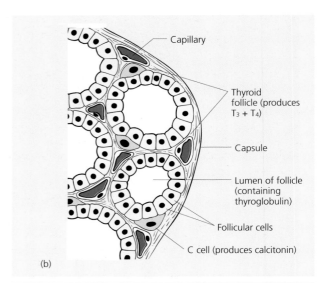

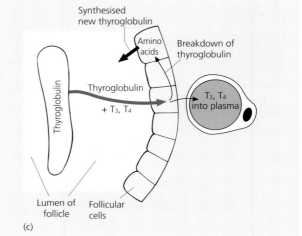

Figure 9.7 The thyroid gland. (a) Anatomical position. (b) A diagram of a section through the gland showing follicles, the glandular follicular cells and the glandular C cells that are associated with the follicles. (c) Synthesis of thyroxine (T_3, T_4) involving the complex protein thyroglobulin within the lumen of a follicle. Note how the hormone is produced and stored within the follicle lumen, but is secreted from the follicular cells after removal of the thyroglobulin

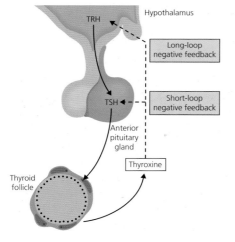

1. Blood thyroxine below its homeostatic range or low metabolic rate stimulates receptors in hypothalamic cells to activate genes to produce enzymes that produce thyroid-releasing hormone (TRH).
2. TRH is transported in the portal vessel, which connects the hypothalamus to the anterior pituitary lobe. TRH stimulates receptors in the anterior pituitary thyrotrophic cells, which stimulate gene activity to produce the enzymes necessary for thyroid-stimulating hormone (TSH) production.
3. TSH combines with receptors in the thyroid cells, activating genes to produce the enzymes that produce thyroxin.
4. Thyroxine is released into blood to re-establish homeostatic levels.
5. Thyroxine above its homeostatic range or high metabolic rate inhibits gene activity the hypothalamus (i.e. long-loop negative feedback) to stop the production and secretion of TRH, and in the anterior pituitary thyrotrophic cells (i.e. short-loop negative feedback) to stop the production and secretion of TSH. Thyroxine levels in the blood fall as it is used up at cellular level.

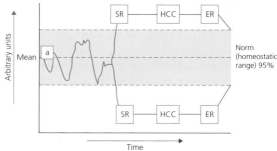

Figure 9.8 Thyroxine control. SR, sensory receptor; HCC, homeostatic control centre; ER, effector response. [a, Represents boxes a_1–a_4 in Figure 1.7, p.11, reflecting the individual variability in the homeostatic range. The blue area represents the norm (homeostatic range) 95%]

Q How is the concentration in blood of thyrotropin (TSH) increased in people who produce insufficient thyroxine?

BOX 9.7 DYSFUNCTIONING OF THE THYROID GLAND

Hyposecretion

Hashimoto's thyroiditis (or disease) is an autoimmune disorder that is the commonest cause of primary hypothyroidism, in which the release of thyroxine (T4) is low despite secretion of thyroid-stimulating hormone (TSH or thyrotropin) because of thyroid function problems; the lack of negative feedback from thyroxine means that TSH release is abnormally high. The use of thyroxine replacement therapy is 'titrated' against TSH concentration as TSH release is normalized by the administered thyroxine. The high levels of TSH can sometimes result in the patient exhibiting goitre as the thyroid increases in size to improve thyroxine secretion. Thus, goitre may appear in both hyperthyroidism and hypothyroidism.

In secondary and tertiary hypothyroidism the disorder relates to other causes, usually hypothalamic, so TSH secretion is low, and hence thyroxine secretion is also low.

In hypothyroidism (Figure 9.9a) the low levels of thyroxine results in a lower level of cellular respiration and therefore low levels of the end-product of cellular respiration, adenosine triphosphate ATP (see Chapters 2, p.36, and 4, p.102). Generation of ATP equates to the metabolic rate of a cell and consequently the basal metabolic rate (BMR) is reduced. This reduction is largely responsible for the signs and symptoms experienced in this condition. The BMR may be only 60% of its homeostatic value, so it is not surprising that cold intolerance is a frequent symptom in people who are hypothyroidic. The lowering of the BMR is also responsible for a slowing down of cognitive processes, for causing a bradycardia, reducing the cardiac output/blood pressure, and for reduced respiratory effort, leading to weight gain and fatigue.

Uncontrolled hypothyroidism in its chronic stages results in the skin becoming thicker and peripheral oedema is present (a condition known as myxoedema). Patients with myxoedema are severely affected and are unable to metabolize sedatives, analgesics and anaesthetic drugs, and the build-up leads to coma. Myxoedematous coma is the life-threatening endstage of hypothyroidism, where the patient suffers hypothermia, cardiovascular imbalances (e.g. hypercholesterolaemia, cardiomyopathy and congestive heart failure), respiratory imbalances (e.g. hypoventilation) and severe metabolic imbalances (e.g. hyponatraemia, hypoglycaemia, hypercapnia, hypoxaemia, lactate acidosis).

See the case of a patient with hypothyroidism, Section VI, p.646.

Hypersecretion

Hyperthyroidism is the name given to a syndrome of excessive secretion of thyroid hormones. A common cause is an autoimmune response that sensitizes the gland to TSH (thyrotropin); this is called Graves disease. The patient exhibits an elevated BMR, readily observable as a raised pulse rate. The person will also feel very warm as a consequence of excessive heat generation. Structural changes can also occur to facial tissues, producing a smooth texture to the skin. Protein deposition behind the eyes may also occur over time, causing the eyes to seemingly bulge forward; this is referred to as exophthalmos (Figure 9.9b).

Treatment is aimed at either surgically removing sections of the thyroid gland (thyroidectomy) to reduce the total secretion rate, using anti-thyroid drugs to prevent hormone synthesis, or using antagonistic drugs to block the actions of the hormones. Radioactive iodine may also be used to damage thyroid cells and reduce their secretory activity.

Calcitonin

Calcitonin is secreted by pockets of cells located within the thyroid gland (Figure 9.7b). Its main role is to promote the uptake of calcium ions by bone cells when plasma calcium concentration is elevated, thus returning blood calcium concentration to within its homeostatic range. As the concentration of calcium declines, the release of calcitonin is reduced. Calcitonin activity forms only one part of the process by which plasma calcium concentration is regulated; its concentration reflects a balance between uptake from the intestine, incorporation or release from bone, and excretion in urine (Figure 9.10).

The parathyroid glands

The parathyroid glands are four small patches of tissue found on the posterior surface of the lobes of the thyroid gland (see Figure 9.7a). They secrete the peptide parathyroid hormone (PTH) when the plasma calcium ion concentration is below its homeostatic range. It acts to stimulate osteoclast cells in bone to release calcium from bone mineral (Figure 9.10). It also promotes the activation of vitamin D within the kidneys. This vitamin is now recognized by many authorities to be a hormone (although it has retained its name), and increases calcium absorption from food contents in the gut.

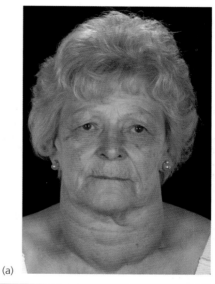

(a)

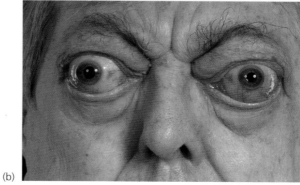

(b)

Figure 9.9 Underactive and overactive thyroid gland. (a) A woman with hypothyroidism. Note the presence of an enlarged, or hypertrophied, thyroid gland (goitre). This is an adaptive response to raise the output of thyroxine. (b) Woman with hyperthyroidism, exemplifying the exophthalmos that can occur with time in the uncontrolled condition. Reproduced with the kind permission of the Medical Illustration Department, Norfolk and Norwich University Hospital NHS Trust

BOX 9.8 DYSFUNCTIONING OF THE PARATHYROID GLAND

Hyposecretion

Since parathyroid hormone (PTH) is responsible for raising plasma calcium concentration, its deficiency will promote a decrease in calcium (hypocalcaemia). The ion influences the threshold for activation of excitable tissues, and hyposecretion of the hormone will therefore lead to increased neural excitability and even a pronounced muscle spasm called tetany (see Box 17.5, p.472). Tetany of the diaphragm muscle is life threatening. Synthetic hormone is available for hormone replacement treatment.

One cause of hyposecretion arises from the location of the gland cells in the thyroid gland. The removal of thyroid tissue to correct hyperthyroidism will more than likely entail the removal of some parathyroid tissue as well. Thus, correcting the thyroid problem can potentially lead to deficient PTH secretion, and therefore lead to difficulties in maintaining calcium homeostasis.

Hypersecretion

Excessive secretion of the hormone promotes demineralization of bone, since its actions are normally to regulate plasma calcium concentration through release of the ion from bone. A common cause of excess PTH is the ectopic production of PTH-like protein by tumours. In this case, the hypercalcaemia may be treated by elevating the blood calcitonin concentration by administering synthetic calcitonin. This in turn will increase uptake of calcium by bones.

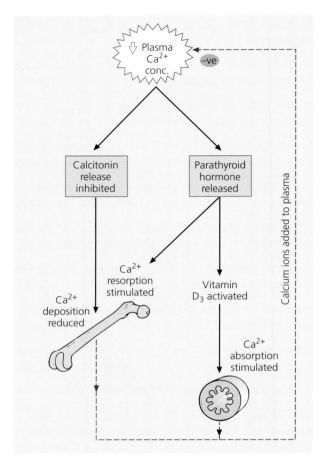

Figure 9.10 Hormonal regulation of calcium ion concentration in blood plasma. The responses to a decreased calcium concentration are shown. Note that the calcium concentration is largely a balance between calcium deposition in, or resorption from, bone and uptake from the bowel. The latter must also compensate for losses in urine

Q How would the responses change if plasma calcium concentration were excessive?

By stimulating directly the release of calcium from bone and by enhancing indirectly the absorption of calcium from the gut, PTH rapidly corrects any deficiency in plasma calcium concentration. Release of the hormone becomes inhibited as the calcium concentration begins to rise above its homeostatic range.

The adrenal glands

As the name suggests, the adrenal glands lie adjacent to the kidneys; in fact they lie on top of them. Each gland can be subdivided into an outer layer, or cortex, and an inner layer, or medulla. Cells in the cortex secrete steroid hormones, and cells in the medulla secrete catecholamine hormones (Figure 9.11).

The adrenal cortex

The cortex secretes a range of steroids that collectively are referred to as corticoids (= derived from the cortex). The steroids can be divided into:

- *glucocorticoids*: have effects on glucose metabolism;
- *mineralocorticoids*: have effects on the electrolyte composition of plasma;
- *gonadocorticoids or sex steroids (androgens/oestrogens)*: the amounts secreted are very small compared with the amounts produced by the gonads.

Glucocorticoids

Glucocorticoids are produced by a layer of the cortex called the zona fasciculata (Figure 9.11). There are a number of glucocorticoids, with similar molecular structures and actions. The most important are cortisol and corticosterone, which have a variety of actions. In particular, they promote the breakdown of protein in skeletal muscle, the synthesis of glucose from the released amino acids, and the production of glycogen from some of the synthesized glucose in the liver. The hormones also mobilize fatty acids from fats stored in adipose tissue, and inhibit the uptake of glucose by many tissues. The net effect is to:

- maintain glycogen stores in the liver that can be mobilized as and when required;
- increase plasma glucose concentration and so raise the availability of glucose for metabolism by various tissues;
- increase free fatty acid concentrations in blood plasma, and so raise their availability for metabolism by tissues.

Glucocorticoids also exert 'permissive' effects that enhance the actions of other hormones, such as adrenaline. Other effects are to stimulate red blood cell production and to reduce inflammation.

Clearly, the glucocorticoids have wide-ranging effects on the body. The actions detailed above would be particularly

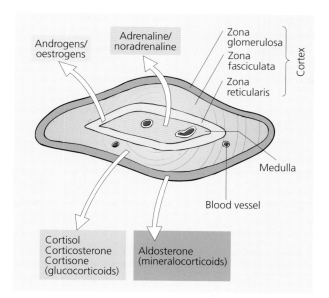

Figure 9.11 Diagram of a cross-section through an adrenal gland to illustrate the cortical zones, the medulla, and the hormones secreted from them

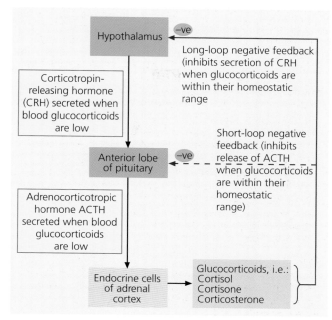

Figure 9.12 Feedback loops in the regulation of the release of glucocorticoid hormones (e.g. cortisol). Compare with that for thyroxine in Figure 9.8

Q What would happen to this control if someone had a corticotropin-producing tumour in the pituitary gland?

useful during times of physical activity and following trauma, when there may be wound healing and a need to re-establish a 'normal' state of homeostasis generally. It is perhaps not surprising that they are released when the body is under stress, including that produced by surgical trauma (see Box 21.6, pp.601–2). They have been called the 'hormones of stress' and our capacity to cope with demands are markedly reduced in their absence.

As noted earlier, the release of glucocorticoids is stimulated by ACTH (often called corticotropin) from the anterior pituitary gland (Figure 9.12). This in turn is released in response to the secretion of corticotropin-releasing hormone from the hypothalamus. The glucocorticoids normally exert inhibition (negative feedback) on the release of both hormones, and therefore provide a high degree of control of their own secretion. The secretion rate can be modulated, however, by neurological inputs to the hypothalamus; this is how perceptions of stress can increase secretion.

Mineralocorticoids

Mineralocorticoids are steroids secreted by cells of the zona glomerulosa of the adrenal cortex (Figure 9.11). The main mineralocorticoid is aldosterone, the release of which is stimulated by sodium deficiency or by an increased plasma potassium concentration. It has an important role in the maintenance of sodium (and hence water) and potassium balance. Its actions are:

- in the kidney, to stimulate sodium reabsorption in exchange for potassium or hydrogen ions, thus conserving sodium but increasing the urinary excretion of potassium/hydrogen ions (these are the main actions of the hormone);
- in sweat and salivary glands, to promote sodium reabsorption from sweat and saliva, thus diluting them and conserving sodium ions;

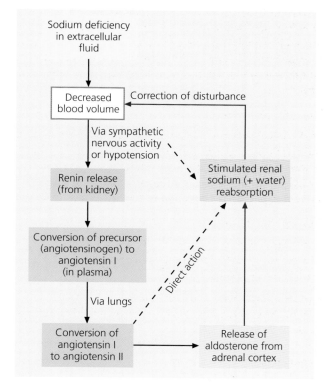

Figure 9.13 The renin–angiotensin–aldosterone axis, and its role in the regulation of sodium balance. Note that aldosterone is only one of the hormones that influences sodium regulation. Angiotensin is also involved in the regulation of arterial blood pressure (see Chapter 12)

Q How would an angiotensin-converting enzyme (ACE) inhibitor drug alter this response?

• in the gut, to stimulate sodium absorption, thus adding sodium to body fluids.

Sodium deficiency results in a reduced extracellular fluid volume (see Box 6.6, p.127); aldosterone release in these cir-

---

BOX 9.9 DYSFUNCTIONING OF THE ADRENAL CORTEX

Hyposecretion of glucocorticoids and mineralocorticoids
Deficiency of cortisol secretion produces Addison's disease. The role of cortisol is to mobilize glucose when necessary, so its deficiency when extra demands are made on the body can decrease blood glucose concentration and lead to lethargy and muscle weakness. Blood pressure may also be lower than usual as the hormone also facilitates other hormones such as adrenaline, for example when standing, so causing dizziness or fainting. Skin changes in Addison's disease, with areas of hyperpigmentation, or dark tanning of both exposed and unexposed parts of the body; this darkening of the skin is most visible on scars, skin folds, lips, pressure points such as the elbows, knees, knuckles and toes, and on mucous membranes. Intervention is by hormone replacement through administration of synthetic steroid.

Hyposecretion of aldosterone can adversely affect sodium levels, although compensatory mechanisms will often ensure that sodium homeostasis is reasonably regulated. However, aldosterone is the body's only potassium-regulating hormone, so plasma potassium concentration will be elevated (hyperkalaemia), leading to disorders of nerve and muscle functions (particularly observable as a bradycardia). Intervention is by administration of synthetic steroid.

Hypersecretion of glucocorticoids and mineralocorticoids
Excess cortisol in the blood (called Cushing's syndrome) arises from a variety of causes, including pituitary adenoma (known as Cushing's disease), adrenal hyperplasia, ectopic ACTH production (e.g. from a small cell lung cancer) or it may be secondary to other treatments (referred to as iatrogenic) such as excessive steroid use. Hypersecretion of cortisol mobilizes fatty acids, causing a redistribution of fat stores, and may produce a round face often called 'moon face'. Excessive oedema is observed, including that of the abdomen (ascites), partly because of the overlap in actions with the mineralocorticoid aldosterone (see below). Red or purple striations may be observable on the abdomen if distension is extreme. The person becomes prone to bruising, and wound healing is usually poor (glucocorticoids suppress leucocytes; this action is exploited in the treatment of inflammation and some types of leukaemia).

Excess aldosterone causes aldosteronism. Primary aldosteronism is excessive secretion of the hormone because of a disorder of the gland itself; secondary aldosteronism is excessive secretion caused by another disorder, such as renal failure (via increased generation of angiotensin). Aldosterone has an important role in the regulation of plasma potassium concentration through its action to promote potassium excretion in urine. Aldosteronism is therefore characterized by low plasma potassium concentration (hypokalaemia), leading to disorders of nerve and muscle functions (particularly observable as tachycardia). Sodium retention will also be observed through the hormone's other actions to promote sodium reabsorption on the kidneys. Aldosterone antagonists may be used to block the actions of the hormone on the kidneys.

Gonadocorticoids
Sex steroids from the cortex are secreted at a very low rate compared with those from the gonads. They are not considered to be significant in sexually mature adults, but they can be problematic when gonadal function is deficient; for example, cortical oestrogens may promote breast development in boys, while androgens may cause voice deepening, hair loss, changes in skin texture, and facial hair in women (a condition called hirsutism – see Figure 16.3, p.451). Under these circumstances, the psychological effects can be profound.

---

cumstances is mediated by increased generation of the hormone angiotensin (Figure 9.13). This peptide hormone is produced from a precursor (a protein called angiotensinogen) found in plasma, although final activation is produced by the actions of angiotensin-converting enzyme (ACE) as blood passes through the lungs. The initial conversion of angiotensinogen is induced by the enzyme renin, released from cells close to the renal glomeruli (called the juxtaglomerular cells; see Figure 15.6a, p.422) during sodium deficiency. The complex link between these hormones is referred to as the renin–angiotensin–aldosterone axis. The axis has further influences on sodium conservation, and has a role in blood pressure control (see Figure 12.29a and associated text, p.349). Reversal of the disturbance reduces the activation of angiotensin, leading to reduced aldosterone secretion.

The stimulation of aldosterone release when plasma potassium concentration is elevated is reversed when the action of the hormone to promote the urinary excretion of this ion corrects the disturbance. Although the mediation of angiotensin in releasing aldosterone when there is sodium deficiency is just one hormonal response to the situation, aldosterone is the only hormone known to have a major influence on potassium homeostasis.

Gonadocorticoids

Androgens and oestrogens are secreted by a layer of the adrenal cortex called the zona reticularis (Figure 9.11). Production by the adrenal gland is slight compared with that of the gonads, and their actions for much of adulthood are probably of little consequence. However, they do have important influences on fetal development, and on prepubertal growth during childhood (Box 9.9).

The adrenal medulla

The adrenal medulla secretes the catecholamine hormones adrenaline and noradrenaline; adrenaline is the main secretion. These hormones are produced and secreted by cells that develop from neurons in the embryo, and so are modified cells of the sympathetic nervous system, hence the overlap in their roles with that part of the nervous system.

The hormones are released when sympathetic nerves to the adrenal glands are activated. Their actions support the activities of this branch of the autonomic nervous system. Particular effects are to promote responses that facilitate physical activity (the fright/fight/flight responses – see Figure 21.6, p.598):

• cardiac function is increased, with greater force of contraction and increased pulse rate;
• selective vasoconstriction and vasodilation are induced, which helps to raise blood pressure and redistribute blood to active tissues;
• sweat production is increased, which helps to dissipate excess heat from increased metabolism;
• bronchodilation is induced, which lowers airway resistance and facilitates alveolar ventilation;
• gut motility is decreased, reducing the demands on gut muscle cells and diverting blood from the gut to active tissues;

- metabolic fuels (glucose and fatty acids) are mobilized to meet the needs of increased metabolic activity.

Sympathetic nerve stimulation is usually transient, and its activity declines once the demand for activity has passed. Hormone release will normally be reduced as a consequence.

The gonads

The testes and ovaries produce steroid (mainly) and peptide hormones. The gonadal steroids produced by males are collectively called androgens, the main one being testosterone. Testosterone is essential for determining the production of spermatozoa (spermatogenesis; see Figures 18.11, p.503, and 18.14, p.505), and is responsible for promoting their capacitation (i.e. bringing to functional capacity).

The gonadal steroids produced by females are of two types: oestrogens, the main ones being oestriol, oestradiol and oestrone, and progestins, the main one being progesterone. Oestrogens and progesterone determine and regulate the menstrual cycle and breast development (see Figures 18.15, p.507 and 18.16, p.508).

The gonads also produce the peptide inhibin, which, although poorly understood, seems to modulate steroid production and gametogenesis.

The roles of these hormones are explained in detail in Chapter 18, but it is worth noting here that the control of their

BOX 9.10 DYSFUNCTIONING OF THE ADRENAL MEDULLA

Hyposecretion

This is unlikely to have a major consequence, since sympathetic nerve activity will normally compensate. One functional disorder of note, however, is that of circulatory shock, in which both nerve activity and hormone release are ineffective, owing to either cardiac dysfunction or profound vasodilation as a consequence of hypoxia or toxins. Although this is not actually caused by hyposecretion of the hormone, it serves to illustrate the need for appropriate activity when required. Adrenaline itself may be administered, but drugs that stimulate catecholamine receptors may also be used (e.g. beta-receptor agonists to raise heart rate, or alpha-receptor agonists to induce vasoconstriction). However, the fact that sympathetic activity and hormone secretion will actually be occurring in this state means that such intervention may have limited success.

Hypersecretion

Sympathetic nerve activity and catecholamine secretion may be sustained in severe distress as a consequence of the limbic–hypothalamic modulation of autonomic nuclei in the brainstem. Such stress-related responses may have long-term costs to the individual (e.g. hypertension may develop arising from the cardiac and vascular actions; see Table 21.2, p.589). Other problems relate to disturbances of gastrointestinal functions, although these are not always easy to separate from those caused by dietary and behavioural responses to prolonged stress.

Intervention is targeted at antagonizing catecholamine receptors (e.g. using beta-blockers to reduce heart rate, or using alpha-receptor antagonists to induce vasodilation).

BOX 9.11 DYSFUNCTIONING OF GONADAL STEROID SECRETION

Hyposecretion

Deficiency of these hormones causes a failure of puberty in adolescents, or lack of fertility in adults (referred to as hypogonadism, because the gonads are underactive). In adult men, lack of testosterone produces castration syndrome, in which there is a heightening of voice tone, changes to skin and facial characteristics, a loss of libido and a 'feminizing' of behaviour as a consequence of reduced secondary sexual characteristics. Adult women may experience some of the masculinizing effects through the actions of adrenal gonadocorticoids (see earlier). Other consequences are loss of libido and changes to the cervix and breasts. The menstrual cycle will be irregular, or may even stop.

The problem may be caused by a disorder of the production of gonadal hormones, or it may reflect inadequate gonadotropin release from the anterior pituitary. In the former case, administration of sex steroid may improve the situation, while in the latter, synthetic gonadotropins may be administered to trigger sex steroid release from the gonads. Giving gonadotropin-releasing hormone to stimulate the pituitary to release gonadotropin has also been used.

Menopause

The declining secretion of oestrogens during the menopause has effects in addition to causing atrophy of the reproductive system, including vasomotor changes ('hot flushes' and sweats) associated with altered autonomic nervous system activities. Psychological effects may also be apparent. The withdrawal of ovarian steroids may facilitate expression of the actions of testosterone, which is produced in small quantities throughout life by the adrenal cortex of both sexes. This androgen can cause the growth and coarsening of facial hair, and a deepening of the voice in postmenopausal women.

In the long term, the most serious consequences for physical health are reductions in the ratio of high- to low-density lipoproteins in blood plasma (see Chapter 5, p.109), which begins to favour the deposition of cholesterol in blood vessels (possibly resulting in strokes and heart disease; see Figures 12.7c,d, p.313, and 12.13a,b, p.324), and the loss of bone matrix and mineral, leading to osteoporosis. Although such changes will be initiated in the perimenopausal period, their progress is gradual, and effects are most likely to be observed many years later. Studies indicate that hormone replacement therapy during the perimenopausal and postmenopausal years prevents, or at least reduces, these changes, although concern has been expressed regarding the possibility of promoting oestrogen-induced tumours.

The menopause appears to have no comparable process in men, but this is a debatable area, especially from the psychological perspective. Biologically, although testosterone secretion declines with age, its metabolism also declines, so plasma concentrations decline only slowly if at all. Sperm production continues well into late adulthood, although the numbers of sperm and their viability may be decreased slightly. Men whose testosterone secretion significantly diminishes may exhibit castration syndrome, a term that reflects the voice heightening and facial changes (a 'softening') that are characteristic of losing the secretion of this hormone through trauma.

Hypersecretion

Both androgens and oestrogens influence cognition and behaviour. In men, excess testosterone is thought to promote aggressive behaviours. In women, excess oestrogens and progesterone may cause irregular menstrual cycles with particularly heavy blood loss. Behavioural changes may also be observed. The long-term health risks of excess oestrogens are the potential for cardiac damage and development of cancerous tumours of the breast and cervix. Long-acting drugs that suppress the release of luteinizing hormone have also been found to be useful to treat endometriosis (growth of endometrial tissue outside the uterus) by suppressing development of the corpus luteum and so preventing progesterone release.

release is via gonadotropins from the anterior pituitary: follicle-stimulating hormone (FSH) and luteinizing hormone (LH). These peptide hormones are named after their effects in females, but are they are chemically identical in both sexes. They are released in response to the presence of gonadotropin-releasing hormones (GnRH) produced by the hypothalamus. Regulation is exerted by negative feedback effects of the gonadal steroids on both the hypothalamus and pituitary (see Figures 18.15, p.507 and 18.16, p.508).

The gut and pancreas
The gut

The gut produces a wide variety of hormones that mediate digestive functions (see Table 10.4, p.240). These are peptides, the main ones being:

- gastrin, produced by cells lining part of the stomach;
- secretin, produced by cells lining the duodenum;
- cholecystokinin–pancreozymin (CCK–PZ), produced by cells lining the duodenum.

Gastrin

Gastrin secretion is stimulated by the presence of food in the pyloric region of the stomach (see Figure 10.9a, p.242). It has a role in gastric acid secretion. Gastrin also stimulates gastric motility, and the muscular contractions mix the chyme and empty the gastric contents into the duodenum. However, its release is inhibited if the acidity of the chyme becomes intense, since this fall in pH acts as the negative feedback signal on the hormone-secreting cells.

Secretin

Secretin was the first hormone to be identified (the term 'hormone' was coined after its discovery). It is secreted by mucosal cells lining the duodenum in response to the presence of acidic chyme (i.e. when chyme has entered the duodenum from the stomach; see Figure 10.9, p.245). The hormone acts to neutralize and then alkalinize the chyme by stimulating the secretion of a bicarbonate-rich fluid from the pancreas. The alkalinity is essential for the action of digestive enzymes in the duodenum. As the acidity falls, the release of secretin declines.

Cholecystokinin-pancreozymin

This hormone's name is a clumsy combination of what was once thought to be two distinctive hormones – cholecystokinin (CCK) and pancreozymin (PZ) – that were discovered independently. The two names relate to the dual actions of the hormone. It is released from mucosal cells lining the duodenum in response to the presence of chyme (see Figure 10.10, p.245). The stimuli seem to be the major foodstuffs of the chyme (i.e. carbohydrates, fats and semi-digested proteins). The hormone then promotes the secretion of digestive enzymes by the pancreas (hence the 'pancreozymin' component of the name). It also has other actions in relation to fat digestion: it promotes the release of bile from the gall bladder, and so facilitates emulsification of fats, and it reduces gastric emptying, and so increases the time that chyme remains in the duodenum ('cholecystic gland' is an old term for the gall bladder, hence the cholecystokinin component of the name).

Table 9.2 Factors influencing the release of insulin and glucagon

Excitatory influences	Homeostatic relevance	Inhibitory influences	Homeostatic relevance
Insulin			
Direct influence of elevated blood glucose concentration	Increased glucose utilization after food intake Promotes glycogenesis	Blood glucose deficit	Reduction of glycogenesis, leaving more glucose available for cellular respiration
Increased parasympathetic nervous activity from hypothalamus to pancreatic beta-cells (in response to elevated blood glucose)	Increased glucose utilization after food intake Promotes glycogenesis	Increased sympathetic nervous activity from hypothalamus to pancreatic beta-cells (in response to stress or exercise)	Reduction of glycogenesis, leaving more glucose available for cellular respiration
Duodenal hormones (e.g. CCK–PZ) in response to glucose present in digestive chyme	Feed-forward release of insulin in preparation for glucose load from gut	Somatostatin (released by direct stimulation of pancreatic delta-cells by insulin)	Fine control of insulin release in presence of stimulatory factors
Glucagon			
Direct influence of blood glucose deficit	Promotion of glycogenolysis and gluconeogenesis to provide glucose for cellular respiration	Direct influence of elevated blood glucose concentration	Decreased glycogenolysis/ gluconeogenesis Increased glucose utilization (via promotion of insulin release)
Increased parasympathetic nervous activity from hypothalamus to pancreatic alpha-cells (in response to blood glucose deficit)	Promotion of glycogenolysis and gluconeogenesis to provide glucose for cellular respiration	Somatostatin (released by direct stimulus of pancreatic delta-cells by glucagon)	Fine control of glucagon release in presence of stimulatory influences

CCK–PZ, cholecystokinin–ancreozymin.

ACTIVITY

The complementary actions of secretin and cholecys-tokinin–pancreozymin (CCK–PZ) on pancreatic secretions are a good example of the level of coordination that can be introduced by hormones. The digestive enzymes released from the pancreas in response to CCK–PZ operate most effectively in an alkaline environment, which is induced by the actions of secretin. Refer to Chapter 10, pp.245–6 and review the enzymes released by the pancreas during digestion. Note how their actions relate to the digestion of carbohydrates, fats and polypeptides, the very substances that stimulate the release of secretin and CCK–PZ.

Other gut hormones

The gut also produces a host of putative hormones; these are substances that seem to have an effect on the organs but have yet to be researched to the extent required for their recognition as hormones. One such substance is a peptide called motilin, which some authorities do consider to have hormone status. Motilin is secreted by cells lining the ileum. It appears to have a role in coordinating the pattern of motility (i.e. contractions) of the ileum as it changes from that observed between meals to a pattern associated with standing waves and peristalsis when chyme is present.

Another example is gastric insulinotropic peptide (GIP), released in response to the presence of monosaccharides in the digestive chyme. Its name reflects the main documented action to act as a tropin and stimulate the release of insulin. This is seen as being anticipatory of a glucose load entering the circulatory system (see below). Its alternative name, gastric inhibitory peptide (GIP), reflects its other action to reduce gastric emptying.

The pancreas

The endocrine tissue of the pancreas is found as discrete clusters of cells, called the islets of Langerhans. These gland cells produce peptide hormones (Table 9.2):

- *insulin*: produced by the beta-cells (β-cells) of the islets;
- *glucagon*: produced by the alpha-cells (α-cells) of the islets;
- *somatostatin*: produced by the delta-cells (δ-cells) of the islets.

Insulin

Insulin release is promoted when blood glucose concentration is elevated beyond its homeostatic range. Insulin acts to stimulate the uptake and utilization of glucose by the liver, skeletal muscle cells and adipocytes. Energy is released by cellular respiration, and glycogen synthesis is promoted to replenish carbohydrate stores. The conversion of glucose into certain amino acids and glycerol promotes further storage of metabolic fuel. Insulin release decreases again as plasma glucose concentration declines. Insulin is the only known hypoglycaemic hormone (i.e. hormone that reduces blood glucose concentration).

Glucagon

In contrast, glucagon release is stimulated by a decrease in the glucose concentration of plasma below its homeostatic range. Its actions are the opposite of those of insulin (i.e. it is a hyperglycaemic agent), promoting the mobilization of glucose via the breakdown of glycogen and the synthesis of glucose from glycerol and amino acids. Glucagon release declines as the plasma glucose concentration increases.

Somatostatin

Somatostatin release is stimulated by the presence of glucagon or insulin in the blood. It seems to act locally in the pancreas as a paracrine secretion, and inhibits the release of the other two hormones when blood glucose is within its normal range (i.e. normoglycaemia) thus preventing excessive secretion. Control of the release of glucagon and insulin is also provided by their actions to promote the other's release (their antagonistic actions will help to prevent excess responses to either).

The thymus

The thymus is a lymphoid gland found in the neck (see Figure 13.4b, p.367). It has an important role in the differentiation of

---

BOX 9.12 DYSFUNCTIONING OF THE PANCREATIC ISLETS

Hyposecretion

Diabetes mellitus is observed when there is a problem with the hormone insulin (see the case study of a child with insulin-dependent diabetes Type 1, Section VI, p.634). The effects are to increase blood glucose concentration (hyperglycaemia), leading to excretion of glucose in the urine (glycosuria) and dehydration. Urinary tract infections may also be observed. Medium- to long-term hyperglycaemia has the potential to damage the eye (retinopathy), the nervous system (neuropathy) and the renal system (renopathy) as a consequence of the direct effects of glucose on tissues and the shift towards fat metabolism that is also observed in this condition. Unstable regulation of blood glucose concentration can also result in episodes of hypoglycaemia, which has behaviour-inducing consequences (frequently aggression), and may induce poor coordination, confusion and even coma as a consequence of poor delivery of glucose to brain cells.

The condition is subdivided into the form in which the individual is incapable of producing the hormone (insulin-dependent diabetes mellitus, IDDM) and the form in which the individual exhibits poor release of the hormone and/or poor tissue responses to it (non-insulin-dependent diabetes mellitus, NIDDM). The former typically occurs in children or adolescents, and the latter during adulthood. (IDDM is sometimes still referred to by the earlier names, Type 1, early-onset or juvenile diabetes; NIDDM may be referred to as Type 2 or late-onset diabetes).

Care for IDDM patients revolves around a need to take insulin as a hormone replacement, and paying particular attention to dietary habits and foods eaten, especially in relation to the timing of insulin administration. The intention is to provide extrinsic control of blood glucose concentration, preventing excessive hyperglycaemia or hypoglycaemia.

Care for NIDDM patients has similar objectives and will also involve dietary advice. However, this form of diabetes may also be treated pharmacologically, depending upon the actual problem. For example, a drug such as tolbutamide may be used to stimulate the pancreas to release its insulin or a metabolic stimulant drug such as metformin may be used to promote metabolism of glucose.

T-lymphocytes as precursor cells from bone marrow pass through the gland. Differentiation is not completely understood, but it is promoted by the peptide hormones thymin, thymosin and thymopoietin, which are released within the thymus. They appear to have similar actions but the mechanism of their control is unknown.

The thymus gland involutes and begins to atrophy early in adulthood, by which time the secondary lymphoid tissues will have a full complement of the T-cells necessary for immunity. This suggests that the hormones perform most of their roles relatively early in life.

The pineal gland

The pineal gland is an outgrowth of neural tissue situated in the roof of the third cerebral ventricle, deep within the brain. Its main secretion is the peptide melatonin. Documented actions of this hormone include the induction of sleep, but it has also been shown to prevent ovulation via an inhibition of the release of GnRH from the hypothalamus (therefore, overproduction of melatonin can delay puberty). Links with the human menstrual cycle have not been established, however. There is some evidence that melatonin influences the secretion of other pituitary hormones, and the rich innervation of the pineal gland by sympathetic neurons would seem to suggest further roles.

One documented role is that of a mediator of the sleep–wake circadian rhythm. The gland receives impulses from the eyes (see Figure 22.6a, p.615), and is postulated to be involved in the light–dark synchronization of the rhythmicity observed for some physiological parameters, presumably via its neural links with the hypothalamus. The role of the hormone in promoting sleep is entirely in keeping with this further role in determining circadian rhythms. The gland calcifies during adulthood, and its activities are thought to become less efficient, thus making circadian rhythms less effective in elderly people.

The gland is also of interest for historical reasons. Its central position in the brain and its unclear functions led to it for many years being postulated to be the 'spiritual' centre of the brain, conveying conscience as a human faculty. There is no evidence for this, although it could also be argued that 'conscience' is an indeterminate faculty.

The placenta

This gland is obviously only functional in pregnant women. The placenta is often considered in its role in providing nutrients, oxygen and other metabolites to the developing fetus, but it also has important endocrine functions. The placenta produces large amounts of oestrogens and progesterone throughout the pregnancy, which help the mother to maintain her pregnancy, promote changes in the mother's physiology that will support fetal development, facilitate breast development, and help to prepare the reproductive tract for the birth process. Oestrogen production by the fetal adrenal gland is also an important source of the hormones. Other placental hormones are:

> ### BOX 9.13 HORMONAL CONTROL OF BREAST DEVELOPMENT IN PREGNANCY, AND LACTATION
>
> Breast development and lactation provide illustrations of altered set points in homeostasis, induced by hormone release that is linked to the need for the development of specific tissues and functions.
>
> **Breast development**
> In this case, we see the roles of increased production of gonadal steroids (although in pregnancy these are released mostly from the placenta), and their interaction with placental lactogen. Progesterone from the placenta promotes the growth of breast alveoli (i.e. the glandular tissue that secretes milk). Oestrogens from the placenta stimulate growth of lactiferous ducts that will transport milk to the nipple. Placental lactogen has a permissive role (i.e. the actions of oestrogen and progesterone on the breast will be effective only in the presence of this hormone). Placental lactogen also inhibits the release of prolactin from the pituitary gland. This hormone has a central role in lactation (see below), and its inhibition by placental lactogen during pregnancy prevents milk secretion from the developing alveoli.
>
> **Lactation**
> Lactation is the process of milk secretion. It is clearly most effective if milk is secreted according to need (i.e. when a baby is suckling). Suckling promotes a number of hormonal responses (see Figure 18.10c, p.499):
>
> - Prolactin release from the pituitary gland is stimulated via neural input to the hypothalamus (remember that the release of hormones from the anterior pituitary gland involves releasing or inhibitory hormones from the hypothalamus). Prolactin causes secretion of milk by the alveoli of the breast.
> - Neural inputs to the hypothalamus also promote the release of oxytocin from the pituitary gland. This hormone contracts the lactiferous ducts and so enables milk to be conveyed to the surface. Oxytocin release stimulated by suckling may also help to contract down the uterus after birth (remember that oxytocin is a vital hormone in labour).
> - Neural inputs to the hypothalamus also cause the pituitary to release less gonadotropin, which then reduces oestrogen release from the ovarian follicles. This may be a mechanism to reduce the likelihood of another pregnancy while the infant is dependent upon the mother, but it is not unfailingly effective.

- *(Human) chorionic gonadotropin (hCG)*: a hormone produced by the early placenta that helps to maintain oestrogen and progesterone production by the corpus luteum within the mother's ovary until the placenta is sufficiently developed in this respect (i.e. hCG peaks at about 3 months postfertilization). The hormone continues to be produced by the placenta for the duration of the pregnancy, albeit at a lower rate than in the first few weeks, but its role in the pregnancy is unclear. The term 'chorionic' indicates that the source of the hormone is from embryonic cells within the placenta (the chorion is one of the extra-embryonic membranes; see Figure 19.8, p.532).
- *Placental lactogen (also called chorionic somatomammotropin)*: involved in breast development during pregnancy (Box 9.13). It is also a metabolic hormone, and alters maternal glucose and fat metabolism. Its release increases during

pregnancy, and it is used clinically as an index of placental function. Again, the term 'chorionic' is of note – the hormone derives from embryonic cells within the placenta.

- *Relaxin*: a hormone that relaxes the symphysis pubis joint in the mother's pelvis, and promotes dilation of the cervix during birth.

These secretions emphasize how maternal physiology is influenced by the placenta, the cells of which are derived partly from the fetus. (Who is controlling whom?) It may be the mother who is supporting the fetus, but fetal secretions are instrumental in ensuring that this occurs. In endocrine terms, the placenta is often referred to as a fetoplacental unit, a name that recognizes that the fetus makes a contribution to the hormonal secretion.

Other hormones

Various other hormonal secretions have been identified, secreted by cells that do not form identifiable glands, but are endocrine nonetheless. Their numbers continue to grow. In addition to those substances now accepted as hormones, a host of others are putative ones. A comprehensive list of all these secretions is not possible, but some of those recognized as hormones are discussed here.

- *Atrial natriuretic factor (ANF)*: a peptide hormone (hence sometimes abbreviated as ANP which stands for atrial natriuretic peptide) that originates from cells lining the atria of the heart and in particular the right atrium. The hormone is named because of its action to increase urinary sodium excretion, but ANF also has an important role in promoting vasodilation, particularly of veins. The hormone is released when an increase in blood volume stretches the atrial wall. Although this could occur transiently, for example when the venous return is increased during exercise, the main role of the hormone is probably in the longer-term regulation of blood volume. Its vasodilatory actions on veins help the circulatory system to accommodate any increase in volume (and therefore avoid arterial hypertension), while the renal actions help to reduce blood volume (by excreting sodium chloride and water; see Chapter 12, p.348).

- *Prostaglandins*: are local eicosanoid hormones; they were named after they were first identified as secretions in seminal fluid from prostate glands. They are produced by most, if not all, body tissues and probably only influence cells in the vicinity of their secretion (i.e. they are paracrine secretions). There are various kinds of prostaglandin, E_2, $F_{2\alpha}$ and PGI_2 being the main ones, and their roles vary with the tissue. For example, prostaglandins help to maintain blood flow to tissues such as the stomach; they influence ion transport mechanisms in the kidney; they contract the cervix after coitus, and the uterus during birth; and they produce pain and inflammation when tissues are damaged (see Chapter 20, p.562). They act either directly or by modulating the actions of other hormones. Thromboxanes are another group of eicosanoids that also act locally; for example, they are part of the clotting factor secretion produced by blood platelets. Leukotrienes are also eicosanoids. One documented action of these is in promoting contraction of bronchial smooth muscle during asthma.

- *Erythropoietin*: a peptide hormone produced by conversion of a precursor (erythropoietinogen) in plasma by the enzyme erythrogenin, which is released from the kidney when blood perfusing the organ is deficient in oxygen. The hormone promotes production of red blood cells (a process called erythropoiesis, hence the hormone name) by bone marrow (see Figure 11.3, p.273).

- *Endothelium-derived relaxing factor (EDRF)*: a substance produced by capillary endothelial cells. It has an important role in the intrinsic regulation of vascular resistance in tissues. Its actions are to stimulate the production of nitrous oxide by the cells, which in turn causes vasodilation.

- *Vitamin D*: it may seem odd to include a vitamin in a chapter on hormones, but many authorities now recognize it as one. Vitamin D, also called cholecalciferol, is obtained either from the diet or from the conversion of a steroid precursor in the skin through the actions of sunlight. However, this must then be converted to an intermediary in the liver, and then into the active form (1,25-dihydroxycalciferol) in the kidneys. In this form, it promotes the uptake of calcium from the intestine. It is the intrinsic production in the skin of a precursor and the conversion to the active form that is observed when calcium concentrations are beginning to decrease which have promoted the view that it is a hormone.

- *Leptin*: a peptide secreted by adipose tissue when adipose cells increase their fat content. It crosses the blood–brain barrier, and acts on centres within the hypothalamus to promote satiety, and to cause a decrease in food intake. Leptins were only discovered during the 1990s, but they have attracted a tremendous amount of interest, not least because they are considered to be one of the regulators of body weight, a homeostatic mechanism that had been very poorly understood.

A host of peptide growth factors have also been identified; for example, epidermal growth factor has a role in regulating cell division by mitosis (not necessarily confined to the epidermis). Neurogenic (or nerve growth) factor has a role in nerve axon growth in the embryo/fetus and infant, and if there is nerve damage. These peptides probably have localized actions, and so are paracrine or autocrine secretions. Although the actions of these and other 'tissue' hormones have been documented, the control of their secretions is generally poorly understood.

SUMMARY

1 Hormones are chemical messengers that provide a means of communication between tissues in different parts of the body, and therefore are part of the coordinating mechanisms of the body.

2 The process of hormone synthesis/release, transportation in extracellular fluid, and interaction with target cells means that responses are slower than those of nerve stimulation, so hormones are generally not involved in responses that must occur rapidly (i.e. within seconds).

3 Hormones are secreted by glands, although not all glandular secretions can be considered to be hormones. Hormone-secreting glands are generally referred to as endocrine glands.

4 Hormones are either peptides, catecholamines (modified amino acids), steroids (modified lipids) or eicosanoids (modified fatty acids). Their diverse actions help to regulate the range of physiological parameters vital for health.

5 Hormones produce a large response by target cells because the cell activation is amplified through the cascade effect of second messenger activation (hormones are the first messenger chemicals).

6 Many hormones are tropins (i.e. they promote the release of further hormones from target gland tissue). Others are released in response to non-hormonal stimuli, and promote a change in those parameters.

7 Hormone release is usually controlled by negative feedback mechanisms. Some glands utilize short-loop control, others long-loop.

8 This chapter identifies over 40 important hormones and the glands that produce them. The stimuli that release them are largely identified, as are the feedback processes (where applicable) that control their secretion.

9 Disorders of hormone function arise from a failure to control hormonal secretion, or from a lack of response of target tissues to the hormone after it is released. Clinical intervention is directed at correcting the secretory defect, replacing the hormone (if it is deficient in blood), preventing/promoting hormone action with appropriate antagonistic/agonistic drugs, or stimulating tissue function by other pharmacological means.

FURTHER READING

Most generic texts on human functioning will include discussion of hormones. Alternatively, a specialist text might be consulted that extends the discussion, e.g.:

Warren, E. (2006) Hypothyroidism. *Practice Nurse* **31**(1): 28–32.

CHAPTER 10

THE DIGESTIVE SYSTEM

INTRODUCTION: RELATION OF THE DIGESTIVE SYSTEM TO CELLULAR HOMEOSTASIS

The digestive system aids intracellular homeostasis by helping to ensure that cells are provided with the 'normal' requirements of molecules necessary to maintain cellular structural and functional components. The importance of a balanced diet was discussed in Chapter 5, which emphasized that the food we consume consists of a diversity of molecules. The bulk of the diet is provided by three main classes of food: carbohydrates, lipids and proteins. These are usually consumed as large, insoluble molecular complexes, and must be reduced in size and made soluble before they can be absorbed into blood, transported to their site of action, and used in cellular metabolism for production of enzymes to enable growth, repair of component parts, production of energy, etc.

The breaking down and increase in solubility of ingested food is called digestion. In addition to the three main classes of food, dietary constituents must also include water, vitamins, minerals and nucleic acids. These substances are already soluble, and are small enough to be absorbed into blood, hence their digestion is unnecessary.

This chapter is concerned with how food intake is regulated, the process of digestion, and the role of the liver in determining the fate of the majority of these endproducts of digestion.

REGULATION OF FOOD INTAKE

Many areas of the brain have been identified as having a role in feeding and satiety. The most important area is the hypothalamus, which has two centres involved in the regulation of food intake: the hunger (or feeding) centre, and the satiety (or cessation of feeding) centre.

The hunger centre is constantly active, unless it is inhibited by input from the satiety centre. There are many theories as to the regulatory factors associated with food intake but it is outside the scope of this book to discuss these theories in detail. However, it is sufficient to say that low levels of glucose and amino acids have been put forward as stimulants to the hunger centre and, conversely, it is said that high levels of these substances act as stimulants to the satiety centre. Some hormones (e.g. noradrenaline, cholecystokinin and glucagon) in the blood are thought to act on the hypothalamus to decrease appetite and increase energy expenditure, while other hormones (e.g. adrenaline, growth hormone releasing factor, glucocorticoids, insulin, somatostatin and progesterone) in the blood act on the hypothalamus to increase appetite and decrease energy expenditure. Psychological factors are also an important consideration, since they can override the usual intake mechanisms; this occurs in obesity, anorexia nervosa and bulimia. The body temperature theory attempts to explain why it is that we tend to eat more in winter, linking this with the colder environmental temperatures that result in a lowering of the body temperature and a stimulation of the hunger centre. The reverse reasoning is given to explain why we tend to eat less in hot summer months. This may partly explain why we tend to gain a little weight in the winter months, but it must be remembered that many other contributory factors are also important. Finally, the gastrointestinal stretch receptor theory has received most recognition in controlling food intake and the cessation of intake (Figure 10.1). This suggests that distension of the stomach and duodenum by the presence of food stimulate stretch receptors in these organs above their 'normal' or baseline firing range. These receptors send sensory impulses to the hypothalamic satiety centre, which in turn inhibits hunger centre activity, bringing about cessation of food intake. Conversely, if the degree of stretching falls below the baseline firing rate, then the sensory information is not sufficient to stimulate the satiety centre output. Thus, the inhibition to the hunger centre is removed, with the result that feeding is promoted.

Currently, there is considerable evidence now for a role of adipose tissue (via the hormone leptin) as a regulator of or

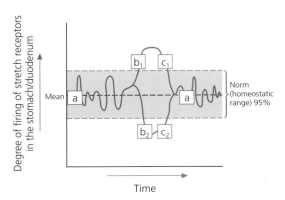

Figure 10.1 The regulation of food intake. (a) 'Normal' level of firing of stretch receptors. Stimulus is not enough to stimulate satiety centre and the hunger centre. b_1, Increased rate of firing of stretch receptors above their baseline level, resulting in sensory input to the satiety centre. This centre inhibits the hunger centre's output, and so causes the cessation of food intake. b_2, Decreased rate of firing of stretch receptors below their baseline level, resulting in a decrease in sensory fibre input to the satiety centre (i.e. insufficient to stimulate it), thus stimulating the hunger centre activity, causing the individual to seek food. c, Restoration of 'normal' stretch receptor activity by appropriate changes in satiety (c_1) and hunger (c_2) centre activity. (a, represents boxes a_1–a_4 in Figure 1.7, p.11, reflecting the individual variability in the homeostatic range)

Q List the theories that attempt to explain the control of food intake.

contributor to regulation of food intake; for further details please see the case study on obesity, Section VI, p.636.

OVERVIEW OF THE ANATOMY AND PHYSIOLOGY OF THE DIGESTIVE SYSTEM

The anatomy and physiology of the human digestive system evolved to convert consumed food into a form that could be used by the cells. The conversion can be divided into five principal physiological processes:

1 *Ingestion (eating)*: the process of taking food into the mouth.
2 *Digestion*: the breakdown of food to render it suitable for absorption.
3 *Absorption*: the passage of the endproducts of digestion from the digestive tract into the transporting (cardiovascular and lymphatic) systems, which distribute these metabolites to the cells that require them.
4 *Assimilation*: the liver's role in maintaining the blood homeostatic level of these metabolites, which is necessary for optimal cellular metabolism.
5 *Defecation (egestion)*: the elimination of indigestible substances, such as fibre, certain excretory products (e.g. bile salts and bile pigments) and unabsorbed substances (e.g. some water and electrolytes) from the body.

The digestive system, as shown in Figure 10.2, is adapted to perform these functions. Thus, regional anatomical differentiation can be identified that facilitates the performance of specialized functions. In particular:

* the structure of the mouth is suited to the chewing and moisturizing of food, and swallowing;

* the stomach provides a large, distensible region for holding food, 'sterilizing' food, and the commencement of protein digestion;
* the small intestine continues the digestive process, and is supported by the release of bile and enzymes from the pancreas. Distal parts of the small intestine are concerned particularly with the absorption of food products;
* the large intestine also exhibits limited absorptive activities. Its main role is to consolidate undigested remains into semi-solid faecal masses. A number of bacteria present within the large intestine also contribute to the digestive process by promoting further breakdown of undigested material;
* the liver assimilates many of the products.

The organs of the digestive system can be divided into two groups (Table 10.1): the main organs of the alimentary or gastrointestinal tract (e.g. the stomach and intestines) and the accessory digestive organs (e.g. the pancreas and liver).

Table 10.1 The main organs and accessory organs of the digestive system

Main organs	Accessory organs
Mouth	Lips, teeth, tongue, salivary glands, palate
Pharynx	
Oesophagus	
Stomach	
Small intestine	Pancreas, gall bladder, liver
Large intestine	

The alimentary tract is a continuous tube about 10 m long extending from the mouth to the anus. The accessory organs (e.g. saliva glands, pancreas, gall bladder and liver) associated with the production and release of digestive secretions are positioned outside the digestive tract. The glandular part of the lining epithelium also produces secretions, which are transported along channels called ducts to their sites of action. Most secretions (except for bile) contain enzymes, which accelerate the process of chemical digestion. For the chemical process to operate efficiently, however, physical churning and softening of foodstuffs must also occur. The processes of both physical and chemical digestion can be identified throughout the tract.

The major regions of the gastrointestinal tract are separated from one another by circular rings of involuntary muscle called sphincters, or by a valve-like structure. The pyloric sphincter, for example, separates the stomach from the small intestine, and the ileocaecal valve separates the terminal region of the small intestine from the first part of the large intestine. The functional significance of these structures is to aid movement of food in one direction along the tract, and to provide a means of control over that movement.

Exposure to pathogens is a potential problem, because the openings of the digestive tract are in contact with the external environment. Lymphatic nodes ('patches') throughout the tract help to remove infectious agents (see Figure 13.4a, p.367). Furthermore, the marked pH changes observed throughout the tract provide another external defence mechanism against potential pathogenic invaders. However, if the

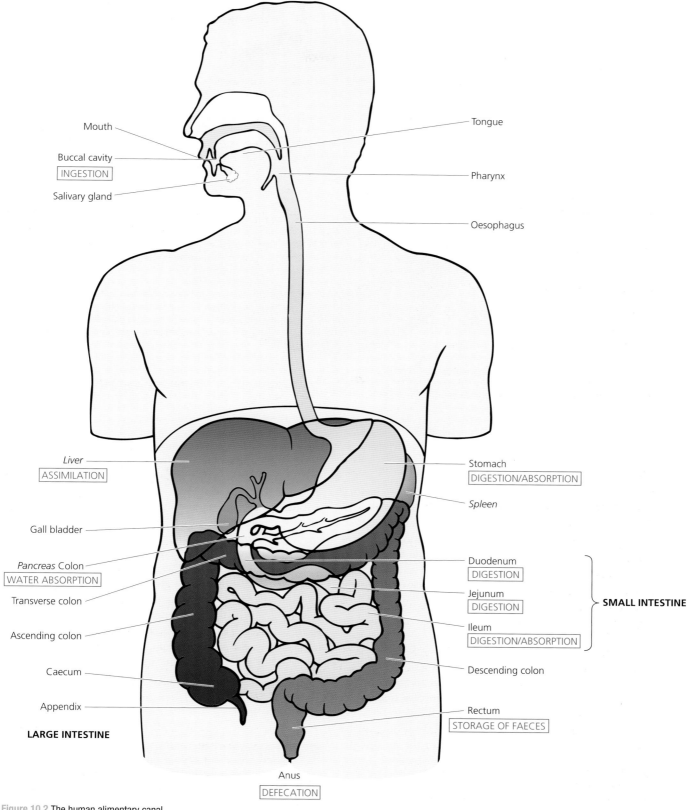

Mouth

Buccal cavity
INGESTION

Salivary gland

Tongue

Pharynx

Oesophagus

Liver
ASSIMILATION

Gall bladder

Pancreas Colon
WATER ABSORPTION

Transverse colon

Ascending colon

Caecum

Appendix

LARGE INTESTINE

Stomach
DIGESTION/ABSORPTION

Spleen

Duodenum
DIGESTION

Jejunum
DIGESTION

Ileum
DIGESTION/ABSORPTION

Descending colon

Rectum
STORAGE OF FAECES

SMALL INTESTINE

Anus
DEFECATION

Figure 10.2 The human alimentary canal

Q *Identify the food, which are digested in (1) the stomach and (2) the small intestine.*

Q *Identify the substances, which are absorbed from (1) the stomach, (2) the ileum and (3) the colon.*

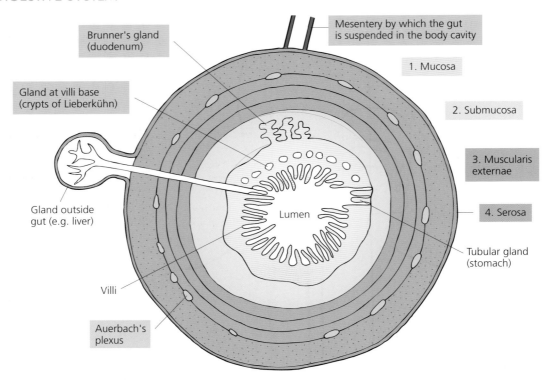

Figure 10.3 Generalized diagram of the structure of the human gut

Q Using boxes 10.16, p.249 and 10.25, p.259, identify a gastrointestinal investigation associated with each main region of the gastrointestinal tract.

invaders survive these mechanisms and gain entry into the blood, then our internal defence mechanisms are activated in an attempt to destroy these organisms.

The remainder of this chapter discusses the individual regions, their associated physical and chemical digestive processes, and the regional homeostatic imbalances (pathologies) and developmental issues regarding this organ system. First, though, it is important that you become familiar with the types of cells and membranes found in the alimentary canal; reference to Figures 2.24–2.26, pp.52–5 may be useful while you are reading this section.

GENERAL HISTOLOGY OF THE GASTROINTESTINAL TRACT

The basic structure of the gastrointestinal tract follows the same pattern from mouth to anus, with some functional adaptations throughout. Figure 10.3 illustrates the generalized histological appearance of the gastrointestinal tact. The tract has four principal layers or coats called tunicae: the mucosa, the submucosa, the muscularis externa and the serosa.

The mucosa

The mucosa is a mucous membrane that forms the innermost lining of the tract. The function of mucous is to lubricate the food to ease its passage. The membrane comprises two layers. The inner glandular epithelial membrane is the layer exposed to

the lumen and thus the contents of the digestive tract. It is glandular simple epithelium (throughout most of the tract), hence it is adapted for secreting watery digestive juices. Most of the digestive glands develop from this inner membrane. It is also involved in absorption, and therefore has adaptations for this process in appropriate areas. The oesophagus (food tube) and anal canal require the additional protection of a stratified (layered) epithelium, as they are exposed too much wear and tear.

The outer membrane, or lamina propria, is a loose connective tissue that supports the glandular epithelium. It accommodates digestive glands, and blood and lymph vessels, providing nutritive and defence functions to the glandular epithelial layer. The propria is attached to a layer of smooth muscle called the muscularis mucosa. This muscle's fibres are subjected to a sustained tonic state of contraction, and are responsible for the folded appearance of the digestive and absorptive surfaces.

BOX 10.1 MUCOUS MEMBRANE ULCERS

The mucous membranes normally have a shiny red appearance. However, a common problem with people who are frequently distressed, or who have a poor state of health, is the presence of small, greyish-white mouth ulcers. (See also Box 10.11.) These are often painful, and as a result may interfere with eating. Local mild antiseptics (e.g. the liquid antiseptic TCP) usually aid healing.

The submucosa

The submucosa contains blood vessels and nerves. The layer also contains a large amount of collagen and elastic fibres. It functions to control the tract's secretory activities, and to bind the mucosa to the third coat, the muscularis externa.

The muscularis externa

In most regions, the muscularis externa consists of an outer sheet of longitudinally arranged involuntary (smooth) muscle fibres and an inner sheet of circularly arranged involuntary muscle fibres. A meshwork of nerves, called Auerbach's (or myenteric) plexus, lies between these sheets of muscle fibres, and is responsible for coordinating their activity. Contraction of these fibres generates the specialized movements of the gastrointestinal tract that move food along the tract, aid the mixing of its contents, and therefore facilitate the digestive process.

The serosa

The serosa is part of a serous membrane called the peritoneum. The serosa of the gut is known as the visceral peritoneum, as it is attached to the surface of the digestive organs. Its counterpart, the parietal peritoneum (not a part of the gut serosa), lines the wall of the abdominal cavity. The fluid-filled space between these serous membranes, called the peritoneal cavity, provides a protective cushioning of the gut during digestion and upon changes in intra-abdominal pressure associated with breathing movements. An extension of the peritoneum forms the mesenteries of the gut. These are outward folds of the serous coat of the small intestine that bind this organ to the posterior abdominal wall. The mesenteries accommodate the blood vessels, lymphatics and neurons that supply this region.

> **ACTIVITY**
>
> Using p.58 in Chapter 2, reflect on your understanding of the anatomy and function of serous membranes.

The regional adaptations of the membranes in the gut are summarized in Table 10.2.

PHYSIOLOGY OF THE DIGESTIVE SYSTEM

Digestion is all those processes involved in breaking down consumable large, complex, insoluble molecules to simple, soluble molecules (known as food!), so that these substances can be absorbed readily into the blood for transport to the cells that utilize them. There are two processes involved in this breakdown:

1 *Physical digestion*: this involves a variety of structural components of the digestive tract, which mechanically reduce the size of the ingested food particle (Figure 10.4a) and moisten

Table 10.2 Regional features of the alimentary canal

Oesophagus

Folded mucosa
Stratified squamous epithelia
Thick muscularis mucosa
Some glands are present
Absence of serosa
Thickest muscularis externa; upper third is voluntary, the mid-third is a mixture of voluntary and involuntary, and the latter third is involuntary
Papillae project into the epithelium

Small intestine

Duodenum
  An abundance of villi compared with jejunum and ileum; villi are short and leaf-shaped
  Goblet cells
  Intestinal folds – plicae
  Brunner's glands
  Crypts of Lieberkühn

Jejunum
  As for duodenum except taller plicae, and villi are tongue-shaped

Ileum
  As for duodenum except fewer plicae, and finger-shaped villi
  Aggregates of lymph nodules – Peyer's patches

Stomach

Large mucosal folds – rugae
Thick muscular wall
Numerous gastric pits
An abundance of exocrine glands in the lamina propria
Parietal cells in the fundus
Oblique layer in the muscularis externae

Large intestine

Appendix
  Lymphatic tissue, with lymphocytes between the crypts
  Narrow lumen

Colon
  No villi
  Long tubular glands
  Few goblet cells
  Thin muscularis externa consisting of three muscular bands – taeniae (giving this region a pouched appearance)
  Large lumen
  Peyer patches project into submucosa

Rectum
  As for colon, except no taeniae, and thick muscularis externa
  Stratified epthelium near the retroanal junction
  Longest glands

Q Why are the epithelia of the oesophagus and colon stratified (i.e. layered)?

Q Why is the muscularis externa of the rectum thick?

BOX 10.2 EMBRYOLOGICAL FORMATION OF THE GUT

The embryo cells flatten during the fourth week of development, and become folded to form an enclosed tube. The lumen of the tube lined with epithelium will form the gut. The epithelium is derived from embryonic endoderm, with the exception of the epithelia lining the anal canal and parts of the mouth cavity, which is of ectodermal origin. The wall layers beyond the endoderm lining are formed from embryonic mesoderm (see Figure 19.5, p.525). Suckling movements are apparent from the twenty-fourth week of gestation, and the fetus takes in a substantial amount of amniotic fluid during the gestational period. The digestive glands along the wall of the digestive tube are formed from endoderm.

The primitive gut is divided into foregut, midgut and hindgut. The foregut comprises the pharynx, oesophagus, stomach and duodenum, and, as far as where the bile and pancreatic ducts drain into the gut, the pancreas and liver. The midgut develops and continues from the duodenum to the jejunum, ileum, caecum and appendix, and up to the transverse colon. The hindgut develops into the remainder of the colon, the rectum and the proximal anal canal. Before birth the gut fills with meconium, which contains digestive secretions.

Developmental abnormalities can occur during the gestation period (see Figure 19.4, p.526); for example, regions of the digestive tube may become stenosed, as in pyloric stenosis (see Box 10.10, p.243).

---

it. The function of physical digestion is to increase the surface area of the food particles to aid chemical digestion.

2 *Chemical digestion*: this involves the breakdown of chemical bonds within molecules too large to be absorbed directly into the blood. Enzymes accelerate (catalyse) this breakdown by promoting hydrolysis of the molecules. Hydrolysis is the chemical breakdown using water, whereby a hydrogen (H) group from the water molecule is added to one of the products of this breakdown, and a hydroxyl (OH) group is added to the other (Figure 10.4b). Figure 10.4b shows that heat is also given off as a result of this process, so the actions of digestive enzymes also contribute to the thermoregulation of cells and extracellular fluid.

Physical and chemical digestion occur simultaneously. For convenience, however, the processes will be described individually for each anatomical region of the gut. Pancreatic and liver functions will also be described separately, but it should be remembered that integration of regional functions determines the final outcome of the digestive/assimilative processes.

A person's nutritional status can be compared with scientific tables of 'ideal' weight for height and build, or can be explored more specifically. The boxed text in this chapter is concerned mainly with the common regional problems associated with the alimentary canal, starting at the mouth and terminating at the anus.

The mouth, pharynx and oesophagus
The mouth

The mouth (oral or buccal) cavity is the opening of the alimentary canal, which aids ingestion. This is the only region that is surrounded by bony skeletal structures (i.e. the upper and lower jaws – the maxilla and mandible, respectively). The muscles associated with these bones are responsible for controlling the overall size of the mouth. The muscular lips or labia guard the opening. The hard and soft palates, the latter tapering backwards, shape the roof of the buccal cavity, terminating in a projection called the uvula. The cheeks outline the sides of the mouth, and the tongue forms the floor. The jaws support the cavity and contain the sockets that accommodate the teeth. The mouth is lined with a mucous stratified epithelial membrane, reflecting the wear and tear associated with this area.

Salivation

Water makes up 90–95% of saliva; the remaining 5–10% comprises dissolved solutes, including:

- ions, such as bicarbonate (HCO_3^-), chloride (Cl^-), phosphate (PO_4^{2-}), sodium (Na^+) and potassium (K^+);

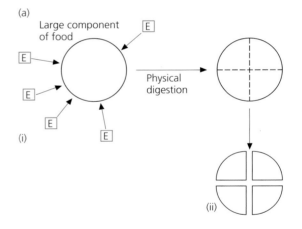

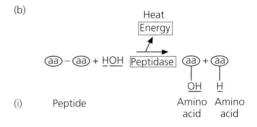

Figure 10.4 (a) Physical digestion – an aid to chemical digestion: (i) before physical digestion, the enzymatic action is limited to the area surrounding the food component; (ii) after physical digestion. Note that the physical and chemical processes occur simultaneously. Physical digestion merely makes chemical digestion more efficient by increasing the available surface area for enzymatic breakdown. (b) Hydrolysis of peptides: during hydrolysis (accelerated by enzymatic action), a water molecule (as H^+ and OH^-) is added to the two breakdown products (i.e. amino acids), breaking the chemical bond (called a peptide bond) that is holding the products together. E, enzyme; aa, amino acid

Q Differentiate between the processes of chemical and physical digestion.

Table 10.3 Homeostatic functions of saliva components

Saliva components	Homeostatic roles
Water	Dissolves food for the appreciation of taste
	Vital for digestion (hydrolysis) and to provide the necessary aqueous medium for the enzyme's maximum breakdown efficiency
Bicarbonates and phosphates	Buffering action keeps the pH within its homeostatic range (6.35–6.85), essential for enzymatic action; pH changes to slightly alkaline during chewing, which is important for maximizing the effects of salivary amylase, and for destroying the enzymes of acidophilic bacteria
Amylase	Initiates carbohydrate digestion
Lysozymes and antibodies	Destroy bacteria, hence prevent infection
Mucin	Forms soluble mucus in the presence of water, which has a lubricating and moisturizing action
Urea	Excretory products of amino acid metabolism
Chloride	Being a cofactor, it aids salivary amylase

Q Name the three pairs of salivary glands.

- the enzyme salivary amylase;
- lysozymes;
- organic substances, such as urea, albumins and globulins (especially gammaglobulins or antibodies, in particular immunoglobulin A);
- mucin, derived from mucus-secreting cells.

Each component has a homeostatic role, as illustrated in Table 10.3.

The pH of saliva is 7–8. Its production varies between 1 and 1.5 L/day. Most is produced from three main pairs of salivary glands (Figure 10.5), called the parotid, submandibular and sublingual glands, whose ducts open into the mouth cavity on either side of the internal surface of the mouth.

The parotid glands are the largest salivary glands, but are responsible for only about 25% of the daily secretion. Their cells are specialized for contributing to the watery and enzyme-rich component of saliva. They are positioned just below and in front of the ears, and their ducts (called Stenson's ducts) open at a point opposite the second upper molar teeth. The glossopharyngeal (IXth cranial) nerve supplies the parotids. Parotid saliva is also rich in antibodies (immunoglobulin A, IgA).

BOX 10.3 MUMPS

The mumps virus (myxovirus) typically attacks the parotid glands. The condition, mumps (or parotitis), is an enlargement and inflammation of the parotid glands. Swelling occurs on one or both sides of the face. Inflammation of these glands cause electrolytes to become concentrated, and may result in salivary stone formation, causing blockage of the glandular ducts, leading to a swelling of the affected gland. Other accompanying symptoms are moderate fever, general discomfort (malaise), and extreme pain in the throat, especially when swallowing.

In about one-third of males infected after puberty, the testes also become inflamed. Usually only one testis is affected, so sterility rarely occurs. The incidence of mumps (along with other childhood diseases) has declined following the availability of a vaccine since 1967 (see Figure 13.27, p.393).

Tumours of the nerve or the blood vessel supplying the glands (particularly the parotid glands) also give rise to painful swelling.

The submandibular glands are positioned under the base of the tongue in the posterior aspects of the mouth. Their ducts (called Wharton's ducts) extend centrally along the floor of the mouth, opening behind the lower central incisors. They are responsible for approximately 70% of the daily production of saliva. Their cells are specialized to function in a similar way to the parotid cells, but they also secrete mucous and so produce a more viscous secretion.

The sublingual glands are the smallest of the paired glands, and are responsible for about 5% of the daily production of saliva. Their cells are mainly mucous-secreting cells, and are responsible for producing a very viscous secretion, with little enzyme present. These glands are positioned under the tongue, and have several Rivinus's ducts, which open onto the floor of the mouth.

The submandibular and sublingual glands are responsible for the spray of saliva that sometimes flows out when one yawns. Both of these pairs of glands are supplied by the facial (VIIth cranial) nerve.

Other salivary glands are also present over the palate and tongue, and upon the inner side of the lips. They respond to mechanical stimulation from the presence of food in the mouth, rather than neural activity to the gland.

Control of salivation

Saliva production by the paired glands is controlled mainly via parasympathetic neurons (see Figure 8.29, p.198). There is

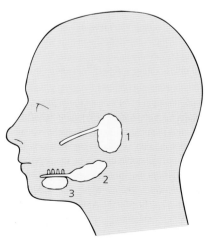

Figure 10.5 Human salivary glands: 1, parotid glands (Stenson's duct); 2, submandibular glands (Wharton's duct); 3, sublingual glands

Q Identify the main constituents of saliva.

BOX 10.4 THE EFFECTS OF DEHYDRATION AND STRESS ON SALIVA SECRETION

Saliva glands cease to secrete watery saliva in states of dehydration, as part of the homeostatic conservation of body water. As a result, the mouth becomes dry and may become coated with a thick viscous saliva secretion; this stimulates the sensation of thirst. Liquid intake restores body fluid volumes to within their homeostatic ranges. A nurse should frequently and repeatedly cleanse the mouth of a patient who is dehydrated, so as to remove this viscous secretion and reduce the unpleasant sensation of thirst.

The tongue may also appear temporarily dry when an individual is anxious, nervous or frightened, as sympathetic nervous system activity inhibits the flow of watery saliva and stimulates a viscous secretion.

ACTIVITY

Differentiate between the actions of parasympathetic and sympathetic innervation on saliva flow and saliva water content. (If you are experiencing difficulty see Figure 8.29 and associated text, pp.197–202).

---

always a constant flow of saliva in moderate amounts, because it has other homeostatic functions in addition to a role in digestion (Table 10.3).

An increase in the basal level of saliva secretion (and stomach secretions) occurs with the sight, smell and touch of food, together with the sound of food preparation, or the anticipation of food intake. This is known as a 'Pavlovian nervous conditioning response', after the Russian psychologist who first described the principle. The stimuli increase salivary flow as a result of conditioned reflexes set up from our association areas and memory regions of the brain. Such responses are important, as they allow the mouth to lubricate food and commence chemical breakdown as soon as it enters. The presence of ingested food stimulates an even greater salivary flow, by stimulating taste buds on the tongue and other regions in the mouth. Any object rolled on the tongue has the same effect. Once the food is swallowed, a large flow continues that cleanses the mouth, 'washing' the teeth and diluting food residues.

The tongue

The tongue is an accessory organ of the digestive system. The tongue's extrinsic muscles are important in moving it from side to side and in and out; its intrinsic muscles are responsible for changing its shape. The superior surface and the sides of the tongue contain projections called papillae. The papillae are associated with the sensation of taste, as they contain the taste buds; the details of taste are discussed in Chapter 7, pp.158–9.

Tongue movements alter the shape and volume of the mouth cavity, and are also vital in forming speech.

Physical digestion in the mouth

Physical digestion reduces the size of the food particles to aid the chemical processes involved in digestion. It involves the action of the jaw muscles, the teeth and the tongue. The size of the mouth opening, together with the biting action of the teeth, is responsible for determining the size of the food particle ingested. Powerful jaw muscles voluntarily control mouth opening, and the size of this opening is restricted by the perimeter of the muscular lips and the joint between the mandible and the cranium. The teeth are considered in detail in Box 10.6 and Figure 10.6. The incisors, or biting teeth, mainly control the size of the particle we take in. The canines are used to a limited extent for tearing and shearing fleshy meat from its bone, although as man's diet and social eating habits have changed, these teeth have become less important in ingestion and have become much less prominent in modern man.

Once the food particles are inside the mouth, the premolars and molars crush and grind them, reducing their size. This is controlled by the jaw muscles, and the mechanical process is termed 'mastication' (chewing). Also important in this chewing process is the involuntary movement of the tongue, which moves food particles around the oral cavity; in doing so, the tongue produces friction between the particles and structures that they rub against and, as a result, the particle are fragmented. Simultaneous with this physical breakdown is the mixing and lubrication of food with saliva. Saliva contains the enzyme amylase, which initiates the chemical breakdown of carbohydrate within the food.

Chemical digestion in the mouth

The chemical breakdown of large, insoluble molecules begins in the mouth. Most dietary carbohydrates are in the form of polysaccharides (see Figures 5.2a, p.108 and Table 5.1, p.107), and salivary amylase ('amyl-' = starch) initiates the breakdown

BOX 10.5 NORMAL AND ABNORMAL APPEARANCES OF THE TONGUE

The visual appearance of the tongue is of concern to many people, but the following appearances are only cosmetically displeasing, as they are considered quite 'normal':

- furring, common in mouth breathers;
- fissuring, common in elderly people (this may be an indication of the wear and tear associated with the ageing process);
- sublingual vein varicosities.

There are, however, many deviations from the tongue's normal, moist, pink appearance, which are indicative of deficiency diseases, such as the pallor associated with anaemia, the smooth, red appearance of a patient with pernicious anaemia, and the 'dry' tongue seen in dehydration. Tongue movements, particularly during swallowing, will be affected adversely as a consequence of certain neural lesions involving areas of the brain, especially the brainstem, which regulates the movements, and the cranial nerves, which supply the tongue.

Superficial inflammation of the tongue, called glossitis ('glossa' = tongue), may be associated with inflammation of the mouth, generally referred to as stomatitis ('stoma' = mouth). Glossitis may arise in people who experience dental caries, gum infection, gastric disorders or mucous membrane infections, and in people who smoke and drink alcohol excessively. Treatment varies with each case, and an important part of treatment is allaying the person's fear of cancer.

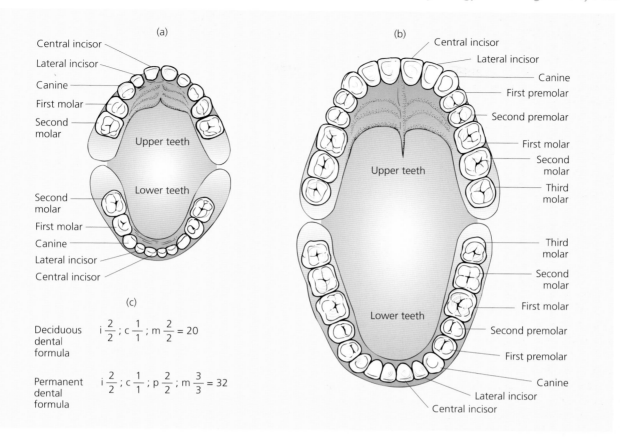

Figure 10.6 Dentition and dental formulae. (a) Deciduous (milk) dentition. (b) Permanent (adult) dentition. (c) Dental formulae include the number of teeth associated with one-half of either the lower or upper jaw

Q How are the various types of teeth adapted to provide specialized functions?

BOX 10.6 TEETH AND THE ORAL CAVITY

The development of teeth, essential for biting and chewing solid food, begins during fetal life, but teeth do not begin to erupt until about 6 months after birth. These are the deciduous (milk) teeth; on average, one tooth erupts each month until all 20 are present (Figure 10.6). The incisors erupt first; these are chisel shaped for biting. The cuspid or canine teeth erupt next; these are used to tear and shred food. The molars are the last to erupt; they are used to crunch and grind food.

Deciduous teeth are shed from about 6–7 years of age, and are replaced with permanent teeth that are normally in place by about 12 years of age, although a further four 'wisdom teeth' may erupt during teenage or early adulthood years. The wisdom teeth may be a source of pressure and pain, as the relative size of the jaw recedes with age. If this is the case, these teeth may be removed surgically.

Excluding the wisdom teeth, there are 28 permanent teeth, composed of four incisors, two canines, four premolars and four molars in each jaw (Figure 10.6). Since there are only 20 deciduous teeth, some permanent teeth do not have deciduous predecessors. Permanent teeth have extensive roots, but they have the same basic structure as the deciduous teeth.

The ageing process is associated with the following changes:

- Tooth enamel and dentine wear down, so cavities are more likely.
- Teeth are lost as a result of periodontal disease and roots that break easily.
- Taste and smell diminish.
- Saliva secretion decreases.

The overall result of these changes is that eating becomes less pleasurable, appetite is reduced, and food is not chewed or lubricated sufficiently, so swallowing becomes difficult for the older person.

A general problem associated with teeth is the accumulation of plaque, which may lead to inflammation of the gums (gingivitis), dental decay and caries formation, leading to loss of teeth. Prevention is necessary, and involves avoiding foods that have a greater tendency for plaque formation, and adequate oral hygiene.

During pregnancy, the gums have a tendency to swell and become spongy. As a consequence, bleeding may occur. This has implications on the dental health of a woman, and for this reason dental care is provided during pregnancy until 1 year after birth. A dental hygienist may also offer advice, such as using a soft toothbrush to reduce the aggravation of the gums.

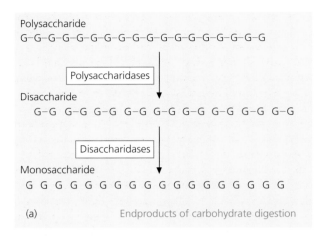

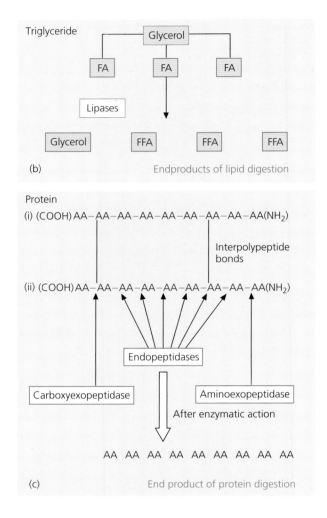

Figure 10.7 Digestive enzymes. Endopeptidases break down the bonds between amino acids other than the terminal bonds. Carboxyexopeptidases are involved in breaking the terminal peptide bond associated with the amino acid which has its carboxyl acid group exposed. Aminoexopeptidases are involved in breaking the terminal peptide bond associated with the amino acid which has its amine group exposed. (a) The mode of action of carbohydrases. (b) The mode of action of lipases on a triglyceride (most dietary fats are in the triglyceride form). (c) The mode of action of proteases; (i) and (ii) are polypeptide chains (protein molecules consist of two or more polypeptide chains). AA, amino acid; (COOH)AA, carboxylic acid terminal amino acid; FA, fatty acid; FFA, free fatty acid; G, monosaccharide (e.g. glucose); (NH$_2$)AA, amino terminal amino acid

Q *Reflect on your understanding of how enzymes are named.*

of the carbohydrate starch by breaking the bonds between the monosaccharide subunits (glucose) from which starch is constructed (Figure 10.7a).

In theory, amylase is capable of converting starch into the disaccharide maltose, which consists of two glucose molecules joined together. However, this takes time. In practice, the food is in the presence of amylase for only 15–30 minutes: food is usually in the stomach within 4–6 seconds of eating it; it remains for a while in areas of the stomach in which gastric acid is not present, thus amylase continues to work. Eventually, the food is passed to acidic areas of the stomach, where the acidity denatures and inactivates the amylase, so at this stage carbohydrate digestion ceases. Thus, the carbohydrate components of the food at this point are starch molecules that have not been in contact with amylase, dextrins (intermediate breakdown products between starch and the disaccharide maltose) and to a small extent maltose itself. No other foods are chemically broken down in the mouth, or on the food's journey to the stomach. As a result of the physical and chemical processes, the food leaving the mouth is reduced to a soft, flexible ball (called a bolus; plural, boli) that is swallowed easily.

ACTIVITY

Reflect on your understanding of the physical and chemical digestive functions of the mouth.

The pharynx and oesophagus

The pharynx, or throat, is a cone-shaped cavity approximately 12 cm long. It is subdivided into:

- *the nasopharynx*: the area behind the nasal passageways concerned with the flow of air through the respiratory pathways;
- *the common pharynx or oropharynx*: contains the tonsils on its lateral walls. The mouth is anterior to this region;
- *the laryngeal pharynx*: the area around the larynx that bifurcates into the larynx (voice box) and oesophagus.

The oesophagus is a collapsible muscular tube approximately 25 cm long running from the pharynx to the stomach, anterior to the thoracic vertebrae, but behind the trachea. The oesophagus penetrates the diaphragm before entering the stomach via the oesophageal hiatus, more commonly called the cardiac sphincter.

The pharynx and the oesophagus are lined with a stratified epithelium (pp. 53–4), as these regions are associated with a great deal of wear and tear during the passage of food.

The swallowing process

The swallowing of food, called deglutition, is aided by the moist consistency of the bolus of food resulting from the presence of saliva and mucous secreted from the lining of the mouth and oesophagus. In addition, the absence of cartilage from the posterior surface of the trachea helps to reduce friction as the food passes down the oesophagus. This is because the anterior surface of the upper section of the oesophagus lies against the posterior surface of the trachea; the presence of cartilage would make swallowing extremely uncomfortable.

The swallowing process involves a triad of responses (Figure 10.8):

1 *The voluntary stage*: the tongue voluntarily moves the bolus of food to the back of the mouth, and then into the oropharynx. This involves the tongue rising and pushing itself against the soft palate (Figure 10.8a).

2 *The involuntary pharyngeal stage*: this begins with the bolus stimulating receptors in the oropharyngeal region, resulting in an involuntary swallowing reflex. Sensory impulses ascend to the deglutition (swallowing) centre of the medulla and lower pons of the brainstem. Parasympathetic motor output causes the soft palate, and its extension the uvula, to move upwards, thus sealing off the nasal passageways and preventing food from entering the nasal cavity (Figure 10.8b). Parasympathetic motor impulses also cause the larynx to move upwards, sealing off the opening of the larynx, called the glottis, with the epiglottis (Figure 10.8c), and widening the space between the laryngeal pharynx and oesophagus. This aids the passage of the bolus. Once food has moved into the oesophagus, breathing is resumed with the opening of the respiratory pathway. Occasionally, when we drink liquids very quickly the sealing of the nasal passageways is too slow and the drink passes into them. Alternatively, food particles may be swallowed so fast that the sealing of the glottis is incomplete and food becomes lodged at the top of the larynx, stimulating the coughing reflex and expelling the irritant particles from the larynx.

3 *The oesophageal stage*: once the bolus has entered the oesophagus, muscular movements (peristalsis) are responsible for its

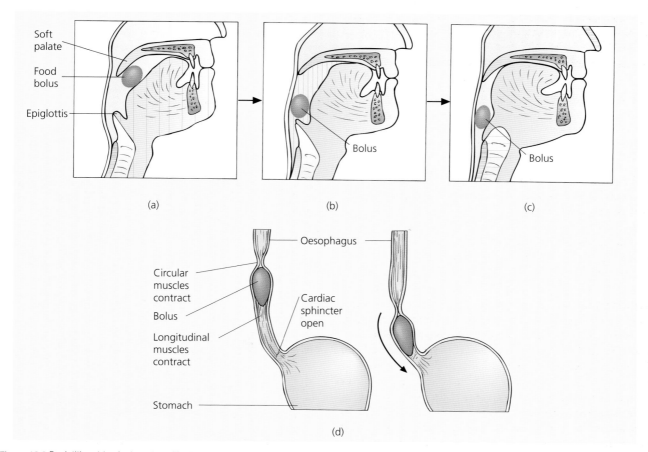

Figure 10.8 Deglutition: (a) voluntary stage (the tongue rises against the palate); (b,c) involuntary pharyngeal stage (nasal and laryngeal passages sealed off via the rising soft palate and epiglottis, respectively); (d) oesophageal stage (peristaltic motion and entry to the stomach)

Q Describe the mechanisms involved in the swallowing reflex.

Table 10.4 Regulation of the alimentary canal's activities

Region	Functional activity	Regulator of function
Mouth	Opening via jaw muscular movement	Mainly by the trigeminal nerve, but also the facial nerve
	Taste	Glossopharyngeal nerve – sensory to posterior third of tongue – and facial nerve – sensory to anterior two-thirds of the tongue
	Mastication	Trigeminal nerve
	Tongue movements	Facial nerve
	Salivary flow	Facial nerve (submandibular and sublingual glands), glossopharyngeal nerve (parotid glands)
Swallowing reflex	Upward movement of soft palate	Facial nerve
	Movement of the epiglottis over the glottis	Vagus nerve
	Oesophageal peristalsis	Facial nerve and mesenteric/Auerbach's plexus
Stomach	Entry via relaxation of the cardiac spincter	Vagus nerve
	Churning	Vagus nerve
	Gastric juice secretion	Vagus nerve; actions of gastrin (gastric and duodenal)
	Exit via the relaxation of the pyloric sphincter	Vagus nerve
Small intestine	Peristalsis, segmentation	Vagus nerve
	Pancreatic juice secretion	CCK–PZ and secretin
	Bile secretion from the gall bladder	CCK–PZ
	Intestinal juice secretion	Vagus nerve
Large intestine	Entry from the small intestine through the ileocaecal valve	Gastrocolic (vagus nerve)
	Peristalsis	Vagus and pelvic nerves
	Exit via:	
	1 Relaxation (opening) of the internal sphincter	Pelvic nerve
	2 Relaxation (opening) of the external sphincter	Controlled voluntarily

CCK-PZ–cholecystokinin–pancreozymin.

Q. Discuss the importance of pH variation in the alimentary canal.

transport to the stomach. Although the main function of peristalsis is to propel the food along the tube, it is inevitable that there will be friction between food boli and the oesophageal surfaces as they 'rub' against each other. This aids physical digestion to a limited extent. Peristaltic movement of food occurs throughout the gastrointestinal tract, from the oesophagus to the final elimination via the anal canal.

The medulla of the brainstem controls the events in the first part of the oesophagus via parasympathetic motor impulses, and may influence gut movements in other sections of the tract. However, a myenteric plexus ('myenteric' = within muscle, 'plexus' = collection of nerve cells) is capable of generating peristaltic movements in the absence of extrinsic stimulation. Figure 10.8d illustrates the peristaltic process. Circular muscle fibres contract immediately behind the bolus, which constricts the oesophagus in this region and forces the bolus downwards. Longitudinal fibres immediately in front of the bolus simultaneously contract, thus shortening and expanding the diameter of the section, and allowing the forward propulsion of the bolus. The coordinated action of these muscular movements provides the appearance of a continuous wave of contraction. Swallowing also promotes the relaxation of the normally contracted cardiac sphincter, and allows passage of the bolus into the stomach.

The duration of swallowing depends upon the consistency of the food (fluid-like foods travel quicker) and the body's position (an upright body position facilitates a more rapid descent). Taking these extremes into consideration, the time for the passage of boli from entering and leaving the oesophagus ranges from 1 to 8 seconds.

Table 10.4 summarizes the regulation of alimentary canal activities.

The stomach

The stomach is a J-shaped muscular organ, located immediately below the diaphragm on the left side of the abdominal cavity. Its size and shape varies according to content (the stomach's folds, or rugae, disappear when the stomach is distended), and according to which part of the respiratory cycle the person is in. Upon inspiration, the diaphragm is pulled down, which displaces the stomach downwards slightly. With expiration, the stomach extends upwards. The opening from the oesophagus, and the exit into the first region of the small intestine, are guarded by the cardiac and pyloric sphincter muscles, respectively. These are normally contracted, thus

BOX 10.7 OESOPHAGEAL IMBALANCES

Dysphagia

Dysphagia is a difficulty in swallowing. It can result from mechanical obstruction of the oesophagus (caused by tumours, strictures, or out-pouching of the wall – diverticular hernia), or a disorder that impairs oesophageal motility, such as functional dysphagia caused by neurological (e.g. Parkinson's disease) or muscular disorders (e.g. dermatomyositis) that interfere with voluntary swallowing or peristalsis.

Management of dysphagia depends upon the cause. Definitive treatments include mechanical dilation of the oesophageal sphincter, and surgical separation of lower oesophageal muscles. The patient is also taught to manage symptoms by eating slowly, eating small meals, taking fluids with meals, and sleeping with the head elevated to prevent regurgitation and aspiration.

Oesophagitis

This is reflux of the stomach contents into the oesophagus, mainly caused by inefficiency of the cardiac sphincter or increased abdominal pressure. The acid that is present naturally in the stomach irritates the cell lining of the oesophagus, causing 'heartburn'. The severity of symptoms becomes worse in older people (Fass *et al.*, 2000). It can be detected by a barium swallow or by gastroscopy (see later).

Oesophageal varices

These often occur secondary to liver cirrhosis, where weak collateral veins around the oesophagus can rupture easily. This can lead to large blood loss, and the patient will present with haematemesis (vomit containing blood). Varices are detected by gastroscopy, and may be banded or compressed (see Box 10.16, p.249).

---

preventing passage of stomach contents. The stomach is held in position by the mesenteries of the peritoneum.

Figure 10.9a illustrates the four main regions of the stomach:

- The cardiac region surrounds the cardiac sphincter muscle.
- The fundic region is the elevated rounded part around and to the left of the cardiac portion.
- The body region occupies most of the stomach; it lies between the fundic and pyloric parts.
- The pyloric region is the most inferior part of the stomach, lying superior to the pyloric sphincter.

Entry of food

The cardiac sphincter relaxes and opens when food is present in the lower oesophagus, allowing entry of boli into the stomach. Simultaneously, the pyloric sphincter, which guards the exit from the stomach, contracts so that food cannot pass immediately into the small intestine without first undergoing gastric digestion.

Physical digestion in the stomach

The stomach 'churns' food using a mechanism peculiar to this organ. A three-dimensional muscular movement is brought about by the presence of an additional oblique muscular layer (Figure 10.9a). This movement increases the efficiency of physically breaking down food boli that have entered this region, and mixes food with the stomach's chemicals, or gastric juice, thus facilitating chemical digestion.

There is regional variation in the peristalsis movements of the stomach. The fundic region exhibits only a few peristaltic waves, as this is the 'storage' area of the stomach; food is not mixed with gastric secretions, so salivary amylase continues to work here. The waves of contraction beginning in the body of the stomach become more vigorous in the inferior regions, and are very forceful in the pylorus region. These latter waves of contraction allow liquidized foods a more rapid exit from the stomach should the pyloric sphincter relax. Contraction of the sphincter, however, normally seals off the exit from the stom-

BOX 10.8 HIATUS HERNIA, PREGNANCY AND HEARTBURN

Hiatus hernia occurs when part of the person's stomach herniates, or distends, through the oesophageal gap (hiatus) in the diaphragm. It may be congenital or may result from an acquired weakness. Often there are no symptoms, but pain and 'heartburn' from the reflux of gastric acid can occur. Correction involves external manipulation of the herniated region back into the abdomen. If this is unsuccessful, then a simple and effective operation can remove the problem.

Heartburn is also a common disorder of pregnancy. Increased levels of the hormone progesterone during pregnancy relax the cardiac sphincter. This slows digestion of food, which may make the woman feel nauseous after meals. Therefore, pregnant women are encouraged to eat smaller meal portions (e.g. five small meals a day instead of the usual three).

---

ach, resulting in the temporary backward movement of the food within the pylorus, producing a more efficient mixing of the gastric contents.

Chemical digestion in the stomach

The stomach's secretion is called gastric juice, and is produced from the compound tubular glands of the gastric pits. About 2–3 L per day are produced. The main function of the secretion is the conversion of the semi-solid boli of food into a semi-liquid chyme. In addition, the gastric juice contains a protease enzyme, which initiates protein breakdown.

Each gastric gland possesses three types of secretory cells (Figure 10.9b) – mucous cells, chief cells and oxyntic cells – which secrete separate components of the gastric juice. Another type of specialized endocrine cell present in the gastric mucosa secretes the hormone gastrin, which stimulates a greater flow of gastric juice. Gastrin is released when food is present in the stomach.

Mucous cells

Normally, the gastric cells are protected by mucous and by intact gastric cell membranes with low permeability to hydrogen irons and tight junctions between the cells. Mucous (or neck) cells are located mainly in the neck of the gland, and secrete the mucous part of the juice. Mucous adheres to the

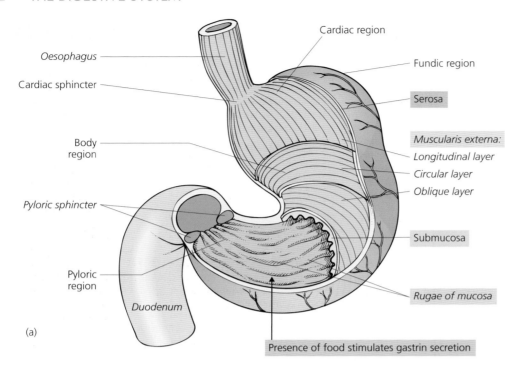

(a)

Oesophagus
Cardiac sphincter
Body region
Pyloric sphincter
Pyloric region
Duodenum

Cardiac region
Fundic region
Serosa
Muscularis externa:
Longitudinal layer
Circular layer
Oblique layer
Submucosa
Rugae of mucosa

Presence of food stimulates gastrin secretion

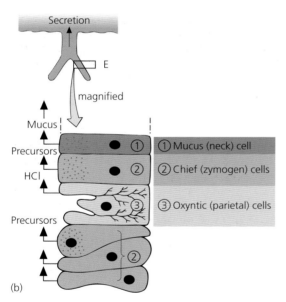

(b)

Secretion
E
magnified
Mucus
Precursors
HCl
Precursors

① Mucus (neck) cell
② Chief (zymogen) cells
③ Oxyntic (parietal) cells

Figure 10.9 (a) The stomach. (b) The gastric (tubular) gland

Q Describe the sphincter functions of the stomach when (1) food is approaching the stomach, (2) food is being digested within the stomach and (3) food has been digested by the stomach.

gastric mucosal surface. It prevents autodigestion of the stomach wall by the hydrochloric acid and proteolytic enzymes present in gastric juice. The mucous layer normally is about 1 mm thick.

Chief cells

Chief (or zymogen) cells produce two enzyme precursors (inactive enzymes), pepsinogen and prorennin. These are activated by the acidic gastric juice to pepsin and rennin, respectively. Both enzymes accelerate protein digestion. Pepsin converts proteins into polypeptides (long chains of amino acids); it is an endopeptidase enzyme, so it breaks the peptide

bonds in places other than at the terminal peptide positions (see Figure 10.7c, p.238). Rennin converts the soluble protein of milk into an insoluble form, in order to retain it in the stomach for longer periods so pepsin can have its proteolytic effects.

Pepsin is responsible for 10–15% of protein digestion; the remainder occurs in the small intestine.

Oxyntic (or parietal) cells

The oxyntic (or parietal) cells contain intracellular channels, called canaliculi, in which hydrochloric acid (HCl) is produced. The initial chemical reactions leading to the production of hydrochloric acid occur in the cytoplasm, but the final reactions occur in the channels away from the cytoplasm. The acid in gastric juice has the following functions:

- activation of the precursor enzymes pepsinogen and prorennin;
- provision of the optimal pH (pH 2–3) for the action of pepsin (and rennin);
- inactivation of salivary amylase;
- destruction (i.e. denaturization) of the enzymes of alkali-liking bacteria present in ingested food (i.e. HCl is bactericidal);
- dissolves splinters of bone that may have been swallowed.

BOX 10.9 LACTATING INFANTS

The digestive system of the newborn cannot synthesize the full range of digestive enzymes necessary for a mixed diet, and gastric secretion is inadequate. The infant is therefore dependent upon milk feeds, and the tongue of babies is in a forward position to facilitate suckling. The relative position of the tongue changes gradually, and digestive enzyme secretion increases in capacity and variety, so the baby becomes able to cope with semi-solid foods.

The reliance of the infant on milk feeds necessitates the production of the gastric enzyme rennin. This coagulates milk protein, and so slows its advance through the stomach, giving more time for its digestion. Rennin is not to be confused with the renal enzyme renin, which stimulates an enzyme cascade that regulates blood pressure (see Figure 12.29a, p.349).

Gastric lipase is another enzyme that is secreted into the gastric juice of infants. This breaks down butterfat molecules in milk. It requires a pH of 5–6 for its actions, however, and so has a limited role in the adult stomach where pH values are generally lower. Adults rely on lipases secreted into the small intestine to digest lipids.

Tooth development begins during fetal life (see Box 10.6).

Parietal cells are also responsible for producing intrinsic factor of Castle. This chemical is essential for the carriage of vitamin B_{12} through the stomach, and for its absorption by the small intestine. People without this factor exhibit the homeostatic imbalance of pernicious (megalocytic) anaemia (see Table 11.6, p.282).

Exit of food

The pyloric sphincter is usually partly open when food is present in the stomach, thus allowing liquid material to pass through very quickly. However, the endproduct of stomach digestion called chyme is semi-liquid and requires the sphincter to be completely open to allow the passage of large quantities per unit time.

Regulation of gastric functions

The secretion of gastric juice is usually related to the presence, or anticipation, of food. Three phases are responsible for controlling the secretion of gastric juice:

1 *The cephalic stage*: this involves parasympathetic nerve stimulation of the stomach via the vagus nerve. It is a conditioned association reflex that occurs when we smell, see or taste food (i.e. it is preparatory for the arrival of food). It is responsible for inducing contractions of stomach muscle, which bring about churning, and an increased rate of gastric juice secretion.

2 *The gastric phase*: the presence of food in the pyloric region of the stomach results in the release of the hormone gastrin, which aids gastric motility (muscular movement) and stimulates the increased secretion of gastric juice.

3 *The intestinal phase*: once food comes into contact with the mucosa of the first region of the small intestine, called the duodenum, a variety of hormones [e.g. cholecystokinin–pancreozymin (CCK–PZ), gastric inhibitory peptide and secretin] is released. Most of these hormones inhibit gastric

BOX 10.10 PYLORIC STENOSIS AND PYLOROSPASM

Pyloric stenosis

This is a major disorder of gastric emptying. The pyloric sphincter grows or hypertrophies, causing a narrowing of the lumen of the stomach's exit, and dilation of the stomach. An extra peristaltic effort is therefore needed to force the gastric contents through the narrowed pyloric sphincter, thus the muscle layers of the stomach may also become hypertrophied.

The condition is more common in small babies. It usually appears by the third week of extrauterine life. Pyloric stenosis is five times more common in males (5 in 1000 births) than in females. The condition is also more common in children with Down syndrome. Pyloric stenosis is inherited as a multifactorial trait; an increase in gastrin secretion by the mother in the last trimester of pregnancy also increases the likelihood of pyloric stenosis in the infant.

The hallmark symptom of pyloric stenosis is projectile vomiting – the spraying of liquid vomit some distance from the infant. The vomiting may lead to malnutrition, dehydration and electrolyte imbalances. Standard treatment for hypertrophied pyloric stenosis in those cases that do not resolve themselves is a pyloromyotomy, in which the muscles of the pyloric sphincters are separated. As part of the care and discharge planning, the patient should be given dietary advice regarding the necessity to take small, frequent meals.

See the case study of a child with hypertrophic pyloric stenosis, Section VI, p.649.

Pylorospasm

In this condition, the muscle fibres of the pyloric sphincter fail to relax normally, so food does not pass easily from the stomach to the duodenum. The stomach becomes overfull, and the infant vomits often to relieve the pressure build-up. Antispasmodic drugs are given to relax the pylorospasm, and the infant is re-fed after vomiting.

motility and gastric secretion, and so delay gastric emptying. This allows more time for digestion (particularly of lipids) in the duodenum. In addition, these hormones help prevent homeostatic imbalances, such as gastric ulcers, occurring in the stomach as a result of excessive gastric acid secretion in the absence of food. Conversely, duodenal gastrin may also be released when the chyme is rich in proteins and polypeptides. This is identical to the stomach's gastrin, and promotes protein digestion of food in the duodenum if there is any remaining following stomach digestion.

The small intestine, pancreas and gall bladder
The small intestine

The small intestine extends from the pyloric sphincter to the ileocaecal valve located at the junction with the large intestine. It is about 6.5 m long, with a diameter of 2.5 cm. The small intestine is a coiled structure occupying a large part of the abdominal cavity. It is suspended by the mesenteries, which carry the nerves, and blood and lymphatic vessels that support this area. The small intestine is the main area of digestion and absorption, and is divided anatomically into three distinct regions (see Figure 10.2, p.231):

• The duodenum is the shortest section of the small intestine, extending from the pyloric sphincter for about 25 cm. It forms a loop inferior to the stomach, and encloses the body

BOX 10.11 GASTRITIS AND PEPTIC ULCERS

Gastritis

This is inflammation of the stomach mucosa, often caused by prolonged exposure to certain substances (e.g. aspirin and other non-steroidal anti-inflammatory drugs, or NSAIDS, and alcohol), that disturb the cell arrangement of gastric mucosa, and increase the permeability of the cell membranes to hydrogen ions. This lowers the cellular pH, and so decreases optimal enzyme functioning. The subsequent cell damage may result in gastric inflammation (gastritis) and bleeding, hypoxia and eventually necrotic areas of gastric mucosa, and can lead to the formation of an ulcer. Patients with arthritis who are prescribed long-term aspirin as an analgesic are often given enteric-coated aspirin; the enteric coat prevents the absorption of aspirin from the stomach.

Treatment for chronic gastritis is a soft, bland diet, and avoidance of irritant foods, smoking and alcohol. Patients are encouraged to minimize anxiety-causing situations that initiate gastric secretion when the stomach is 'empty'.

Diagnosis can be made by gastroscopy. *Helicobacter pylori* (*H. pylori*) bacteria are often present on biopsy.

Peptic ulcers

Peptic ulcers are breaks in the protective mucosal lining caused by gastric secretions. They may be gastric, duodenal or (occasionally) oesophageal in origin. The presence of ulcers is a sign of a homeostatic imbalance associated with either excessive secretion of gastric juice, reduced resistance of the gastric mucosa to the secretion, or the presence of a short stomach, but the most common cause is infection of the affected region with *H. pylori*. Other contributory causal factors are:

- hereditary tendency;
- use of steroids, as these decrease mucosal resistance;
- habitual use of NSAIDs, alcohol and heavy smoking;
- a 'stress' or 'type A' personality (although this is now controversial);
- chronic diseases, such as emphysema, rheumatoid arthritis or cirrhosis.

Although both gastric and duodenal ulcers are classified as 'peptic' ulcers, they have different symptoms. For example, the boring/burning pain of gastric ulcer comes soon after eating and is not relieved by eating more food, whereas duodenal ulcer pain comes approximately 2 hours after a meal, when chyme exits the stomach, and is relieved temporarily by further eating because this stops gastric emptying for a while.

Diagnosis can be made by gastroscopy. *H. pylori* bacteria are often present on biopsy.

Principles of correction are based upon the patient eating an easily digestible meal, using antacid preparations to neutralize the gastric acids, or using other drugs to diminish gastric secretions and/or motility. For gastric ulcers, mucous secretion can be increased by the administration of carbenoxolone (a liquorice derivative).

BOX 10.12 NAUSEA AND VOMITING

Nausea

Nausea is an unpleasant sensation that may occur as a result of an emotional disturbance, indigestion, gastritis, or unpleasant sights and smells. Nausea may be accompanied by autonomic nervous stimulation, resulting in one or more of pallor, sweating, and a sudden secretion of saliva into the mouth.

Vomiting

Vomiting (emesis) is forceful expulsion (regurgitation or antiperistalsis) of the contents of the gastrointestinal tract, usually preceded by nausea and excessive salivation. It is a reflex resulting in:

1 Closure of the larynx via the epiglottis, sealing the glottis.
2 Closure of the nasal passageways in order to prevent the entrance of the vomitus.
3 Forceful contraction of the diaphragm and abdominal wall muscles.
4 Closure of the pyloric sphincter, which increases the stomach pressure, causing gastric regurgitation.

The responses are determined by neural output from the vomiting centre of the medulla of the brainstem. The centre sends motor impulses to the above areas to initiate the act, in response to sensory impulses from one (or more) of the following:

- gastrointestinal irritation by chemicals, microorganisms, or handling of the viscera during surgery, thus acting crudely as a 'protective' response to remove the initiating stressor;
- cerebral tumour or raised intracranial pressure;
- higher cerebral centres in response to intense fear, anxiety, unpleasant smells, etc.;
- impulses from the vestibular apparatus (balance organ of the ear), for example in seasickness;
- some drugs, e.g. morphine, digitalis and emetics (e.g. ipecacuanha); thus the principle of pharmacological correction is the use of anti-emetic drugs;
- general anaesthetics.

Examination of the products of the vomit (called vomitus) is indicative of the associated aetiological factor. For example, the presence of blood may indicate gastric (peptic) ulceration, whereas the presence of undigested food could indicate an obstruction to the pyloric sphincter.

The consequences of vomiting, particularly if chronic, are reduction of nutrient uptake, and a change in body fluid composition. There is a loss of fluid and electrolytes. The loss of gastric acid can result in metabolic alkalosis, although chronic vomiting may induce a metabolic acidosis because the body uses fat as an energy source to compensate for reduced carbohydrate intake.

Weight loss and nutritional disturbances occur if vomiting is prolonged. In addition, inhalation of vomit can lead to aspiration pneumonia, and ultimately death. To prevent any potential vomitus from being inhaled, the unconscious patient must be placed in a semi-prone position to encourage vomitus to be 'drained out' via gravity.

The principles of correction of nausea and vomiting vary according to the aetiology (e.g. the avoidance of gastric irritants such as alcohol). The secondary consequences may also require correction, including fluid replacement and/or buffer therapy (see Box 6.1, p.121).

ACTIVITY

Reflect on your understanding of the chemical and physical digestive processes of the stomach.

ACTIVITY

Regarding the H^+ content of blood, differentiate between metabolic acidosis and metabolic alkalosis (see pp.128–33).

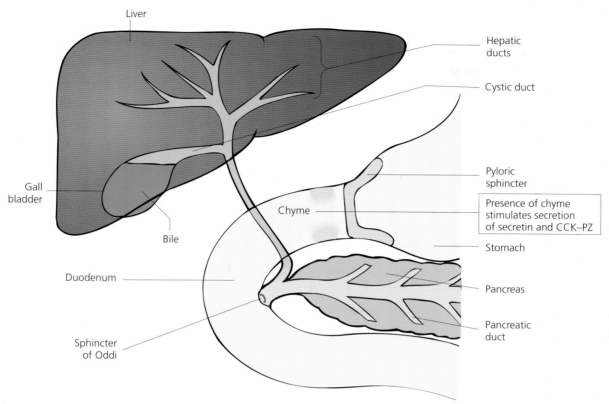

Figure 10.10 The relationship between the stomach, liver and pancreas. CCK–PZ, cholecystokinin–pancreozymin

Q What is the hallmark symptom of infantile pyloric stenosis?

Q Describe the mechanisms involved in the gastrocolic reflex.

of the pancreas. The united ducts from the gall bladder and the pancreas empty into the duodenum via the circular ring of involuntary muscle called the sphincter of Oddi (Figure 10.10).

- The jejunum is about 2.7 m long. It extends from the duodenum to the final part of the small intestine, or the ileum. The duodenum and jejunum are both concerned mainly with digestion.
- The ileum is about 3.6 m long. It connects the small intestine with the large intestine, or caecum, via the ileocaecal valve. It is the main area of absorption.

The mucosal epithelium of the small intestine has circular folds, or plicae. Projecting from these plicae are finger-like projections called villi. The villi bear further projections called microvilli. These folds and projections increase the surface area available for digestion of the chyme and for the process of absorption. At the base of the villi are intestinal glands called crypts of Lieberkühn. These are responsible for secreting the intestinal juice. Brunner's glands in the duodenal submucosa produce alkaline mucus, which, together with pancreatic and bile salts, neutralizes the acidic chyme as it enters the duodenum from the stomach. The pH actually becomes slightly alkaline, which is conducive to the activation of pancreatic precursor enzymes and the optimal functioning of enzymes within the intestines. Mucous partly protects the intestinal

wall from autodigestion by the multiple enzymes (particularly the proteases) secreted into the intestine.

The pancreas

The pancreas is a soft, tapering gland. Its head lies within the loop of duodenum, and the whole structure positions itself inferior and horizontal to the stomach (Figure 10.10). The pancreas is about 12–15 cm long and 2.5 cm thick. It contains both exocrine and endocrine secretory cells. Exocrine (or acini) cells have a role in digestion. They are responsible for secreting precursor and active digestive enzymes into the duodenum via the pancreatic duct. Other acini cells produce the bicarbonate-rich, alkaline fluid into which the enzymes are secreted before being released into the duodenum.

Endocrine cells (islets of Langerhans) include:

- alpha-cells, which produce the hormone glucagon;
- beta-cells, which produce the hormone insulin;
- delta-cells, which produce the hormone somatostatin.

ACTIVITY

Refer to the Figure 2.30, p.55 and Tables 10.6, p.248 and 9.2, p.222 respectively and distinguish between the terms 'exocrine' and 'endocrine' in relation to the function of the pancreas.

BOX 10.13 PANCREATITIS

Pancreatitis (inflammation of the pancreas) is relatively rare and potentially serious; it carries a 10–15% mortality rate (McArdle, 2000). Pancreatitis may be acute or chronic. In acute pancreatitis, the more severe condition, which may be associated with heavy alcohol intake or biliary tract obstruction, the pancreatic cells release the enzyme trypsin instead of its precursor trypsinogen; the trypsin begins to digest the pancreatic cells. Patients with chronic pancreatitis are 16 times more likely to develop pancreatic cancer than other people (Chowdhury and Rayford, 2000).

The patient will often present with abdominal pain, and investigations are often made on abdominal ultrasound and blood amylase analysis (amylase is one of the digestive enzymes normally produced by the pancreas). A raised amylase (over 1000 IU/L in the last 48 hours) is indicative of pancreatitis.

Patients usually respond to treatment, but recurrent attacks often occur. Treatment involves narcotics (e.g. Demerol) to relieve the pain; oral foods are withheld, and gastric suction is instituted to 'rest' the gland. Parenteral fluids are given to restore blood volume. Cimetidine may be administered to prevent stimulus of the pancreas. Surgical drainage may be necessary.

Common laboratory tests of pancreatic function are summarized in Table 10.5.

BOX 10.14 AGEING AND THE ASSOCIATED GLANDS OF DIGESTION

The following are associated with the ageing process:

- fibrosis, fatty acid deposits, and pancreatic atrophy;
- decrease in secretions of digestive enzymes;
- no changes occur to the gall bladder or bile duct, but there is an increased prevalence of gallstones (Box 10.15).

These hormones are important in blood sugar regulation. Insulin lowers blood glucose (it is a hypoglycaemic agent), whereas glucagon raises the blood glucose level (it is a hyperglycaemic agent). Somatostatin has a paracrine (or dual) role, and inhibits insulin and glucagon secretion when the blood glucose concentration is within its homeostatic range. Somatostatin also inhibits the secretion of pancreatic enzymes.

The pancreas is referred to as a 'mixed gland', since it has both endocrine and exocrine tissue. Its exocrine (digestive) roles are described below, and its endocrine (hormone) roles are considered in more detail in Table 9.2, p.222 and Box 9.12, p.223.

The gall bladder

This pear-shaped organ is about 7–9 cm long. It is attached to the undersurface of the liver. Its function is to store and concentrate bile, and to secrete it into the bile ducts, which unite with the pancreatic duct and enter the duodenum via the sphincter of Oddi (Figure 10.10). Bile is synthesized within the liver.

Physical digestion in the small intestine

The principal movement within the small intestine is called segmentation (Figure 10.11). This mechanism involves a series of isolated contractions in alternating localized positions. The contractions of circular muscle fibres constrict the tube, segmenting the food chyme into smaller masses. Next, the muscle fibres within the individual segments contract, with the result that further smaller masses are produced. As the muscle fibres relax, the larger segments are reformed. The overall results are that food particles are broken mechanically into smaller particles, and there is a thorough mixing of the food with digestive juices.

Segmentation stops periodically, and a wave of peristalsis then moves the food further along the intestine. This movement also contributes to the physical breakdown of food, as friction occurs between the food and the intestinal wall. Peristaltic movement is weaker in this region than in the oesophagus and stomach, so food is retained in the small intestine for longer, reflecting the time required for digestion to be completed.

Bile

Bile is a yellow-green alkaline (pH 7.6–8.6) fluid. The liver produces about 80–100 mL of bile daily. It is transported to the gall bladder by the hepatic and cystic ducts (Figure 10.10). Bile is stored and concentrated in this organ until it is required in the small intestine. Bile is mainly a watery secretion; other components include bile salts, bile pigments, cholesterol, lecithin, mucus and several ions. It has two principal functions: physical digestion and excretion.

Physical digestion by bile

Bile is frequently not recognized as being involved in physical digestion because it is a chemical secretion. Bile salts (sodium taurocholate and sodium glycocholate) and lecithin, however, are responsible for emulsification, i.e. the reduction of large globules of fat (lipids exist as globules in a watery intestinal chyme solution) into small droplets. This process falls more under the broad heading of physical breakdown since no enzymes are involved. The increased surface area produced by

Table 10.5 Common laboratory tests of pancreatic function

Test	Normal range	Clinical significance
Serum amylase	60–180 Somogyi units/mL	↑ levels with pancreatic inflammation
Serum	1.5 Somogyi units/mL	↑ levels with pancreatic inflammation (may be elevated with other conditions; differentiates with amylase isoenzyme study)
Urine amylase	35–260 Somogyi units/hour	↑ levels with pancreatic inflammation
Stool fat	2.5 g/25 hour	Measures fatty acids; decreased pancreatic lipase increases stool fat

Somogyi units: a measure of the level of activity of amylase in blood serum, as analysed by the Somogyi method.

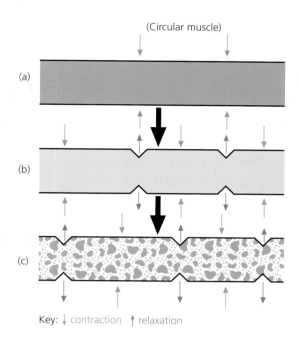

(Circular muscle)

(a)

(b)

(c)

Key: ↓ contraction ↑ relaxation

Figure 10.11 Segmentation: (a) semi-liquid chyme in one mass; (b) chyme segmented via isolated contraction of circular muscle fibres; (c) chyme segmented further as other areas contract. Note that relaxation is an inevitable consequence of contraction

Q How does segmentation differ from peristalsis?

emulsification aids the actions of digestive enzymes (lipases) to speed up the chemical breakdown of lipids. The emulsification process is rather like pouring cooking oil into water. As the large globule of oil first enters the water, it disperses into smaller fat droplets, increasing the total surface area. Bile also prevents the droplets coalescing into larger ones, which oil droplets in water eventually do.

After bile salts have performed their digestive function, they are involved in another homeostatic function by aiding the absorption of long-chain fatty acids (see later). Most of the salts are reabsorbed in the process and recycled by the liver into bile. Bile salts also contribute to the alkaline medium within the intestine, which buffers the acidic chyme and produces a pH at which intestinal enzymes operate with maximum efficiency.

Excretory function of bile

The bile pigments, bilirubin ('rubro-' = red) and biliverdin ('verd-' = green), are produced by the liver from the breakdown of haemoglobin released when old erythrocytes are destroyed. The liver removes the iron and protein (globin) part of haemoglobin; these are then homeostatically recycled (see later). The remaining parts of haemoglobin comprise the bile pigments, the principal one being bilirubin. When the bile is secreted into the intestine, this pigment is converted into urobilinogen and stercobilin. The former is absorbed into blood and then transported to the kidneys where it is converted into urochrome, which is responsible for the yellow colour of urine. Stercobilin remains in the intestine, where it is responsible for colouring the faeces. These components of faeces and urine are genuine excretory products, as they have been involved in cellular metabolism (which differentiates them from the indigestible material present in faeces).

ACTIVITY

Describe how bile contributes to physical digestion within the small intestine.

Chemical digestion in the small intestine

Before reading this section, you may find it useful to review the structures of the main food groups since digestion is concerned with reducing complex molecules to simpler constituents (see Chapter 5, pp.105–12). Chyme entering the small intestine consists of a mixture of nutrients (Table 10.6). These include:

- *Carbohydrates*: various polysaccharides arising from partially digested starches. Some disaccharides, such as maltose, may

---

BOX 10.15 GALLSTONES (CHOLELITHIASIS)

The production of stone-like concretions of the gall bladder in a person is a result of either:

- inadequate bile salts or lecithin in the bile, which results in multiple-faceted stones, composed of calcium and bile pigments;
- excessive cholesterol, resulting in its precipitation out of solution and crystallization. These cholesterol crystals coalesce; they are responsible for 85% of all gall stones.

Gall stones often go undetected in the body, but as they increase in size, they may be responsible for minimal, intermittent or complete obstruction to the flow of bile from the gall bladder into the duct system (Agrawal and Jonnalagadda, 2000).

The more common situation is partial obstruction of the outlet from the gall bladder, resulting in a heartburn pain or discomfort (called biliary colic) after eating, when digestive enzymes, notably cholecystokinin–pancreozymin (CCK–PZ), are released and contract the gall bladder. The inflammation produced is called cholecystitis, after the old name of the gall bladder, the cholecystic gland. If the stone becomes mobile and lodges itself, there is intense pain and fever, with the yellow coloration of the skin characteristic of obstructive jaundice appearing in due course. Complete obstruction of the flow may even be fatal. Bile pigment accumulation in the blood may cause intense itching of the affected area. Frequent bathing and the use of a soothing lotion, such as calamine, is sometimes helpful to the patient.

Investigations performed to detect gall stones may include X-ray, intravenous cholangiogram, endoscopic retrograde cholangiopancreatography (ERCP), or laparotomy (see Box 10.16).

Correction involves administering gall-stone-dissolving drugs (e.g. chenodeoxycholic acid) or fragmentation of stones using high-frequency sound waves (called lithotripsy). Surgical removal of the gall stones may be necessary if non-invasive treatments are ineffective; often, a cholecystectomy will be performed to remove the gall bladder and the stone inside.

Table 10.6 Actions of the enzymes of the human alimentary tract

Enzyme/enzyme precursor	Site of secretion	Site of action	Substrate acted upon	Products of action
Salivary amylase	Mouth	Mouth, oesophagus	Starch	Maltose disaccharides, dextrins – (mainly)
Pepsinogen → pepsin	Stomach	Stomach	Proteins	Polypeptides
Pancreatic amylase	Pancreas	Small intestine	Starch	Disaccharides (maltose)
Enterokinase	Small intestine	Small intestine	Trypsinogen	Trypsin
Trypsinogen → trypsin	Pancreas	Small intestine	Polypeptides/chymotrypsinogen	Peptides/chymotrypsin
Chymotrypsinogen → chymotrypsin	Pancreas	Small intestine	Polypeptides	Peptides
Carboxypeptidases	Pancreas	Small intestine	Peptides	Smaller peptides
Aminopeptidases	Pancreas	Small intestine	Peptides	Smaller peptides
Lipase	Pancreas	Small intestine	Triglycerides	Diglycerides, monoglycerides, fatty acids, glycerol
Disaccharidases (maltase, sucrase, lactase)	Small intestine	Small intestine	Disaccharides (maltose, sucrose, lactose)	Monosaccharides (glucose, fructose, galactose)
Peptidases	Small intestine	Small intestine	Oligopeptides	Amino acids
Nucleotidases	Small intestine	Small intestine	Nucleotides	Sugar – deoxyribose, phosphate, organic bases

be present, reflecting some success on the part of salivary amylase activity. In addition, depending upon the food that was consumed, other disaccharides may be present, such as lactose (milk sugar) and sucrose (cane or table sugar). The monosaccharides glucose, fructose (fruit sugar) and galactose (grape sugar) may also have been taken in.

- *Fats*: these are not chemically digested up to this point; they enter the small intestine in their consumed chemical form (i.e. mainly triglycerides).
- *Polypeptides*: present as a result of the proteolytic actions of gastric pepsin.
- *Vitamins, minerals and water*: together with monosaccharides, these are not digested because they are small enough to be absorbed across the gut wall. The other components of chyme must be digested chemically; the small intestine initiates and completes these processes via secretions of the pancreas and the intestinal mucosa.

Digestive secretions of the pancreas

About 1200–1500 mL of pancreatic juice are produced and secreted daily. Water is the main constituent of this clear, colourless secretion. Other constituents include pancreatic salts, 'protein'-digesting enzymes, carbohydrate-digesting enzymes, fat-digesting enzymes, and nucleic-acid-digesting enzymes. Pancreatic salts, the most common of which is sodium bicarbonate, contribute to the alkalinity (pH 7.1–8.2) of pancreatic juice. We have already described the neutralizing effects of the juice, bile salts and intestinal secretions on gastric acid as it enters the duodenum.

Pancreatic juice contains two endopeptidases, 'protein'-digesting or, more accurately, polypeptide-digesting, enzymes. (i.e. enzymes that act on peptide bonds within the protein molecule), called trypsin and chymotrypsin. Figure 10.12 illustrates how both are secreted into the duodenum as the pre-

cursors trypsinogen and chymotrypsinogen, respectively. These are activated rapidly within the duodenum. An enzyme called enterokinase secreted from the duodenal mucosa activates trypsinogen. Once trypsin is produced, this activates further conversion of trypsinogen into trypsin (an example of a positive feedback response), and converts chymotrypsinogen into its active form, chymotrypsin. Being endopeptidases, they break down large polypeptide fragments into smaller and smaller subunits called peptides (see Figure 10.7c, p.238).

A further role of trypsin is the activation of another pancreatic precursor, procarboxypolypeptidase. Once activated, this

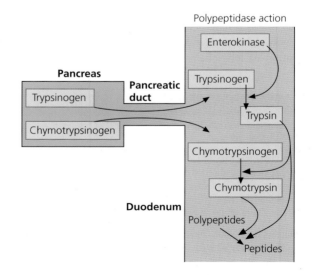

Figure 10.12 Action of trypsin/chymotrypsin (endopeptidases)

Q Which hormones stimulate the release of pancreatic juice?

Q (1) List the enzymes associated with the pancreas, and (2) identify their substrates and the breakdown products.

operates as an exopeptidase (an enzyme that acts on peptide bonds at the end of a protein/polypeptide molecule), breaking down the terminal peptide bond and exposing the carboxylic acid part of the amino acid molecule (see Figure 10.7c, p.238). Exopeptidases remove terminal amino acids one at a time from the ends of the chain, until a dipeptide (two amino acids connected by a peptide bond) is formed.

- *Carbohydrate-digesting enzyme, or pancreatic amylase*: breaks down remaining polysaccharides into the disaccharide sugar maltose (Table 10.6).
- *Fat-digesting enzyme, or pancreatic lipase (together with intestinal lipase)*: detaches fatty acids from glycerol one at a time (remember that a triglyceride molecule consists of three fatty acids attached to a glycerol molecule; see Figure 5.2c, p.108). A mixture of triglycerides, diglycerides, monoglycerides, glycerol and free fatty acids may therefore be found in the duodenum (see Figure 10.7b, p.238). Lipases continue their breakdown actions until all the fatty acids are removed from the ingested lipids.
- *Nucleic acid-digesting enzymes, or nucleases*: these include ribonucleases, which act on RNA, deoxyribonucleases, which act on DNA, and nucleotidases, which act on DNA fragments (Table 10.6). These enzymes are essential, since all foods consumed are of cellular origin and will usually contain nuclear components. Thus, we must break down the

components present, rendering them into a form that can be utilized within our own cells for the synthesis of our own nucleic acids during cell division.

Digestive secretions of the intestinal mucosa

Intestinal juice, called succus entericus, is a clear, yellow, alkaline (pH 7.6) fluid produced at a rate of 2–3 L/day from Brunner's glands in the duodenum and from the crypts of Lieberkühn in the ileum. The juice is mostly of a watery constitution, but it also includes a variety of digestive enzymes (Table 10.6). These enzymes are concerned with the final chemical breakdown of ingested foods. They include:

- *'Protein'-digesting enzymes (more correctly termed peptidases)*: a variety of dipeptidases are present in intestinal juice. These enzymes are responsible for breaking down dipeptides into individual amino acids. At this point, protein digestion is complete, and the endproducts of protein digestion, amino acids, can now be absorbed into the circulation.
- *Carbohydrate-digesting enzymes (or disaccharidases)*: this group includes three enzymes that are responsible for digesting disaccharides (molecules of two simple sugar units) into their constituent monosaccharides. The enzymes are named after the disaccharide that they break down: maltase converts the disaccharide maltose into its two constituent glucose molecules, lactase breaks down lactose into glucose and

---

BOX 10.16 MINIMAL ACCESS SURGERY: ENDOSCOPY

'Open' surgical procedures may have a major impact on the maintenance of homeostasis, and recovery may take many months. An alternative approach that has a lesser impact on homeostasis is referred to as 'minimal access surgery'. The access to body cavities is enabled by use of an endoscope ('endo-' = inside, '-scopy' = looking) to view internal structures. The equipment used will vary according to the cavity to be examined; the term 'endoscopy' tends to be used in association with the procedure for examining the gastrointestinal tract and specific names are given to other procedures:

Procedure	Organ visualized
Oesophagoscopy	Oesophagus
Gastroscopy	Stomach
Duodenoscopy	Early duodenum
Oesophogastroduodenoscopy	(The collective term for the above)
Colonoscopy	Rectum and colon
Laproscopy	Abdominal cavity

This chapter cannot explore all of these procedures. Instead this box will focus on upper gastrointestinal endoscopes (termed oesophogastroduodenoscopy).

Oesophogastroduodenoscopy (OGD) allows visualization of the oesophagus, stomach and proximal duodenum, the performance of certain surgical procedures, and the removal of tissue samples for biopsy. A flexible endoscope ('gastroscope'; 'gastro-' = stomach) is passed via the mouth into the oesophagus, stomach or proximal duodenum. The passage of the endoscope is monitored. The tip can be bent in several directions, and channels incorporated into the endoscope are used to suction secretions, to flush the tip, and to take samples of tissue for biopsy, as necessary. The endoscope may also be used to dilate constrictions, remove unwanted objects, and to arrest bleeding.

Common disorders that are diagnosed, and/or treated, using OGD include:

- Oesophageal carcinoma – a tumour in the oesophagus that is linked with smoking, high alcohol intake and a history of oesophageal trauma or gastro-oesophageal reflux. The majority of tumours appear in the lower two-thirds of the oesophagus.
- Oesophageal varices (see Box 10.7, p.241).
- Carcinoma of the stomach. The majorities of such tumours are located in the pyloric (i.e. lower) region. Patients often present late with anorexia and pain, and generally there is a poor prognosis.
- Gastritis (see Box 10.11, p.244).
- Ulceration (see Box 10.11, p.244).

The duodenum is the location where the bile duct and the pancreatic duct empty into the gut through the sphincter of Oddi. A form of OGD, referred to as endoscopic retrograde cholangiopancreatography (ERCP), uses a side-viewing endoscope so the sphincter of Oddi (see Figure 10.10, p.245) can be viewed. It is performed under X-ray, as radio-opaque dye is introduced into the bile duct to locate any blockages. Small stones can often be removed via this method. A wire can be introduced down the scope, which is inserted past the stone, then a basket or balloon on the end of the wire can be opened, and the wire withdrawn. This procedure can drag the stone into the duodenum, where it can be passed normally. If the bile duct has become blocked, a sphincterotomy can be performed, in which the end of the duct is cut and enlarged. Stents can also be inserted into the bile or pancreatic duct to allow free drainage of contents, correcting any narrowing. Other common disorders that are diagnosed, and/or treated, using ERCP include pancreatitis (see Box 10.13) and cancer of the pancreas.

galactose, and sucrase converts sucrose into glucose and fructose. Carbohydrate digestion is now complete, and monosaccharides can be absorbed into blood.

- *Fat-digesting enzymes (or lipases)*: these operate in the same way as pancreatic lipases (i.e. they remove fatty acids from glycerol). The breakdown products of fats are now absorbed into the blood and lymphatic circulation.
- *Intestinal nucleases*: these share the breakdown functions with pancreatic nucleases; they break down nucleic acids within the food chyme.

Regulation of the functions of the small intestine

The control of intestinal motility and secretions is mainly hormonal. However, parasympathetic neurons (via vagus, splanchnic and pelvic nerves) also play a part. The presence of food, and the resultant mechanical stimulation of the intestinal walls by food, causes a release of a variety of hormones, the main ones of which are:

- *Secretin:* released in response to the presence of an acidic chyme in the duodenum; causes the release of an alkali-rich pancreatic juice in order to buffer this acidity.
- *Cholecystokinin–pancreozymin* (CCK–PZ): stimulates the release of bile from the gall bladder and an enzyme-rich pancreatic juice. The stimulus for its release is a nutrient-rich chyme in the duodenum, in particular the presence of fats (note the role of bile in fat digestion).
- *Motilin:* responsible for stimulating a more forceful contraction of the intestinal muscles. It is thought to have a role in promoting a greater movement of food along the tract, particularly in the small intestine.

The secretion of intestinal 'juice' is thought to result from the mechanical contact of food with the intestinal mucosa. It is uncertain whether the mechanism of release is controlled hormonally or neurally. The intestine is also a rich source of putative hormones (i.e. substances such as bombesin with demonstrable action but which have yet to be accepted as genuine mediators of intestinal function).

Absorption

Absorption is the process whereby the endproducts of digestion and the ingested 'soluble' nutrients, which do not need to be broken down, are transported from the lumen of the alimentary tract into the body's transporting systems. Most nutrients are absorbed directly into blood, although long-chain fatty acids are absorbed into the lymphatic circulation. The ileum accounts for 90% of absorption, and is anatomically adapted for this process (Figure 10.13). Adaptations include:

- a large surface area. The ileum is very long (approximately 6.5 m), and the surface area of its lining is increased by many circular folds (plicae) and the finger-like projections, villi and microvilli;
- a very thin absorptive epithelium. The mucosal membrane is a simple columnar epithelium. This is constantly being dam-

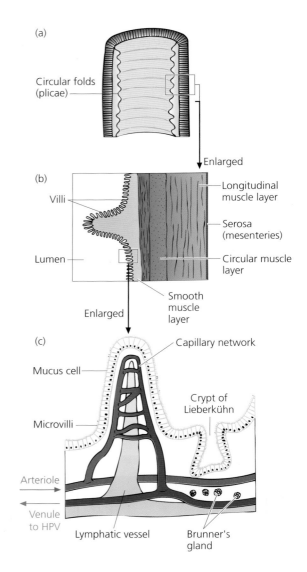

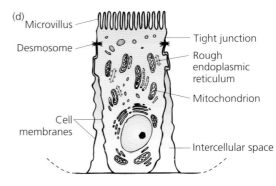

Figure 10.13 Villi: (a) longitudinal section of duodenum showing circular folds; (b) vertical section through one circular fold; (c) vertical section through one villus; (d) enlarged intestinal cell. HPV, hepatic portal vein

Q List the enzymes associated with pancreatic and intestinal juices, and identify their substrates and the breakdown products from these.

aged and worn away, so cells must be mitotically active (especially at the bases of the villi) in order to replace the cell loss;

- an extensive blood and lymphatic supply to the villi;
- a small extracellular space between the absorptive cell and the blood capillaries and lymphatic vessels;
- the walls of the blood and lymphatic vessels consist of a squamous (i.e. thin) endothelium.

The mouth, stomach and large intestine absorb the remaining 10% of the endproducts of digestion.

Nutrient absorption in the ileum

Absorption of materials occurs specifically through the epithelial membranes of villi. The process depends upon mechanisms involving facilitated and passive diffusion, osmosis, active transport and pinocytosis. These mechanisms were discussed in pages 28–33 and summarized in Table 2.2, p.27), and you are advised to refamiliarize yourself with these processes. Figure 10.14 summarizes the main processes involved in absorption.

BOX 10.17 ABSORPTION OF GLYCERYL TRINITRATE

Oral absorption is clinically useful. For example, the drug glyceryl trinitrate (GTN), used to treat angina, is absorbed sublingually (under the tongue), providing quick entry to the blood. The result is a rapid dilation of coronary blood vessels, leading to an improved delivery of arterial oxygen to the cardiac muscle, and so removing the ischaemic pain of angina.

Substances absorbed by the stomach include glucose, salts, a little water, and vitamin B_{12}. Alcohol is absorbed mainly in the small intestine (80%) and the stomach absorbs the remainder, hence its rapid effects and the obvious concern is of today's 'binge-drinking' culture in the UK. A large intake of protein decreases the rate of alcohol absorption from the stomach. Absorption by the large intestine, particularly the colon, is mainly that of water, although most of this is absorbed by the ileum.

There are two stages to the absorption process. First, the nutrient components must enter the luminal side (i.e. the apical membrane) of the epithelial cell, which involves a variety of

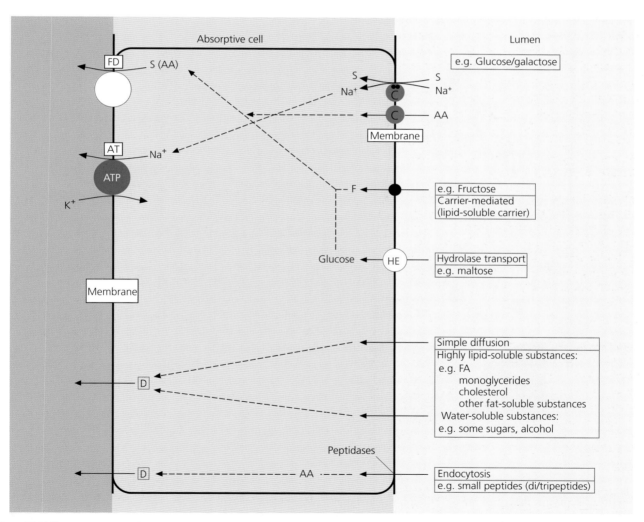

Figure 10.14 The transport mechanism of absorption in the ileum. AA, amino acid; C, carrier; D, diffusion; FA, fatty acid; FD, facilitated diffusion; HE, hydrolysing enzyme; S, sugar, AT, active transport

Q *How does passive diffusion differ from facilitated diffusion?*

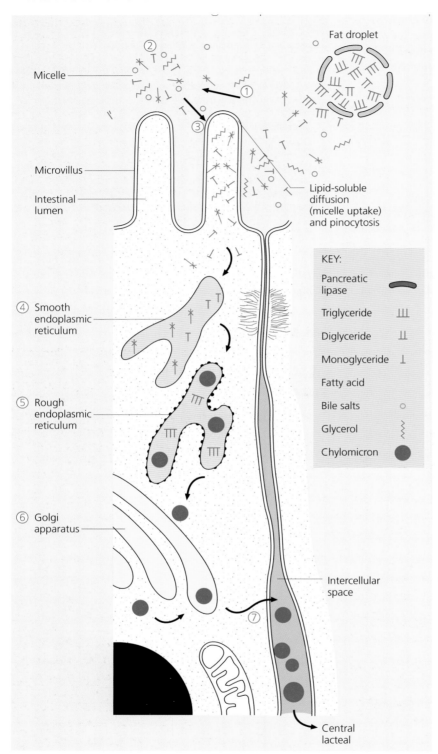

Figure 10.15 Transport of lipids from intestinal lumen through absorptive cells and into the interstitial space. Products of fat (triglyceride) digestion – monoglycerides, fatty acids and glycerol ① – form micelles ② with the bile salts in solution. They enter the absorptive cell by pinocytosis ③ across the microvillus membrane. Within the cell, the products accumulate in the smooth endoplasmic reticulum ④, from which they are passed to the rough endoplasmic reticulum ⑤. There, they are resynthesized into triglycerides and, together with a smaller amount of phospholipids and cholesterol, are stored in the Golgi complex as chylomicrons ⑥ – droplets about 150 nm in diameter. These then leave the cell ⑦

Q Identify the path of flow of long-chain fatty acids through the cardiovascular system from their entrance in the neck region to the liver.

different mechanisms, described below. Second, the materials must leave via the lamina propria (i.e. basolateral membrane) surface of the mucosal epithelial cell into the blood capillaries and central lymphatics, or lacteals. This relies mainly on passive diffusion.

Monosaccharide absorption

Fructose is transported into the epithelial cell by carrier-mediated facilitated diffusion. Glucose and galactose are transported in a similar way, but they are co-transported with sodium. Glucose and sodium share the same carrier protein, which contains two specific receptor sites (one for glucose, the other for sodium), both of which must be occupied before transport can take place. Monosaccharide absorption is completed by the terminal part of the ileum.

Amino acid absorption

This occurs mainly in the duodenum and jejunum. Facilitated diffusion co-transporting with sodium is the mechanism involved. Occasionally, dipeptides and tripeptides are absorbed into epithelial cells by pinocytosis, and the final stages of digestion occur within those cells.

Fatty acid absorption

There are two mechanisms for the absorption of fatty acids, depending on the length of the fatty acid chain. Short-chain fatty acids (i.e. those with fewer than 10–12 carbon atoms) pass into the epithelial cell and then into the circulation by simple diffusion because of their high lipid solubility. This accounts for approximately 20% of fat transported. Most dietary fats, however, contain long-chain fatty acids (those with more than 12 carbons atoms); these must combine with fat-soluble vitamins (A, D, E and K), glycerol, monoglycerides and bile salts to form a micelle-like structure, which is pinocytosed into the epithelial cell (Figure 10.15). Once inside the cell, the micelle breaks down into its component parts. The

bile salts and fat-soluble vitamins diffuse into the blood; the free fatty acids are combined with glycerol and monoglycerides to form triglycerides. Thus, the initial digestion of dietary fats is simply to facilitate the formation of this micelle so that fats, fat-soluble vitamins, and bile salts can collectively pass over the apical membrane of the epithelial cell.

Within the epithelial cell, the triglycerides become coated with a lipoprotein coat to form water-soluble structures called chylomicrons. These diffuse into the lymphatic minor drainage vessels or lacteals of a villus, and are transported via the lymphatic system into the thoracic lymphatic duct, which drains into the circulation at the junction of the left subclavian and left jugular veins in the neck (see Figure 13.3a, p.366). Finally, they arrive at the liver through the hepatic artery.

Cells that metabolize these substances contain lipoproteases, to break down the coat of the chylomicron, and triglyceridases, to release individual fatty acids.

The digestion and absorption of the three major nutrients of the diet are summarized in Figure 10.16.

ACTIVITY

Describe how endproducts of digestion are absorbed from the gut and taken to the liver.

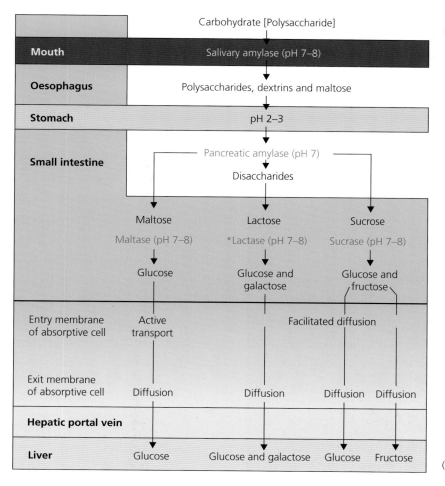

Figure 10.16 Summary of digestion and absorption: (a) carbohydrate; (b) protein; (c) fat

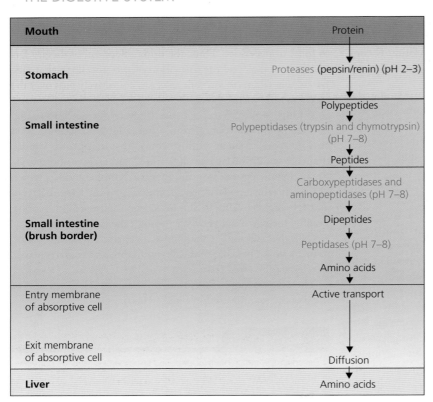

(b)

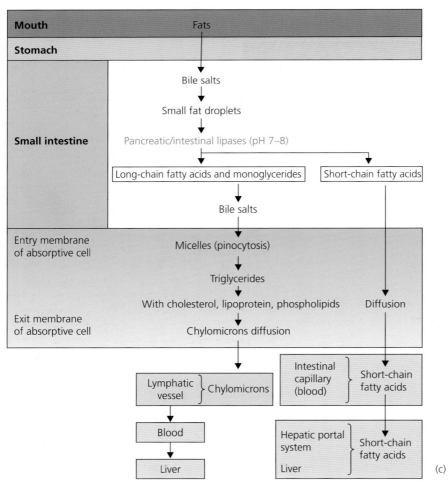

(c)

Figure 10.16 *Continued* Summary of digestion and absorption: (a) carbohydrate; (b) protein; (c) fat

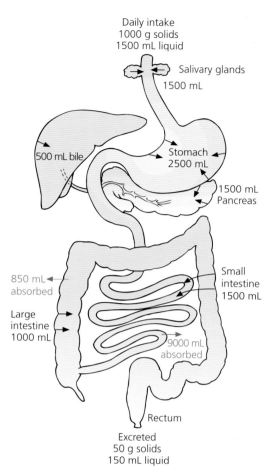

Figure 10.17 Water fluxes in the human alimentary canal, in millilitres. Figures vary with the condition and size of the subject

Q *How much water is absorbed each day?*

Absorption of water-soluble vitamins (B and C complexes)

These are absorbed by diffusion, although for vitamin B_{12} conjugation with the stomach's intrinsic factor of Castle is necessary.

Water absorption

About 10 L of water a day are absorbed. Of this, 1–2 L are from ingested (i.e. liquid and solid) sources (depending on thirst and social habits), and the remainder is from the accumulation of gastrointestinal secretions. As Figure 10.17 illustrates, the main area of absorption is the small intestine, which absorbs 9 L/day; the remainder is absorbed in the colon of the large intestine in order to consolidate the faeces. The absorption of water into intestinal epithelial cells, and then into the blood capillaries lining the villi, is via osmosis, which is promoted by the absorption of electrolytes and digested foods.

Absorption of electrolytes

Electrolytes are absorbed from gastrointestinal secretions and ingested components; they help to maintain electrolyte home-

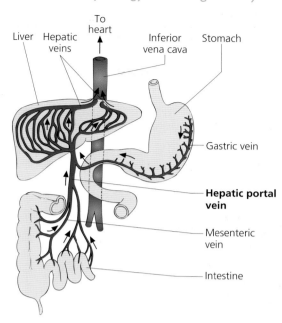

Figure 10.18 The hepatic portal system. Blood is carried directly from the stomach and intestines to the liver via the mesenteric, gastric and hepatic portal veins. Hepatic veins then convey it to the heart by way of the inferior vena cava

Q. *Structurally what differentiates the portal vessels in the body from arteries and veins?*

ostasis. In addition to active transport, electrolytes can also move in and out of cells by diffusion. Parathyroid hormone and, in particular, vitamin D are important in regulating the active transport of calcium from the gut (see Figure 9.10, p.217). Iron, magnesium, phosphate and potassium absorption is dependent upon active transport methods. Negatively charged ions (anions), such as chloride, iodide and nitrates, passively follow positive ions (cations), such as sodium.

Absorbed products pass via capillaries into venules, which drain from the intestinal wall into larger veins. These then link up with veins from other areas of absorption (stomach and colon) to form the hepatic portal vein. This large vessel carries the endproducts of digestion directly to the liver (Figure 10.18). All the absorbed components take this route, except for long-chain fatty acids, which pass to the liver via the hepatic artery after being drained into the lymphatic system, as discussed earlier. The liver assimilates the products, and has a role in the homeostatic control of the blood concentrations of some components. Some products of digestion or liver synthesis are then transported in blood to specific cells of the body that require them to sustain their intracellular homeostatic processes.

The large intestine

The large intestine extends from the ileocaecal valve to the external sphincter muscle of the anus, and is about 1.5–2 m long. It has a wider diameter (about 6.5 cm) than the small intestine, hence its name. The longitudinal muscle layer forms

BOX 10.18 SURGICAL LESIONS AND GASTROENTERITIS

Disorders of the small intestine commonly arise through surgical lesions, or as a consequence of inflammation of the stomach and the intestines (a condition called gastroenteritis). There is no appreciable difference in digestive and absorptive functions when quite a large amount (up to 50%) of the intestine is surgically removed. However, if less than 25% remains, digestion and absorption are so reduced that the patient can only survive via parenteral feeding (i.e. infusion of nutrients into a large vein).

Diarrhoea, vomiting, high temperature, and signs of dehydration characterize gastroenteritis. There are four main causes of gastroenteritis:

- infection (e.g. cholera, dysentery);
- metabolic and/or absorptive homeostatic imbalances (e.g. indigestion following excessive starch intake, diarrhoea following too much protein, and conditions such as coeliac disease that exhibit an inability to digest fat);
- emotional and nervous conditions (e.g. 'nervous diarrhoea');
- various other causes, such as allergies or tumours, although the latter occur most commonly in the colon.

Principles of correction depends on the aetiological factors, but generally food is withdrawn for a day or so, and drinking water is encouraged. Antibiotics and other drugs may not be given until the cause is established, since they may mask the cause of inflammation.

three bands, called taeniae, which are maintained in a tonic state of contraction, giving this part of the intestine a 'pouched' appearance. Structurally, the large intestine has four main areas: the caecum, colon, rectum and anal canal.

The caecum is the first pouch. Inferiorly, it leads to a blind-ended tube of lymphatic tissue called the appendix.

The colon consists initially of the ascending colon, which is superior to the caecum on the right abdominal side. The ascending colon passes vertically to the transverse colon, which lies just under the inferior surface of the liver (as the hepatic flexure). This extends across the abdominal cavity until it becomes the descending colon on the left side of the abdomen. After descending, the colon becomes the sigmoid colon, which projects to become the third principal part, the rectum.

BOX 10.19 DIVERTICULOSIS AND DIVERTICULITIS

Diverticulosis occurs when a small protrusion of the mucous membrane bulges out (herniates) through a weak part of the bowel's muscular wall, usually in the large intestine. Although the causes of diverticuli are unknown, diverticulosis tends to occur in older people with a long history of constipation; it is associated with a low-fibre diet (Camilleri *et al.*, 2000). An increase in dietary fibre intake frequently relieves symptoms; however, if the condition is extensive, or long-standing, and perhaps giving rise to symptoms of obstruction, it is often dealt with by removing the affected area of the bowel.

The diverticuli are usually numerous and become filled with stagnant faecal matter. Diverticulitis occurs when these pouches become infected. Acute diverticulitis (i.e. inflammation of the diverticuli) may proceed to abscess formation or peritonitis, and requires prompt surgical treatment. Chronic diverticulosis requires investigation to exclude the possibility of other conditions.

The investigations performed to detect diverticular disease include barium X-ray, and sigmoidoscopy to exclude carcinoma of the bowel.

BOX 10.20 APPENDICITIS

Inflammation or abscess formation occurs if stools, foreign bodies, tumour of the caecum, or a kinking of the beginning of the large intestine blocks the opening to the appendix. The inflammation that follows the obstruction is characterized by fever, and hence a high white cell (neutrophil) count. Localized pain is usually followed by loss of appetite, nausea and vomiting. The infection may cause oedema and ischaemia, and may progress to gangrene and perforation within 2–36 hours, producing inflammation of the peritoneum (peritonitis) as the faecal matter penetrates and irritates the abdominal cavity.

Correction is essentially an early surgical removal of the appendix (appendicectomy), since it is safer to operate than risk rupture, peritonitis and gangrene.

The rectum is about 16–20 cm long, and lies anterior to the sacrum and coccyx bones. Its terminal 2–3 cm become the fourth principal part of the large intestine, the anal canal.

The anal canal is richly supplied with arteries and veins. Its opening to the exterior is called the anus, which is regulated by two sphincter muscles. The internal sphincter muscle is controlled involuntarily, whereas the external sphincter is under voluntary control.

Homeostatic functions of the large intestine

Homeostatic functions of the large intestine include:

- storage of indigestible food until it is eliminated from the body;

BOX 10.21 HAEMORRHOIDS

Haemorrhoids, commonly known as piles, are dilated, enlarged and often inflamed venous vessels of the lower rectum and anal canal. External piles are dilations of the inferior rectal plexuses. They originate in the anal canal, and in many cases present with no symptoms, except an occasional burning sensation when a constipated motion is passed. Internal piles are dilations of the superior/middle rectal plexuses that occur in the part of the bowel and anal canal covered with mucous membrane. They may remain in the anal orifice, producing slight and intermittent bleeding on occasion, which can cause considerable pain, bleeding and itching. Extreme pain is associated with a dilated vein becoming thrombosed and inflamed. Most cases are caused by constipation and straining at stool, so avoiding constipation is an important preventive measure. A diet high in fibre is important, as stools are bulkier and of a softer consistency, which allows an easier passage through the intestine. Piles are also common in pregnancy because of the rise in intra-abdominal pressure, which can cause venous engorgement by compressing the gut.

Detection is by rectal examination, proctoscopy and/or sigmoidoscopy.

If the bowel is kept open with an appropriate diet and bland laxatives, then small piles usually subside. For more serious cases, an injection of an irritant fluid into the haemorrhoids may be necessary, causing scarring and obstruction to the distended vein. Surgical closure is seldom necessary. The most widely used principle of correction for bleeding piles that consistently cause severe pain is ligation of the pile. This cuts off the blood supply, and in a few days the pile dries up and falls off. Infrared photocoagulation, using high-energy light beams, may also be used to coagulate the haemorrhoids.

BOX 10.22 DIARRHOEA

Diarrhoea

Diarrhoea usually occurs when the intestinal movements are too rapid for adequate absorption of water, resulting in a large amount of water being eliminated. Diarrhoea can occur in bowel infections through food poisoning, certain foods in the diet, malabsorption syndromes, with use of laxatives or treatments such as radiotherapy and antibiotic therapy, and even anxiety (nervous diarrhoea) can increase bowel movements.

The causes of diarrhoea are summarized in Table 10.7.

Severe diarrhoea results in distressing pain and tenderness around the anal ring, a large loss of water and electrolytes (particularly sodium and potassium bicarbonate), resulting in dehydration and potential electrolyte imbalances (e.g. hypokalaemia – low blood potassium – and the loss of alkaline digestive juices of the intestine may cause metabolic acidosis; see Figure 6.5, p.133)

Although bowel problems may not be central to the patient's need for care, they can aggravate the primary problem if allowed to develop. The presence of diarrhoea is an important healthcare observation, and additional data obtained from further observations and questioning the patient can ascertain any associated evidence such as:

- frequency of bowel actions;
- the state of hydration, and food and fluid intake;
- the smell of the patient's breath;
- the condition of the patient's tongue;
- activity levels;
- quantity and consistency of stool passed (e.g. patients with high-fibre diets will produce large, soft stools, which should float in the lavatory);
- stool containing undigested food (occurs in conditions of intestinal hurry);

- colour of stool (a very bright red blood content may indicate damage to the rectal blood vessels, tarry black stools may indicate bleeding from the gastric or upper intestinal regions and pale stools may be the result of obstructive jaundice);
- heavy digestive bleeds are likely to be associated with other symptoms of blood loss (e.g. pallor, increased, but weakened pulse, low blood pressure and in the extreme case shock);
- odour of stool (a change may occur with malabsorption states);
- pain on passing stools (may indicate the presence of haemorrhoids, anal fissure or constipation);
- stool containing mucus (may signify an inflammatory condition in the gut). Inflammatory bowel disease is characterized by inflammation of the mucous lining of the gut with blood and mucus present in diarrhoea. A patient suffering from a severe inflammatory bowel disease may have 40 or more diarrhoea bowel evacuations in a 24-hour period; consequently they may sometimes experience sleep loss and severe restriction of activities of daily living.

An understanding of the facts gained from observation, combined with the knowledge of the underlying pathophysiology, allows the healthcare practitioner greater opportunities to make accurate decisions, for example, when to involve specialist medical staff.

Principles of correction depend upon the cause. However, routine treatment of simple cases is usually based on kaolin or chalk mixtures, which absorb toxins and allay intestinal irritation. Antibiotic therapy may also be used. Since there is fluid loss, sweetened drinks with a little salt are useful in restoring water and electrolyte balance. Severe diarrhoea may require intravenous infusion of a suitable solution (see Chapter 6, pp.134–135).

- secretion of mucus, which ensures lubrication of the faeces and eases the elimination process. Mucus also contributes to the alkaline pH of this region, because it contains HCO_3^- ions;
- absorption of most of the remaining water, electrolytes and some vitamins. The amount of water absorbed depends upon the length of time that the residue of food remains in the colon. Of this residue, 70% is eliminated within 72 hours of ingestion; the remainder may stay in the colon for a week or longer. The longer it stays there, the more water will be absorbed.

Symbiotic bacteria within the colon produce vitamin K and some of the vitamin B complexes (B_1, B_2 and folic acid). The small amounts of vitamin synthesized are not nutritionally significant, unless the individual has a diet that is deficient in these vital nutrients, in which case this may be regarded as a crude homeostatic mechanism for the maintenance of these vitamins in blood. The small amount of vitamin B_{12} produced in this region is also insignificant, as the vitamin is absorbed only in the small intestine, thus any produced or remaining in the colon is eliminated.

Bacteria also ferment any remaining carbohydrates, releasing gases (carbon dioxide, hydrogen and methane),

---

Table 10.7 Causes of diarrhoea and constipation

Diarrhoea	Constipation
Foods rich in spices, fruits such as gooseberries and prunes, high alcohol intake	Deficiency in dietary fibre
Distress	Depression and dementia
Drugs, e.g. antibiotics, iron preparations, laxatives	Drugs such as narcotic opiates (codeine, morphine, etc.), some antihypertensives (e.g. methyldopa), anticholinergics, and aluminium antacids
Neoplasms: malignant growths may result in a change in bowel habit, such as alternating periods of diarrhoea and constipation	Neoplasms: change in bowel habits brought about by intestinal growths can lead to alternating bouts of diarrhoea and constipation
Inflammation conditions of the gut, e.g. ulcerative colitis, irritable bowl syndrome, Crohn's disease (this increases peristaltic motions)	Inactivity
Malabsorption syndrome	Weak pelvic floor musculature
Pathogenic infective organisms, such as *Salmonella*, usually as a result of ingestion of contaminated foods; other symptoms include abdominal pain and nausea	Dehydration
Diverticulosis	Haemorrhoids
Thyrotoxicosis	Hyperthyroidism

BOX 10.23 CONSTIPATION

Constipation refers to a failure or difficulty with the passage of hard stools. It is the opposite of diarrhoea, in that the faeces are hard because of the absorption of most of the water, usually as a consequence of food residues remaining in the colon for long periods of time (e.g. when there is little fibre in the diet).

Constipation provides few external clues to its presence, and the healthcare practitioner usually relies on the recent history of bowel activity to identify the condition. Arguably, an average of one bowel evacuation per 24-hour is normal, so if a person goes 3 days without evacuation then there is a potential for constipation. The patients at risk of constipation are patients with inadequate food intake, reduced mobility, altered level of consciousness or a combination of these. It is not surprising that the elderly form a high risk category for this condition (Camilleri *et al.*, 2000); however, everyone at some time in their lives experiences constipation, and one should not be overly concerned about this. Conversely, if the condition becomes a chronic problem, then this is usually indicative of underlying pathology, such as bowel obstruction or poor bowel motility, as a consequence of chronic hypokalaemia (as occurs with certain diuretic drug therapies), chronic hypercalcaemia (as occurs with parathyroid hormone-secreting tumours) or use of analgesics such as morphine.

Other signs to help the practitioner's diagnosis of constipation include the abdominal distension because of food retention and pain because the faeces become difficult to eliminate, confusion, nausea and presence or absence of anorexia. In addition, halitosis, a furred tongue, headache, irritability and flatulence may also occur. The passage of hard stools may also result in the development of haemorrhoids (see Box 10.21).

The causes of constipation are summarized in Table 10.7.

The principles of correction of constipation involve the use of mild laxatives that induce defecation, and treatment of the underlying pathology. The management of constipation is a common routine hospital function.

The patient should be encouraged to adopt a comfortable squatting position, where possible; this is much more efficient for the process of defecation because sitting on a bed pan is uncomfortable and therefore does not aid defecation. The following preparations are commonly used in the hospital environment:

- oral or rectal lubricants (e.g. orally administered liquid paraffin or rectally administered glycine suppositories) serve to soften the faeces. Frequent use should be avoided, since the lubricants may interfere with the absorption of fat-soluble vitamins (A, D, E and K);
- gut stimulants (aperients; e.g. senna derivatives, bisacodyl and cascara) irritate the mucosa of the colon, and thus aid defecation;
- osmotic aperients [e.g. orally administered magnesium sulphate (milk of magnesia) or phosphate and lactulose administered as enemas] draw water into the lumen of the gut and the surrounding blood capillaries, causing a large watery stool;
- bulking agents (e.g. methylcellulose derivatives such as dietary fibre, Normacol or Celevac), reduce the mouth-to-anus transit time by attracting water to the gut contents, thus providing a bulky, relatively soft stool;
- manual evacuation of faeces: if the above methods fail to manage constipation, then manual removal may be performed in extreme circumstances. The patient will need an analgesic or sedative before this potentially painful and embarrassing procedure.

Constipation during pregnancy

Constipation is considered a minor disorder of pregnancy. It usually occurs as a result of the effects of progesterone on the smooth muscle of the gut. This reduces the peristaltic action and, together with increased water reabsorption of the colon, increases the risk of constipation. Pregnant women are encouraged to keep to a diet rich in fruit and vegetables, and to increase their fluid intake. Bran foods are also recommended.

---

which contribute to flatulence. The amount of flatulence varies according to the amount and type of food consumed (e.g. baked beans and onions increase the rate of fermentation and so lead to increased flatulence). Bacteria also break down any remaining proteins and fatty acids in the gut, and convert bilirubin into urobilinogen and stercobilirubin, which are responsible for the characteristic colours of the urine and faeces, respectively (see also Figure 11.7, p.279).

The caecum and ascending colon continue to absorb water, and the semi-liquid chyme is converted to semi-solid faeces. Components of the faeces include:

- water;
- inorganic salts;
- bacteria and components of bacterial decomposition;
- alimentary canal cells that have sloughed off;
- small amounts of the endproducts of digestion that have not yet been absorbed;
- excretory products (bile salts, bile pigments and mucus);
- indigestible remains (cellulose and vegetable fibres, known as roughage or fibre). Fibre is vital for correct bowel function and as such it has a protective role against bowel disease. Fibre absorbs and holds water, electrolytes and bile salts. Holding water ensures that the stool has an easy passage. The colon's absorption of water prevents the faeces from being too wet. The absorption of electrolyte and bile salts in the fibre itself aids the elimination of these substances.

Refined foods are those in which the fibre is largely removed or cooked sufficiently to change it to digestible carbohydrates and thus produce a higher degree of nutrition efficiency with less waste material. The refining of food is common in the Western world and has resulted in an increasing incidence of digestive disorders such as chronic cancers and diverticular disease. The latter is a condition in which the mucous lining of the bowel is pushed through the muscle wall into pouches that can become inflamed (called diverticulitis; see Box 10.19).

Rectal distension as a consequence of the accumulation of faecal matter stimulates rectal wall receptors, which send sensory neuronal input to the sacral region of the spinal cord,

BOX 10.24 PERITONITIS

Sluggish colonic movement is conducive to bacterial growth. These bacteria are potentially pathogenic if released into other areas of the body; for example if released into the abdominal cavity via intestinal perforation, or rupture of abdominal organs, such as the appendix, they may cause life-threatening acute inflammation of the peritoneum (peritonitis). Long-term antibiotic therapy results in a loss of these symbiotic bacteria, and encourages the colonization of this area with other potentially pathogenic antibiotic-resistant bacteria. A less serious form of peritonitis can result from the rubbing together of inflamed peritoneal membranes.

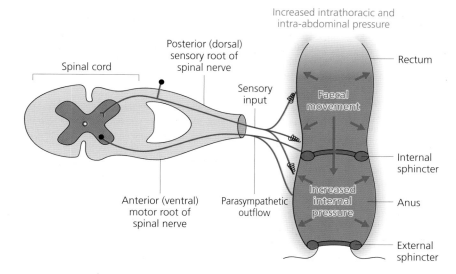

Figure 10.19 Defecation

resulting in parasympathetic output from the spinal cord to the rectum and anal canal, thus completing the reflex arc. Simultaneously, impulses pass via the spinal cord to the cerebral cortex, which means that we can voluntarily inhibit defecation, if necessary, through the control of the external sphincters (Figure 10.19). Defecation results from longitudinal muscle contraction, which causes a reduction in the length of the rectum, thus increasing the pressure within it. This increased pressure, together with voluntary contractions of diaphragmatic and abdominal muscles, forces the internal sphincter open; the faeces are expelled through the anus via the voluntarily relaxed external anal sphincter muscle (which is usually in a state of tonic contraction). The degree of rectal muscle contraction and straining required depends on the consistency of the faeces.

The gastrocolonic reflex is an important stimulus for defecation. This autonomic neural reflex occurs two to three times daily, usually following meals, and increases peristaltic wave activity to move food along the colon. This is more noticeable after breakfast because it is eaten when the stomach is empty. The gastrocolonic reflex results in an increased contraction of the terminal ileum, relaxing the ileocaecal valve and stimulating

BOX 10.25 LOWER GASTROINTESTINAL ENDOSCOPY

Lower gastrointestinal endoscopy includes colonoscopy and flexible sigmoidoscopy. This technique has replaced diagnostic laparotomy. Colonoscopy allows viewing of the large intestine. A flexible colonoscope, similar in design to the endoscope, can reach approximately 175 cm, while a flexible sigmoidoscope can view up to 60 cm of the bowel. This is useful in detecting abnormalities that occur mainly in the descending colon, rectum and anal canal (79% of cancers in the large intestine affect these regions; Davies *et al.*, 1998). These instruments are inserted into the anus, and pushed carefully along the bowel, guided by images projected onto a television screen. Similar to oesophapogastroduodenoscopy (OGD), treatment such as the removal of polyps can be performed and biopsies can be taken.

To view the colon effectively the colon must be empty of faeces. Picolax may be given the day before to completely clear faecal residue and an enema may be given on the day of the procedure.

The anal canal and rectum can also be viewed by rigid sigmoidoscopy. Carbon dioxide gas can be passed into the lower descending colon to view the mucosa. Proctoscopy can also examine the anorectal region.

The techniques of colonoscopy and flexible sigmoidoscopy carry risks of perforation, especially in a gut wall that has already been weakened by inflammation or disease.

Laparoscopy

Whereas OGD and colonoscopy utilize an orifice of the body to access the lumen of the gut, laparoscopy entails making an access into the abdominal (peritoneal) cavity. This involves the use of a rigid endoscope (a laparoscope) that is admitted into the peritoneal cavity via a guide inserted into an incision (called a port) in the abdominal wall. Images transmitted to a TV monitor facilitate the visualization of the peritoneal cavity through the anterior abdominal wall.

Laparoscopy may be used for diagnostic purposes, for example to look for lesions, adhesions, or growths that might explain the occurrence of abdominal pain. It may also be used for surgical removal of tissue, or for repair. Tissues removed or treated surgically relate to most of those organs that are accessible within the abdominal cavity. Surgical procedures commonly undertaken by laparoscopy include:

- *Cholecystectomy*: removal of the gall bladder, perhaps because of extensive stone formation.
- *Urolithectomy*: removal of stones from within the kidney.
- *Nephrectomy*: removal of a kidney, perhaps because of the presence of a tumour.
- *Hysterectomy*: removal of the uterus, perhaps because of the presence of a carcinoma.

BOX 10.26 INFLAMMATORY BOWEL DISEASE AND FAECAL INCONTINENCE

Inflammatory bowel disease

This term encompasses the two inflammatory conditions ulcerative colitis and Crohn's disease, which are believed to be different versions of the same autoimmune disease (O'Keefe, 2000). These conditions are characterized by spells of inflammation. In ulcerative colitis, the mucosa and submucosa of the large intestine are affected. In Crohn's disease, all layers of the tissue structure are affected, and inflamed segments can occur anywhere in the gastrointestinal tract. The inflammatory events caused by exacerbations of Crohn's disease can lead to fistula formation and narrowing, while the risk of colorectal cancer is increased by ulcerative colitis. Both conditions cause weight loss, diarrhoea, passage of blood and pain; the absorption of nutrients is impeded.

Detection of inflammatory bowel disease is performed by examination of diarrhoea, endoscopic examination and ultrasound to detect any abscesses.

Principles of correction depend on the severity of the symptoms. It is often treated with sulfasalazine (a combination of sulfa drugs and aspirin). Steroids are also given to suppress the inflammatory response and alleviate the cramping pain. Broad-spectrum antibiotics are prescribed if bacterial infection is suspected. If the condition becomes chronic and severe, then the patient is admitted to hospital and intravenous are fluids administered.

If there is persistent severe disease, or the risk of carcinoma is high, surgical intervention may be required, such as removal of part or the entire colon (called colectomy), or externalization of the ileum (called ileostomy), which bypasses the colon.

Faecal incontinence

Defecation is a reflex response to rectal distension. Faecal incontinence is an inappropriate emptying of the bowel, and may result from any of the following:

- severe fluid diarrhoea, because the sphincters are adapted to retain semi-solids or solid material and are inefficient at retaining fluids;
- fluid leakage around an impacted mass of hard faeces;
- profuse fluid discharge from some kinds of rectal growth.

Faecal incontinence is more common in older people. These people also have a greater risk of cerebrovascular accidents (strokes), following the sharp rise in blood pressure associated with exertion during elimination, especially during constipation. Older people also commonly exhibit deterioration of cerebral and spinal cord functions, which may result in defecation as soon as rectal distension occurs (Norton and Chelvanayagam, 2000).

Principles of correction vary. Rehabilitation through education removes the problem for some people. For others, the problem is incurable, in which case management may involve the use of incontinence pads and rubber sheeting.

---

colonic peristalsis. This reflex, therefore, allows filling of the colon; consequently, a mass movement of food residue occurs. The person becomes aware of this only when the faeces enter the rectum.

ACTIVITY

Describe the mechanism involved in defecation.

The liver

The liver is the largest gland in the body. The bulk of the liver occupies the right upper quadrant, or hypochondrium, of the

BOX 10.27 AGEING AND THE GASTROINTESTINAL TRACT

Voluntary control of the external anal sphincter muscle is learned as an infant through potty training. The delay to achieving this is due largely to the need for a maturation of the brainstem area involved, although psychological factors may also be operative.

The ageing process is associated with the following changes to the gastrointestinal tract:

- the motility and volume of the stomach, and the acid content of gastric juice, are reduced;
- intestinal villi become shorter and more convoluted;
- intestinal absorption, motility and blood flow all decrease, impairing nutrient absorption;
- the endproducts of digestion are absorbed more slowly, and in smaller amounts;
- rectal muscle mass atrophies (shrinks), and the anal sphincter weakens;
- constipation is common, and is related to immobility and a low-fibre diet.

abdominal cavity under cover of the lower ribs, which function to protect it (see Figure 1.4, p.7). On the left side of the abdomen, the liver lies superior to the upper part of the stomach, the presence of which explains why the bulk of the liver is on the right. Above the liver is the diaphragm, anterior to it is the anterior abdominal wall, and below it are the stomach, gall bladder, bile ducts, duodenum, right colonic flexure of the colon, the right kidney and the adrenal glands (Figure 10.2).

The liver is soft, and is extremely red because of its rich blood supply (approximately one-fifth of its weight is blood). Lacerations of the liver are dangerous, as the individual bleeds profusely and such injuries are difficult to repair.

Anatomy of the liver

The liver is covered almost entirely by peritoneum. It has two main lobes – a large right lobe and a smaller left lobe – separated by ligaments. The right lobe is associated with two further lobes called the inferior quadrate and posterior caudate lobes. The hepatic portal vein from the gastrointestinal tract enters the liver on its lower surface, and subdivides into smaller and smaller vessels, which finally enter a connecting (or anastomosing) system of smaller blood spaces called sinusoids.

The lobes of the liver are composed of microscopic structural and functional units known as the liver lobules (Figure 10.20a). A hexagonal capsule of connective tissue, called Glisson's capsule, surrounds each lobule. Internally, each lobule consists of chains or cords of cells referred to as hepatocytes. The cords are arranged radially around a central vein. Between the cords are the blood and bile sinusoids, which are equivalent to the circulatory capillaries of other tissues; they allow an exchange of substances between hepatocytes, blood and bile channels.

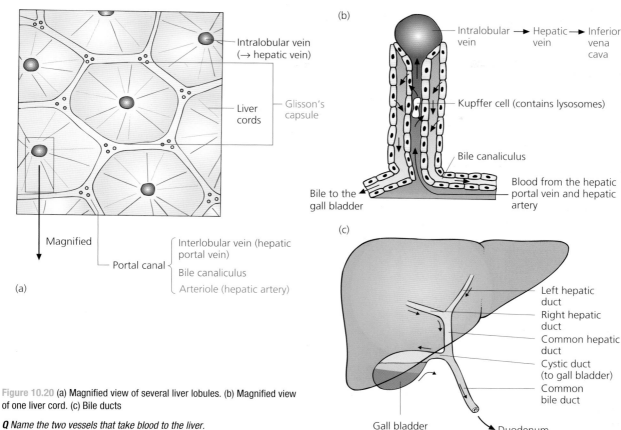

Figure 10.20 (a) Magnified view of several liver lobules. (b) Magnified view of one liver cord. (c) Bile ducts

Q Name the two vessels that take blood to the liver.

The blood sinusoids carry hepatic arterial (from an interlobular arteriole) and hepatic portal (from interlobular veins) blood from the edge of each corner of the hexagonal capsule to the central vein.

ACTIVITY

Using Figure 10.18, remind yourself of the origins of the hepatic portal vein.

Of the hepatic circulation, 80% of the blood is from the portal vein and 20% is from the hepatic artery, so these sinusoids contain a mixture of nutrient-rich (portal) venous blood and oxygen-rich arterial blood. Oxygen, nutrients and some poisons, such as alcohol, are extracted by the hepatocytes for assimilation or detoxification (see below). Also present within the sinusoids are reticuloendothelial (Kupffer) cells, which destroy bacteria and old erythrocytes and leucocytes. Sinusoidal blood drains into the intralobular (central) vein, which is a tributary of the hepatic vein that drains blood from the liver into the inferior vena cava and thence to the heart.

Bile channels are used in the transport of bile produced from the hepatocytes lining them. The flow of bile is in the opposite direction to that of blood, and so flows towards one of the small bile channels (bile canaliculi) at the corners of the hexagonal capsule (Figure 10.20b).

The corners of each liver lobule thus contain branches of the hepatic artery, the hepatic portal vein and a bile canaliculus. This collection of vessels is sometimes referred to as a hepatic triad (Figure 10.20a). Bile canaliculi drain into the right and left hepatic ducts, which then form the common hepatic duct. This transports the bile into the gall bladder via the cystic duct (Figure 10.20c). Bile is stored and concentrated in this bladder until the duodenum requires it. Bile production and the regulation of its release were discussed earlier in this chapter.

Homeostatic roles of the liver

The liver is an extremely important homeostatic organ. It is vital in the intermediate metabolism of many endproducts of digestion and has a homeostatic role as an assimilatory organ. It also has an exocrine role in the secretion of bile, which is conveyed to the gall bladder.

Assimilation

The liver is part of the reticuloendothelial system, which is involved in breaking down worn-out erythrocytes (see Figure 11.7, p.279) and removing the useful components of haemoglobin. For example, iron is extracted and used to maintain its homeostatic range within blood, in order to support the metabolic reactions that require it, such as the production of 'new'

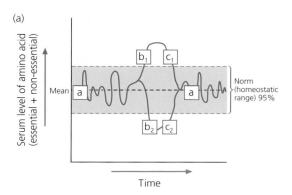

(a)

Figure 10.21 (a) The liver's utilization of the endproducts of globin breakdown: a, homeostatic pool of serum amino acids. b_1, Amino acids above their homeostatic range as a result of post-absorption of a protein-rich meal and/or excessive haemolysis (breakdown) of erythrocytes. b_2, Amino acids below their homeostatic range because of insufficient dietary protein. c_1, Restoration of serum non-essential amino acids levels by deamination of the excess into urea (ornithine cycle) and energy (glycolysis and Krebs cycle). c_2, Increased non-essential amino acids by transamination of excess of some amino acids into those below their homeostatic range and/or proteolytic breakdown and/or increased dietary intake, and increased essential amino acids via increased dietary intake. (b) Summary of the metabolic pathway for amino acids. (a, Represents boxes a_1–a_4 in Figure 1.7, p.11, reflecting the individual variability in the homeostatic range)

Q When does transamination occur?

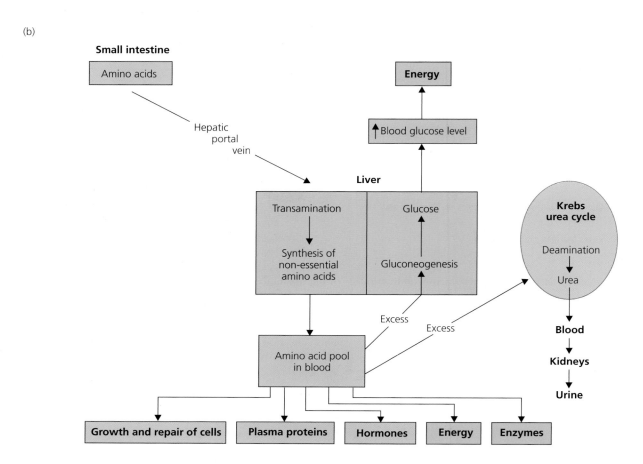

(b)

erythrocytes to replace the loss of 'old' ones. The globin part of the haemoglobin molecule is converted into its constituent amino acids, which are added to the essential and non-essential amino acid pools within the blood to help maintain their individual homeostatic values. If some of the non-essential amino acids are already within their homeostatic range, they can be converted (or transaminated) into other non-essential amino acids if necessary (Figure 10.21a). Conversely, if these amino acids are already within their homeostatic range, the excess may be broken down (or deaminated) into urea by the ornithine cycle of reactions and into glucose-like compounds, which are use to produce energy via glycolysis and the Krebs

cycle (see Figure 4.9, p.101). Figure 10.21b summarizes the metabolic pathway for amino acids.

Excess glucose molecules are taken from blood sinusoids into the hepatocytes to maintain blood glucose concentrations homeostatically (Figure 10.22a). As a consequence, the intracellular glucose within the hepatocytes may rise above its homeostatic range; this excess must be removed. Some of the excess is used in cellular respiration to sustain normal metabolic processes; the remainder is converted into the storage component glycogen by a process called glycogenesis. If there is still an intracellular excess of glucose when the cell stores of glycogen are full, it is converted into glycerol and hence to fat

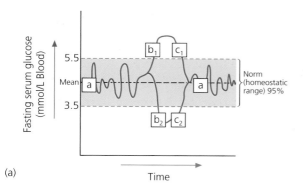

(a)

Figure 10.22 (a) The role of the liver in blood glucose regulation. (b) Normal blood glucose level. b_1, Elevation post-absorption of a meal. b_2, Decreased glucose levels owing to greater cellular uptake for increased metabolism. c_1, Glucose in excess of its homeostatic range taken into hepatocytes and skeletal muscle cells mediated by effects of insulin. Consequently, intracellular levels rise; this excess is used in cellular respiration and in promoting a glucose store in the form of glycogen (glycogenesis). If glycogen stores are full, then the excess glucose is converted into fat (lipogenesis) within fat stores throughout the body. c_2, Depressed glucose levels in the blood are corrected by measures such as glycogenolysis (i.e. glycogen is converted to glucose). If levels remain low, lipolysis (fat breakdown) and proteolysis (protein breakdown) occur. The latter occurs only in severe starvation states. c_2, Events mediated by glucagon, somatomedin, adrenaline, noradrenaline, thyroxine and the sympathetic nervous system act to increase glucose availability. (b) Summary of the metabolic pathway for monosaccharides (glucose, galactose and fructose). (a, Represents boxes a_1–a_4 in Figure 1.7, p.11, reflecting the individual variability in the homeostatic range)

Q Explain the paracrine role of somatostatin (refer to chapter 9 for help).

(b)

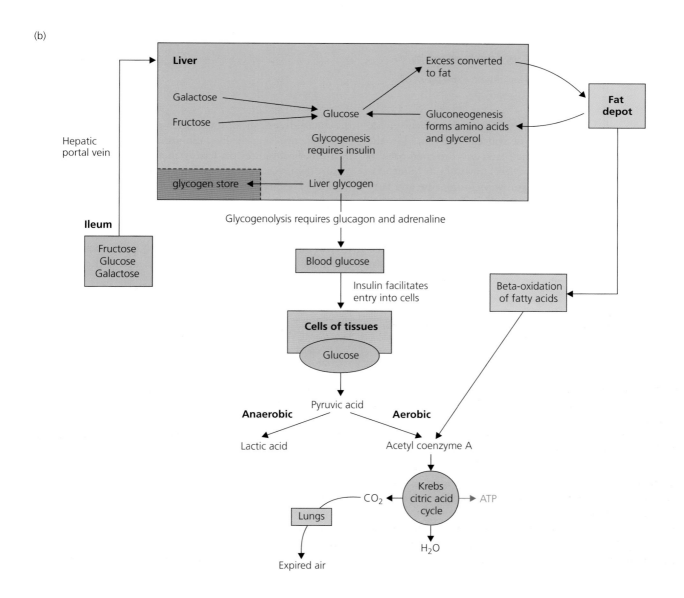

(c)

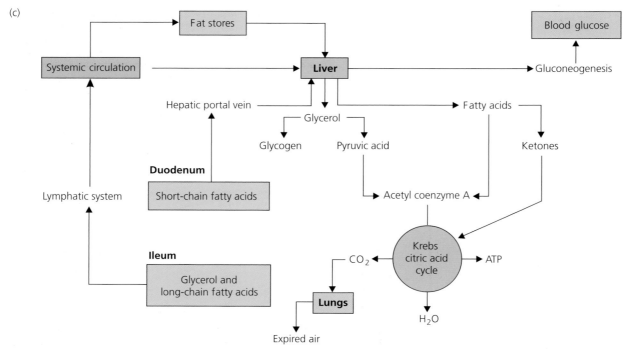

Figure 10.22 *Continued* (c) Summary of the metabolic pathway for fats

Q. What general name is given to enzymes involved in lipid digestion?

by a process called lipogenesis. Note that these mechanisms are reversible, so when blood glucose concentrations are low the glucose stores (first glycogen, then fats) are converted back to glucose to raise the blood glucose level to within its homeostatic parameters. The metabolic pathways for glucose and fatty acids are summarized in Figure 10.22b,c.

The fat-soluble vitamins (A, D, E and K), and the minerals iron (Fe) and copper (Cu), are stored by hepatocytes when the absorption of a meal produces blood levels in excess of their individual homeostatic ranges. Excess water-soluble vitamins (C and B complexes), water and other minerals pass through

the sinusoids, except for those taken into hepatocytes for their metabolic needs, as the liver cannot store them, transfer them into other substances or destroy them. The body's excretory organs then remove these excesses in order to maintain their individual homeostatic levels (Figure 10.23).

Excess fatty acids and glycerol are converted into glucose only if hypoglycaemia is present and there are inadequate glycogen stores. Otherwise, these substances pass through the liver to the storage regions of the body (i.e. the adipose tissues under the skin and surrounding organs such as the heart and kidneys).

BOX 10.28 THE LIVER AND ALCOHOL

Alcohol undergoes detoxification in the liver. The enzyme alcohol dehydrogenase speeds up the detoxification (oxidation) process that converts alcohol to acetaldehyde. This chemical is converted to acetyl coenzyme A, which is used in the same way as it is when it is produced from carbohydrates, fats and proteins, i.e. it is used to produce energy (ATP) via the Krebs cycle (see Figure 4.9, p.101).

Individuals vary in their ability to metabolize alcohol, and alcoholics can metabolize more since continued exposure accelerates the enzymes involved in chemical breakdown. The Health Education Authority recommends that men should drink no more than 21 units of alcohol per and women should drink no more than 14 units per week. One unit of alcohol is equivalent to half a pint of beer, or one 175 mL glass of wine, or a single measure of spirit.

Over-consumption of alcohol stimulates the formation of collagen, which damages cellular organelles; the resultant fibrosis impedes the passage of substances between blood and the liver cells. Such damage

is reversible at first, if alcohol is removed. However, if overindulgence is continued, the person may develop cirrhosis (irreversible scarring leading to portal hypertension, Figure 10.24, and loss of hepatocytes) and/or jaundice (Figure 10.25) may occur, both of which may be fatal.

Cirrhosis may also arise from chronic progressive inflammation caused by a parasitic infection. Cirrhosis is classified depending upon the cause. The scarred tissue impairs liver function as fibrosed or adiposed connective tissue cells replace the normal functional liver cells. Other complications arise, such as congestion of the hepatic portal vein, abdominal oedema, uncontrolled bleeding, and an increased sensitivity to drugs.

Control primarily involves preventing further damage (e.g. by the avoidance of alcohol intake in alcoholic cirrhosis) and taking vitamin supplements to ensure optimal conditions for tissue repair, regeneration and function. Liver transplants can be successful for the treatment of end-stage liver disease.

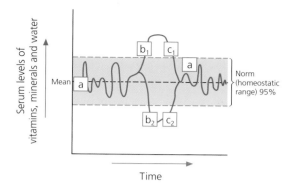

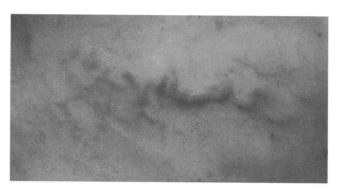

Figure 10.23 The role of the liver in vitamin, mineral and water regulation. (a) Normal levels of vitamins, minerals and water pre-absorption. b_1, Increased levels of vitamins, minerals and water above their homeostatic ranges following dietary intake. b_2, Decreased levels of vitamins, minerals and water below their homeostatic ranges as these nutrients are used in metabolism. c_1, Excess fat-soluble vitamins (A, D, E and K) and minerals (iron and copper) are stored in hepatocytes. Excess water-soluble vitamins (C and B complexes), other minerals and water pass through the liver to the excretory organs in order to restore their homeostatic ranges. c_2, Corrective measures to restore these nutrients to within their serum homeostatic ranges (i.e. the liver releases its stores of fat-soluble vitamins, iron and copper). Water-soluble vitamins, other minerals and water must be consumed to restore their homeostatic ranges. (a, Represents boxes a_1–a_4 in Figure 1.7, p.11, reflecting the individual variability in the homeostatic range)

Q *Describe the secretory, storage and detoxification assimilative roles of the liver.*

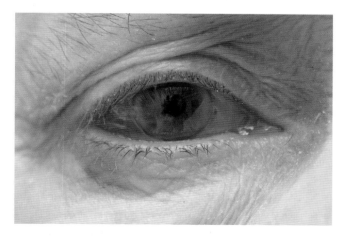

Figure 10.24 Cirrhosis. Abnormal blood flow pattern in the liver caused by cirrhosis resulting in portal hypertension. The increased pressure is transferred to collateral dilated venous channels seen here on the patient's abdomen. Reproduced with the kind permission of the Medical Illustration Department, Norfolk and Norwich University Hospital NHS Trust

Figure 10.25 Ischaemic hepatitis which is indicated by jaundice around the eyes. Reproduced with the kind permission of the Medical Illustration Department, Norfolk and Norwich University Hospital NHS Trust

Secretory functions

The liver secretes bile salts, which are important in emulsification (described earlier) and the absorption of fats, phospho-

lipids and lipoproteins. The anticoagulant heparin, and the plasma proteins, are also produced and secreted by the liver.

Detoxification/deactivation functions

The liver contains detoxifying enzymes, which are responsible for transforming poisons such as alcohol into harmless substances. Similarly, ammonia produced when excess amino acids are deaminated to provide energy is converted into urea. Moderate amounts of urea are harmless to the body, and the kidneys and the sweat glands easily excrete the excess. The liver also deactivates various hormones, thus reducing their blood concentrations and hence their physiological activities.

Storage functions

In addition to the storage of the various nutrients, the liver also stores some poisons (e.g. the insecticide DDT) that cannot be broken down and excreted.

Other functions

Because liver cells have hundreds of enzymes, the organ is responsible for at least as many important homeostatic functions, some of which remain to be identified. For example, the liver, together with the kidneys, is involved in the activation of vitamin D, and it contributes indirectly to the regulation of blood pressure by synthesizing angiotensinogen, the precursor of the hormone angiotensin.

As a result of the liver being involved in a large number of metabolic reactions, it is inevitable that many of these give off heat. Thus, the liver is an important contributor to thermoregulation.

The common laboratory tests of liver function are summarized in Table 10.8.

ACTIVITY

Identify a homeostatic failure associated with each region of the gut. Suggest the principles of correction associated with the failures you have named.

BOX 10.29 DEVELOPMENT OF THE LIVER

The liver is responsible for approximately 55% of the total body weight at birth, and is largely responsible for the protuberant abdomen of infancy. As growth rate slows during childhood, there is a corresponding decline in metabolism and, as a result, the liver becomes proportionately smaller; in the adult, the liver represents approximately 2.5% of the body weight. As a result of the ageing process, the size and weight of the liver decrease, and blood flow to the liver decreases, decreasing the efficiency of drug metabolism.

BOX 10.30 HEPATITIS

Hepatitis is an inflammation of the liver that may arise as a result of poisoning from various drugs or, more commonly, from one of five types of viral infection. *Hepatitis A virus* (HAV) (previously known as infectious hepatitis) tends to occur as local outbreaks, and is transmitted by the faecal–oral route (i.e. faecal contamination of food). An attack usually starts with the appearance of jaundice and bile-coloured urine, following signs of toxaemia, loss of appetite and fever. It does not cause lasting liver damage, and most patients recover in 4–6 weeks.

Hepatitis B virus (HBV) (formerly known as serum hepatitis) may be transmitted through contaminated syringes and transfusion equipment, or by other body secretions, such as tears, saliva or semen. The virus may produce chronic liver inflammation, which can persist throughout the person's lifetime. HBV is a hazard that must be considered during blood transfusion, renal dialysis and transplant surgery. Infected patients are also at increased risk of cirrhosis. Even when recovery is complete, patients can remain carriers of the virus.

Hepatitis C virus (HCV) is similar to HBV, and is often transmitted through blood transfusion. *Hepatitis D virus* (HDV) and *Hepatitis E virus* (HEV) have also been identified.

These infections can all cause acute hepatitis; HBV and HCV can also cause chronic hepatitis.

There is no specific treatment for acute viral hepatitis. In most patients the disease is self-limiting with full recovery. A low-fat, high-carbohydrate diet is beneficial if bile flow is obstructed. Physical activity may be restricted. Interferon alpha can be useful in the treatment of chronic hepatitis B and hepatitis C, and thymosin may be a promising new treatment for hepatitis B.

To prevent transmission of hepatitis A, washing the hands and using gloves for disposing of bed pans and faecal matter are imperative. The administration of immunoglobulins before exposure or early in the incubation period can prevent hepatitis A and hepatitis B. Vaccines are available to protect against hepatitis A and hepatitis B infections. Prophylaxis is recommended for healthcare workers and others who are at risk of contact with infected body fluids, particularly children (Jefferson *et al.*, 2001).

Table 10.8 Common laboratory tests for liver function

Test	Homeostatic range	Clinical significance
Serum enzymes		
Alkaline phosphatase	13–39 U/mL	↑ With biliary obstruction and cholestatic hepatitis
Aspartate amino transferase	5–40 U/mL	↑ With hepatocellular injury
Lactate dehydrogenase (LDH)	200–500 U/mL	↑ Isoenzyme LDH_5 with hypoxic and primary liver injury
Bilirubin metabolism		
Serum bilirubin		
Indirect (unconjugated)	< 0.8 mg/dL	↑ With haemolysis
Direct (conjugated)	< 0.2–0.4 mg/dL	↑ With hepatocellular injury or obstruction
Total	< 1.0 mg/dL	↑ With biliary obstruction
Urine bilirubin	0	↓ With biliary obstruction
Urine urobilinogen	0–4 mg/24 hours	↑ With haemolysis
Serum proteins		
Albumin	3.5–5.5 g/dL	↓ With hepatocellular injury
Globulin	2.5–3.5 g/dL	↑ With hepatitis
Total	6–7 g/dL	
Transferrin	250–300 µg/dL	Liver damage with ↓ values, iron deficiency with ↓ values
Blood clotting functions		
Prothrombin time	11.5–14 seconds	↑ With chronic liver disease (e.g. cirrhosis) or vitamin K deficiency
Partial thromboplastin time	25–40 seconds	↑ With sever liver disease or heparin therapy

Table 10.9 Dukes staging of colorectal cancer

Dukes stage	Severity of the cancer
A	Only mucosa and submucosa affected
B	Muscle wall involved, but no lymph node involvement
C	Lymph nodes have been infiltrated
D	Metastases present, or severe spread – cure impossible

Information from http://www.cancerhelp.org.uk

BOX 10.31 COMMON CANCERS OF THE GASTROINTESTINAL TRACT

Oesophageal carcinoma

A tumour in the oesophagus is usually linked with smoking, high alcohol intake and a history of oesophageal trauma or gastro-oesophageal reflux. The patient tends to present late with dysphagia (difficulty in swallowing). The majority of tumours appear in the lower two-thirds of the oesophagus, and can be detected by gastroscopy, computerized axial tomography (CAT) or computed tomography (CT) scan and ultrasound.

Carcinoma of the stomach

Most tumours are located at the pyloric region, and have a poor overall prognosis. Patients often present late with anorexia and pain. Diagnosis can be made from biopsy during gastroscopy.

Carcinoma of the liver

Secondary tumours occur most frequently in the liver, although primary lesions also occur, usually in the right lobe, which can infiltrate the portal vein, causing portal hypertension. Secondary deposits can occur anywhere in the liver. Spread is possible into nearby lymph nodes or pleura. As the liver enlarges, its capsule stretches, causing pain.

Blood tests and biopsy can detect the carcinoma. Ultrasound or CT scan can indicate the extent of the lesion.

Cancer of the pancreas

Cancer of the pancreas is a common cancer experienced in both men and women. It is often found in the head region of the organ. Frequently, the patient experiences jaundice and weight loss. An obstruction of the bile duct may be cleared by endoscopic retrograde cholangiopancreatography (see Box 10.16, p.249), but this condition carries a poor prognosis for the patient, as spread is common.

Colorectal cancer

This type of malignancy is now very common and is linked to a low-fibre diet. A higher risk of colonic cancer is evident in ulcerative colitis. As in carcinoma of the stomach, patients often present late, as symptoms are often vague and unthreatening, such as a change in bowel habit. Endoscopy can be employed to detect a mass and ultrasound or CT scanning can search for any spread to surrounding tissues. The system of Dukes staging is often used to class the severity of the carcinoma once it has been detected (Table 10.9).

SUMMARY

1 Provided that a balanced diet is ingested, the digestive system ensures that cells receive the nutrients (metabolites) necessary for their correct functioning (metabolism).
2 Digestion is the breakdown of food. It involves physical processes (provided mainly by specialized gut movements), and chemical processes (i.e. hydrolysis). Chemical digestion is accelerated by specific enzymatic actions.
3 Hydrolysis converts large, insoluble molecules into small, soluble molecules, which can be absorbed into the blood.
4 The digestive system consists of an alimentary canal and several accessory organs.
5 Various regions of the canal are adapted to perform specialized functions:
  a The mouth is adapted to receive food, initiate digestive processes, and perform a limited amount of absorption. It also serves as the organ of speech.
  b The salivary glands secrete saliva, which moistens food, helps bind food particles together, initiates carbohydrate digestion, makes taste possible, and helps cleanse the mouth, gums and teeth.
  c The pharynx and oesophagus act as passageways for boli of food.
  d The stomach receives boli of food, mixes them with gastric juice, initiates protein digestion, performs limited absorption duties and passes chyme into the small intestine.
  e The small intestine receives secretions from the pancreas and the gall bladder, completes digestion of food, absorbs most of the end-products of digestion and transports the indigestible remains to the large intestine.
  f The large intestine absorbs water and electrolytes, and stores and expels the faeces.
  g Fibre is important for correct bowel function and provides protection against bowel disease. Lack of fluid or fibre in the diet and a lack of exercise are important factors in constipation.
  h The pancreas is a mixed gland, having both endocrine and exocrine tissue. Its exocrine secretion, pancreatic juice, contains many enzymes that, together with intestinal juice and bile components, complete the digestive process.
  i The gall bladder receives bile from the liver, and stores and concen-

trates it until it is required by the small intestine. Bile is involved in emulsification.
  j The liver assimilates most of the absorbed nutrients in order to prevent nutrients being in excess of their homeostatic ranges within blood, and to synthesize other vital biochemicals.
6 Food is moved through the alimentary canal principally by peristalsis.
7 Homeostatic imbalances can result from:
  a malnutrition (i.e. insufficient intake of nutrients, or from an overindulgence of nutrients);
  b disturbances in the ability to chew or swallow food. In the mouth, such disturbances can result from poor functioning of the mucous membranes, teeth, gums, tongue or salivary glands;
  c problems affecting pharyngeal or oesophageal function, including tonsillitis, hiatus hernia and oesophageal diverticulosis;
  d disorders of the stomach, the symptoms of which are often exacerbated by the high acidity of gastric juice. Disorders may arise because of localized inflammation (e.g. gastritis), and ulceration of the gastric mucosa is a relatively common disorder. Nausea and vomiting are frequently associated with stomach disorders;
  e disorders of the small intestine, which commonly relate to disturbances in enzyme or mucous secretion, or in absorption. Since many digestive enzymes originate from the pancreas, pancreatic infections (pancreatitis) or blockage of ducts (as in cystic fibrosis) will disturb the digestive process. More commonly, however, disorders arise through surgical lesions or as a consequence of gastroenteritis;
  f disorders of the large intestine, which are relatively common, and include inflammation, which may be localized as in appendicitis, ulcerative colitis and diverticulitis. Rectal function disturbance as a result of blood vessel congestion (haemorrhoids) is also relatively common;
  g disorders of the liver, which may compromise the utilization of the products of digestion and the production of bile.
8 Mucus in diarrhoea is sign of excessive inflammation of the bowel's mucous membranes that results in all the production of mucus, as occurs in inflammatory bowel disease.
9 Blood in the stools may indicate a bleed somewhere within the colon, if fresh, or a bleed within the stomach or ileum, if darker, colon or rectal–anal regions.

REFERENCES

Agrawal, S. and Jonnalagadda, S. (2000) Gallstones, from gallbladder to gut: management options for diverse complications. *Postgraduate Medicine* **108**(30): 143–53.

Camilleri, M., Lee, J.S., Viramontes, B., Bharucha, A.E. and Tangalos, E.G. (2000) Progress in geriatrics. Insights into the pathophysiology and mechanisms of constipation, irritable bowel syndrome, and diverticulosis in older people. *Journal of the American Geriatrics Society* **48**(9): 1142–50.

Chowdhury, P. and Rayford, P.L. (2000) Smoking and pancreatic disorders. *European Journal of Gastroenterology and Hepatology* **12**(8): 869–77.

Davies, P., Button, C. and Foster, M. (1998) Rectal bleeding. *Nursing Times* **16**: 46–9.

Fass, R., Pulliam, G., Johnson, C., Garewal, H.S. and Sampliner, R.E. (2000) Symptom severity and oesophageal chemosensitivity to acid in older and young patients with gastro-oesophageal reflux. *Age and Ageing* **29**(2): 125–30.

Jefferson, T., Demicheli, V., Deeks, J., MacMillan, A., Sassi, F. and Pratt, M. (2001) Vaccines for preventing hepatitis B in health-care workers. *The Cochrane Library*, Issue 1. Oxford: Update Software.

McArdle, J. (2000) The biological and nursing implications of pancreatitis. *Nursing Standard* **14**: 46–51.

Norton, C. and Chelvanayagam, S. (2000) A nursing assessment tool for adults with fecal incontinence. *Journal of WOCN* **27**(5): 279–91.

O'Keefe, T. (2000) Irritable bowel syndrome (IBS): holistic treatment approach. *Positive Health* (59): 35–7.

CHAPTER 11

THE CARDIOVASCULAR SYSTEM 1: BLOOD

INTRODUCTION

The circulating blood acts as an intermediary between the external environment (outside the body) and the internal environment (tissue fluid and cells). Figure 11.1 illustrates the constant interchange between the external environment and body fluids for the maintenance of extracellular and intracellular homeostasis. The importance of blood as an intermediary tissue cannot be overemphasized: any area of the body deprived of the contents of circulating blood will be subjected to functional impairment, resulting in tissue death within a matter of minutes if the circulation is not restored. A number of homeostatic functions can therefore be ascribed to blood and the circulatory system in relation to the composition of the internal environment, but also in relation to defence of tissues.

Respiratory gases

The blood transports oxygen from the lungs to cells for the process of cellular respiration (i.e. the energy-producing process involving the breakdown of food). Carbon dioxide is a product of cellular respiration, and the excess (i.e. level above its homeostatic range) must be removed from the cells to prevent a pH imbalance. Carbon dioxide diffuses into blood, which then transports it to the lungs for excretion. This removal from the blood is necessary to prevent homeostatic imbalances also occurring in this body fluid (see pp.128–33 for short-term, intermediate and long-term regulation of acid–base homeostasis of body fluid).

Metabolic wastes

Metabolic wastes are generally considered to be substances that cannot be metabolized by cells. They also include useful substances in excess of their homeostatic ranges that cannot be stored, destroyed, or transferred into other metabolites. The blood transports these substances from the tissues to the excretory organs for removal from the body, in order to prevent consequential build-up to toxic levels (see Figure 6.3, p.126).

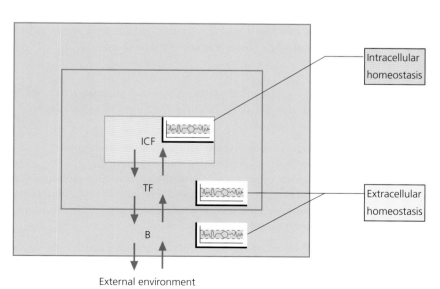

External environment

Figure 11.1 The interchange between external and internal environments in order to maintain homeostasis. Component intake must match component output in order to achieve extracellular and thus intracellular homeostasis. B, blood; ICF, intracellular fluid; TF, tissue fluid

Q Suggest why the composition of blood is important for intracellular homeostasis.

Nutrients

The endproducts of digestion are transported to the liver for processing or assimilation (see Figures 10.16, pp.253–4 and 10.18, p.255). Nutrients from storage areas (e.g. fats from adipose tissue and proteins from muscle tissue) are transported to cells requiring them for their own metabolic processes. Fats and proteins can be used to produce energy in cells when the body has depleted its carbohydrate reserves, and may also be assimilated into other cellular processes.

Regulatory materials

Hormones and enzymes and are taken from their sites of production to their target cells (see Tables 9.1, p.211, and 10.6, p.248, respectively).

pH and electrolyte composition

Buffer chemicals in blood and intracellular fluid contribute to the homeostatic regulation of body fluid pH (acid–base) balance and, to some extent, the electrolyte composition of the body fluids. Acid–base regulation is essential for the optimum functioning of enzymes, and hence metabolism, within these fluid compartments. Blood is slightly alkaline (mean pH 7.4), while cells are slightly acidic (mean pH 6.8).

ACTIVITY

Refer to previous chapters to reflect on your understanding of the following: the liver's role in assimilation (Chapter 10, pp.260–5), enzymes as the 'key chemicals of life' (Chapter 1, p.8 and Chapter 4, pp.97–9), and the role of genes in the process of protein (enzyme) synthesis (Chapter 2, pp.39–41).

Thermoregulation

Cells must release heat generated by metabolism in order to prevent intracellular imbalances, since optimal enzyme action occurs within a narrow temperature range. The removal of heat from cells by blood may cause blood temperature to rise above its homeostatic range. This occurs when cellular metabolism is high, as in strenuous exercise, fever and illness, and times of distress. The excess heat is distributed to the skin surface, where it is dissipated (see Figure 16.7, p.456). Alternatively, heat may be redistributed to areas of the body that require warming, when their regional temperatures have fallen below their homeostatic ranges. Normally the temperature of blood is about 38°C; the normal body temperature varies between different sites in the body (see Figure 16.8, p.456).

Haemostasis

Blood clotting helps preserve body fluid homeostasis by restricting fluid loss through damaged vessels or injury sites, a process called haemostasis (see Figure 11.15, p.291). This helps prevent excessive loss of extracellular fluids, which could seriously affect blood pressure and cardiovascular function.

BOX 11.1 ELECTROLYTE DISTURBANCES

Blood electrolyte disturbances in individuals are a reflection of intracellular imbalances (see Table 1.3, p.11 for normal values). For example, hyponatraemia (sodium deficiency in the blood) can be a result of severe diarrhoea and vomiting (often abbreviated as D&V). It causes a reduction in extracellular fluid volume, resulting in hypotension (low blood pressure), weakness, dizziness, mental confusion and fainting because of the diminished transport of metabolites to the cells. Details of electrolyte disturbances can be found in Chapter 6, pp.127–8.

Cellular defence mechanisms

White blood cells and antibodies in the blood are instrumental in defending the body against potential disease-causing microbes (pathogens) and their poisonous chemical secretions (toxins). These processes are described in more detail in Chapter 13. The blood also transports toxic substances to the liver and kidneys, where they are detoxified and excreted.

Blood is in constant interaction with tissues, hence its functions will clearly overlap with those of various tissues and organs (Box 11.1). Many of these roles, such as pH regulation, temperature regulation and gas transport are described elsewhere in the appropriate chapters. Blood is a tissue in its own right, however, and its cellular components and capacity to be transformed from a liquid to a semi-solid clot will be described in this chapter.

OVERVIEW OF THE COMPOSITION OF BLOOD

The volume of blood circulating in the cardiovascular system averages 5–6 L in males and 4–5 L in females. It accounts for approximately 8% of the total body weight. Blood appears to be a uniform (homogeneous), dark red, viscous liquid that, if left to stand for a few minutes, normally clots or solidifies. Microscopic investigation reveals, however, that blood is a mixture of cell types, suspended in a fluid compartment called plasma. Plasma and red blood cells account for about 55% and 44% of a blood sample, respectively. The remaining 1% consists of white blood cells and platelets (Figure 11.2).

Plasma

The blood contains some 2.5–3 L of plasma, a pale yellow fluid of which 90% is water. The remaining constituents of plasma include:

- plasma proteins (albumins, globulins, fibrinogen);
- regulatory chemicals (enzymes, hormones);
- various other organic chemicals, including nutrients (e.g. glucose, amino acids, fatty acids and glycerol), cholesterol, and waste products of metabolism (e.g. urea and creatinine);
- inorganic substances (electrolytes).

These components give plasma a greater density and viscosity than water. The dissolved proteins make this fluid sticky, cohesive and resistant to flow.

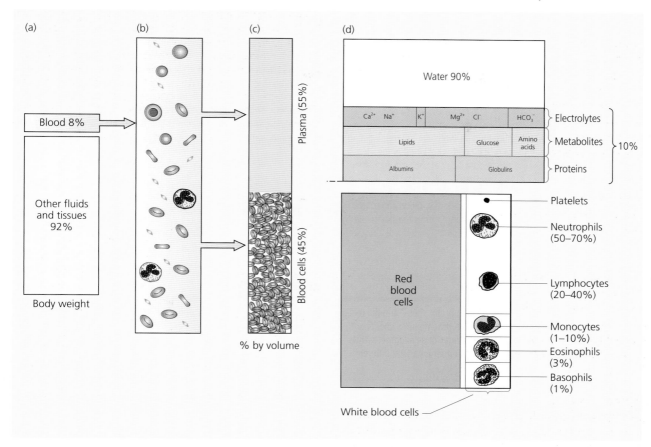

Figure 11.2 The homeostatic composition of body fluids and blood: (a) body fluids; (b) whole blood; (c) centrifuged blood; (d) separate components of blood. Percentages are of white blood cells

Q Name the cellular elements of blood.

ACTIVITY

Define the following terms: (1) organic; (2) inorganic; (3) density; (4) viscosity.

Blood cells

The cellular components of blood are:

- *Red blood cells (erythrocytes; 'erythro-' = red)*: transport respiratory gases (and hydrogen ions to and from cells, and define the person's blood group.
- *White blood cells (leucocytes; 'leuco-' = white)*: important components of the body's immune system, concerned with defending the body against pathogens and their toxin secretions.
- *Platelets (thrombocytes; 'thrombus' = clot)*: of fundamental importance in blood clotting. Their homeostatic role is in haemostasis (i.e. they prevent blood loss, and thus help maintain body fluid balance following injury to a blood vessel).

Blood production

Blood production (haemopoiesis) occurs in three stages, according to the individual's period of growth and development. These are referred to as the mesoblastic, hepatosplenic and myeloid stages.

The mesoblastic stage

The first blood cells to be produced in the unborn child originate from the embryonic mesodermal cells that migrate to the yolk sac, where they form 'blood islands' (see Figure 19.5, p.527). These become hollow tubes that secrete a plasma-like fluid from their walls. Proliferation of cells lining these tubes forms the early cells of the circulation. These nucleated cells (called megaloblasts of Ehrlich) contain the pigment haemoglobin; their sole purpose is to transport oxygen to the developing embryonic tissue cells. Blood production from these cells is sufficient for the first few weeks of embryonic life, but is inadequate to support further development.

The hepatosplenic stage

This stage of blood production begins at about the sixth week of gestation; it is mainly responsible for the relatively large size

BOX 11.2 TAKING A BLOOD SAMPLE

Owing to the interdependence of body parts (see Figures 1.5, p.9 and 1.6, p.10), if any part of the body is functionally abnormal then this is almost always reflected in the composition of blood. Taking blood samples for laboratory analysis is called venepuncture. This is a straightforward procedure that involves withdrawing a specimen of blood from a vein using a hypodermic needle and a syringe. Blood is usually taken from the median cubital vein, which is anatomically anterior to the elbow (see Figure 12.19b, p.331) A tourniquet is wrapped around the arm above the venepuncture site to cause the build-up of blood in the vein. If the patient repeatedly makes a fist, the visibility of the vein increases, enhancing the success rate of the procedure.

A small specimen of blood may be taken from a finger stick (e.g. in people with diabetes mellitus who need to check their blood sugar levels during the day). In babies, taking a blood sample from the heel is less stressful and more straightforward than taking it from the arm. The heel stick specimen (analysed by the Guthrie test) is used to check for neonatal abnormalities such as phenylketonuria, galactosaemia and hypothyroidism.

Healthcare workers need to exercise care to avoid infection with pathogens, such as human immunodeficiency virus (HIV) and hepatitis B virus (HBV), when handling blood, other body fluids, and potentially contaminated items such as needles, syringes, intravenous equipment and linen. The UK Department of Health (2000) suggests the following precautions when handling such products:

- Wear protective gloves, plastic aprons, masks and, where appropriate, gowns and eye goggles.
- Dispose of used items such as 'sharps' (i.e. anything capable of inflicting cuts, scratches or punctures).

ACTIVITY

Use Appendix C to look up the meaning of the prefix 'mes-' and the root '-derm'. Using a medical/nursing/healthcare practitioner's dictionary, differentiate between the embryo and fetal stages of development. Note that a blast is an embryonic cell that has not undergone final differentiation.

ACTIVITY

Refer to Figures 3.8, p.70, and 3.17, p.80 to identify the bones mentioned above.

BOX 11.3 HAEMOPOIESIS

All blood cells originate from a common stem cell called the haematocytoblast (Figure 11.3). These stem cells are a result of cell specialization, since they are differentiated from other cells within the body once the particular genes for blood cell development are expressed. Once this initial specialization has taken place, producing the common stem cell, the cells divide mitotically and specialize further into red blood cells, white blood cells or platelets. This differentiation of the stem cell into blood cells is again by specific gene expression. Furthermore, once a cell has become specialized, it cannot be transformed into another cell (blood cell or otherwise).

of the liver between the seventh and ninth weeks of gestation. It is necessary because the fetus is growing rapidly and its tissues require a correspondingly greater blood supply to sustain this activity. The liver ('hepato-') and spleen ('-splenic') become the main contributors of this enhanced blood production, although the thymus is also involved. The liver becomes the major haemopoietic site between weeks 13 and 17 of gestation, and continues to produce blood until the later stages of pregnancy.

The myeloid stage

The term 'myeloid' refers to the activities of immature blood cells (called precursor cells) in bone marrow. The bone marrow becomes active in blood cell production from the fifth month onwards, establishing itself as the major haemopoietic organ of the fetus at about 7 months. Production from this site continues throughout life. At birth, all the marrow is active in blood production; it is called red active marrow, because although it produces all blood cells, the extensive number of erythrocytes colours it red. As the infant grows, the active red marrow of the long bones is replaced by yellow inactive (or fatty, lymphoidal) marrow. The tibia and radius bones of the limbs are the first bones to lose this haemopoietic ability, followed by the femur and then the humerus. In the young adult, the active marrow is found in the flat bones, such as the cranium, ribs, sternum and pelvis, and in the vertebrae. The liver, spleen and the yellow inactive marrow are, however, capable of reverting back to their erythrocyte production function when erythrocyte numbers are deficient in severe anaemias, and so act as homeostatic regulators.

The marrow's haemopoietic functions can be divided into erythropoiesis (red cell production), leucopoiesis (white cell production) and thrombopoiesis (platelet production). These processes will be discussed later.

COMPOSITION AND PHYSIOLOGY OF THE BLOOD

Plasma

Plasma forms approximately half of the total blood volume, and one-fifth of the total volume of extracellular fluid (male value, 52–83 mL/kg; female value, 50–75 mL/kg). Plasma and tissue fluids are very similar in composition, except for the total amount of protein present. This is not surprising, as the membrane of a blood capillary (i.e. tiny blood vessel) separates these two fluids and is permeable to most substances. Tissue fluid is derived from plasma at the arterial side of the capillary, and returns to the plasma at the venous side (see Figure 6.2, p.124). However, despite this interchange of plasma and tissue fluid, there remain some differences in their composition.

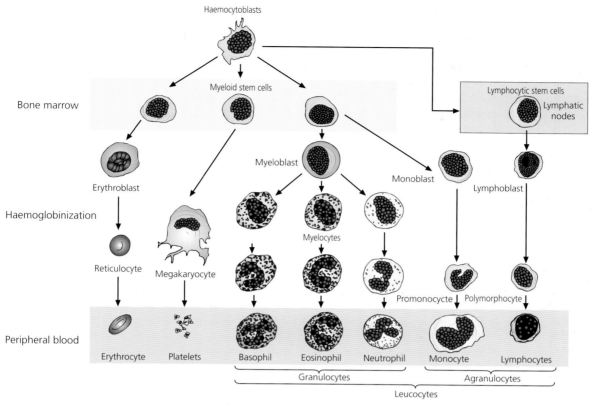

Figure 11.3 Haemopoiesis: the origin and differentiation of blood cells

Q *Distinguish between neutrophils and eosinophils, and erythropoiesis and leucopoiesis.*

Q *What do the granules represent in granulocytes?*

BOX 11.4 HAEMATOLOGY

The study of blood is called haematology. It involves estimating:

- the number of cells and values of non-cellular blood components, and comparing these with the homeostatic ranges expected;
- the shape (morphology) and size of the cellular components, using a stained blood film.

Full complete blood count

A full complete blood count (FBC or CBC) screens for anaemia, various infections, and blood-clotting disorders; it is also very important in pregnancy, especially with pre-eclampsia and HELLP syndrome (see Box 12.27, p.352. It includes counts of the red blood cells (RBCs), white blood cells (WBCs) and platelets, a differential white cell count, and an estimate of the haematocrit and haemoglobin values (see Box 11.10, p.282). Figure 11.4 shows an example of a laboratory slip used in clinical blood analysis.

Bone marrow biopsy

This clinical test may confirm a diagnosis suggested by clinical examination and blood investigations. It provides information about the homeostatic status of haemopoiesis, the number of the respective cellular components, and the presence of abnormal cells, as found in metastatic cancers and Hodgkin's disease.

The biopsy procedure involves puncturing the bone with a needle, then taking (i.e. aspirating) a specimen of the bone marrow with a syringe. The iliac crest and sternum are common sites of biopsy in adults, and the tibia is a common site in children, since these areas have relatively thin layers of bone above the marrow. Alternatively, small sections of bone may be removed using a trephine needle. The procedure is unpleasant for the patient because of the pressure that needs to be applied to penetrate the bone. Local anaesthetic is used to ensure no pain is perceived; a general anaesthetic may be used in children.

BOX 11.5 CHANGES TO BLOOD COMPOSITION DURING PREGNANCY

During pregnancy, there is a maximum rise in plasma volume and red blood cell volume of 50% and 20%, respectively; this is called haemodilution. Plasma volume begins to increase in the first trimester (trimester = period of 3 months), then increases rapidly during the second trimester, with a further slight increase in the third trimester. Red cell volume begins to increase in the second trimester, with the greatest increase in the third trimester.

Because of the different pace of the changes in plasma and red cell volumes, the haemoglobin and packed cell volumes reduce progressively until approximately 30 weeks' gestation. After 30 weeks' gestation, there is a reversal as the increase in red cell volume outweighs the plasma volume.

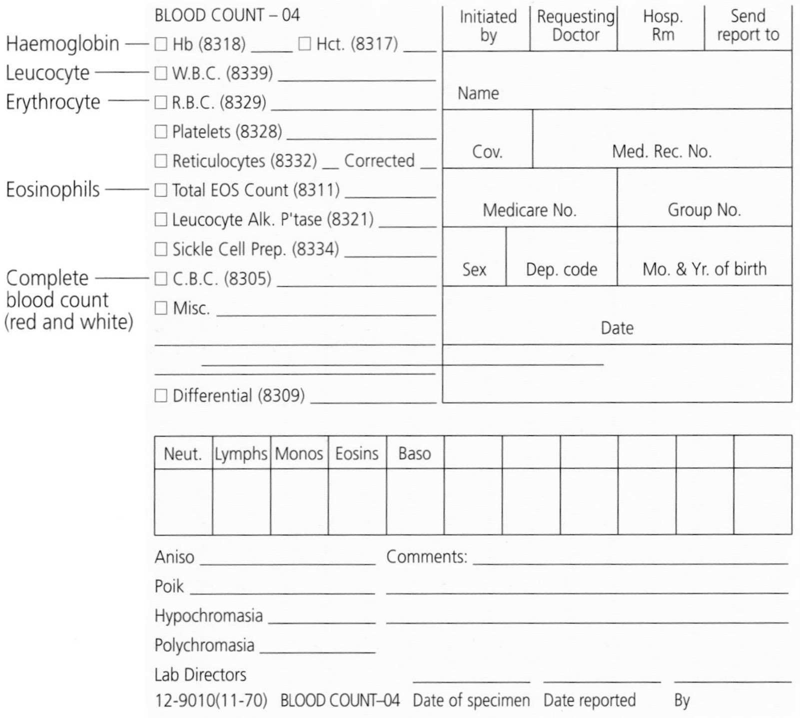

BLOOD COUNT – 04		Initiated by	Requesting Doctor	Hosp. Rm	Send report to

Haemoglobin — ☐ Hb (8318) _____ ☐ Hct. (8317) ___

Leucocyte ——— ☐ W.B.C. (8339) _____

Erythrocyte ——— ☐ R.B.C. (8329) _____   Name

☐ Platelets (8328) _____

☐ Reticulocytes (8332) __ Corrected __   Cov.   Med. Rec. No.

Eosinophils ——— ☐ Total EOS Count (8311) _____

☐ Leucocyte Alk. P'tase (8321) _____   Medicare No.   Group No.

☐ Sickle Cell Prep. (8334) _____

Complete ——— ☐ C.B.C. (8305) _____   Sex | Dep. code | Mo. & Yr. of birth
blood count
(red and white) ☐ Misc. _____   Date

_____

☐ Differential (8309) _____

Neut.	Lymphs	Monos	Eosins	Baso			

Aniso _____   Comments: _____

Poik _____   _____

Hypochromasia _____   _____

Polychromasia _____

Lab Directors

12-9010(11-70) BLOOD COUNT–04 Date of specimen | Date reported | By

Figure 11.4 A laboratory slip requesting blood analysis

Q Distinguish between whole blood, serum and plasma.

Q What is the blood volume of a healthy adult female?

One of the most noticeable differences is in the concentration of the respiratory gases. Plasma has a higher concentration of oxygen, while tissue fluid has a higher concentration of carbon dioxide. As a result, oxygen diffuses from blood into tissue fluid, and carbon dioxide diffuses into the plasma. Diffusion, as discussed in Chapter 2, pp.28–9, could be expected to result in a uniform distribution of the gases, but this is not the case, because cells are constantly removing and using oxygen from tissue fluid, and supplying carbon dioxide to it, in order to maintain cell homeostasis. Thus, diffusion is a working concept to explain the movement of molecules down their concentration gradients. Another notable difference between plasma and tissue fluid is the large presence of dissolved proteins in the plasma (70 g/L compared with 20 g/L in tissue fluid). Plasma proteins are macromolecules that are too large to pass through pores in the capillary membranes, and thus generally in health do not pass into tissue fluid. Intracellular fluid has a different composition from plasma and tissue fluid because of the selectively permeable properties of cell membranes (see Chapter 2, pp.27–8, and Table 6.1, p.122).

Plasma proteins

Plasma contains three principal types of proteins: albumins, globulins and fibrinogen. The latter is a protein involved in blood clotting. The plasma also contains other proteins associated with clotting (e.g. a globulin called prothrombin). Most plasma proteins are produced in the liver.

Albumins

Approximately 70% of the solutes found in plasma are proteins. Albumins comprise about 55–60% of this protein component, and thus are important determinants of the viscosity of blood

(i.e. the plasma proteins slow down the flow rate of blood). Albumins osmotically draw water (and its dissolved components) from the tissue fluid back into the venous side of the blood capillary, and so facilitate the capillary exchange process. This helps to maintain the blood volume and hence blood pressure. Other plasma proteins, being macromolecules, also contribute to the viscosity and osmotic potential of blood. Albumins also have important transport functions: for example, they bind to calcium and bilirubin, thus maintaining the homeostatic concentration of these 'free' chemicals in body fluids (both are physiologically active only when unbound). Albumins also bind to certain drugs (e.g. aspirin). Although largely retained in plasma, a small amount of albumin is found in the tissue fluid, where it has similar properties to that in plasma.

Globulins

Globulins comprise about 33–38% of the plasma proteins. They are much larger molecules than albumins. Globulins are subdivided into the following fractions:

* *Gamma globulins*. Consist mainly of most of the known antibodies, and so are produced in the circulation and the lymphatic systems in response to an 'antigenic insult' (see Figure 13.20, p.385). Their role is to protect the body from pathogens and their toxins, hence their alternative name, 'immunoglobulins'. Globulins are used as a basis for therapeutic administrations (e.g. anti-tetanus injections consist of an antibody-rich gamma globulin fraction of horse serum).
* *Alpha globulins*. These have several transport functions. They bind to smaller proteins, and certain electrolytes, and so prevent these substances from passing out in the urine.
* *Beta globulins*. These also have several transport functions.

Table 11.1 Chemical composition, description and homeostatic functions of plasma components

Component	Description	Homeostatic function
Water	Liquid portion of blood; constitutes approximately 90% of the plasma Water is derived from absorption from the digestive tract and from cellular respiration	Transports components below, blood cells and heat
Solutes Proteins	Constitutes approximately 7% of the plasma Produced by the liver	General Provides blood with viscosity, a factor related to the homeostatic regulation of blood pressure Exerts considerable osmotic pressure to maintain water balance between blood and tissues, hence homeostatically regulates blood volume and thus blood pressure
Albumins		Binding functions Transport lipids
Globulins	Group to which antibodies belong	Gammaglobulins (antibodies) attack pathogens Include an important blood-clotting precursor molecule (prothrombin) Important in transport of ions, hormones and lipids
Fibrinogen	Produced by the liver	Homeostatic role in blood clotting, when it is converted into insoluble fibrin
Non-protein nitrogen-containing substances	Include urea, uric acid, creatinine, and ammonium salts	Byproducts of protein metabolism; these are excreted to prevent toxic build-up
Food substances	Products of digestion passed into blood for distribution to all body cells; products include amino acids (from proteins), glucose (from carbohydrates), fatty acids and glycerol (from lipids), and vitamins	Used for energy production, growth, repair and maintenance of cells
Regulatory substances	Enzymes and hormones	Enzymes catalyse chemical reactions to a rate compatible with life Hormones regulate metabolism
Respiratory gases	Oxygen and carbon dioxide	Oxygen has a homeostatic role in cellular respiration (Krebs cycle) Carbon dioxide is important in the regulation of pH of body fluids
Electrolytes	Inorganic salts Positive ions (cations) include Na^+, K^+, Ca^{2+} Negative ions (anions) include Cl^-, HCO_3^-	Help to maintain osmotic pressure, normal pH, and physiological balance between tissues and blood

Q. Describe the origin and functions of plasma proteins.

Some contain specific metal-combining groups (e.g. transferrin is a protein that transports iron) and some carry fat-soluble vitamins. Others contribute to the blood clotting process.

Fibrinogen and prothrombin

Fibrinogen and prothrombin (a beta-globulin) act as precursors of the active clotting proteins, fibrin and thrombin, respectively (see wound healing later).

General roles of plasma proteins

In addition to the specific functions mentioned above, plasma proteins have some more generalized roles. In the 'normal', slightly alkaline plasma, proteins carry a negative charge. As ions, they are capable of 'mopping up' positively charged hydrogen ions when these are in excess of their homeostatic range (e.g. as occurs when the metabolic rate is increased). This important buffering action contributes to the homeostatic maintenance of blood pH, which is essential for optimum enzymatic activity.

Plasma proteins also act as a protein reservoir (i.e. they can be used in times of chronic dietary protein deficiency). However, this may lead to protein depletion in the plasma (hypoproteinaemia), which has consequences for fluid distribution.

Table 11.1 summarizes the homeostatic functions of plasma constituents.

Cellular components of blood

The cellular components of blood make up about 45% of whole blood (see Figure 11.2c, p.271). The three principal cell types (as described earlier) are erythrocytes, leucocytes and thrombocytes (platelets). Table 11.3 summarizes the homeostatic functions of blood cells.

BOX 11.6 SERUM ANALYSIS

Plasma is frequently the subject of clinical biochemical analysis as an indication of a person's state of health (Figure 11.5). Table 1.3, p.11 shows the homeostatic ranges of various organic and inorganic components within plasma. Deviations from these values are indicative of an individual's fluctuating physiological condition, or may be a sign of underlying pathology. Thus, such levels are used as aids to diagnose specific disorders. Analysis of plasma components could be potentially difficult, as samples coagulate (clot) within a matter of minutes after taking them. Therefore, anticoagulants are added to samples to prevent clotting. The remaining plasma-like fluid (called serum) is then analysed for components.

Homeostatic failures of the plasma proteins

Albumin deficiency (hypoalbuminaemia) occurs when there is damage to the glomerular capillaries of the kidneys (see Figure 15.6, p.427), which results in albumin being filtered and passing out in the urine. Albumin synthesis by the liver is such that its deficiency results only when there are large amounts of albumin lost from the body, or when inadequate dietary amino acids prevent its synthesis. This condition, together with other hypoproteinaemias, causes a decrease in the plasma osmotic pressure, resulting in an accumulation of the tissue fluid called oedema. There are other causes of oedema; for example, healthcare profession-

als and carers will often see gravitational oedema of the lower limbs in static elderly patients. Liver diseases, protein malnutrition, inflammation and allergic reactions cause such deficiencies in plasma proteins.

Gamma-globulin excess (hypergammaglobulinaemia) is indicative of chronic infection states, collagen diseases and parasitic infections, and reflects the increased antibody production in these conditions. Gamma-globulin deficiency (agammaglobulinaemia) may occur as a congenital disease (congenital = present at birth) and in patients who are subjected to recurrent infection, and so reflects a failure or decline in antibody response to infection.

Fibrinogen excess (hyperfibrinogenaemia) occurs in pathological acute infections, and in pregnancy. Increased fibrinogen levels result in a faster erythrocyte sedimentation rate (ESR; see Box 11.10). Fibrinogen and prothrombin deficiencies (hypofibrinogenaemia and hypoprothrombinaemia, respectively) cause longer bleeding and clotting times. Hypofibrinogenaemia occurs in liver diseases, such as cirrhosis, and can also cause problems in pregnancy.

Clinical correction of such disorders involves plasma transfusions. An immune response in the recipient is avoided by infusing 'conditioned' plasma (i.e. plasma minus the antibodies it may contain). Table 11.2 summarizes the clinical use of infused plasma components in re-establishing a patient's plasma homeostatic balance.

Figure 11.5 Clinical analysis of plasma components using homeostatic principles. (a) Homeostatic dynamism. Value fluctuating above and below the mean within the component's homeostatic range (see Table 11.2). The fluctuation is a result of the component entering and leaving the plasma. For example, some plasma components such as nutrients leave blood at the arterial side of the capillary bed, while others, such as metabolic wastes, enter the blood at the arterial side of the capillary bed. Consequently the component's level fluctuates. b_1, Plasma component in excess of its homeostatic range. The excess could be indicative of a clinical condition (e.g. the presence of the cardiac-specific enzyme creatinine phosphokinase above serum baseline level, which occurs after a myocardial infarction – heart attack). Alternatively, the excess may be indicative of a 'normal' temporary change in the plasma level of the component (e.g. elevated glucose concentration after absorption of a carbohydrate-rich meal). b_2, A decrease in the component level below its homeostatic range. This could be indicative of a clinical condition (e.g. low levels of plasma proteins might be indicative of liver damage, as occurs in tissue fibrosis due to cirrhosis), since the hepatocytes produce plasma proteins, and fibrosis impairs this synthesis. Alternatively, the low levels could be a 'normal' temporary change (e.g. hypoglycaemia, which occurs 1 hour after the absorption of a carbohydrate-rich meal because of the long-duration effects of the hypoglycaemic agent insulin). (c) Clinical intervention, or the body's normal

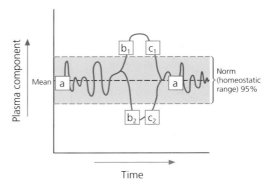

negative homeostatic feedback mechanisms, which correct the temporary pathological and normal physiological homeostatic imbalances, respectively. (a, Represents boxes a_1–a_4 in Figure 1.7, p.11, reflecting the individual variability in the homeostatic range)

Q List seven functions of the circulating blood.

Erythrocytes

Structure

Microscopically, red cells appear as biconcave discs. Each cell has a doughnut shape, having a thick outer margin and a very thin middle region. Erythrocytes are approximately 7.2 μm in diameter and are 2.2 μm thick; the central portion narrows to 0.8 μm (Figure 11.6b, p.278). The biconcavity provides a large surface area with respect to volume (compared with a spherically shaped cell). The biconcavity provides a large surface area with respect to volume (compared with a spherically shaped cell), thus maximizing the available membrane surface for the exchange of respiratory gases. This structural adaptation also gives these cells greater flexibility, enabling them to pass through capillaries that are even narrower than the diam-

eter of the erythrocyte. The membrane, as with all cellular membranes, contains surface chemical markers called antigens. Some of the blood cell antigens, namely A, B and D (rhesus) types, together with specific plasma antibodies, determine an individual's ABO and rhesus blood group (described later).

The cytoplasm of the erythrocyte consists mainly of the red pigment haemoglobin. This pigment accounts for approximately 95% of the intracellular protein, and is responsible for approximately one-third of the cell's mass. Its main functions are the transportation of respiratory gases (primarily oxygen) and the regulation of blood pH (when haemoglobin is not transporting respiratory gases, it has a buffering action).

Table 11.4 illustrates the clinical importance of homeostatic values concerning the erythrocyte.

Table 11.2 Plasma components for clinical use in redressing plasma component homeostasis*

Plasma component	Clinical homeostatic correction
Plasma protein fraction	Plasma replacement
	Blood volume expansion
Human albumin	Albumin replacement in hypoalbuminaemia, e.g. in nephrosis
Fresh frozen plasma	Clotting factor deficiencies, e.g. in liver disease
Cryoprecipitate (factor VIII, fibrinogen)	Classical haemophilia (haemophilia A)
	Von Willebrand's disease
	Fibrinogen deficiency
Factor VIII concentrate and freeze-dried factor VIII	Classical haemophilia A
Factor IX concentrate	Christmas disease (haemophilia B)
Human immunoglobulin (Ig)	Hypogammaglobulinaemia, e.g. to produce passive immunity to viral diseases such as rubella (German measles)
Human-specific globulin (antibodies)	To produce passive immunity to rare, life-threatening disease, e.g. tetanus

*Applying principles shown in Figure 11.5.

Table 11.3 Various types of blood cells. A differential white cell count is taken by examining a stained blood smear; the values in this table represent the numbers of each type encountered in a sample of 100 leucocytes.

Leucocytes	Blood cell		Diameter (µm)	Number/mm³ (homeostatic range)	Differential white cell count (%)	Homeostatic function
		Erythrocytes	7.0–7.7	4.2–6.2 million		Transportation of respiratory gases (particularly oxygen) Buffer in acid–base regulation
Granulocytes		Neutrophils	9–14	3000–6750	60–65	Phagocytic – engulf pathogens or debris in tissues
		Eosinophils	10–14	100–360	2–4	Phagocytic – engulf items in tissues that are labelled with antigens (combat allergies)
		Basophils	8–10	25–90	0.5–1.0	Enter damaged tissue release histamine (combat allergies)
Agranulocytes		Lymphocytes	6–12	1000–2700	20–35	Cells of the lymphatic system provide defence against specific pathogens or toxins
		Monocytes	10–15	150–70	3–8	Mobile and fixed macrophages, engulf pathogens or debris
		Thrombocytes	2–4	150 000–400 000		Blood clotting

Reproduced from Craigwyle, M.B.L. (1975) *A Colour Atlas of Histology*. London: Wolfe Medical Publications.

Q Give a function for each of the following: (1) basophils, (2) fixed macrophages, and (3) megakaryocytes.

Production of erythrocytes

The number of red blood cells remains similar throughout life, but they have a lifespan of 100–120 days, and so their production must match their loss in order to homeostatically control the number of red cells present. Approximately 1% of circulating red cells are replaced daily; this may seem a small proportion, but it actually means that three million erythrocytes enter the circulation every second.

Figure 11.3 simplifies the processes involved in erythropoiesis. The main characteristic changes for the development of a mature erythrocyte take about 1 week. During this time,

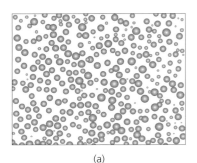

(a)

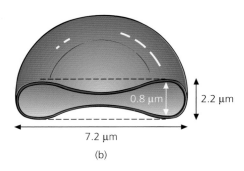

(b)

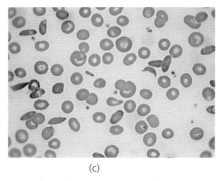

(c)

Figure 11.6 The structure of erythrocytes: (a) when viewed in a standard blood smear, erythrocytes appear as two-dimensional doughnut-shaped objects; (b) in cross-section, erythrocytes appear as three-dimensional. The biconcavity produces a greater surface area for the process of gaseous exchange. The dashed line represents the smaller surface area of a spherical cell. (c) Peripheral blood taken from a patient with sickle cell disease. Reproduced with the kind permission of Lakhani *et al.*, *Basic Pathology*, 3rd edn. Hodder, London

Q Under what physiological conditions is erythropoietin released?

Table 11.4 Clinical importance of the homeostatic ranges concerning erythrocytes

Measure	
Erythrocytic count	
Infant	
Adult male	4.5–6.5 million/mm³
Adult female	4.5–5 million/mm³
Packed cell volume (PCV) (haematocrit)	
Infant	
Adult male	0.47 (47%)
Adult female	0.42 (42%)
Haemoglobin (Hb)	
Adult male	13–18 g/mL
Adult female	11.5–16.6 g/mL

Q Why is circulating blood not white?

the cell gradually becomes smaller and smaller. The nucleus 'ripens', with the loss of the nucleoli and the condensation of nuclear material. The cytoplasm 'ripens' due to the process of haemoglobinization. Some of the organelles and inclusions (e.g. nucleus, mitochondria and ribosomes) are removed to increase the available space for haemoglobin. Mature erythrocytes therefore cannot divide or produce proteins, and they are dependent upon anaerobic respiration for their ATP source. This form of respiration (see Figure 4.8, p.100) produces much less energy from glucose breakdown. Perhaps red cells come to the end of their lives when their ATP level falls below the requirements necessary to maintain their homeostatic roles and, consequently, metabolism is reduced so much that it becomes incompatible for the continued existence of the cell.

There are many factors that regulate the maturation process. These can be divided broadly into those that stimulate erythropoiesis (e.g. hypoxia and hypersecretion of the metabolic hormones: thyroid-stimulating hormone, thyroxine, adrenocorticotropic hormone, growth hormone and androgens) and those that inhibit erythropoiesis (e.g. an oxygen-carrying capacity of the blood above or within its homeostatic range, and an undersecretion of the hormones mentioned above).

The process of erythropoiesis is controlled by the release of a factor called erythrogenin from the kidney tissue in response to hypoxia. This factor converts a precursor protein in plasma,

Table 11.5 Dietary components necessary for erythropoiesis

Dietary component	Homeostatic important in erythropoiesis
Protein	Synthesis of globin part of haemoglobin Synthesis of other cellular proteins, including conjugated molecules, e.g. lipoproteins, glycoproteins
Iron	Contained in the haem part of haemoglobin
Vitamin B$_{12}$ and folic acid	Synthesis of DNA
Vitamin C	Facilitates the absorption of iron Important in normal folic acid metabolism
Vitamin B$_6$, riboflavin, and vitamin E	Important for normal erythropoiesis, since deficiency of these substances has been associated with anaemia
Copper and cobalt	Copper is essential for haemoglobin synthesis Cobalt is important in vitamin B$_{12}$ synthesis Therefore, these trace elements may have a role in human erythropoiesis

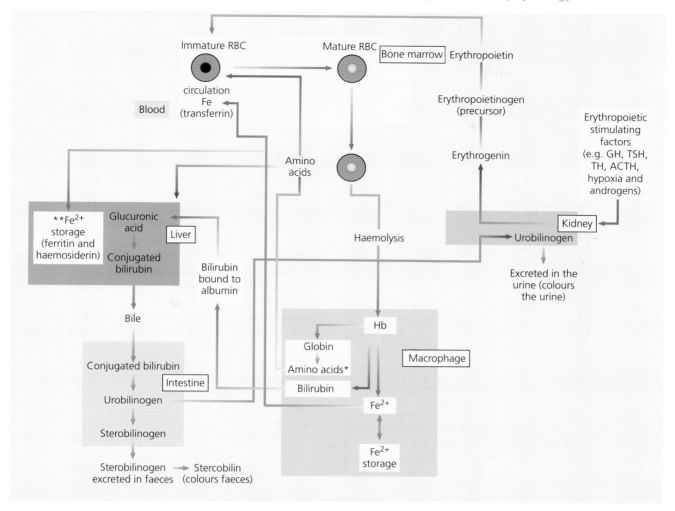

Figure 11.7 Production and destruction of erythrocytes: a homeostatic process. This diagram indicates the normal pathways for recycling the amino acids and iron (Fe) content of old or damaged erythrocytes, and the pathway associated with red cell production. ACTH, adrenocorticotropic hormone; GH, growth hormone; Hb, haemoglobin; RBC, red blood cell; TH, thyroid hormone; TSH, thyroid-stimulating hormone; *, transamination (deamination if the amino acid pool is above the homeostatic range); **, occurs if circulatory iron is in excess of its homeostatic range

Q Describe the process of red blood cell breakdown.

BOX 11.7 BLOOD DOPING

Some athletes have used blood doping and the administration of erythropoietin in an attempt to improve their performance, particularly during endurance events. This involves removing blood cells from the body, storing them for 4–5 weeks, then reintroducing them into the body a couple of days before the athletic event to increase the oxygen-carrying capacity of blood. Blood doping is banned by the International Olympics Committee because of the extra workload it enforces on the heart because of the increased viscosity of blood resulting from the addition of extra erythrocytes.

BOX 11.8 ABNORMAL RED CELLS

It is still a mystery as to how tissues recognize aged red cells, but we do know that the spleen is involved. An enlarged spleen (referred to as splenomegaly) is observed in conditions associated with abnormal red cells e.g. sickle cell anaemia.

erythropoietinogen, into erythropoietin, which activates the erythropoietic tissues to increase red cell production and release them into the circulation (Figure 11.7). At sea level, the atmospheric oxygen conditions are sufficient to meet the metabolic demands of humans. When erythrocyte production exceeds the homeostatic range (e.g. values greater than 6.5 million/mm^3 for men and 5 million/mm^3 for women; Table 11.4), production is inhibited because the secretion of erythrogenin is prevented. This is an example of a negative feedback mechanism. As time passes, the numbers of erythrocytes return to their normal homeostatic levels, because cells are still being destroyed at their normal rate of breakdown. At this point (within the homeostatic range), production must begin again at a rate that matches that of destruction, in order to maintain the 'normal' levels. The levels of erythropoietin then rise owing to erythrogenin secretion and its activation of erythropoietinogen. Erythropoietin release is, therefore, controlled tightly

BOX 11.9 JAUNDICE AND NEONATAL EXCRETION OF CONJUGATED BILIRUBIN

The conjugation of bilirubin by liver cells is used diagnostically in determining whether jaundice, a retention of bilirubin in the body, is caused by a liver problem or something else. In this way, the ratio of conjugated to free bilirubin in bile is an important assessment.

Bacterial cultures take time to establish in the gut of a neonate. Consequently, the conjugated bilirubin is not converted to stercobilin in the bowel, but is excreted intact, hence the different faecal colour observed in neonates.

within its 'normal' parameters. A change outside these parameters occurs, for example, when erythrocyte destruction becomes greater than production, resulting in low levels of erythrocytes, as is observed in haemolytic diseases.

Table 11.5 summarizes the dietary components essential for erythropoiesis to occur.

Destruction of erythrocytes

When red cells are about 100–120 days old, they are removed from the circulation by the reticuloendothelial system (i.e. the spleen, liver, subcutaneous tissue and lymph nodes), where phagocytes ingest and destroy the old erythrocytes.

ACTIVITY

Before continuing, we suggest you study the sections 'Structure of haemoglobin' (Chapter 14, pp.413–14) and 'Carriage of oxygen' (see Chapter 14, p.414). You may also wish to refamiliarize yourself with the intracellular digestion role of lysosomes (see Figure 2.10, p.34), since this organelle is vitally important in phagocytosis of red cells.

Haemoglobin undergoes an elaborate breakdown process. Its most valuable components are conserved and re-utilized. The remainder is excreted in faeces and urine.

The stages involved in the breakdown of haemoglobin (Figure 11.7) are as follows:

1 The haem component of haemoglobin consists of a porphyrin ring compound, with a ferrous (Fe^{2+}) ion at the centre of each ring (see Figure 14.10, p.414). Once ingested by macrophages, this ring is opened by oxidation, forming a straight-chain molecule consisting of the components of haem and globin, called choleglobin.

2 Iron and globin are removed from choleglobin, converting it into bilirubin (red bile pigment). Iron and globin are useful substances, and are re-utilized by the body. Some of the iron is used for the resynthesis of haemoglobin and other iron-containing compounds. However, if the iron released from the haemoglobin causes its availability to go above the homeostatic range, the excess is transferred into iron storage compounds called ferritin and haemosiderin. Thus, an increased haemosiderin concentration (above its normal range) in the liver and the spleen is indicative of diseases in which there is excessive red cell breakdown (haemolysis). Iron is released from such stores when there is insufficient in the blood to meet metabolic needs. The globin molecule is hydrolysed (broken down with water) into its constituent amino acids, which enter the amino acid body fluid 'pools' from which haemoglobin is resynthesized.

3 Some bilirubin becomes bound tightly to albumin. This complex passes into liver cells. Other free or unbound bilirubin, being lipid soluble, passes into the liver cells with ease.

BOX 11.10 CLINICAL TESTS

Reticulocyte count

Erythrocyte imbalances are result from a mismatch between erythrocyte production and destruction. In order to investigate such imbalances, a reticulocyte count is taken. Reticulocytes are immature erythrocytes that account for 0.5–1.5% of the erythrocyte population in a normal blood sample. Reticulocyte counts of less than 0.5% indicate that blood production cannot match the loss of erythrocytes; this occurs in patients with pernicious anaemia and iron-deficiency anaemia, and during radiation therapy. Low reticulocyte counts may also be caused by a deficiency of erythrogenin and/or erythropoietinogen and/or erythropoietin. If the count is above 1.5%, erythrocyte production is greater than destruction. This occurs in response to a number of conditions, including haemolytic anaemia, leukaemia and carcinoma. High reticulocyte counts, however, may also indicate a good red bone marrow response to previous blood loss, or to iron therapy in someone who has been iron deficient (Figure 11.8).

Erythrocyte sedimentation rate

The erythrocyte sedimentation rate (ESR) is the rate at which red blood cells in a vertical tube containing an anticoagulant fall under gravity out of suspension, and then settle on the bottom of the tube. This tendency to sediment is dependent on the relative concentration of the plasma components and plasma viscosity. The ESR is determined by measuring the length of the column of clear plasma above the red blood cells after 1 hour. The homeostatic range is 1–5 mm/hour for men and 5–15 mm/hour for women.

The ESR is raised in inflammatory diseases, some forms of cancers, and pregnancy. Values in excess of 100 mm/hour are found in chronic infections, such as tuberculosis. It is still unclear why such a condition should alter the ESR.

Haematocrit

The packed cell volume is measured following the use of a centrifuge to concentrate red blood cells at the bottom of a sample tube. The conversion of this to a percentage that red cells comprise the blood column is called the haematocrit. Measuring the packed cell volume (or haematocrit) as a percentage of whole blood is another routine clinical test. A haematocrit value of 40 means that 40% of the total volume blood is composed of red blood cells. The normal range of the haematocrit is 40–54% (mean 47%) in adult males and 38–46% (mean 42%) in adult females. Thus, red cells account for nearly half the volume of whole blood. Higher numbers of erythrocytes exist in men (5.4 million/mm³) than in women (4.8 million/mm³) because of the need to transport more oxygen to support the male's greater metabolic rate.

The higher red cell count and haematocrit value in males is associated with the presence of testosterone. This hormone stimulates synthesis of erythropoietin by the bone marrow and kidney. Lower values in females during their reproductive years may also result from excessive loss of blood during the menstrual flow. A haematocrit value of 15% is extremely low, and a value of 65% is extremely high; such values reflect the homeostatic imbalances of severe anaemia and polycythaemia, respectively.

Figure 11.8 The homeostatic and clinical control of the number of erythrocytes, using a reticulocyte count as an indicator of the red cell number. The reticulocyte count is the percentage of reticulocytes within the total number of erythrocytes. (a) Normal homeostatic levels of reticulocytes. This indicates that the erythrocyte homeostatic range is being achieved (i.e. red cell production rate matches destruction rate). b_1, Reticulocyte count is beyond the homeostatic range (i.e. > 1.5% of mature erythrocytes), indicating that production is greater than destruction of red cells, resulting in polycythaemia. The excessive production can be considered a normal physiological reaction in response to altitude hypoxia, which results in hypersecretion of the hormone erythropoietin. Alternatively, polycythaemia may be indicative of a pathological homeostatic imbalance, as experienced with cancers of erythropoietic sites and/or kidney cells, resulting in hypersecretion of erythrogenin. b_2, Reticulocyte count is below the homeostatic range (0.5%), indicating that production is less than destruction. The low levels may be indicative of pathological homeostatic imbalances, such as anaemias (Table 11.6 and part b of this figure), liver or kidney diseases that cause hyposecretion of erythrogenin, resulting in less erythropoietin reaching the erythropoietic sites, or conditions that cause a hyposecretion of the hormone precursor erythropoietinogen. c_1, Clinical correction of pathological

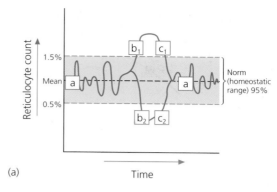

polycythaemia involves 'bleeding' therapy. c_2, Clinical correction of red cell deficiency involves red cell infusions. (a, Represents boxes a_1–a_4 in Figure 1.7, p.11, reflecting the individual variability in the homeostatic range.) (b) Presenting symptoms and systemic effects of anaemia. Reproduced with the kind permission of Lakhani *et al.*, *Basic Pathology*, 3rd edn Hodder, London

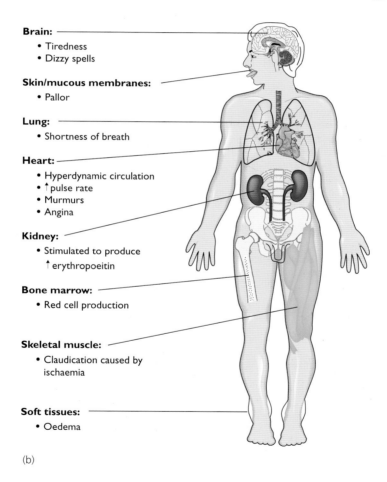

Brain:
- Tiredness
- Dizzy spells

Skin/mucous membranes:
- Pallor

Lung:
- Shortness of breath

Heart:
- Hyperdynamic circulation
- ↑ pulse rate
- Murmurs
- Angina

Kidney:
- Stimulated to produce ↑ erythropoeitin

Bone marrow:
- Red cell production

Skeletal muscle:
- Claudication caused by ischaemia

Soft tissues:
- Oedema

(b)

The bilirubin–albumin complex within the liver cells is combined to form a complex called conjugated bilirubin. This water-soluble complex facilitates the conjugated bilirubin excretion. Together with other substances, such as bile salts, bilirubin and conjugated bilirubin form bile, which is secreted from the liver to the gall bladder, where it is stored and concentrated. From the gall bladder, the bile is passed to the intestine, where it aids the physical digestion (emulsifica-

tion) of lipids. Within the intestines, bilirubin is reduced to urobilinogen by bacterial action. Some urobilinogen is reabsorbed into the circulation and is re-utilized by the liver, although some is excreted in the urine, contributing to its colour. The urobilinogen remaining in the intestines is converted via gut bacteria into stercobilinogen, and is excreted in the faeces. Stercobilinogen exposed to the air is oxidized to stercobilin, which is responsible for the colour of faeces.

BOX 11.11 HAEMOGLOBIN AND IRON DEFICIENCY ANAEMIAS

Haemoglobin values of below 13.5 g/dL in adult males, 11.5 g/dL in adult females, and 11 g/dL from 3 months to puberty indicate anaemia. A value of 15 g/dL is the lower normal limit at birth. The newborn has a relatively high amount of haemoglobin, including the form required for intrauterine life, referred to as fetal haemoglobin (Hb-F; see Chapter 14, p.414).

The severity of symptoms will depend upon the level of haemoglobin and the length of time over which the problem has developed. For example, adults with chronic anaemia do not normally experience health problems until the haemoglobin values are below 8 g/dL; an older person in whom blood supply and respiratory efficiency are compromised may have symptoms with values of 11 g/dL.

Iron-deficiency anaemia results from a homeostatic imbalance between iron requirements and supply. Normally, very little iron is lost from the body, although significant amounts may be lost in women who frequently experience heavy menstrual flow. Modern diets in the UK are generally sufficient to replace the iron that is lost, although iron-deficiency anaemia is not unusual in people whose diets lack iron. Iron-deficiency anaemia is commonly seen in communities when babies are weaned late and given a diet deficient in iron. Absorption of iron from many diets may not be sufficient to maintain optimal iron nutrition, especially in developing countries where diets contain inhibitors that bind iron and prevent it being absorbed. Healthcare practitioners should be alert to the vulnerable groups, so they can give culturally sensitive nutritional information.

Table 11.6 Classification of anaemia

Increased blood loss	
Haemorrhage	Acute, e.g. road traffic accident
	Chronic, e.g. menstruation, peptic ulcer
Haemolysis	Intracellular cause, e.g. abnormal haemoglobin variant such as sickle cell anaemia, thalassaemia
	Extracellular cause, e.g. bacteria, drugs, severe infection
Decreased blood production	
Nutritional deficiency, poor absorption of nutrients	Lack of iron results in small red blood cells (microcytic anaemia) with reduced haemoglobin
	Lack of vitamin B_{12} results in macrocytic or megaloblastic anaemia (so-called because of abnormal red blood cells precursors); vitamin B_{12} can also be deficient due to a lack of the stomach's intrinsic factor of Castle, which aids its absorption, and thus occurs when the stomach lining atrophies after a gastrectomy
	Folate may not match the demand, e.g. in pregnancy
Bone marrow failure (aplastic anaemia)	Primary, e.g. congenital
	Secondary, e.g. acquired (e.g. ionizing radiation), cytotoxic drugs (e.g. bulsulfan), bone cancer

BOX 11.12 ANAEMIA AND HAEMOPOIETIC GROWTH FACTOR

Haemopoietic growth factor is a chemical similar to erythropoietin that promotes blood cell synthesis in bone marrow. It is made available through recombinant DNA technology. It has tremendous potential for treating patients who have diminished ability to produce blood cells. Recombinant or genetically engineered erythropoietin (epoietin) is extremely effective in alleviating the extreme tiredness and breathlessness in people with chronic kidney disease. The use of epoietin potentially also has benefits for anaemic patients with associated chronic inflammatory diseases, such as arthritis.

Anaemia

Anaemia is a sign of a disease, rather a disease in itself. It is defined as a low oxygen-carrying capacity of blood and occurs when the number of erythrocytes, or the amount of haemoglobin, is below its homeostatic range. Erythrocytes and haemoglobin are at first reduced equally, but as the bone marrow replaces lost erythrocytes, blood investigations may reveal either a shortage of red cells (and hence pigment), or an adequate number of red cells with abnormally low levels of pigment present (i.e. each cell is deficient in haemoglobin).

Anaemia is classified according to its causal factors, and is divided broadly into conditions that are a consequence of an increased blood loss and those that are due to a decreased blood production (Table 11.6).

In general, irrespective of its type, anaemia affects all organ systems. It is characterized particularly by signs and symptoms of oxygen shortage at peripheral tissues, including:

- pallor of the skin, especially noticeable on the lips and eyelids, where the outer layer of the skin is relatively thin;

- a feeling of tiredness and listlessness;
- a full, soft pulse, with pulse and respiratory rates increasing unduly on slight exertion;
- a tendency for the ankles to swell, owing to peripheral oedema;
- appearance of central nervous system symptoms (only in severe anaemia), such as tinnitus (ringing in the ears), headaches, spots before the eyes, fainting and giddiness.

Minor signs aid differential diagnosis. For example, haemolytic anaemias, when red cell destruction is excessive, often show the classical jaundice appearance because of the deposition of bile pigments in skin (bilirubin is excessive because of the faster breakdown of haemoglobin). However, standard laboratory tests based on the number, size and morphology of erythrocytes, and cellular haemoglobin contents, are required for accurate diagnosis. It is important that the underlying cause is identified, as this forms the basis of correction. For example, iron-deficiency anaemia is treated with digestible iron salts (such as ferrous sulphate tablets), while simultaneously ensuring that the patient eats an appropriate diet. Severe anaemias may require blood transfusions, although this has the associated risk of fluid overload, unless the anaemia is caused by acute haemorrhage, as occurs in traumatic accidents or major surgery.

Concentrated (packed) red cells are preferable to whole blood transfusions, in order to restore the oxygen-carrying capacity of blood without greatly disturbing the blood volume. Washed red cells may be administered to remove antigenic substances (e.g. plasma proteins) attached to the erythrocytes. Frozen preparations may also be used, because freezing lowers

BOX 11.13 BLEEDING POLYCYTHAEMIC PATIENTS

The causes of polycythaemia are largely unknown, but various hormones are known to affect the rate of erythropoiesis. Polycythaemia, therefore, may be a clinical sign of certain endocrine disorders (e.g. the hypersecretion of cortisol in Cushing's syndrome).

True polycythaemia is one of the very few diseases for which bleeding is still employed as a principle of correction of a homeostatic imbalance. Modern methods include the insertion of a wide-bore needle into a vein; this has superseded the traditional methods of vein cutting, or applying blood-sucking leeches.

the leucocyte and thrombocyte content and eliminates pathogenic organisms.

Polycythaemia

Blood with an increase of 2–3 million red cells/mm³ above the normal homeostatic range is considered to be polycythaemic ('poly-' = many, 'cyte' = cell, '-aemia' = of blood). The presence of excessive cells increases the blood viscosity, and therefore slows the flow rate of blood. This increases the risk of intrinsic blood clotting (described later) and its potential consequences, such as ischaemic attacks and thrombotic infarctions. Polycythaemia occurs in dehydrated patients, as all body fluids are concentrated, with the result that erythrocytes become relatively more numerous in any measured quantity of blood, or in situations of chronic oxygen shortage.

There are various pathological conditions of the heart, circulation, lungs and bone marrow that cause the body to manufacture extra erythrocytes. In order to carry sufficient quantities of oxygen to support metabolic demands, sometimes twice the normal amount of red cells is produced. An increase in erythrocytes also occurs during prolonged hypoxia (deficiency of oxygen in the tissues) when living at high altitudes. This is referred to as physiological polycythaemia, and it occurs as a homeostatic adaptation, whereby it becomes 'normal' and necessary to have a large number of red cells as a compensatory mechanism for the low levels of atmospheric oxygen. Polycythaemia therefore is not always a sign of pathology, but may be a consequence of the homeostatic set points being reset. Mountaineers and people living above 10 000–12 000 feet may have haematocrit values as high as 65%.

ACTIVITY

Reflect on your understanding of the clinical tests haematocrit, erythrocyte sedimentation rate, and complete blood count. Read the article by Provan and Weatherall (2000) about acquired anaemias and polycythaemia.

Leucocytes

Structure

Leucocytes are nucleated and do not contain haemoglobin so, in contrast to red blood cells, they appear 'white'. Leucocytes fall into two main groups: granulocytes (neutrophils, eosinophils and basophils) and agranulocytes (lymphocytes and monocytes). The cytoplasm of granulocytes contains granules; that of agranulocytes does not. Granulocytes are classified according to their reactions to staining techniques and their size. All granulocytes have a lobed nucleus, whereas agranulocytes possess spherical (lymphocytes) or kidney-shaped (monocytes) nuclei.

White cells are far less numerous than red cells and platelets, with an average of 5000–9000/mm³. The range represents a large variation in the number of leucocytes within individuals. The numbers vary even on an hour-to-hour basis, according to various accompanying physiological and psychological factors, such as exercise and emotions. A greater fluctuation arises in response to underlying pathology.

Homeostatic functions of leucocytes

White cells are components of the immune system. As they circulate in blood vessels, they are 'looking' for signs of pathogenic invasion in adjacent tissues. Leucocytes are attracted chemically (a process called chemotaxis) to the site of inflammation by, for example, the toxic secretions of pathogens and components of the inflammatory and immune responses. This chemotaxic response attracts the white cells to the invaders, damaged tissues and other white blood cells. The movement of the leucocytes across capillary membranes is called diapedesis. In this way, most white cells are located in the peripheral tissues, since there is no human tissue that is not susceptible to pathogenic invasion; the mucous membranes and the skin are under constant threat, whereas deeper body tissues are less threatened. Thus, white cells present in blood represent only a small fraction of the total population of leucocytes. The generalized homeostatic function of white cells is to protect the body by combating microbes and non-self substances (collectively called antigens) using two processes: phagocytosis (see Figure 13.10, p.378) and antibody production (see Figures 13.20, p.385 and 13.21, p.387). The entire collection of leucocytes has the sole purpose of defending the body against pathogenic invasion, including the removal of toxins, waste products of microbial metabolism and abnormal or damaged cells.

The homeostatic ranges and a summary of the homeostatic functions of leucocytes are shown in Table 11.3, p.277.

Classification

The granular components within granulocytes contain potent enzymes and chemicals that kill bacteria. Neutrophils account for the largest proportion (about 60–65%) of the circulating leucocyte population. They are so-called because they are difficult to stain with either acidic or basic dyes, but neutral dyes stain their granules purple (see Table 11.3, p.277). Neutrophils have a distinctive lobed nucleus, hence the alternative name polymorphonucleocytes ('polymorph-' = many forms). Neutrophils are 9–14 µm in diameter, and are very mobile. They are the first cell type to arrive at a site of injury; they are also the most active phagocytes in response to tissue destruction by bacteria. Large numbers of neutrophils are destroyed in any bacterial infection. These, together with dead bacterial cells and their contents, form the pus that occurs at the injured site. Some bacterial toxins are fever-producing substances (called pyrogens). It is thought that they activate neutrophils to produce further pyrogens that cross the blood–brain barrier and affect the temperature-regulating centre within the hypothalamus of the brain.

Eosinophils represent about 2–4% of the circulating white cells. They are generally only slightly larger than neutrophils. Eosinophils have bilobed nuclei, and easily take up acidic dyes like eosin, hence the name (see Table 11.3, p.277). Eosinophils are mobile and phagocytic, but not as phagocytic as neutrophils and monocytes. Eosinophils phagocytose bacteria more readily if the bacteria are coated with antibodies. These white cells also combat irritants that cause allergies, so their numbers gradually increase in allergic reactions and parasitic infections. Their granules contain lysosome enzymes and, by their involvement with antibody-mediated (i.e. immunoglobulin E, IgE) immune responses, they function to neutralize and limit the effects of inflammatory substances, such as histamine and bradykinin, produced by damaged tissue. Eosinophils especially collect at the site of allergic reactions (e.g. in the respiratory mucous membranes in hay fever and asthma). Eosinophils and neutrophils are often collectively called microphages to avoid confusion with the larger phagocytes (macrophages) found in the blood and peripheral tissues.

Basophils account for about 0.5–1% of circulating white blood cells. Their granules stain easily with basic dyes, hence the name (see Table 11.3, p.277). Basophils are important in allergic reactions. They become mast cells in inflamed tissues, and secrete their granular contents (heparin, serotonin and histamine), which exaggerate the inflammation response at this site. Other chemicals released by activated basophils attract eosinophils and further basophils to the affected area. Basophils bind to their surface-specific IgE antibodies, which are released in response to allergic irritants. Secretion and breakdown of basophil granules occur upon subsequent exposure to the antigen, for which the bound IgE is specific (see Figure 13.24, p.391). Basophils release histamine and are involved in hypersensitive reactions to allergens (i.e. antigens that cause allergies). Histamine is a vasodilator; large quantities may cause a decrease in blood pressure, with a resultant increase in the heart rate. Itching and pain are also associated with hypersecretion of histamine.

Lymphocytes account for 20–35% of the leucocyte population. Most are found outside the blood within the lymphatic system, although they may appear in blood, especially when there is an infection. Morphologically, they are divided into large (10–15 μm) and small (8–10 μm) lymphocytes. The smaller cells are approximately the same size as red cells, and their nucleus occupies most of the cytoplasm (see Table 11.3, p.277). Functionally, lymphocytes are subdivided into T- and B-lymphocytes. These cells also have a number of subdivisions, which are discussed in Chapter 13. To summarize, T-lymphocytes attack the microbes directly in the cellular immune response (see Figure 13.18, p.384) and B-lymphocytes differentiate into large 'plasma' cells characterized by the production of vast quantities of rough endoplasmic reticulum (see Figure

13.20, p.385). These cells produce and secrete the antibodies (gamma-globulins) that attach to antigenic material. There is a high degree of specificity with regard to antibody–antigen binding (see Figures 13.13 and 13.14, p.380). Once formed, the covered or bound antigen (e.g. microbe or bacterial toxin) cannot come into contact with any other chemical in the body; as a result, the antigen is rendered harmless to body tissues. Antigen–antibody binding therefore helps combat infection, and gives the body immunity to some diseases.

Monocytes account for 3–8% of circulating leucocytes. These cells are easily recognizable under the microscope because of their large size (they are approximately 10–18 μm in diameter, nearly twice the size of a red cell) and distinctive kidney-shaped nuclei. These characteristics are illustrated in Table 11.3, p.277. There are different categories of monocytes:

- Free monocytes ('mobile' macrophages) are found outside the blood. They are extremely mobile, and so have an abundance of mitochondria. They arrive at the site of injury very quickly and are phagocytic. Macrophages release chemicals that attract other macrophages, phagocytes and fibroblasts to the inflamed area. Fibroblasts secrete a fibrous material that 'walls off' the injured area. Macrophages (and granulocytes) respond to a diverse range of stimuli, unlike lymphocytes, which respond to specific antigens (microbes and their antigens). Monocytes entering the infected tissues are called 'wandering' or 'scavenger' macrophages, as they clean up the debris following injury.
- Immobile (fixed) monocytes are found in most connective tissues. They are slower to respond, and take longer to reach the site of invasion. Despite this, they destroy more microbes because of the vast quantities that enter the site of infection.

The monocytes that migrate into reticulendothelial tissues (bone marrow, spleen, liver and lymph nodes) develop into larger specialized cells (e.g. the liver's Kupffer cells; see Figure 10.20b, p.261). These survive for long periods, and are important in the destruction of aged erythrocytes. Others migrate into skin becoming 'fixed' in position, and contribute to the non-specific defences of that organ.

Production and destruction of leucocytes

Leucopoiesis is the general term used for the production of all white cells. The process is subdivided, and other terms are employed to describe specific leucocyte production and maturation. These include granulopoiesis (synthesis of granulocytes), lymphopoiesis (synthesis of lymphocytes), and monopoiesis (synthesis of monocytes). The developmental processes associated with leucopoiesis are summarized in Figure 11.3, p.273.

Granulopoiesis occurs in the red active bone marrow. The formation of the nucleus, the loss of some organelles such as the mitochondria, and the formation of cytoplasmic granules characterize the development processes. Although the homeostatic regulation of granulopoiesis has yet to be identified, it is known that the maturation process takes about 14 days. Approximately 50% of these newly formed mature cells adhere closely to the endothelial lining of blood vessels; these are

BOX 11.14 DIFFERENTIAL WHITE BLOOD COUNT

A differential white cell count is taken by examining a stained blood smear. The values obtained represent the number of each type of leucocyte encountered in a sample of 100 white cells. It confirms which specific white cell imbalance is present, and it is therefore a diagnostic aid for certain clinical conditions:

- Neutrophil leucocytosis occurs in acute bacterial infection (e.g. appendicitis, pneumonia), and inflammatory reactions associated with tissue cell death (e.g. cerebrovascular accident, or stroke, and myocardial infarction, or heart attack).
- Lymphocytosis occurs in chronic infection, such as measles, mumps or hepatitis.
- Eosinophilia occurs in allergic reactions and in parasitic invasion of the body.

Figure 11.9 illustrates the homeostatic and clinical control of the leucocyte population.

Table 11.7 shows the classification of homeostatic imbalances associated with blood cells. Slight temporary increases in leucocytes occur during digestion, and an increase of longer duration exists in pregnancy. The latter requires the homeostatic set points to be changed to accommodate the altered metabolic requirements. In most situations, however, leucocytosis implies a normal protective reaction to a variety of potential pathological conditions, especially in response to inflammation or infection. In any infection, leucocytosis representing an increase from 9000 to 15 000/mm^3 is a good sign, indicating that white cells are responding to the challenge. Conversely, no increase, or an inadequate increase, in leucocytes is an unfavourable sign. Once the infection subsides, the number of leucocytes returns to the normal homeostatic parameters.

Figure 11.9 The homeostatic and clinical control of the number of leucocytes. (a) Homeostatic levels of the number of leucocytes (i.e. production rate = destruction rate. b$_1$, Leucocytosis: white cells in excess of their homeostatic range. The excess can be a result of the homeostatic set points being changed in response to altered states of health (e.g. pregnancy), in which case the excess can be considered a normal adaptation to changing metabolic demands. Alternatively, the excess may be an indication of a protective response to infection and/or an underlying pathology. A differential white cell count indicates which leucocytic imbalance is present. The differential white cell count is an important diagnostic aid (see Tables 11.8 and 11.9). b$_2$, Leucopenia: white cells below the homeostatic range. Leucopenia can be a lack of all white cells, or a result of inadequate levels of specific white cells (Table 11.7). c$_1$, Clinical correction of leucocytosis includes chemotherapy and radiotherapy. Bone marrow transplantation may be required for those patients experiencing very high-dose chemotherapy, as this destroys all residual leucocytes. c$_2$, Clinical correction of agranulocytosis includes removal of the aetiological factor (e.g. rapid withdrawal of offending drugs, such as sulphonamides and antihistamine), and injections of hydrocortisone or adrenocorticotropic hormone (ACTH).

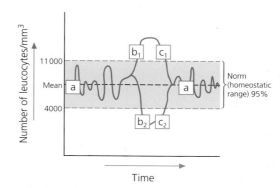

Granulocyte transfusions are still at the experimental stage and are used when antibiotic therapy is ineffective in controlling severe infections in patients with bone marrow neutropenia. (a, Represents boxes a$_1$–a$_4$ in Figure 1.7, p.11, reflecting the individual variability in the homeostatic range)

Table 11.7 Classification of homeostatic imbalances of blood cells

Blood cells	Excess (may indicate)	Deficiency (may indicate)
Leucocytes		
General	Leucocytosis	Leucopenia
Granulocytes	Neutrophilia (bacterial infection, burns, stress, inflammation, myocardial infarction)	Neutropenia (radiation exposure, drug toxicity, cytotoxic drug therapy, vitamin B$_{12}$ deficiency, systemic lupus erythematosus)
	Basophilia (allergic reaction, leukaemia, cancer, hypothyroidism)	Basopenia (pregnancy, ovulation, stress, hyperthyroidism)
	Eosinophilia (allergic reaction, parasitic infection, autoimmune disease)	Eosinopenia (drug toxicity, stress)
Non-granulocytes	Lymphocytosis (some leukaemias and viral infections, particularly Epstein–Barr virus and agents of glandular fever)	Lymphopenia (prolonged illness, malignant disease, e.g. Hodgkin's disease, immunosuppression cytotoxic therapy, treatment with cortisol)
	Monocytosis (viral or fungal infection, tuberculosis, some leukaemias, other chronic diseases)	Monopenia (bone marrow depression, treatment with cortisol)
Thrombocytes	Thrombocytosis (drugs, e.g. sulphonamides)	Thrombocytopenia (infections, some autoimmune diseases)
Erythrocytes	Polycythaemia	Anaemia (see Table 11.6)

Q *Differentiate between a physiological and a pathological polycythaemia.*

Q *Give two conditions that are associated with examples of thrombocytosis and thrombocytopenia.*

BOX 11.15 LEUKAEMIA

Leukaemia is a group of diseases characterized by gross excessive activity of the leucopoietic organs (bone marrow, spleen, lymph glands). Leukaemia is frequently called 'cancer of the blood' because of the vast quantities of circulating leucocytes. These proliferating white blood cells crowd out other cells produced in the marrow, so symptoms usually include a deficiency in red blood cells and platelets (i.e. anaemia and thrombocytopenia, respectively). The causes of leukaemia are largely unknown, although a few have been identified. For example, some people have a genetic predisposition that is triggered by environmental factors, such as radiation or viruses. Leukaemias are classified according to the cell type involved (Table 11.8) and according to the rate of development, i.e. acute and chronic leukaemias.

The most common cause of death from leukaemia is internal haemorrhaging, especially within the brain. Another frequent cause of death is uncontrolled infection owing to the lack of mature, or normal, leucocytes. In this case, leucocyte production is so fast that the cells do not mature and are dysfunctional. Treatment is aimed at correcting this abnormal accumulation of white cells using radiotherapy and anti-leukaemic (cytotoxic) drugs. Partial or complete remission may be induced, lasting perhaps for as long as 15 years. Table 11.9 compares the typical results of a differential white cell count of a normal person and a patient with leukaemia.

BOX 11.16 GRANULOCYTE COLONY-STIMULATING FACTORS AND BONE MARROW TRANSPLANT

Granulocyte colony-stimulating factors (GCSFs) are administered to cancer patients who are taking non-specific cytotoxic drugs that kill cancer cells but also damage surrounding bone marrow cells in the process. The GCSFs help to promote replacement of these marrow cells.

The GCSFs and epoietin (see Box 11.12, p.282) are also given to patients who have received bone marrow transplants to improve the outcome of the procedure.

Bone marrow transplants are an exciting addition to the therapeutic possibilities for haematological disease. Transplant may be used to treat patients with aplastic anaemias, haemolytic anaemias, sickle cell disease, acute leukaemia, Hodgkin's and non-Hodgkin's disease, thalassaemia, infrequent congenital immune deficiency and haemopoietic disorders, and breast, ovarian and testicular cancers. The transplant involves the intravenous transfer of red bone marrow stem cells from the healthy donor to the recipient. The aim is to provide a normal haemopoi-

etic function. The transplanted cells travel immediately to the marrow spaces that have been emptied by disease (e.g. in aplastic anaemia); in patients with cancer, the defective red bone marrow first must be destroyed by high doses of chemotherapy and whole-body radiation. Although a transplant is the best chance of a cure for such patients, it has potential risks. The donor cells proliferate in the marrow, releasing functional cells into the peripheral circulation. Complete marrow recovery may take 6–8 weeks.

The major barrier to the success of bone marrow transplant is the antigenic differences between donor and recipient. Identical twins are ideal donors for each other as they have identical human leucocyte antigen (HLA); therefore bone marrow transplants between identical twins are nearly always successful. More commonly, the donor is an HLA-identical brother, sister or parent; these transplants are often successful. If the patient and donor are not HLA-identical, immunosuppression is necessary.

BOX 11.17 LEUCOPENIA

A marked reduction of white blood cells – leucopenia – is usually known as a neutropenia, since the most significant reduction is usually the neutrophil population. Neutropenia is usually a consequence of bone marrow depression, often as a result of the toxic side-effects of drugs (e.g. chlorpromazine or the sulphonamides) in people with high sensitivity. It may also arise as a consequence of a radiotherapy and anti-cancer drug therapy. It is also associated with overwhelming infections, such as

malaria, typhoid fever and hyposplenism (a condition in which the spleen destroys neutrophils at an accelerated rate).

Management of leucopoenia is by the withdrawal of any possible offending drugs; if the granulocyte count is very low, the patient is protected from obvious sources of infection. The aim of treatment is to abolish the factor responsible for the bone marrow depression. Spontaneous restoration of marrow function often occurs in 2–3 weeks.

Table 11.8 Types of leukaemia and the cells involved

Type	Cells involved
Myeloid (myelocytic, myeloblastic)	Granulocytes
Lymphocytic (lymphoblastic)	Lymphocytes
Monocytic	Monocytes

Table 11.9 Typical results for a differential leucocyte count

Leucocytes	Normal	Leukaemia patient
Neutrophils	65	3
Monocytes	8	1
Lymphocytes	24	96
Eosinophils	2	–
Basophils	1	–

Values are percentage of total leucocyte population in blood from a normal person and blood from a patient with leukaemia.

referred to as marginating cells. The remaining granulocytes circulate in the blood. Within a matter of hours, however, some of these circulating cells enter the tissues requiring their services; these never return to blood.

Some agranulocytes (i.e. lymphocytes and monocytes) are produced in the red bone marrow, but other areas, however, are also involved. For example, before birth, and for a few months after birth, some lymphocytes (T-cells) are produced in the thymus gland. Subsequently, most lymphocytes (T- and B-cells) and monocytes are formed within the lymph nodes and other lymphatic tissue, such as the spleen, adenoids, tonsils and appendix (see Figure 13.4a, p.367).

The lifespan of a leucocyte is the shortest of all the cellular components of blood. While red cells live for 100–120 days and platelets for 5–9 days, in a healthy body white cells will survive for only 4–5 days. Neutrophils have an even shorter

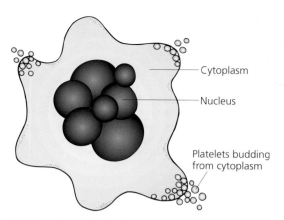

Figure 11.10 A megakaryocyte, showing platelet budding

Q Where do megakaryocytes originate?

lifespan – 12 hours or less – when they are actively phagocytosing bacteria, as the bacterial antigens interfere with metabolism and accelerate cell death.

Homeostatic failures affecting the leucocyte population

Leucocytosis and leucopenia are general terms used to indicate leucocyte levels above and below, respectively, the homeostatic range. The suffixes '-osis' and '-penia' are used to indicate a specific leucocytic excess or deficiency, respectively (e.g. granulocytosis or granulocytopenia).

Thrombocytes

Structure

Thrombocytes (platelets) are more numerous than leucocytes, but less numerous than erythrocytes; there are approximately 250 000/mm³. Thrombocytes are the smallest cellular components of blood, being only 2–4 μm in diameter. They do not have a nucleus; microscopically, they appear as a disc-shaped structure with a colourless cytoplasm. Their membranes are the sites of many enzymatic reactions, and contain specific receptors for collagen and the hormones serotonin and adrenaline. These receptors enable platelets to respond to tissue damage and trauma. Microfilaments in the cytoplasm are composed of a contractile protein called platelet actomyosin (i.e. analogous to actin/myosin in muscle cells). These filaments function in

the haemostatic process of clot retraction (see later). Thrombocytes possess numerous cytoplasmic granules that contain enzymes (or factors) that are released when platelets aggregate together and/or are lysed. These enzymes are important in the homeostatic function of blood coagulation.

Production and destruction of thrombocytes

Thrombocytes are formed in the red marrow, lungs and, to some extent, the spleen and liver, by the fragmentation (platelet budding) of very large cells called megakaryocytes (Figures 11.3, p.273 and 11.10). The rate of platelet production (called thrombopoiesis) is regulated tightly between the two interchangeable platelet 'pools' of the circulation and spleen. The feedback mechanism for thrombopoiesis and this interchange has yet to be identified. However, it must be stimulated by a low platelet count (thrombocytopenia). A platelet's lifespan is about 5–9 days, after which it is destroyed by specialized macrophages of the liver and spleen.

WOUND HEALING

Wound healing is a remarkable process. Without it, surgery would be impossible; furthermore, the more surgery advances, the greater becomes the problem of wound healing. The problems are numerous for patients with systemic ischaemia, infection, pre-existing medical conditions such as jaundice and diabetes mellitus, or malnutrition, and patients taking anti-inflammatory and steroidal drugs, but the requirements are the same: a safely healed wound after surgery.

Wound assessment has traditionally been the responsibility of nursing staff, and has tended to be subjective, often relying on anecdotal evidence that frequently fails to report accurate information. It is our view that accurate wound assessment and management are dependent on an understanding of the biochemistry of healing, the factors that delay the process, and the optimal conditions required at the wound surface to maximize healing.

A wound may be defined as 'an interruption to the continuity of the external surface of the body, which may be due to accidental injury, planned surgery, thermal injury, pressure, or disease process such as leg ulceration or carcinoma' and wound healing as 'the physiological process by which the body

Figure 11.11 Repair, regeneration and restoration of a tissue's structural and functional integrity following injury. a, Structural and functional integrity of body tissues intact. b, Compromised structural and functional integrity of the body's tissues owing to tissue loss. c, Speedy and complete repair and regeneration with complete restoration of the functional integrity of body tissues. Labile tissues, such as the skin, undergo mitosis throughout life, and therefore have excellent repair capabilities. d_1/d_2, Partial repair and regeneration, with only partial restoration of the functional integrity of body tissues following injury. Stable tissues, such as the liver, normally exhibit little mitotic activity during adult life but are capable of increasing the rate of cell division if they are damaged. Although such tissues may heal, their complex architecture may not regenerate, and they may not necessarily be restored to full function. e, Minor repair and regeneration, with loss of functional integrity of tissue

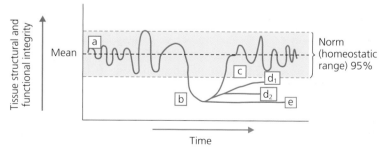

following injury, resulting in scarring of the damaged area. Permanent tissues, such as the brain, spinal cord and skeletal muscle, exhibit little mitotic activity during adult life. They are so complex that little repair, other than scarring, can be achieved following injury. (a, Represents boxes a_1–a_4 in Figure 1.7, p.11, reflecting the individual variability in the homeostatic range)

Table 11.10 Role of nutrients in the process of wound healing. Note that nutrients are intracellular metabolites and/or products of metabolism

Intracellular metabolites/products vital for wound-healing process		Role of nutrients in providing intracellular products vital for wound healing	Nutrient deficiency: the effect on wound healing
Macronutrients			
Proteins			
General role of proteins		Metabolism of cell membranes Enzyme synthesis	Prolonged inflammation Impairs fibroplasia
Specific role of an amino acid	Cysteine	Important role in collagen synthesis	Delays collagen synthesis Delays angiogenesis Delays wound remodelling
Lipids			
General roles of lipids		Concentrated energy source Metabolism of cell membranes	
Specific role of a fatty acid	Linoleic acid	Maintains integrity and function of cellular unit membranes Prostaglandin precursor	Rare
Carbohydrates			
General role of carbohydrates		Energy source for all cells	
Specific role of glucose		Primary energy fuel for metabolism of leucocytes and fibroblasts	Gluconeogenesis from protein metabolism resulting in protein energy malnutrition in patients with severe injuries
Micronutrients			
Vitamins			
General role of vitamins		Cofactors, therefore important for general metabolism and maintenance of health	
Specific roles of some vitamins	Vitamin C	Cofactor for several amino acids Antioxidant factor enhances wound healing	Wounds healing inefficiently Increases likelihood of pressure sore development
	Vitamin B complex	Involved in collagen cross-linkages	Rare
	Vitamin A	Epithelial proliferation/migration *Collagen cross-linkages	Rare
	Vitamin E	Antioxidant may work with vitamin C	Rare
	Vitamin K	Coagulation (see text)	
Minerals			
General role of minerals		Cofactors, therefore important for general metabolism and maintenance of health	
Specific roles of minerals Iron		*Cofactor important in collagen synthesis	Anaemia, therefore delays the wound-healing process Decreased collagen synthesis/cell proliferation
Zinc		*Cofactor important in collagen synthesis, protein synthesis	Decreased wound-healing processes
Copper		*Cofactor important in collagen cross-linkages	
Calcium		*Remodelling of collagen	
Magnesium		*Synthesis of collagen	

*Important in remodelling of collagen; deficiencies lead to decreased collagen cross-linkages, therefore reducing strength of scar tissue.

replaces and restores the function of damaged tissue' (Clancy and McVicar, 2002).

Skin is predominantly affected. Other tissue (e.g. muscle) may be torn, bones fractured and blood flow disrupted during a major procedure such as open-heart surgery. This section considers only the healing of skin wounds but the healing process following injury to the skin is a good illustration of the basic processes of healing. Bone healing is a modification on this and is discussed in Chapter 3, pp.66–8.

The extent of tissue injury or tissue death (necrosis) depends largely on the intensity and duration of the exposure to the injurious agent, as well as the type of tissue involved (Clancy and McVicar, 2002). Thus, the homeostatic responses of tissue repair, regeneration and replacement are necessary following tissue injury or tissue death to maintain the numbers of cells within their homeostatic limits, and so as not to compromise cell, tissue and organ system functional integrity. Tissues can be divided into three categories according to their repair, regeneration and restoration capabilities (Figure 11.11).

Figure 11.12 The interdependency of organ systems in providing intracellular metabolites and products necessary for wound healing. Intracellular metabolites include micronutrients (Table 11.10). Intracellular products include macronutrients (Table 11.10) and products of metabolism that are important in the healing process, including serotonin (released from basophils), histamine (released from basophils, platelets and cells that have been damaged), prostaglandins and kinins (released from cells that have been damaged), clotting factors (released from cells that have been damaged, and from platelets), antibodies (released from B-lymphocytes), collagen and elastin (released from fibrocytes), macrophage-attracting substances (e.g. complement; released from liver cells), prothrombin and fibrinogen (released from liver cells), cytotoxic substances (released from T-lymphocytes), and mitotic growth factors (released from cells that have no contact inhibition). (a, Represents boxes a_1–a_4 in Figure 1.7, p.11, reflecting the individual variability in the homeostatic range)

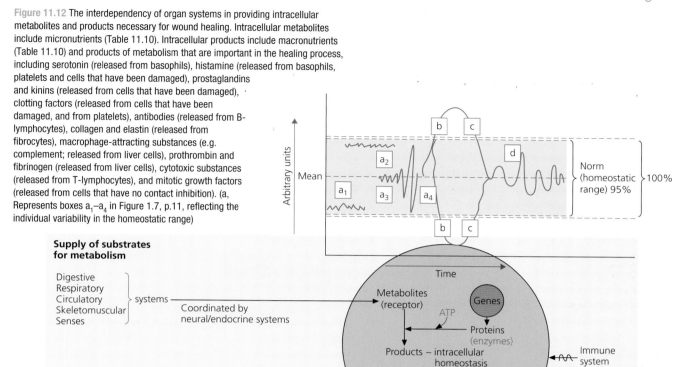

BOX 11.18 CLASSIFICATION OF WOUNDS

Wounds are conventionally classified as either superficial (non-bleeding) or deep (bleeding). Damage to the epidermis will not result in bleeding, since this layer does not contain blood vessels. Its main function is to form a protective covering from the external environment. Wound healing of this tissue involves the replacement of cells known as the germinating layer, since the layers above it are derived from the mitotic activity of this layer (Figure 11.13a).

Damage to the deeper dermal layer results in a bleeding wound, since blood vessels are present in this layer of the skin (Figure 11.13b). This type of injury involves a more complicated type of wound healing. The initial homeostatic responses are involved in repairing and regenerating damaged blood vessels, thus restoring transport of the vital factors essential for the wound-healing process of the tissue above it (i.e. the epidermal cells). Of course, if blood vessels are damaged directly, blood will also be lost at the site of the injury, by either escaping to the outside or being retained in the tissue as a bruise (haematoma). Wound healing of connective soft tissues follows a similar process. It involves the for-

mation of new epithelium and contraction of healthy granulation tissue beneath to form a fibrous scar.

There are two basic types of wound healing: primary and secondary intentions. Healing by primary intention (or closure) is the most common type of healing following surgery. It occurs when the tissue edges are maintained in apposition. The lower layers are stitched with a dissolvable suture, and the skin is either sutured or clipped together (Figure 11.14a). This should be achieved in all incised surgical wounds and primarily sutured fresh traumatic lacerations. The wound heals quickly with minimal scarring.

In secondary intention healing, the wound edges are distant from each other. The cavity fills via granulation tissue from the lowest part of the wound upwards, with the epithelial layer being the last to grow (Figure 11.14b). This type of wound closure is sometimes achieved in full-thickness burns, chronic leg ulceration, after surgical excision of necrotic tissue and when the wound is infected.

A wound may also be categorized as clean, bacterially contaminated, or infected.

Chapter 1 discussed the importance of the interdependency of organ systems in maintaining intracellular homeostasis (see Figures 1.5, p.9 and 1.6, p.10). This interdependence is vital in producing the optimal physico-biochemical conditions required at the wound surface to maximize the healing process. For example:

- efficient digestive functioning provides essential intracellular nutrients (metabolites and products of metabolism) for

repair, regeneration and restoration of tissue integrity following injury (Table 11.10 and Figure 11.12);
- efficient circulatory functioning is necessary to transport leucocytes (to protect the integrity of undamaged cells), nutrients, oxygen and biochemicals important to the wound-healing process to the site of tissue damage;
- the lymphatics prevent the accumulation of tissue fluid via their drainage facilities, and so minimize the discomfort

(oedema and associated pain) that can accompany inflammation as a result of fluid compression on surrounding soft tissues;

* the excretory organs remove cellular/chemical debris from the damaged site. This decreases the likelihood of septicaemia (the presence of a large number of bacteria and their toxins) and toxaemia (poisoning of the blood by absorption of bacterial toxins), particularly during injury accompanied by an infection;

* the coordinators (neural/hormonal mediators) of body functions direct the systemic interactions listed above involved in providing the optimal physico-biochemical conditions for the wound-healing process.

Therefore, it should not come as any surprise that an inefficiency of one component part of the body leads to functional disturbances of other parts. For example, if cardiovascular function is compromised (e.g. in progressive atherosclerosis), as occurs in older people and in people with diabetes mellitus, wound healing is delayed because of inadequate cardiovascular homeostatic responses to tissue damage.

Local and general responses to injury

The homeostatic responses to injury are divided into two types of response:

* *Local responses*: responses in the injured tissues (the focus of this chapter).
* *General responses*: responses elicited in the rest of the body by the local response. These responses can be referred to as 'shock'. Many forms of shock exist, each of which describes the pattern of responses to a particular injury or 'antigenic insult'; for example, cardiogenic shock is a response to heart failure, haemorrhagic shock is a response to haemorrhage, traumatic shock is a response to trauma and septic or endotoxic shock is a response to infection (Clancy and McVicar, 1996).

BOX 11.19 ASSESSMENT OF WOUNDS

Careful assessment of the patient's wound by the nurse (and other healthcare practitioners) is vital in identifying the specific stage/phase of the healing process, since treatment may vary at each stage/phase. Poor wound management often results from an incorrect identification of the stage of wound healing or a failure to detect any variation from the normal process. The characteristics associated with healing, therefore, are a vital part of the healthcare process involved in wound care. Clinical observation skills are important in identifying prolonged inflammation, infection, necrotic tissue, unhealthy granulation tissue, ischaemia, delayed epithelialization, skin maceration, sensitivities and allergies. Observational skills also are required to identify nutritional and fluid imbalances and whether the patient is in pain. Other factors that need to be included are the patient's coping processes, and psychological factors and their effects on healing.

ACTIVITY

Before continuing read about the structure and associated functions of the skin in Chapter 16, pp.446–54.

The wound-healing process

The healing process occurs as a set of homeostatic responses brought about by trauma. The process can be divided conveniently into four main stages: the vascular, inflammation, proliferation and maturation stages. Substages or phases exist within the main stages (e.g. the platelet and blood coagulation phases of the vascular stage). There is, however, considerable overlap between the stages/phases, and in the time required by an individual to progress to the next stage/phase of healing.

The vascular stage

The vascular stage comprises five principal phases: the vascular, platelet, coagulation, clot retraction and clot destruction phases. The process is summarized in Figure 11.15.

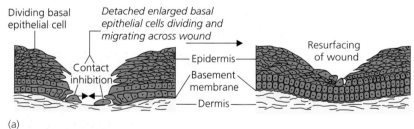

Dividing basal epithelial cell
Detached enlarged basal epithelial cells dividing and migrating across wound
Resurfacing of wound
Contact inhibition
Epidermis
Basement membrane
Dermis
(a)

Blood clot in wound
Basement membrane
Basal epithelial cell migrating across wound
White blood cell
Bundle of collagenous fibres
Fibroblast
Monocyte
Scab formation
'New' tissue
Dilated blood vessel   *Damaged blood vessel*
(b)

Figure 11.13 (a) Epidermal wound healing following superficial injury (e.g. a mild abrasion of the skin). Basal (germinating) cells divide and migrate across a superficial wound. (b) Epidermal wound healing following injury to deep layers of the skin (e.g. a surgical incision). This involves generation of a new blood supply (angiogenesis) before the division and migration of basal (germinating) cells across the surface of the wound

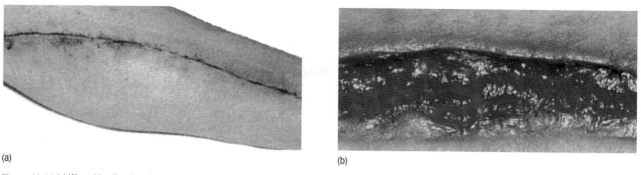

(a)

(b)

Figure 11.14 (a) Wound healing by primary intention or closure (e.g. as occurs with surgical incision). The wound is closed to eliminate the dead space, and is held together by sutures or clips. There is minimal granulation and a low risk of scarring. If scarring is present, it fades with time and disappears when wound healing is matured. Primary closure is not appropriate for infected or long-standing wounds. (b) Wound healing by secondary intention or closure (e.g. as occurs with leg ulceration when there is a lot of tissue lost or when there is a risk of infection). The wound is left open to heal by granulation. Cosmetically, the results are comparable to primary intention wound healing

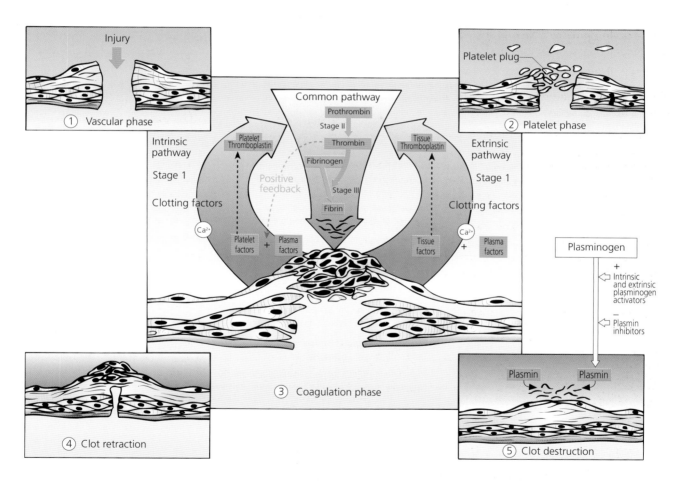

Figure 11.15 The clotting mechanism. (Details of plasma and platelet clotting factors are discussed in the text and in Table 11.11.) 1, Vascular phase: vessels go into spasm in the damaged smooth muscle, which decreases blood flow. 2, Platelet phase: thrombocytes accumulate and adhere to the damaged vessels, forming the platelet plug. 3, Coagulation phase: activation of clotting and clot formation. 4, Clot retraction: contraction of the blood clot. 5, Clot destruction: enzymatic (plasmin) destruction of the clot. +, stimulatory; −, inhibitory

Q *Why does whole blood fail to clot when calcium ions are removed?*

Q *What are the outcomes of the first, second and third stages of clotting?*

The vascular phase

Seconds after damage to blood vessels, the muscular wall (the tunica media; see Figure 12.12a p.332) contracts, a process called vasoconstriction ('vaso-' = vessel). This muscle spasm decreases blood flow and therefore minimizes blood loss for up to 30 minutes, thus aiding other homeostatic responses within the haemostatic response (responses associated with arresting bleeding). In addition to the vascular stage of haemostasis, the platelet and blood coagulation phases also act to prevent blood loss. These mechanisms are adequate as homeostatic controls in preventing blood loss if the damage is to small blood vessels. If larger blood vessels are involved (resulting in mass haemorrhage), these mechanisms are inadequate.

The platelet phase

The platelets (thrombocytes) that come into contact with the damaged vessel enlarge. They become irregular in shape, and extremely sticky, adhering to the collagen fibres of the vessel wall. These thrombocytes secrete substances (e.g. thromboxane A2, or TXA2) that activate more platelets, causing them to stick to the original platelets. The aggregation and attachment of platelets forms a platelet plug almost immediately after the damage. The plug becomes strengthened by fibrin threads formed during the coagulation process and is extremely effective in preventing blood loss from small vessels.

The blood coagulation phase

Coagulation is a complicated metabolic pathway involving many interdependent enzyme-controlled reactions. Collectively, these reactions are called the clotting cascade. This cascade is a multiplicative process; proenzymes (inactive enzymes) interact such that the conversion of one proenzyme creates an enzyme that activates a second proenzyme, which activates a third proenzyme, and so on, in a chain reaction that increases in magnitude with each step. Many clotting factors are involved (Table 11.11), including plasma factors (numbered I–XIII) and platelet factors (labelled Pf1–4). The cascade occurs rapidly once stimulated; when blood is taken in a blood test, or when a vessel is damaged, blood is converted quickly from its usual liquefied state into a gel-like clot. The process is

Table 11.11 The homeostatic importance of coagulation factors

Coagulation factors	Homeostatic importance
Plasma coagulation factors	
I Fibrinogen	Important factor in stage III of clotting, in which it is converted to fibrin
II Prothrombin	Important in stage II of clotting, in which it is converted into thrombin
III Thromboplastin (thrombokinase)	In extrinsic pathway, referred to as extrinsic thromboplastin; formed from tissue thromboplastin In intrinsic pathway, referred to as intrinsic thromboplastin; formed from platelet disintegration Formation of thromboplastin signifies the end of stage I
IV Calcium ions	Involved in all three stages of clotting Removal of calcium in the plasma prevents coagulation
V Proaccelerin (labile) factor	Required for stages I and II of extrinsic and intrinsic pathways
VI No longer used in coagulation therapy	
VII Serum prothrombin accelerator (stable) factor	Required in stage I extrinsic pathway
VIII Anti-haemophilic factor	Required for stage I of intrinsic pathway Deficiency causes classical haemophilia A
IX Christmas factor (plasma thromboplastin) component	Required for stage I of intrinsic pathway Deficiency causes haemophilia B
X Stuart factor (Stuart–Prower factor)	Required for stages I and II of extrinsic and intrinsic pathways Deficiency results in nose bleeds, bleeding into joints, or bleeding into soft tissues
XI Plasma thromboplastin antecedent	Required for stage I of intrinsic pathway Deficiency causes haemophilia C
XII Hageman factor	Required for stage I of intrinsic pathway
XIII Fibrin stabilizing factor	Required for stage III of clotting
NB. Vitamin K is required for the synthesis of factors II, VII, IX ad X. Vitamin K deficiency often leads to uncontrolled bleeding	
Platelet coagulation factors	
Platelet factor 1 – Pf1	Essentially the same as plasma coagulation factor V
Platelet factor 2 – Pf2	Accelerates formation of thrombin in stage 1 intrinsic pathway and the conversion of fibrinogen to fibrin
Platelet factor 3 – Pf3	Required for stage I of intrinsic pathway
Platelet factor 4 – Pf4	Binds heparin, an anticoagulant during clotting

initiated within 30 seconds of damage, and completed after several minutes. The coagulation phase can be summarized as a sequence of three stages:

1 *Stage I*: damage tissues release a collection of enzymes collectively called thromboplastin or thrombokinase.
2 *Stage II*: thromboplastin converts inactive plasma prothrombin into active thrombin.
3 *Stage III*: thrombin converts the soluble plasma protein fibrinogen into insoluble fibrin, which forms the threads of the clot.

The initiating enzymes (thromboplastin) are released from damaged tissue cells, triggering the extrinsic coagulation pathway, and/or in plasma following the lysis of platelets, which triggers the intrinsic coagulation pathway. The extrinsic pathway is initiated by the release of a tissue factor (an enzyme) from damaged peripheral cells and/or damaged capillary endothelial cells. This enzyme, together with certain plasma factors (IV, V, VII and X), forms extrinsic or tissue thromboplastin, which is equivalent to stage I of the clotting cascade (Figure 11.15). The second stage utilizes extrinsic thromboplastin to convert prothrombin into thrombin. The third stage is then promoted, with the conversion of fibrinogen into fibrin by the action of thrombin and plasma factors IV and XIII. Most steps in the extrinsic mechanism also require the presence of calcium ions.

The intrinsic pathway is normally activated when there is damage to the internal lining of the blood vessels. It is also activated by the presence of a rough surface, such as fatty plaques or calcium deposits attached to the internal lining of the blood vessel (see Figure 12.13a, p.324). This stimulus removes the normal repulsion activities between platelets and endothelial cells lining the blood vessels, with the result that platelets adhere to the rough surface. The aggregation and clumping of platelets bring about their lysis, releasing platelet coagulation factors (Pf1–4) into the plasma. The clumping reaction is sometimes all that is necessary to plug a lightly damaged area.

Stage I of the intrinsic pathway involves four platelet factors (Pf1–4) and seven plasma factors (IV, V, VIII, IX, X, XI and XII) to form intrinsic thromboplastin. Most factor activations require the presence of calcium. The second and third stages are the same for both intrinsic and extrinsic pathways, and involve the conversion of prothrombin into thrombin by thromboplastin, and the conversion of fibrinogen to fibrin. Both also require the presence of calcium ions.

Thrombin is a key chemical because of its further involvement in the third stage. Thus, it also stimulates more platelets to adhere to one another, resulting in a further lysis of platelets, and thus the consequential release of further platelet factors. The more thrombin that is released, the more platelet factors are released, resulting in more thrombin production, hence greater clot formation. This cyclical process is therefore a positive feedback mechanism. It ensures continual platelet lysis until the clot is formed so that the healing process can proceed appropriately. For example, the tissue damage that accompanies bleeding activates both extrinsic and intrinsic pathways to maximize clot formation and arrest bleeding.

The clot retraction phase

Once the fibrin meshwork has been formed, the platelets and erythrocytes stick to its strands. The platelets contract, with the result that the entire clot retracts, bringing the torn edges closer together, stabilizing and consolidating the injury. The clot plugs the damaged vessel to prevent further blood loss, and the retraction makes it easier for fibroblasts, smooth muscle cells, and endothelial cells to perform their homeostatic repair functions.

The clot destruction phase

Once the area is repaired, the clot is dissolved via the process of fibrinolysis, which involves tissue factors (intrinsic and extrinsic) that activate the precursor plasminogen into the clot-dissolving enzyme plasmin.

ACTIVITY

List the three stages of the clotting reaction. Describe the role of extrinsic and intrinsic thromboplastin.

The inflammation stage

This is the part of the non-specific response to infection: when a tissue is damaged via mechanical, thermal or chemical causes, or in response to a hypersensitive reaction or a pathogenic invasion, the body reacts in the same way. The tissue soon shows the four classic signs of inflammation (Figure 11.16), which provide a reassurance that normal homeostatic responses have been activated following injury. These signs are redness, an increase in tissue temperature, swelling, and pain and discomfort. These signs may be followed by an additional loss of function. The first three responses are characteristic of changes in the microcirculation in the injured tissue. The redness (erythema) results from vasodilation of the arterioles (smallest arteries); heat results from increased blood flow; and swelling (oedema) is caused by an increase in the extravascular

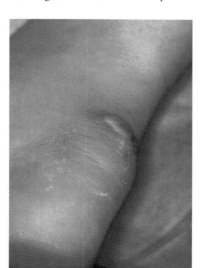

Figure 11.16 Wound showing the classical signs of inflammation (see also Figures, 13.1b, p.360, 13.3c, p.366 and 13.10c, p378)

Q List the classical signs of inflammation.

fluid content of the injured tissues. This post-traumatic oedema is promoted by an increase in microvascular permeability; the consequential loss of blood components is called exudation.

The permeability changes are in response to the secretion from the site of injury of cellular products of metabolism (see Figure 11.12, p.289), such as:

- histamine, released from mast cells (basophils), platelets and damaged cells at the site of injury;
- serotonin and heparin, released from mast cells;
- kinins and prostaglandins, released from injured cells.

The role of the exudate is to promote the entrance of proteins and phagocytic white cells into the wound from the plasma. Generally, the proteins in the tissue fluid create a colloidal osmotic pressure, promoting fluid leakage from plasma, resulting in the accumulation of tissue fluid (McVicar and Clancy, 1997). The increased blood flow to the area, and the accumulation of fluid in the soft tissues, eventually exerts pressure on sensory nerve endings, making the wound feel uncomfortable and/or painful. Pain is also a result of the presence of kinins and prostaglandins, which stimulate pain receptors (see Figure 20.1, p.526).

The next part of the process of inflammation involves the removal of debris and microorganisms. Phagocytes, such as neutrophils and macrophages, dispose of damaged tissue cells, foreign material and microorganisms via phagocytosis (see Figures 13.10, p.378, and 13.17, p.383). This process is facilitated by the presence in the exudate of other white cells (T- and B-lymphocytes) and various proteinaceous components, collectively called complement. Complement facilitates the phagocytic and lymphocytic responses to either prevent or fight infection (see Figure 13.15b,d, p.381).

ACTIVITY

Refer to Chapter 13, pp.375–88 for the details associated with the phagocytic response, the lymphocytic responses, and the role of complement.

To summarize, neutrophils are attracted into the wound first, usually within a few hours of injury; they are followed by macrophages. The activity of lymphocytes essentially cleanses the wound bed. Macrophages arriving at the site secrete growth factors, prostaglandins and complement factors, which aid antibody–antigen complexing. Since these chemicals promote healing, macrophages are usually present during all stages of wound healing. In clean wounds, the inflammatory phase lasts approximately 36 hours; in necrotic or infected wounds, the process is prolonged.

The biochemical constitution of the exudate reflects the intensity and duration of the injurious agent. For example:

- serous exudate has low protein content, indicating that there is superficial and minimal damage, as occurs with blistering of the skin;

BOX 11.20 INFLAMMATION

The process of inflammation is considered beneficial since it involves the homeostatic responses that restore tissue homeostatic integrity by neutralizing and destroying antigens locally at the site of injury. The process is referred to as a biological emergency response, since there is a latent stage of approximately 12 hours before any obvious healing begins. Therefore, during the inflammatory process the patient may feel generally ill. Signs and symptoms may include fever, loss of appetite, and tiredness. The process of wound healing may also instigate harmful effects, such as:

- oedema in vital organs, such as the lungs, heart and brain. Cerebral oedema is a common cause of raised intracranial pressures in head injury;
- autolysis (self-destruction) of local body tissues, due to the release of lysozymes from the large numbers of phagocytes presents in the exudate;
- complications caused by the lodging of antigen–antibody complexes.

The detrimental aspects of inflammation means that wound healing can be encouraged to go to completion faster if it can be reduced when healing is sufficiently progressed. Suppression of inflammatory responses by the hormone cortisol is an aspect of the stress response following trauma (see Chapter 21, p.599).

ACTIVITY

Refer to Chapter 13, in particular Figure 13.15, p.381 to review the antigen–antibody complexing process.

- fibrinous exudate indicates damage of a more intense nature, since this type of wound requires the development of a protective fibrin clot. The material must be removed if a scar is not to form;
- haemorrhagic exudate has the same biochemical constitution as a fibrous exudate, with the additional presence of erythrocytes, indicating that the injury has damaged blood vessels;
- purulent exudates are wounds that contain pus (a mixture of living and dead body cells, dead microbes, cell debris such as proteinaceous fibres and bacteria toxins). Such an exudate is detrimental to the healing process.

The proliferation stage

Following the vascular and inflammatory stages, replacement, repair and regeneration of injured cells must occur. This stage is referred to as proliferation, during which the wound is filled with new connective tissue. The three processes involved are granulation, contraction and epithelialization.

Granulation

The filling of the deep wound with tissue during proliferation is usually referred to as granulation (see Figure 11.13b, p.290). Initially, this process involves the creation of new capillaries (a process called angiogenesis) in the wound bed to support the mitotic activity that provides replacement cells.

BOX 11.21 ANGIOGENESIS

The importance of an adequate blood supply in granulation is illustrated by the slow rate of healing induced by circulatory deficiencies in conditions such as diabetes mellitus. Granulation is also slowed in elderly people, partly because of reduced cardiovascular efficiency, but also because rates of cell division and cell metabolism decline with age.

Angiogenesis is stimulated by the tissue hypoxia that is caused by the disruption of blood flow at the time of injury. Capillary 'buds' develop from the periphery of the wound and grow into the site at about 0.5 mm/day. Macrophage activity (arising from the process of inflammation) may stimulate this process. In addition, macrophages stimulate the production and multiplication of fibroblasts; these cells migrate along the fibrin threads (produced in the vascular phase), lay down a ground substance, and begin the secretion of collagen that supports the granulation tissue and will ultimately form the scar of the wound.

The characteristics of healthy and unhealthy granulation tissue are summarized in Figure 11.17.

Wound contraction

Following the deposition of connective tissue, the fibroblasts that have congregated at the wound margins develop contractile proteins and use their properties to pull the edges of the wound together, thus reducing the size of the wound (see also 'The clot retraction phase' above).

Wound epithelialization

The proliferating, migrating new epithelial cells from the wound edge, and, in skin, remnants of hair follicles, sweat and sebaceous glands, move across the surface of the wound until the wound is closed. It is not understood completely why cells should begin to migrate, but it is thought that the loss of contact between neighbouring cells causes the movement, (i.e. 'contact inhibition' is removed) (see Figure 11.13a, p.290). This concept has been refined in recent years, and it is clear that cells adjoining each other communicate and modulate each others' behaviour. Movement stops when others surround the cell, although these cells however must be of the same 'type' (e.g. cancer cells appear to lose contact inhibition). Once the migrated cells have formed a new germinating layer, they will divide, and new epidermal strata will be formed. Newly formed epithelial cells have a translucent appearance; they are usually whitish-pink (Figure 11.17c) and are 'raised' to some degree in relation to the surrounding tissue. The signs of inflammation should subside; thus the amount of wound exudate decreases and becomes more manageable.

Complete healing is possible only once the epithelial cells have completely bridged the surface of the wound. Any scab over the wound will slough away, and the new epidermis will become toughened by the production of the protein keratin. The whole process normally takes place over 24–48 hours after injury, except when there is substantial tissue loss when epithelialization may continue for up to a year or more.

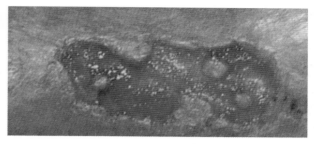
(a)

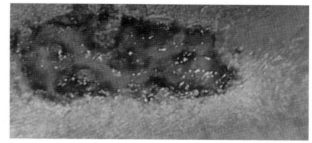
(b)

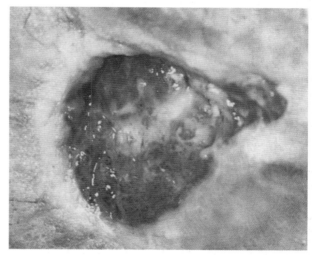
(c)

Figure 11.17 (a) Wound showing signs of healthy granulation. Note that the wound has a bright red, moist, shiny appearance. (b) Wound showing signs of unhealthy granulation. Note that the wound has a dark red colour (in parts), and a dehydrated and dull appearance. (c) Wound showing the process of epithelialization. Note the pinkish-white skin around the edges of the wound

The maturation stage

Once the granulation, wound contraction and epithelialization phases are completed, the final stage of wound healing – maturation – occurs. This stage can take from 24 hours to 2 years to complete, depending upon the severity of the wound and tissue involved. In the maturation phase, the fibrocytes begin to disappear. Collagen fibres form a mesh, strengthening the tissue, and become indistinguishable from the surrounding area in both colour and texture. The original clot is removed by the action of plasmin (see Figure 11.15, p.291; see also 'The clot destruction phase' above).

BOX 11.22 COMMON WOUND HEALING THERAPIES

Some common therapies used in wound care are: biotherapy, hydrotherapy, hyperbaric oxygen, therapeutic light, laser therapy, ultrasound and electrical stimulation.

Biotherapy

Growth factors and living skin equivalent are two forms of biotherapy used for a wound that needs healing. Growth factors stimulate cell proliferation, and therefore coordinate healing in the wound bed. There are various growth factors secreted at specific times as the wound heals and if either one is not produced, secreted or removed at the appropriate time from tissues in the wound healing is compromised.

Platelet-derived growth factor (PDGF) is known as the 'Master Factor' since this plays a central role in attracting and activating cell division of phagocytes (neutrophils, monocytes) and fibroblasts. Fibrocytes are responsible for collagen formation and therefore important in the process of granulation. It is generally claimed that clinically synthetic PDGF-based products such as becaplermin (Regranex gel, 0.01%) increase wound closure rates by over 40%, provided that there is an adequate vascular supply so that proper wound bed preparation can take place. The gel is recommended for use on lower limb diabetic neuropathic ulcers that involve tissues at and below the hypodermis (subcutaneous) level. Other growth factors include:

- *Transforming growth factor beta* (TGF-beta): controls movement of cells to the inflammatory 'beds' and stimulates extracellular matrix formation.
- *Basic fibroblast growth factor* (b-FGF): incites angiogenesis.
- *Insulin-like growth factor* (IGF): enhances collagen production.
- *Epidermal growth factor* (EGF): stimulates epidermal regeneration.

Living skin cell equivalents (e.g. Dermagraft) replace the dermis consist of neonatal fibroblasts seeded on a dissolvable polyglactin suture matrix scaffolding, which serve as an extracellular medium. The fibroblasts produce, secrete and fill the matrix provide an interactive wound covering where growth factors and other molecules may enhance healing of burns and diabetic foot ulcers.

Hydrotherapy

Most forms of hydrotherapy are delivered by pulsatile lavage to clean and debride wounds by combining pulse irrigation with suction. Normal saline solution (at room temperature) is typically used for pulsatile lavage. It is applied with a spray gun, so the solution is delivered under pressure to the wound bed, and concurrently the contaminated fluid is aspirated. Pulsatile lavage may be used on all wounds. In clean wounds and slow healing wounds it enhances granulation tissue formation. In infected and necrotic wounds it removes necrotic tissue and other contaminants.

Another form of hydrotherapy is whirlpool therapy. This involves part of the body being immersed in a water tank, which is heated to a prescribed temperature according to the wound. For example a neutral or local skin temperature (35.5°C) is required for arterial wounds. The aim of this temperature modification is to regulate tissue metabolism in an ischaemic limb. A tepid temperature is used with the treatment (of between 2 and 5 minutes) for venous ulcers, since the oedema associated with such wounds may increase with warm or hot whirlpools for any extended periods of time. Whirlpools are particularly useful in softening tissues, improving blood flow to the area, and hence the delivery of oxygen, nutrients and wound healing chemicals, and removing debris through improving drainage. This therapy is also a form of exercise therapy in patients with open wounds.

Hyperbaric oxygen (HBO) is the delivery of 100% oxygen through a sealed, total-body chamber for decompression therapy for deep sea divers or a small-chamber therapy used for limbs. Total-body chambers increase the amount of dissolved oxygen in the blood to maximize wound healing. The use of total-body chambers hit the headlines in media in 2004 when it was used in an attempt to speed up the healing of footballer Wayne Rooney's broken foot (metatarsal to be more precise) for the finals of the European Championship. There is a growing amount of evidence of the value of HBO in treating patients with venous ulcers and diabetic foot ulcers, which are not responsive to other more traditional therapies. The use of HBO increases a free radical called nitric oxide, which is an important (natural) physiological mediator of vasodilation and neurotransmission, and which plays vital roles in diabetic wound healing.

Therapeutic light

Ultraviolet (UV) radiation or energy has been used as a form of therapeutic light treatment of slow healing and infected wounds. There are three bands of UV radiation: UVA, UVB and UVC. The first two bands of UV are used for the treatment of chronic, slow-healing wounds, necrotic wounds and infected or heavily contaminated wounds. The UVA and UVB bands of energy increase leucocyte accumulation and lysosome activity. The UV energy stimulates the production of cytokines and interleukin-1, both of which play an important part in the process of epithelialization. UVC is used for treating patients with infected wounds, because the energy kills a broad spectrum of microorganisms.

Laser therapy

Laser therapy promotes wound closure and nerve regeneration and is used to provide pain relief.

Ultrasound

Ultrasound is used for treating patients with open and closed wounds and is indicated to enhance wound healing, increase blood flow, decrease inflammation and decrease pain.

Electrical stimulation

High- or low-voltage electrical stimulation is used to increase healing of chronic pressure ulcers. The stimulation is used to enhance blood flow, promote angiogenesis, increase oxygenation, destroy microbes, provide pain relief and promote cell migration.

As the scar tissue matures, its blood supply decreases, and the tissue contracts, causing the scar to become flatter, paler and smoother. Mature scar tissues contain no hairs, or sebaceous or sweat glands.

In summary, wound healing following injury is a dynamic process involving the precise coordination of a number of homeostatic responses at a cellular and biochemical level. These responses are, only as a matter of convenience, divided into a number of stages and phases of wound healing.

BLOOD GROUPINGS

People are classified into one of several blood groups. This depends on the presence or absence of genetically determined antigens, the erythrocyte membrane, and antibodies called agglutinins or isoantibodies in the plasma.

The ABO system

The ABO grouping is based upon two antigens (in blood groups these are referred to as agglutinogens) called A and B,

BOX 11.23 HOMEOSTATIC FAILURES OF THE CLOTTING MECHANISM

Read this box in conjunction with Figure 11.18.

Thrombocyte imbalances

Thrombocytosis is an abnormally high platelet count. This is a common sign of many diseases, including certain leukaemias, such as myeloid leukaemia, and is observed immediately after a splenectomy ('-ectomy' = removal).

Thrombocytopenia is a deficiency of platelets. This may be caused by either a decrease in platelet production or an increased rate of destruction. The latter may be a result of thrombocytes being crowded out of the bone marrow in some bone diseases, such as certain leukaemias, pernicious anaemia or malignant tumours. The thrombocyte concentration may also be reduced by X-irradiation, radioactive isotopes, cytotoxic drugs and other drugs, such as sulphonamides and phenylbutazone. Thrombocytopenia is evident in patients with various types of purpura, a condition characterized by small multiple haemorrhagic spots (petechiae) or large, blotchy areas on the skin and mucous membranes. Purpura is also a complication of other blood diseases, such as leukaemias and severe anaemias, and may result from antibiotic and corticosteroid therapies.

Clotting factor imbalances

The cascade of enzymatic conversions during clotting means that a disorder that affects any individual clotting factor disrupts the whole clotting mechanism. Many clinical conditions can therefore result in clotting abnormalities, particularly those that disrupt calcium and vitamin K metabolism. Calcium ions are important in most of the cascade reactions, so calcium imbalance has a direct effect on coagulation. Vitamin K is required for the synthesis of five clotting factors (including prothrombin), and its deficiency results in a breakdown of the common pathway. Deficiency can be caused by to insufficient dietary intake, malabsorption problems or incorrect utilization. Dietary deficiencies are uncommon, as gut bacteria usually supply the individual with sufficient levels of this vitamin. Deficiencies can occur, however, if these bacteria are interfered with (e.g. after sterilizing treatments of the bowel). Malabsorption of vitamin K is the most common cause of depressed circulating levels. The vitamin requires bile salts for its absorption; thus low circulating levels can occur in liver diseases, in prolonged biliary tract obstruction, and in any other disease that impairs fat absorption (e.g. coeliac disease). Pancreatic disease and chronic diarrhoea may also be responsible for vitamin K deficiency. Conversely, levels in excess of the homeostatic range of vitamin K or calcium may result in inappropriate clot formation (thrombosis).

Increased fragility of capillary walls

Increased fragility of capillary walls results in bleeding, appearing as bruising under the skin, even when there is minimal damage. The main causal factors are thrombocytopenia and autoimmune diseases, and the use of some drugs, such as penicillin and aspirin.

Plaques

Hyperactivity of the clotting mechanism may result from a roughened or irregular surface within the cardiovascular system, causing platelet aggregation and/or lysis. In aggregation, platelets stick to the roughened inner (endothelial) coat of intact vessels. This adhesion may result from the presence of endothelial fatty streaks (precursors of atherosclerotic plaques) or calcium deposits. The presence of fatty streaks and calcium deposits is essentially a consequence of the ageing process and the result of a modern lifestyle. The presence of either may cause intravascular thrombosis.

Thrombosis

A clot is called a thrombus when it forms within an intact vessel. Once formed, the clot progressively enlarges, obliterating more and more of the lumen. This may progress until the clot severely impairs blood flow to the tissue's cells. If the oxygen supply is not restored, cells surrounding the area of the clot will die (necrosis). This is referred to as an infarction. Alternatively, a part of the clot may break off (dislodged thrombi are called emboli) and become lodged in small blood vessels, producing ischaemic changes and infarction at those sites. The lungs are common embolic sites, where the emboli will produce a pulmonary infarction.

Clotting can occur in the heart and arteries, but it is more common in the veins because here the blood is relatively slow moving. The leg or pelvic veins are the most common sites of venous thrombosis, and these carry a risk of subsequent pulmonary embolism. Venous thrombosis is promoted under various circumstances (e.g. after childbirth) and following abdominal operations; it is one of the reasons for encouraging early mobility in surgical patients. Thrombosis may also result from some blood conditions (including anaemia), infections, venous stagnation (as in varicose veins), prolonged bed rest enforced by operation or illness, inflammation, and degeneration of the vessel wall. Venous stagnation may be prevented by limb exercises or, clinically, by the use of elastic stockings or intermittent pneumatic compression of the limbs.

Common arterial clotting sites are the vessels of the heart, leading to coronary-thrombosis-induced heart attack (myocardial infarction, or MI), and the brain's cerebral vessels, leading to a stroke (cerebral vascular accident, or CVA). Pulmonary infarctions (caused by pulmonary embolism), MIs and CVAs have high mortality rates (see Liu *et al.*, 2001).

Deteriorating blood vessels in older people may promote thrombosis within the retinal artery, with the resultant loss of vision, or thrombosis of leg arteries, resulting in gangrene of the foot. As a result of research that established a link between long-haul flights and thrombosis, international airlines have come under pressure to do more to prevent passengers form developing blood clots due to the cramped conditions. The UK government has instructed airlines to issue health warnings with long-haul flight tickets informing passengers of the risks of developing potentially fatal in-flight thrombosis.

Blood clotting is a continuous process in blood vessels, since roughened surfaces are constantly being formed (fatty streaks have been identified upon autopsies of children as young as 6 years old). However, coagulation is always corrected homeostatically by the body's own clot-preventing (e.g. heparin) and clot-dissolving mechanisms (e.g. prostacyclins); thus heparin and prostacyclins are endogenous protective mechanisms against intravascular thrombosis.

The clinical correction of clotting hyperactivity involves the administration of anticoagulants, which prevent clotting, or factors that enhance thrombus dissolution.

Anticoagulants

Blood clotting may be inhibited by preventing the production of normal clotting factors, or preventing the normal function of clotting factors.

- Heparin directly inhibits the conversion of prothrombin to thrombin, and so is a fast-acting anticoagulant. The liver, mast cells and tissues secrete heparin as required, but damage to blood vessels may also cause the liver to reduce its secretion, and so remove this inhibitor to the clotting process. Heparin administration is useful in preventing postoperative thrombosis. It is vital for patients on haemodialysis and those who are undergoing open-heart surgery, and some other operations, in order to prevent potentially fatal clot formation. Heparin is ineffective if it is given orally, since proteolytic enzymes of the digestive system break it down, so it has to be administered intravenously (i.e. into the veins) to have an effect. It is extracted for clinical use from the lungs and bowels of slaughtered cattle.
- Prostacyclin (a prostaglandin) is also an endogenous anticoagulant

continued

BOX 11.23 HOMEOSTATIC FAILURES OF THE CLOTTING MECHANISM *(continued)*

that is secreted from the lining of healthy vessels. It inhibits platelet aggregation and in health is likely to be important in preventing coagulation because of platelet–vessel wall interactions. It is thus a potential anti-thrombotic agent for clinical use. The drug dipyridamole enhances the action of prostacyclins.

- Vitamin K antagonists (e.g. warfarin, phenindione and dicoumarol) are given orally to patients susceptible to thrombosis as a preventive measure. These drugs work by lowering the concentrations of prothrombin and clotting factors II, VIII, IX and X in plasma but the effects will only be apparent after a few days once pre-existing factors have been lost from plasma.
- Various calcium-binding compounds may be added to sample blood as anticoagulants (e.g. ethylenediaminetetraacetic acid, EDTA; acid citrate dextrose, ACD) to prevent clotting in donated blood for blood banks and laboratories. These compounds reduce the ionic calcium in plasma, and so prevent the conversion of prothrombin into thrombin.
- Non-steroidal anti-inflammatory drugs (NSAIDs; e.g. aspirin, phenylbutazone) prolong the bleeding time by preventing platelet interactions through inhibiting TXA2 (see 'The platelet phase', p.292).

It is important that people taking anticoagulants are monitored carefully for bleeding, and that they have regular prothrombin time measurements for blood tests. The prothrombin time is estimated when thromboplastin is added to a blood sample, providing the ideal conditions for a clot to form quickly if adequate prothrombin is present. Many drugs, including aspirin, should not be taken during anticoagulant therapy, unless prescribed specifically, as they may alter the coagulation status of the patient. Discharge planning by the nurse should include education about the drug and its effects, especially for patients that are bleeding. Patients need to carry an anticoagulant card, and to tell all healthcare professionals they deal with that they are taking anticoagulants. Where possible, they should avoid hazards at work and during leisure activities.

Thrombus dissolution
Thrombus dissolution therapy involves the administration of fibrolytic

enzymes (e.g. streptokinase, urokinase), which promote endogenous plasmin production. Streptokinase was the first thrombolytic agent to be identified (in 1982) for dissolving clots in the coronary arteries. It is also now used extensively for removing pulmonary and deep-vein clots. Streptococcal bacteria produce this enzyme. However, it must be used with caution, as extensive tissue damage will result if the drug gains access to extravascular sites.

Haemophilia
Haemophilia affects 0.01% of the population. It is frequently called the 'bleeding disease' because people with haemophilia are at risk of excessive bleeding if accidental blood vessel damage occurs, or if they are subjected to factors that precipitate bleeding. Even an overindulgence of alcohol or penicillin may produce internal haemorrhage. In haemophilia, the gene necessary for the production of specific clotting factors is lacking, defective or not expressed. This gene is on the X chromosome, and the condition occurs predominantly in males. Patients with the disorder are prone to repeated episodes of severe and prolonged bleeding at any site, particularly into muscles and joints with little evidence of trauma.

Haemophilia A is the most common type of haemophilia; it is associated with the absence of (or an abnormal) clotting factor VIII. Haemophilia B is known as 'Christmas disease'; it is a result of the inactivation of clotting factor IX (also known as Christmas factor).

Correction of bleeding conditions
Short-term correction for uncontrolled bleeding involves the application of thrombin, a fibrin spray or a rough surface, such as gauze, as these encourage clotting at a wound. Long-term control involves the administration of the deficient aetiological factor (e.g. factor VIII for the treatment of classical haemophilia A). Major injuries and operations require special measures, such as plasma transfusions and the administration of concentrated anti-haemophilic factors, in order to reduce or control the symptoms.

See the case study of a woman with deep vein thrombosis in Section VI, p.651.

BOX 11.24 BLOOD GROUPS

There are over 35 blood groups. The groups are designated letters (e.g. MN, Sc), or they are named after the person who identified them (e.g. Lewis, Duffy, Kidd). Although these groups are of immense importance in forensic medicine, only two principal blood group systems, the ABO and rhesus systems are clinically important. This is because transfusion of an inappropriate type of blood can promote clumping (agglutination) of red cells in the recipient and should be avoided at all cost.

BOX 11.25 ABO AGGLUTININS

The anti-A and anti-B agglutinins are antibodies of the IgM type. They appear at, or just after, birth, and they exist throughout life, although their production may decline or disappear during old age. Their occurrence in the blood is not understood, since they are produced even in the absence of contact with the non-self antigen.

---

and two agglutinins called anti-A (alpha, α) or anti-B (beta, β). The agglutinogens are attached to the membrane of the erythrocytes, and the agglutinins (isoantibodies) are found in the plasma.

The four blood groups associated with the ABO system are groups A, B, AB and O. Their frequencies exhibit ethnic variation, but in England they are 43%, 8%, 3% and 46%, respectively. People of group A have the A agglutinogen group; group B have B agglutinogens; group AB have both A and B agglutinogens; and group O do not possess either agglutinogen (i.e. O = zero, 0; Figure 11.19). If you follow the simple rule

that the group is named after the agglutinogens present, then you will be able to predict which plasma agglutinins (if any) will also be present. This is because there are only two agglutinins, anti-A and anti-B, and these interact (agglutinate) with opposing agglutinogens A and B, respectively. It is essential to have different agglutinins and agglutinogens in order to prevent auto-crossreactions that would cause agglutination and haemolysis, as shown in Figure 11.19b. This reaction could be fatal if the clump of erythrocytes blocked a blood vessel to a vital organ, such as the heart.

Figure 11.18 The homeostatic and clinical controls of blood clotting. a, Normal ability to coagulate blood (i.e. thrombocyte and clotting factors are within their homeostatic ranges). b_1, Increased clotting. This may be caused by other homeostatic imbalances, such as hyperlipidaemia or hypercalcaemia, responsible for an increased tendency for atherosclerotic plaque and calcium deposit formation, respectively; both precipitate blood clotting. Alternatively, the increased clotting ability may be a result of a normal physiological homeostatic mechanism (haemostasis) that goes into operation when a blood vessel is damaged. b_2, Decreased ability to produce blood clots. This may be caused by a homeostatic imbalance of the factors involved in blood clotting such as hypocalcaemia, hypoprothrombinaemia, hypofibrinogenaemia or inadequate levels of vitamin K or factor VIII (haemophilia, etc.). c_1, Clinical correction involves thrombolytic enzyme (streptokinase or urokinase) therapy. c_2, Clinical correction of prolonged bouts of bleeding involves the administration of the deficient aetiological factors (e.g. factor VIII therapy in classical haemophilia A). (a, Represents boxes a_1–a_4 in Figure 1.7, p.11, reflecting the individual variability in the homeostatic range)

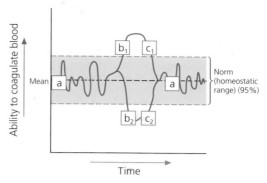

Q How could an enzyme, such as streptokinase, assist in preventing unwanted clotting and removing clots already formed?

(a)

Genotype	AA	AO	BB	BO	AB	OO
Blood group (phenotype)	A		B		AB	O
Agglutinogens	A		B		A B	Neither
Agglutinins	**Anti-B**		**Anti-A**		Neither	Agglutinins **Anti-A** and **Anti-B**

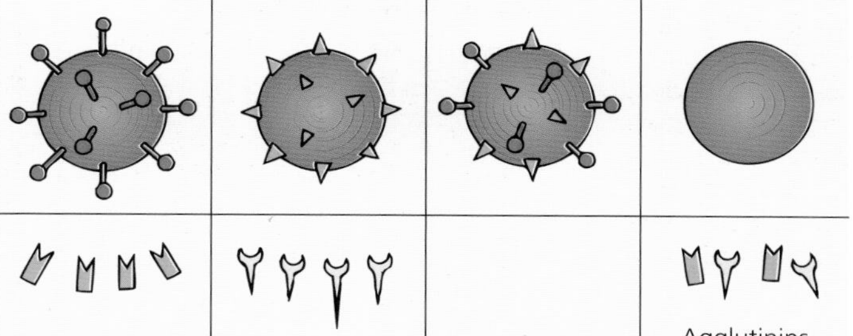

Figure 11.19 (a) Blood grouping. The blood group depends upon the presence of antigens (agglutinogens) on the surface of red cells. This is determined by alleles A, B and O. The plasma contains antibodies (agglutinins) that will react with 'foreign' agglutinogens (i.e. a reaction takes place when the agglutinogens are of the same variety of agglutinins). (b) Cross-reactions (incompatible transfusions) occur when the plasma agglutinins (antibodies) encounter complementary erythrocyte agglutinogens (antigens). The result is extensive clumping (agglutination) of the affected red cells, and subsequent haemolysis. (c) ABO transfusion combinations. ✓, compatible transfusion; ×, incompatible transfusion

Q What are the frequencies within the UK population of blood groups: A, B, AB and O?

Q Distinguish between agglutinogens and agglutinins.

Q Which antibodies are present in blood group A?

(b)

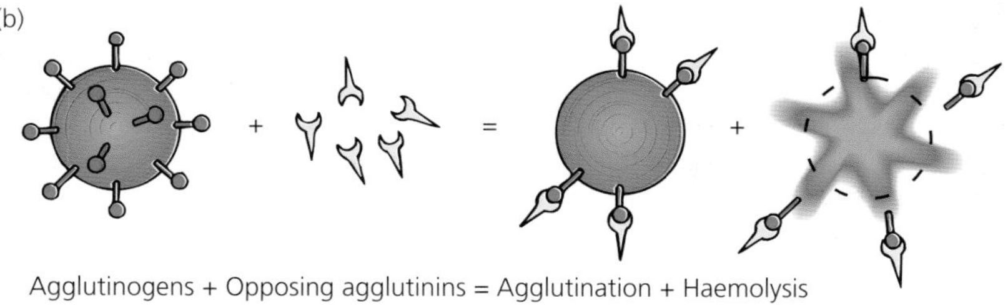

Agglutinogens + Opposing agglutinins = Agglutination + Haemolysis
(e.g. A)   (e.g. Anti-A)

(c)

Donor groups	A	B	AB	O
Recipient group				
A	✓	✗	✗	✓
B	✗	✓	✗	✓
AB	✓	✓	✓	✓
O	✗	✗	✗	✓

Key: ✓ = Compatible transfusion   ✗ = Incompatible transfusion

BOX 11.26 CROSS-MATCHING BLOOD AND BLOOD TRANSFUSIONS

Before the patient receives a transfusion of blood cells, a specimen of blood is obtained for cross-matching with that of the donor. Stringent procedures are followed in identifying the patient's blood to ensure that the transfused blood is compatible. Mistakes do still occur, however, and vigilance and adherence to checking procedures and policies is essential for safe practice.

These principles are important when considering the essentials of successful blood transfusions. It is important to remember, however, that it is the effect of the recipient's plasma agglutinins on the donor's erythrocyte agglutinogens that may cause problems. This is because of the vast numbers of red blood cells (i.e. 5 million/mm^3) with their attached antigens that are transferred. The donor's plasma agglutinins are ignored, since the greater volume of fluid of the recipient soon dilutes them. Thus, agglutination will occur whenever recipient agglutinins and donor agglutinogens of the same type are mixed. Such blood is said to be incompatible; Figure 11.19c shows which transfusion combinations can be successful. For example, blood group A can be transfused into its own blood group.

However, it cannot be transfused into blood group B, since the recipient has plasma anti-A agglutinins, which would react against the donor's agglutinogens (i.e. agglutination will occur). Group A can also be a donor to blood group AB, since AB individuals do not possess either anti-A or anti-B agglutinins. Group AB individuals are known as 'universal recipients' because they can receive blood from any other blood group. Blood groups A, B and AB cannot be donors for blood group O because O recipients have agglutinins anti-A and anti-B, and the A, B and AB groups possess at least one agglutinogen. Conversely, group O individuals are 'universal donors': they can give blood to any other blood group, since they do not have agglutinogens A or B on their surface, and antibody–antigen reactions with the transfused blood will therefore not be initiated.

The use of the term 'universal' has now fallen into disuse, since this term means all possible circumstances and takes no account of blood group systems other than the ABO. Usually, blood of the same group within the ABO system will be used to prevent any possibility of mixing incompatible bloods.

ACTIVITY

Before reading this section, familiarize yourself with the terms 'genotype', 'phenotype', 'alleles', 'allelic variation', 'homozygous' and 'heterozygous'.

BOX 11.27 BLOOD TRANSFUSIONS: RHESUS BLOOD GROUPS

Unlike the situation with the ABO system, the plasma of rhesus-negative individuals does not normally contain rhesus antibodies (agglutinins). However, transfusion of rhesus-positive erythrocytes into a rhesus-negative recipient may stimulate a response in the recipient with the release of anti-D (anti-rhesus) agglutinins. These agglutinins cause agglutination and haemolysis of the transfused cells. When considering transfusions, therefore, the rhesus factor must also be taken into consideration in order to minimize the risks of incompatible transfusions and their fatal outcomes.

Inheritance of the ABO blood groups

Chromosome 9 contains the alleles A, B and O that determine the ABO blood group. Alleles A and B are co-dominant to each other; both are dominant to the recessive allele O. Individuals have two alleles (there are two copies of chromosome 9) and so there are six genotypes that determine the four blood group phenotypes of the ABO system (Figure 11.19a):

- Blood group A is derived from homozygous dominant A (i.e. AA alleles) or heterozygous A (i.e. AO alleles) genotypes.
- Group B is derived from either the homozygous B (i.e. BB alleles) or the heterozygous B (i.e. BO alleles) genotypes.
- Individuals with blood group AB have both A and B alleles.
- Group O people are homozygous for O alleles, which are incapable of coding for agglutinogens.

The rhesus blood group and its inheritance

The rhesus system is so-called because it was first identified in the rhesus monkey. People are classified as having rhesus-positive (Rh-positive) or rhesus-negative (Rh-negative) blood, according to the presence or absence of the rhesus antigen (in fact there are numerous subtypes of this antigen but they are very rare or not clinically important). About 85% of the UK population is rhesus positive (i.e. they possess the rhesus agglutinogen, called the rhesus or D factor) on the surface of their red cells. The remaining 15% of the population are rhesus negative (i.e. they do not possess the rhesus agglutinogen). The dominant rhesus (D) gene found on chromosome 1 controls

ACTIVITY

Using Figure 11.19, explain the rationale of the following:

Blood group A can donate to groups A and AB, and receive blood from groups A and O.

Blood group O can donate to all other groups, but can receive blood only from group O.

Blood group B can donate blood to group B and AB, and receive blood from groups B and O.

Blood group AB can donate only to group AB, but can receive from all other groups.

Blood group O negative is used as a universal donor in UK accident and emergency departments when a patient has had a significant blood loss.

Blood group O positive cannot donate blood to group O negative.

the presence of the agglutinogen. With two copies of chromosome 1 (i.e. two alleles), the three possible genotypes responsible for determining the rhesus groupings are:

- Homozygous dominant (DD) and heterozygous (Dd): these people will be rhesus positive.

	Father	Mother
Parent genotypes	DD	dd
Gametes	D and D	d and d
Offspring genotypes	Dd Dd	Dd Dd
Offspring blood groups (phenotypes)	Rh+ Rh+	Rh+ Rh+

	Father	Mother
Parent genotypes	Dd	dd
Gametes	D and d	d and d
Offspring genotypes	Dd Dd	dd dd
Offspring blood groups (phenotypes)	Rh+ Rh+	Rh− Rh−

(a)

Figure 11.20 (a) The inheritance of rhesus-positive (Rh+) offspring. There is a 75% chance of producing a rhesus-positive child from a rhesus-positive father and a rhesus-negative (Rh−) mother, because the father could be homozygous dominant (DD) or heterozygous (Dd). Thus, both possibilities have to be taken into consideration when calculating the probability of producing a rhesus-positive child from these two parental phenotypes. (b) Pregnancy and rhesus incompatibility

Q What accounts for the symptoms of haemolytic disease of the newborn (HDNB), and how can this be prevented?

Q Why is the firstborn baby unlikely to have HDNB?

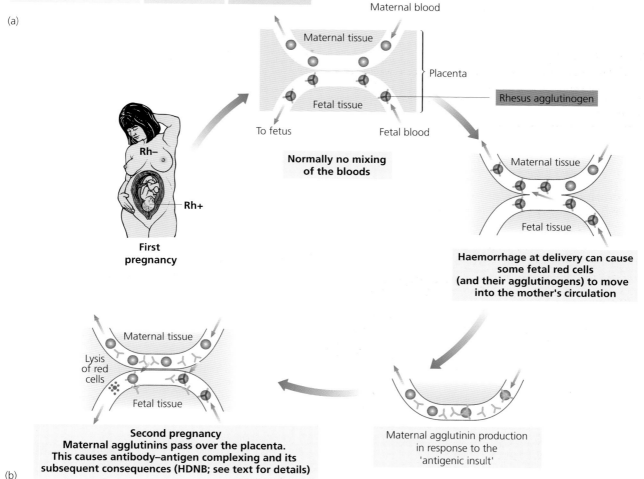

(b)

• Homozygous recessive (dd): this genotype is not capable of coding for the rhesus agglutinogen, so these people will be rhesus negative.

Scientists investigating the problems affecting the availability of an adequate supply of stored blood are experimenting with the possibility of interconverting blood groups. Early attempts have been successful in converting blood group B into group O. In the future, such interconversions may abolish the problem of regional blood shortages.

BOX 11.28 THE RHESUS FACTOR –HAEMOLYTIC DISEASE OF THE NEWBORN

Complications may occur if a rhesus-negative mother bears a rhesus-positive fetus, which is possible since the genotype of the fetus may be different from that of the mother. Genetically, there is a 75% chance of this occurring if the father is rhesus positive (Figure 11.20a).

Under normal circumstances in pregnancy, there is no mixing of fetal and maternal bloods, although the two circulations are in very close proximity within the placental unit. During childbirth, however, severe contractions of the uterus wall may squeeze some fetal rhesus-positive erythrocytes into the maternal circulation (Figure 11.20b). The fetal agglutinins passed into the maternal circulation do not pose a risk to the mother, as the large maternal blood volume dilutes their effects many-fold.

Maternal anti-D agglutinins are not produced in significant amounts against this 'antigenic insult' until after the delivery, and so the first infant is not affected. The small agglutinins (gamma immunoglobulin, IgG), however, are capable of crossing the placental membranes and entering the blood of subsequent fetuses. If the fetus is rhesus positive, then the anti-D antibodies will cause a transfusion reaction. This is referred to as haemolytic disease of the newborn (HDNB). This disease can be monitored *in utero* by amniocentesis, which samples amniotic fluid (for bilirubin assessment), and by fetoscopy, which obtains fetal blood samples for blood analysis. However, both processes carry a risk of miscarriage.

Without treatment, HDNB may result in stillbirth or neonatal death soon after delivery. Premature delivery may be induced after 7–8 months of development. Before this time, and in severe cases, the fetus can also be treated successfully by intrauterine transfusions. Neonates with HDNB have anaemia coupled with jaundice because the resultant rhesus antibody–antigen reactions cause excessive haemolysis (resulting in anaemia), and the metabolized pigment (now bilirubin) becomes deposited in the skin, mucous membranes and the eyes (leading to jaundice).

Correction after birth depends upon the severity of the condition. It may involve an exchange transfusion, whereby the neonate's entire rhesus-positive blood is replaced with rhesus-negative blood (which will not respond to any agglutinins present). The transfused blood will eventually be replaced by the baby's own rhesus-positive blood, by which time the signs and symptoms of anaemia and jaundice will have disappeared. Milder forms of jaundice may not require an exchange transfusion, and principles of correction will then involve the application of artificial ultraviolet light. The ultraviolet light converts the fat-soluble bilirubin into water-soluble biliverdin, which is excreted in the urine.

There is no equivalent haemolytic disease of the newborn with reference to the ABO system. This is because the anti-A and anti-B antibodies are of the immunoglobulin M (IgM) type, not IgG, and so are too large to pass through the placental membranes. However, problems can occur if there is damage to the maternal–fetal placental unit.

Rhesus immunization

If a risk of HDNB is known, the potential problem is avoidable by rhesus immunization (i.e. administration of anti-D). Anti-D destroys any fetal cells that may have passed into the maternal blood before they have time to stimulate the mother's own immune response. Anti-D is given in the following cases:

- when a rhesus-negative woman has become reactive (sensitized) to rhesus-positive blood cells, and who has given birth to a rhesus-positive baby;
- to prevent sensitization of a rhesus-negative woman before giving birth;
- to a rhesus-negative women having an abortion, unless it is shown that the fetus is rhesus negative;
- to a rhesus-negative woman who has not become reactive to rhesus-positive blood cells, following an incident during pregnancy that may lead to bleeding across the placenta (the afterbirth) or of the fetus;
- to prevent sensitization of a rhesus-negative woman who has been given, for any reason, blood components containing rhesus-positive red blood cells.

Anti-D should not be injected intravenously since it may cause a severe reaction. Injection should be intramuscular, so that the antibody enters the blood at a much slower rate. Care should be taken to draw back the plunger of the syringe before injecting, in order to ensure that the needle is not in a blood vessel. Injection should be within 72 hours of birth, whenever possible, to have the best effects; however, if an incident occurs during pregnancy, then the injection should be given at the time of the incident to be most effective. After 72 hours, the mother's immune system may begin to respond significantly to any fetal blood cells.

The use of anti-D may interfere with the response of other vaccines, especially MMR (measles, mumps and rubella) and varicella (chickenpox) vaccines. Such vaccinations should be given at least 3 weeks before, or at least 3 months after, anti-D.

SUMMARY

1 Blood is the fluid that, under normal circumstances, is contained within the cardiovascular system. Its main components are plasma and erythrocytes.

2 Additional components found in smaller concentrations are other cellular elements – leucocytes and thrombocytes – and non-cellular materials dissolved in the plasma. The latter include organic substances (nutrients, enzyme, hormone, urea, etc.) and inorganic substances (cationic and anionic electrolytes).

3 All components of blood must be maintained within their homeostatic parameters to maintain blood volume (hence blood pressure), interchange materials vital to maintain intracellular homeostasis and combat pathogenic infection.

4 Deviations in the homeostatic ranges of blood constituents, together with the presence of abnormal constituents (e.g. cytoplasmic chemicals, such as cardiac-specific enzymes) make serum analysis one of the most important clinical diagnostic tools.

5 Wound healing involves a number of homeostatic responses at cellular and biochemical levels.

6 Haemostasis (blood clotting) is a homeostatic mechanism that prevents the loss of blood when a blood vessel is damaged. It involves the activation of both extrinsic and intrinsic pathways.

7 Intravascular thrombosis is a result of the activation of the intrinsic clotting mechanism.

8 Thrombocytes (platelets) have an essential role in activating the enzyme-controlled clotting cascade.

9 Different blood groups are associated with genetically determined differences in antigens on erythrocyte membranes and antibodies in blood serum.

10 The ABO and rhesus blood grouping systems are used to classify blood donated for transfusion. Matching of blood types for transfusion is important to prevent agglutination (clumping) of red blood cells. The rhesus antigen must also be considered if a pregnant woman is rhesus negative as she may produce antibodies if her blood makes contact with that of a rhesus-positive fetus.

REFERENCES

Clancy, J. and McVicar, A.J. (1996) Shock: a failure to maintain cardiovascular homeostasis. *British Journal of Theatre Nursing* **6**(6): 19–25.

Clancy, J. and McVicar, A.J. (2002) *Physiology and Anatomy. A Homeostatic Approach,* 2nd edn. London: Arnold.

Department of Health (2000) *The NHS Performance Guide 1999–2000.* London: HMSO.

Liu, M., Counsell, C., and Sandercock, P. (2001) Anticoagulation for preventing recurrence following ischaemic stroke or transient ischaemic attack. *The Cochrane Library*, Issue 1. Oxford: Update Software.

McVicar, A.J. and Clancy, J. (1997) The physiological basis of fluid therapy. *Professional Nurse* **12**(8): 19–25.

Provan, D. and Weatherall, D. (2000) Haematology. Red cells II: acquired anaemias and polycythaemia. *Lancet* **355**(9211): 1260–8.

FURTHER READING

Clancy, J. and McVicar, A.J. (1996) Homeostasis: the key concept in physiological control. *British Journal of Theatre Nursing* **6**(2): 17–24.

Clancy, J. and McVicar, A.J. (1997) Wound healing: a series of homeostatic responses. *British Journal of Theatre Nursing* **7**(4): 25–33.

Hutten, B.A. and Prins, M.H. (2001) Duration of treatment with vitamin K antagonists in symptomatic venous thromboembolism. *The Cochrane Library*. Oxford: Update Software.

CHAPTER 12

THE CARDIOVASCULAR SYSTEM 2: THE HEART AND CIRCULATION

INTRODUCTION: RELATION OF THE CARDIOVASCULAR SYSTEM TO CELLULAR HOMEOSTASIS

The cardiovascular system consists of the heart and the blood vessels of the body. The relation of this system to cellular homeostasis is that it delivers nutrients, oxygen, hormones, etc. to the cells of the body, and removes 'waste' products of metabolism from them, so preventing toxicity. The cardiovascular system, however, requires the cooperative functioning of other systems in order to maintain blood composition and so preserve intracellular homeostasis. For example, the digestive and excretory organs are instrumental in maintaining the homeostatic constitution of blood, and the autonomic nervous system and endocrine system coordinate cardiovascular (and other system) functions. Each cooperative component is a homeostatic control system, and a disturbance in one results in malfunction of another as a consequence of the interdependency of organ system function, as discussed in Chapter 1, pp.8–10.

Cardiovascular function must be adaptable if adequate blood flow to the tissues is to be maintained during the varying metabolic demands, that occur during surgery, trauma, times of distress and when resting or exercising, since there is only a limited volume of blood available in the body. Blood may be directed to where it is needed most, and away from the less active areas, but at all times there must be an adequate blood flow to the most vital organs (brain and heart), since these high-priority tissues are particularly sensitive to reduced blood supply.

The cardiovascular system, therefore, provides the transport 'hardware' that keeps blood continuously circulating to fulfil intracellular homeostatic requirements. The heart (= 'cardio-') is the transport system's pump; the delivery routes are the hollow blood vessels (= 'vascular') leading from, and eventually back to, the heart (Figure 12.1). The blood is the transport medium (see Figure 11.1, p.269)

The essential principles underlying the homeostasis of blood composition were described in Chapter 11. This chapter describes:

- specific aspects of the heart, including its size, location, functional anatomy, coronary circulation, conduction system and related electrocardiography, the cardiac cycle, and cardiac output;
- the functional anatomy of the arterial, capillary and venous systems, the routes of circulation, and the homeostatic control of blood pressure;
- some common examples of cardiovascular homeostatic failures and their principles of correction.

ACTIVITY

Reflect on your understanding of how cardiovascular function aids the maintenance of intracellular homeostasis.

OVERVIEW OF THE ANATOMY AND PHYSIOLOGY OF THE CARDIOVASCULAR SYSTEM 1: THE HEART

The main role of the heart is to promote the flow of blood throughout the body in one direction. It also produces a hormone that is important in maintaining blood volume and hence blood pressure. Flow of blood is promoted by the generation of a pressure gradient, and the pumping action of the heart is responsible for elevating blood pressure sufficiently to maintain an adequate blood supply to the tissues.

The volume of blood removed from the heart by this pumping action must match the volume of blood entering the heart during the 'filling' phase of the pump cycle; otherwise the heart will become congested (see Box 12.16, p.338). This in turn relates to the physical activity being performed by the body: an increase in activity reduces the time taken for blood to circulate around the body, so the heart must pump more blood per unit time. The heart, then, has to be versatile, with a variable pumping rate according to the needs of the body. The control of the heart pump is described later. This section outlines the basic structure and functioning of the heart in relation to the unidirectional flow of blood through it.

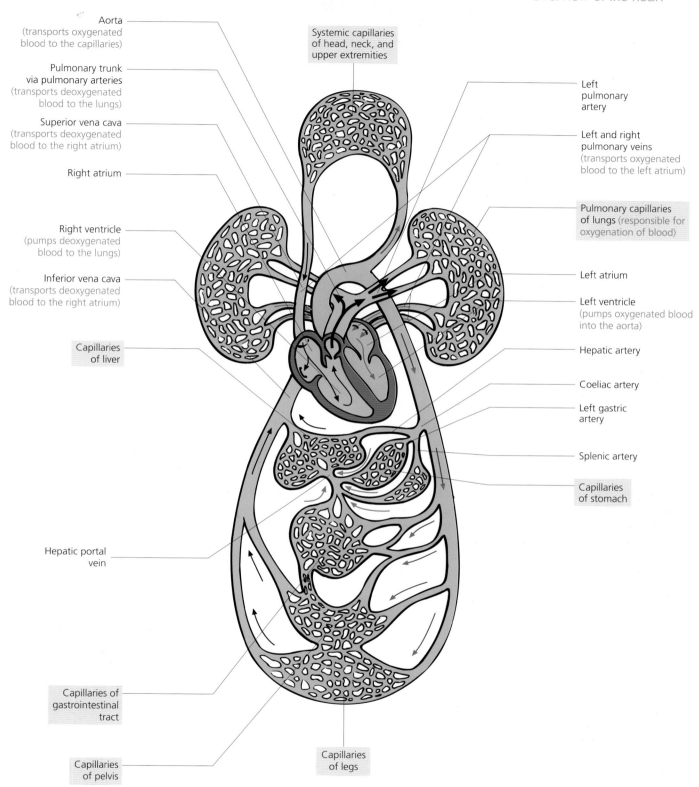

Figure 12.1 Circulatory routes. Red (arterial) and black (venous) arrows show systemic circulation; thick black arrows in the pulmonary blood vessels show pulmonary circulation; thin green arrows indicate hepatic portal circulation

Q Describe the route taken by blood as it moves from the right atrium to the kidneys and back to the right atrium.

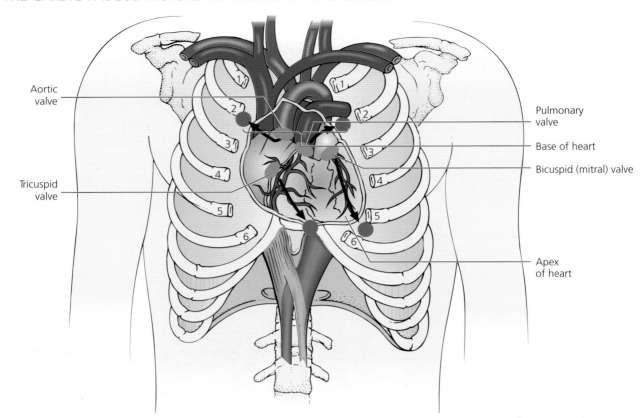

Aortic valve

Tricuspid valve

Pulmonary valve

Base of heart

Bicuspid (mitral) valve

Apex of heart

Figure 12.2 Location of the heart, heart valves (green spots) and auscultation sites (red spots) for heart sounds. The heart is located within the mediastinum, which is the middle region of the thoracic cavity

Heart size and location

Figure 12.2 shows that the heart is located obliquely (since the heart tips slightly to the left) between the lungs, and is enclosed within the medial cavity of the thorax, called the mediastinum. It lies anterior to the vertebral column and posterior to the sternum. The heart weighs approximately 250–350 g; its size is often compared with the person's closed fist to demonstrate the approximate, but variable, dimensions. The heart's broad 'base', formed by the upper chambers, or atria, is about 9 cm wide, and projects superiorly and posteriorly towards the right shoulder, extending some 12–14 cm within the second or third intercostal space. The organ is fixed by vessels at its base, thus allowing its more pointed apex to move upwards on contraction. The apex, formed by the tip of the lower chambers, or ventricles, of the heart (particularly the left ventricle), is directed inferiorly and anteriorly towards the left hip. It rests on a muscle called the diaphragm, which separates the thoracic and abdominal regions of the body's trunk. The apical heartbeat, produced by contraction of the heart muscle, can be felt on the left side of the chest about 8 cm from the sternum between the fifth and sixth intercostal spaces. Approximately two-thirds of the heart is located to the left of the sternum.

The upper border of the heart, formed by the atrial chambers, is where the great vessels, called the aorta, vena cavae and pulmonary artery, enter and leave the heart.

Functional anatomy of the heart

The heart is a four-chambered structure enclosed within a supportive and protective membrane called the pericardium. The walls of the heart are composed mainly of a specialized form of muscle called cardiac muscle (or myocardium). The chambers of the heart are separated by walls of tissue called septa. Communication between the atria and ventricles is provided by valve structures.

The pericardium

The pericardium ('peri-' = around) is a membranous sac comprising two layers: the fibrous pericardium and the serous pericardium (Figure 12.3). The former is a tough, dense connective tissue layer that protects the heart and anchors it to the diaphragm, great vessels and sternum. Although the fibrous pericardium holds the heart in position, it is flexible enough to allow sufficient movement, so that the heart can contract vigorously and rapidly when the need arises. The serous pericardium is a thinner, more delicate membrane that forms a double layer around the heart. The outer (or parietal) layer lines the inner surface of the fibrous pericardium. The inner (or visceral) layer (also called the epicardium, meaning 'upon the heart') is attached to the muscle layer of the heart. Between these two serous layers is the pericardial cavity, which is a thin potential space containing a film of watery fluid. The

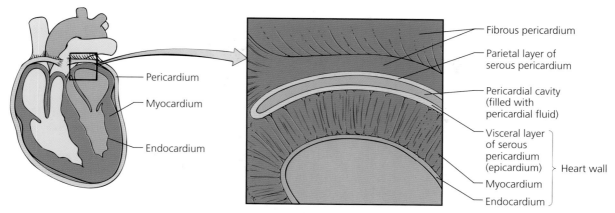

Figure 12.3 The pericardial layers and the heart wall

BOX 12.1 CARDIAC TAMPONADE AND PERICARDITIS

An excessive build-up of the pericardial fluid or extensive bleeding into the pericardium (see Figure 12.7d, p.313) is potentially life-threatening because of the consequential compression (cardiac tamponade) on the heart tissue, which can stop the heart beating. This excess fluid or blood needs to be removed (aspirated) to prevent this. The causes of tamponade are varied, but analysis of the aspirated fluid aids diagnosis. Aspiration alone may be enough, but surgery may be required if the underlying cause is trauma or aneurysm.

Both deficiency and excessive build-up of pericardial fluid can lead to inflammation of the pericardium, a condition known as pericarditis. This is often associated with a painful 'pericardial friction rub' (which can be heard by a stethoscope examination) of the parietal and visceral pericardial membranes.

tension produced by this film holds the two layers together. The fluid also prevents friction between the membranes when the heart contracts.

The heart wall

The wall of the heart consists of three layers: the epicardium (a component of the pericardium), the myocardium ('myo-' = muscle), and the endocardium ('endo-' = inner) (Figure 12.3).

The myocardium

The myocardium forms the bulk of the heart wall. Upon contraction, it is responsible for pumping blood into the vessels of the circulatory system. The structure of cardiac muscle is discussed later. The external surface of the myocardium is lined by epicardium and the internal surface by endocardium.

The endocardium

The endocardium is continuous with the endothelial lining of blood vessels leaving and entering the heart; it also covers the valves between the heart chambers. It is a smooth, glistening, white sheet of squamous endothelium, which rests on a thin sheet of connective tissue. Its smooth surface prevents activation of the blood-clotting cascade. The presence of fat, calcium

or fibrin deposits roughens the endocardium and enhances the likelihood of blood clotting.

ACTIVITY

Reflect on your understanding of the clotting mechanism described in Chapter 11, pp.290–3 and summarized in Figure 11.15, p.291). Identify the clotting pathway (intrinsic or extrinsic) that instigates the common coagulation pathway to promote intravascular thrombosis.

The heart chambers

The interior of the heart is divided into four hollow chambers that receive circulating blood. The two upper chambers are called atria (singular, atrium), and the two lower chambers are called ventricles (Figure 12.4). An internal partition divides the heart longitudinally and forms the interatrial and interventricular septa (singular, septum), which separate the two atria and two ventricles, respectively. The interatrial septum possesses an oval depression called the fossa ovalis. This structure corresponds to the location of the foramen ovale ('foramen' = window), an opening in the fetal heart that diverts blood away from the lungs since the placenta, rather than the lungs, provides the route for gaseous exchange in the fetus (see Box 12.3, p.311).

Each atrium is separated from its respective ventricle by an atrioventricular valve (AV). The atria are the receiving chambers for blood returning to the heart from the circulation. They are small and thin-walled, since they need to contract only minimally to push the blood a short distance to the ventricles (very little pressure is generated within the atria during their contraction). Flow into the ventricles is also encouraged by gravity. The ventricles are the discharging chambers and form the actual pumps of the heart; accordingly, ventricular walls are thicker than atrial walls since they must generate a greater pressure to promote adequate output. However, the muscular wall of the right ventricle is thinner than that of the left, since the right ventricular pump is responsible for circulat-

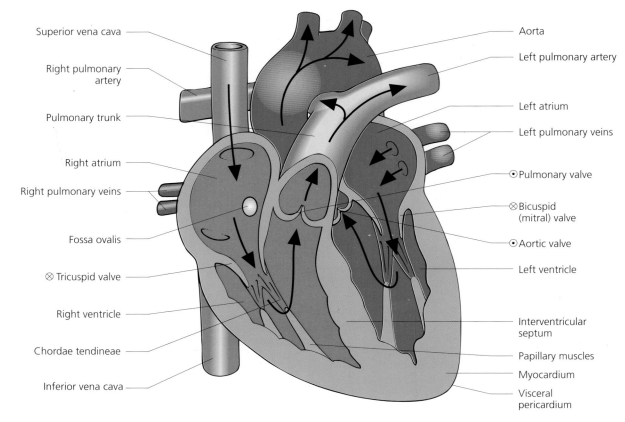

Superior vena cava

Right pulmonary artery

Pulmonary trunk

Right atrium

Right pulmonary veins

Fossa ovalis

⊗ Tricuspid valve

Right ventricle

Chordae tendineae

Inferior vena cava

Aorta

Left pulmonary artery

Left atrium

Left pulmonary veins

⊙ Pulmonary valve

⊗ Bicuspid (mitral) valve

⊙ Aortic valve

Left ventricle

Interventricular septum

Papillary muscles

Myocardium

Visceral pericardium

Figure 12.4 Frontal section of the heart

Q Describe the path of blood flow through the heart.

Q Identify which vessels returned (1) the deoxygenated blood to the heart and (2) the oxygenated blood to the heart

ing blood in the low-resistance circulation of the lungs, whereas the left ventricular pump is responsible for circulating blood to the rest of the body and must generate a much higher pressure to maintain this.

The heart valves

Blood flow through the heart and the circulatory system must be unidirectional if haemodynamic efficiency is to be maintained. Valves in the heart (and in the larger veins; see later) maintain this one-way flow. There are four heart valves: the paired AV and semilunar valves (Figures 12.2 and 12.4); these open and close passively in response to differences in blood pressure on the two sides of the valve.

The atrioventricular valves

The AV valve between the right atrium and the right ventricle is often called the tricuspid valve because it contains three cusps or flaps. Similarly, the AV valve between the left atrium and the left ventricle is the bicuspid (or mitral valve) because it consists of two cusps (and because of its resemblance to a bishop's mitre). The cusps are fibrous connective tissue covered with endocardium that extends from the chamber walls; their pointed ends project into the ventricles. White collagen fibres called the chordae tendineae, or 'heart strings',

anchor the cusps to small papillary muscles within the ventricles.

The tendineae keep the valve flaps pointing in the direction of blood flow, so that the AV valve opens when blood is passed from atrium to ventricle. At this point, the papillary muscles relax and the chordae tendineae slacken, allowing the valves to open (Figure 12.5a). Upon ventricular contraction (i.e. systole, see later – cardiac cycle), however, blood is pumped out of the ventricle into an artery; any blood tending to pass back towards the atria drives the valve cusps upwards until they close the opening. Papillary muscles also contract, which tightens the chordae tendineae and prevents the flaps from inverting into the atria (Figure 12.5b).

The semilunar valves

The semilunar valves are so-called because of their half-moon shaped cusps. Aortic and pulmonary semilunar valves are located at the bases of the large arteries, the aorta and pulmonary artery, which leave the left and right ventricles, respectively. Their role is to encourage unidirectional flow from ventricle to artery. The mechanism of action is different from that of the AV valves. Upon ventricle contraction, the semilunar valves are forced open, and their cusps become flattened against the arterial wall as blood is ejected (Figure 12.5c).

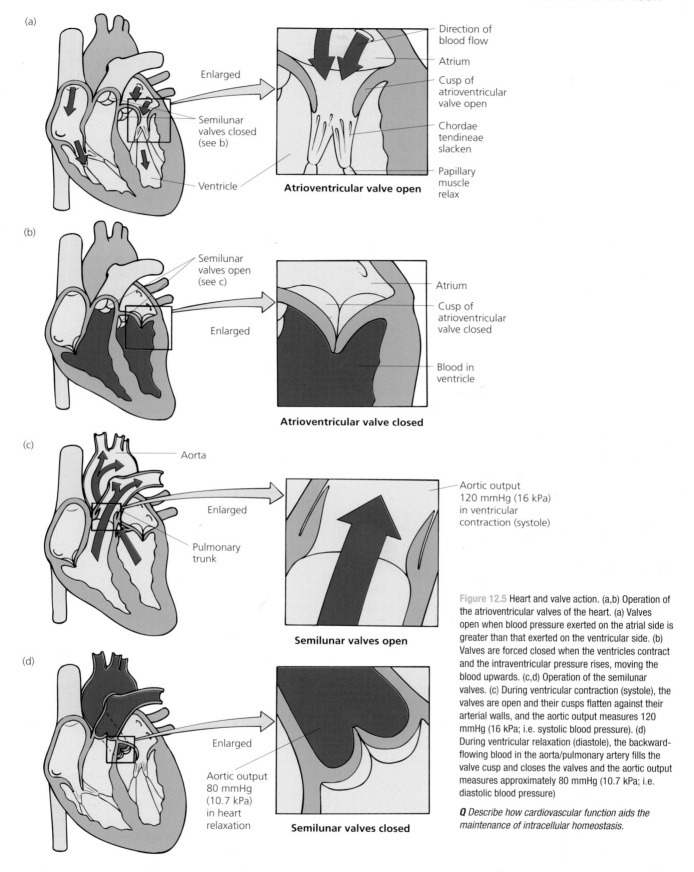

(a)

Enlarged

Semilunar
valves closed
(see b)

Ventricle

Direction of
blood flow

Atrium

Cusp of
atrioventricular
valve open

Chordae
tendineae
slacken

Papillary
muscle
relax

Atrioventricular valve open

(b)

Semilunar
valves open
(see c)

Enlarged

Atrium

Cusp of
atrioventricular
valve closed

Blood in
ventricle

Atrioventricular valve closed

(c)

Aorta

Enlarged

Pulmonary
trunk

Aortic output
120 mmHg (16 kPa)
in ventricular
contraction (systole)

Semilunar valves open

(d)

Enlarged

Aortic output
80 mmHg
(10.7 kPa)
in heart
relaxation

Semilunar valves closed

Figure 12.5 Heart and valve action. (a,b) Operation of
the atrioventricular valves of the heart. (a) Valves
open when blood pressure exerted on the atrial side is
greater than that exerted on the ventricular side. (b)
Valves are forced closed when the ventricles contract
and the intraventricular pressure rises, moving the
blood upwards. (c,d) Operation of the semilunar
valves. (c) During ventricular contraction (systole), the
valves are open and their cusps flatten against their
arterial walls, and the aortic output measures 120
mmHg (16 kPa; i.e. systolic blood pressure). (d)
During ventricular relaxation (diastole), the backward-
flowing blood in the aorta/pulmonary artery fills the
valve cusp and closes the valves and the aortic output
measures approximately 80 mmHg (10.7 kPa; i.e.
diastolic blood pressure)

Q *Describe how cardiovascular function aids the
maintenance of intracellular homeostasis.*

Upon ventricular relaxation (i.e. diastole, see later – cardiac cycle), pressure within the ventricle falls; blood is no longer propelled forward, but begins to flow backwards. This causes the cusps to close, which prevents backward flow into the ventricles (Figure 12.5d).

Path of blood flow through the heart

The right atrium receives deoxygenated blood (i.e. blood that has given up some of its oxygen as it passes through tissues) from all parts of the body except the lungs. The left atrium receives oxygenated blood from the lungs. However, both atria receive blood simultaneously as the two sides of the heart must operate in a synchronized way if flow through the heart is to be efficient. For convenience it is useful to consider the path of blood flowing through the heart as a sequence, from right to left side.

Blood enters the right atrium via three vessels:

* *the superior vena cava*: returns blood from structures above the heart (i.e. head, neck and arms);
* *the inferior vena cava*: returns blood from structures below the heart (i.e. the trunk and legs);
* *the coronary sinus*: collects blood from most of the vessels supplying the heart wall.

Relaxation of the atrium muscle enlarges the chamber and creates a suction pressure that draws blood into the right atrium (the entrances of the above vessels are not guarded by valves). This atrium delivers blood to the right ventricle upon opening of the tricuspid valve. The right ventricle then pumps blood to the lungs via the pulmonary 'trunk' vessel through the opened pulmonary (semilunar) valve; simultaneously, the tricuspid valve closes to prevent backflow. The pulmonary trunk divides into right and left pulmonary arteries, which take the blood to the right and left lungs, respectively. Oxygenation of blood takes place in lung tissue, and the blood is transported to the left atrium via the four pulmonary veins (two from each lung).

Blood flows into the left atrium upon its relaxation, which again creates a suction pressure. Most of the blood passes passively through the opened bicuspid valve into the left ventricle. The rest of the blood then passes actively through the valve via the contraction of the left atrium. Shortly after this, the ventricles contract pumping blood into the aorta through the opened aortic (semilunar) valve; simultaneously, the mitral valve closes to prevent backflow. From the aorta, some blood passes into the first branch of the aorta – the coronary arteries – while the remainder is carried into the aortic arch, thoracic aorta and abdominal aorta. Vessels branching from the aorta transport blood to all body parts to sustain intracellular homeostasis (see Figure 12.1, p.305).

Heart sounds

Listening to the heart sounds through a stethoscope (called auscultation) is performed by specialized healthcare practitioners (e.g. doctors, emergency-care practitioners, cardiac nurses), and this is important to observe the normal and abnormal heart sounds. Upon listening one does not hear the opening of the valves, since this is a silent, relatively slow developing process. Valve closure is more sudden, however, and the sudden pressure differentials that develop across the valve produce vibrations of the valve and the surrounding fluid. The sounds given off travel in all directions through the chest; these are best heard at the surface of the chest in locations that differ slightly from the actual location of the valves (see Figure 12.2, p.306). Four sounds are recognized in any single cycle of events, though the first two are most prominent:

* When ventricles first contract, the closure of the AV valves produces a long, booming sound, since the vibration is low in pitch and is of relatively long duration. This is the first heart (or Korotkoff) sound, and is described as 'lub'.
* The second heart sound – 'dup' – is caused by the closure of the semilunar valves at the beginning of ventricular relaxation. This sound is a relatively rapid 'snap', since valve closure is extremely fast; thus the surroundings vibrate for only a short period of time. If the aortic valve closes just before the pulmonary valve the second sound can be split into two sounds. This split second sound is common in healthy young people when they breathe in. Inspiration causes an increased filling of the right ventricle and hence raises the volume ejected when the ventricle contracts (referred to as the ventricular stroke volume). This takes longer to eject (during ventricular contraction or systole) and so the pulmonary valve closure is delayed, slightly delaying the resultant sound.
* A third sound caused by the entry of blood (at the start of the heart's relaxation or diastole) into the relaxed ventricles through the AV is also a common occurrence in young people.
* A fourth sound is audible just before the first and this is caused by the atrial contraction or systole.

Coronary circulation

The heart chambers are continuously bathed with blood, which provides nourishment to the endocardial cells. The myocardial and pericardial cells, however, are too far away to receive nutrients from this blood source. Nutrition is provided by a number of blood vessels, which comprise the coronary circulation. Numerous vessels pierce the myocardium and carry blood to the vicinity of the myocardial and pericardial cells. This arrangement is essential, since the oxygen consumption of the heart muscle is greater than that of any other tissue because of its constant pumping action. At rest, the oxygen consumption is 8 mL/100 g of heart tissue per minute. The supply of blood via the coronary circulation accounts for 1/20th of the total output from the heart, even though the heart represents only 1/200th of the body's weight. The main coronary vessels – the right and left coronary arteries – branch from the aorta just superior to the aortic valve. They lie on the heart's surface (the epicardium), encircling the heart in an atrioventricular groove. These vessels reminded early anatomists of a crown, or corona, hence the name (Figure 12.7a). Their branches and sub-branches penetrate deep into the cardiac muscle.

BOX 12.2 HEART MURMURS AND TREATMENT OF HEART VALVE DYSFUNCTION

A heart murmur is an abnormal rushing or gurgling noise heard before, between or after the normal heart sounds, or a sound that masks the normal heart sounds. Young healthy people during strenuous exercise or in pregnancy may produce a benign (harmless) murmur occasionally, and this is due to the turbulence of the blood leaving the heart. However, most murmurs, especially at rest, indicate a heart valve disorder.

Certain infectious diseases of the endocardium can damage heart valves, which are made up of this tissue. Endocardial damage can be congenital (inherited or through nature–nurture interactions) or acquired (nurture or environmental). The acquired forms cause inflammation (ischaemia), degenerative or infectious alterations of valve structure and hence function. The usual cause of acquired valve dysfunction is inflammation of the endocardium, secondary to acute rheumatic fever (hence why most such patients are now elderly following rheumatic fever in childhood), which usually follows a streptococcal infection of the throat. These bacteria stimulate an immunological response, in which antibodies attack the bacteria but inflame the connective tissue of the heart valves. This can cause the cusps of the valve to stick together, thus narrowing their openings (a process called stenosis). Subsequent damage to the edges of the cusps impairs closure, and backward flow occurs. The valve is now said to be 'leaky' or incompetent. Although stenosis (Figure 12.6b,c) and incompetence (Figure 12.6a,d) may coexist, often one predominates. These valve disorders create turbulence in blood flow and produce the extra sound called murmurs. Given that there are four valves and each one is capable of stenosis and incompetence, a total of eight valve disorders is possible, resulting in eight heart murmurs. (For more information on heart murmurs including systolic and diastolic murmurs, murmurs in children and murmurs in pathologies at the heart see the website http://www.patient.co.uk/showdoc/40000504)

The pumping efficiency of the heart declines and, as a consequence, the workload of the heart is increased. However, a severe valve deformity is necessary for there to be a serious impairment to the pumping efficiency. In such cases, the heart ultimately becomes weakened, which can cause heart failure. It is the mitral valve that is usually affected, since pressure differentials developed by the left ventricle are greater than those across the tricuspid valve are. Mitral incompetence occurs in 10–15% of the population (Nagle and O'Keefe, 2000).

Treatment of heart valve dysfunction

A patient with valve dysfunction is strongly advised to reduce their dietary salt intake, and is treated with drugs such as cardiac glycosides, diuretics and antibiotics until the faulty valve needs to be replaced surgically with a synthetic or animal (usually pig or cow) heart valve (Huether and McCance, 2006):

- *Dietary salt restriction*: a low sodium chloride intake is associated with a reduction in blood volume.
- *Cardiac glycosides (e.g. digoxin)*: increase the force of myocardial contraction and reduce the oxygen consumption of the heart.
- *Diuretics (e.g.furosemide)*: inhibit sodium chloride (NaCl) reabsorption in the loop of Henle (see Figure 15.7, p.430 and Box 15.10, p.431), where NaCl absorption is high, and so greatly increase urine production (and so reduce blood volume). These diuretics are used for patients with pulmonary oedema caused by moderate to severe heart failure, and for reducing peripheral and pulmonary oedema. For patients with mild forms of heart failure and hypertension, distal tubule diuretics such as bendroflumethiazide are commonly used; NaCl reabsorption in the distal tubule is less and so urinary changes are more moderate (and the drugs are also potassium-sparing).
- *Antibiotics*: penicillin is the drug of choice in the prevention of endocarditis, for patients with heart valve defects or prosthetic valves. A broad-spectrum antibiotic (e.g. amoxicillin) is most commonly used, as it is active against Gram-positive and Gram-negative bacteria as well as strains of *Escherichia coli*, *Haemophilus influenzae* and *Salmonella* species. For patients who are allergic to penicillin a combination of vancomycin and gentamicin might be used.

If however, the mitral stenosis, or the insufficiency is severe, this requires one of the following surgical interventions:

- *Open commissurotomy*: this involves the separation of the fused cusps of the stenosed valve, during open-heart surgery.
- *Mitral annuloplasty*: this involves the reduction of a dilated annulus, which is contributing to the backflow of blood. The reduction is achieved by sutures or by the insertion of a prosthetic ring.
- *Mitral valve replacement*: during this procedure the mitral valve cusps, chordate tendineae and papillary muscles are excised (surgically removed) and replaced by a mechanical prosthesis (Huether and McCance, 2006).

BOX 12.3 CONGENITAL HEART DEFECTS

Most congenital cardiac imbalances result from teratogenic influences during early stages of pregnancy when the heart is developing. Some of these defects are mentioned in Chapter 19 (see Figure 19.4, p.526 and Table 19.2, p.534). Such defects account for approximately one-half of all infant deaths arising from congenital abnormalities. The most frequent are septal defects and patent ductus arteriosus (a vessel between the pulmonary artery and aorta that allows blood to bypass the lungs in the fetus). Failure of closure of the foramen ovale soon after birth results in an atrial septal defect (ASD), commonly referred to as a 'hole in the heart'.

Since blood passes from the right side of the heart to the lungs for oxygenation, cardiac defects involving right-to-left shunts (e.g. tetralogy of Fallot, transposition of the aorta and pulmonary arterial trunk) prevent complete oxygenation of the blood. Significant defects cause cyanosis (a blue coloration of the skin and mucous membranes caused by low oxygen content of blood). This may be treated initially with oxygen therapy depending upon the severity of the cyanosis, and later with corrective surgical techniques to abolish the shunts and/or vessel abnormalities.

In conditions comprising left-to-right shunts (e.g. patent ductus arteriosus, patent foramen ovalis, atrial and ventricular septal defects) the heart compensates to improve the oxygen supply to the body by increasing its cardiac output, usually via a rise in the heart rate. If the desired oxygenation is not reached the heart can enlarge and fail through increased pulmonary blood flow, leading to congestive heart failure if not corrected. Correction involves controlling the consequential pulmonary oedema, providing respiratory support, and restricting fluids. Furosemide, a loop diuretic, may be prescribed if the imbalance does not correct itself, in order to reduce blood volume and cardiac congestion (see Box 12.16, p.338). Surgical correction may be necessary.

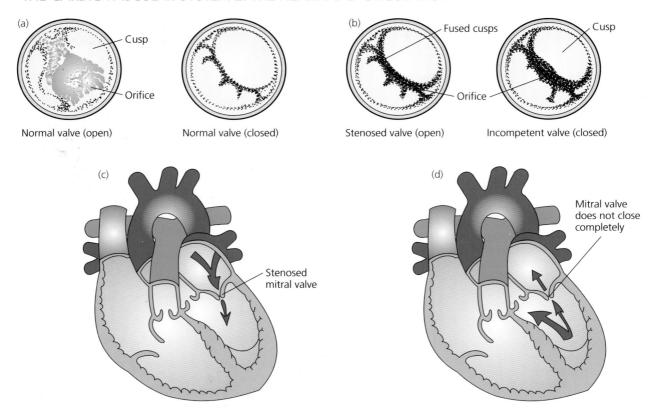

Figure 12.6 Valve stenosis and incompetence. (a) Normal position of valve in opened and closed positions. (b) Stenosed opened valve and closed incompetent valve. (c) In mitral stenosis, the valve is unable to open sufficiently during left atrial emptying, resulting in improper filling of the left ventricle. The left atrial wall has to work harder, hence its muscle wall thickens (hypertrophy). (d) In mitral incompetence, the valve does not close properly. During left ventricular emptying, some blood is returned to the left atria

The right coronary arterial branches are the marginal artery, which supplies the lateral part of the right side of the heart, including the right atrium, and the posterior interventricular artery, which extends to the apex serving the posterior ventricular walls.

The left coronary arterial branches are the left anterior descending branch, which serves the interventricular septum and the anterior wall of both ventricles, and the circumflex branch, which supplies the left atrium and the posterior left ventricular wall.

Coronary vessels deliver most blood when the heart is relaxed. They are largely ineffective during ventricular contraction, as they are compressed by the contracting myocardium, and their entrances from the aorta are blocked partly by the cusps of the opened aortic valve.

Having supplied the heart tissue, blood is collected from the left ventricle via the cardiac veins, which merge to form the coronary sinus. This empties into the posterior aspects of the right atrium. The sinus comprises the great cardiac vein, the middle cardiac vein and the small cardiac vein (Figure 12.7b).

Blood from the right side of the heart is collected via the anterior cardiac vein, which empties directly into the anterior aspects of the right atrium. Blood returning to the atrium will have very little oxygen – less than any other venous blood in the body, since the active heart muscle extracts more oxygen from the blood it receives than do other tissues.

Factors that influence coronary blood flow are:

- *The demand of cardiac muscle for oxygen*: the removal of oxygen from the coronary circulation at rest is approximately three times greater than in normal circulation; in times of increased oxygen demand (e.g. exercise, the stress of impending surgery), the additional oxygen required is supplied by an increased coronary blood flow. The change in blood flow is directly proportional to the oxygen requirements. The mechanism is intrinsic to the tissue (i.e. the tissue regulates it), but the metabolic stimulus to provide the additional blood has yet to be identified.
- *Neural mechanisms*: the autonomic nervous system indirectly affects coronary blood flow. Parasympathetic stimulation decreases the heart rate, resulting in decreased cardiac oxygen consumption, therefore decreasing coronary flow.

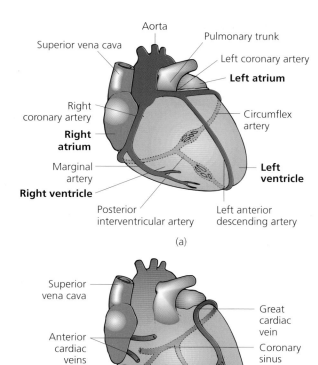

(a)

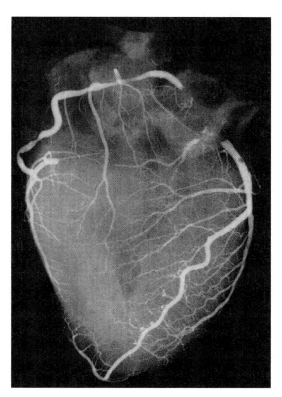

(b)

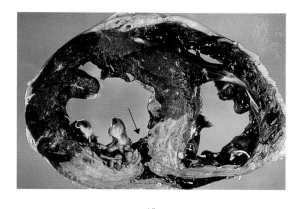

(d)

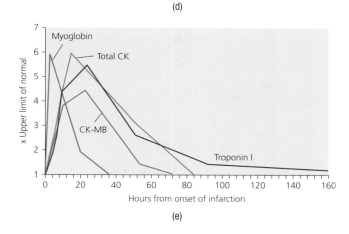

(c)

Figure 12.7 Coronary circulation. (a) Arterial supply. (b) Venous drainage. (c) Coronary arteriogram showing main coronary arteries and numerous collateral vessels to compensate for the flow disruption of the left anterior descending artery (reprinted with the permission of Lakhani *et al.*, *Basic Pathology*. 3rd edn, Hodder, London). (d) Left anterior descending artery infarction. Heart sliced through the right and left ventricle is stained to demonstrate infarction in the area supplied by the left anterior descending artery. The left ventricular wall is ruptured (arrow), allowing blood into the pericardial space. (Slice viewed from below, right ventricle at the right of the photograph) Reproduced with the kind permission of Lakhani *et al.*, *Basic Pathology*. 3rd edn. Hodder, London.
(e) Serum cardiac enzymes following an acute myocardial infarction: the relative timing, rate, peak values and duration of cardiac marker elevation above the upper limit of normal caddie serum markers following an anterior myocardial infarction. Creatine kinase (CK); CK-MB, CK myocardial band

BOX 12.4 CORONARY ARTERIAL DISEASE

Ischaemic heart disease is a homeostatic imbalance that reflects myocardial oxygen insufficiency, arising from a narrowed or occluded coronary artery. Some people with the disease have no signs or symptoms; others experience angina pectoris (chest pain), and some suffer an acute coronary syndrome that can range from unstable angina to a heart attack (myocardial infarction). Atherosclerotic plaques may cause narrowing and occlusion, or plaques may become complicated by a thrombotic narrowing (see Box 12.8, p.323). If the narrowing progresses slowly, a collateral (alternative) arterial supply grows, effectively acting as a homeostatic control to replace the malfunctioned vessel. If, however, a sudden severe narrowing or occlusion occurs, the collateral circulation has insufficient time to develop, and consequently myocardial infarction may occur.

Angina pectoris literally means 'choked chest'. It may result from a variety of causes:

- increased physical demands on the heart that cannot be met by the coronary circulation;
- stress-induced spasms of the coronary arteries;
- high blood pressure (hypertension) which increases excessively the oxygen demands of the heart;
- fever, which elevates cardiac activity and hence its oxygen needs;
- hyperthyroidism (i.e. excessive release of thyroid hormones), which increases cardiac activity;
- aortic stenosis;
- atherosclerosis.

Myocardial infarction

A myocardial infarction, or 'coronary', occurs when the coronary arteries become completely occluded, cutting off blood flow to the tissue beyond the occlusion, which results in the death of the myocardial tissue. A thrombus or embolus (i.e. a homeostatic failure of the clotting process) may cause occlusion in one of the coronary arteries. The after-effects depend partly on the size and location of the necrotic area. In chronic ischaemic heart disease, small infarcts may give rise to myocardial weakness, angina, 'silent' myocardial infarction, or heart failure. If the ischaemic heart disease is acute, then one or more large arteries are occluded, and the atheroma is usually complicated by thrombosis. Consequently, a large infarct results, and death may occur as a result of acute heart failure, ventricular fibrillation (see Figure 12.10f, p.318), rupture of the ventricular wall, or pulmonary or cerebral embolism (leading to respiratory or cerebral failure).

See the case study of a woman with a myocardial infarction, Section VI, p.654.

Risk factors

Some risk factors for coronary arterial disease (CAD) are:

- modifiable by altering the diet, (i.e. managing conditions that have a direct link to CAD, such as diabetes mellitus). Similarly, people who are overweight can reduce weight; those with high cholesterol may reduce their blood cholesterol levels;
- modifiable by changing other lifestyle habits, such as stopping smoking, changing type A personality behaviour or adopting a moderate exercise programme (which actually reverses the process of CAD);
- not modifiable (i.e. beyond our control). These factors include genetic predisposition, age and gender. Adult men are more likely than adult women to develop CAD, but after the age of 70 years, the risks are roughly equal. The nurse's and other healthcare practitioner's role in health education and health promotion is vital as a preventive measure and in minimizing the reoccurrence of CAD;
- controllable with medication (e.g. antihypertensive drugs).

Diagnosis

Electrocardiogram (ECG) analysis (see Box 12.6, p.319) and serum cardiac-specific enzyme levels are used to diagnose CAD (see Figure 12.7e). Cardiac catheterization with coronary angiocardiography is an invasive procedure used to visualize the coronary arteries and assess the degree of the occlusion (Figure 12.7c). It is also used to:

- measure pressures in the chambers of the heart and blood vessels;
- assess cardiac output (the quantity of blood ejected by the left ventricle per minute) and diastolic properties of the left ventricle;
- measure the flow of blood through the heart and blood vessels, and the oxygen content of the blood;
- assess the status of heart valves and conduction system;
- identify the exact location of septal and valve defects;
- inject clot-dissolving drugs (e.g. streptokinase) into a coronary artery to dissolve an obstructing thrombus.

The procedure involves inserting a long, flexible radio-opaque cardiac catheter into a peripheral vein (for right heart catheterization) or peripheral artery (for left heart catheterization), and guiding it under X-ray observance. A radio-opaque dye is then injected into the blood vessels or heart chambers.

Treatment

Failure of myocardial homeostasis requires clinical intervention to re-establish it. Vasodilator drugs (e.g. glyceryl trinitrate) are given for angina to increase coronary flow, or beta-blockers (e.g. atenolol) may be used to reduce the oxygen requirements of the myocardium. An infarcted patient may be given oxygen therapy, aspirin, cholesterol-lowering drugs, and/or clot-dissolving agents, or may require a coronary bypass operation to remedy cardiac integrity (i.e. if a large area of the myocardium is affected and/or major vessels are occluded).

Coronary arterial bypass grafting

This is a surgical procedure in which a blood vessel from another part of the body is grafted to a coronary artery, so as to bypass the blocked area. The grafted blood vessel is sutured between the aorta and the unblocked portion of the coronary artery.

Percutaneous transluminal coronary angioplasty (PTCA)

This non-surgical procedure involves inserting a balloon catheter into an artery of an arm or leg, and then gently guiding it into a coronary artery. Angiograms are taken to locate fatty plaques, the catheter is advanced to the point of obstruction, and a balloon-like device is inflated with air to squash the plaque against the vessel wall. A special device resembling a spring coil (called a 'stent') is placed permanently in the artery to keep the artery patent (open), thus permitting blood to circulate. This is inserted in order to prevent the recurrence of the stenosis of the opened arteries.

Conversely, sympathetic stimulation increases the heart rate and myocardial contractility, increasing oxygen consumption, and increasing coronary flow.

- *Aortic pressure*: this is the principal factor that determines the rate of blood flow to the cardiac muscle, since the aortic pressure is produced by the heart itself. Any increase in aortic pressure generated by the contraction of the heart results in increased coronary blood flow.

The conduction system

Before considering the conduction system of the heart, it is important that you understand the anatomy and functioning of cardiac muscle, and its differences from skeletal muscle.

Myocardial muscle fibres have anatomical features that reflect their unique function of pumping blood; otherwise, their structure is similar to skeletal muscle cells. Both are striated in appearance, and their contractions are associated with the sliding filament mechanism (see Figure 17.6, p.471). Cardiac fibres, however, are small, fat and branched, and usu-

ACTIVITY

Distinguish between the clinical conditions of myocardial ischaemia and myocardial infarction see the case study of a woman with a myocardial infarction, Section VI, p.654. Read the article by Cucherat *et al.* (2001) for a discussion of angioplasty and intravenous thrombolysis for acute myocardial infarctions.

ally have one nucleus, whereas skeletal muscle cells are taller and cylindrical, and have many nuclei. Adjacent cardiac cells are interconnected via intercalated discs and cross-bridges, unlike the independent skeletal muscle fibres. The intercalated discs contain anchoring structures (called desmosomes) that prevent separation of adjacent cells upon their contraction, and minute gap junctions that allow direct transmission of electrical impulses (depolarization) across the whole heart. The structure of cardiac muscle allows the entire myocardium to behave as a single unit or 'functional syncytium', but also ensures that the organ is contracted in different planes, unlike the linear contraction observed in skeletal muscle fibres.

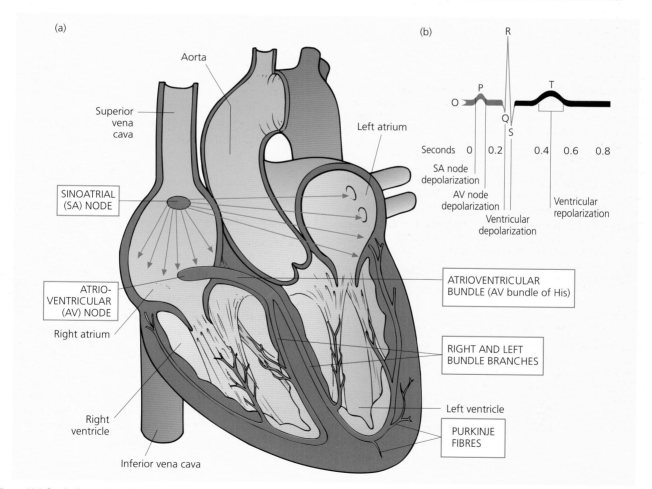

Figure 12.8 Conduction system of the heart and corresponding electrocardiogram. (a) Location of the nodes and bundles of the conduction system. Arrows indicate the flow of action potentials through the atria. (b) Normal electrocardiogram of a single heartbeat. AV atrioventricular; SA, sinoatrial

Q Describe what is meant by the 'vagal brake'?

Q Compare the intrinsic rhythm of the SA node with that of other components of the heart's conduction system.

Compared with skeletal muscle, myocardial cells also have more mitochondria, constituting 25% of the volume of the muscle fibres (2% in skeletal muscle). This is because heart muscle cells require more adenosine triphosphate (ATP) for their continual demands of contraction. Both muscle types use a variety of 'fuel' molecules for respiration, although cardiac cells are more adaptable and can readily switch metabolic pathways to use whatever nutrient is available. The main problem associated with myocardial insufficiency, therefore, lies with a lack of oxygen, not fuel molecules.

The orderly and coordinated myocardial contraction, which produces efficient emptying of the heart chambers, is controlled by an intrinsic regulatory mechanism – the cardiac conduction system. This is composed of a number of patches (called nodes) and conducting fibres of specialized muscle tissue called:

* the sinoatrial (SA) node;
* the atrioventricular (AV) node;
* the atrioventricular (AV) bundle (or bundle of His), and its left and right bundle branches;
* the Purkinje fibres (Figure 12.8a).

The specialized myocardial cells of the nodes are self-excitatory (i.e. they spontaneously and rhythmically generate the electrical activity that results in their contraction). The resting rate of self-excitation of the SA node of an adult is faster than other members of the conducting system; hence it is called the pacemaker. The impulse that will eventually cause the heart to contract is therefore initiated within the SA node tissue located in the right atrium, just below the opening of the superior vena cava. The impulse spreads from the SA node to atrial myocardial cells, causing their neural excitation and subsequent contraction. It then enters the AV node located at the base of the interatrial septum. This is the last region of the atria to be stimulated; its slower conducting properties give the atria time to empty their blood into the ventricles, before the ventricles begin their contraction. The atria therefore finish their contraction before the ventricles begin theirs, which facilitates unidirectional blood flow. Once through the AV node, the impulse travels quickly through the rest of the conduction system, beginning with the bundle of His. This extends down to the heart apex as the right and left bundle branches, which distribute electrical impulses over the medial surfaces of the ventricles. Ventricular contraction is finally stimulated by the Purkinje fibres, which emerge from the bundle branches and carry the neural impulses to the lateral ventricular myocardial cells.

Although the rate of the heartbeat is determined by the intrinsic properties of the SA node, this may be altered by the autonomic nervous system, or by blood-borne hormones such as thyroxine or adrenaline. The ability of the SA node to generate impulses in the absence of such external stimuli is referred to as autorhythmicity, and results from spontaneous changes in the permeability of cell membranes to potassium and sodium (see Figure 8.21, p.188). The gradual stimulation (depolarization) of the membrane reaches threshold forming

BOX 12.5 ECTOPIC BEATS

Stimulants, such as caffeine and nicotine, when used in excessive amounts may increase the excitability of the conduction system to such a degree that ectopic beats result in abnormal contractions. Other triggers of ectopic beats are electrolyte imbalances, hypoxia and toxic reactions to drugs, such as digitalis.

an electrical impulse (action potential; see Chapter 8, pp.186–9 for explanation of action potentials), which is transmitted through the rest of the conducting system, resulting in myocardial contraction. Following the action potential, the SA node cell membranes return to their initial resting value and are gradually stimulated again. This repetitive, self-excitatory mechanism causes the rhythmical and repetitive muscle contraction associated with heart activity. Although the SA node is the pacemaker, autorhythmicity is also displayed in other parts of the conduction system. For example, in isolation from the SA node, the AV node discharges at a rhythmical rate of 40–60 action potentials per minute, while the rest of the system discharges at a rate of 15–40 beats per minute (bpm). In life, these tissues rarely have the opportunity to generate action potentials because they are stimulated by impulses from the SA node before they reach their own threshold levels. If, for some reason, the SA node is inactivated, the tissue with the next fastest autorhythmical rate (i.e. the AV node) takes over pacing. This site is then called an ectopic pacemaker; it may pace the heart for some period of time.

ACTIVITY

Draw a labelled diagram of the heart, including its conduction system.

The electrocardiogram

The action potentials of myocardial cells are electrical changes that can be recorded as they move through the myocardium. This recording is known as the electrocardiogram or ECG. The ECG is recorded by placing electrodes on the arms and legs (limb leads) and at six positions on the chest (chest leads). The ECG amplifies the heart's electrical activity and produces 12 different recordings from different combinations of limb and chest leads. Each chest and limb electrode records slightly different electrical activity, because it is in a different position relative to the heart (Figure 12.9). By comparing these records with one another, and with normal records, the practitioner can check specific nodal, conducting and contractile properties, and determine whether the heart is enlarged or certain region is damaged.

Patients that are admitted to clinical areas with acute coronary problems can be monitored using either three or five leads attached to their chest. The electrical readout is presented on a

(a)

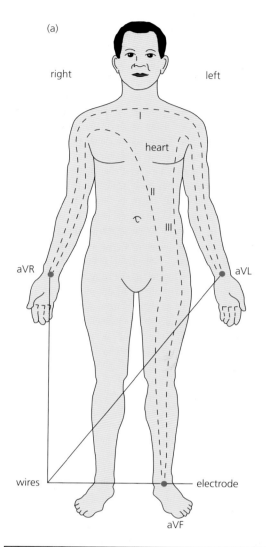

(b)

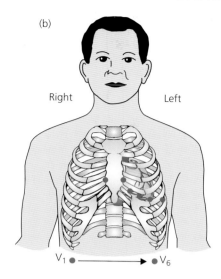

Figure 12.9 A 12-lead electrocardiogram (EGC). (a) Limb leads. Bipolar: lead I measures voltage difference between left and right arms; lead II measures voltage difference between left leg and right arm; lead III measures voltage difference between left leg and left arm. Unipolar: aVR measures voltage difference between zero and right arm; aVL measures voltage difference between zero and left arm; aVF measures voltage difference between zero and left leg. (b) Chest leads. V_1 and V_2, right ventricle; V_3 and V_4, septum and part of left ventricle; V_5 and V_6, rest of left ventricle. Red dots, lead positions. Note: clavicles not shown. (c) Sinus rhythm. The rate in this example is about 80 beats per minute (bpm). The P wave and ORS morphology are normal. The PR interval is normal (0.16 second). The QRS duration is normal. The frontal plane QRS axis is normal. An isolated T wave inversion in one of the inferior leads is normal

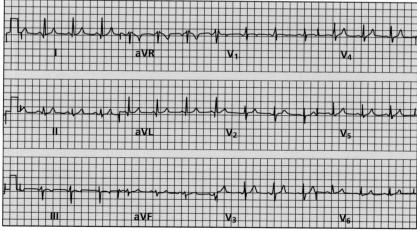

Sinus rhythm twelve-lead ECG

small screen by the bed, or may be conveyed to the central monitor. Cardiac monitors are used for observing the heart rate and rhythm. Although certain changes in the shape of the ECG waves and intervals can be seen on the screen (e.g. ST segment elevation), unlike the 12-lead ECG the cardiac monitor does not pinpoint areas of myocardial damage.

Figure 12.8b illustrates the important features of an ECG analysed with the leads in one of the standard configurations (lead II right arm to left leg). The three clearly recognizable events, or waves, normally accompanying each heart cycle are:

1   A small P wave upward deflection. This corresponds to atrial electrical stimulation (depolarization). The upward swing of the P wave represents SA node depolarization; the downward deflection represents AV node depolarization. Events to initiate the actual contraction process introduce a slight delay and the atria contract about 100 milliseconds after the P wave begins (i.e. mechanical events follow electrical activity). The PQ interval before the next appearance of electrical activity occurs as the impulse disappears down the Bundle of His.

2   The QRS complex signifies ventricular depolarization. The complex begins as a downward deflection, continues as a large upright triangular wave, and ends as a downward wave at its base. Shortly after the QRS complex begins the ventricles start to contract. The relatively strong electrical signal reflects the comparatively larger mass of ventricular muscle compared with that of the atria.

3   The smaller, dome-shaped T wave is indicative of ventricular electrical recovery (or repolarization), and occurs just before the ventricles start to relax. The T wave is smaller and wider than the QRS complex because repolarization occurs more slowly than depolarization There is no deflection corresponding to atrial repolarization, since it occurs during the ventricular depolarization period and the electrical event is hidden by the QRS complex.

Cardiac biomarkers

It was briefly discussed in Box 4.2 (p.98) that specific cell enzymes may become detectable in blood and if, for example, the cardiac cells are damaged, specific serum cardiac biomarkers are detectable. The relative timing, rate of rise, peak values, and duration of cardiac enzyme biomarker elevation are important diagnostic aids of the timing of an acute myocardial infarction (MI, see Figure 12.7e):

*   Myoglobin is an oxygen-carrying protein, comparable to haemoglobin, that is normally present in cardiac and skeletal muscle (hence, it is not cardiac specific). This tiny molecule is released very quickly from myocardial cells that have undergone an infarction. Myoglobin becomes elevated within 1 hour following death of myocardial cells, with peak values reached within 4–8 hours.
*   Creatine kinase (CK, formerly CPK – creatinine phosphokinase kinase) is an enzyme found in muscle cells. As in other cell types, muscle cells use ATP as their main energy source, but muscle cells also use creatinine phosphate as another storage form of energy; the enzyme CK releases the phosphate and so converts adenosine diphosphate (ADP) to ATP. The CK in blood exceeds its normal range within 4–8 hours of a MI and declines to normal values within 2–3 days. There are three isoenzymes of CK (isoenzymes are structural isomers of the molecule – see Chapter 4, p.96),

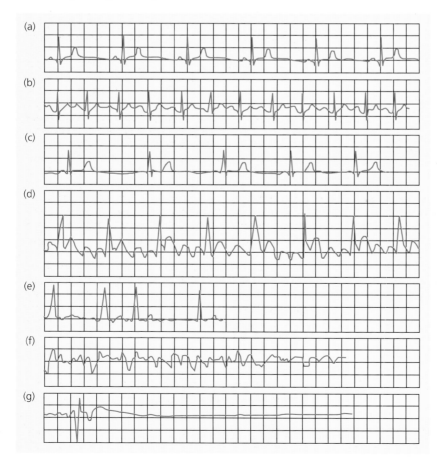

Figure 12.10 Cardiac arrhythmias. (a) Sinus rhythm (included for reference). (b) Sinus tachycardia: the heart rate at rest is > 100 bpm. (c) Sinus bradycardia. The heart rate at rest is < 60 bpm. (d) Atrial flutter: the characteristic atrial 'saw tooth' waves appear at a regular interval and at a rate of 250–400/minute. (e) Atrial fibrillation (AF): atrial waves are rapid, small and irregular. (f) Ventricular fibrillation (VF): ventricular rhythm is rapid and chaotic. (g) Asystole: ventricular standstill

Q What do the wave and interval components of the ECG represent?

Q Describe what is meant by the term 'sinus rhythm'.

Q Identify the conditions that cause sinus tachycardia.

Q What is the treatment for sinus bradycardia?

Q How many atrial impulses reach the ventricles?

Q List three cause of AF.

Q Identify the treatment for a patient undergoing VF.

Q Identify two causes of asystole, and the treatment for the condition.

BOX 12.6 ELECTROCARDIOGRAM (ECG) ANALYSIS, STRESS TESTING, ARRHYTHMIAS AND CARDIAC BIOMARKERS

An ECG analysis involves measuring voltage changes (i.e. the relative heights of the wave deflection) and determining the duration and temporal relationships between the various components. That is, small electrical signals associated with specific waves may mean that the mass of heart muscle associated with that wave has decreased (e.g. small P waves may represent atrial atrophy). Conversely, large electrical signals (large amount of depolarization) of specific waves may indicate heart muscle enlargement (e.g. larger-than-normal QRS complexes may indicate ventricular hypertrophy, as occurs in semilunar valve stenosis). An enlarged Q wave may indicate a myocardial infarction and an enlarged R wave generally indicates enlarged ventricles. The size and shape of the T wave may be affected by any condition that slows ventricular repolarization. A flatter-than-normal T wave occurs when the heart muscle is receiving insufficient oxygen (e.g. in coronary arterial disease). An enlarged T wave may indicate hyperkalaemia (increased blood potassium levels), which may be a result of surgical or medical treatment (e.g. the unwanted side effects of certain drugs).

Reading an ECG also involves the examination of time-spans between waves (called intervals or segments). For example, the PQ interval (also called the PR interval, because the Q deflection may not always be obvious) is the time between the start of atrial depolarization and the onset of ventricular depolarization. If this exceeds 0.2 seconds, it may indicate damage along the conduction system or within the AV node. For example, in coronary arterial disease and rheumatic fever, scar tissue may form in the heart. As the impulse detours around the scar tissue, the PQ interval lengthens. The QT interval (i.e. the period required for ventricles to undergo a single depolarization and repolarization cycle) approximates to the duration of a ventricular contraction. A conduction imbalance, poor coronary blood flow, or myocardial damage may extend the interval. In addition an ST segment elevation can indicate acute myocardial damage.

Stress test

A stress test evaluates the heart's electrical response to the stress of physical exercise. During strenuous exercise (unlike when a person is at rest), the coronary arteries, if narrowed, are unable to meet the heart's increased need for oxygen, creating changes that can be noted on the ECG. These include ST segment elevation, and Q wave changes.

The ECG, together with other heart investigations, is therefore useful in diagnosing, and in following the course of recovery from, myocardial damage as occurs in myocardial infarction. ECGs are also used to monitor fetal welfare. Because it also identifies the sequence of events, it is also useful in the diagnosis of abnormal cardiac rhythms (arrhythmias).

Arrhythmias

The heart rate varies with changing activities. In exercise, an increased heart rate is considered quite normal, since the homeostatic set points are altered to accommodate the increased metabolic demands of the tissues to prevent intracellular homeostatic imbalances. However, if the heart rate is persistently and markedly increased or decreased at rest, but still in sinus rhythm (i.e. each P wave is followed by a QRS complex), this usually signals conduction malfunctions – sinus tachycardia (Figure 12.10b) and sinus bradycardia (Figure 12.10c), respectively. Sinus tachycardia is a heart rate beyond its homeostatic parameters ('tachy-' = fast); sinus bradycardia is a heart rate below its homeostatic parameters ('brady-' = slow). Clinically, tachycardia and bradycardia refer to resting heart rates of > 100 and < 60 beats per minute, respectively. A sinus tachycardia can be a physiological response to fever, exercise, anxiety or pain; it may accompany shock, left ventricular failure, cardiac tamponade, hyperthyroidism or pulmonary embolism, or it may be a response to sympathetic stimulating drugs. A sinus bradycardia may be normal in athletes; it may also accompany hypothermia, or it may be caused by increased vagal tone due to bowel straining, vomiting or pain, or be a response to beta-blocking drugs.

The rhythm disturbances detected can indicate what course of action is necessary to re-establish homeostatic function. For example, if the pulse falls to as low as 40 beats per minute (as occurs in sinus bradycardia or complete heart block of the conduction system), and drugs fail to help the condition, this requires an insertion of an artificial pacemaker. This battery-driven device stimulates the ventricles at a set rate nearer to that of a healthy heart. The battery can last up to 15 years; however most are replaced between 5 and 10 years.

In atrial flutter, the atria contract abnormally rapidly (about 200–300 times per minute) (Figure 12.10d). The characteristic atrial waves ('saw tooth' according to appearance) occur at regular intervals, and at a rate of 240–400 per minute; only every second to fourth atrial impulse reaches the ventricles. Atrial flutter may arise as a result of heart failure, pericarditis, heart valve disease, pulmonary embolism or hypoxia. It is usually treated with propranolol or quinidine, or by direct current shock (cardioversion).

Atrial fibrillation (AF) is a rapid, irregular contraction of atrial fibres approximately 400–500 times per minute (Figure 12.10e). The arrhythmia may appear intermittently, or as a chronic rhythm. In AF, the pumping effectiveness of the heart is reduced by 20–30%, which is still compatible with life though palpitations can be distressing and fatigue excessive. The causes of this condition include congestive cardiac failure, mitral stenosis, postcoronary artery bypass or valve replacement surgery, pulmonary embolism, chronic obstructive lung disease, hyperthyroidism and hypoxia.

Ventricular fibrillation (VF) is a rapid, irregular contraction of the ventricular fibres (Figure 12.10f). If the ventricles are fibrillating, they are useless as pumps as the coordination with filling from the atria is lost. Unless the heart is defibrillated quickly, then the circulation stops and brain death occurs. Cardiopulmonary resuscitation is necessary. Defibrillation involves exposing the heart to strong electrical shocks that interrupt the chaotic twitching of the heart by depolarizing the entire myocardium, in the hope that the SA node will resume activities again and the normal (or sinus) rhythm will be re-established. The UK Resuscitation Council publishes guidelines for managing all types of cardiac arrest/defibrillation in accordance with UK Resuscitation Council (2005) guidelines is as follows: a single 150–360 J biphasic or 360 J monophasic shock followed by cardiopulmonary resuscitation for 2 minutes. Adrenaline is given every 3–5 minutes; amiodarone may be given if the initial three shocks are unsuccessful.

Asystole occurs when the ventricles are at a standstill (i.e. no QRS complexes; Figure 12.10g). The causes include myocardial ischaemia or infarction, aortic valve disease, hyperkalaemia and acute respiratory failure. A patient undergoing asystole requires cardiopulmonary resuscitation with the administration of adrenaline and atropine. Treatment is repeated if necessary.

---

with the MB isoenzymes (CK-MB) being highly specific for injury to myocardial cells.

- Troponin I and cardiac troponin T are proteins which form the part of the calcium-binding complex of the thin myofilaments of myocardial tissue (see Figures 17.6, p.471 and

12.7e, p.313) Hence, troponins are extremely specific markers of cardiac damage and are important diagnostic indicators of an acute MI. Normally troponin I levels are <0.35 µg/L; cardiac troponin is less than 0.1 µg/L. Troponins rise (although troponin T is not illustrated in

Figure 12.7e) more slowly than myoglobin in blood, but the change is similar to that of CK-MB and may be useful for a diagnosis of MI up to 3–4 days following the incident. Thus, cardiac troponin serum assays are more reliable markers than other cardiac enzymes since they are more capable of detecting episodes of MI in which cell damage is below that detected by CK-MB levels.

A differential diagnosis of cardiac diseases is made via the different levels of delegated troponins. For example:

- a diagnosis of an MI uses the definition criterion of troponin I levels < 0.5 ng/mL (if combined with ST elevation on the ECG – this is classified as an acute MI);
- the diagnosis of acute coronary syndrome with troponin elevation includes a definition criterion of troponin I levels of between 0.05 and 0.5 ng/mL; whereas
- acute coronary syndrome with normal troponins (also known as unstable angina) have a diagnostic criterion of troponin I level of up to 0.04 ng/mL.

In addition, as long as tissue injury continues, the troponin I levels remain high. Troponin I levels rise rapidly and are detectable within 1 hour of myocardial cell injury. Troponin I levels are not detectable in individuals without cardiac injury, although troponin T many increase in the absence of cardiac damage, for example in sustained vigorous exercise, or if the patient is on cardiotoxic drugs such as doxorubicin. See the case study of a woman with a myocardial infarction, Section VI, p.654.

Extrinsic innervation of the heart

Although external nerve stimulation is not required for heart contraction, the autonomic nervous system modifies the activity of the intrinsic conduction system. The regulatory significance of this effect is discussed later. This section is concerned with the anatomy of the nerve supply to the heart. The general anatomy and tissue innervation of the autonomic nervous system is detailed in Chapter 8, pp.197–202 and summarized in Figure 8.29, p.198.

The medulla oblongata of the brainstem contains two 'cardiac centres' that control autonomic nerve activity to the heart. The cardiac accelerator centre controls sympathetic nerve activity to the heart, and the cardiac inhibitory centre controls parasympathetic nerve activity to the heart (Figure 12.11).

Neurons from both centres innervate collections of nerve cells (ganglia) within the heart wall, from which the neurons innervate the SA and AV nodes and some of the heart muscle. Sympathetic stimulation (as occurs in exercise and the stress response) accelerates the heart rate, and increases the force of myocardial contraction. Conversely, parasympathetic stimulation decreases the heart rate, but has little or no effect on the force of myocardial contraction.

OVERVIEW OF THE ANATOMY AND PHYSIOLOGY OF THE CARDIOVASCULAR SYSTEM 2: BLOOD VESSELS AND CIRCULATION

The regulation of cardiovascular function and the preservation of intracellular homeostasis involve an interaction between the cardiovascular system, circulatory components, tissue fluid and other organ systems mentioned in the introduction to this chapter. Blood is transported in the systemic and pulmonary circulatory systems via a network of specialized vessels:

- arteries and arterioles transport blood away from the heart;
- capillaries exchange materials between blood and cells;
- venules and veins return blood to the heart.

This section examines the structure and function of the vessels that constitute the vascular system.

BOX 12.7 MYOCARDIAL PRESERVATION DURING CARDIAC SURGERY AND INTEROPERATIVE AUTOTRANSFUSION

During cardiac surgery ischaemic damage to the heart must be minimized and the myocardium preserved. Previously, for cardiac surgery to be performed it was necessary to immobilize the heart, empty the chambers and induce ventricular asystole. To achieve this, cooling of the heart used a cardioplegia solution and cardiopulmonary bypass. Surgical advances and the development of 'minimal access surgery' have enabled cardiac surgeons to develop new techniques, which avoid using cardioplegia and cardiopulmonary bypass. One recent development is minimal access coronary artery bypass grafting; the surgery is performed on the beating heart, thus avoiding the need to immobilize the heart. Advances in minimal access surgery mean that many cardiac procedures are now being performed in this way.

Autotransfusion or autologous blood transfusion describes the collection and donation of blood from and to the same patient. The two most common ways this can be achieved are that the patient donates their own blood preoperatively to receive it later during surgery or during the postoperative period. Second, blood can be collected during the surgery and processed to return red cells to the patient during the perioperative period.

In intraoperative autotransfusion salvaged blood is sucked from the operative site using a sterile closed system through a filter containing a mixture of normal saline and heparin; this prevents the blood from clotting within the filter and the centrifuge system. Once there is sufficient blood loss (this varies depending on the system used), the blood can be processed. The blood is transferred into a centrifuge system where it is washed in normal saline; this process separates the non-cellular, cellular and biochemical debris from the red blood cells and eliminates 95–99% of unwanted contamination. The debris might include bone or tissue fragments, fatty lipids, fatty acids, fibrinolytic factors and plasma. The salvaged red blood cells are transferred into a blood transfusion bag and then through a blood-giving set back to the patient. Intraoperative autotransfusion is commonly used in major vascular surgery, for example aortic aneurysm repair, cardiac surgery, trauma and orthopaedic surgery, and in situations where there is an anticipated blood loss of greater than 20% of the patient's blood volume. Contraindications to autotransfusion include presence of bowel contents, the presence of tumour cells, urine and some irrigating fluids.

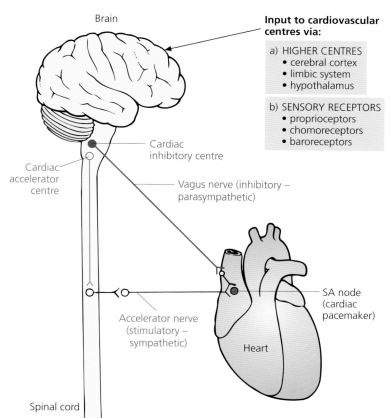

Brain

Input to cardiovascular centres via:

a) HIGHER CENTRES
- cerebral cortex
- limbic system
- hypothalamus

b) SENSORY RECEPTORS
- proprioceptors
- chomoreceptors
- baroreceptors

Cardiac inhibitory centre

Cardiac accelerator centre

Vagus nerve (inhibitory – parasympathetic)

SA node (cardiac pacemaker)

Accelerator nerve (stimulatory – sympathetic)

Heart

Spinal cord

Figure 12.11 Neural pathways for controlling the heart rate. SA, sinoatrial

Q *Compare the effects of parasympathetic and sympathetic stimulation on the heart's conduction system.*

Structure and function of blood vessels

Blood vessel structure varies according to the function, but all vessels, except capillaries, have the same basic structure of three distinctive layers (coats or tunicae; Figure 12.12a):

- *The tunica interna (the innermost coat)*: consists of a single layer of flattened cells. This endothelial lining in vessels larger than 1 mm in diameter is supported by connective tissue dominated by elastic fibres (Figure 12.12b,c). Capillaries are composed only of this layer, with few or no elastic fibres, so as to aid the rapid exchange of water and solutes between the tissue fluid and blood plasma.
- *The tunica media (the middle coat)*: consists predominantly of smooth muscle fibres supported by a layer of collagen and elastin fibres.
- *The tunica externa (the outer connective tissue sheath)*: consists principally of elastin and collagen fibres.

The relative thickness and fibre composition of each layer varies according to the vessel's function (Figure 12.12b,c). The middle layer shows the greatest variation. It is absent in capillaries, for example, but in large arteries close to the heart it is composed mainly of elastin tissue. In addition to elastic properties, arteries (especially the arterioles) have contractile functions due to their smooth muscle layer being innervated by the sympathetic nervous system. Contraction squeezes the wall around the vessel, a process called vasoconstriction, since the muscle fibres are arranged in rings around the vessel. Conversely, when sympathetic stimulation is suppressed, the muscle fibres relax, causing the arterial lumen to increase in diameter, a process called vasodilation.

The arterial system

The characteristics of arteries are that they always transport blood away from the heart, and they usually carry oxygenated blood. The exceptions to the latter are the pulmonary arteries in the adult circulation, which carry deoxygenated blood from the right ventricle to the lungs, and the umbilical arteries in the fetal circulation, which carry deoxygenated blood from the fetus to the placenta.

Arteries are classified as elastic arteries, muscular arteries and arterioles, according to their size and function.

Elastic arteries

These large vessels have diameters of up to 25 mm. The aorta, pulmonary trunk and their major branches are elastic arteries. The tunica media contains considerably more elastic fibres than muscle fibres. Elastic fibres are also present in the other layers (Figure 12.12b,c). These fibres facilitate arterial stretching to accommodate the extra blood volume and pressure instigated by ventricular contraction and arterial recoiling upon ventricular relaxation. Consequently, blood flows continuously, even when the ventricles are filling during the relaxation period and output from the heart has momentarily ceased.

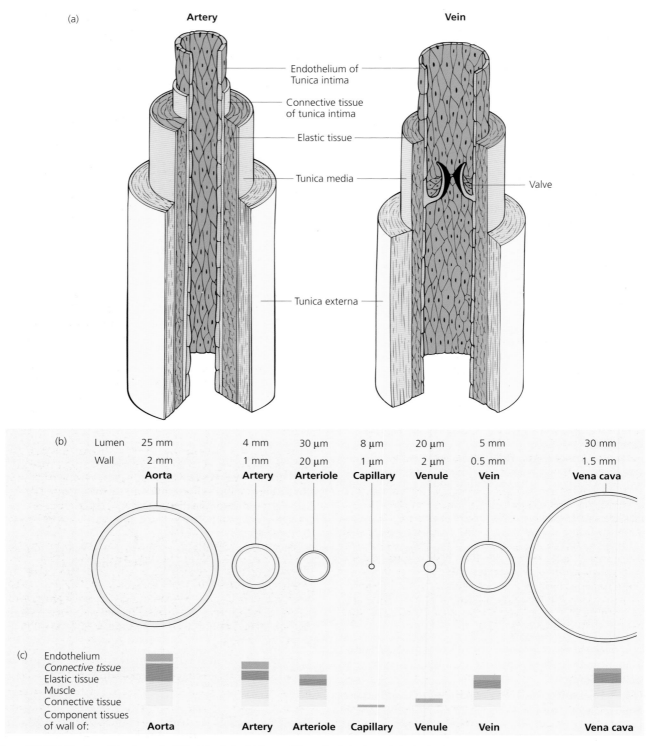

Figure 12.12 (a) Structure of blood vessels. (b) Variation in the thickness of the walls of blood vessels in the circulatory system. (c) Variation in components of the walls of the various blood vessels in the circulatory system

Q Identify the structure and composition of the walls of arteries and veins. How are they similar? How do they differ?

Despite their muscle content, elastic arteries have relatively ineffective vasoconstrictory powers.

Elastic arteries are the 'conduction arteries', since they conduct blood away from the heart to the muscular arteries.

Muscular arteries

Elastic arteries give rise to relatively more muscular arteries, sometimes referred to as 'distributing arteries' because these medium-sized vessels of 1–4 mm in diameter distribute blood

BOX 12.8 ARTERIOSCLEROSIS AND ATHEROSCLEROSIS

Several types of arteriosclerosis ('hardening of the arteries') exist, some more dangerous than others. Arteriosclerosis associated with ageing is a progressive, degenerate arterial imbalance, in which the artery walls gradually lose elastic and muscle fibres. These vessels become stiff, hard and relatively inelastic, and eventually their lumen is narrowed as they become infiltrated with collagen and calcium. Because of the lack of distensibility, arteriosclerotic vessels are less able to change their radius and lumen size; hence blood pressure peaks are much higher. This exposes their walls to greater stresses, and increases the risk of cerebrovascular accidents and myocardial infarctions. The risks are elevated further if the patient is also hypertensive from additional factors.

Atherosclerosis

Atherosclerosis is a type of arteriosclerosis characterized by the deposition of lipids, cholesterol compounds, excessive smooth muscle and fibroblastic cells in the form of atheromatous plaques in the blood vessel wall. (Figure 12.13a). Plaques grow and spread along the arterial wall, forming a swelling that protrudes into the lumen, thus compromising blood flow to the affected organs. The origin of plaques is debatable, although vascular 'fatty streaks', if not absorbed (a homeostatic control process), are thought to be precursors. Streaks are evident in autopsies of children as young as 6 years old, and may be of genetic and/or environmental origin. Arteries most commonly affected are identified in Figure 12.13d. Atherosclerosis is therefore an obvious cause of coronary artery disease (see Box 12.4, p.314), cerebral vascular accidents, and tissue ischaemia in peripheral vascular disease.

Atherosclerosis predisposes the person to other imbalances, such as:

* thrombosis: the endothelial lining over the plaque breaks down, and circulating platelets are activated and stimulate the clotting cascade; the developing thrombus (or emboli) may cause ischaemia, infarction and gangrene (Figure 12.13b,c);
* aneurysm formation: local dilation of the wall called an aneurysm weakens the arterial wall; rupture of this causes haemorrhaging.

Atherosclerosis has a multifactorial aetiology. The risk factors of smoking and hypertension may have their own adverse effects by damaging the endothelium (i.e. the inner lining of blood vessels). For example, with smoking, nicotine increases platelet adhesion, and carbon monoxide may increase the permeability of the arterial endothelium, thus increasing plaque formation. Research has also demonstrated a positive relationship between elevated serum cholesterol levels (due to a change to the normal ratio of high-density lipoprotein to low-density lipoprotein in favour of the latter; see Chapter 5, pp.109–10 and Table 12.1) and the instance of atherosclerosis, especially associated with coronary arterial disease (Pradka, 2000).

Table 12.1 Interpretation of blood cholesterol screening results

Less than 5.2 mmol/L
This is the required level suggested by doctors. The threat of heart disease is low, provided that other risk factors* are also low.

*Other known risk factors in heart disease include: smoking, high blood pressure, diabetes mellitus Type 2, obesity, lack of exercise, too much alcohol

Between 5.2 and 6.5 mmol/L
This result indicate moderate risk group. This range is characteristic of people in the UK. The individual should be advised on healthy eating. In addition, other risk factors should be highlighted. If appropriate, the individual should stop smoking, and reduce alcohol intake and weight. These values need to be checked for improvement in 6 months' time.

Between 6.5 to 7.8 mmol/L
Values indicates a high level of cholesterol. Individuals are advised to visit their doctor for advice.

7.9 mmol/L and over
This value is too high a level of cholesterol and need urgent consideration and attention. High levels of cholesterol may be inherited within a family, and it is generally appropriate for parents, sisters, brothers and children to be tested. The individual must visit the doctor for advice.

Note: A single test hardly ever provides a completely certain result, even with good equipment and in a professional hands. A high result should be checked by general practitioners.

The information above is based upon the European Atherosclerosis Society guidelines.

Consequently, an inappropriate diet, smoking and a lack of exercise are important contributory factors that modify the underlying pathophysiology associated with atheroma (Clancy and McVicar, 1998). Such interactions are major risk factors in the incidence of coronary heart disease in the UK. Care is directed at the consequences of atheroma, but also at encouraging people to reappraise their lifestyle and so reduce the risk of heart disease.

The incidence of atherosclerosis increases with advancing years. It is more common in men than women, until the time of menopause; then the sex distribution of atherosclerosis becomes equal. Family history of arterial disease (both genetic and environmental factors), stressful lifestyle, personality type A (although the existence of such personalities is now contested), characterized by aggressive restless behaviour, and diabetes mellitus are all associated with increased incidence of atherosclerosis.

to peripheral tissues. They are often named according to the tissue or part of the body that they supply (see 'Blood vessel nomenclature', p.329). The vessels have a thick tunica media that contains considerably more smooth muscle fibres than elastin fibres. They are therefore less distensible than elastic arteries, but are capable of greater vasoconstriction and vasodilation, adjusting blood flow to suit the needs of the structures supplied.

Arterioles

Arterioles are the smallest arteries, having an average diameter of 20–30 µm. They deliver blood to the capillary vessels within tissues. Those arterioles nearest to the muscular arteries have similar tunica components, whereas smaller arterioles change their characteristics. Those nearest the capillaries are composed of an endothelial coat and an incomplete layer of smooth muscle; these muscle fibres enable the arteriolar diameter to be altered, and hence regulate blood flow through their dependent tissues (Figure 12.14). Relaxation of specialized regions – the precapillary sphincters (which consist of a few circular muscle fibres) – close to the arteriolar–capillary junction may cause the capillary bed to become fully perfused with blood. Partial sphincter contraction reduces blood flow, and total contraction causes capillary shutdown. Arteriolar and sphincter diameters are controlled by smooth muscle contraction, induced extrinsically by the sympathetic nervous system, or

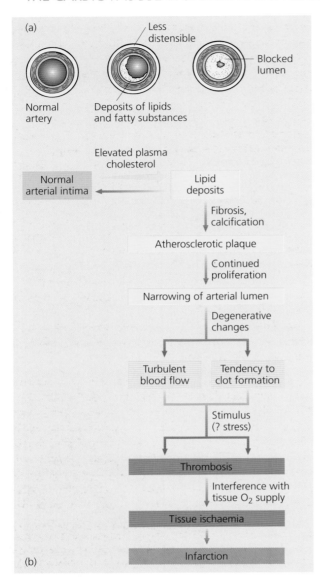

(a)

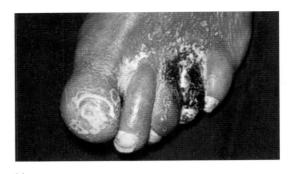

(c)

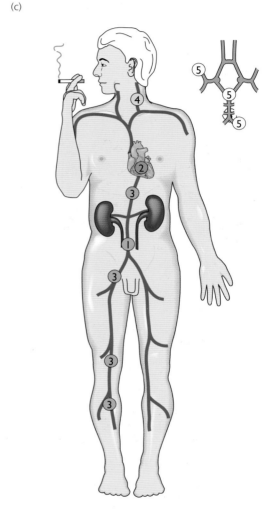

(d)

Figure 12.13 (a) Atherosclerotic vessel changes. (b) Mechanism producing atherosclerosis and tissue infarction. (c) Gangrenous toe caused by ischaemia from blocked peripheral vessels (reprinted with the permission of Abrahams *et al.*, *Illustrated Clinical Anatomy*, Hodder, London). (d) Distribution of atheroma. Sites in order of frequency: 1, abdominal aorta; 2, proximal coronary arteries; 3, descending thoracic aorta, femoral and popliteal arteries; 4, internal carotid artery; 5, vertebral/basilar/middle cerebral arteries (reproduced with the kind permission of Lakhani *et al.*, *Basic Pathology*, 3rd edn. Hodder, London)

Q Explain how circulatory function is altered by atherosclerosis.

intrinsically (called autoregulation) in response to changes in tissue fluid composition. An example of the latter is the central nervous system ischaemic response, in which cerebral hypoxia (lack of oxygen in brain tissue) causes dilation of the cerebral arterioles.

Capillaries

Capillaries form the part of the circulation often referred to as the microcirculation, since they average only 8 μm in diameter. They are located close to almost all body cells, but their distribution varies according to the activity of the tissues they serve. For example, high-activity sites, such as muscle, liver, kidney, lung and nervous tissues, have a rich distribution, whereas lower-activity sites, such as tendons and ligaments, have a poor distribution. The skin's epidermis, the cornea of the eye, and cartilage tissue are devoid of capillaries, and cells of these tissues have very low rates of metabolism.

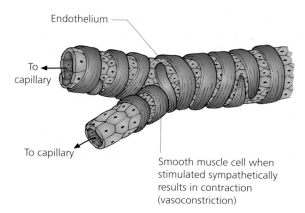

Endothelium

To capillary

To capillary

Smooth muscle cell when stimulated sympathetically results in contraction (vasoconstriction)

Figure 12.14 Structure of an arteriole

Q *How do arterioles affect capillary blood flow?*

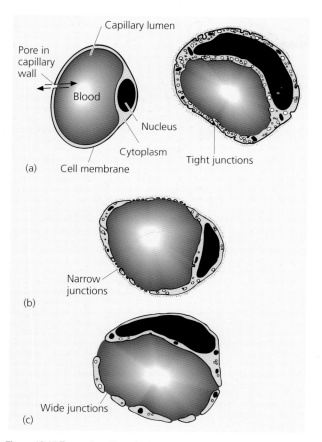

Capillary lumen

Pore in capillary wall

Blood

Nucleus

Cytoplasm

Tight junctions

(a)   Cell membrane

Narrow junctions

(b)

Wide junctions

(c)

Figure 12.15 Types of capillary. (a) Continuous – connected by tight junctions (e.g. found in muscle). (b) Fenestrated – allows external diffusion (e.g. found in kidney glomeruli and brain choroid plexus). (c) Discontinuous – maximizes exchange of materials (e.g. found in adrenal glands)

A typical capillary consists of a tube of endothelial cells sitting on a basement membrane. In most regions, this tube forms a complete lining, with the endothelial cells being connected by tight junctions; these are referred to as continuous capillaries. Fenestrated capillaries are located in those few areas

where extensive fluid exchange occurs (e.g. in the kidney glomeruli, and in the brain's choroid plexus). Discontinuous capillaries are located in the liver (sinusoids), bone marrow and adrenal glands, where they form flattened, irregular passageways that slow the blood flow through these tissues to maximize the period of absorption and secretion across the capillary walls (Figure 12.15).

The prime homeostatic function of capillaries is to permit the exchange of metabolites and wastes between blood and tissue cells; thus they are sometimes called the 'exchange vessels'. For efficient exchange, it is necessary to have:

- *a short distance for substances to diffuse through*: the structure and location of capillaries is admirably suited for exchange, since they comprise a single layer of cells that are in close proximity to tissue cells. The thick walls of arteries and veins present too great a barrier for this process to be efficient;
- *a large surface area*: the total cross-sectional area of the capillaries throughout the body is many thousands times more than that of the aorta;
- *a steady but slow rate of blood flow*: the capillary flow velocity is about 700 times lower than that in the aorta because of the narrowness of these vessels.

Capillaries function as a part of interconnected networks known as a capillary plexus or capillary bed (Figure 12.16a). A single arteriole gives rises to dozens of capillaries, which in turn collect to form several venules. The capillary entrance is guarded by precapillary sphincters, which control flow, as discussed earlier. Blood flow in arteries is pulsatile, related to the pulse in arterial blood pressure, but blood flow through capillaries between arterioles and venules is usually at a near-constant rate. Blood flow can vary between individual capillaries, however. Each precapillary sphincter's cycle of alternate contraction and relaxation occurs perhaps a dozen times a minute. The activities of various sphincters within the tissue mean that blood may reach the venules by one route at a certain time, and by a different route at another time (Figure 12.16).

Other mechanisms that modify circulatory supply to capillaries include:

- *Collateral circulation*: capillary networks may be supplied by more than one artery. The union of the branches of two or more artery supplies to the same region is called an arterial anastomosis. Such vessels could be considered an evolutionary homeostatic adaptation, since blockage of one arterial supply to a capillary bed, caused by disease, injury or surgery, is compensated for by another route of supply, thus guaranteeing a reliable blood supply to tissues (e.g. the cerebral circulation; see Chapter 8, p.182). The alternative route of blood flow is known as a collateral circulation (see Figure 12.7c, p.313). Arteries that do not anastomose are known as 'end arteries'. Obstruction to an end artery interrupts the blood supply to the old segment of an organ, producing death (necrosis) of a segment (see Box 12.4, p.314).
- *Arteriovenous anastomoses (AV shunts)*: these vascular 'short circuits' result from a fusion of arterioles and venules, and

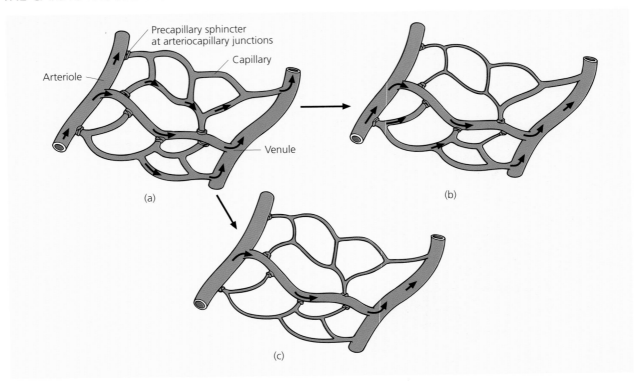

Figure 12.16 The organization of a capillary plexus. (a) Structure of a capillary plexus. (b) and (c) Two possible alterations in the pattern of flow through the capillary plexus as vasomotion occurs

Q. Arterioles provide the main means of varying resistance to blood flow through tissues. Identify three other factors that influence how easily blood flows through a vessel.

are opened when the smooth muscle of arterioles contracts, causing the capillary bed to be bypassed. Relaxation of this muscular component encourages flow through the capillary bed, rather than through the anastomoses. Rates of blood flow through the low-resistance shunts can be very high, so they are found in tissues in which such rates are sometimes appropriate. In the skin, for example, they act as a thermoregulatory mechanism by facilitating the conservation or loss of body heat (see Figure 16.10, p.459).

The venous system

The venous system is the collection or drainage system that takes blood from capillary beds (when blood has exchanged substances with tissue fluid) towards the heart (see Figure 12.1, p.305). En route from the venous side of the capillary network, vessels increase in diameter, their walls thicken, and they progress from the smallest veins (venules) to the largest veins (vena cavae).

Venules

Capillaries merge to form venules, which range from 8 to 100 μm in diameter. The smallest postcapillary venules consist almost entirely of a lining endothelium with a few surrounding fibroblast cells. They are, therefore, extremely porous and inflammatory substances and leucocytes move easily through

their walls from blood to the site of injury via the process of diapedesis (see Figure 11.13b, p.290). As the venules approach veins, a sparse tunica media and tunica externa become apparent.

Veins

Venules merge to form veins. These vessels have the three tunicae found in arteries (see Figure 12.12a, p.322). Their walls are thinner, however, particularly the tunica media, since they have less elastic tissue and smooth muscle. Their lumens are larger for a given external diameter (Figure 12.12a,b, p.322), and they offer less resistance to blood flow. This is important because the pressure of blood within the venous circulation is low and provides little force to circulate blood. Veins are, however, still distensible enough to adapt to variations in volume or pressure of blood passing through them. In fact, the thin walls and large lumens mean that about two-thirds of the total blood volume is found within the venous system at any time, which is why veins are referred to as the capacitance vessels or blood (vein) reservoirs (Figure 12.17).

The following adaptations within this low-pressure system aid the return of blood to the heart:

- *Large-diameter lumens*: this means that veins have little resistance to blood flow. The diameter is influenced by the sympathetic nervous system (i.e. changes in sympathetic tone increase or decrease the pooling capacity of the vessel).

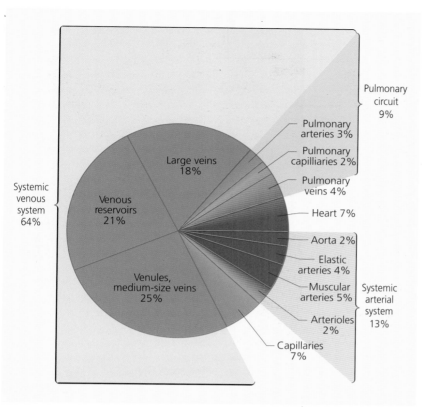

Figure 12.17 The distribution of blood within the circulatory system

- *Valves*: these are internal folds of the endothelial lining of large veins that resemble the semilunar valves of the heart in structure and function. They are present in the deep veins of the limbs; since the upward flow of blood is opposed by gravity, these veins are compressed by surrounding skeletal muscles (skeletomuscular pumps), which ensure unidirectional flow (Figure 12.18a,b).
- *Large veins, such as the vena cavae*: these are responsive to the pressure changes in the thoracic cavity that occur during the respiratory cycle, thus assisting venous return to the heart by acting as a thoracoabdominal pump.

Venous sinuses

Venous sinuses are specialized flattened veins consisting of tunica interna supported by surrounding tissues rather than other tunicae. They may form relatively large spaces where blood collects before passing on, for example the coronary sinus or the sinuses between the layers of the dura mater around the brain.

Blood reservoirs

Two-thirds of the total blood volume at any time is normally found within the systemic veins; whereas arteries contain about 13%, pulmonary vessels 9%, the heart 7%, and capillaries the remainder (Figure 12.17). The veins are known as the blood capacitance vessels or blood reservoirs, since they serve as storage depots for blood that can be moved quickly to other parts of the body if the need arises. For example, during strenuous exercise, the vasomotor centre ('vas-' = vessel, 'motor' = excitatory nerve supply) of the medulla oblongata of the brainstem

---

BOX 12.9 VARICOSE VEINS

Valve damage may be congenital or acquired, as occurs if the venous system is exposed to high pressure for long periods (e.g. in venous hypertension, pregnancy, abdominal tumours, obesity) and in standing for long, extended periods. The resultant 'leaky' or incompetent valve allows backflow of blood, causing pooling of blood distal to the valve (Figure 12.18c); such varicose veins can become long and tortuous. Consequently, fluid may leak into the surrounding tissues, producing oedema. The affected vein and tissue around it may become inflamed and painfully tender, and varicose ulcers may develop.

Areas in the vicinity of the varicose veins may ache because the diffusion of oxygen and nutrients following oedema is reduced. These veins are liable to haemorrhage if knocked, but the patient's main complaint is usually of their appearance. Veins close to the surface of the legs (especially the saphenous vein) are highly susceptible to varicosities (Figure 12.18d). Deeper veins are not usually as vulnerable, because surrounding skeletal muscle prevents their walls from stretching excessively.

There is no cure for this condition, but an operation can be performed that strips out the affected vein, with ligatures to the supplying veins. Non-surgical intervention includes wearing support tights or stockings, thus assisting venous return by maintaining pressure on the legs. Deep breathing also assists venous return. Preventive measures include sitting down at intervals throughout the day with the feet raised on a stool. Crossing the legs while sitting down should be avoided, since this stops blood flow through the vessel behind the knee.

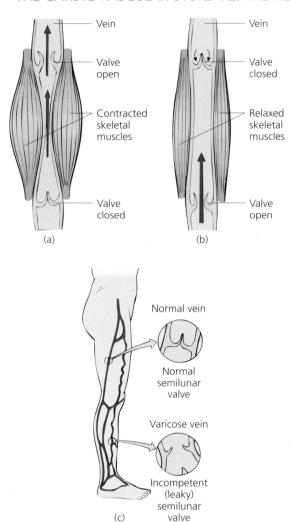

(a)

(b)

(c)

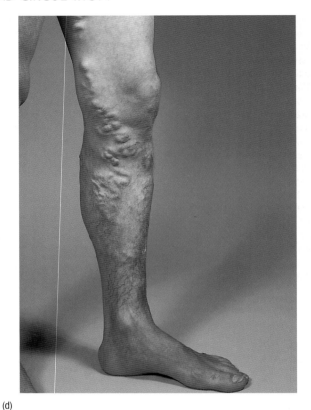

(d)

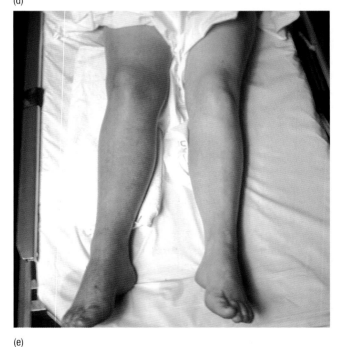

(e)

Figure 12.18 Operation of skeletomuscular pumps and vein valves in returning blood to the heart. (a) When skeletal muscles contract and press against the flexible veins, the valves proximal to the area of contraction are forced open and blood is propelled towards the heart. The back-flowing blood closes the valves distal to the point of contraction. (b) When skeletal muscles relax, the valves proximal to the muscle close to prevent backward flow. The distal valves open, creating an upward suction pressure and forcing blood upwards. (c) Varicose veins. Veins near the surface of the body (especially in the legs) may bulge and cause venous valves to leak. The enlarged vein is said to be 'varicose'. (d) A varicose great saphenous vein distended with blood, because the valves of the communicating gains are incompetent (i.e. leaky). (e) Deep vein thrombosis – note swollen right leg. (d,e) Reproduced with the kind permission of Abrahams *et al.*, from *Illustrated Clinical Anatomy*, Hodder, London

Q How do varicose veins develop? What complications may arise from varicose veins?

increases its sympathetic output to major veins, causing their vasoconstriction. In this way, the vessels act as venous blood reservoirs since constriction diverts blood away from them and so increases the cardiac output. Consequently, the volume of blood within the capillary beds of skeletal muscles increases, enabling the tissues to obtain more oxygen and nutrients, and so manufacture the ATP necessary for the increased muscle contraction. Other factors affecting the vasomotor centre are identified in Figure 12.22d, p.340.

Routes of circulation

The heart operates as a double pump, since it has left and right ventricular pumps that serve two distinctive circulatory circuits – the systemic circulation and the pulmonary circulation

BOX 12.10 ANEURYSM

An aneurysm is a localized, permanent, thin, weakened section of the vessel wall that bulges outward, forming a balloon-like sac. Abdominal aortic aneurysms account for approximately 75% of all aneurysms (Huether and McCance, 2006). Those occurring in the aorta are often caused by atherosclerosis, and are associated with hypertension (high blood pressure). Other common causes are syphilis, congenital blood vessel defects, and trauma. Elective surgery is the usual treatment, and can be very effective. If untreated, the aneurysm enlarges and the blood vessel wall becomes so thin that it bursts. If an aortic aneurysm ruptures, the results are disastrous unless immediate advanced life support and specialist surgery are available.

The Berry aneurysm, which affects vessels of the circle of Willis (an anastomosis of arteries at the base of the brain), results from a congenital vessel defect. Rupture leads to subarachnoid or intercerebral haemorrhage. This condition is also associated with hypertension. Signs and symptoms of a stroke occur when cerebral aneurysms leak. Clot-stabilizing drugs and a number of clinical measures are used to reduce intracranial pressure before surgical intervention.

(see Figure 12.1, p.305). The systemic circulation routes oxygenated blood through a long-loop circuit, from the left ventricle of the heart (via the force created by the left ventricular pump), through the aorta and its branches, to all body cells other than those of lung tissue. Blood is returned to the right atrium via the vena cavae and coronary sinus. The roles of this circuit are to transport metabolites (e.g. oxygen and nutrients), and to remove 'waste' products of metabolism (e.g. excess carbon dioxide and water) from tissue cells. The pulmonary circulation routes deoxygenated blood through a short-loop circuit from the right ventricle of the heart (via the force created by the right ventricular pump), through the pulmonary trunk, which bifurcates into the left and right pulmonary arteries, taking blood to their respective lungs for gas exchange.

The systemic circulation of the adult can be subdivided functionally, according to the organs supplied: the coronary circulation (discussed earlier), the renal circulation (see Figures 15.2b, p.423, 15.3, p.424 and 15.7, p.430) cerebral circulation (see Figure 8.17, p.182), the cutaneous circulation (see Figure 16.10, p.458), the skeletomuscular circulation (Figure 17.2, p.465), the hepatoportal circulation (see below and Figure 10.18, p.255), and the pulmonary circulation (see Figures 12.1, p.305 and 14.4, p.401).

The hepatoportal circulation consists of the hepatic artery, which supplies the liver with oxygenated blood, and the hepatic portal vein, which supplies nutrients directly from the digestive organs (this is deoxygenated blood). The hepatic vein drains blood from the liver into the inferior vena cava.

A portal vein is one that carries blood from one capillary bed directly to another, without passing through the heart and being redistributed by arteries. There are a few examples in the body, (e.g. the vascular connection between the hypothalamus and the anterior pituitary gland; see Figure 9.5, p.214 and associated text), but the hepatic portal vein is the largest. This vein receives blood from veins draining the stomach, intestines and spleen (via the superior mesenteric vein and splenic vein), the pancreas (via the pancreatic vein and branches of the splenic vein), the colon (mainly via the inferior mesenteric vein) and the gall bladder (via the cystic vein).

Blood entering the lungs via the pulmonary circulation undergoes gaseous exchange. A pair of pulmonary veins eventually merge from each lung, routing blood back into the heart's left atrium. These vessels are the only veins (in the adult) that carry oxygenated blood. The role of the pulmonary circuitry, therefore, is to transport deoxygenated blood to the lungs for oxygenation and carbon dioxide excretion.

Blood vessel nomenclature

Blood vessel nomenclature is complex and outside the intentions of this book. Accordingly, blood vessels are only named in this book where appropriate, and chapters have only highlighted the important circulations and vessels associated with the homeostatic roles of particular organ systems. Suffice to say, the name of a blood vessel usually gives a clue to its appearance and/or distribution (Figure 12.19). Thus, if you become familiar with the major skeletomuscular and neural 'landmarks', there should be few surprises. You should note the following, however:

- The peripheral distribution of arteries and veins on the left and right sides are almost the same, except near the heart, where large vessels (i.e. the vena cavae and pulmonary veins) connect to the atria and other vessels (i.e. pulmonary trunk and aorta) connect to the ventricles.
- A single vessel may change its name as it passes specific boundaries (e.g. the aorta is subdivided into the ascending aorta, aortic arch, and thoracic and abdominal aorta). This makes accurate anatomical descriptions possible where vessels extend to the periphery.

CARDIAC PHYSIOLOGY

The heart is an extremely active organ, beating approximately 30 million times, and ejecting some 2.1 million litres of blood, every year. The previous section outlined the physiological basis for the coordinated contraction of the heart, the structure and function of blood vessels, and the specific routes of circulation. This section examines the details of cardiac physiology associated with the events of each heart beat, the homeostatic control of cardiac output, and how cardiac parameters may be varied to meet changing peripheral demands.

Cardiac cycle

The cardiac cycle represents the events associated with the flow of blood through the heart during one heartbeat. Since alternate myocardial contraction and relaxation mainly achieve the

ACTIVITY

Re-familiarize yourself with the names of the chambers of the heart, and the names of the autonomic nerves that supply the heart and their origins in the brainstem.

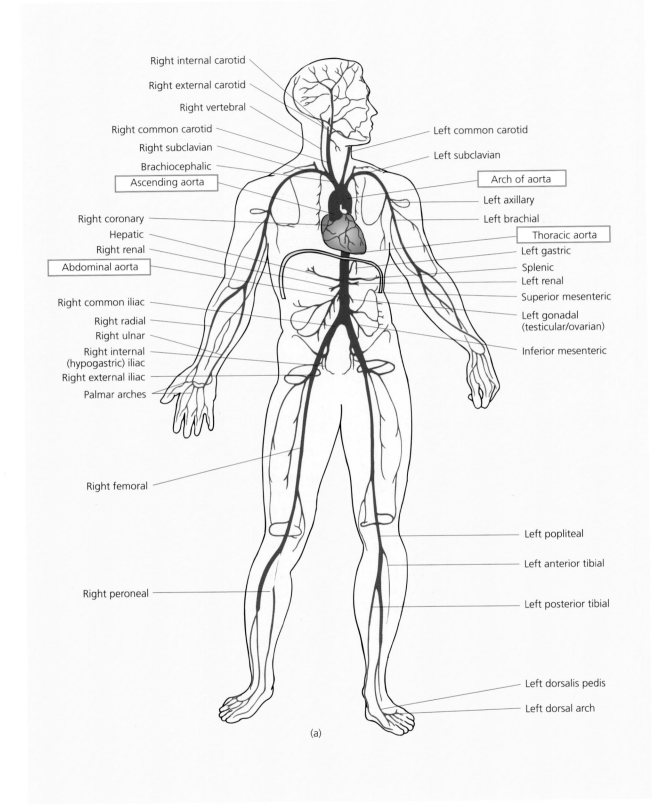

Right internal carotid
Right external carotid
Right vertebral
Right common carotid
Right subclavian
Brachiocephalic
Ascending aorta

Right coronary
Hepatic
Right renal
Abdominal aorta

Right common iliac
Right radial
Right ulnar
Right internal (hypogastric) iliac
Right external iliac
Palmar arches

Right femoral

Right peroneal

Left common carotid
Left subclavian

Arch of aorta
Left axillary
Left brachial
Thoracic aorta
Left gastric
Splenic
Left renal
Superior mesenteric
Left gonadal (testicular/ovarian)
Inferior mesenteric

Left popliteal

Left anterior tibial

Left posterior tibial

Left dorsalis pedis
Left dorsal arch

(a)

Figure 12.19 Major blood vessels of the systemic circulation: (a) arteries; (b) veins

Q Describe the route taken by blood as it moves from the hepatic portal vein to the hepatic vein.

Q Describe the route taken by blood as it moves from the left ventricle to the right external carotid.

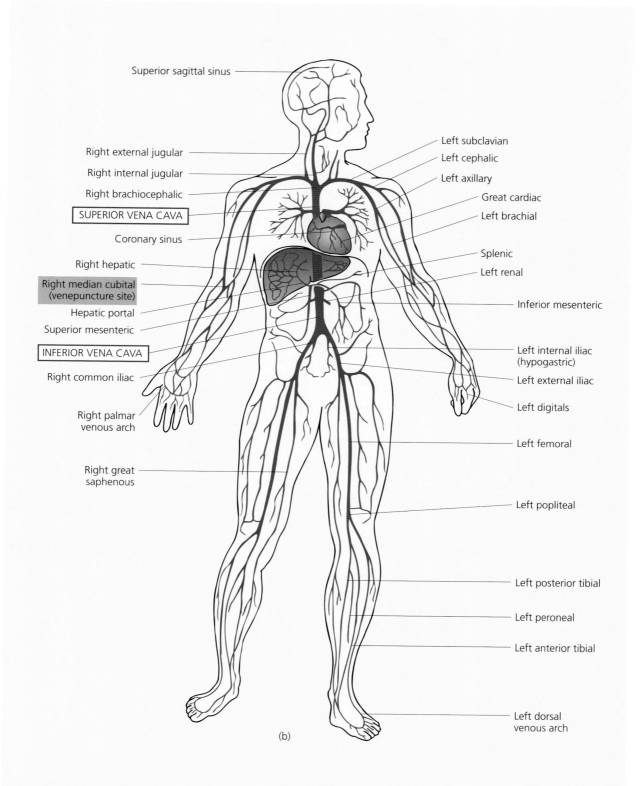

Superior sagittal sinus

Right external jugular

Right internal jugular

Right brachiocephalic

SUPERIOR VENA CAVA

Coronary sinus

Right hepatic

Right median cubital
(venepuncture site)

Hepatic portal

Superior mesenteric

INFERIOR VENA CAVA

Right common iliac

Right palmar
venous arch

Right great
saphenous

Left subclavian

Left cephalic

Left axillary

Great cardiac

Left brachial

Splenic

Left renal

Inferior mesenteric

Left internal iliac
(hypogastric)

Left external iliac

Left digitals

Left femoral

Left popliteal

Left posterior tibial

Left peroneal

Left anterior tibial

Left dorsal
venous arch

(b)

movement of blood, the cycle employs the terms 'systole' (period of contraction) and 'diastole' (period of relaxation). Systolic contraction ejects blood from atria into adjacent ventricles, and from ventricles into the arterial trunks (i.e. pulmonary and aortic trunks). Diastolic relaxation is the period in which the heart chambers become filled with blood. Thus, the cardiac cycle is conveniently split into four phases: atrial and ventricular diastole, and atrial and ventricular systole. Since the sequence of events in the right and left sides of the heart is the same, we use the traditional approach of describing the cardiac cycle in terms of left-sided events (Figure 12.20).

The main difference from the right-sided events is that the pressure generated by the left ventricle during systole is considerably higher than that generated by the right ventricle. This is because the total resistance to flow in the systemic circulation is greater than in the pulmonary circulation, so less pressure is required to promote circulation of the blood through the lungs; this is reflected by the relative thickness of the ventricular walls. Despite these pressure differences, the ventricles eject the same amount of blood with each contraction.

Our explanation of the cardiac cycle begins with the heart in total relaxation, when both atria and ventricles are relaxed, and it is mid- to late diastole (i.e. the chambers are almost filled with blood).

Period of ventricular filling (mid- to late diastole)

Pressure within the heart is low at this point, so pulmonary venous blood flows passively into the left atrium. As blood enters, the atrial pressure becomes greater than ventricular pressure. Consequently, the AV (bicuspid) valve opens into the left ventricle, and blood passes from the atrium to the ventricle throughout the diastolic period. The semilunar (aortic) valve is closed, since the pressure in the aorta is greater than the left ventricular pressure (Figure 12.20, interval 1a). About 70–80% of the ventricular filling occurs during diastole. Towards the end of this period, the tissue of the SA node discharges spontaneously and a wave of electrical excitation spreads throughout the atria (i.e. atrial depolarization corresponding to the P wave of the ECG). The subsequent atrial myocardial contraction, or atrial systole, accounts for the final 20–30% of ventricular filling (Figure 12.20, interval 1b). The amount of blood within the ventricles at the end of ventricular diastole is called the ventricular end diastolic volume (VEDV). Atrial systole and ventricular diastole therefore occur simultaneously. Throughout diastole, the pressure in the aorta falls, since blood is moving throughout the systemic circuitry but is not being replenished by blood ejected from the left ventricle.

Ventricular systole

Following contraction, the atria go into diastole. The wave of depolarization is passed from the AV node to the conduction system provided by the bundles of His, and then progresses throughout the Purkinje system. This need for ventricular systole to be slightly delayed after atrial systole highlights the importance of the electrical resistance provided by the AV node, noted earlier. Ventricular depolarization (corresponding

to the QRS complex of the ECG) induces ventricular myocardial contraction, or ventricular systole. This causes the left ventricular pressure to rise sharply, closing the AV (bicuspid) valve and preventing backflow into the left atrium. For a split second, the ventricle is a completely sealed chamber; this brief period is sometimes referred to as the isovolumetric ventricular contraction phase (Figure 12.20, interval 2a), and is responsible for the rapid increase in the pressure within the ventricle. This phase ends as the ventricular pressure becomes greater than that in the aorta, when the semilunar (aortic) valve opens and ventricular ejection occurs (on the right side of the heart the right ventricle simultaneously ejects its blood into the pulmonary arterial trunk). The ejection is initially rapid, but then tapers off. The ejection of blood from the left ventricle (Figure 12.20, interval 2b) causes the pressure in the aorta to reach approximately 120 mmHg (= 15.8 kPa; 1 kPa = 7.6 mmHg; see Appendix B). The left atrial pressure rises slowly throughout the ventricular ejection period, because of the continued flow of blood into it from the pulmonary veins.

Early diastole

During this brief phase (i.e. following the T wave on the ECG), the ventricular myocardium relaxes, causing the left ventricular pressure to decrease to a value below the aortic pressure. This results in a backward flow of blood in the aortic trunk, which causes closure of the semilunar (aortic) valve. Closure of the aortic valve causes a very brief rise in the aortic pressure, known as the dicrotic notch (Figure 12.20).

After closure of the semilunar (aortic) valve, the AV (bicuspid) valve remains closed for a fraction of a second, thus once again the left ventricle is a sealed chamber. The ventricular blood volume at this phase of ventricular relaxation is referred to as the end systolic volume (ESV), and the relaxation phase as isovolumetric ventricular relaxation (Figure 12.20, interval 3). Pressure within the ventricle falls sharply. This stage ends when the left atrial pressure rises (as a result of atrial filling) above the ventricular pressure, thus causing the AV valve to open and the ventricular filling phase begins once again. Atrial pressure falls to its lowest point, and ventricular pressure begins to rise, completing the cycle.

At an average heart rate of 70 bpm, each cardiac cycle takes about 0.8 seconds; atrial systole accounts for 0.1 seconds and ventricular systole for 0.3 seconds; the remaining 0.4 seconds

Figure 12.20 Summary of events occurring in the heart during the cardiac cycle. (a) Events in the left side of the heart. An electrocardiogram (ECG) tracing is superimposed on the graph (top) so that pressure and volume changes can be related to electrical events occurring at any point. Time occurrence of heart sounds is also indicated. (b) Events of phases 1–3 of the cardiac cycle depicted in diagrammatic views of the heart

Q List the 'stages' of the cardiac cycle, and describe briefly the electrical events (as recorded by the ECG) that precede each mechanical event.

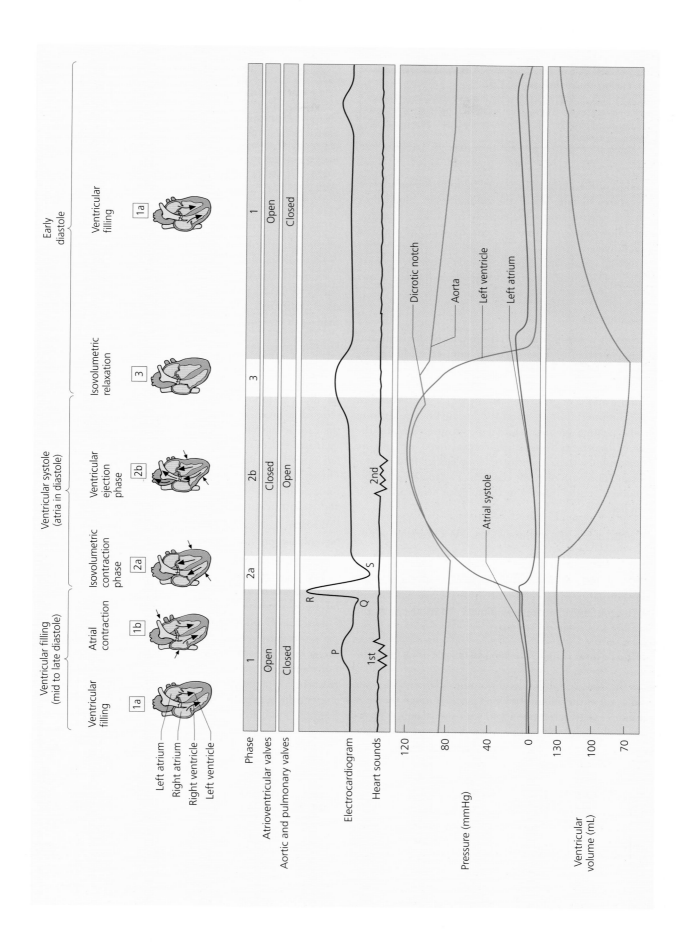

Ventricular filling
(mid to late diastole)

Ventricular systole
(atria in diastole)

Early
diastole

Left atrium
Right atrium
Right ventricle
Left ventricle

Ventricular
filling

Atrial
contraction

Isovolumetric
contraction
phase

Ventricular
ejection
phase

Isovolumetric
relaxation

Ventricular
filling

| 1a | 1b | 2a | 2b | 3 | 1a |

Phase	1	2a	2b	3	1
Atrioventricular valves	Open		Closed		Open
Aortic and pulmonary valves	Closed		Open		Closed

Electrocardiogram

P R Q S

Heart sounds

1st 2nd

Pressure (mmHg)

120
80
40
0

Dicrotic notch
Aorta
Left ventricle
Left atrium
Atrial systole

Ventricular
volume (mL)

130
100
70

ACTIVITY

Find the four heart valves in Figure 12.4, p.308.
Using Figure 12.5, (p.309), describe when these valves open and close during the passage of blood through the heart, and how they ensure that blood flows in one direction. At what point on the chest is the heartbeat palpated most readily?

BOX 12.11 CARDIAC OUTPUT CHANGES DURING PREGNANCY

Blood volume and the cardiac output at rest rise by approximately 40% during pregnancy. The most significant rise in cardiac output occurs during the first trimester. It peaks around 30 weeks, and is maintained for the rest of the pregnancy. The extra demands are due to mum having an additional organ to perfuse, namely the placenta. The rising levels of oestrogen and progesterone in pregnancy also contribute to the increase in cardiac output as they cause a fall in peripheral vascular resistance

is the period of total heart relaxation (diastole). There are two salient features to note about the cardiac cycle: blood flow through the heart is controlled entirely by pressure changes, and blood flows along pressure gradients through the available opening, provided by the valves. These pressure changes reflect the alternating systolic and diastolic periods, cause the opening and closing of the heart valves, and keep blood flowing in one direction.

Cardiodynamics

Cardiodynamics investigates the movements of the heart and the forces generated by cardiac contraction. In so doing, the components can be identified that comprise the cardiac output. This is the quantity of blood ejected by the left ventricle each minute and is of great clinical interest. It is expressed in litres per minute (L/minute), and is calculated by multiplying the stroke volume (volume ejected per contraction) by the number of heartbeats (ventricular contractions) per minute (i.e. stroke volume is the quantity of blood ejected into the systemic circulation with each left ventricular systole). Generally, this volume is related directly to the force of ventricular contraction; i.e.

$$\text{Cardiac output (CO)} = \text{stroke volume (SV)} \times \text{heart rate (HR)}$$

The cardiac output, therefore, provides a useful indicator of ventricular homeostatic efficiency over a period of time. During 'normal' resting conditions, the average adult heart rate is 70 bpm, and the stroke volume is 70 mL/beat, so the cardiac output is about 5 L/minute:

$$\text{CO} = \text{SV} \times \text{HR} = 70 \times 70 = 4900 \text{ mL/minute} = 4.9 \text{ L/minute}$$

Since the average adult blood volume is about 5 L, this means that the entire volume of blood passes through the heart every minute. Cardiac output varies with the changing metabolic demands of the body, rising when the heart rate or stroke volume increases, and falling when the heart rate or stroke volume decreases. The output can increase up to 25 L/minute in a normal, fit person performing strenuous exercise, and up to 35 L/minute in a well-trained athlete; for comparison this means that the entire blood volume passes through the heart five to seven times every minute (i.e. around once every 10 seconds). The increase above the resting cardiac output is termed the cardiac reserve and is important because it enables us to meet the increased metabolic demands during periods of activity. People with severe heart disease may have little or no cardiac reserve, which limits their ability to perform even the

simple task of daily living, such as washing and dressing.

To understand how the cardiac output changes, we need to examine its contributory factors. For convenience, the regulation of the heart rate and stroke volume will be considered separately, although alterations in cardiac output usually reflect changes in both aspects of cardiac function.

Regulation of the heart rate

The resting stroke volume under healthy conditions tends to be relatively constant. However, when blood volume drops rapidly (e.g. following a haemorrhage) or when the heart is seriously weakened, as in MI, the stroke volume declines and the cardiac output and blood pressure are maintained by an increased heart rate. The SA node initiates contraction, and if left to itself would set a constant heart rate of 90–100 bpm. However, tissues require different volumes of blood flow under different conditions (e.g. stress) – neural stimulation and endocrine activity (see Figure 21.6, p.598) influence the heart rate.

Neural mechanisms

The most important extrinsic influence affecting heart rate is the autonomic nervous system. The heart is innervated from the cardiac centres in the medulla oblongata of the brainstem by both sympathetic and parasympathetic divisions (see Figure 12.11, p.321) via cardiac (or accelerator) and vagal nerves, respectively. When activated sympathetically, noradrenaline is released at its cardiac synapses (i.e. SA node, AV node and portions of the myocardium) and binds to beta-1 receptors. The sympathetic nervous system is activated when the person is exposed to physical stressors (e.g. exercise or hospital admission) and certain emotional conditions (e.g. sexual arousal, or the anxiety or fear associated with the outcome of a surgical operation). This excitatory neurotransmitter increases the heart rate and the force of myocardial contraction. The additional contraction prevents a decline of the stroke volume as would happen if only the heart rate was increased; the reduction of the diastolic period as a consequence of the more rapid rate reduces the filling of the ventricle, but by increasing the force of contraction the ventricle empties more efficiently and so maintains, or even increases, the stroke volume (ordinarily the ventricle does not actually empty during systole – an ESV remains and it is this that is drawn upon).

Conversely, the activation of the parasympathetic neurons in certain emotional conditions, such as severe depression, and/or in normal circumstances when stress thresholds are not achieved, releases acetylcholine at their cardiac synapses. Acetylcholine binds to muscarinic (alpha) receptors; it is an inhibitory neurotransmitter that hyperpolarizes the membrane of the SA cells by opening potassium channels, which stabilizes the membrane, reduces its rate of spontaneous depolarization in autorhythmic fibres, and so decreases the heart rate.

Both autonomic divisions are active under resting conditions, and so both acetylcholine and noradrenaline are normally released at the cardiac synapses. The predominant influence, however, is inhibitory (i.e. the parasympathetic nervous system via the vagus nerve exerts a 'vagal tone' or vagal brake' on the inherent rate of discharge of the SA node, which is about 100 bpm, slowing the heart rate to 70–72 bpm). With maximum stimulation by the parasympathetic division, the heart can slow to 20 or 30 bpm, or even stop momentarily. Conversely, during exercise the predominant influence is excitatory, and so sympathetic innervation dominates. With maximum sympathetic stimulation, the heart rate may reach 200 bpm in a 20-year-old. At such a high heart rate, the stroke volume is lower than at rest because of the very short filling time. The maximum heart rate declines with age. As a rule, subtracting the person's age from 220 provides a good estimate of their maximum heart rate.

The autonomic nervous system thus makes delicate adjustments in cardiovascular function to meet the demands of other systems.

The atrial reflex

The atrial (or Bainbridge) reflex involves a combination of intrinsic and neural (extrinsic) modifications of the heart rate, which consequently affect the cardiac output. Intrinsically, an increased return of venous blood to the heart, observed when lying down or during exercise, stretches the right atrial wall. This causes a greater cardiac output, because atrial stretch receptors respond by externally stimulating an increased sympathetic activity, thus causing the SA node cells to depolarize faster, and increasing the heart rate by 10–15%.

Endocrine control of the heart rate

Adrenaline and noradrenaline secreted from the medulla of the adrenal gland by its sympathetic activation mimic the cardiac effects of the excitatory neurotransmitter noradrenaline, and so quickly enhance the heart rate and the force of myocardial contraction. Exercise, stress and excitement cause the adrenal medulla to release more hormones. Endocrine secretions of the thyroid gland (thyroxine), when released in large quantities, cause a slower but more sustained rise in the heart rate; tachycardia is a sign of hyperthyroidism (excessive thyroid hormone). Endocrine secretions also enhance the cardiac effects of adrenaline and noradrenaline.

Intracellular and extracellular ionic homeostasis must be maintained for normal heart function (e.g. sodium and potassium are crucial for the production of action potentials in nerve and muscle fibres). It is therefore not surprising that ionic imbalances, as a result of hormonal actions becoming compromised, can quickly affect the pump effectiveness of the heart. In particular, the relative concentrations of potassium, calcium and sodium have a large effect on cardiac function:

- Hypernatraemia (excess blood sodium) inhibits the transport of calcium into cardiac cells, thereby reducing contractility, since calcium is the trigger for muscle contraction.
- Hyperkalaemia (excess blood potassium) lowers the resting electrical potential of the cells, bringing them closer to threshold, which may result in cardiac excitation and increased heart rate. However, large excess prevents repolarization (i.e. electrical recovery), and therefore restimulation of the membrane, leading to heart block and cardiac arrest. Hypokalaemia (insufficient blood potassium) produces a feeble heart beat thereby instigating life-threatening arrhythmia.
- A moderate increase in extracellular and intracellular calcium speeds the heart rate and strengthens the heartbeat.

Other factors that influence cardiac function are age and gender, exercise and temperature.

Age and gender

The normal resting heart rates varies throughout the lifespan (Table 12.2). The resting heart rate of an adult female is 72–80 bpm; this is higher than the resting heart rate of an adult male (64–72 bpm), reflecting gender differences in heart size and hence stroke volume.

Exercise

Sympathetic stimulation increases the heart rate during exercise. The resting heart rate of a trained athlete is, however, substantially lower (about 40–60 bpm) than in a less physically fit person, since the athlete has a well-developed myocardium that is better equipped to pump more blood per contraction (i.e. the stroke volume is increased). Similarly, the heart rate

---

BOX 12.12 DRUGS AND THE HEART RATE

Cardiovascular drugs affect the heart rate and blood pressure and hence knowledge of this is necessary when healthcare professionals are evaluating a patient's reactions to such drugs. Drugs that increase the heart rate are called positive chronotrophic drugs ('chronos-' = time). These are sympathetic agonists (i.e. mimic/stimulate sympathetic stimulation of the heart), and include drugs such as isoprenaline, adrenaline and atropine. Drugs that decrease the heart rate are called negative chronotrophic drugs. These are sympathetic antagonists (i.e. they block/reduce sympathetic stimulation of the heart) and include drugs such as the beta-blockers (e.g. propranolol). These drugs are commonly used to treat angina, thyrotoxicosis and anxiety states. Digoxin is a drug that slows (i.e. negative chronotrophic action) and strengthens the heartbeat (i.e. positive inotropic affect; see Box 12.14), and is used for cardiac irregularities such as heart murmurs (see Box 12.2, p.311).

Care must be taken not to allow the heart rate to fall below 60 bpm. Bradycardia is a sign of digoxin toxicity, and the healthcare practitioner should check the patient's heart rate before administering digoxin. Patients that have been administered this drug (especially if elderly) should be observed for coupled heartbeats, confusion and nausea.

Table 12.2 Normal resting heart rate throughout the lifespan

Developmental age	Heart rate (bpm)
Fetus (8–9 months gestation age)	140–150
Newborn	120–130
1 year	110
2–5 years	115–110
5–10 years	110–90
10 years to adult	90–60
Adult	80–50

Adapted from Whaley, L.F. and Wong, D.L. (1995) *Nursing Care of Infants and Children.* St Louis: Mosby.

BOX 12.13 SURGERY AND HYPOTHERMIC REDUCED HEART RATES

During surgical repair of certain heart abnormalities, it is helpful to slow the patient's heart rate by hypothermia, in which the person's body is deliberately cooled to a low body 'core' temperature. The hypothermia slows metabolism, which reduces the oxygen needs of the tissues, allowing the heart and brain to withstand short periods of interrupted or reduced blood flow during the surgical procedure (Clancy *et al.*, 2002).

necessary to maintain an increased cardiac output during exercise will also be lower in a trained athlete.

Temperature

A raised body temperature, as occurs during fever or strenuous exercise, increases the heart rate by causing the SA and AV nodes to discharge more frequently. Conversely, a decrease in body temperature, such as that caused by prolonged exposure to a cold environment, depresses the heart rate.

Homeostatic regulation of the stroke volume

Remember that the stroke volume is the volume of blood pumped out of the ventricles per contraction, and thus represents the difference between the end diastolic volume (EDV), which is the amount of blood that collects in a ventricle during diastole or relaxation (left ventricular EDV is about 120 mL), and the ESV, which is the amount of blood remaining in the ventricle after ventricular systole or contraction (left ventricular ESV is about 50 mL). The resting stroke volume, therefore, approximates to 70 mL:

$$SV \text{ (mL/beat)} = EDV \text{ (120 mL)} - ESV \text{ (50 mL)} = 70 \text{ mL/beat}$$

Consequently, a change in the EDV and/or the ESV will alter the stroke volume.

The end diastolic volume and the intrinsic regulation of stroke volume

The volume of blood within the ventricle at the end of diastole is also referred to as the preload, and depends upon two inter-related factors:

- The venous return (i.e. the volume of blood entering the heart, and hence the ventricles during ventricular diastole. This alters in response to changes in the cardiac output, the peripheral circulation, and other mechanisms that alter the

rate of blood flow through the vena cavae (the main veins returning blood to the heart from all body tissues).
- The filling time (i.e. the duration of ventricular diastole). This depends entirely on the heart rate. When the heart rate exceeds 160 bpm, stroke volume usually declines because of the short filling time. At such rapid heart rates, EDV is less, and the preload is lower. People who have slow resting heart rates usually have large resting stroke volumes, because filling time is prolonged and the preload is larger.

The intrinsic control of stroke volume is illustrated by the

ACTIVITY

What happens to the resting heart rate, EDV and stroke volume in a bradycardic patient?

responses of the heart to changes in venous return. If the venous return (hence venous pressure) is suddenly increased, more blood flows into the heart. Consequently, the increased EDV stretches the myocardium further. This additional stretch of the muscle fibres promotes a more forceful contraction when the myocardium is stimulated, and results in a greater volume being ejected. The 'more in – more out principle' is referred to as the Frank–Starling law of the heart. In this way, venous return changes the ventricular EDV, and hence the stroke volume, and therefore cardiac output, since:

$$\text{Cardiac output} = \text{stroke volume} - \text{heart rate}$$

Cardiac output and venous return will then remain in balance. Factors that alter the venous return are discussed later.

The end systolic volume and autonomic regulation of stroke volume

The stroke volume is also altered by autonomic-associated changes to the volume of blood left in the ventricle after systole. Sympathetic neurons, as discussed previously, release the neurotransmitter noradrenaline when activated, and stimulate the secretion of adrenaline from the adrenal glands. These chemicals have two important effects on the heart: the heart rate is increased causing shorter filling times (i.e. reduction of EDV), and the force and degree of myocardial contractility are enhanced. When stimulated, the heart ejects more blood because the ventricle empties more efficiently, thus decreasing the ESV.

The interrelationship between the EDV and ESV is particularly noticeable during exercise, when sympathetic activity is pronounced. Thus, the increased venous return and the increased contractility of the heart act to produce a large increase in stroke volume (up to about 120 mL/beat).

Reducing the ESV might be expected to reduce the EDV, as blood fills a more efficiently emptied ventricle. However, moderately increased heart rates during exercise actually cause the EDV to remain fairly normal because of the increased rate of

BOX 12.14 INOTROPIC AGENTS AND MYOCARDIAL CONTRACTILITY

Substances that increase myocardial contractility are called positive inotropic agents, whereas those that decrease contractility are called negative inotropic agents. Positive inotropic agents, such as adrenaline and noradrenaline, often promote calcium inflow during cardiac action potentials, which strengthens the force of the myocardial contraction. In addition, increased calcium levels in the extracellular fluid and the drug digitalis all have positive inotropic effects. Conversely, the inhibition of the sympathetic nervous system, via anoxia, acidosis, some anaesthetics (e.g. halothane) and increased potassium levels in the extracellular fluid, have negative inotropic effects. A class of drugs called calcium channel blockers exerts a negative inotropic effect by reducing calcium inflow, thereby decreasing the strength of the heartbeat.

BOX 12.15 CLINICAL ASSESSMENT OF THE CARDIAC OUTPUT

Cardiac output can be assessed by direct or indirect means. Indirect methods may include measuring related variables, such as the urinary output, or peripheral toe and limb temperatures, and 'capillary refill time – CRT'. CRT is more contemporary and may be more appropriate – less than 2 seconds is normal and can be measured either peripherally or centrally. These variables are used to classify the cardiac output as being high, normal or low. However, a more accurate, and repeatable measurement, such as:

- *Thermodilution*: this involves inserting a triple-lumen Swan–Ganz catheter, with a thermistor (temperature sensor) located at its tip, into a peripheral vein, and advancing it to the right atrium. A bolus of cold saline of known temperature is injected into the catheter. As the saline and right atrial blood mix, the temperature changes; this is sensed by the thermistor, which records when the bolus passes its tip. The actual temperature recorded will depend upon the time taken for the bolus to reach the thermistor and the volume of blood into which the cold saline was dispersed. The data can then be used to calculate the cardiac output.
- *Imaging*: recent technology has largely superseded thermodilution by using imaging techniques to assess the output. This methodology is non-invasive and also provides moment-to-moment evaluation of changes.

venous return that is observed. However, heart rates above moderate levels reduce filling times, and decrease the EDV. Thus, stroke volume peaks at a heart rate of approximately 175 bpm; further rises in heart rate are accompanied by a decrease in stroke volume.

ACTIVITY

Reflect on your understanding of the Frank–Starling law of the heart, and the chronotrophic and inotropic actions of drugs. Using a pharmacology textbook and/or discussing with an anaesthetist, identify some common drugs with these actions.

Afterload

Ejection of blood from the heart begins when the pressure in the right ventricle (about 8 mmHg) supersedes the diastolic pressure in the pulmonary trunk and the pressure in the left ventricle supersedes the diastolic pressure in the aorta (80 mmHg or 10.53 kPa).

At these points, the higher pressure in the ventricles causes blood to push the semilunar valves open. The pressure that must be overcome before these valves can be opened is termed the afterload. At any given preload (EDV; see above), an increase in the afterload causes stroke volume to decrease, and more blood remains in the ventricles at the end of systole. Hypertension and atherosclerosis increase the afterload. The ventricle responds by increasing the wall thickness so as to produce better contractility, but this is eventually detrimental (Box 12.16).

CIRCULATORY PHYSIOLOGY

Having read the previous sections, you should now be aware that:

- the heart is a muscular pump;
- the arteries are the conduction and distribution vessels;
- the arterioles are precapillary resistance vessels;
- the capillaries are the exchange vessels;
- the veins are the blood reservoirs and drainage vessels.

In order to understand how the supply of blood to a tissue is regulated to maintain cellular, tissue and organ system homeostatic processes, we need to consider three interrelated physical aspects of circulation: blood flow, blood pressure and peripheral resistance. The last two aspects influence the rate of blood flow. Changes in cardiac output and peripheral resistance collectively determine how blood pressure is regulated.

Blood flow

Blood flow is the quantity of blood that passes through a vessel in a given period of time. Blood circulates in the systemic and pulmonary circuits, and the rate of flow is dependent upon two factors: arterial blood pressure and the peripheral resistance (i.e. opposition to blood flow) provided by blood vessels and blood viscosity.

The flow rate of any fluid is proportional to the pressure applied to that fluid. Thus, fluid flows from high-pressure to low-pressure regions, and the greater the pressure differential, the faster the movement. Flow only continues, however, if the pressure exceeds the opposing forces of resistance. Therefore, the rate of flow is inversely proportional to the resistance since for a given pressure, i.e. the higher the resistance, the lower the flow rate:

Blood flow = blood pressure differential/resistance to flow

The nature of the vessel's lining also influences blood flow. A smooth endothelial lining is associated with an even (or lamina) flow, whereas a roughened endothelium caused by calcium, fatty deposits, or thrombus formation, etc., causes

BOX 12.16 HEART FAILURE AND CARDIOMYOPATHIES

Heart failure

The venous return and the normal myocardial pumping activity largely determine the cardiac output. If the pumping is compromised (despite a satisfactory venous return), it may result in the cardiac output not being able to meet the metabolic demands of the body. In such circumstances, the terms heart failure, cardiac failure or pump failure are used. Since the heart has two ventricular pumps, it is possible to have left heart failure (as occurs in left-sided myocardial infarction, mitral or aortic valve incompetence, aortic stenosis and systemic hypertension), and right heart failure (as occurs in pulmonary diseases). When both sides of the heart fail, the term 'congestive heart failure' is used.

In left ventricular failure, the output is less than the volume received from the right heart. The left ventricle therefore become congested with blood, causing imbalances in:

- the chambers and vessels preceding the left ventricle (i.e. an increased volume, hence pressure, occurs in the left atrium, pulmonary veins, and capillaries). The latter may cause pulmonary oedema, which compromises gaseous exchange; if severe, this can be life threatening. A back-up of blood will also cause congestion of the right ventricle;
- the vessels and tissues after the left ventricle (i.e. the decreased cardiac output reduces tissue perfusion, the severity of which is related directly to the depressed cardiac output). Renal function may be impaired, causing fluid retention, which exacerbates the cardiac congestion. Other symptoms exhibited include:
  - dyspnoea (shortness of breath or difficulty in breathing) on exertion, which is caused by low cardiac output failing to provide adequate oxygenation of the tissue cells, plus the increased venous return pooling in the pulmonary circulation, causing pulmonary oedema resulting in a decrease in gaseous exchange;
  - orthopnoea (difficulty in breathing when lying down) occurs because of the effects of the sudden increase in the venous return (which occurs when lying down) not being ejected from the left side of the heart. Blood pools in the pulmonary circulation therefore restricting vital capacity. Sitting the patient up in bed or in a chair decreases venous return because of changes in hydrostatic pressure, and can relieve the problem. This position also improves chest expansion, hence vital capacity, therefore potentially improving gaseous exchange;
  - paroxysmal nocturnal dyspnoea (difficulty in breathing during the night);
  - fatigue, owing to the lack of metabolites reaching the cells.

Correction is aimed at the underlying cause. Diamorphine (BNF, 2008) is often administered to treat left heart failure accompanied by pulmonary oedema, because of its vasodilator effects, as well as its analgesic and opiate properties. An intra-aortic balloon may also sometimes be used to treat left heart failure. This device decreases afterload, decreases preload, increases coronary arterial perfusion, and increases systemic blood pressure. The mortality rate of left heart failure, despite treatment, is 60–80% (Huether and McCance, 2006).

In right heart failure, the right ventricular output is less than the volume returned from the systemic circulation; congestion therefore occurs behind the right ventricle in the systemic venous circulation. Consequently, oedema occurs at various peripheral sites, such as the feet, ankles and wrist, and the sacrum when lying, which may predispose the patient to the formation of pressure ulcers. The liver and spleen become distended, thus compromising their functions. Most commonly, right-sided heart failure occurs as a result of left-sided heart failure, because of the increased back pressure in the pulmonary circulation.

Correction therefore begins with treatment of the underlying left heart failure or pulmonary disease. The goal is to reduce pulmonary hypertension and increase oxygen arterial content. Thus, oxygen is administered continuously. Diuretics (e.g. furosemide) in conjunction with restricted water and sodium intake decrease venous blood volume (preload). Myocardial contractility is increased with digoxin. Bed rest reduces myocardial oxygen demand, and promotes diuresis by increasing renal perfusion.

Short-term homeostatic control mechanisms compensate in acute heart failure. Long-term homeostatic controls compensate in chronic heart failure. Acute failure, as occurs in myocardial infarction, means that the damaged ventricular myocardium cannot pump out its returning blood, leading to decreased cardiac output, heart congestion and an increased right atrial pressure.

The decreased cardiac output induces a decreased arterial pressure, which stimulates the baroreceptor reflex and promotes appropriate vasomotor sympathetic activity (see main text). This precipitates an increased myocardial contractility and vessel vasoconstriction, which improves the arterial pressure, but makes more demands on the damaged ventricle. Increased venous return further increases atrial pressure, which increases the ventricular end diastolic volumes and thus the force of contraction (Frank–Starling effect). In addition, sympathetic activity redistributes blood flow away from non-essential organs (e.g. guts, kidney and skin) to vital organs (brain and heart).

In chronic heart failure, another compensatory mechanism occurs (i.e. oedema at the expense of plasma volume), which further decreasing the cardiac output.

The renin–angiotensin system, sympathetic activity and the secretion of aldosterone and antidiuretic hormone are activated by the reduced blood pressure (see main text). Such responses provoke the compensated heart failure mechanisms (i.e. by increasing blood volume, increasing venous return and increasing the force of contraction – Frank–Starling effect), all of which aid the restoration of the cardiac output. In severe failure, these mechanisms can increase blood volume so much that the myocardium is pushed beyond its physiological parameters of contraction, resulting in ventricular congestion, and consequently an enlarged heart. A vicious circle of positive feedback ensues, which, if not corrected, eventually results in death. This is known as decompensated heart failure.

Correction involves the administration of drugs such as cardiac glycosides (e.g. digitalis) that increase the force of ventricular contraction, thus improving its emptying, thereby increasing cardiac output and improving renal function (Hood et al. 2001). In addition, they decrease the heart rate, which extends the diastolic period, thus increasing myocardial oxygen supply (recall that, unlike other tissues, coronary blood flow is higher during diastole than during systole, when myocardial vessels may be crushed by the contraction).

Cardiomyopathies

Cardiomyopathy is a degenerative condition of myocardial cells, whereby the myocardium becomes thin and weak, the ventricles enlarge, and the muscle tone becomes incapable of maintaining an adequate cardiac output; consequently heart failure results. Cardiomyopathies occur frequently secondary to other imbalances, such as chronic alcoholism, coronary arterial disease, pathogenic infections and multiple sclerosis. They also occur as primary imbalances, as there are several inherited forms of the condition. Correction is aimed at removing the underlying primary causal factor (e.g. avoiding alcohol in alcoholic cardiomyopathy). However, this is not always possible, as in the inherited cases, when correction necessitates a heart transplant.

irregular (or turbulent) flow. Laminar flow is silent, whereas turbulent flow may be heard using a stethoscope.

Initial pressure regulation occurs within the tissues themselves, since blood flow through capillaries is under local autoregulatory control (i.e. if peripheral tissues become ischaemic, then local arteries and precapillary sphincters dilate and so increase blood flow and oxygen availability). The central nervous system ischaemic response is of particular note. It occurs immediately to minimize the period of cerebral ischaemia, as brain cells can be damaged irreversibly if deprived of oxygen for only a few minutes. Cells respond to ischaemic conditions by releasing carbon dioxide, lactic acid, adenosine, potassium and hydrogen ions, and other metabolites. These substances are responsible for the dilation of blood vessels. Consequently, the increased blood flow to the tissues aids restoration of oxygen levels to within the homeostatic range. This intrinsic mechanism is important for meeting the nutritional demands of active tissues, such as muscle, in times of strenuous exercise.

Blood pressure

Blood circulates because the heart pump establishes a pressure gradient. Blood pressure is determined largely by the hydrostatic (water) pressure exerted by the blood on the walls of blood vessels. The highest average pressure, created by the left ventricular pump, is observed in the aortic arch before its coronary branches, where it is about 95 mmHg (12.5 kPa); the lowest average pressure is at the junction of the superior and inferior

vena cavae, where it is about 3–5 mmHg (0.39–0.66 kPa). The average pressure is most important, since the left ventricle pumps blood in a pulsating manner and tissue flow generally varies accordingly. The systemic arterial pressure in a resting young adult moves between about 120 mmHg and 80 mmHg (15.79 kPa and 10.53 kPa). The higher value is observed following ejection of blood from the left ventricle during systole, and is therefore called the systolic pressure. The lower value is that observed at the end of diastole, and is therefore called the diastolic pressure. Figure 12.21 illustrates how blood pressure declines unevenly throughout the cardiovascular system: the difference between the blood pressure at the base of the aortic arch and the right atrium represents the maximum driving force for the circulation (i.e. the circulatory pressure). Bearing in mind the relatively small pressures of the venous system, arterial pressure approximates to the circulatory pressure and so is most widely assessed in practice. Unless stated otherwise, the term 'blood pressure' refers to the pressure in the large arteries.

Peripheral resistance

Resistance refers to the impedance (or opposition) to blood flow created by the amount of friction the blood encounters as it passes through the vessels. The term 'peripheral resistance' is

---

ACTIVITY

Suggest why the maintenance of arterial blood pressure is so important to intracellular homeostasis.

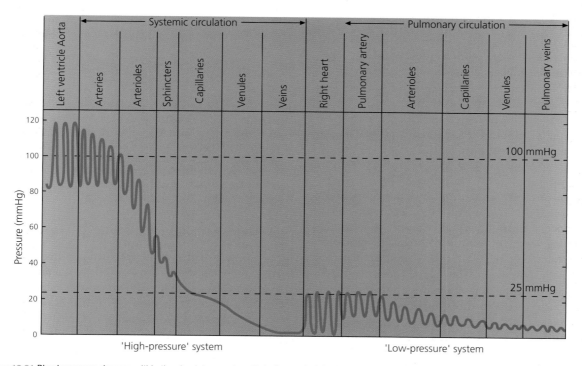

Figure 12.21 Blood pressure changes within the circulatory system. Note the gradual decline in circulatory pressures within the systemic circuit, and the elimination of the pulse pressure oscillations in the arterioles

Q *Which blood vessels are known as (1) the distributing vessels, (2) the precapillary resistance vessels, (2) the exchange vessels and (4) the capacitance vessels?*

BOX 12.17 OBESITY AND HIGH BLOOD PRESSURE

High blood pressure (hypertension) and obesity frequently coexist, both conditions attracting considerable morbidity. In dealing with a hypertensive patient whom the health carer considers overweight, it is important to establish whether the patient is aware that they are overweight, and whether the patient understands the types of problems that they be associated with this (see the case study on obesity, Section VI, p.636). Current evidence suggests that it is fat within the abdomen that is most significant as it produces factors such as renin that affect blood pressure. There is, therefore, a debate whether the measurement of abdominal body fat (rather than the body mass index) provides a more accurate indicator of obesity, for example by measuring waist circumference or the saggital (cross-sectional) abdominal diameter. Behavioural change is an extremely difficult undertaking, and patients need to be ready to change before advice is likely to be heeded. Once a patient is at this stage, having a strategy to assist weight loss is more likely to see an effective outcome (Holmwood, 2000).

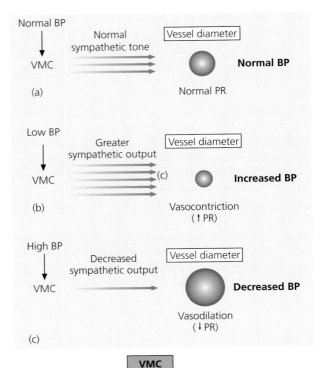

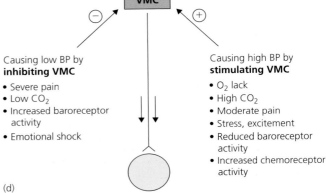

Figure 12.22 Vasomotor centre control of blood pressure via changing the peripheral resistance of arterioles. (a) Normal blood pressure (i.e. within homeostatic range). (b) Low blood pressure (i.e. below homeostatic range) results in vasoconstriction to increase the blood pressure. (c) High blood pressure (i.e. above homeostatic range) results in vasodilation to decrease the blood pressure. (d) Factors affecting a vasomotor centre. BP, blood pressure; PR, peripheral resistance; VMC, vasomotor centre

generally used, since most friction is encountered in the small vessels of the peripheral circulation. Resistance is related to blood viscosity, the length of the blood vessels, and the diameter of the blood vessels.

The viscosity (thickness) of blood depends mostly on the ratio of red blood cells to plasma (fluid) volume, and to a smaller extent on the concentration of plasma proteins. The relationship between vessel length and resistance is simple: the longer the vessel, the greater the resistance. In a healthy person, the viscosity and length of vessels normally remains unchanged, and thus may be considered as constant variables. Arterial blood pressure is then dependent primarily on the diameter of blood vessels. Homeostatic imbalances, such as polycythaemia, dehydration and hyperproteinaemia, increase blood viscosity, resistance and hence pressure. Imbalances such as anaemia, haemorrhage and hypoproteinaemias decrease blood viscosity, resistance and blood pressure.

In health, changes in the diameter of blood vessels provide the main means of varying peripheral resistance. The relationship between the diameter of blood vessels and resistance is also simple: the smaller the diameter, the greater the resistance to blood flow.

Normally, the peripheral resistance primarily reflects the resistance due to arterioles (i.e. located between the large arteries and capillary beds), in particular their diameter, and is influenced by neural and hormonal mechanisms, although tissues have varying degrees of intrinsic control. The vasomotor centre of the brainstem's medulla regulates arteriolar diameter via its sympathetic innervation. The normal background level of vasomotor activity sets the vasomotor or sympathetic tone of arterioles, which determines the peripheral resistance under resting conditions (Figure 12.22a). Thus, greater vasomotor sympathetic outflow increases the resistance due to arteriolar vasoconstriction (Figure 12.22b), and reduction in sympathetic output decreases the peripheral resistance by inducing vasodilatation (Figure 12.22c). Factors affecting vasomotor activity are discussed later in this chapter.

'Normal' blood pressure

There is no such value as a normal blood pressure reading for the population as a whole. However, there is a normal value for any particular individual, but even that value will vary according to the different metabolic demands of night and day activities (i.e. circadian rhythms), and the developmental age. Multiple factors have an influence on blood pressure, and it is not surprising that people have significantly different but 'normal' blood pressure values. Thus, it is usual to refer to a 'normal range' of blood pressure rather than to a single value.

Table 12.3 Average blood pressures associated with developmental age

Age (years)	Systolic pressure (mm Hg)	Diastolic pressure (mm Hg)
Newborn	80	45
10	105	70
20	120	80
40	125	85
60	135	88

BOX 12.18 BLOOD PRESSURE IN CHILDREN

The systolic blood pressure rises with age, averaging approximately 90 mmHg at 1 year of age to approximately 105 mmHg at 10 years. (Please note: variation occurs because of differing growth rates and sizes.) It is important that the healthcare practitioner when taking a child's blood pressure uses the right size cuff for their age (e.g. neonate, 2–5 cm cuff width; infant of 1–4 years, 6 cm cuff width; children 4–8 years, 9 cm cuff width). The wrong size cuff will result in inaccurate results.

Common parameters affecting blood pressure include:

- *Age*: there is a direct relationship between advancing years and increasing blood pressure (Table 12.3).
- *Gender*: the average blood pressure of a 20-year old adult male is expressed as 120/80 mmHg. Female values are slightly less, because women generally have lower blood pressures than men.
- *Race*: in Western societies, blood pressure values tend to increase with advancing years; a contributory factor to this is the high levels of fat in the diet. This is not universal (e.g.

South Sea Islanders show little, if any, increase in the mean blood pressure with increasing age). The elevation in blood pressure with age may be related to genetic and/or environmental factors, and is likely to be a result of arteriosclerosis (see Box 12.8, p.323).

ACTIVITY

Suggest why, in general, there are gender differences associated with blood pressure.

Pulse and pulse pressure

Pulses

The alternate expansion and elastic recoil of an artery with each left ventricular systole is called the pulse and may be felt where the artery lies superficially, and over a bony or firm surface, and so can be palpated; the pulse rate is equivalent to the heart rate. Pulses are taken by the observer's middle three fingers (not the thumb because the observer's own pulse can be palpated there) at pulse sites. The strongest pulse is in the arteries closest to the heart. It weakens progressively as it passes through the arterial tree, disappearing altogether within the capillary networks.

The most common and accurate pulse under normal circumstances to be examined is the radial pulse. However, accuracy diminishes when the blood pressure drops too low or the

BOX 12.19 TAKING BLOOD PRESSURE

The measurement of blood pressure is routinely undertaken in adults, and is advocated in children aged 8 years and over, as part of a cardiovascular assessment. The frequency of the recording will depend upon the patient's condition, the reason for admission, and the result of the reading. It is therefore essential that the technique is performed accurately, on the same arm each time, and that the patient is prepared before the procedure. Ideally, the patient will not have been exerted or smoked in the preceding 30 minutes, since these activities increase the reading. The patient must also be relaxed, since anxiety causes an increase in the blood pressure. Ideally, the patient should be allowed to settle into their new environment for at least 30 minutes before the procedure. In an emergency admission, this is inappropriate, and the blood pressure result will frequently be required as soon as possible, and perhaps dictate the patient's treatment.

The patient should be seated comfortably, or lying if they are unable to sit, with the arm supported on a pillow at a level of the heart. Tight clothing should be removed. Arterial pressure is measured using a sphygmomanometer (Figure 12.23). This involves putting an appropriately sized inflatable cuff around the (usually) left upper arm to record blood pressure in the brachial artery (opposite the heart; the pressure measurement is taken to be a measure of aortic pressure). Measurement may be manual or electronic.

Manual measurement
A stethoscope is placed over the artery distal to the cuff. The cuff is inflated until a pressure is reached that exceeds the systolic value for the person's age, level of fitness, etc. (i.e. the pressure should be enough to

compress completely the brachial artery and thus stop blood flow). The radial and brachial artery can be palpated as the cuff is inflated. The observer should be at eye level with the mercury manometer, and the stethoscope placed over the brachial artery (just below the cuff). When the pulse disappears, the cuff is inflated a further 30 mmHg (3.95 kPa). This will be sufficient to ascertain the systolic pressure, which may require cuff inflation to only 150 mmHg.

The cuff is released slowly while listening for audible sounds that indicate flow of blood through the artery and the systolic and diastolic pressures. Upon deflating, the first (Korotkoff) sound is heard through the stethoscope. This 'tapping' sound is sharp and clear, and results from the movement of blood through the no longer occluded vessel. The mercury column reading at this point corresponds to the systolic blood pressure (i.e. the force at which blood is pumped against the walls during left ventricular contraction). As the cuff pressure falls further, the sound changes to a 'blowing' or 'swishing' noise, then suddenly becomes muffled and faint. It then disappears, as blood movement beyond the previously sealed vessel is no longer impeded. The muffling point estimates the diastolic pressure (i.e. the force of blood in arteries during ventricular diastole) but if difficult to ascertain then the disappearance point is used.

Electronic measurement
Electronic equipment (e.g. Dynamap) is now used much more commonly than mercury sphygmomanometers in a large number of clinical settings. However, not all Health Authorities are contemporary. In addition, there is still a place for manual methods with some patients, for example, those with irregular heartbeats.

(a)

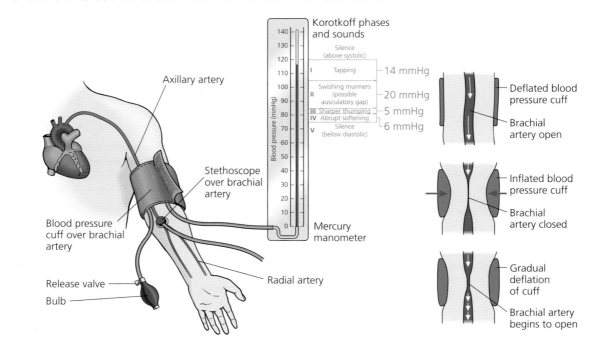

Korotkoff phases and sounds

	Silence (above systolic)	
I	Tapping	14 mmHg
II	Swishing murmers (possible ausculatory gap)	20 mmHg
III	Sharper thumping	5 mmHg
IV	Abrupt softening	6 mmHg
V	Silence (below diastolic)	

Axillary artery

Stethoscope over brachial artery

Blood pressure cuff over brachial artery

Release valve

Bulb

Radial artery

Mercury manometer

Deflated blood pressure cuff

Brachial artery open

Inflated blood pressure cuff

Brachial artery closed

Gradual deflation of cuff

Brachial artery begins to open

Figure 12.23 (a) Conditions employed in measuring blood pressure. Equipment: correct-sized cuff; manometer on level surface; stethoscope beneath the cuff. Patient sitting/lying comfortably with arm supported by pillow. Healthcare professional at eye level with the manometre. (b) Common blood pressure measurement errors

Q *What is the equivalent in kPa of 150 mm Hg? (Use the conversion rate mentioned earlier in this chapter.)*

(b) Blood pressure measurement inaccuracies

Artificial high reading	**Artificial low reading**
• Artery below heart level • Cuff too short/too narrow • Overinflation of cuff/deflation too slow • Reinflation without rest • Tight clothing on upper arm	• Artery above heart level • Cuff too long • Deflation too fast

arm is obese, which then makes feeling (palpation) of the pulse more difficult.

In adults and infants over the age of 2 years, other areas (Figure 12.24) include:

- The temporal pulse is located on each side of the head just in front of the upper margin of the ears.
- The carotid (neck) pulse is used in cardiopulmonary resuscitation and is located in the soft tissue on each side of the larynx. Using this site on conscious patients may sometimes be necessary (for example, when the radial pulse is obscure); however, its use must be explained to the patient so they will not be worried. The carotid pulse must be felt with only gentle pressure, since the carotid arteries supply to the brain and therefore their blood flow rate must not be hindered.
- The apical (apex of the heart) pulse measurements is an alternative to the radial pulse to record the number of left ventricle contractions per minute. The observer listens through the chest wall with a stethoscope to the heart itself, counting the sounds per minute. The apex beat is located by placing the diaphragm of a stethoscope over the space between the left fifth and sixth ribs close to the mid-clavicular line. The apical pulse is advocated in children from birth to 24 months because during this period, the

pulse rate is quite viable and can be influenced considerably by crying, activity and feeding. The apical pulse rate is also used in the assessment of adults with irregular heart rates and/or where measurements are pulse deficit is required.
- The brachial (arm) pulse is felt against the humerus, along the inner aspect of the upper arm, beneath the brachial muscle.
- The femoral pulse, used when embarrassment of the patient is not an issue (e.g. cardiac procedures), is felt approximately halfway across the groin.
- The pedal pulses are important for assessing blood supply to the leg and foot and should be used in any limb vascular disease and during surgery if the patient has been using support bandages or splintage materials.
- Other pulses include the popliteal (behind the knee) pulse, the posterior tibial pulse, and dorsalis pedis pulse (in the foot).

The first pulse usually to be examined is the right radial pulse. If appropriate, the timing of the left radial and femoral pulses may then be compared with that of the right radial pulse as this provides information on the comparative health of vessels in the arterial system. Delayed pulsation normally occurs because of a proximal stenosis somewhere, particularly of the aorta (called coarctation).

hyperthyroidism and excessive catecholamines. It is also a compensatory mechanism for improving the tissue blood supply when a patient is in shock. Bradycardia occurs when the impulse from the heart's pacemaker (i.e. SA node) does not always reach the ventricles (as in heart block) and the ventricular contraction rate slows down. Causes of bradycardia include hypothermia, hypothyroidism, raised intracranial pressure, acute ischaemia and infarction of the sinus node, chronic degenerative changes (e.g. fibrosis) of the atrium and sinus node, and in response to drug therapy with beta-blockers, digitalis and other anti-arrhythmic drugs. Extreme bradycardia and tachycardia result in inadequate filling of coronary arteries, which can lead to myocardial starvation and infarction. A lack of oxygen to the brain initially leads to confusion and disorientation, and can give rise to brain damage.

The normal maximum heart rate (above which normal filling of the heart can not take place) is about 175 bpm. At this maximum the cardiac cycle is reduced to 0.33 seconds (normal = 0.8 seconds). The systolic (contraction) period is 0.2 seconds and diastolic (relaxation) periods 0.13 seconds. To attain an adequate filling during diastole requires a minimum diastolic phase of about 0.12 seconds, therefore a heart rate of above 180 bpm would reduce the diastolic phase below this minimum and the cardiac output would be decreased.

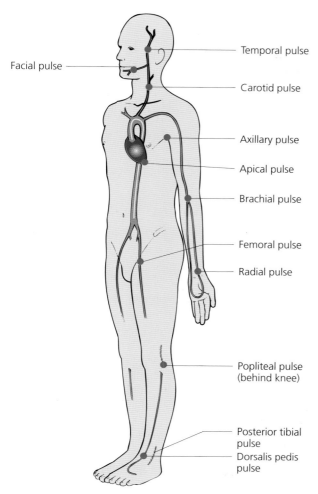

Figure 12.24 Pulse points. Each pulse point is named after the artery with which it is associated

Q Explain what causes a pulse in an artery.

ACTIVITY

What terms are used to denote an abnormally fast heart rate and an abnormally slow heart rate? Name a class of drugs that is used to decrease the heart rate.

When assessing a person's pulse, three factors should be observed: rate, strength and rhythm.

Rate

The pulse rate is calculated most accurately by counting the beats felt within 60 seconds. Pulse rates may vary as a result of age, level of fitness, posture, temperature, stage within the perioperative period or change in health status.

The resting pulse rate should be between 60 and 80 bpm, when an adult patient is lying quietly in bed. The pulse rate equates to the heart rate and so is raised during exercise, fear and excitement. The accurate recording and reporting of an abnormally fast or slow heart rate is essential. It will often indicate a sudden change in a person's condition that needs to be assessed and possibly treated. Tachycardia is a fast pulse rate of 100 bpm or more and a bradycardia is a lower rate, usually below 50 bpm. Tachycardia occurs during systemic infections, exercise, fever, emotion, pregnancy, anaemia, cardiac failure,

Strength

The strength or volume of the pulse is important because it can give an indication of heart function, cardiac output and probable blood pressure. The strength of the pulse relies upon the force of left ventricle contraction and the stroke volume. There is a clear relationship between palpable pulse sites and systolic blood pressures, e.g. the radial pulse is greater than 80 mmHg (10.6 kPa), the femoral is greater than 70 mmHg (9.3 kPa), and the carotid is greater than 60 mmHg (8.0 kPa). A weak pulse is indicative of poor stroke volume (Box 12.21), or perhaps blood vessel occlusion through arteriosclerosis proximal to the pulse site.

Rhythm

The rhythm of the pulse is the pattern in which the beats occur. In healthy people, the pattern is regular because the chambers of the heart are contracted in a coordinated manner. An irregular pulse may suggest an underlying disorder (Box 12.21).

Some healthcare professionals use the brachial or temporal pulse with the younger child (particularly if they are uncooperative) since they are more accurate. For the older cooperative child the radial pulses are used. Measuring the carotid pulse in

BOX 12.20 PULSE RATES IN CHILDREN

In children, their pulse is regular; there is a slight acceleration during the inspiration and a slight deceleration during expiration. This is due to the effect of breathing movements on venous return and the effect usually disappears in adults though it can persist. It is not considered an important deviation.

The cardiovascular system in children must adapt to its changing metabolism and the increased demands placed on it as a result of growth of all parts of the body. In children a pulse range falls gradually from between 110 and 160 bpm at less than 1 year of age to 60–100 bpm in children older than 12 years.

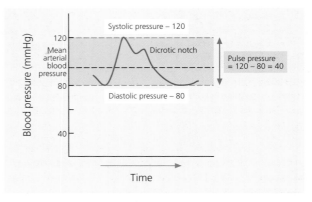

Figure 12.25 Arterial blood pressure: systolic, diastolic and pulse pressures

Q *What are the primary determinants of blood pressure?*

children is not acceptable because it carries a specific risk of reducing the blood supply to the brain, and should not therefore be used in children of any age (Box 12.24, p.347).

Fast heart rates can be caused by a complication of congenital heart defects or by heart failure (see Boxes 12.3, p.311 and 12.16, p.338, respectively).

Pulse and mean pressures

The pulse rate should not be confused with the pulse pressure, which comprises the difference between systolic and diastolic pressures; in a young adult male, this approximates to 40 mmHg (5.26 kPa) (Figure 12.25). The pulse pressure provides information about the condition of blood vessels. Homeostatic imbalances, such as arteriosclerosis (hardening of the vessels) and patent ductus arteriosus (a vessel in the fetus), record higher pulse pressures.

The mean arterial pressure lies between the systolic and diastolic values (Figure 12.25), and is calculated by adding one-third of the pulse pressure to the diastolic pressure. Both the mean arterial and pulse pressure values become smaller with increasing distance from the heart. The former decreases because of the friction that blood encounters within blood vessels, the latter because vessels become less elastic. The pressure

oscillations disappear in the arterioles (see Figure 12.21, p.339), but arteriolar vessels containing precapillary sphincters cause the mean pressure to remain steady at about 25–30 mmHg (3.29–3.95 kPa). As blood passes through the capillary beds, the pressure falls from 25–30 mmHg (3.3–4.0 kPa) at their arterial side to 15–18 mmHg (1.97–2.37 kPa) at their venous side. The decline aids capillary exchange of plasma constituents with tissue fluid (see later).

Venous pressure

Whereas arterial pressure determines the rate of blood flow to tissues, venous pressure influences venous return to the heart, which in turn is an important determinant of the cardiac out-

ACTIVITY

Identify the common locations where the pulse point is felt most easily.

BOX 12.21 PULSE IRREGULARITY

Most individuals experience an occasional irregularity perceived as a 'missed pulse' or 'dropped beat'. This is often the result of occasional ventricular ectopic (an 'extra beat', followed by a compensatory pause). Palpitations (heartbeats felt by the patient on the chest wall) are often normal, as occurs during extreme exercise or occasional extra heartbeats; however, they may also be associated with arrhythmias. Incidences should be reported but might not be treated. A regularly occurring irregularity may be detected as a cyclical event that could be the result of a heart block. Otherwise, an irregular pulse rate may be the result of atrial fibrillation (see Box 12.6, p.319), the most common irregular cardiac rhythm. It occurs in 2–4% of the adult population over the age of 60 years.

Pulse strength reflects a change in systolic blood pressure, as a consequence of altered stroke volume.

- The force of contraction will decrease in diseases such as left heart failure, since the heart muscle is unable to achieve the full stroke volume. A surplus of blood may be retained inside the heart at the end of each

ventricular systolic period. Therefore, the output is reduced to the arteries (the forward problem) and a backlog of blood unable to enter the ventricles because they are already partly filled and hence can only accept a smaller volume of blood from the veins (the backward problem).
- The stroke volume also decreases in hypovolaemic shock, where the circulating blood volume is less than normal as a consequence of bleeding. A weak, fast pulse is feature of shock, dehydration and exhaustion: weak (often described as a 'thready' pulse) because of low stroke volume and fast because the heart tries to compensate by pumping faster, which is part of the sympathetic response. In such cases, it may be necessary to feel the carotid or femoral pulse.
- Hyperthyroidism and heart block can increase the force of contraction.

Cardiac arrest should not be diagnosed simply because a radial pulse cannot be felt. In contrast, patients with infection, stress or anaemia, or after exercise, may have a very strong, 'bounding' pulse. An inconsistent pulse pressure within each beat may indicate Corrigan's (or 'water hammer') pulse, found in children with aortic valve incompetence.

BOX 12.22 JUGULAR VENOUS PRESSURE AND CENTRAL VENOUS PRESSURE

Observation of the jugular vein in the neck gives a crude indication of the venous pressure; for example raised jugular venous pressure (JVP) may indicate venous congestion secondary to cardiac failure. The central venous pressure (CVP) is the most frequently monitored venous pressure. This is the pressure in the central veins (the superior and inferior vena cavae) as they enter the heart. As the tip of the catheter used to measure CVP lies in the right atria, CVP is equivalent to right atrial pressure. The catheter is radio-opaque, and its position is confirmed by a chest X-ray. If the tricuspid valve is normal, the CVP equals the end diastolic pressure in the right ventricle and, as such, is an index of right ventricular function. Impaired right ventricular function would lead to a back pressure that would raise the pressure in the atrium and hence give a higher CVP reading.

The volume of blood returning to the heart (venous return) is the other major determinant of the CVP. Changes in circulatory fluid volume and the venomotor tone will alter the venous return: an increase in a circulatory fluid volume or venomotor tone will increase the venous return and give a higher CVP reading, and vice versa. One of the major clinical advantages of measuring CVP is that it monitors the circulating blood volume, so it is used to manage fluid replacement therapy in hypovolaemia, which may occur after burns, haemorrhage or surgery. Sequential measurements give an indication of adequate fluid replacement therapy and help prevent fluid overload.

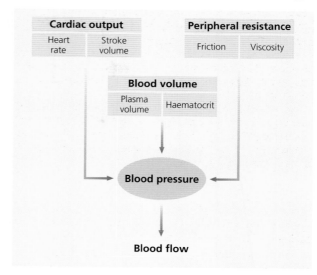

Figure 12.26 Factors influencing blood pressure and blood flow

Q What are the contributory factors of the cardiac output?

Q How does the heart rate affect the cardiac output?

put. Venous blood pressure is less than one-tenth of arterial pressure. When a person is standing up, the venous pressure must overcome gravitational forces so that blood returns and flows within the inferior vena cava. This is made possible with the aid of three factors: valves, muscular pumps produced by muscle contraction in the limbs, and thoracoabdominal pumps, produced by pressure reductions in the thorax and pressure changes in the abdomen during breathing movements.

In exercise, the combined function of these factors is to increase venous return to its maximum, so as to enable an increase in cardiac output to a level required for the continuance of the exercise.

Homeostatic control of arterial blood pressure

Although variations in blood viscosity may affect blood pressure, such variations are not normally observed. The three principal factors influencing blood pressure are the cardiac output, the peripheral resistance, and the blood volume (Figure 12.26). The factors are related by the equation:

$$\text{Blood pressure} = \text{cardiac output} \times \text{total peripheral resistance}$$

Cardiac output

Cardiac output is the volume of blood ejected into the aorta each minute. Blood pressure varies directly with cardiac output (i.e. an increase in cardiac output increases blood pressure, and vice versa). Recall that:

* cardiac output = stroke volume × heart rate, so changes in either will alter blood pressure;

* cardiac output is regulated partly by the cardiac accelerator and inhibitory centres of the brainstem's medulla via sympathetic and parasympathetic output, respectively (see earlier, p.334);
* hormones (e.g. adrenaline, thyroxine), ions (e.g. potassium, sodium, calcium), physical and emotional factors (e.g. depression), temperature, gender and age all affect the heart rate, the heart's force of contraction (stroke volume) and, therefore, cardiac output (see earlier).

Peripheral resistance

Peripheral resistance in a normal healthy person is the major opposition to blood flow through peripheral vessels, and is determined largely by the diameter of the vessels. Peripheral resistance is regulated by the activity of the sympathetic nervous system, which promotes constriction and dilation of arterioles (see Figure 12.22, p.340), or by the release of vasoconstrictor hormones.

Blood volume

Blood pressure varies directly with blood volume.

BOX 12.23 IMBALANCES OF BLOOD VOLUME AND BLOOD PRESSURE

The average volume of blood in a human body is 5 L. Homeostatic imbalances, such as haemorrhage, may decrease blood pressure by excessively decreasing the blood volume. Conversely, imbalances such as sodium retention induced by aldosteronism (excess of the hormone aldosterone) increase blood pressure by promoting water retention thereby increasing blood volume, and hence return of blood to the heart. Accompanying the larger volume of blood is a greater stretch on the arterial wall, which in turn increases the elastic recoil, which contributes to the higher blood pressure.

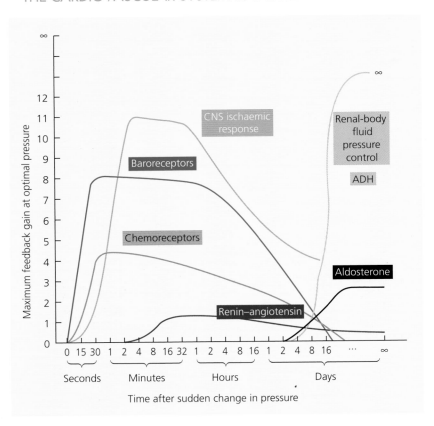

Figure 12.27 Arterial pressure control mechanisms at different times after the onset of an arterial pressure imbalance. Green boxes, short-term controls; blue boxes, long-term controls

Q How do angiotensin-converting enzyme (ACE) inhibitors affect blood pressure? Using the BNF or a pharmacology textbook, name three commonly used ACE inhibitors

The interrelationships between cardiac output, peripheral resistance and blood volume determine cardiovascular functioning, and their control stabilizes blood pressure to within its homeostatic parameters at rest and during exercise, when these parameters are modified to increase blood pressure to its altered homeostatic set points. To maintain cellular homeostasis, blood pressure must be regulated tightly, since pressure changes (especially a decrease) influence the transport of metabolites and waste products of metabolism to and from cells.

Figure 12.27 illustrates a number of short-term and long-term homeostatic regulators of blood pressure. As discussed in Chapter 1, p.13, short-term controls act to restore homeostatic equilibrium quickly. If they fail, long-term controls must respond and if these fail to redress homeostasis then illness occurs. Blood pressure controls are important in preventing its inappropriate elevation (hypertension), which can cause mechanical damage to vessels of the heart, brain and kidneys, or its reduction (hypotension), which can cause inadequate blood supply or ischaemia, and hence lead to necrotic changes to tissues. Short-term controls are neural responses; these adjust cardiac output and peripheral resistance to stabilize blood pressure and hence tissue blood flow. Various vasoconstrictor hormones support this action, but their effects are slower to be initiated. Long-term controls change the blood volume, which alters the cardiac output and hence blood pressure. These regulators are mainly hormonal responses, which

again highlights the distinction between these two coordination systems: the nervous system responds and acts immediately to homeostatic imbalances, while the endocrine system is comparatively slower to respond and its courses of action are of a longer duration.

Short-term homeostatic control of blood pressure

Neural mechanisms provide the immediate responses to changes in blood pressure (and blood gas concentration). This immediacy prevents fainting from an inadequate blood supply to the brain, for example when a person stands upright very quickly (gravity causes a pooling of blood below the heart on standing, which reduces the cardiac output).

Reductions in cardiac output (including those imbalances that decrease blood volume) promote vasoconstriction of blood vessels, except those of the heart and brain, which can be considered a homeostatic adaptive mechanism that maintains blood flow to these vital organs. In these instances, blood pressure is controlled especially by sympathetic activity, which is stimulated by afferent information from stretch receptors (baroreceptors) within the circulatory system and/or chemoreceptors of vessels or higher centres in the brain. Chemoreceptors detect changes in blood gas composition (oxygen, carbon dioxide) or blood pH (concentration of hydrogen ions). These reflexes are mediated by the brainstem's medulla vasomotor centre, and act to control arteriolar diameter (Figure 12.28).

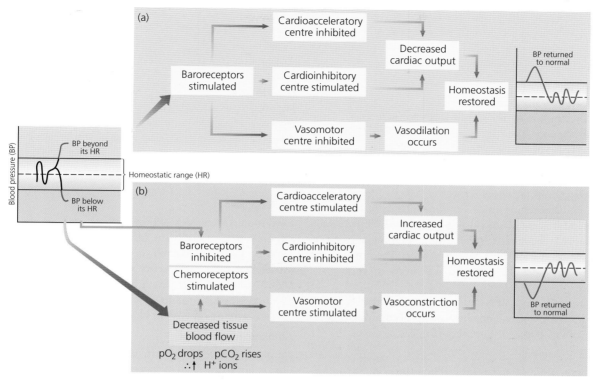

Figure 12.28 Reflexes that assist in the regulation of blood pressure. (a) The baroreceptor reflexes. (b) The chemoreceptor and baroreceptor reflexes. BP, blood pressure

Q Which division of the autonomic nervous system causes an increased blood pressure?

Baroreceptor reflexes

Baroreceptors are specialized mechanoreceptors that respond to systemic blood pressure changes. Arterial baroreceptors are located mainly in the aortic sinus, carotid sinus, and within the large arteries of the neck and thorax; they therefore monitor blood pressure at the beginning of the systemic circuit. Atrial baroreceptors monitor blood pressure at the end of this circuit. The atrial reflex differs from the aortic and carotid reflexes in that they monitor stretch within the heart rather than in blood vessels. For example, an increase in right atrial blood pressure means that blood is arriving faster than it is being pumped out of the ventricle. Atrial baroreceptors respond by stimulating the cardiac accelerator centre, which increases the cardiac output, which in turn removes the potential congestion in the right atrium, thus returning the atrial pressure to normal. In contrast, arterial baroreceptors are high-pressure receptors. When there is an increase in systemic blood pressure, they have a number of effects. First, they stimulate the cardiac inhibitory centre and hence parasympathetic vagal nerve activity, which depresses the heart rate and so reduces cardiac output. Second, they inhibit the cardiac accelerator centre, and so reduce sympathetic activity to the heart. This makes the influence of vagal nerve activity even more effective. Finally, they inhibit vasomotor centre activity, causing peripheral vasodilation, which reduces peripheral resistance. Collectively, such responses result in a compensatory decrease in blood pressure (Figure 12.28a).

Conversely, if there is a decrease in blood pressure, then arterial baroreceptors promote the opposite response by decreasing vagal nerve activity, and promoting sympathetic activity to the heart and blood vessels, causing an increase in cardiac output and peripheral vasoconstriction. The consequence of such responses is a compensatory increase in blood pressure (Figure 12.28b).

The central role of baroreceptors is to protect the circulation against short-term (second-to-second) changes in blood

---

BOX 12.24 CAROTID SINUS SYNCOPE AND CAROTID SINUS MASSAGE

Because of the anatomical position of the carotid sinus (i.e. close to the anterior surface of the neck), it is possible to stimulate the baroreceptors by putting external pressure on this region of the neck. Anything that stretches or puts pressure on the carotid sinus (e.g. hyperextending the head, wearing a tight collar, or carrying a heavy shoulder load) may slow the heart rate and cause carotid sinus syncope (i.e. fainting due to inappropriate stimulation of the carotid sinus baroreceptors).

Physicians sometimes use carotid sinus massage to manipulate cardiac function. This involves carefully massaging the neck over the carotid sinus to slow the heart rate. Such a technique is useful in patients with paroxysmal supraventricular tachycardia, a type of tachycardia that origins in the atria.

In chronic hypertension ('chronic' = persisting for some years), the baroreceptors seem to be reset to maintain pressure at a higher set point.

pressure, such as those that may occur with changing posture. Figure 12.27 illustrates their immediacy of response to blood pressure changes, and their ineffectiveness in protecting against sustained blood pressure changes.

Chemoreceptor reflex

Chemoreceptors are located in the aortic arch, carotid sinus (specifically known as the aortic and carotid bodies), large arteries in the neck, and the central nervous system (see Figure 14.14, p.418). They are sensitive to low levels of oxygen (especially those outside the central nervous system), and are even more sensitive to high levels of carbon dioxide (hypercapnia) and hydrogen ions (acidosis).

These imbalances are usually a consequence of low blood pressure and inadequate blood flow (Figure 12.28b). In such circumstances, chemoreceptors transmit impulses to the cardiovascular centres of the brainstem, which in turn increase blood pressure and blood flow to the heart to correct the imbalance.

The rate and depth of breathing are also increased, which facilitates gas exchange. The chemoreceptors are discussed in more detail in Chapter 14, pp.417–18.

Higher centre control

Higher brain centres, such as the cerebral cortex and hypothalamus, although not involved routinely in blood pressure regulation, can modify arterial blood pressure via the medulla centre of the brainstem in response to strong emotions. For example, during the 'fight, flight and fright' response and sexual excitement, the hypothalamus and cerebral cortex stimulate the vasomotor sympathetic reflex, bringing about vasoconstriction and an accompanying increase in arterial pressure. In addition, sympathetic stimulation causes the secretion of catecholamines (adrenaline and noradrenaline) from the adrenal medulla. These hormones mimic and prolong many of the sympathetic responses of Selye's general adaptation syndrome's alarm stage (see Chapter 21, pp.596–600), including persistent vasoconstriction and the consequential protracted increase in blood pressure.

Long-term control of blood pressure

As stated previously, some hormones, such as adrenaline and noradrenaline, act as short-term homeostatic regulators of blood pressure by influencing cardiac function and peripheral resistance. Others, such as angiotensin II, erythropoietin, aldosterone, atrial natriuretic factor or peptide (ANF; also known as atrial natriuretic peptide, ANP), antidiuretic hormone (ADH) and cortisol are longer-term regulators, which act by influencing blood volume and/or peripheral resistance (Figures 12.28 and 12.29).

Angiotensin II

Angiotensin II, a powerful vasoconstrictor, is produced by activation of a plasma precursor, angiotensinogen, by the enzyme renin, which converts angiotensinogen to angiotensin I, and angiotensin-converting enzyme (ACE), which converts angiotensin I to angiotensin II. Renin is secreted from special-ized kidney cells that detect a fall in blood pressure or in response to vasoconstrictor activity to this area. ACE is found in the lungs, and is activated by the presence of angiotensin I. Angiotensin II also stimulates the secretion of aldosterone and ADH (see below). Aldosterone stimulates the renal retention of sodium and hence water. In addition, angiotensin stimulates the hypothalamic thirst centre, so the person seeks fluid intake. The high levels of aldosterone (and ADH) ensure that much of any sodium/water consumed will be retained, hence elevating blood volume and blood pressure (Figure 12.29a). Renin is not secreted when the blood pressure and blood volume is high.

Erythropoietin

Erythropoietin is secreted by kidney cells as an indirect response to a decrease in blood pressure, and as a direct response to a considerable decrease in the oxygen-carrying capacity of blood, as occurs when one ascends to altitude before acclimatization. Erythropoietin stimulates erythrocyte production, which results in an increased blood pressure and oxygen-carrying capacity of blood (Figure 12.29a).

Atrial natriuretic factor

An increase in venous return, as experienced when blood volume is high, causes an overstretching of the atrial wall, which stimulates the release of ANF (also known as ANP, see above). As Figure 12.29 demonstrates, this hormone decreases blood volume and blood pressure by promoting sodium and water losses via the kidneys, stimulating peripheral vasodilation, antagonizing the effects of adrenaline/noradrenaline, aldosterone and ADH, and decreasing thirst. As blood volume and pressure are restored there is less stretch and, hence, a decrease secretion of this factor – yet another example of negative feedback control.

Antidiuretic hormone

Antidiuretic hormone (ADH, vasopressin) is produced by the hypothalamus and released from the posterior pituitary in response to low blood pressure (via arterial baroreceptor stimulation) and/or an excessive increase in the osmotic concentration of plasma as a consequence of dehydration (via hypothalamic osmoreceptors). The hormone causes intense vasoconstriction (hence the name 'vasopressin') and water conservation by the kidneys, which help to reverse changes in blood pressure (Figure 12.29a). High blood pressure has the opposite effects.

Cortisol

Cortisol is secreted from the adrenal cortex in higher volumes during the stress response. This hormone reduces the permeability of the capillary wall to prevent water from leaving the circulation thereby aiding the stabilization of blood volume.

Role of the kidneys in the regulation of blood pressure

The kidneys are long-term homeostatic regulators of blood pressure, influencing it via their ability to alter blood volume. For example, when blood volume and blood pressure rise, the

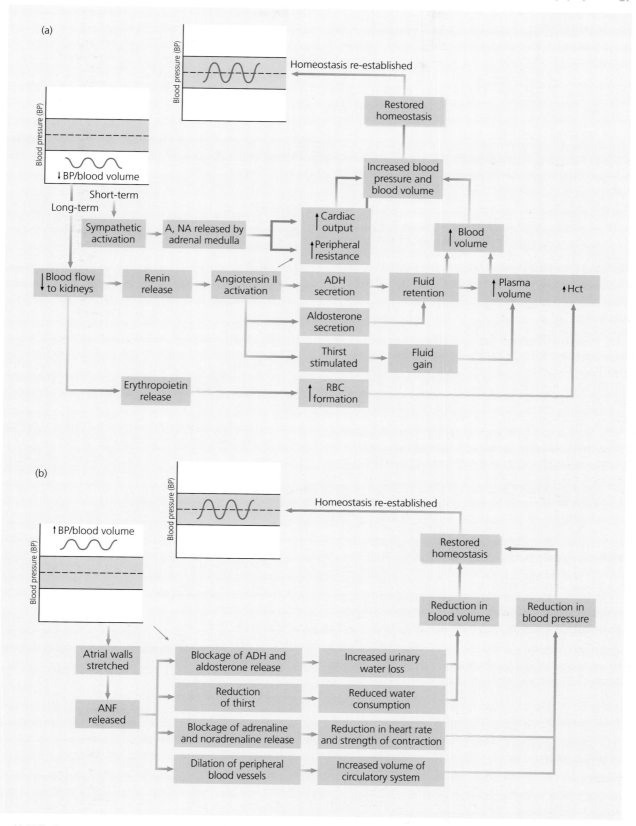

Figure 12.29 The homeostatic regulation of blood pressure (BP) and blood volume. (a) Factors that compensate for decreased blood volume and pressure. (b) Factors that compensate for increased blood volume and pressure. Hct, haematocrit; A, adrenaline; NA, noradrenaline; ANF, atrial natriuretic factor (also known as ANP); ADH, antidiuretic hormone; RBC, red blood cell; ↑, increased; ↓, decreased.

ACTIVITY

List and explain briefly the short-term and long-term regulators of blood pressure following haemorrhage.

kidneys produce more urine, thus decreasing blood volume and causing blood pressure to fall. Conversely, when blood pressure and blood volume are low, the kidneys produce little urine, conserving water and returning it to the circulation, increasing blood volume and blood pressure. These mechanisms are responses to the endocrine secretions discussed earlier, especially aldosterone and ADH. The near-constancy of blood volume in the adult is an indication of their effectiveness.

BOX 12.25 HOMEOSTATIC FAILURES OF THE CIRCULATION

We have already focused on imbalances in which there is insufficient oxygen supply to the myocardium (e.g. coronary arterial disease resulting in coronary ischaemia and myocardial infarction), and inadequate blood flow to the cells (e.g. atherosclerosis and arteriosclerosis). This box focuses on an inability to maintain arterial pressure (e.g. hypertension and hypotension), and further imbalances in which there is an inadequate blood flow to the cells (e.g. shock). A general guide used to indicate high or low blood pressure is the value of 100 mmHg (13.3 kPa): if the diastolic goes above this value it suggests hypertension, and if the systolic goes below it suggests hypotension.

Hypertension
Hypertension is a circulatory imbalance in which a persistent resting systolic pressure is greater than 140 mmHg (18.6 Pa) (in elderly people greater than 160 mmHg or 21.3 kPa) and diastolic pressure is over 90 mmHg (11.8 kPa). Clinicians are concerned with blood pressure readings, because a significantly increased mortality exists in people who have hypertension. The risk increases rapidly with increasing pressure, and the patient is most at risk from a cerebral vascular accident (CVA) and/or myocardial infarction (MI).

Hypertension may occur when the muscle and elastic components of arterial walls are replaced by fibrous tissue (see Box 12.8, p.323). Consequently, the walls of small and medium arteries become thick, hard and inflexible, and their lumens are narrowed. Large arteries, however, may lose their elasticity and dilate, resulting in an exacerbated pulsating flow. At the bends and branches of the arterial tree, there is an increased tendency for blood clotting, as platelets and fibrin are deposited. Blood vessels most commonly affected are cerebral, coronary and renal vessels, thus CVAs, MIs and renal diseases are common clinical manifestations of hypertension (see Figure 12.13d, p.324).

In 85–90% of individuals with hypertension there is no identifiable medical cause, since it is almost certainly multifactorial and is likely to be produced by a combination of nature–nurture interactions (i.e. genetic and environmental factors – see below). This form of hypertension is referred to as 'primary' (or essential) hypertension. The condition begins as an intermittent process during the late 30s to early 50s. However, occasionally there is an abrupt onset and this usually results in rapid deterioration of these patients. The condition gradually becoming 'fixed' that is, if it cannot be controlled by eliminating risk factors.

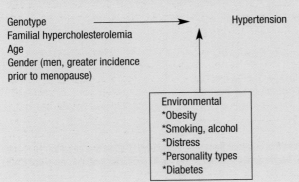

Family lifestyle
Diet (high cholesterol, high salt and low fibre)

Key: *Indicates factors that some authors classify as a modifiable environmental factors. However, the authors of this text believe that it is not that straightforward as the Human Genome Project has now identified genes associated with these factors and hence these factors perhaps should also be included under the subheading of genotype. For example, to date three genes have been attributed to the occurrence of obesity, and if all three have been inherited then the reduced metabolism will be such that the individual is likely to remain obese despite attempts at dieting. Conversely, a person who has not inherited an obesity gene can modify their diet accordingly to remove this environmentally induced risk factor for causing developing hypertension. The impact of smoking, and alcohol consumption is also not purely environmentally induced, since these behaviours have been associated with addictive genes. Diabetes mellitus and personality types have also been linked to the inheritance of susceptibility genes and, as is the case with obesity, could be modifiable and non-modifiable factors.

In 10–15% of all cases, hypertension results from other imbalances, and so is called secondary hypertension. Causes include:

- excessive renin release, as occurs with kidney damage, leading to excessive angiotensin generation, and hence an increase in peripheral resistance;
- hypersecretion of aldosterone (Conn's syndrome) and cortisol, and hence an excessive blood volume, as occurs in people with:
  - hypothalamic and/or pituitary tumours, which cause excessive release of adrenocorticotropic hormone (ACTH) i.e. the stimulant for the secretion of aldosterone and cortisol from the adrenal cortex;
  - an adrenal cortical tumour that displays an excessive reaction to ACTH;
  - failure in the negative feedback mechanisms that control ACTH and adrenal steroid release;
- hypersecretion of ADH due to hypothalamic tumours, or a failure in the feedback mechanisms. Excessive release of ADH exerts its hypertensive effects by increasing peripheral resistance, and by promoting water retention;
- atherosclerosis (see Box 12.8, p.323 and Figure 12.13, p.324).

Hypertension is usually asymptomatic, and it is often referred to as the 'silent killer' since, being asymptomatic, it remains untreated. The risk of premature morbidity and mortality years is positively correlated with increases in systolic and diastolic pressures.

Malignant hypertension occurs in a patient when there is a persistent diastolic pressure exceeding 130 mmHg (17.3 kPa). It may be irreversible and can lead to kidney failure and death within a few years. The result of persistent hypertension can be an accommodation of three complications:

1 Cardiac hypertrophy leading ultimately to congestive cardiac failure.
2 Arteriosclerosis (which aggravates high blood pressure problems).
3 Cardiovascular and cerebrovascular accidents.

BOX 12.25 *Continued*

Correction involves pharmacological and non-pharmacological therapy aimed at the primary imbalance, or at compensation for the imbalance, for example:

- *Pharmacological treatment*: many cardiac drugs have an affect on both the heart rate and blood pressure. These drugs have already been discussed.
  - Negative chronotropic, such as beta-blocker, drugs (e.g. atenolol, methyldopa) provide a reduction of the heart rate, hence the cardiac output and thus a lowering of the blood pressure (Box 12.26).
  - Diuretics (e.g. furosemide) decrease blood pressure by increasing urine output. Such drugs inhibit the renal reabsorption of sodium (mostly in the second convoluted tube of the kidney nephrons; see Figure 15.7, p.430). The extra sodium excreted takes with it extra water (via osmosis), and this water loss decreases the blood volume, one of the important factors in the maintenance of blood pressure. Some drugs also have a vasodilator affect outside the kidney, and therefore have a role in decreasing blood pressure.
  - angiotensin-converting enzyme (ACE) inhibitors (e.g. captopril) decrease the blood pressure by preventing the formation of angiotensin, hence blocking its vasoconstriction effects. The result is a reduction in peripheral resistance and thus a drop in blood pressure (Figure 12.29a).
- *Non-pharmacological treatment*: these treatments for hypertension are widely practised, and in most cases should be tried before starting a drug regime. Initiatives such as weight loss, salt restriction, decreasing alcohol intake and stopping smoking might help to relieve hypertension. Relaxation techniques and biofeedback decrease sympathetic activity, reducing cardiac output, and promote a decreased peripheral resistance, and have been successful in some cases. If hypertension is diagnosed and treated effectively (usually involving drug therapy), there is no reason why much of the cardiovascular-related disease cannot be prevented.

ACTIVITY

Using the information in Box 12.14, p.337 the reader should be able to differentiate between inotropic and chronotropic drugs.

Hypotension

Hypotension is a circulatory imbalance in which the patient has a sustained systolic blood pressure below 100 mmHg (13.15 kPa). Acute hypotension is one of the most important indicators of circulatory shock (see Box 12.28, p.354). Chronic hypotension may be associated with:

- poor nutrition, resulting in anaemia and hypoproteinaemias;
- Addison's disease (i.e. an inadequate secretion of cortisol and aldosterone from the adrenal glands, leading to diminished blood volume and cardiac function);
- hypothyroidism (i.e. an inadequate secretion of thyroid hormones, leading to reduced cardiac function);
- severe tissue wasting, as occurs in cancer patients, resulting in lowered peripheral resistance and blood pooling.

Hypotension produces an inadequate blood supply to the brain, which may result in unconsciousness. Depending upon the cause, this may be brief (fainting) or prolonged, severe as a characteristic of shock (Box 12.28, p.354) or be extreme of which leads to death.

Postural hypotension is a low blood pressure accompanying changing position from lying to sitting or standing; however, rapid compensatory mechanisms guarantee that for most people this is not a problem. The frequency of postural hypotension increases in older individuals, who suffer a temporary hypotension, hence dizziness, when they rise suddenly from a lying or sitting position, which may also result in a transient loss of consciousness (called syncope). This happens because of a decreased sensitivity of the baroreceptor reflex as a natural consequence of ageing. The healthcare practitioner should be aware of this when mobilizing elderly patients, when changing their position, such as when getting them up from a bed onto a chair or from a chair to a standing position. These postural changes should be done slowly and in small stages, allowing time for the blood pressure to adjust with after each stage. Communication is of paramount importance; the healthcare practitioner should always allow the patient to decide the speed of the move and the chance to signal any symptoms of low blood pressure, such as feeling faint or dizzy.

When hypotension is the result of autonomic neuropathy (e.g. owing to poorly controlled diabetes mellitus) or overriding of autonomic reflexes during drug treatment for hypertension, the healthcare practitioner may be asked to perform postural blood pressure recording. The (mean) blood pressure is recorded in the same arm, first with the patient lying down and then in a standing position. If a difference exists between the systolic pressures, the patient is said to have a postural fall in blood pressure (postural hypotension). It is particularly significant if the difference is 20 mmHg (2.63 kPa) or more, and can indicate a large-volume fluid loss. Correction of hypotension as always is aimed at removing the underlying cause, and using antihypotensive drug therapy and cardiac stimulants (Box 12.8, p.323).

BOX 12.26 SURGERY, POTENTIAL CARDIOVASCULAR MALFUNCTION AND THEIR TREATMENTS

It is common for cardiac dysrhythmias and hypotension to occur under anaesthesia. Anaesthetic agents can produce depression of the heart rate and of the motor tone of the peripheral vessels. The homeostatic mechanisms mentioned in the main text are largely responsible for the maintenance of normal blood pressure in a fit person during surgery. However, in cases where deeper anaesthesia is used, or in elderly people, or people with other predisposing problems, these mechanisms may be unable to regulate the blood pressure within the normal homeostatic range.

Blood pressure checks are paramount postoperatively in order for the patient full recovery. Hypotension may also indicate blood loss (internally or externally) and should be reported and acted on immediately.

Adrenoceptor agonists

Drugs that mimic the action of the sympathetic nervous system (sympathomimetics, e.g., adrenaline, noradrenaline, isoprenaline and dopamine) cause vasoconstriction. They also have varying effects on the heart. Adrenaline influences alpha- and beta-receptors, and affects both the heart and peripheral vessels.

- *Adrenaline*: acts on both the alpha- and beta-adrenoceptors in the sympathetic nervous system. Alpha actions cause coronary and peripheral vasoconstriction, while the beta action causes an increase in heart rate, increased myocardial contractility and coronary vasodilation. Adrenaline is used in cardiac arrest to stimulate the heart without causing peripheral vasodilation and a resulting fall in blood pressure. It is used to preserve coronary and cerebral blood flow. (Note: nicotine enhances the secretion of adrenaline from the adrenal medulla, and so causes vasoconstriction, hence its link with hypertension.)

BOX 12.26 *Continued*

- *Noradrenaline*: mainly affects alpha-receptors and the vascular system, causing an increase in peripheral resistance.
- *Isoprenaline*: works by selectively stimulating the beta-receptors. It causes the rate and force of the heartbeat to increase (thus increasing myocardial oxygen demand); it also relaxes smooth muscle causing vasodilatation.
- *Dopamine*: when given by intravenous infusion, stimulates the cardiac beta-adrenoceptors. It is also given in low doses to increase renal perfusion, causing selective renal vasoconstriction and an increase in the blood pressure, ultimately increasing urine production. The dose is critical: high doses can induce vasoconstriction and exacerbate heart failure; it is therefore important that it is used when invasive haemodynamic monitoring of the patient is in place.

Alpha-adrenoceptor blocking drugs

These drugs reduce arteriolar and venous tone, causing a fall in peripheral resistance, hypotension and a fall in central venous pressure. They reverse the effects of adrenaline and noradrenaline at the smooth muscle receptor sites and so cause vasodilation. Extra intravenous fluids need to be given to maintain the circulation following administration of these drugs.

Intraoperatively phentolamine is used in a number if different ways. It promotes vasodilation in cardiopulmonary bypass surgery, it antagonizes vasoconstriction in situations such as cardiogenic shock, and it also acts as a myocardial stimulant by blocking the actions of adrenaline and noradrenaline on peripheral vessels causing vasodilation. There is a resulting fall in blood pressure and central venous pressure; therefore, extra intravenous fluid is required to maintain circulation.

Alpha-receptor blocking drugs are also used in the treatment of peripheral vascular decease in order to increase blood flow to ischaemic tissues. These drugs increase blood flow to the skin rather than to the muscles, and thus are sometimes used to assist in the treatment of varicose ulcers. Drugs can also affect the smooth muscle in the blood vessel wall directly; for example glyceryl trinitrate (GTN) is a potent vasodilator that relaxes the vascular muscle and is particularly effective in the treatment of angina.

Beta-adrenoceptor blocking drugs

These drugs competitively block the beta-receptors. These drugs have varying lipid solubility and cardioselectivity and are effective in reducing blood pressure and angina:

- *Atenolol*: usually the drug of choice for prophylaxis of angina; it is a cardioselective beta-blocking drug and acts by slowing the heart rate and reducing the myocardial demand for oxygen. It is effective in the treatment of cardiac dysrhythmias and hypertension.
- *Propranolol*: acts by antagonizing the beta effects of isoprenaline on the heart and bronchi. There is a fall in heart rate and cardiac output, and myocardial oxygen consumption is reduced. Propranolol is used to effectively control ectopic heartbeats; it is also useful when treating arrhythmias caused by an overdose of digitalis. It is useful in controlling supraventricular tachycardia, tachycardia resulting from the use of hypotensive drugs, and excess adrenaline, and to reduce myocardial oxygen consumption, thus reducing the incidence of angina.
- *Labetalol*: is both an alpha- and beta-adrenoceptor blocker. It is useful in reducing myocardial oxygen consumption and in causing peripheral vasodilatation. Because the alpha-blocking effects are milder and have a shorter duration, the effects of the drug are similar to beta-adrenoceptor blocking drugs. It is commonly used during elective surgery to create a moderate reduction in blood pressure.

In depression and grief, the higher centres decrease the vasomotor sympathetic reflex; the resultant decrease in blood pressure can cause fainting. The hypothalamus also mediates the redistribution of blood flow and changes in cardiovascular dynamics associated with exercise and changes in body temperature.

ACTIVITY

Explain how circulatory function is altered by (1) hypertension, (2) hypotension, (3) aneurysms and (4) haemorrhage.

BOX 12.27 PRE-ECLAMPSIA AND HELLP SYNDROME

Pre-eclampsia is the development of hypertension with proteinuria and oedema, or both, induced by pregnancy after the 20th week of gestation.

Total peripheral resistance decreases by about 25% in normal pregnancy. In pre-eclampsia, the woman's total peripheral resistance increases – this appears to be the main cause for the elevation in blood pressure seen in this condition – and the normal cardiac output rise of 40% achieved in pregnancy rises even further. The failure of the total peripheral resistance to decrease is thought to be a consequence of the maternal circulatory system being unable to respond appropriately to the fetal trophoblast cells within the forming placenta. The spiral arterioles of the placenta fail to dilate, and maternal blood is forced through these constricted arterioles, which consequently raises the blood pressure.

Management of this condition is possible when it is mild. If the condition becomes increasingly severe (i.e. the blood pressure continues to rise, proteinuria increases, and blood coagulation levels decrease) the only treatment is to deliver the fetus. The condition then usually resolves over 48–72 hours.

Pre-eclampsia reflects itself in changes in the blood. Biochemical tests are performed regularly in women with pre-eclampsia. A rare condition that may present is haemolysis, elevated liver enzymes and low platelets (HELLP) syndrome. This presents with right upper quadrant pain, jaundice and nausea. The seriousness of HELLP should not be underestimated, and is considered to be an indication for delivery.

Local regulation of blood pressure

Blood flow to tissues must be regulated tightly since it is responsible for:

- absorption of nutrients from the gastrointestinal tract;
- gaseous exchange in the lungs;
- transport of oxygen, nutrients, hormones, etc. to tissue cells throughout the body;
- the removal of waste products of metabolism from cells;
- processing of blood by the kidneys and other excretory organs.

The flow of blood to specific tissues reflects the metabolic demands of that tissue. At rest, for example, skeletal muscles receive approximately 20% of the total blood volume each minute. During exercise, blood is redistributed from other areas (e.g. kidneys and abdominal organs), so that skeletal muscles receive a higher proportion of the (increased) cardiac output to cater for their increased metabolic demands (Figure 12.30).

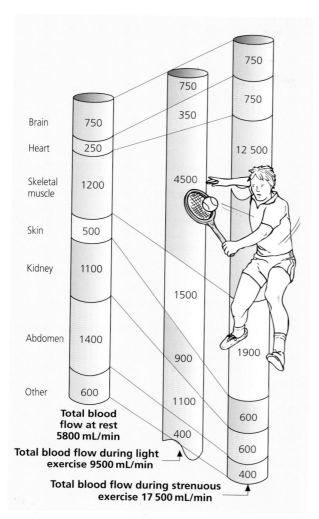

Figure 12.30 Distribution of blood flow to selected body organs at rest, during light exercise, and during strenuous exercise

Q Explain how an athlete's low resting heart rate does not compromise cardiac function.

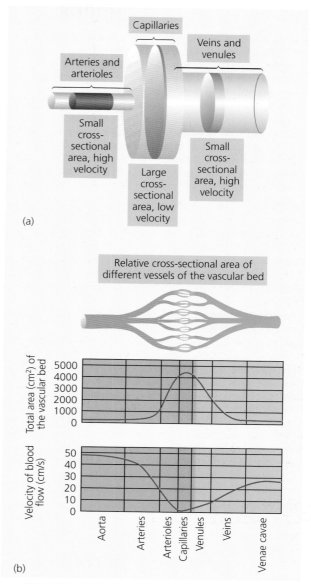

Figure 12.31 Relationship between cross-sectional area of blood vessels and velocity of blood flow. (a) Relative cross-sectional areas of arteries, capillaries and veins. (b) Relationship between blood flow velocity and total cross-sectional area in various blood vessels of the systemic circulation

Vasodilators produce local dilation of arterioles and relaxation of precapillary sphincters, independent of the centrally mediated autonomic responses discussed earlier, the result of which is an increased flow of blood into the capillary beds. Vasoconstrictors have the opposite effect. This local regulation of blood pressure and flow is termed 'autoregulation'. It is the major regulator of regional blood flow in the brain, and as such is termed 'cerebral autoregulation'. Even though the total blood flow to the brain remains almost constant, regardless of the degree of physical or mental activity, blood distribution to various parts of the brain changes dramatically with different activities.

Velocity of blood flow

The speed at which blood flows varies throughout the systemic/pulmonary circulations and with the specific stages of the cardiac cycle. The greatest velocity is recorded in the aorta during ventricular systole. Furthermore, since velocity is related inversely to the cross-sectional area of blood vessels, the

flow rate decreases as the aorta branches, being slowest within the capillary beds; this is essential, as the capillaries are the exchange vessels (Figure 12.31a). Flow speeds up again in the venous system as blood collects from the different tissues and is returned to the heart (Figure 12.31b).

Tissue autoregulation – local regulation of blood flow

Tissue autoregulation of blood flow is independent of systemic control, but is proportional to the tissue's requirements, being regulated by local conditions. Flow is, therefore, increased automatically in response to:

- nutrients and oxygen levels falling below their homeostatic range (i.e. when they fail to meet the demands of the tissue);

BOX 12.28 SHOCK

Circulatory shock is any condition in which blood vessels are inadequately filled, thereby producing a tissue blood flow that is inadequate for cellular homeostatic requirements. The lack of cellular metabolites results in intracellular imbalances (e.g. insufficient oxygen produces hypoxia and promotes anaerobic respiration; the persistent build-up of 'waste' products causes cell death, and organ damage ensues). Shock is classified as hypovolaemic (due to low blood volume), cardiogenic (of cardiac origin), vascular (of blood vessel origin), neurogenic (of neural origin), anaphylactic (as a consequence of an allergic reaction) or septic, which is a leading cause of admission to critical care units.

Hypovolaemic shock ('hypo-' = low, '-volaemic' = blood volume) is the most common form of this imbalance. Causes include:

- severe acute haemorrhage, where bleeding can either be arterial, venous or capillary. Arterial bleeds are more serious, since blood is lost from a high-pressure system in pulses; speed is of the essence to control this loss before the patient either bleeds to death or the resultant shock becomes irreversible. Bleeding may be internal (within body cavities, or as bruising into tissues) or external (into the external environment);
- extensive superficial burns (when there is excessive loss of tissue fluid, leading to further exudation from the blood plasma);
- severe vomiting and diarrhoea (when excessive loss of gut fluid promotes further secretion from the blood plasma).

In hypovolaemia, there is:

- increased heart rate, which acts to improve cardiac output and redress this homeostatic balance. The resultant rapid, 'thready' pulse is an initial sign of the condition (the 'thready' nature of the pulse reflects a diminished pulse pressure);
- intense vasoconstriction, which acts to re-establish blood volume by forcing blood from blood reservoirs (spleen, liver, etc.) into the circulation to enhance venous return, and by increasing peripheral resistance, both of which stabilize blood pressure. If blood loss continues, blood pressure drops sharply as compensatory mechanisms are exceeded; this is serious, and is a late sign of shock.

Figure 12.32 illustrates the homeostatic controls involved in redressing the blood volume after haemorrhage.

Other forms of shock:

- *Cardiogenic shock*: when the hearts as a pump fails to sustain a normal stroke volume and hence there is a sudden reduction in cardiac output. A common clause of cardiogenic shock is myocardial infarction.
- *Vasogenic shock*: when the cause is the vascular system itself. In this type of shock, blood volume is normal and constant, and inadequate circulation results from a huge drop in peripheral resistance as a consequence of extreme vasodilation, leading to pooling in the large veins. Consequently, a decrease in venous return, cardiac output and arterial pressure results. There are several forms of vascular shock. The most common causes of this imbalance are loss of vasomotor (neural) tone, and septicaemia as a consequence of a severe Gram-negative bacterial infection (bacterial toxins are potent vasodilators). Extensive peripheral vasodilation also occurs in anaphylactic shock, a dangerous allergic reaction (see Figure 13.24, p.391 and Box 13.16, p.388).
- *Neurogenic shock*: may occur as a result of a sudden acute pain and/or severe emotional experience. Both stimulate a parasympathetic (vagal) slowing of the heart rate, thereby reducing the cardiac output and arterial pressure. Venous pooling of blood may reduce the venous return. These changes decrease cerebral flow, which may cause a temporary loss of consciousness (fainting), a phenomenon known as a 'vasovagal attack'. For further reading, see Clancy and McVicar (1996).

There are similarities in the cardiovascular symptoms of shock regardless of cause. Apart from the thready pulse noted earlier, indicative signs are usually a cold and clammy skin – cold because of vasoconstriction induced by sympathetic nerve responses to the falling blood pressure, and clammy because sympathetic nerves also promote sweating (this sign is paradoxical in shock, being more suited to hyperthermia). Variation may initially be seen with anaphylactic and septic since vasodilation is the cause of these forms; the skin at first may be flushed. If untreated shock quickly becomes irreversible and fatal, probably as a consequence of sustained tissue hypoxia.

- carbon dioxide levels above the homeostatic range. This is the most powerful trigger to autoregulation, and could be viewed as resulting from an accumulation of this metabolic product owing to inadequate blood flow;
- the release of metabolically active substances from cells, such as lactic acid, kinins, prostaglandins, potassium and hydrogen ions, which will occur if blood flow to the tissue is inadequate;
- the presence of inflammatory chemicals, such as histamine, which promote the protective inflammatory response when the tissue is damaged.

These stimuli cause immediate arteriolar vasodilation and relaxation of precapillary sphincters, thus causing an increased blood flow to the tissues concerned. Autoregulation is considered to be both a short-term and a long-term regulator of blood flow, which acts to redress homeostasis in particular tissues. Cerebral blood flow in particular is regulated by one of the most precise autoregulatory mechanisms in the body. Brain tissue, however, is particularly sensitive to increased carbon dioxide (and the consequential decreased pH), and excessive carbon dioxide levels may remove the brain's autoregulatory response, resulting in severe brain damage. Oxygen deficit is a less potent stimulus, even though neurons are totally intolerant of ischaemic conditions. Oxygen deficit, however, increases the presence of many of the metabolites noted above, and regulatory mechanisms protect the area from damage by responding to the changing levels of these metabolites.

Blood flow through capillary networks is intermittent because of the contraction and relaxation of the smooth muscle fibres of the arterioles and precapillary sphincters of true capillaries.

Capillary dynamics related to cellular homeostasis

Body fluids are compartmentalized into intracellular and extracellular fluids. Extracellular fluid is subdivided further into plasma and interstitial (tissue) fluid. Within the extracellular fluid compartment, the exchange of fluid between plasma and tissue fluid is important since it brings nutrients into the proximity of cell membranes and aids the removal of substances

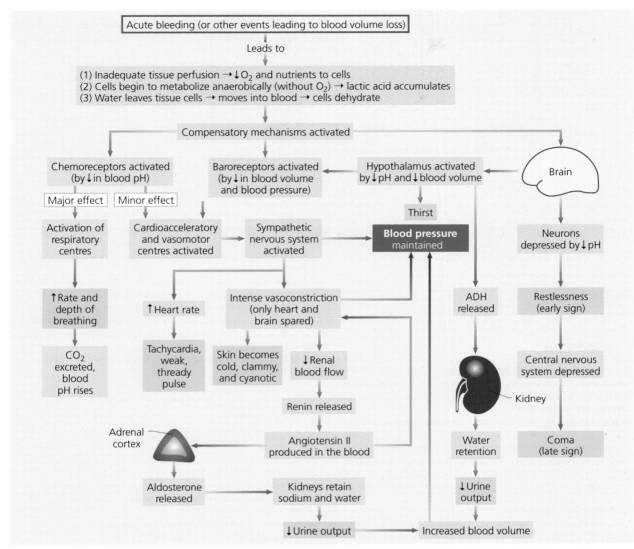

Figure 12.32 Events and signs of hypovolaemic shock. Conditions shown in the blue boxes are clinical indications of shock. ADH, antidiuretic hormone

Q Define 'shock', and list the major types of shock.

secreted by cells ('wastes', hormones, etc.) in the opposite direction. Such exchanges are essential if solutes are to enter and exit intracellular fluid efficiently. In order to prevent excessive loss of fluid from plasma (which would induce hypovolaemia), or an excessive build-up of tissue fluid (oedema), a similar volume of fluid must be returned to plasma as was extruded from it.

The movement of water and some of its dissolved solutes between plasma and tissue fluid occurs at the capillary level. Water is driven out of the plasma largely because the hydrostatic pressure of the arterial end of the capillary is higher than the osmotic (referred to as the oncotic or colloidal) pressure generated by plasma proteins. The hydrostatic pressure decreases along the length of the vessel as water is moved (exuded) into the tissue fluid, and is eventually exceeded by the plasma oncotic pressure. Proteins are largely retained within

capillaries because of their macromolecular size (although small proteins can be transferred across capillary membranes). Net pressure at the venous end of the capillaries thus favours the return of fluid into the capillary (a small volume of exudate is returned to the circulation via lymph vessels that drain the interstitial spaces). Plasma protein concentration is, therefore, another important factor in the homeostatic maintenance of a normal circulatory blood volume.

ACTIVITY

Identify the forces (i.e. pressures) that determine the exchange of water and nutrients between blood and tissue fluid across the walls of the capillaries.

Table 12.4 Cardiopulmonary resuscitation

Procedure	Physiological rationale underpinning action
Assess environment and note time	Beware falling masonry, electric current, traffic, etc. (may cause further injury to patient/rescuer)
	Time important to assess risk of cerebral hypoxia
Assess patient, including level of consciousness	Patient may be asleep, fainted, drunk, etc.
	Other injuries may be present that could be exacerbated
	Skin colour may indicate hypoxia, CO poisoning, etc.
	Damage could occur if patient is resuscitated when not required
Call for help	Spontaneous recovery unlikely, medical assistance (ALS) required, two rescuers better than one (CPR is exhausting)
Assess other injuries	Trauma to face/neck/chest could impair resuscitation attempts
	Take care to not cause further damage
Position patient flat	Patient must be supine on hard surface so effective airway maintenance and chest compressions can be undertaken
Assess airway	Any blockage will prevent air from entering or leaving lungs
Remove airway obstruction/finger sweep	Clearing blockages, e.g. vomit/food/foreign objects/loose dentures, will allow passage of air through airway
Open airway using jaw-thrust or chin-lift technique	When unconscious, lack of muscle tone causes tongue to occlude airway; this technique lifts tongue away from back of throat
	Beware of hyperextending neck
Assess breathing	Breathing movements may be difficult to see, so look/listen/feel
	Ventilating an already breathing patient will cause damage
	Assess for at least 5 seconds, as normal respiratory rate is about 12–16 breaths/minute
Breathe exhaled air into patient (whilst pinching nose in adult/child)	Expired air contains 14% oxygen, which will adequately oxygenate unconscious patient
	Pinch nose to prevent escape of gas
Release nose pinch	To allow escape of air from patient's air passages and lungs with minimum resistance
Assess circulation by checking pulse (carotid in adult, brachial in infant)	Assesses whether any cardiac output is occurring
	These pulse sites best reflect left ventricular activity
Apply precordial thump ONLY If cardiac arrest is witnessed AND if ALS available	Precordial thump can induce cardiac arrhythmias, which will require ALS
Place hands on sternum with arms straight and elbows locked	Anatomical location of heart
	Pressure is delivered most efficiently when the force is not absorbed by bending the arms or dissipated laterally
	Injury to other vital organs and rib fractures may occur with incorrect hand position
Commence external chest compression	Action mimics ventricular systole by opening pulmonary and aortic valves, and closing atrioventricular valves (cardiac pump theory), and by increasing pressure in thorax, resulting in blood being squeezed out of lungs (thoracic pump theory)
Release pressure between compressions	Action allows diastolic filling of heart chambers
	Decrease in thoracic pressure also draws blood into lungs
Apply rhythmic compressions and ventilation at a ratio of 15:2 (or 5:1)	Rate of compression must be sufficient to mimic normal heart rate (adult 70–80 bpm, infant 100 bpm)
	Be aware of the time taken to ventilate
	Ratio of 5:1 preferable as this reduces the interval between each ventilation
Continue until help arrives	At best, CPR provides only 25% of normal cardiac output, which is sufficient to maintain oxygenation of vital organs in unconscious patient
	As spontaneous recovery is unlikely, circulation of artificially oxygenated blood must continue until arrival of ALS
Place patient in recovery position (should cardiopulmonary function return)	Prevents patient from rolling on to back and allows airway maintenance
	Close monitoring of patient is essential
	Be aware of other injuries

ALS, advanced life support; bpm, beats per minute; CO, carbon monoxide; CPR, cardiopulmonary resuscitation.

Exercise: a change in cardiovascular homeostatic set points

A number of interrelated changes occur during a steady or low rate of aerobic (isotonic) exercise. For example, the oxygen consumption of exercising skeletal muscles is increased, facilitated by precapillary sphincter relaxation in these tissues as a response to their changing metabolic requirements. Consequently, blood flow increases (see Figure 12.30, p.353),

and blood is returned to the veins at an increased rate. The increased venous return to the heart results from a greater activity in the skeletal muscular 'pumps', which force blood along the peripheral veins. The accompanying increased breathing rate also increases blood flow into the vena cava via the suction pressure created by the thoracoabdominal pumps. A greater venous return to the heart results in an increased cardiac output by mechanisms associated with Frank–Starling and Bainbridge reflexes, and increased sympathetic activity

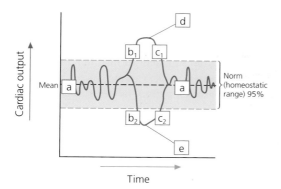

Figure 12.33 Cardiac output: an expression of cardiovascular function. a, Cardiac output fluctuating within its normal homeostatic parameters. b_1, Increased cardiac output as occurs normally, when the homeostatic parameters are reset (e.g. exercise), and abnormally, when indicating a homeostatic imbalance, such as right-to-left cardiac shunts (e.g. tetralogy of Fallot, transposition of the great vessels), aortic stenosis (and its associated left ventricular hypertrophy), and tachycardia. b_2, Decreased cardiac output, as occurs with homeostatic imbalances, such as the left-to-right cardiac shunts (atrial septal defects, ventricular septal defects, patent ductus arteriosus), cardiomyopathies, bradycardia, heart failure and incompetent valves. c_1, c_2, Correction varies according to the imbalance (e.g. oxygen therapy for a cyanosed patient, drugs or pacemaker to correct conduction imbalances, and surgical techniques to correct structural defects). d, Re-established homeostasis of cardiac output. e, Homeostatic failure of cardiac output. (a, Represents boxes a_1–a_4 in Figure 1.7, p.11, reflecting the individual variability in the homeostatic range)

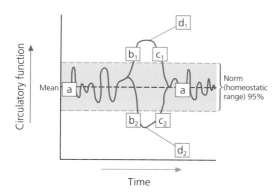

Figure 12.34 Circulation: an expression of cardiovascular function. a, Circulatory function fluctuating within its homeostatic range. b_1, Increased circulatory flow, as occurs normally with increased oxygen supply to the myocardium and muscle cells when the homeostatic flow parameters are reset, as in exercise, and abnormally, as occurs in hypertension. b_2, Decreased circulatory flow, as occurs in the homeostatic imbalances of hypotension, ischaemic disease, myocardial infarctions, cerebrovascular accidents and thrombotic changes in vessels. c_1, Clinical correction is dependent upon the underlying imbalance (i.e. antihypertensive therapy used in hypertension may be via diuretics, beta-blockers, calcium channel blockers or relaxation therapies). c_2, Clinical correction of the imbalance (e.g. hypotension is treated with antihypotensive drugs) or by treating the underlying cause of the imbalance (e.g. thyroxine administration in hypothyroidism); myocardial ischaemia is treated with glycerol trinitrate, angioplasty or streptokinase therapy; tissue ischaemia is treated with peripheral vasodilators. d, Continued imbalance because of the irreversibility of the underlying cause, for example (d_1) prolonged hypertension leading to cerebrovascular accident, myocardial infarction, renal failure, etc., or (d_2) prolonged hypotension leading to death due to cerebral ischaemia/infarction. (a, Represents boxes a_1–a_4 in Figure 1.7, p.11, reflecting the individual variability in the homeostatic range)

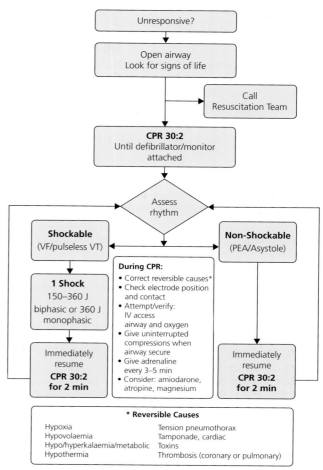

Figure 12.35 Resuscitation Council UK (2005) Guidelines. Reproduced with the kind permission of Resuscitation Council. CPR, cardiopulmonary resuscitation; IV, intravenous; PEA, pulseless electrical activity; VF, ventricular fibrillation; VT, ventricular tachycardia

(Figure 12.33). As long as the increased cardiac output can supply the increased demand, then arterial pressure will be maintained, despite the increase in muscle blood flow (Figure 12.34). Indeed, the increased cardiac output observed during exercise actually causes an increase in systemic blood pressure as a consequence of an elevated systolic blood pressure; diastolic pressure is little changed.

There are minimal alterations in blood flow distribution to accommodate low levels of exercise, although skeletal and cardiac muscles, together with the skin, exhibit a small increase. The increased skeletal muscular flow is via the release of local metabolic factors mentioned (see text), which relax precapillary sphincters at these sites. The increased skin blood flow is via hypothalamic–vasomotor centre responses to an increase in body temperature, which causes vasodilation of the skin arterioles and promotes the removal of the excess heat generated by the body. Severe exercise promotes additional physiological adjustments to accommodate the massive increase in the peripheral distribution of blood to skeletal muscles. In addition to metabolic factors, these include:

- sympathetic stimulation of the cardiac accelerator centre, which accounts for a cardiac output increase of up to 20–35 L/minute, depending on the person's fitness;
- redistribution of blood flow to skeletal muscles via a shutdown of blood flow to 'non-essential' organs (e.g. kidneys, gut) by vasomotor sympathetic stimulation to their arterioles, and an increased blood flow to skeletal muscle, heart and lungs via reduced vasomotor sympathetic activity to their vasculature.

With training, cardiovascular fitness is improved by the increased myocardial bulk that develops. This increases the stroke volume and hence cardiac output; a trained athlete thus has a lower heart rate for a given cardiac output compared with an untrained person. Sebastian Coe, the famous 1500-m runner of the 1980s, claimed to have a resting heart rate of just 36 bpm (compared with the adult average of 72 bpm). This would still have been sufficient to maintain blood flow to his tissues, due to his large stroke volume. Such a heart rate associated with a non-athletic person, however, is clinically referred to as a bradycardia, since the accompanying lower stroke volume would be insufficient to deliver blood to the surrounding tissues.

ACTIVITY

Consider the steps involved in cardiopulmonary resuscitation (CPR) listed in Table 12.4. Would you carry them out in that order? If not, arrange them into an appropriate sequence. For each procedure, provide the physiological rationale for that particular action.

SUMMARY

1. The cardiovascular system is the body's transport network, and is adapted to maintain intracellular and extracellular homeostasis.
2. The cardiovascular system comprises a double circulation (i.e. pulmonary and systemic circuits). The pulmonary circuit oxygenates blood to within its homeostatic parameters. The systemic circuit delivers oxygen, nutrients, etc. to tissue cells throughout the body to maintain their intracellular homeostasis.
3. The heart has two ventricular pumps: the right pump supplies the pulmonary circuit; the left pump supplies the systemic circuit.
4. The heart wall comprises three layers (epicardium, myocardium and endocardium) and four chambers (paired upper atria and lower ventricles).
5. Valves ensure unidirectional flow through the heart and venous system.
6. The heart sounds 'lub-dup' correspond to the closing of the AV and semilunar valves, respectively, during the functional cycle of cardiac contraction. Heart murmurs are evidence of stenotic or incompetent valves.
7. Coronary vessels deliver blood to the myocardium. Their partial or complete occlusion compromises myocardial function, and leads to the homeostatic imbalances of angina and/or MI.
8. The cardiac cycle describes the sequence of events that occurs with each heartbeat. The cycle consists principally of diastolic (relaxing and filling) and systolic (contracting and emptying) stages.
9. The cardiac output, a clinically important homeostatic parameter, is calculated by multiplying the heart rate by the stroke volume. Changes in either will change the cardiac output.
10. The heart rate is controlled intrinsically and modified extrinsically by the autonomic nervous system and the endocrine system. It varies according to age, gender, temperature and level of activity.
11. The normal adult pulse rate is 65–72 bpm.
12. A weak rapid pulse is a characteristic of shock.
13. The stroke volume varies according to changes in the venous return, which alter the stretch within the chambers (Frank–Starling law), to the period of ventricular filling, and to autonomic neural activity.
14. Most blood vessels share a common structure, consisting of three tunicae (interna, media and externa). Their microstructure, however, is adapted for their specific homeostatic functions.
15. The path of blood flow is from the heart to arteries (elastic, muscular, distributing vessels), to arterioles (smallest arteries), to capillaries (exchange vessels), to venules (smallest veins) and to veins (drainage vessels and blood reservoirs). The veins take blood back to the heart.
16. Blood flow is calculated by dividing the blood pressure differential between arterial and venous vessels by the peripheral resistance provided by the vasculature, particularly arterioles. Blood pressure provides the force necessary to produce blood flow along the vessels.
17. Arterial blood pressure is calculated by multiplying the cardiac output by the total peripheral resistance.
18. Arterial blood pressure is measured by a sphygmomanometer. It is expressed as systolic and diastolic values. Blood pressure increases with age and with homeostatic imbalances, such as arteriosclerosis, hypertension, etc., and decreases with imbalances, such as hypotension, shock, heart failure, etc.
19. The mean arterial pressure is calculated by adding one-third of the pulse pressure to the diastolic pressure.
20. It is important to use a cuff that is the correct size for adults and correct for the children's age; the wrong size cuff will give in accurate results.
21. Blood pressure is normally maintained within its homeostatic range via a number of short-term and long-term blood pressure homeostatic controls. These can be divided broadly into neural and endocrine mechanisms, respectively.
22. Cardiovascular homeostatic parameters are reset in 'normal' homeostatic adaptive states, such as exercise and pregnancy.
23. The medulla oblongata of the brainstem contains the cardiac centres and the vasomotor centres. These centres control cardiovascular function.
24. Cardiovascular malfunctions may be classified as cardiac and circulatory homeostatic imbalances. It cannot be overemphasized, however, that neither malfunction exists in isolation without compromising the other's homeostatic function, together with the homeostatic functions of other tissues and organs, because of the interdependence of organ system functioning. Consequently, a vast array of clinical problems ranging from the less severe (e.g. temporary ischaemic pain) to the very severe (e.g. cerebrovascular accident, kidney failure and pulmonary failure), present themselves when cardiovascular function is impaired.

REFERENCES

Clancy, J. and McVicar, A.J. (1996) Shock: a failure to maintain cardiovascular homeostasis. *British Journal of Theatre Nursing* **6**(6): 19–25.

Clancy, J. and McVicar, A.J. (1998) Homeostasis and nature – nurture interactions: a framework for integrating the life sciences. In Hinchliffe, S.S.M., Norman, S.E. and Schober, J.E. (eds) *Nursing Practice and Health*, 3rd edn. London: Arnold.

Clancy, J., McVicar, A.J. and Baird, N. (2002) *Perioperative Practice. Fundamentals of Homeostasis*. London: Routledge.

Cucherat, M., Bonnefoy, E. and Tremeau, G. (2001) Primary angioplasty versus intravenous thrombolysis for acute myocardial infarction. *The Cochran Library*, Issue 1. Oxford: Update Software.

Holmwood, C. (2000) Overweight and hypertensive. *Australian Family Physician* **29**(6): 559–63.

Hood, W.B. Jr, Dans, A., Guyatt, G.H., Jaeschke, R. and McMurray J. (2001) Digitalis for treatment of congestive heart failure in patients in sinus rhythm. *The Cochran Library*, Issue 1. Oxford: Update Software.

Huether, S.E. and McCance, K.L. (2006). ***Pathophysiology*, 5th edn** – *The Biologic Basis for Disease in Adults and Children*. London: Mosby.

Joint Formulary Committee (2008) *British National Formulary*, 48 edn. London: British Medical Association and Royal Pharmaceutical Society of Great Britain.

Nagle, B.M. and O'Keefe, L.M. (2000) Closing in on mitral valve disease. *Nursing* **29**(4): 32–7.

Pradka, L.R. (2000) Lipids and their role in coronary heart disease: what they do and how to manage them. *Nursing Clinics of North America* **35**(4): 981–91.

Clancy, J., McVicar, A.J. and Baird, N. (2001) *Fundamentals of Homeostasis for Perioperative Practitioners*. London: Routledge.

Department of Health (2002) *National Service Framework for Coronary Heart Disease*. London: Department of Health.

Fleury, J. and Keller, C. (2000) Assessment. Cardiovascular risk assessment in elderly individuals. *Journal of Gerontological Nursing* **26**(5): 30–7.

Goh, T.H. (2000) Common congenital heart defects: the value of early detection. *Australian Family Physician* **29**(5): 429–62.

Knight, M., Duley, L., Henderson-Smart, D.J. and King J.F. (2001) Antiplatelet agents for preventing and treating pre-eclampsia. *The Cochrane Library*, Issue 1. Oxford: Update Software.

Liu, M., Counsell, C. and Sandercock, P. (2001) Anticoagulation for preventing recurrence following ischaemic stroke or transient ischaemic attack. *The Cochran Library*, Issue 1. Oxford: Update Software.

Marcus, G.M., Michaels, A.D., De Marco, T. *et al.* (2004) Usefulness of the third heart sound in predicting an elevated level of B-type natriuretic peptide. *American Journal of Cardiology* **93**: 1312–13.

Sowers, J.R. and Lester, M. (2000) Hypertension, hormones, and aging. *Journal of Laboratory and Clinical Medicine* **135**(5): 379–86.

Swierczynski, D. (2000) A taste of their own medicine. Diagnosis: heart murmur. *Men's Health* **15**(9): 62–66.

Wigginton, M. (2001) Expanded ECGs: easy as V4, V5, V6. *Nursing* **31**(1): 50–1.

Williams, M.J. Eds. Clancy, J. and McVicar, A.J. (2001) Know your heart. *British Journal of Perioperative Nursing* **11**(6): 270–7.

Yu, H.H., Pasternak, R.C. and Ginsburg, G.S. (2000) Lipid management for patients with CAD, part 1: what to expect, when to start: consider an aggressive strategy for prevention of cardiac events. *Journal of Critical Illness* **15**(5): 247–62.

FURTHER READING

Blumenthal, J.A., Sherwood, A., Gullette, E.C.D. *et al.* (2000) Exercise and weight loss reduce blood pressure in men and women with mild hypertension: effects on cardiovascular, metabolic, and hemodynamic functioning. *Archives of Internal Medicine* **160**(13): 1947–58, 2068–9.

Clancy, J. and McVicar, A.J. (1996) The essentials of cardiovascular physiology. *British Journal of Theatre Nursing* **6**(4): 19–27.

USEFUL WEBSITES

British Hypertension Society: http://www.bhsoc.org

http://www.patient.co.uk (an extremely useful website for any human pathology)

Heart Auscultation: http://www.patient.co.uk/showdoc/40000504.

CHAPTER 13

THE LYMPHATIC SYSTEM, IMMUNITY AND MICROBIOLOGY

INTRODUCTION

Relation of the lymphatic system to cellular homeostasis

Blood distributes oxygen and other metabolites to the body cells, and removes cellular waste products. Cells are bathed in tissue (interstitial) fluid, which acts as an intermediary fluid between blood and cells (refer back to Figure 11.1, p.269). The lymphatic system is an extensive, branched tubular network that aligns itself with the blood's circulation, and it is adapted for the prevention of tissue fluid accumulation (Figure 13.1a). Excess fluid is returned to the circulation, so the lymphatic system is important in the homeostatic maintenance of all body fluids. Swollen lymph nodes are a sign that this function is compromised and potentially also an infection is present (Figure 13.1b). The system also acts as an intermediary between the digestive and circulatory systems (i.e. following absorption of a meal, it transports long-chain fatty acids and fat-soluble vitamins such as A, D, E and K). In addition, the lymphatic system has immunological defence functions, filtering and destroying potential environmental hazards. Figure 13.1 summarizes the homeostatic functions of the lymphatic system.

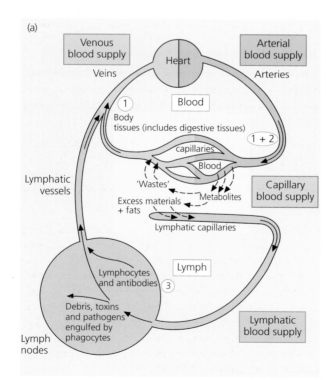

(a)

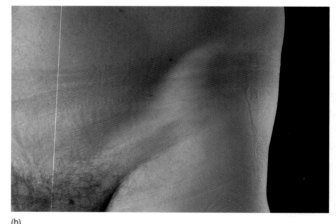

(b)

Figure 13.1 (a) Summary of the homeostatic functions associated with the lymphatic system: 1, regulation of body fluids; 2, fat and fat-soluble vitamins (A, D, E and K) absorption; 3, defence functions. (b) Patient exhibiting inflammation (note the swelling) of the left groin lymph nodes during an infection. Reproduced with the kind permission of the Medical Illustration Department, Norfolk and Norwich University Hospital NHS Trust

Q Using the text and this figure, describe the homeostatic functions of the lymphatic system.

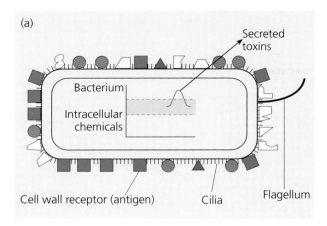

(a)

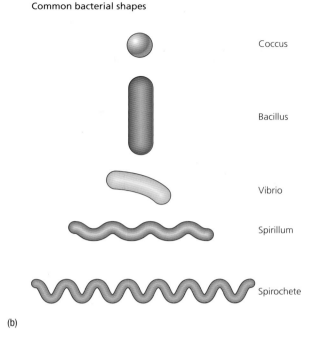

Common bacterial shapes

Coccus

Bacillus

Vibrio

Spirillum

Spirochete

(b)

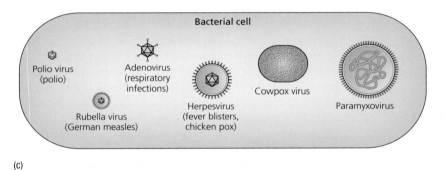

(c)

Figure 13.2 (a) The immunogen is the bacterium, which may have many antigens (i.e. cell-wall receptors). (b) A comparison of the size of common microbes. (c) Classification of bacteria based on morphology

Q Differentiate between the following: (1) immunogen, (2) antigen and (3) pathogen.

Relation of the immune system to cellular homeostasis

The human body's external and internal (or immunological) defences act continually to maintain cellular homeostasis by combating harmful environmental agents. Agents that frequently trigger an immune response are:

- disease-causing microorganisms called pathogens or immunogens (e.g. bacteria and viruses; see section on microbiology and Boxes 13.1 and 13.2);
- membrane surface receptors (antigens) of pathogens (Figure 13.2a);
- pathogenic secretions (e.g. bacterial toxins, which are also antigenic; Figure 13.2a);
- environmental pollutants, such as dust particles (pollutants are in abundance, even, potentially, in operating theatre areas).

Resistance comprises complementary non-specific and specific defence mechanisms. Non-specific resistance is the immunity present at birth. It includes mechanisms that provide immediate but general protection against the invasion of a wide range of pathogens, such as bacteria, viruses, fungi and parasites. These defence mechanisms are the same for everyone, hence the term 'non-specific'. They include:

- external physical and chemical barriers, such as the skin, and chemical barriers, such as the acidity of the stomach;
- internal (bodily) reactions, including the phagocytic response, which provide immunological surveillance against pathogenic microbes and microbial toxins.

Specific resistance is the immunity that is acquired during life upon exposure to harmful agents (termed antigenic insults); it thus develops more slowly. It develops mostly after birth, when an individual becomes exposed to potential environmental hazards. The body system responsible for immunity is the lymphatic system. Specific immunity is the lymphocytic response. It involves activating specific lymphocytes (lymph cells), and stimulating them to release their secretions (cytotoxic substances and antibodies) in response to 'foreign' substances (antigens) entering the body.

BOX 13.1 WHY HEALTHCARE PROFESSIONALS NEED TO UNDERSTAND IMMUNITY

An understanding of immunological homeostasis is important for health-care professionals, since the human body's defences are continually operating to maintain intracellular integrity by waging warfare on harmful environmental agents. These noxious agents are in abundance in hospitals, even in the 'sterile' clinical areas of an operating theatre.

At the turn of the century, of all the patients entering hospital without an infection, 10% would contract a hospital-acquired infection, and at any one time about 20% of all patients in hospital were suffering from a hospital-acquired infection (May, 2000; Salvage 2000). Today, even with all the advances in hygiene the patient is still at risk of acquiring the much publicized methicillin-resistant *Staphylococcus aureus* (MRSA) and *Clostridium difficile* infections. The prevention of such an occurrence is a key nursing and health carer practitioner's responsibility and was one of the main reasons why the 'Modern Matron' was reintroduced to the British National Health Service.

Healthcare practice requires a swift response to dynamic changes associated with the patient's condition (e.g. as with the progressive nature of wound development), wound healing and the stages of infection and fever. All need continued involvement in reassessing, modifying care plans and implementing care according to the patient's changing needs. In relation to the operating theatre, staff must constantly support, monitor and anticipate the side-effects and complications of trauma caused by injury either outside the theatre or by surgery itself.

Aseptic technique is a procedure associated with specific tasks, such as wound dressing, but awareness of the importance of hand washing, cleanliness and prevention of infection to yourself, others and vulnerable patients, is far more important in all healthcare activities and as a result is high on the current government agenda.

Both non-specific and specific immunities are adapted to maintain the equilibrium of the body's internal environment.

The immunity role of the lymphatic system forms the main focus of this chapter, which first continues with an overview of microbiology, including those organisms (pathogens) that cause illness.

OVERVIEW OF MICROBIOLOGY

Microbiology is the study of microbes. A microbe (also called microorganism) is any organism that is visible only with a microscope. These are the smallest, simplest and most numerous organisms on earth.

Classification

Microorganisms existed from before humans. Countless microbes do not normally cause disease in humans, living in a state of either commensalism, where there is little or no benefit or harm to humans, or in mutualism, where there is some benefit gained by both microbes and humans. This non-harmful equilibrium occurs when the human's immunity works well, but these organisms can cause infection when immunity is compromised or fails. This transformed characteristic is shared by numerous microbes, which can bring about infectious disease in the immunocompromised individual, and thus, these organisms are often called pathogens.

Microbes are either autotrophic or heterotrophic. Autotrophic organisms (plants) synthesize food themselves (i.e. 'auto-'), whereas heterotrophic organisms (animals) rely upon other organisms for their food. Some microorganisms live in seclusion, for example, an amoeba (a protozoon) typically lives alone, cruising through the water. Others, however, such as fungi, live in colonies to assist each other to stay alive.

Microorganisms reproduce asexually or sexually. The former term means some microbes divide into two identical pieces, whereas the latter term is used for organisms that need the deoxyribonucleic acid (DNA) of two microbes to produce a new microorganism. Microbes that hold their genes (comprising DNA) in a congregated mass, which floats within the cytoplasm and not inside a nucleus, are termed prokaryotes. Whereas microorganisms that hold their genes in a nucleus are termed eukaryotes. On average, eukaryotic cells are a few hundred times larger than prokaryotic cells.

Most prokaryotes are bacteria – the simplest of organisms – and are very small compared to other cells (although compared to a virus they are large; Figure 13.2b) since they have no organized nucleus, and usually they do not contain most of the usual organelles (i.e. no endoplasmic reticulum, Golgi complex, mitochondria, lysosomes, etc. (see Figure 2.3, p.24 and Table 2.1, p.25). However, they usually possess ribosomes since like any cell or organism their chemical reactions are dependent upon enzymes as biological catalysts and ribosomes are the site of enzyme production (see Figure 2.14, p.41). Prokaryotes cannot perform cell division (mitosis or meiosis) like other cells and microbiologists do not know exactly how they reproduce, but it is not through usual methods.

Eukaryotes have organized DNA in a well-defined nucleus and hence they are able to create cellular organelles. Some eukaryotes can produce the flagellum (a tail-like structure to help it move; see Figure 2.11ci–ii, p.38). They may also be able to produce cilia (little hairs that help scoot the cell through the water). Eukaryotes are self-sufficient organisms and this is thought to have aided them to evolve innovative levels of differentiation and specialization. These organisms are limited in size by their surface area-to-volume ratio, although some eukaryotic cells can grow very large because substances pass into them by diffusion. For example, some eukaryotic slime moulds can swell their size up to a metre wide. The cells of these eukaryotes are multinucleated and this why they can grow very large.

Types of microbes
Viruses

Viruses are the smallest infection-causing microbes found on earth (size between 0.01 and 0.1 μm). The most common viruses found in water are rotavirus and poliovirus (Figure 13.2b). Some microbiologists dispute that viruses cannot be classified as living organisms as they cannot reproduce independently, do not contain functional parts (organelles) found in 'normal' cells, and they are unresponsive to environmental changes.

Viruses need to infect a viral-specific host cell (e.g. animal or plant cells, or other microorganisms) since cannot replicate. The virus is relies upon the host cell to reproduce it. For this reason, viruses are termed obligate intracellular parasites. Outside of the host they are lifeless particles termed virions. They do not need food but they possess a few essential structures:

- They contain a tiny quantity of either DNA or ribonucleic acid (RNA). The nucleic acid is considered the core of the virus.
- Viruses are enclosed by a protein coat (called the capsid), which protects the nucleic acid. The capsid's chemistry helps the virus infect specific host cells by attaching to the host membrane receptor sites.
- Some viruses have a second coat (called the envelope), which is composed of lipids and proteins rather like the way a typical cell membrane is structured. This second coat can also aid a virus penetration into systems unnoticed and help them invade new host cells.

Diseases caused by viruses include the common cold, flu, and common childhood infections such as chicken pox and measles.

Classification of viruses

Viruses are basically classified according to three basic shapes.

1 *Helical*: this group are tube-like viruses as their protein coat (capsid) coils like a garden hose around the centralized core.
2 *Polyhedra*: this group includes the classic virus shape that looks like a 12-sided geometrical shape (i.e. dodecahedron). These viruses have a hard shell of capsomeres (pieces of a capsid). There is a variation of the polyhedral virus known as a globular-shaped virus, which is a polyhedral virion inside a spherical envelope.
3 *Complex*: these viruses have the geometric head but also long projections or 'legs'.

Bacteriophages

Bacteriophages are viruses that infect bacteria. They are used in gene technology to transfer foreign DNA into the nucleic acid of bacterial cells. The bacterium then obtains the capability to perform the function of that particular gene and make a specific enzyme and hence change the metabolism of the cell.

Slime moulds

Slime moulds are autonomous organisms and are not to be confused with fungal moulds, although frequently they act like fungi. Slime moulds comprise two major forms, cellular and acellular moulds.

- Cellular slime moulds are thousands of individual cells that coexist together at the food source. Some do the eating; others reproduce while some build special structures.

- Acellular slime moulds (called plasmodial slime moulds) being multinucleated unicellular organisms can be up to a metre across. The slime moulds 'creep' across the floor of forests digesting everything in their vicinity. Upon reproduction, slime moulds release a variety of spores.

Bacteria

Bacteria are tiny microbes (size between 0.1 and 10 μm). Commonly known species of bacteria are *Salmonella* and *Escherichia coli* (*E. coli*). Bacteria are the simplest of organisms that perform the characteristic of life – reproduction. Bacteria were among the earliest forms of life on earth. The photosynthetic cyanobacteria paved the way for today's algae and plants, and the fossils of this group of bacteria date back more than 3 billion years.

Bacteria exist everywhere – in the air, the soil, the water, in yoghurts, in bread, and in plants and animals, including humans. Thus the human mouth contains in excess of 500 bacterial species. These organisms ideally grow in moist conditions and can live in a large variety of temperatures. In optimal conditions they can reproduce extremely rapidly, producing millions of offspring in a few hours. However, bacteria cannot reproduce in acid conditions (i.e. low pH values). Some bacteria can form protective spores that are resilient to drying and heating. When favourable conditions return, these spores germinate and an active vegetative cell is released.

Bacteria are single cells (i.e. unicellular) although some bacteria can be found in pairs, chains and clusters. Some are mobile by the action of flagella, which may appear singly or in groups spread randomly over the cell surface. Some bacteria possess fimbriae (fringe-like protuberances) that enable them to stick together. Others secrete sticky chemicals on their cell wall, which is situated beyond their cell membrane, and this protects the organism and helps bacteria to stick to other substrates, as well as to other bacteria. Being prokaryotic bacteria do not have any organelles, just cell particulates called ribosomes to enable them to produce enzymes that control their chemical reactions.

Bacteria genes form a tangle known as a nucleoid. Bacterial DNA possesses small loops of DNA (called plasmids) that can be transported from one cell to another, either in the action of sex or by bacteriophage viruses. This ability to transfer genes makes them extremely adaptable for developing antibiotic resistance and these adaptable genes may be multiplied extremely quickly through bacterial populations. Genetic engineering technology has capitalized on this to insert new genes into bacteria.

Bacteria have numerous functions only some of which are mentioned in this text. Some are harmless and live inside animals (e.g. stomachs of cows). These bacteria produce cellulase, an enzyme that breaks down cellulose into sugars, which is useful as otherwise cows could not digest grass and plants. Other bacteria are pathogenic and cause diseases like botulism and serious diseases such as: tuberculosis (TB), tetanus or meningitis. Many bacteria are involved in the decomposition of dead plants and animals.

Classification of bacteria

Bacteria classification is based on their shape or morphology (see Figure 13.2c).

1 *Rod-shaped*: these bacteria multiply making chains like a set of linked sausages.
2 *Lobed or comma-shaped*.
3 *Spiral-shaped*: these bacteria twist a little in the shape of a corkscrew.
4 *Spherical*: these bacteria usually form chains of cells like a row of circles.

In addition to morphology, bacteria have also been classified historically on the basis of their biochemistry and the environmental conditions under which they live. The more recent launch of molecular biology has resulted in the classification of bacteria on the basis of similarities among DNA sequences. Many bacteria are also classified by whether they are Gram-positive or Gram-negative. Gram-positive organisms remain stained with methyl violet after washing with acetone; this reflects differences in the cell walls of the bacteria.

Fungi

Fungi are a large and diverse group of eukaryotic, non-photosynthetic, spore-forming organisms. Fungi are enveloped by a rigid cell wall. The production of energy takes place in mitochondria. Fungal cells have a complex arrangement of internal membranes.

These organisms can be divided into two main groups: filamentous fungi (including moulds and macrofungi such as mushrooms) and yeasts:

• Moulds are multicellular fungi (usually found in damp places) while mushrooms/toadstools are a compilation of strands (called hyphae) living beneath the ground. The hyphae are the 'fungus in action', decomposing leaves or rotting bark; upon reproducing they develop a stalk and cap. Some moulds are problematic, for example producing 'athlete's foot'.
• Yeasts are unicellular fungi. Many are beneficial, for example in bread-making. Some are infectious, for example *Candida* species are responsible for candidiasis (thrush). Some yeasts cause even more serious infections in compromised patients such as those with acquired immune deficiency syndrome (AIDS); see the case study on a young man with symptomatic HIV/AIDS, Section VI, p.656).

Protozoa (protists)

Protozoa are a large collection of eukaryotic, unicellular organisms. Examples include amoebae. Protozoa are very mobile and live on solid nutrients located in water. These organisms do not possess the rigid cell wall found in bacteria. Protozoan size (between 1 and 20 µm) and structure vary, ranging from the simple fluid organization of *Amoeba* to *Paramecium* which contains a fixed shape, and a complex internal organization with specialized organelles. Protozoa have advanced structures that are not associated with other microbes and as such these organisms may be the underpinning organisms from which multicellular organisms have evolved.

Prions

Prions are chemicals, not microorganisms (they do not have the characteristics of living organisms – namely, reproduction) but are worth mentioning here because they can be transmitted from one animal to another and trigger illness. For example, prions are thought to be responsible for 'mad cow' disease (bovine spongiform encephalitis, BSE) and the comparable

---

BOX 13.2 HELPFUL AND HARMFUL MICROBES

Helpful microbes
Some bacteria live symbiotically (i.e. for mutual benefit) in the guts of animals and humans; for example, bacteria in the large intestine of humans utilize the indigestible remains of the human diet, and in return produce vitamins B and K, which are absorbed and utilized.

Other bacteria produce anti-bacterial chemicals (presumably for their own defence) and these are useful to us as antibiotics, for example penicillin and streptomycin. Antibiotics damage bacterial cell walls and this helps our white blood cells to destroy the bacteria. Antibiotics are ineffective against viruses but a doctor may also prescribe an antibiotic if you have a viral infection as a preventative measure against acquiring a secondary bacterial infection.

Some bacteria aid the breakdown of dead organic matter in the soil and, consequently, are a part of the food web in many environments. Nitrogen-fixing bacteria live in the roots of plants and help plants absorb nitrogen from the soil. Nitrogen is important constituents of plant protein and hence is important for the growth of the plant. Because it is also an important constituent of plants enzymes, these tiny bacteria give such plants an advantage for their survival.

Harmful microbes: *Amoeba* to *Paramecium*
Many bacteria cause disease in humans, animals, and plants, and are

noted earlier and elsewhere in this book, but many are harmless and useful. However, the same cannot be said for viruses as their lifecycle makes them pathogenic to their host species. Examples of viruses that are harmful to humans include rabies, pneumonia, meningitis and human immunodeficiency virus (HIV). Immunocompromised animals are more easily infected as they have reduced immune functions. For example younger organisms will have a lowered acquired immunity so are more susceptible than older organisms that have usually been exposed to many environmental antigenic insults as a consequence of their relatively long-term exposure to their environment. However, immunity of elderly people is compromised and so tolerance to antigenic insults is much lower.

Unfortunately, humans appear to be accidentally increasing the pathogenicity of some microorganisms. Antibiotic administration has been the means of treating infection for many, many years and some organisms are now showing signs of having evolved tolerance and so can maintain a subclinical presence in the body. These bacteria in time reproduce, and are responsible for producing an infection, and there is a chance that antibiotics will not work again. Examples are the bacterium methicillin-resistant *Staphylococcus aureus* (MRSA) and the protozoon *Clostridium difficile* (*C. diff.*) that continue to be problematic in hospital environments.

human Creutzfeldt–Jakob disease (CJD variants). Both are fatal diseases in which the brain tissue breaks down.

Biotechnology

Biotechnology is the scientific experimentation with microbes. The use of microbes and their homeostatic components (for example, microbial receptors, genes, enzymes and products of metabolism; see Figure 1.6, p.10) is a way of producing medicines to prevent illnesses, treat illnesses, and to save human lives. Microbiologists have studied how microorganisms behave in plants, animals and humans and in collaboration with immunologists have developed techniques to boost human immunity. Microbiologists are also working with microbes to reduce the negative impact humans have on the environment, for example bacteria that break down oil in water.

Unfortunately, the disadvantage of biotechnology is that techniques are used for harmful reasons, for example production of fatal chemical compounds. Fortunately, the United Nations have developed a treaty on the basis that the majority of the world has chosen not to develop diseases for use in biological warfare since they understand how hazardous and unmanageable these diseases could be.

Effective microbial technology

Effective microbial (EM) technology is now a major science, helping in the production of sustainable practices for agriculture, animal husbandry, organic farming, environmental stewardship, human health and hygiene, and much more. For example, EM technology in agriculture is effective in organic farming, as an alternative to chemical fertilizers. This technology has also been incorporated into livestock, aquaculture and community health services such as waste treatment. Domestically, EM has been introduced, for example, into composting household waste. Some yoghurt-based drinks also contain probiotic bacteria that are claimed to have health benefits – how much needs to be consumed to give such qualities is still under debate.

Household tap water contains microbes, which after a few days will colonize the surfaces with which they are in contact. These colonies form biofilms, which contribute greatly to the microbial contamination of drinking water. Biofilm microbes exhibit an enhanced tolerance against biocides (chemicals that destroy life) and are difficult to remove, especially from non-accessible surfaces and so may recontaminate the water system following disinfection.

Antimicrobial drugs

The use of use of antimicrobial drugs should be fully understood to provide effective and appropriate treatment, prior to their use. Selection of the most appropriate drug can be partly achieved through knowledge of the organism responsible for the infection. The classification of bacteria (see text earlier) is based on their shape (e.g. cocci are spherical, bacilli are rod-shaped) or according to their Gram-positive or Gram-negative properties.

Microbial drugs work in several different ways in order to inhibit bacterial growth. For example:

- *Nitroimidazoles* inhibit nucleic acid synthesis. Metronidazole (a nitroimidazole drug) is active against most anaerobic bacteria and some protozoa. It is used in the treatment of postoperative anaerobic infections and peritonitis. Because it has no action against aerobic organisms it is used as a combined treatment with other antimicrobial drugs.
- *Penicillins, cephalosporins and vancomycin* inhibit cell wall synthesis. The penicillins (e.g. benzylpenicillin) are effective against Gram-positive organisms, such as *Staphylococcus aureus*, which commonly causes wound infections, pneumonia and septicaemia. In situations where the infection is caused by penicillin-resistant staphylococci, flucloxacillin is often used, as it is resistant to the penicillinase produced by resistant bacteria. Cefuroxime belongs to the group of cephalosporin antibiotics; it is given by injection and often used as a prophylactic in surgery and in conjunction with metronidazole. It is effective in combating serious infection where other antibiotics are ineffective. As infections are becoming more resistant to antimicrobial treatments more powerful drugs are being developed. Vancomycin is a bactericidal antibiotic that is active against most Gram-positive organisms. It is important in the treatment of patients with septicaemia or endocarditis caused by methicillin-resistant *Staphylococcus aureus*.
- *Aminoglycosides* inhibit protein (hence enzyme) synthesis. Aminoglycoside drugs such as gentamicin are used to treat acute life threatening Gram-negative infections, such as *Pseudomonas aeruginosa*, until antibiotic sensitivity is known.

OVERVIEW OF THE ANATOMY AND PHYSIOLOGY OF THE LYMPHATIC SYSTEM

Lymphatic vessels and the lymphatic circulation

The lymphatic capillaries are thin, closed-ended vessels present in all body tissues, except in the spleen and in those areas not serviced directly by the circulation (e.g. cornea of the eye), the central nervous system and bone marrow. The lymphatics of the skin travel in loose subcutaneous adipose tissue, generally following veins, whereas visceral lymphatics generally follow arteries, forming networks (called plexuses) around them. Lymph (the tissue fluid inside the lymphatics) is produced at a rate of about 1.5 mL/minute throughout the body. The lymphatics merge, forming larger vessels, the largest of which drain into two large ducts called the right lymphatic duct and the thoracic duct.

These ducts empty their contents into blood within the neck region, at the junction of the left subclavian and jugular veins (Figure 13.3a,b). By preventing tissue fluid accumulation, this drainage helps to ensure that a constant blood volume and composition is maintained. Approximately 2–4 L of interstitial fluids accumulate and return to the blood in 24 hours. This results in a constant turnover of tissue fluid. If, however, the return of lymph is blocked, as in the case of tumour compression, then tissue fluid accumulates (oedema) distal to the obstruction.

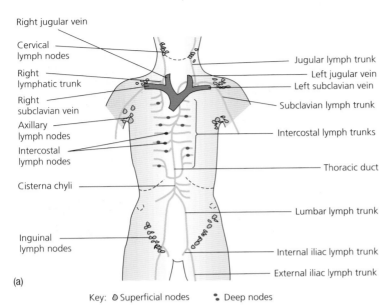

Right jugular vein
Cervical lymph nodes
Right lymphatic trunk
Right subclavian vein
Axillary lymph nodes
Intercostal lymph nodes
Cisterna chyli
Inguinal lymph nodes

Jugular lymph trunk
Left jugular vein
Left subclavian vein
Subclavian lymph trunk
Intercostal lymph trunks
Thoracic duct
Lumbar lymph trunk
Internal iliac lymph trunk
External iliac lymph trunk

(a)

Key: ◎ Superficial nodes   ⦂ Deep nodes

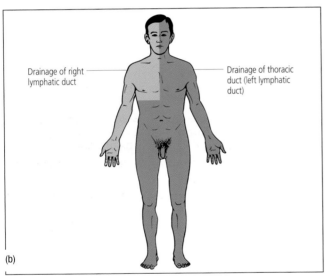

Drainage of right lymphatic duct

Drainage of thoracic duct (left lymphatic duct)

(b)

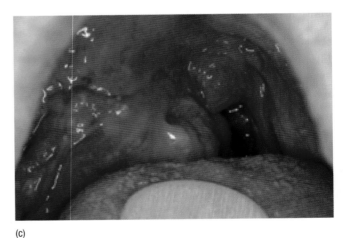

(c)

Figure 13.3 (a) The main vessels and nodes of the lymphatic system. (b) Lymphatic drainage into the circulation. The right lymphatic duct drains the right side of the head and neck, and the right arm. The thoracic lymphatic duct drains the rest of the body. (c) Patient exhibiting right-sided tonsillitis. Reproduced with the kind permission of the Medical Illustration Department, Norfolk and Norwich University Hospital NHS Trust

Q Outline the clinical importance of lymph nodes.

BOX 13.3 LYMPHOEDEMA FOLLOWING SURGICAL REMOVAL OF BREAST CANCER

Upon surgical removal of the axillary lymph glands, such as in the treatment of breast cancer, the disruption of lymph drainage from the limb means that the patient frequently has arm oedema (lymphoedema; see 2.17d, p.46). The patient may experience problems such as heavy, painful arms and skin tightness and swelling, causing an alteration of body image in addition to the breast surgery; in some patients there is a consequential loss of self-esteem. Management of the lymphoedema consists of skin care, massage and compression, advice on activities, exercise and psychological support.

Return of lymph to the circulation

The flow rate of lymph is very slow compared with blood. Two factors control lymph flow rate, and hence its return to blood:

* *Tissue pressure*: when tissue fluid pressure (i.e. volume), rises above its homeostatic range, there is a greater formation of lymph, which enhances its flow rate and drains the excess fluid.

* *Lymphatic pump*: lymph vessels have valves that promote unidirectional movement towards the neck region, so lymph can be returned to the blood circulation. The flow of lymph is encouraged via the compression exerted by muscles and other tissues surrounding the lymphatic vessels. These muscles and tissues are referred to as the 'lymphatic pumps'. Increased metabolic rate (such as experienced during exercise and stress) increases the efficiency of lymphatic pumps. This

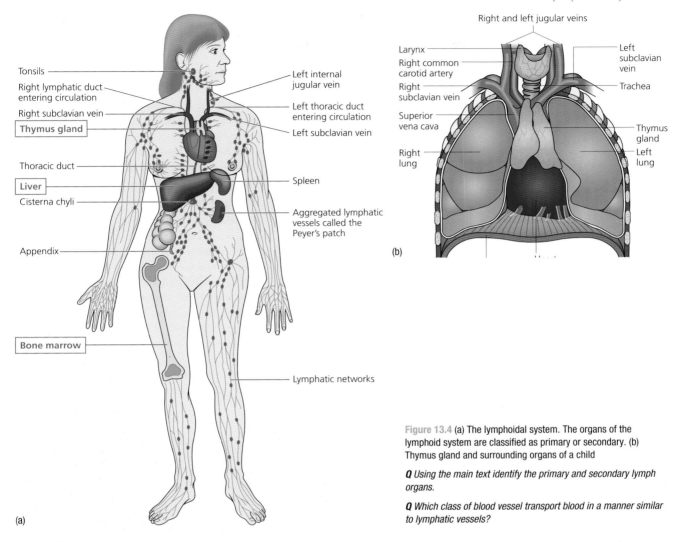

Figure 13.4 (a) The lymphoidal system. The organs of the lymphoid system are classified as primary or secondary. (b) Thymus gland and surrounding organs of a child

Q Using the main text identify the primary and secondary lymph organs.

Q Which class of blood vessel transport blood in a manner similar to lymphatic vessels?

is a homeostatic necessity, since an increased metabolic rate is associated with a larger blood flow to the highly metabolizing cells, resulting in greater tissue fluid formation. Consequently, greater lymph formation results, producing a greater flow rate of lymph to maintain blood volume, hence blood pressure.

The lymphoidal system

In addition to fluid and solutes of the tissue fluid, lymph contains specialized cells (T- and B-lymphocytes; see later) that form an important part of the mechanism by which the body defends itself against infection by microbes. The cells are found in various organs that comprise the lymphoidal system, which may be classified as primary or secondary (Figure 13.4). It is the primary organs (bone marrow, thymus and fetal liver)

that produce the lymphocytes. These then travel to the secondary organs (spleen, lymph nodes, and other lymphoidal tissue throughout the body).

Lymph nodes

Lymphatic nodes are oval-shaped masses of lymphatic tissue encapsulated by dense, connective tissue. The organ consists of:

- *cortex:* contains B-lymphocytes aggregated into primary follicles. Following an antigenic insult (i.e. presence of non-self chemicals), these follicles develop into a focus of active growth or proliferation, and are then termed secondary follicles. These follicles are in intimate contact with the antigen-presenting cells of the system;
- *paracortex:* contains T-lymphocytes;
- *medulla:* contains T- and B-lymphocytes.

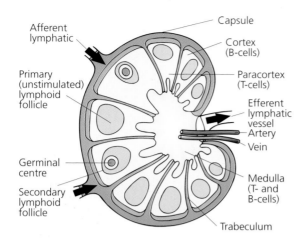

Figure 13.5 Structure of a lymph node

Q Why are lymph nodes associated with the spleen, thymus and gut considered to be organs of the lymphatic system?

The roles of the T- and B-lymphocytes are described later. Each node has internal extensions of fibrous capsule, called trabeculae, which dip through the outer cortex and inner medullar regions of the node (Figure 13.5). Nodes can exist individually, located randomly (e.g. the urogenital and respiratory mucous membranes), or they can exist as multiple nodular complexes located at specific sites (e.g. the tonsils, and Peyer's patches, appendix, spleen and thymus gland) (see Figure 13.4a).

Afferent vessels transport lymph into the node sinuses (a series of irregular channels), after which it circulates into one or two outgoing (efferent) vessels located at the exit. Efferent vessels are wider than afferent vessels; they contain valves that open away from the nodes and encourage the flow of lymph in one direction.

Nodular filtering action: a homeostatic function

Antigens (any immune-activating chemical) become entrapped in the lymph nodes as they filter the lymph passing through the lymphatic network during its passage from the periphery to the thoracic ducts. They are destroyed via:

- phagocytosis by white blood cells called macrophages (see Chapter 11, pp.283–5);
- secretion of cytotoxic chemicals (e.g. interleukin, interferon) by T-lymphocytes;
- antibodies produced and secreted by B-lymphocytes.

The thymus gland

The thymus is positioned in the upper thorax above and in front of the heart, between the lungs, and behind the sternum. It extends back into the root of the neck (see Figure 13.4b).

The size of the thymus increases until puberty. It begins to involute during adolescence, and by middle age it has returned to its size at birth (see Figure 13.4a,b for a comparison of child and adult sizes). Despite this reduction in size during adulthood, evidence suggests that the thymus continues to function throughout life. However, the effectiveness of its lymphocytes in response to antigenic insults declines.

Structure of the thymus

The thymus is a bilobed gland encapsulated by fibrous tissue. Each lobe has a peripheral cortex and a central medulla. The cortex consists of small, medium and large, tightly packed lymphocytes; the medulla comprises mainly epithelial cells and diffused scattered lymphocytes. Internal capsular extensions (trabeculae) divide the organ into lobules, which consist of an irregular branching framework of epithelial cells responsible for the production of thymus secretions and lymphocytes.

Homeostatic functions of the thymus

The thymus is primarily responsible for the production and support of T-cells. Such cells originate in the bone marrow, where stem cells differentiate into specialized lymphocytes in a process called lymphopoiesis. The majority of these cells enter the thymus, where they develop in the cortex into stem T-lymphocytes. These undergo cell division (mitosis), and upon maturation move into the medulla. These mature cells remain in systemic blood, enter systemic blood, and are transported to lymphoidal tissue, or remain in the thymus gland, to become the future generations of T-lymphocytes.

Epithelial cells of the gland also produce thymosin, a hormone responsible for the maturation of the thymus and other lymphoidal tissue.

BOX 13.4 DI GEORGE SYNDROME

The role of the thymus to produce T-lymphocytes means that children suffering from Di George syndrome, who are born without a thymus, are highly susceptible to those infections usually defended by T-cells. Death may occur unless a healthy thymus graft is transplanted. Children may also be born with B-cell deficiencies and so are subject to infections usually defended primarily by antibodies. These children require repeated injection of serum antibodies from healthy donors.

The spleen

The adult spleen is the largest collection of lymphoid tissue in the body. It is approximately 12 cm long, 7 cm wide and 2.5 cm thick, and weighs about 150 g. The spleen is positioned in the left of the abdomen, lying between the stomach and diaphragm (Figure 13.4a).

Structure of the spleen

Anteriorly, the spleen's encapsulated surface is covered with peritoneum. The organ's oval shape is determined by structures that are in close proximity (Figures 13.4a and 13.6a). It contains a number of surface features including:

- a gastric impression (the organ's soft consistency enables its shape to change according to the stomach's contents);
- a renal impression;
- a colon impression;
- a smooth, convex diaphragmatic surface, that conforms to the concave surface of the adjacent diaphragm.

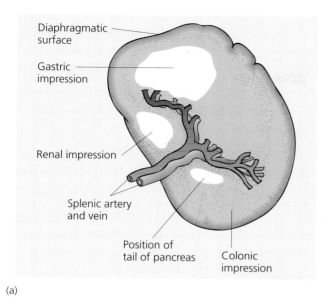

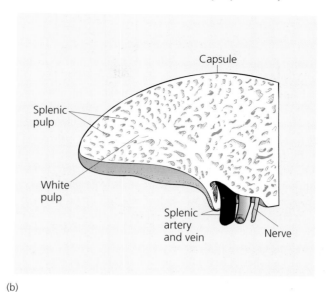

(a)

(b)

Figure 13.6 (a) The spleen: the oval shape is determined by the structures in close proximity to it. (b) Section of the spleen

The organ is divided into an outer red pulp, which contains sinuses filled with blood, and a centrally located white pulp consisting of lymphatic tissue. The latter contains lymphocytes and macrophages. Entering and leaving the spleen are the splenic artery and vein, efferent lymphatics (vessels leaving the spleen) and a nerve supply (Figure 13.6b). Blood in the splenic artery flows into the spleen's sinuses; these have pores between the lining endothelial cells, allowing blood to come into close association with the pulp cells.

Homeostatic functions of the spleen

The spleen performs the same functions for blood that lymph nodes perform for lymph and is involved with:

- *phagocytosis:* because the spleen is part of the reticuloendothelial system, it has phagocytes that are involved with the breakdown of red blood cells (erythrocytes). The breakdown products bilirubin, iron and globin are released from haemoglobin (see Figure 11.7, p.279), and are passed to the liver by splenic and portal veins. Leucocytes, thrombocytes and

microbes are also phagocytosed in the spleen. The spleen has no afferent lymphatics, so it is not exposed to infections spread via the lymphatic system;
- *development of lymphocytes:* the spleen produces T-lymphocytes and, in particular, B-lymphocytes.

In addition to these immunological functions, the spleen acts as a blood reservoir, releasing blood on demand (e.g. following severe haemorrhage). This release is controlled by the sympathetic nervous system and is a homeostatic mechanism that helps to maintain the composition of body fluids.

ACTIVITY

Before studying the next section, reflect on your understanding of the meaning of 'immunity', and the difference between the specific and non-specific immune responses. Suggest why the spleen-, thymus- and gut-associated lymph nodes are considered organs of the lymphatic system.

BOX 13.5 HOMEOSTATIC IMBALANCES OF THE SPLEEN AND THYMUS

Splenomegaly (enlargement of the spleen) usually occurs secondary to other conditions, such as circulatory disorders and infections, or cirrhosis of the liver.

Hyperactivity of the spleen increases its phagocytic activities and leads to a reduced blood cell count (i.e. anaemia, thrombocytopenia and leucopenia). Surgical removal – splenectomy – is the only known cure for this condition.

Rupture of the spleen because of its soft consistency is quite common in traumatic injuries, such as broken ribs. Rupture causes severe intraperitoneal haemorrhage, and may lead to shock (see Figure 12.32, p.355). Following diagnosis, the condition is stabilized with blood transfusion. Splenectomy is performed to prevent the patient bleeding to death.

Once bleeding has been controlled the person soon recovers. A missing or non-functional spleen produces hyposplenism when people may be more prone to microbial infection, for example special immunization programmes are recommended. However, it does not normally pose a serious problem. Healthcare professionals can anticipate and prevent the anxiety of 'How long can I live without my spleen?' by explaining that blood cells, especially white cells, produced in other areas of the body (e.g. bone marrow, liver) take over, and that there is a mass of other lymphatic tissue to cope with the spleen's former immunological role.

Hypertrophy of the thymus is associated with autoimmune disease of the thyroid (thyrotoxicosis).

PHYSIOLOGY OF THE LYMPHATIC SYSTEM: LYMPH FORMATION

Chapter 6, pp.124–6 discussed how positive filtration pressures in blood capillaries cause the secretion (exudation) of fluid from plasma, resulting in the formation of tissue fluid, and how negative filtration pressures at the venous ends of capillaries ensure that tissue fluid is returned to the blood. Figure 6.2 (p.124), summarizes this capillary exchange process. The return, however, cannot compensate totally for the loss, thus there is a potential for the accumulation of tissue fluid. In addition, because capillary walls are slightly permeable to protein, there is a slow but steady loss of small blood proteins to tissue fluid. These proteins cannot be returned to the circulation across capillary walls, since there is insufficient fluid pressure to move them in that direction.

The lymphatics drain the tissue fluid that is in excess of its homeostatic range, and so returns the contents, such as proteins, to the blood. The endothelial cells of lymphatic vessels are not bound tightly, but they overlap; the regions of overlap function as one-way valves. These permit the entry of fluid (and the small exuded proteins) into the vessels, but prevent their return to the interstitial spaces. Accumulation of tissue fluid causes the tissues to swell; the increased tissue fluid pressure opens the endothelial valves further, so more fluid can flow into the lymph capillaries. The larger capillaries also contain semilunar valves. These are quite close together and each causes the vessel to bulge, giving the lymphatic system a beaded appearance (see Figure 13.4a, p.367). As discussed earlier, these valves aid normal lymphatic flow. On its return journey to blood, lymph flows through one or more lymph nodes. Their homeostatic function is to filter the lymph of potential antigenic material, and then destroy pathogens and their toxins (described later).

The large thoracic duct receives lymph from vessels below the diaphragm, from the left half of the head, neck and chest,

---

BOX 13.6 HOMEOSTATIC IMBALANCES OF THE LYMPHATIC SYSTEM

There are multiple clinical conditions associated with lymphatic homeostatic imbalances. This box considers two ways in which lymphatic function can be jeopardized: the spread of disease, leading to lymphatic infections and/or tumours, and lymphatic obstruction.

Spread of disease

Lymph capillaries drain tissue fluid, which may contain pathogens and tumour cells. If these are not phagocytosed, they may settle and multiply in the first lymph node they encounter, thus producing localized infection (see Figure 13.3c, p.366, tonsillitis) or tumours. Alternatively, subsequent to proliferation, they may spread to other lymph nodes, blood or other parts of the body, using the body's transporting systems. Consequently, each new site of infection or (metastatic) tumour becomes a further source of infection or malignant cells via the same routes, thus producing infections or tumours elsewhere, such as in tonsillitis, appendicitis, glandular fever, lymphoma, thymoma and splenomas. Breast cancer frequently shows lymphatic spread.

Inflammation of the lymphatic vessels (lymphangitis) may cause the vessel to be visible in the superficial vessels as a red streak tracking to the next set of lymph nodes (e.g. from an infected toe to the nodes at the back of the knee).

Infections and tumours, and the presence of excessive amounts of abnormal material such as bacteria and their toxins, can cause lymph node and lymph organ enlargement (Figure 13.7). With a 'sore throat' or a 'cold', the cervical (neck) lymph nodes enlarge in response to the infection. Lay people often claim that their 'glands are up', but please note that lymph nodes are not glands, as they do not secrete. Glands are 'up' because the nodes are actively producing lymphocytes to defend against the incoming antigens. The nodes only become swollen and painful when the immunogen (e.g. bacteria) has infected the node and the person's defence mechanisms are compromised.

The enlargement is reversed when the infection subsides (either naturally or by using clinical intervention, e.g. antibiotic therapy), and/or the tumour or abnormal particle is destroyed or moved on (see Figure 2.17c, p.46, cancer before and after surgery). Reinfections, new tumours or reintroduced abnormal particles, however, result in tissue fibrosis and a continued enlargement. Lymphatic organs that become chronically inflamed are associated with abscess formation and may require surgical removal to reduce the incidence and severity of subsequent infections.

Cancerous lymph nodes, as well as feeling large, are firm, non-tender and fixed to underlying structures. In contrast, infected lymph nodes that are enlarged due to infection are not firm, are moveable, and are very tender. The cancerous nodes often become the sites of metastatic cancer.

Lymphatic obstruction

Tumours, depending upon their site and growth, can cause obstruction inside lymphatic vessels or inside nodes. In addition, if external to the lymphatic vessel, they may cause sufficient external pressure to restrict lymph flow. Surgery to remove lymph node cancers and to prevent metastases can also result in lymphatic obstruction. The accumulation of lymph as a result of the obstruction to lymph flow results in a swelling, called lymphoedema, the extent of which depends upon the size of the obstructed vessel (see Figure 2.17d, p.46). Lymphoedema also occurs as a consequence of local inflammation, and the subsequent lymphatic fibrosis, which enhances this condition. Other causes of lymphoedema include damage from surgery, radiotherapy or parasitic disease, such as filariasis (infestation with tiny thread-like worms).

Lymphoidal tumours are classified as Hodgkin's and non-Hodgkin's lymphomas. Hodgkin's lymphoma, a malignant disease, is initially a homeostatic imbalance of cell division (hyperplasia) in the superficial lymph glands, which metastasize to other lymphoidal tissues throughout the body. Although white blood cell counts are elevated, the cells are immature. Specific complications include a deficiency of cell-mediated immunity and thus an increased susceptibility to microbial infections. This disease was formerly always fatal; however, isolated bouts of radiotherapy, or combined radiochemotherapy, have considerably improved the prospects of securing remission for long periods. The effectiveness of treatment depends largely on the stage of disease when the treatment is begun.

Non-Hodgkin's tumours occur in the lymphoidal tissue and bone marrow, and are classified as low grade or high grade. Low-grade lymphomas are well-differentiated tumours that progress slowly; death occurs usually after several years. High-grade lymphomas are poorly differentiated tumours that progress rapidly; death occurs in weeks or months.

Thymomas (thymus tumours) and splenomas (spleen tumours) are rare. Node and organ enlargement caused by tumour growth usually necessitates surgical removal, since complications may arise because of growth interfering with the functions of adjacent structures.

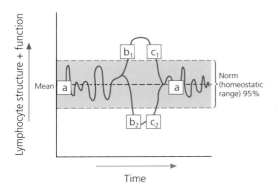

Figure 13.7 Lymphocytic structure and function: a homeostatic process. (a) Normal lymphocytic function and structure. b_1, Hyperplasia of lymphatic tissue and organs. Tumours are examples of permanent failures of hyperplasia, such as lymphomas (Hodgkin's and non-Hodgkin's), thymoma (rare, but occurs in myasthenia gravis) and splenomas (hypersplenism). Pathogenic infections are examples of temporary hyperplasia, such as tonsillitis (bacterial infection), glandular fever (viral infection) and splenomegaly (secondary infected site). These are signs that the immune system is attempting to restore homeostasis. b_2, Homeostatic failures associated with hypoplasia of lymphoidal tissue and organs, such as hyposplenism (missing or functionless spleen). c_1, Clinical correction involves radiotherapy, chemotherapy, surgical removal (only cure for hypersplenism) or, more commonly, a combination of the above to remove permanent hyperplastic failures. Correction of temporary hyperplastic failures depends upon type of infection (e.g. antibiotic therapy for tonsillitis or rest for glandular fever). c_1, Correction involves special immunization programmes. (a, Represents boxes a_1–a_4, p.11, reflecting the individual variability in the homeostatic range)

and empties into the venous system, close to the junction of the left internal jugular and left subclavian veins. The smaller right lymphatic duct ends at a comparable location on the right side. It drains lymph from the right side of the body above the diaphragm (see Figure 13.3a,b, p.366).

The lymphatic system is therefore a homeostatic mechanism for the maintenance of body fluid composition and volume. Clinical conditions that inhibit such a return may influence fluid distribution to such an extent that death can occur in less than 24 hours if the balance is not restored.

ACTIVITY

Describe the relationship between plasma, tissue fluid and lymph. Which factors promote the flow of lymph?

PHYSIOLOGY OF THE IMMUNE SYSTEM: THE IMMUNE RESPONSES AND DEFENCE MECHANISMS

There are many ways that harmful microbes can spread:

- *Person-to-person*: by the mixing of: blood (e.g. by sharing needles), saliva (e.g. by kissing) or, for very infectious diseases, through the air (e.g. by coughing or sneezing).
- *By food*: bacteria may survive in food if it is inadequately cooked or if it is reheated, and can give you food poisoning.
- *By water*: contaminated water may spread diseases, such as typhoid or cholera.
- *By insects* many diseases are spread by insects. Bubonic plague (Black Death), for example, is carried by fleas living on rats, and malaria is carried by mosquitoes in certain parts of the world.

How can we protect ourselves against infectious diseases? The following section is concerned with:

- how the external defences are adapted to prevent the entry of environmental hazards into the body;
- how the internal defences operate following external defence failure;

- how immunization, monoclonal antibodies and transplantation are used for the benefit of the individual;
- what happens when the immune mechanisms malfunction.

The human body has many natural defences that help prevent harmful microbes entering and causing harm. Our external and internal defence mechanisms both exhibit non-specific (i.e. common) and specific responses. Non-specific immunity has two roles: to prevent the entry of any pathogenic agents into the body, and to prevent the spread of those agents that have successfully gained entrance to the body. The role of specific immunity goes beyond this by mounting a coordinated response against infection by an individual type of microbe (i.e. a specific antigen).

External defence mechanisms

The non-specific components of the external defence mechanisms include (Figure 13.8):

- skin and mucous membranes;
- digestive reflexes and secretions;
- tears;
- lysozymes;
- urination and defecation;
- placenta and mammary glands;
- memory and stress response.

Skin and mucous membranes

The skin and mucous membranes are the body's first line of resistance. Both act as physical barriers that prevent pathogenic agents from entering their target tissues. For example, the viruses that cause hepatitis must gain access to liver cells. These organisms, however, must first penetrate external barriers to enter blood, which then transports them to their target sites.

The intact skin is the most effective external barrier of the body. It provides a watertight barricade, protecting the internal organs (viscera) from infection. The effectiveness becomes apparent only when there is widespread damage to the skin. For example, with serious burns, infection becomes a real danger, and infection prevention and control are major considerations in treating burns patients.

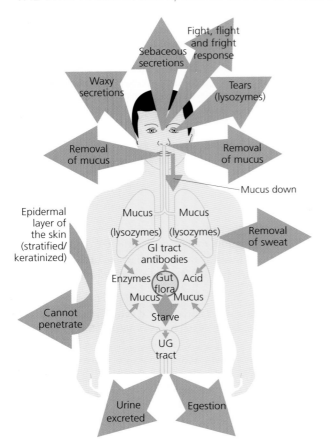

Figure 13.8 The physical and chemical barriers of natural immunity and potential sites of infection. GI, gastrointestinal; UG, urogenital

Q Describe how the acid and alkali pH along the gastrointestinal tract is related to providing immunity.

BOX 13.7 INFECTIONS: A FAILURE OF THE EXTERNAL BARRIERS

When the epidermis and the blood vessels in the dermis are damaged by cuts (see Figures 11.13, p.290 and 11.17, p.295) and burns, the person is potentially exposed to pathogenic infection, in particular staphylococcal infections, since the natural habitats of *Staphylococcus* (a type of bacterium) include hair follicles and sweat glands. Other environmental pathogens may also seize the opportunity (e.g. it is common for tetanus-causing bacteria to be introduced into the circulation via gardening injuries). Since skin wounds are common, tetanus immunization programmes have been developed to prevent this type of infection. Blood clots produce a scab if the skin is cut, which stops bacteria from invading using the open wound and, of course, stops the bleeding.

When adhesive tape is removed from the skin, it removes much of the stratum corneum, thus making the skin much more permeable at that site. The use of detergents and organic solvents, such as white spirit and turps, also increases the permeability of the skin. These chemicals dissolve components of the lipid matrix between cells and allow fluid to enter the spaces, which act as channels for the diffusion of water-soluble substances.

Prolonged soaking in water changes the character of the skin's surface. The epidermal cells 'swell' as they take up more water and the properties of the barrier change. Skin infections are therefore much more frequent in people whose skin is regularly soaked in water. Perhaps a contributory factor for this type of infection is the washing away of protective secretions.

surface each day. These characteristics make this tissue a formidable physical barrier for the entrance of potential pathogenic materials, and bacteria rarely penetrate the intact healthy epidermis. In addition, new epidermal cells are continually being formed because the skin is constantly subjected to abrasion and injury. The epidermis is normally renewed every 15–30 days. A potential risk for access of microbes arises when there is a reduced blood supply to the skin as erosion of the skin tissue occurs, and any tissue breakdown occurs more quickly.

Chemical factors

The epidermal surface contains sweat and sebaceous glands. Sweat and sebum secretions are acidic (pH 5.5) in nature, which discourages the growth of alkali-liking microbes whose enzymes cannot operate in such conditions. The acidic pH, however, encourages growth of microbes whose enzymes favour this environment. However, these organisms must still penetrate the stratified epidermis if they are to cause infection in the organs of the body. Sweat and sebum also contain bactericidal chemicals (i.e. chemicals that kill bacteria), antibodies and lysozymes, which contribute to the skin's functions of protection and defence. Sebum, for example, inhibits the growth of certain bacteria, such as *Streptococcus*, which are the main cause of sore throats.

Perspiration (sweating) actively removes some microbes from the skin's surface. Changing climatic conditions can, however, alter the skin's resistance to certain infections. For example, hot, humid environments, in which sweat evaporation is limited, encourage fungal infections, such as athlete's foot.

The skin contains two principal layers: the outer epidermis and the inner dermis. Together, they provide physical and chemical protection.

ACTIVITY

Before going any further, use Figures 16.1, p.447 and 16.5, p.452 to review the structure and functions of skin.

Physical factors

The epidermis is a stratified epithelium. The stratum corneum (outer layer) is toughened by cells containing the waterproofing protein keratin, which provides the primary barrier to the loss of water and other hydrophilic (water-liking) substances from the body. The lipid matrix in which cells are embedded is not penetrated easily by hydrophilic substances (i.e. water does not pass through lipids). Also, proteins inside cells attract and hold on to those molecules. This restricts water loss from the body. Consequently, the surface of the skin is normally fairly dry, and only a small amount of water is lost from the

Skin derivatives, such as hair and nails, protect the epidermis from mechanical abrasion and consequential damage from hazardous stimuli. Ceruminous secretion (earwax) also acts as an external barrier to microbes.

The skin's interactive roles with the body's specific immune responses are discussed later.

Mucous membranes line those body cavities that are open to the external environment. The principal cavities concerned are the respiratory, digestive and urogenital tracts. Mucus is a viscous secretion that prevents membrane desiccation (drying out); its adhesive properties trap microbes, and so prevent their spread. In some regions, cilia remove the entrapped materials from the body. For example, respiratory epithelia move mucus (and inhaled noxious agents) to the throat. This stimulates coughing or sneezing reflexes to remove the mucoidal mixture to the external environment (unfortunately, this is also a highly effective way of spreading infection), or the mucus is simply swallowed and gastrointestinal secretions usually destroy any microbes present (see below).

The pH of mucus, and the presence of lysozymes and antibodies, contributes to epithelial defence functions. Mucous membranes, however, are less effective than the skin at inhibiting microbial penetration. Infection is therefore more frequent in body cavities that are open to the external environment. Common microbial infections of the respiratory, digestive and urogenital mucous membranes include colds, influenza, gastroenteritis and sexually transmitted infections.

Digestive reflexes and secretions

Information from our sensory taste buds and olfactory sensory receptors regarding the palpability of food will either enhance our desire to eat or lead us to reject it. In the digestive tract, reflex diarrhoea and vomiting (D&V) expel unwanted invaders and hence protect the epithelia.

After swallowing, the vomiting reflex is a mechanism of rejection of food and its microbial content. The vomiting centre of the brain, located in the medulla oblongata, receives signals from receptors in the upper respiratory tract and the chemoreceptor trigger zone in the medulla oblongata itself. Receptors in the upper digestive tract monitor the volume and composition of ingested products, whereas cells in the medulla are sensitive to blood-borne chemicals, including drugs such as apomorphine.

The vomiting reflex triggers the relaxation of the stomach and retroperistalsis ('retro-' = reverse) of the small intestine. These events hold substances in the stomach. Simultaneously, the glottis closes, closing off the respiratory tract. Contractions of the abdominal muscles and diaphragm squeeze the stomach and expel its contents through the oesophagus and into the mouth. The pressure in the stomach drives the part of the oesophagus that usually lies in the abdomen up into the thorax, causing the cardiac sphincter function to be lost (see Figure 10.9, p.242). The vomiting reflex is accompanied by a generalized activation of sympathetic nervous system, which causes increased salivation, sweating, tachycardia and cutaneous vasoconstriction.

Irritation of the lower digestive tract causes secretion and contractile activity that promotes expulsion of irritants via the rectum, as in diarrhoea. Irritants include bacterial toxins (e.g. cholera toxin) and plant products used as laxatives (e.g. senna). Cells of the gastrointestinal epithelium are constantly shed, thus this epithelium must undergo constant renewal to sustain its homeostatic function. These cells are digested; the products are absorbed and reused in cell metabolism. The rapid replacement of gastric cells in the stomach may be an important way to protect the stomach against erosion-producing ulcers.

The main digestive secretions are:

- *Saliva*: in addition to its digestive properties, saliva has defence functions, including:
  - washing and cleansing the teeth, gums and mouth, thus removing food particles that otherwise would encourage bacterial growth and the consequential formation of acids, which may lead to dental caries, loss of teeth, or gum abscess;
  - discouraging the growth of acidophilic (acid-liking) microbes by inactivating their enzymes through saliva being alkaline (pH 7.2–8);
  - containing antibodies (salivary immunoglobulin A, IgA) that helps destroy microbes, or coats them and prevents them accessing the mucosal membranes.
- *Gastric juice*: food (and the inevitable presence of microbes) is swallowed and passed to the stomach. In this region, gastric acid (pH 2–3) destroys alkalophilic (alkali-liking) microbes and bacterial toxins. Conversely, the stomach's pH encourages growth of acidophilic microbes that have escaped the pH effects of saliva (e.g. the bacterium *Helicobacter*).
- *Intestinal juice*: the intestinal alkaline fluid (pH 7–8) destroys acidophilic microbes that escape from the stomach into the duodenum.

Digestive secretions therefore have important external defence properties by destroying (denaturing) microbial enzymes, and so promoting microbial death. Gastrointestinal tract infections such as gastroenteritis occur when these defence functions are overwhelmed.

Lachrymal secretions (tears)

Lachrymal secretions are continually secreted and blinking spreads them over the eye surface. This continual washing action helps to dilute microbes and keep them from settling on the surface of the eye. Tears only become evident, however, when they are secreted in excess. Hypersecretion may be caused by the presence of large microbial colonies or irritants on the eye surface, or when the individual is overcome by severe emotions.

Enzymes and antibodies (called IgA) in tears break down microbes to stop them entering the body; however, if they are unsuccessful in preventing the entrance of entrapped dust particles and microbes, these are directed towards the nasal passageways via the lachrymal ducts. Respiratory and digestive defences then usually destroy pathogenic materials.

Lysozymes

Lysozymes are a variety of catalytic enzymes (nucleases, proteases, lipases, carbohydrases, etc.) that are capable of 'digesting' potential pathogens. Lysozymes are abundant in tissue fluids, tears, saliva and nasal secretions, so their effects are widespread.

Urination and defecation

Urine and faecal matter are potential media for the growth of pathogenic organisms, although urine is sterile when first produced. Frequent urination and defecation, especially the latter, helps to prevent excessive growth of these colonies.

Placenta and lactation

The development of the placenta during pregnancy and the process of lactation following birth provide further routes of potential pathogenic invasion of the fetus and newborn, and possibly the mother.

Memory and stress response

Once the individual has become conditioned to identify potential environmental threats (e.g. the expected presence of pathogenic microbes or corrosive acids) then memory and the stress response are involved in avoiding such potential hazards.

> ### ACTIVITY
>
> Identify how each external defence mechanism attempts to prevent the entry of environmental hazards ('antigenic insults').

Internal non-specific defence mechanisms

External defences are mainly non-specific but non-specific immune responses are also observed internally; these include the inflammatory and phagocytic and chemical responses to antigens. Internal defences also include the specific immune responses (called the lymphocytic response) that act against specific antigens. These will be described later.

Inflammation

Inflammation has both protective and defensive roles, and acts to restore tissue homeostasis by neutralizing and destroying antigens at the site of an injury. Inflammation is an internal defence mechanism representing a coordinated non-specific response to tissue injury (i.e. the processes involved are the same in response to any antigenic insult or wound damage). The appearance of the inflamed area, however, depends upon two factors:

- *Strength of environmental hazard (or stimulus) applied*: the weakest stimulus produces a reflex vasoconstriction, causing the inflamed area to pale, whereas stronger stimuli produce vasodilation of capillary networks, then arterioles, bringing a flush to the tissue. The strongest stimulus produces a raised wheal around the lesion or wound. Such inflammation is

> ### BOX 13.8 FEVER ASSOCIATED WITH INFECTION AND INFLAMMATION
>
> Fever commonly occurs during infection and inflammation. Many bacterial toxins elevate body temperature, sometimes by causing the release of fever-causing cytokines (cyte = cell; kine = excite/move) – chemicals released to promote activity of defence cells, collectively called pyrogens (note, fever = pyrexia). Elevated body temperature intensifies the actions of interferons, inhibits the growth of some microbes, and speeds up body reactions that aid repair.

usually associated with redness, pain, heat and swelling. The injured site may lose its functions, but this depends upon the actual site and the extent of the injury.

- *Pathogenicity*: the presence of microbes with a greater pathogenicity in the wound (i.e. ability to cause disease) causes a greater degree of inflammation.

The body reacts in the same way regardless of whether a tissue is damaged via mechanical, thermal or chemical causes, or in response to a hypersensitive reaction or a pathogenic invasion. The tissue soon shows the four classic signs of inflammation (see Figure 11.16, p.293 and Figures 13.1b, p.360, 13.3c, p.366 and 13.10b, p.378), which provide reassurance that normal homeostatic responses have been activated following injury. These signs are redness, increase in tissue temperature, swelling, discomfort and/or pain. An additional sign of loss of function may follow these responses. These are discussed under the subheading 'The inflammation stage' in Chapter 11, pp.293–4.

> ### ACTIVITY
>
> Refer to Chapter 16, p.460 for a definition of fever and for details of how the hypothalamic thermostat is reset.

The role of the exudate producing the inflamed area is to promote the entrance of proteins and various phagocytic white cells into the wound from the plasma. Generally, the proteins in the tissue fluid create a colloidal osmotic pressure, promoting fluid leakage from plasma, resulting in the accumulation of tissue fluid (McVicar and Clancy, 1997). The increased blood flow to the area (and the accumulation of fluid in the soft tissues) eventually exerts pressure on sensory nerve endings, making the wound feel uncomfortable and/or painful. Specifically, proteins such as prothrombin and fibrinogen stimulate the clotting process – a homeostatic response discussed in Chapter 11 (see Figure 11.15, p.291) that creates a physical protective barrier between the external and internal environments of the body. The resulting clot thus acts to isolate the area and prevent the spreading of antigenic material.

The biochemical constitution of the exudate reflects the intensity and duration of the injurious agent, for example:

- serous exudate has low protein content. Such exudate indicates that there is superficial and minimal damage (e.g. blistering of the skin);

BOX 13.9 ABSCESSES AND ULCERS

If pus cannot be drained out of an inflamed area, the result is an abscess (i.e. an excessive build-up of pus in a confined space; see Figure 13.28, p.395). Abscesses include pimples and boils. When superficial inflamed tissue is removed from the surface of an organ or tissue, the opening sore is called an ulcer. People with diabetes mellitus or advanced atherosclerosis are susceptible to ulcers in the tissues of the legs. These 'diabetic ulcers' develop because poor oxygen and nutrient supplies to the tissues cause them to become susceptible to very mild injuries and/or infectious processes. Stasis (venous) leg ulcers arise because of incompetent venous return, and may coexist with diabetic ulcers in obese diabetic patients.

- fibrinous exudate indicates damage of a more intense nature, since this type of wound requires the development of a protective fibrin clot. Such material must be removed to prevent the formation of a scar;
- haemorrhagic exudate has the same biochemical constitution as a fibrinous exudate, with the additional presence of red blood cells, indicating that the injury has damaged blood vessels;
- purulent exudates are wounds that contain pus (a mixture of living and dead cells of the body, dead microbes, cell debris such as proteinaceous fibres, and bacterial toxins). Such an exudate is detrimental to the healing process.

ACTIVITY

Reflect on the function of leucocytes and blood coagulation role in wound healing, as detailed in Chapter 11, pp.287–95.

Although the process of inflammation is considered beneficial, since it involves homeostatic responses that restore tissue integrity by neutralizing and destroying antigens locally at the site of injury, the patient may nevertheless feel generally ill. Signs and symptoms may include fever, loss of appetite, and tiredness. The process of wound healing may also instigate harmful effects, such as:

- oedema of vital organs, such as the lungs, heart and brain. Cerebral oedema is a common cause of raised intracranial pressures in head injury patients;
- autolysis (self-destruction) of local body tissues, owing to the release of lysozymes from the large numbers of phagocytes present in the exudate;
- complications caused by the lodging of the antigen–antibody complex (discussed later).

The next process of inflammation involves the removal of debris and microbes. Phagocytes, such as neutrophils and macrophages, dispose of damaged body cells, foreign material, and microbes via the process of phagocytosis. This process is facilitated by the presence in the exudate of other white cells, T- and B-lymphocytes and complement (discussed later). Complement facilitates the phagocytic and lymphocytic responses to either prevent and/or fight infection.

To summarize, neutrophils are attracted into the wound first, usually within a few hours of injury; they are soon followed by macrophages. The activity of lymphocytes essentially cleanses the wound bed. Macrophages secrete growth factors, prostaglandins and complement, and, since these chemicals promote healing, these cells are usually present during all stages of wound healing. Eosinophils, another type of white blood cell, become involved if the antigenic materials are coated with antibodies of the IgG and IgE classifications (see later, Figure 13.24a, p.391). In clean wounds, the inflammatory phase lasts for about 36 hours; however, the process is prolonged in necrotic or infected wounds.

Antigenic materials, such as foreign protein, microbes and microbial toxins, which have accumulated and/or been presented to phagocytes at the site of inflammation, also stimulate the body's specific defences.

Non-specific responses: phagocytosis

Microbes that have penetrated external defences must be kept in check by internal mechanisms. When pathogenic agents penetrate the external defence mechanisms, they encounter white blood cells and their antimicrobial chemicals. White blood cells (called phagocytes) ingest bacteria they encounter in extracellular compartments (blood, interstitium, and in the lymphatics). Some white blood cells (B-lymphocytes) produce antibodies that destroy microbes (see later). If an area of the body becomes infected, many white blood cells aggregate in that area to attack the microbes that have invaded.

Phagocytosis is the body's first line of cellular defence against microbial invasion. The process is sometimes so efficient that microbes are removed as potential sources of infection before the lymphocytes have become aware of their presence.

Two broad classes of phagocytes exist: microphages and macrophages ('micro-' = small, 'macro-' = large).

Microphages

These phagocytes, white blood cells called neutrophils and eosinophils, circulate and police the body by entering injured peripheral tissues. Neutrophils have the greater phagocytosing capacity, since they are more abundant and more mobile than eosinophils (see Table 11.3, p.277).

Macrophages

These phagocytes, also called monocytes, are classified as 'wandering' or 'fixed' macrophages. The former migrate to areas of infection, and the latter are permanent residents of specific tissues, such as the reticuloendothelial (Kupffer) cells of the liver (see Figure 10.20b, p.261). The term 'fixed' is misleading, since these cells can be transported to nearby damaged tissue.

Phagocytic giant cells can be produced if several phagocytes accumulate together. This occurs in response to large and highly active antigenic material, and increases the capacity of such cells to destroy the material. Phagocytosis is greatly enhanced if the particles are coated (opsonized) with specific antibodies, and enhanced even further by certain components of the complement system (see below).

Phagocytosis as a homeostatic process

Before phagocytosis begins, mobile microphages and macrophages must move through capillary walls (a process called diapedesis) to the vicinity of antigenic material. For convenience, the process of phagocytosis is divided into four stages (Figure 13.10).

Chemotaxis

Chemicals released from pathogens (e.g. bacterial toxins), lymphocytes (e.g. macrophage-attracting substances), and damaged tissue and surrounding tissues (e.g. histamines) attract phagocytes to the area by a process called chemotaxis. Microorganisms are not entirely defenceless against phagocytic cells. Some microbial toxins kill phagocytes, which contribute to the microbe's own homeostatic defences (e.g. some microbial toxins kill phagocytes).

Adherence

Adherence involves a firm contact being made between the phagocyte's plasma membrane and the antigen. Phagocytes have a number of membrane chemicals, which have sticky properties that aid microbial adherence. Complement also promotes this process. Adherence sometimes proves to be a difficult process, but it is facilitated by trapping the microbe against a roughened surface (e.g. a blood clot) or a solid surface (e.g. blood vessel). This activity is referred to as non-immune (or surface) phagocytosis.

Ingestion and intracellular digestion

Phagocytes employ cytoplasmic streaming to produce cell membrane projections called pseudopodia, which engulf, or ingest, the material to be digested or phagocytosed. The engulfed antigen becomes surrounded by a membrane-lined vacuole, or phagosome, which becomes cytoplasmically bound. Lysosomes coalesce with it, forming a larger structure called a phagolysosome or a secondary lysosome. Lysozymes are released into the vesicle; these enzymes (lipases, proteases, nucleases, etc.) break down complex microbial components into simple molecules. These chemicals pass into the cytoplasm of the phagocyte to be utilized in its metabolism. Lactic acid, another component of lysosomes, provides the pH most suitable for lysosomal enzyme activity.

Some microbes (e.g. tuberculin bacilli) are not entirely defenceless to this process, since they may divide actively within phagocyte vacuoles and destroy phagocytes intracellularly. Others (e.g. human immunodeficiency virus, HIV) remain dormant within phagocytes before exerting their effects. Problems can also arise if the phagocytosed antigens cannot be 'digested' (e.g. asbestos), thereby accumulating inside the cell.

Disposal

Inevitably, some microbial components cannot be degraded, since human genes cannot produce all of the enzymes necessary for total microbial destruction. Indigestible or residual material remains vacuolated within the phagocyte until they are ejected from the cell by exocytosis.

Some toxin-producing microbes are not necessarily killed by phagocytosis, but may become killers of the phagocytes themselves through secretion of toxins. Others (e.g. tuberculin bacilli) even divide within phagolysosomes and destroy the phagocytes from inside the cells. Yet other microorganisms (e.g. HIV) remain dormant within phagocytes for long periods before exerting their effects. Further problems can arise if the phagocytosed antigen cannot be broken down (e.g. coal dust), thereby causing its accumulation inside the cells. These phagocytes then produce an abundance of lysosomes, which fuse with the phagosome in an attempt to destroy the particles. Eventually, phagocytic autolysis (literally self-destruction) occurs when lysozymes are released inside the cells.

An increase in cellular respiration accompanies the process of phagocytosis. Consequently, hydrogen peroxide is produced, which is toxic to many bacteria; it therefore contributes to the body's defence operations. Some bacteria counteract this effect by producing an enzyme, catalase, which converts peroxide into water and oxygen. Needless to say, this enzyme production is a useful homeostatic adaptation, which gives these bacteria a degree of resistance.

Non-specific defence: the chemical environment

The microbe also comes under attack from a hostile internal environment which comprises antimicrobial proteins. Blood and tissue fluid contain three main types of antimicrobial proteins that inhibit microbial growth:

- *Complement*: a group of normally inactive proteins (precursors) located in blood and on cell membranes make up the complement system. When activated, these proteins 'complement' certain immune, allergic and inflammatory reactions.
- *Transferrins*: these iron-binding proteins inhibit the growth of certain bacteria by reducing the amount of available iron.
- *Interferon*: macrophages, lymphocytes and fibroblasts infected with viruses produce a group of proteins called interferons. These chemicals are released from infected cells and move to neighbouring uninfected cells, whereby they bind to surface receptors, stimulating the synthesis of antiviral proteins that interfere with viral replication. This inhibition of replication is essential since viruses can cause disease only if they replicate within body (host) cells. Interferons are an important defence against many different viruses (Figure 13.9).

The specific immune response

In addition to surviving the above non-specific defences, pathogens must also deal simultaneously with the specific (lymphocytic) immune responses. In summary, the non-specific

---

ACTIVITY

Review the details associated with the non-specific phagocytic response. Make notes on the functions of complement in response to bacterial invasion. Before considering cell-mediated and antibody-mediated reactions, use Figure 13.11 and Figure 11.3, p.273, to familiarize yourself with the embryological origin of T- and B-cells, and use a healthcare dictionary to familiarize yourself with the following terms: cytotoxic, cytokines, mast cells, interleukin, toxin, toxoid, antibody, passive immunity, active immunity, diphtheria, tetanus, poliomyelitis and meningitis.

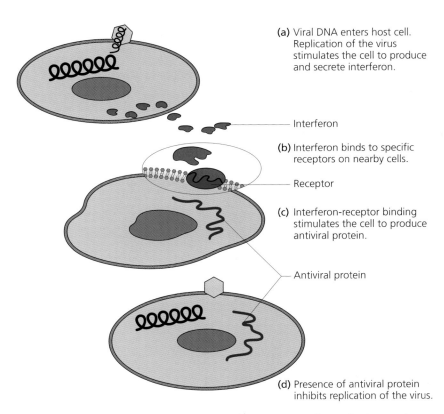

(a) Viral DNA enters host cell. Replication of the virus stimulates the cell to produce and secrete interferon.

Figure 13.9 **Interferon activation**

Interferon

(b) Interferon binds to specific receptors on nearby cells.

Receptor

(c) Interferon-receptor binding stimulates the cell to produce antiviral protein.

Antiviral protein

(d) Presence of antiviral protein inhibits replication of the virus.

mechanisms have common actions against all antigenic insults, whereas lymphocytic responses confer specific immunity against particular antigenic insults. Such responses have two closely allied components:

- A component involved in the production of specific T-lymphocytes, some of which attach themselves to antigenic materials to destroy them. This response is particularly effective against the antigens of fungi, intracellular viruses, parasites, foreign tissue transplants and cancer cells. It is referred to as cellular, or cell-mediated, immunity, since it relies mainly on the secretion by these cells of cytotoxic chemicals and other substances, including lysozymes, macrophage-attracting substances and interferon. Interferon is released specifically when the antigen is a virus. It is important in controlling viral infections by preventing their replication inside host cells. Thus, since antibodies cannot enter cells, interferon succeeds where antibodies fail.
- A component involved in the production and secretion of specific antibodies into the circulation. Antibodies are produced by B-lymphocytes in an attempt to destroy specific antigens present in body fluids and extracellular pathogens that multiply in body fluid but rarely enter body cells (i.e. primarily bacteria). Thus, if antigen 1 penetrates the external defences, antibody 1 is produced against it, whereas if antigen 2 enters the body, antibody 2 is produced, etc. These cells confer humoral, or antibody-mediated, immunity, which is particularly effective against bacteria and viral antigens.

Often, however, the pathogen provokes both types of immune responses. Thus, lymphocytes have an essential role in identifying foreign or abnormal cells and antigens, and distinguishing these from normal cells and tissues. If they fail to do so, the consequences may be uncontrolled proliferation of bacteria, viruses and even aberrant cells of the body itself (i.e. cancer), or destruction of apparently normal cells (i.e. autoimmune disorders).

Before we consider cell-mediated and antibody-mediated reactions, we will discuss the origin of the cells involved, and the structures of antigens and antibodies.

Lymphocyte production and destruction: a homeostatic process

Embryological T-cells (responsible for cellular immunity) and B-cells (responsible for humoral immunity) are derived from bone marrow lymphocytic stem cells, which have originated from common stem cells within the bone marrow (Figure 13.11). The majority of lymphocytic stem cells migrate to the thymus gland, where they are processed into T-lymphocytes. Processing bestows immunological competence (i.e. cells develop the capacity and ability to differentiate into cells that perform specific immune reactions). Competence is endowed by the thymus shortly after birth, and for a few months post-delivery. Removal of the gland before processing impairs the development of cell-mediated immune responses.

Competent T-cells leave the thymus and become embedded in lymphoidal tissue of the fetal liver, spleen, lymph nodes and the gut-associated lymphoidal tissue (adenoids, tonsils, appendix, etc.). Thymosin, a hormone, and other thymus secretions stimulate further T-cell development.

The remaining lymphatic stem cells are destined to become B-cells. They are processed in the bone marrow, and then

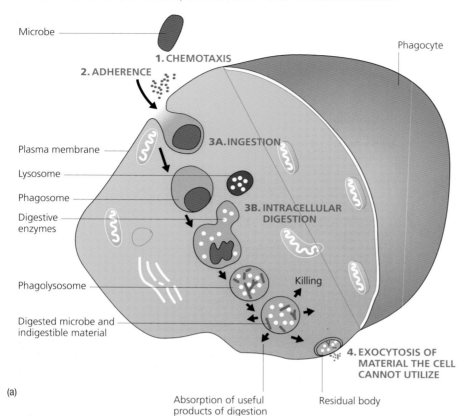

Microbe

1. CHEMOTAXIS

2. ADHERENCE

Phagocyte

3A. INGESTION

Plasma membrane

Lysosome

Phagosome

Digestive enzymes

3B. INTRACELLULAR DIGESTION

Phagolysosome

Killing

Digested microbe and indigestible material

4. EXOCYTOSIS OF MATERIAL THE CELL CANNOT UTILIZE

(a)

Absorption of useful products of digestion

Residual body

Figure 13.10 (a) Phagocytosis: 1, chemotaxis; 2, adhesion; 3a, ingestion; 3b, intracellular digestion; 4 disposal (exocytosis). (b) Chemotaxis and the classic signs of inflammation

Q Phagocytes move through capillary walls by squeezing between adjacent endothelial cells. Is this process known as (1) adhesion, (2) chemotaxis, (3) perforation or (4) diapedesis?

Q List the classic signs of inflammation.

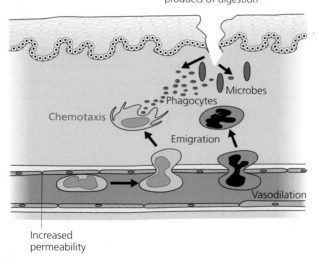

Microbes

Phagocytes

Chemotaxis

Emigration

Vasodilation

Increased permeability

(b)

BOX 13.10 IMMUNITY IN YOUNG AND OLDER PEOPLE

Newborn babies are more susceptible to infection and diseases, since they need to develop their immature specific immunological responses by exposure to environmental insults. The ageing process is associated with increased destruction and decreased production rates of leucocytes. It is, therefore, not surprising that elderly people are also more susceptible to infections and diseases. A lack of gastric juice is more common in old people, which potentially makes them more susceptible to pathogens in the diet.

---

migrate to the lymphoid tissue mentioned above. The presence of both T- and B-cells means that these tissues are now capable of stimulating both cellular and humoral immunities in response to antigenic insults. Consequently, the thymus gland and bone marrow sites are called the primary lymphoidal organs, whereas other lymphoidal tissues are called the secondary lymphoidal organs.

In adults, lymphocyte production (called lymphopoiesis) is maintained in the bone marrow and lymphatic tissue. Lymphocytes have long lifespans compared with most body cells; approximately 80% survive for 4 years, and some live for 20 years or more. Cell production must match destruction to maintain the homeostatic functions of the immune system.

Antigens

Materials that induce specific immune reactions are called antigens. They are not usually normal constituents of the body. Sometimes, however, the distinction between self and non-self fails, and antibodies attack the body's own antigens in a variety of conditions known as autoimmune diseases. Antigens consist of a variety of chemicals. They are usually large, conjugated proteins, such as nucleoproteins, lipoproteins or glycoproteins. Others are lipids and polysaccharides.

Foreign cells, such as bacteria, viruses, fungi and transplanted cells, are sometimes referred to as immunogens. These have antigens as a part of their structure. The immune response against immunogens is a reaction to their cellular antigens, which may be:

• plasma membrane receptors (see Figure 13.2, p.361);
• cell surface structures, such as cilia, flagella, etc;
• secretions, such as bacterial toxins;

Figure 13.11 Lymphocyte development and circulation

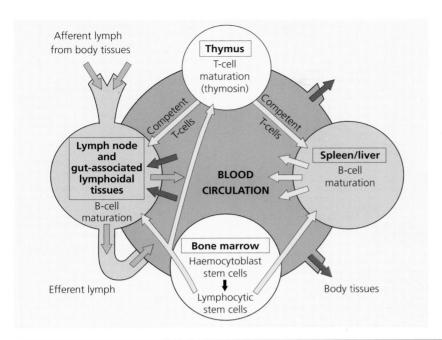

BOX 13.11 TISSUE TYPING AND IMMUNOSUPPRESSANT THERAPY

As discussed in Chapter 11, the antigens on erythrocytes are used to categorize the patient's blood group status (see Figures 11.19, p.299 and 11.20, p.301). Antigens of other body cells (called histocompatibility antigens) are used to determine the patient's tissue type, which is controlled by the genes that are inherited from the biological parents. Transplanted tissues and organs from other people or animals thus possess non-self antigenic material, and recipients therefore produce cell-mediated and antibody-mediated immune responses against transplanted antigens, which may cause transplant rejection. Tissue typing and immunosuppressant therapy minimize the possibility of rejection.

Tissue typing

Tissue typing involves matching the donor and recipient human lymphocytic antigens (HLA). Several-hundred genes at the HLA loci on chromosome 6 determine histocompatibility antigens. Great variations of HLA therefore exist and, since there are thousands of possible genetic, and thus antigenic, combinations, a complete match is extremely unlikely. The closer the HLA match between donor and recipient, the greater the likelihood of transplant success; a nationwide computerized registry helps in this process. Doctors select the most histocompatible and needy organ transplant recipients whenever donor organs become available. Despite national and international cooperation to match donors with recipients, immune rejection is still the main hazard in transplantation. Tissues with a similar genetic make-up are less likely to be rejected. Thus, for example, the graft types are:

- autografts (grafts from the person's own body tissues) have no non-self antigens and are not rejected;
- isografts (grafting from individuals with 'identical' genetic make-up; i.e. identical or monozygotic twins) have little risk of rejection;
- allografts or homografts (grafting between members of the same species, but not genetically identical individuals) have a higher rate of rejection;
- xenografts or heterografts (grafting between species) have the highest rate of rejection.

Tissue typing can also be used to identify biological parents in paternity suits.

Immunosuppressant therapy

Immunosuppressant drugs are also of value in treating severe hypersensitivity states and autoimmune conditions, and to minimize the risk of transplant rejection. Subsequent to transplantation, patients receive immunosuppressant therapy in an attempt to prevent rejection. These drugs are aimed at T-lymphocytes, since these cells are the most active in rejection (Pace, 2000). Unfortunately, immunosuppressants are non-specific, and suppression of the patient's natural defences to otherwise trivial pathogens may result in infection or disease, which may threaten life of the recipient. For example:

- Corticosteroids (e.g. prednisone, hydrocortisone) are used to prevent transplant rejections, in the treatment of severe allergies, and for autoimmune conditions. They operate by gradually destroying lymphoid tissue, which directly depletes T- and B-cells. Their main action, however, is to decrease the activities of phagocytic cells. Thus, they may make the recipients more susceptible to infections.
- Cytotoxic drugs (e.g. methotrexate, 6-mercaptopurine) are used to inhibit replication of lymphocytes. In addition, they also inhibit mitosis of other cells (e.g. in the bone marrow, gastrointestinal tract and skin cells). Consequently, these drugs can produce undesirable side-effects, such as thrombocytopenia, anaemia, leucopenia, hair loss, skin disorders and gastrointestinal upsets.
- Cyclosporin inhibits secretion of interleukin-2 by helper T-cells, but has only a minimal effect on B-cells. Thus, the risk of rejection is diminished while retaining resistance to some diseases.
- Anti-lymphocytic serum (ALS) depletes T-cells, but also damages other lymphocytes, making the recipient more susceptible to infection. Immunizing horses or rabbits with human lymphocytes produces the serum. It has, however, a limited use in preventing the rejection of transplanted organs.

- non-microbial antigens, such as incompatible blood cells, and transplanted tissues or organs, and allergic substances (called allergens), such as pollen grain, fur, feathers, wheat, food additives, etc. Allergens cause the production of specialized antibodies in hypersensitive or allergic immune responses (see Box 13.16, p.389).

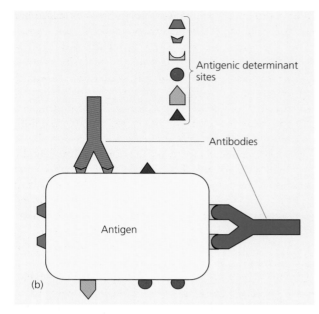

Figure 13.12 Relationship of an antigen to antibodies

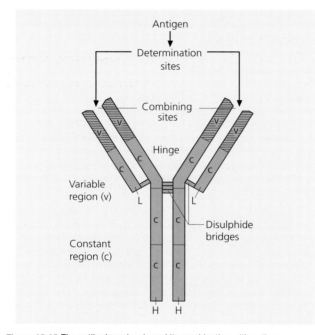

Figure 13.13 The antibody molecule and its combination with antigen

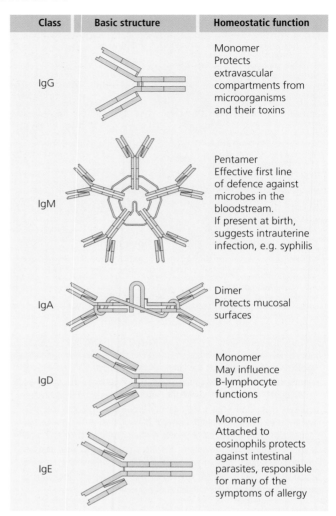

Class	Basic structure	Homeostatic function
IgG		Monomer Protects extravascular compartments from microorganisms and their toxins
IgM		Pentamer Effective first line of defence against microbes in the bloodstream. If present at birth, suggests intrauterine infection, e.g. syphilis
IgA		Dimer Protects mucosal surfaces
IgD		Monomer May influence B-lymphocyte functions
IgE		Monomer Attached to eosinophils protects against intestinal parasites, responsible for many of the symptoms of allergy

Figure 13.14 The structure and function of antibodies

Q Which antibodies can pass over the placenta?

- Immunogenicity is the ability to stimulate the production of specific antibodies and/or the proliferation of specific T-cells.
- Reactivity is the ability of the antigen to react specifically with relevant antibodies or cells it provoked.

Complete antigens possess both important features. Antibodies target an antigen's exposed surface, known as the antigenic determinant site (Figure 13.12). The number of sites is known as the valence. Complete antigens are multivalent, e.g. the antigen of individual microorganisms may have thousands of sites; just two sites are needed to induce antibody formation so small variations in the organism are unlikely to make it 'invisible' to the immune system.

Partial antigens do not stimulate antibody production as they have only one antigenic site. Thus, such antigens have reactivity but not immunogenicity.

Antibodies

Antibodies are produced and secreted in response to the presence of antigens (antigenic insults). They are found in all

Once past the body's non-specific defences, antigens become targeted by the lymphatic tissue by one of three routes:

- Most antigens that enter the blood via an injured blood vessel locate themselves in the spleen.
- Antigens that penetrate the skin enter lymphatic vessels and pass to the lymphatic nodes.
- Antigens that penetrate mucus membranes lodge themselves in the mucosa-associated lymphoid tissue (MALT).

Non-self materials are classified according to whether they promote immunogenicity and/or reactivity:

bodily tissues, although their greatest presence is within blood. Antibodies are very large proteins called gamma-globulins; since they are a part of the immune response, they are often referred to as immunoglobulins (Igs). Major categories include IgG (Ig gamma), IgA (Ig alpha), IgM (Ig mu), IgD (Ig delta) and IgE (Ig epsilon).

Since antibodies are proteins, they consist of polypeptide chains. Most consist of two pairs: a pair of 'heavy' chains (chains of more than 400 amino acids), and a pair of 'light' chains (consisting of 200 amino acids). The partner of each pair is identical: each half therefore consists of a heavy and a light chain and these are joined together by disulphide (sulphur–sulphur) bonds (Figure 13.13). Within each chain there are two distinct regions:

- The constant region is identical in the number, type and sequencing of its constituent amino acids in all antibodies of the same class (i.e. IgG, IgM, etc.; discussed later). However, this region differs between antibody categories, and is thus responsible for distinguishing between the different types of immunoglobulins and their biological functions.
- The variable region differs for each antibody, even for those of the same category, allowing antibodies to recognize and specifically attach themselves to particular antigens. The combining site, at which the antibody molecule combines with the antigen, is located in a relatively small area of the variable region, and is formed by both the light and heavy chains.

Binding to an antigen converts the normal T-shaped antibody molecule into a Y-configuration, and it is this transformation that activates the antibody. Each 'arm' of the Y-configuration contains a combining site; flexibility at the hinge region permits the two combining sites to bind with the antigens in different configurations.

The shape of the combining region will be complementary to the particular determination site on the antigen, and different antibodies will recognize different determination sites on antigens with different structures. This 'lock and key' binding of antibody and antigen sites gives immune responses their specificity. Most antibodies are single molecules (monomers) with just two combining sites for the attachment of antigens; they are said to be bivalent. IgM and IgA antibodies have a higher valency, because they are, respectively, pentamers (i.e. consist of five molecules joined together) and dimers (two molecules joined together) of the basic divalent unit.

The structures and homeostatic functions of immunoglobulins are summarized in Figure 13.14. The combining sites of the antibodies interact with antigens to form macromolecular complexes in a variety of ways, which neutralize, agglutinate, precipitate, lyse or opsonize the antigen (Figure 13.15). Others

---

ACTIVITY

Describe the structure of an antibody.

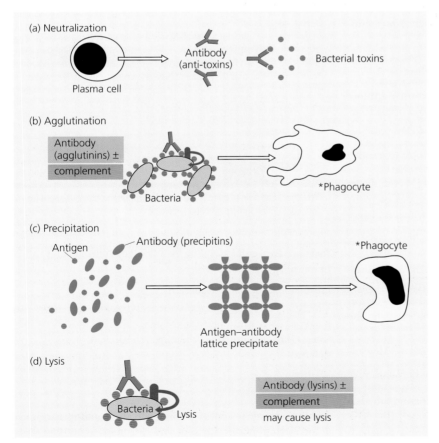

(a) Neutralization

Plasma cell → Antibody (anti-toxins) → Bacterial toxins

(b) Agglutination

Antibody (agglutinins) ± complement

Bacteria → *Phagocyte

(c) Precipitation

Antigen — Antibody (precipitins) → Antigen–antibody lattice precipitate → *Phagocyte

(d) Lysis

Bacteria → Lysis

Antibody (lysins) ± complement may cause lysis

Figure 13.15 Antibody–antigen complexing. Key: *, phagocytic cell (e.g. neutrophil, macrophage); +, presence; –, absence

***Q** How does the antibody–antigen complex cause elimination of an antigen?*

BOX 13.12 CANCER AND MONOCLONAL ANTIBODY THERAPY

Cancer cells possess specific surface antigens characteristic of tumours. The immune system usually recognizes these as being non-self, and thus attempts to destroy them; this is called immunological surveillance. Although sensitized macrophages are involved in the response, there is general agreement that cell-mediated responses are especially involved in tumour destruction. Sensitized killer cells (see later, p.383) react with tumour-specific antigens, initiating their lysis. Some cancer cells, however, employ the phenomenon of 'immunological escape'. Explanations accounting for such an 'escape' include:

- Some tumour cells shed their specific antigens, and therefore evade the initial recognition necessary for immunological surveillance.
- Decreased immune functioning makes people more susceptible to cancer, which supports the increased incidences of cancer observed with the use of immunosuppressive therapy in transplant patients, in people suffering from chronic distress and in older people.

Cancer cells are long-living ('immortal') and divide rapidly, and scientists have been able to fuse individual B-cells with rapidly dividing tumour cells to produce large numbers of hybridoma cells that are plentiful long-term sources of antibodies specific against one antigen, hence the term 'monoclonal' ('mono-' = single). Such antibodies are of diagnostic importance in allergies, pregnancy, and diseases such as rabies, some sexually transmitted diseases and hepatitis. They have also been used to detect cancer at an early stage, and to ascertain the extent of metastasis. The use of highly specific antibodies offers greater sensitivity, speed and specificity than conventional diagnostic tests. They are used independently, or in combination with radioactivity or chemotherapy, in the treatment of cancer. The clinical application of monoclonal antibodies to prevent cancers is an exciting discovery, since such antibodies selectively locate and destroy cancer cells but cause little or no damage to surrounding healthy cells. This treatment, therefore, overcomes some of the major adverse effects of isolated chemotherapy and radiotherapy.

The use of monoclonal antibody vaccines may also prove to be useful in counteracting tissue and organ transplant rejection, and in treating autoimmune diseases. For further reading, see Kosits and Callaghan (2000).

---

prevent the adhesion necessary for microbes to penetrate the skin and mucous membranes.

Neutralization

Bacterial toxins cause disease by binding to specific cells. Neutralization involves antibodies, called anti-toxins, including some IgGs, that bind to the determination sites of the toxin chemicals, thus neutralizing their toxicity. This interaction may alter the toxin's shape, thus removing its specific binding properties and preventing its interaction with cell membranes, or it may destroy the antigen by increasing its susceptibility to phagocytosis.

Agglutination

Some specialized antibodies (of IgG and IgM types) are called agglutinins which, together with complement, cause immunogens to clump together (see earlier, for a discussion of the functions of complement). This is referred to as agglutination; it makes bacteria more susceptible to phagocytosis.

Precipitation

Some specialized antibodies (also IgG and IgM types) are called precipitants as they react with soluble antigens via many cross-linkages to form an insoluble precipitate, which is phagocytosed more readily.

Lysis

Some IgG and IgM antibodies called lysins attach to immunogen surface antigens and directly cause cellular rupture (lysis), hence causing their death. Alternatively, antibody–antigen formation enhances the fixation of complement, which also results in lysis.

Opsonization

Microbes, such as bacteria, have structures ('slippery' plasma membranes) that probably are (homeostatic) adaptations to prevent phagocytosis. Opsonization is the coating of such microbes with antibodies (opsonins include some IgEs, IgGs and IgMs) and some complement proteins. This roughens

BOX 13.13 THE COMMON COLD AND IGE

The common cold (clinically known as coryza) originates from a viral infection; multiple variants of the virus are known to cause it. The viral particles become attached to IgE, which results in lysis of basophils and the release of histamine (see Figure 13.24a, p.391) and prostaglandins. These chemicals cause inflammation of the nasal passageways and excessive production of nasal secretions, leading to symptoms such as a running nose, coughing and sneezing. When the epithelium becomes inflamed in response to an infection, the swollen tissues and extra secretions obstruct the flow of air through the nasal passageways, which makes breathing difficult.

Allergens (i.e. antigens that stimulate an allergic reaction) also operate on IgE in this manner (see later). These protective symptoms of the cold are the means by which the viruses are passed on from one person to the next. Associated symptoms with a common cold include hyperthermia (raised temperature), chest infection and shortness of breath. These secondary complications are caused not by the virus, but by secondary bacterial infection or by a hypersensitive response, such as occurs in asthma.

ACTIVITY

You should be able to identify the specific immunoglobulins that are toxins, agglutinins, precipitins and lysins.

---

their surfaces, enhancing the likelihood of adhesion and subsequent phagocytosis.

Prevention of bacterial adhesion

The IgAs present in mucus, sweat and digestive secretions coat bacteria, decreasing their capacity for attachment to body surfaces, thus minimizing their penetration of our external defences.

Activating the lymphocytic response: a homeostatic process

Very few antigens appear to bind directly to antigen-reactive T- or B-lymphocytes. Instead, some are inserted on the surface

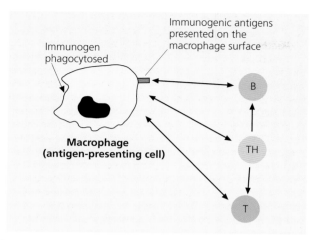

Figure 13.16 Lymphocyte response. B, B-cells; T, T-cells; TH, T-helper cells

Q A decrease in the number of T-cells would affect which type of immunity?

of macrophages following phagocytosis and presented to the lymphocytes; these are known as antigen-presenting cells (APCs; Figures 13.16 and 13.17). A much more important group of APCs is the (non-phagocytic) dendritic cells. These cell types are distributed widely in tissues throughout the body, and appear to trap the antigen, thereby preventing its spread, and then initiate local immune responses. Dendritic cells of the lymph nodes and spleen trap circulating antigens in the lymph and blood, and present them to the resident lymphocytes. Similarly, dendritic cells present in non-lymphoidal tissues trap the antigens, then the complex moves towards the lymphoid tissues. The structure of the spleen and lymph nodes is such that the APCs and lymphocytes are in very close contact. Immunogen antigens, such as those associated with incompatible blood transfusions, transplanted organs, cancers or

'self' antigens that have changed, also sensitize T-lymphocytes. A lymph node under antigenic stimulation shows T- and B-cell proliferation, and thus becomes enlarged in the process.

Upon contact with antigen, the macrophages secrete a chemical called interleukin-1, which is a cytokine previously known as lymphokine, since it increases the activity of lymphocytes; see 'Killer T-cells' below). This is responsible for promoting lymphoidal T- and B-cell multiplication. Proliferation stimulates further macrophage activity and hence further proliferation (i.e. positive feedback mechanism). Macrophages, dendritic cells, and T- and B-lymphocytes thus cooperate to provide immunity against antigenic insults (Figure 13.17).

T-lymphocytes and cell-mediated immunity

There are thousands of different T-cells, each capable of responding to the presence of an antigen, but only those programmed specifically to react with the specific antigen present are activated. Sensitized T-lymphocytes divide, giving rise to clones (i.e. cells that are identical to one another and to their parent cells; Figure 13.18). The major difference is that the parent cells cannot destroy immunogens, but mainly the clones can. Clones include:

* killer T-cells;
* helper T-cells;
* suppressor T-cells;
* delayed hypersensitivity T-cells;
* amplifier T-cells;
* memory T-cells;
* natural killer (NK) lymphocytes.

Killer T-cells

Killer (or cytotoxic or null) cells become attached to antigens. They destroy foreign cells by secreting cytokines, cytolymphotoxins, interferons and lysozymes (see earlier). Cytokines are a

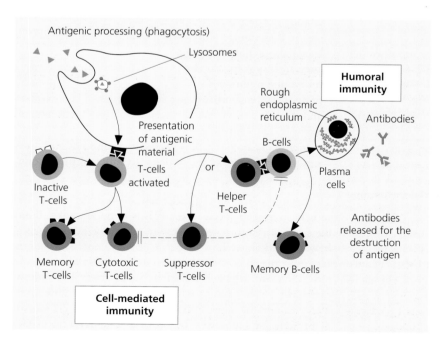

Figure 13.17 Interactions between macrophages, T-cells and B-cells.

Q Does complement activation (1) attract phagocytes, (2) enhance phagocytosis, (3) stimulate inflammation or (4) all of the above?

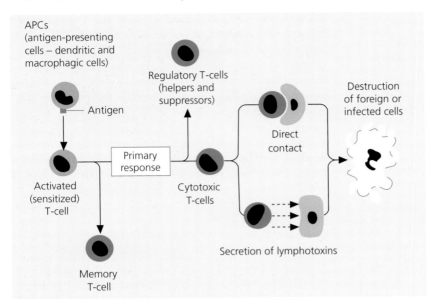

Figure 13.18 Cell-mediated immunity

Q A rise in the level of interferon in the body would suggest what kind of infection?

BOX 13.14 CYTOTOXIC THERAPY

Cytotoxic therapy is the use of cytotoxic substances (see text) to treat medical conditions.

- Interferons were the first cytotoxic substances found to be effective against human cancer.
- Interferon-alpha is used for the treatment of Kaposi's sarcoma, a cancer that often occurs in people with acquired immune deficiency syndrome (AIDS). Its antiviral uses also make it beneficial in the treatment of genital herpes and hepatitis B and C.
- Betaseron (an interferon-beta) slows the progression of multiple sclerosis (MS) and lessens the frequency and severity of MS attacks.
- Of the interleukins, the one most widely used to fight cancer is interleukin-2 which causes proliferation of killer cells.

---

group of local, powerful protein hormones; they give most of the protection provided by killer cells but act in a variety of ways. They include:

- transfer factors (these recruit lymphocytes by transforming non-sensitized T-lymphocytes into sensitized T-cells);
- macrophage-chemotaxis factor (this attracts macrophages, and thus intensifies phagocytosis of the antigen);
- macrophage-activating factor (this directly increases the phagocytic activity of macrophages);
- migration inhibitory factor (this prevents the migration of macrophages, and thus encourages their continued presence at the site of infection);
- mitogenic factor (this induces rapid division of uncommitted or non-sensitized T-cells).

Cytolymphotoxins destroy immunogens directly, by producing 'holes' in their plasma membrane, resulting in their lysis. Interferons are antiviral agents (see earlier) that enhance killer cell activity, resulting in the destruction of the viral-loaded host cells.

The stimulation of killer T-cells is known as cell-mediated immunity, since their secretions are toxic to immunogens (for-

eign cells). Normally, individual immunogens/antigens stimulate both cellular and humoral immune responses but one type usually predominates, depending upon the invading immunogen. Some killer T-cell secretions also promote non-specific responses, and can result in the loss of healthy 'self' tissue in the locality.

Helper T-cells

Helper T-lymphocytes assist plasma cells (derived from B-lymphocytes following their activation by antigen) to secrete antibodies. In addition, helper cells secrete the chemical interleukin-2, which amplifies the proliferation of killer cells. Before this, however, interleukin-2 must be activated by interleukin-1, secreted from macrophages, thus demonstrating the interdependency of white cell types in controlling the homeostatic functions of defence. Interleukins also:

- amplify inflammatory and macrophage responses;
- elevate body temperature, which interferes with the rate of bacterial cell multiplication;
- aid scar tissue formation by increasing fibroblast activity during wound healing;
- promote adrenocorticotropic hormone (ACTH) secretion and the subsequent release of the metabolic hormones collectively called cortisol;
- stimulate mast cell (i.e. cells that secrete histamine and other substances as a part of the response to antigens) production.

Suppressor T-cells

These lymphocytes restrain killer cell and B-cell activities, and so help to moderate responses. This is important, as it limits the effect of cytotoxic secretions on 'self' tissue in the locality. It was noted above how helper T-cells promote lymphocyte activities: the interaction between suppressor and helper T-cells, therefore, regulates the immune response. The ratio of these cells can be used to indicate the presence or absence of infection, and the stage of infection. For example, a 2:1 ratio of helper cells to suppressor T-cells occurs when there are no

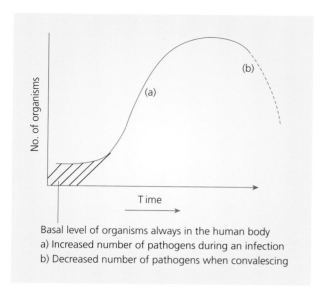

Basal level of organisms always in the human body
a) Increased number of pathogens during an infection
b) Decreased number of pathogens when convalescing

Figure 13.19 The multiplication of pathogens during an infection and when the patient is convalescing

Q Identify the ratio of killer cells to suppressor cells at the points labelled (a) and (b) on this figure.

signs of infection. Early in the infection cycle, however, a higher ratio of helper cells (and hence killer cells, B-cells and their antibodies) to suppressor cells exists, which promotes the removal of non-self antigens. Conversely, several weeks later, a high suppressor cell to helper cell ratio (and hence killer and plasma B-cells, and their corresponding antibodies) is

observed, and the immunological response declines because the person is recovering from the illness or infection.

Delayed hypersensitivity T-cells

These cells secrete various cytokines, including migration-inhibitory and macrophage-activating factors (see earlier), in response to the presence of allergens. Destruction of the allergens at their site of entry means that these cells have key roles in delaying or preventing allergic (hypersensitive) reactions.

Amplifier T-cells

Amplifier lymphocytes somehow exaggerate the activities of helper cell, suppressor cell and B-cell descendants. There are specific amplifier cells for helper cells and others for suppressor cells, etc.

Memory T-cells

Memory cells retain the ability to recognize previously encountered non-self antigens, so that second and subsequent exposures lead to a rapid 'secondary' immune response (Figures 13.19 and 13.20). They may survive for many years and so immunity of this kind is conferred for a long time, and often for life. Production of memory cells in response to administered antigen (together with B-cells and antibodies that also persist in blood; see below) forms the basis of immunization programmes.

ACTIVITY

Using Table 13.1, describe why children need to be immunized only once for measles, mumps, rubella and TB (see Box 13.17, p.394).

Figure 13.20 Humoral immunity

Q How is the body able to distinguish between self-antigens and foreign antigens?

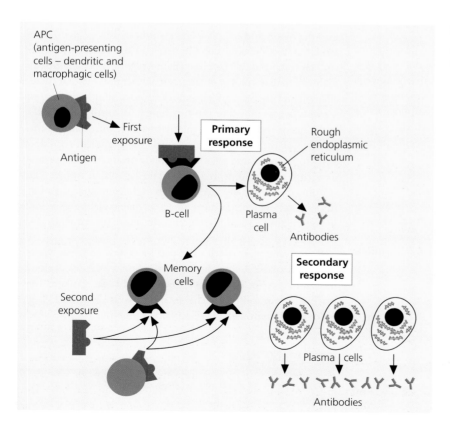

Table 13.1 Childhood immunization programme

Age of immunization	Vaccine
2 months	Diphtheria, tetanus, pertussis, polio and *Haemophilus influenzae* type b (DTaP/IPV/Hib)
	Pneumococcal (PCV)
3 months	Diphtheria, tetanus, pertussis, polio and *Haemophilus influenzae* type b (DTaP/IPV/Hib)
	Pneumococcal (PCV)
	Meningitis C (Men C)
4 months	Diphtheria, tetanus, pertussis, polio and *Haemophilus influenzae* type b (DTaP/IPV/Hib)
	Pneumococcal (PCV)
	Meningitis C (Men C)
Approximately 12 months	*Haemophilus influenzae* type b
	Meningitis C (Men C) (Hib/Men C)
Approximately 13 months	Measles, mumps and rubella (MMR)
3 years 4 months to 5 years	Diphtheria, tetanus, pertussis, polio (DTaP/IPV)
	Measles, mumps and rubella (MMR)
13–18 years	Diphtheria, tetanus, polio (Td/IPV)

Note:
1   A minority of children experience the following reactions, post- immunization.
  (i)   redness and swelling at the site of injection;
  (ii) babies may appear grumpy and grizzly;
  (ii) sickness;
  (iii) diarrhoea;
  (iv) loss of appetite;
  (v)   fever may develop within 2 days and injection. Paracetamol syrup (e.g. Calpol) is given to reduce the fever and extra fluids to prevent dehydration.
2   One to three weeks post-MMR injection the child may not feel well and have a high temperature for a few days. A rash and swelling around the jaw may also be present; symptoms disappear within a few days. The child is not infectious, and paracetamol syrup may be given.

Q *What is immunization, and how does it work?*

Natural killer lymphocytes

NK cells are similar to killer T cells, in the sense that they lyse or break down target cells. The difference is that NK cells directly destroy those cells with altered surface membrane antigens without the need to interact with other lymphocytes or antibodies. They respond to specific antigens and so NK cells are considered to be the first line of defence in specific immunity.

Interim summary

Specific and non-specific defences are therefore coordinated by physical interactions, and by the release of chemical messengers. In addition to lymphocytic secretions, monocytes and macrophages also secrete monokines, such as the tissue tumour necrotic factor. This protein is responsible for:

• slowing down tumour growth;
• killing sensitive tumour cells;
• stimulating the production of granulocytes (white blood cells);
• promoting the activity of phagocytic granulocytes, called eosinophils;
• increasing T-cell sensitivity to interleukin chemicals.

See the case study on a woman with breast cancer, Section VI, p.630.

BOX 13.15 CANCER AND NK CELLS

Since it is believed that cancerous cells have abnormal surfaces, it is possible that secretion of interferon by natural killer (NK) cells plays a prime role in destroying virally infected or damaged cells that might otherwise form tumours. Cancer patients have a reduced number of NK cells; interestingly, the level of decrease corresponds to the severity of disease.

Skin and T-cell interactions

The epidermal cells of skin have active integrative roles with the body's specific immune responses. For example, when antigens penetrate the keratinized cell layer of the epidermis, they bind to cells called Langerhans cells. These cells present the antigenic material to epidermal T-helper cells, activating them. Langerhan cells also interact with epidermal suppressor T-cells, but usually the helper cells predominate, and instigate the destruction of the antigenic substances. If, however, Langerhans cells are destroyed (e.g. by ultraviolet radiation) or are bypassed, then these antigens react directly with suppressor cells, causing their predominance.

Humoral immunity: B-cells and antibody production

The body contains thousands of specialized B-cells, which carry (or express) on their surface antibody molecules that act as receptors for antigens. Each antibody is capable of responding only to a specific antigen (the structure of antibodies was described earlier). When a B-cell is exposed to an antigen, small B-lymphocytes (influenced by interleukin from activated macrophages) become larger plasma cells containing a mass of rough endoplasmic reticulum (Figure 13.20). These cells produce and secrete into the blood and lymph specific antibody (i.e. protein) of the same type as that expressed originally on the surface of the parent cell (even though B-cells remain in lymph). The antibodies then circulate to the site of antigenic invasion. Note that there is a lag phase between antigen exposure and antibody production. Various factors influence this timeframe: for example, the differentiation of the B-cell into the plasma cell, the relative pathogenicity of the organism concerned, the organism's mode of entry to the body and whether antibody production is a primary or secondary immune response. The lag phase can be catastrophic if an organism has very high pathogenicity, for example Ebola virus (which produces a haemorrhagic disease), since the infection rapidly gains hold often with severe consequences (e.g. Ebola infection can kill within a few days).

Within the plasma cell's lifespan (4–5 days to a few weeks), they are capable of producing approximately 2000 antibody molecules per second; their high metabolic rate explains their brief existence. Some B-cells do not possess the genetic capability to differentiate. These remain as memory B-cells, which,

ACTIVITY

Make notes on the specialized and distinctive roles of T- and B-lymphocytes.

together with memory T-cells, are programmed to recognize an original antigen on its second and subsequent invasion of the body. They therefore also contribute to the secondary immune response, described below.

Primary and secondary immune responses

The role of T-lymphocytes in the primary response was noted earlier. For B-cells, those transformed into plasma cells also initiate antibody production in the primary immune response. The speed of this response is determined by the time it takes for antigenic activation of the appropriate B-cell, and for that specific B-cell's multiplication and differentiation. Consequently, there is a gradual sustained rise in circulating antibody concentration, peaking about 1–2 weeks after the initial exposure. Antibody concentration subsequently declines, assuming that the person is no longer exposed to those antigens. The decline in antibody production parallels the death of the plasma cells, which have a limited lifespan because of their high rate of metabolism. If the person recovers from a microbial infection upon first exposure without having to use medication, then it is because the primary immune response has provided sufficient defence to aid recovery. If, however, the primary response has not provided sufficient defence, then an illness 'drags on', and using medication (such as antibiotics) facilitates recovery.

Memory B-cells also may differentiate into plasma cells and become antibody producing, but only upon the second exposure to the original antigen. Memory cells have long lifespans, with some surviving 20 years or more. This secondary (anamnestic or memory) response occurs immediately on second contact with an antigen during this period, with antibodies being secreted rapidly in vast quantities. Peak values are higher and occur much more quickly than in the primary immune response. Figure 13.21 highlights the principal differences between primary and secondary immune responses. The secondary response is usually so swift that signs or symptoms of the illness are either very mild or absent, since the microbe is destroyed quickly and efficiently. The immediate antibody upsurge of the response may have pathological consequences, however, particularly if normal cells are also destroyed, since this could trigger a massive, widespread inflammatory response.

ACTIVITY

Differentiate between the specific and non-specific immune responses.

In summary, immunity is a set of reactions stimulated in response to the invasion of the body by non-self substances or antigens (Figure 13.22). The response is said to be:

Figure 13.21 The primary and secondary antibody responses and clones expansion

Q *Identify the principal differences between the primary and secondary immune responses.*

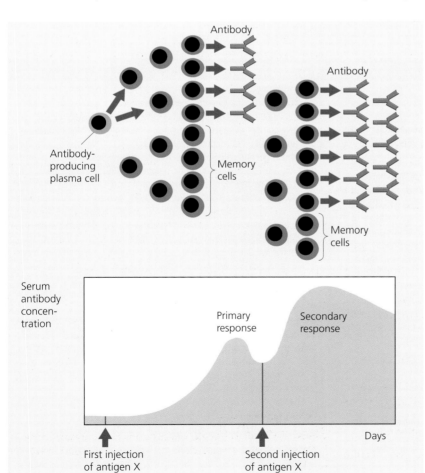

Antibody

Antibody

Antibody-producing plasma cell

Memory cells

Memory cells

Memory cells

Serum antibody concentration

Primary response

Secondary response

Days

First injection of antigen X

Second injection of antigen X

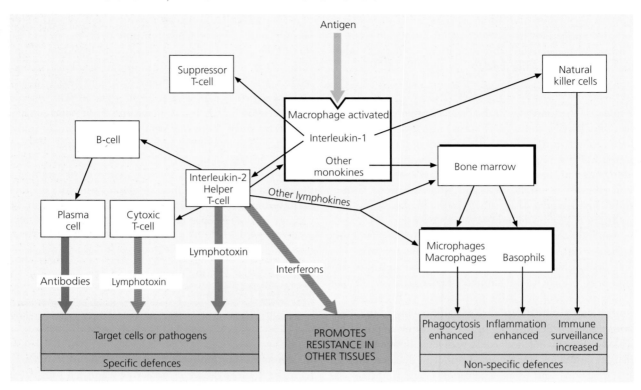

Figure 13.22 Summary of cellular and chemical interactions associated with the immune response

Q How would a lack of T-helper cells affect the humoral mediated immune response?

BOX 13.16 IMMUNE DEFICIENCY DISEASES AND HYPERSENSITIVE RESPONSES

Immune deficiency diseases

Individuals who either lack, or have defective, immune system components are said to have immune deficiencies. Some of these are acquired via transmission, such as acquired immune deficiency syndrome (AIDS), and some are inherited (such as severe immune deficiency syndrome, SCIDS).

Acquired immune deficiency syndrome

AIDS develops subsequent to infection by human immunodeficiency virus (HIV). Typically, the initial infection stimulates antibody production; IgMs are produced up to 1 month, while IgGs appear approximately 1 month post-infection, and continue to rise throughout the remainder of the year. These antibodies are produced in response to the HIV core proteins (Figure 13.23). Interestingly, the inappropriately named 'AIDS test' identifies these antibody markers of HIV infection (perhaps it should therefore be referred to as the 'anti-HIV test', since it is not a test for AIDS, or even HIV directly). Eventually, however, HIV depresses the body's immune system, primarily by invading helper T-cells (as its main host cell), thus inhibiting their central role in immunity. In this way, one homeostatic imbalance of T-cell deficiency leads to a failure of other interdependent homeostatic functions, for example:

- reduced antibody production, since helper cells stimulate immunoglobulin secretion by plasma cells;
- fewer killer T-cells, since helper cells secrete interleukin-2, which stimulates killer cell proliferation.

Monocytes and macrophages are also infected by HIV. The virus mainly remains dormant in these cells, but it decreases the host cell's secretion of interleukin-1, which is needed for the stimulation of interleukin-2 release. Suppressor T-cells are relatively unaffected by HIV.

Overall, HIV infection grossly impairs the person's normal immune functions, and consequently normally harmless microbes can initiate potentially fatal infections; the impairment of the host's defences allows the development of cancer and opportunistic infections of various kinds. The appearance of an opportunistic (or indicator) disease signifies that the person now has AIDS. The two most common diseases that kill AIDS patients are *Pneumocystis carinii* pneumonia (PCP) and Kaposi's sarcoma (KS). The former is a rare form of pneumonia, caused by a unicellular fungus, whereas KS is a rare, malignant skin cancer. Patients with AIDS are also prone to infections of the central nervous system, which eventually produce neurological imbalances such as AIDS dementia.

To date, AIDS appears to be invariably fatal. At present, treatment consists of fighting infections as they occur, experimenting with antiviral medication, and, more recently, via the use of immune system stimulants.

The triggers for the conversions of an HIV infection to early symptoms of AIDS (previously called AIDS-related complex, ARC, though this term is not so widely used now), and from ARC to AIDS, remain a mystery. Each transition has different signs and symptoms, owing to different homeostatic imbalances. The presence of these imbalances at specific times may perhaps help to explain why HIV infection leads to ARC or AIDS. For further reading, see Haddad *et al.* (2001) and Darbyshire *et al.* (2001): these articles discuss the current treatments and educational support for people with AIDS.

See the case study of the young man with symptomatic HIV/AIDS, Section VI, p.656.

Severe combined immunodeficiency

Severe combined immunodeficiency (SCID) is an inherited failure to develop cellular and humoral immunities, either as a consequence of a

BOX 13.16 *Continued*

lack of both T-cells and B-cells, or because the cells are inactive. Consequently, even mild infections can be fatal. Bone marrow transplants from a compatible donor, usually a very close (i.e. genetically similar) relative, have been used to colonize the patient's lymphatic tissue with functional lymphocytes. Although the immunodeficient child cannot reject the bone marrow tissue, the bone marrow can reject the child, since it contains immunologically active lymphocytes that react against the child's tissues.

Hypersensitivity responses

Hypersensitivity occurs either because the body is exposed to an excessive amount of antigen, so the antibody is secreted in too high a quantity, or because the antibodies and T-cells are directed against the body's own tissues (called autoimmune diseases). There are four main types of hypersensitive reactions:

- type I (anaphylaxis) reactions;
- type II (cytotoxic) reactions;
- type III (antibody-mediated) reactions;
- type IV (cell-mediated) reactions.

Type I reactions

An allergy is a hyperimmune response to an antigen (called an allergen in this case) to which most people have no noticeable responses. The symptoms of allergies, such as hay fever and asthma, following exposure to allergens (pollen, antibiotics, etc.) are dramatic and occasionally lethal (see below). People who are sensitive produce IgEs that bind to the surface receptors of mast cells and basophils (Figure 13.24a). These cells are found in and underneath the mucous membranes in the nose, throat, eyes and lungs. Binding causes the person to produce an allergic response, since such an interaction causes cells to release the chemical mediators of anaphylaxis (e.g. histamine, serotonin and prostaglandins). These are responsible for increasing blood capillary permeability, increasing smooth muscle contraction, and increasing secretion of mucus. Consequently, the person may experience oedema, erythema or redness, breathing difficulties and a runny nose, along with other inflammatory responses. Sensitive patients should therefore avoid histamine contained in foods.

Eosinophil counts are elevated during an allergic response, as a homeostatic adaptive response, since these cells are thought to exert anti-inflammatory effects by absorbing histamine.

Anaphylactic reactions, such as hay fever and bronchial asthma, may remain localized. Others are considered systemic (e.g. acute anaphylaxis) and may produce circulatory shock (in this case called anaphylactic shock) and asphyxia, both of which can be fatal without clinical intervention.

Some sensitized people can become accustomed to allergens if they are presented with them gradually and in increasing dosages (i.e. they become desensitised). Children often 'outgrow' allergies for this reason. Since only some people are allergic, this suggests that the tendency to produce IgEs in response to specific allergens may be determined genetically.

An example of a type I reaction that occurs within a few minutes of being sensitized is the response to chemicals in latex gloves. Latex is the sap from the Brazilian rubber tree and contains proteins and resins. The proteins cause allergic reactions in people who have a genetic susceptibility. Thus susceptible healthcare practitioners and patients are at risk in the perioperative environment. Approximately 4% of the UK workforce suffers occupational exposure to natural rubber latex (NRL), of this group 6% might be at risk of developing a latex sensitivity (Moore, 2000).

In the hospital environment powdered gloves are not worn routinely now and they are certainly not used in the sterile environment. The powder acts as a carrier for the latex proteins; hence when powdered gloves are worn more latex protein comes into contact with the skin, where it is subsequently absorbed. Upon removal of the gloves, the powder and proteins are released into the surrounding air where they can be inhaled, causing rhinitis, asthma and conjunctivitis. Inhalation and subsequent absorption into the circulation via the mucous membranes present a greater risk of systemic reaction (Charous, 2000).

Specific screening for NRL sensitivity should be considered for all patients, although this may be impractical and unrealistic. Therefore consideration must be given for facilitating best practice in the clinical setting. During pre-assessment surgical patients who are high risk of having NRL sensitivity should be offered clinical testing for this allergy. All sensitivities and details of their NRL allergy should be documented and all personnel involved in the care of the patient must be informed. Arrangements can then be made for the operating theatre to be cleaned and left free until the patient arrives, and the patient should be the first on the operating list. All equipment used, should, as far as possible be NRL free, although with over 40 000 products in use in the perioperative environment this may not be achievable. Products that are not NRL free must be covered with a barrier material and there should be limited access of staff to the operating theatre. Emergency drugs should also be readily available for use should the patient have and anaphylactic reaction.

In some circumstances such as with emergency patients, the perioperative practitioner may not always have prior knowledge that the patient is NRL sensitive, and these patients could have an anaphylactic reaction to NRL in the perioperative environment; therefore, all equipment used for resuscitation purposes should be latex free.

The problem of NRL allergy is growing and manufacturers of medical equipment are now producing latex-free products; however, until there is a totally NRL-free perioperative environment, the perioperative practitioner must minimize the risk of sensitization for patients and colleagues by following their local policy and guidelines.

Type II reactions

Cytotoxic reactions involve IgG, IgM or IgA antibodies, which bind to antigens on body (mainly blood) cells. This interaction activates the complement system, which causes:

- mast cell secretion of histamine and kinins, which cause local vasodilation and an increased permeability of capillary walls. They are also responsible for bronchoconstriction, which gives rise to inadequate gaseous exchange in the lung;
- the chemical attraction of neutrophils to the site of inflammation, enhancing phagocytosis by activating macrophages. Complement enzymes attached to the antigens and to antibodies identify the cells to be phagocytosed.

Affected cells are phagocytosed and/or destroyed (e.g. in ABO blood transfusions, the recipient's phagocytes lyse incompatible blood cells; see Figure 11.19, p.299). Drugs such as methyldopa may also cause haemolytic anaemia in susceptible people, because the drug coats erythrocytes and promotes immune attack. Similarly, bacterial endotoxins, such as those released from *Salmonella*, also cause erythrocyte haemolysis. Cytotoxic reactions may also result in the chronic failure of transplanted organs, which may become necrotic because of thrombosis of the donated organ. This is caused by an antibody response to the endothelium of the donated organ's blood vessels, causing it to be damaged and resulting in the adherence of platelets and thrombus formation.

Type III reactions

Type III reactions cause antibody – antigen complexes to be deposited in various tissues, for example in joints, causing arthritis, in the heart, causing myocarditis, and in renal glomeruli, causing glomerulonephritis.

BOX 13.16 *Continued*

The complement system in the presence of IgG or IgM may also be activated. A localized type III reaction (Arthus reaction) occurs when antigens are injected: a local vasculitis and inflammatory response occurs as a result of immunoglobulins forming complexes with the injected antigens. This sometimes occurs in diabetic people who have developed IgG antibodies against an antigenic component of their insulin preparations.

Type IV reactions

Cell-mediated (delayed-type) reactions involve T-cells, and are often not apparent for a day or more. They become apparent when allergens bind to tissue cells, causing them to be ingested by macrophages; the antigens are then presented to the T-cells. Consequently, T-cell proliferation is responsible for the destruction of allergens. An example of a type IV reaction is a positive tuberculosis (Mantoux) skin test.

The symptoms of hypersensitive reactions can develop within minutes of the allergic or anaphylactic response. It is important to understand that hypersensitive reactions are normal homeostatic protective responses, which, if excessive (i.e. in severe cases), can result in extensive peripheral vasodilation, producing a fall in blood pressure and possible circulatory collapse. Localized allergic reactions (such as those created by pollen exposure in hay fever sufferers) produce unpleasant but less severe symptoms.

Adrenaline administration counteracts some of the responses to histamine and antihistamine drugs. Treatment of severe anaphylaxis involves antihistamine and corticosteroid injections, in addition to respiratory and/or circulatory support.

Autoimmune diseases

Self-antigens do not normally initiate immune responses. However, our own body cells are sometimes destroyed by autoimmune responses. This type of reactivity may be important in the normal homeostatic control of body function (e.g. in wound healing by removing dead tissues and cells). At other times, autoimmune responses are less beneficial. When autoimmunity noticeably damages otherwise healthy tissues, it causes autoimmune diseases, such as:

- *Diabetes mellitus*: autoantibodies may destroy the beta islets of Langerhans, thus causing the hypoinsulinism associated with Type I or insulin-dependent diabetes mellitus.
- *Hashimoto's thyroiditis*: anti-thyroid antibodies may impair the activity of a person with thyroid gland.
- *Myasthenia gravis*: autoantibodies interfere with the function of motor end plates at neuromuscular synapses, preventing the transmission of nerve impulses to motor muscles. They do so by decreasing the sensitivity of muscle membrane receptors to the neurotransmitter chemical acetylcholine, or by destroying the neurotransmitter itself. These patients have weak muscles that fatigue easily and eventually may become paralysed.
- *Rheumatoid arthritis* (rheumatoid disease) autoantibodies to certain immunoglobulins result in deposition of complexes within the synovial joints, eventually leading to destructive changes. Other tissues such as the lungs and blood vessels may also be affected.

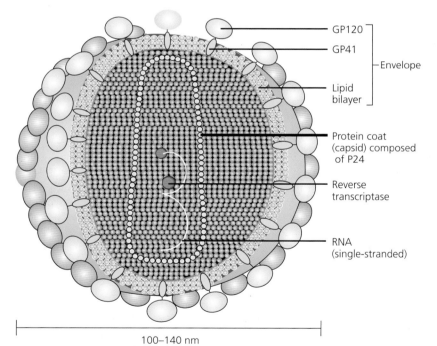

Figure 13.23 Structure of Human immunodeficiency virus (HIV)

Q How do retroviruses differ from 'normal' viruses?

GP120
GP41
Envelope
Lipid bilayer
Protein coat (capsid) composed of P24
Reverse transcriptase
RNA (single-stranded)

100–140 nm

- xenophobic (i.e. the body distinguishes between self and non-self antigenic materials);
- highly specific for different antigenic insults;
- adaptive (i.e. an antigenic invasion produces a response to the environmental, antigenic, insult);
- anamnestic (i.e. there is a memory component of the immune response, allowing both primary and secondary responses to occur).

Immunological competence

Immunological competence is the ability to produce an immune response to an antigenic insult. Cellular immunity

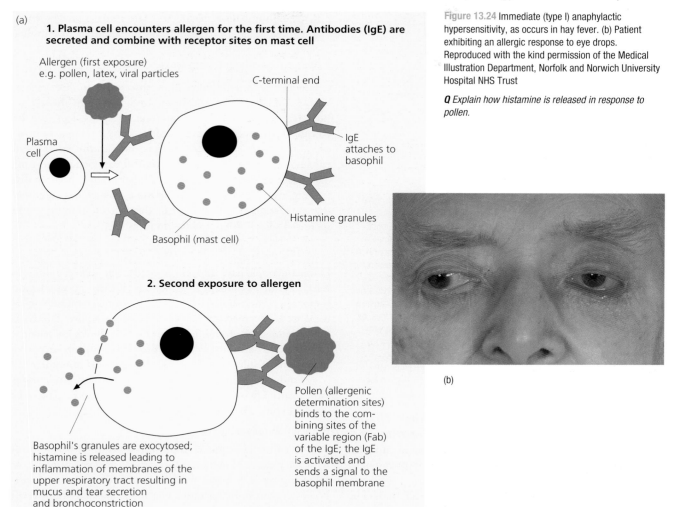

(a)

1. Plasma cell encounters allergen for the first time. Antibodies (IgE) are secreted and combine with receptor sites on mast cell

Allergen (first exposure)
e.g. pollen, latex, viral particles

Plasma cell

C-terminal end

IgE attaches to basophil

Histamine granules

Basophil (mast cell)

2. Second exposure to allergen

Basophil's granules are exocytosed; histamine is released leading to inflammation of membranes of the upper respiratory tract resulting in mucus and tear secretion and bronchoconstriction

Pollen (allergenic determination sites) binds to the combining sites of the variable region (Fab) of the IgE; the IgE is activated and sends a signal to the basophil membrane

(b)

Figure 13.24 Immediate (type I) anaphylactic hypersensitivity, as occurs in hay fever. (b) Patient exhibiting an allergic response to eye drops. Reproduced with the kind permission of the Medical Illustration Department, Norfolk and Norwich University Hospital NHS Trust

Q *Explain how histamine is released in response to pollen.*

occurs from approximately the third month of gestation, but active humoral (antibody) immunity appears much later. The fetus, however, receives IgGs from the maternal circulation until delivery, although this is referred to as passive immunity, since it is not an immunological response of fetal tissue. In the seventh month of gestatory development, the fetus develops IgA and IgM immunological competence if exposed to the relevant antigens. The mother also provides IgAs in breast milk, postnatally. This passive immunity gives resistance for approximately 3 months after birth, until the liver eventually destroys the transferred antibodies. Since there is no anamnestic (memory) immune response in the baby, during this period the infant is vulnerable to infection; routine primary immunization programmes are thus commenced at 2 months of age. This ensures that the acquisition of active immunity against pathogens that have the potential to produce serious diseases, such as diphthe-

ria, tetanus, poliomyelitis and meningitis (see Table 13.1, p.386 and Figure 13.26). This active immunity is long-lasting.

The levels of IgA, IgD and IgE antibodies begin to rise 1 month after birth, and reach half the adult level by 3 years of age. During childhood, the antibody titres rise gradually towards adult levels and the population of memory B- and T-cells increases progressively as one encounters different antigens, until their decline as a consequence of the ageing process.

Stress and immunity

It is generally accepted that distress depresses the immune responses. Interleukin-1, secreted from macrophages, stimulates the secretion of ACTH from the pituitary gland; this has a direct action on lowering antibody production and stimulating the secretion of glucocorticoids from the adrenal glands. These steroidal hormones therefore have anti-inflammatory effects, and their long-term secretion inhibits the immune response, lowering resistance to disease (Figure 13.25). These inhibitory mechanisms are as follows:

- Depression or cessation of the immune response. Glucocorticoid hormones inhibit mast cell activity and so

ACTIVITY

Discuss in broad terms the homeostatic failures associated with the immune system.

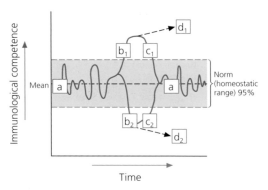

Figure 13.25 Immunological competence: a homeostatic process. (a) Normal homeostatic sensitivity and functioning of the immune system's component parts (i.e. cellular/humoral responses). b_1, Hypersensitive immune response. This can be a temporary hypersensitive response to an overexposure to immunogen and non-immunogen antigens (e.g. as occurs in the secondary immune response), so that signs and symptoms are mild or do not appear, or it can be a pathological hypersensitive response reflecting a homeostatic imbalance, such as occurs in allergies, tissue rejection following transplantation, and autoimmune diseases). b_2, Hyposensitive immune response. This can be a temporary response that does not necessarily reflect an infection or illness, as occurs in acute bouts of distress, or a pathological response, as occurs with immune deficiency syndromes and chronic bouts of distress. c_1, c_2, Normal function restored. d_1, Terminal autoimmune allergic reaction (shock). d_2, Terminal immunological deficiency syndromes, such as acquired immune deficiency syndrome (AIDS). (a, Represents boxes a_1–a_4, p.11, reflecting the individual variability in the homeostatic range)

decrease the availability of histamine, the initiator of inflammation. Capillaries remain impermeable to protein, which reduces the availability of fibrinogen, complement and other cellular defences important in the inflammatory response. This inhibition can halt inflammation.

• Inhibition of interleukin production and secretion. This depresses the stimulation of killer cell proliferation and other responses associated with interleukins.

• Reduced number of phagocytes. This impairs phagocytosis, and the antigenic processing and presentation to lymphocytes.
• Reduced number of lymphocytes.

Consequently, one becomes more susceptible to diseases (i.e. 'diseases of adaptation', according to Selye's stress theory; see Box 21.5, p.599) when the immune system is depressed by chronic distress (known as 'unhealthy stress'). It appears, however, that some stress (i.e. eustress, or 'healthy stress') can enhance immune responses. Eustressful experiences are time dependent and generally short lived, before they become distressing, which could explain why most research has identified the association between distress, the loss of immunity and increased susceptibility to infectious disease.

The acquisition of immunity

Different people have different resistance and susceptibilities to infections, depending on the efficiency of their immunological responses. The subjectivity of a person's immunological response is governed by their unique genetic ability (known as innate immunity which is inherited from the biological parents) to respond to harmful agents, and their environmental exposure to antigenic insults, which is referred to acquired immunity.

An individual can acquire immunity to infectious diseases either naturally or artificially, both of which can be passive or active (Figure 13.26).

Passive naturally acquired immunity

Passive naturally acquired immunity is acquired before birth with the passage of maternal antibodies across the placenta, or following birth in breast-fed babies with the passage of antibodies present in breast milk. The actual antibody transferred by the mother depends upon her own immunological resistance and competence. Passive immunity is short lived, since

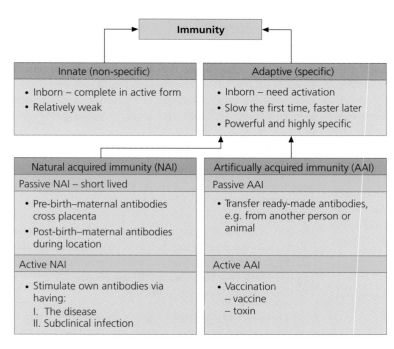

Figure 13.26 Types of immunity

Q What defences, present at birth, provide the body with the defence capability known as the non-specific response resistance?

the child's lymphocytes are not activated, and the maternally derived antibodies are not replaced as they are metabolized.

Another important use of passive immunization is the prevention of rhesus incompatibility in pregnancy by injection of anti-D antibody (see Box 11.28, p.302, and Figure 11.20b, p.301).

Active naturally acquired immunity

This form of immunity involves activating the body to produce its own antibodies. It is acquired by:

• having the disease: this process has been explored in depth in this chapter. During an illness, B-lymphocytes differentiate into plasma cells, which produce and secrete antibodies, usually in sufficient quantities to overcome the potentially infecting antigenic insult. Upon recovery and during convalescence, lymphocytes retain the ability to produce these specific antibodies against the antigens encountered previously, since there is a memory component associated with immunity;

• having a subclinical infection: in this situation, the infection is not severe enough to cause clinical manifestation (i.e. signs and symptoms) of disease. It does, however, stimulate B-lymphocyte activity.

Passive artificially acquired immunity

Passive artificial immunity is acquired by giving people ready-made antibodies using human or animal sera (see Box 13.17 and Table 13.1, p.386). Antibodies are obtained from convalescing individuals, or from horses that have been artificially immunized. The anti-serum (i.e. serum containing antibodies) is administered to prevent the development of a disease in people who are later exposed to the infection, or therapeutically after the disease has developed.

The antibody-containing serum from other species, however, can manifest itself as a dangerous hyperimmune response (anaphylactic reaction) in susceptible individuals.

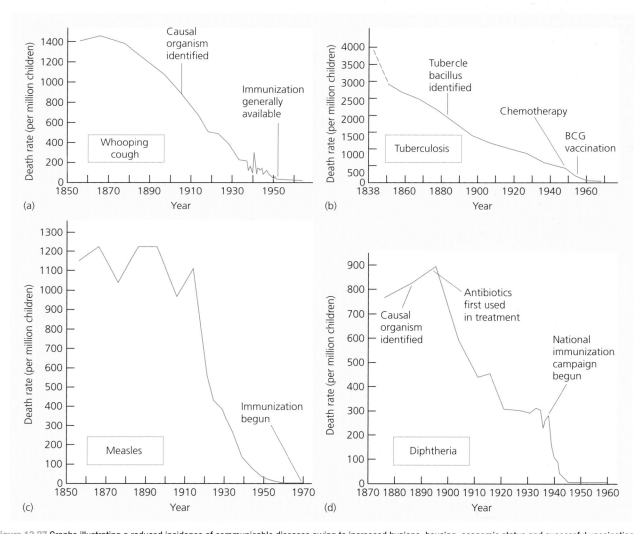

Figure 13.27 Graphs illustrating a reduced incidence of communicable diseases owing to increased hygiene, housing, economic status and successful vaccination programmes. (a) Whooping cough: death rates of children under 15 years in England and Wales. (b) Respiratory tuberculosis: death rates of children under 15 years in England and Wales. (c) Measles: death rates of children under 15 years in England and Wales. (d) Diphtheria: death rates of children under 15 years in England and Wales

Q *Suggest why some immunization programmes (e.g. whooping cough) confer lifelong immunity and others (e.g. tetanus) relatively short-lived immunity.*

BOX 13.17 IMMUNIZATION PROGRAMMES AND CHILDHOOD IMMUNIZATION

Immunization prepares our bodies to fight against diseases in case we come into contact with them in the future. The anamnestic response forms the basis of immunization programmes (i.e. the initial immunization sensitizes the body, so that if the immunogen is encountered in the future through infection, or a booster dose of the antigen is administered, then the body experiences the anamnestic response). Some immunizations have to be given more than once to build up immunity (protection) or to keep the level of antibodies 'topped up'. This 'top-up' is called a booster. Booster dosages are required because antibodies and memory cells have a limited metabolic lifespan, and therefore the antigen must be given periodically to maintain high antibody titres. In some instances there is controversy over side-effects of immunizations (see below); however the success of public health measures and immunization programmes in the UK has made some conditions rare, and this has led to a decline in the uptake of immunization by children, and the incidence of diseases such as measles has since increased.

A child should not be immunized if he or she has:

- pyrexia;
- had a hypersensitive reaction to another immunization or after eating eggs;
- a bleeding disorder;
- been taking immunosuppressants (given after organ transplant or for malignant disease) or high-dose steroids;
- HIV or AIDS;
- had, or is having, treatment for cancer.

Specialist advice is needed before immunizing children who have had convulsions (fits) in the past.

All immunizations (except polio) are given with a small needle into the child's upper arm, buttock or thigh.

DTP-Hib vaccine

This vaccine protects against three different diseases – diphtheria, tetanus and pertussis (whooping cough) – and against infection by the bacteria *Haemophilus influenzae* type b (Hib). The vaccine is administered at 2–4 months; further tetanus and diphtheria boosters are given between 13 and 18 years. The DT part is administered as a booster at 3–5 years.

Diphtheria rarely occurs in the UK. The condition starts with a sore throat, and can progress rapidly to cause problems with breathing. It can damage the heart and the nervous system. In severe cases, it can be fatal.

Tetanus bacteria (*Clostridium tetani*) are found in soil. They come into the body through a cut or burn. This is a painful disease that affects the muscles and can cause breathing problems. If untreated, it can be fatal.

Whooping cough (pertussis, caused by *Bordetella pertussis*) can be very distressing. The patient becomes exhausted by extensive bouts of coughing, which frequently cause vomiting and choking. In severe cases, pertussis can be fatal.

Infection by Hib is can cause a number of serious conditions, including meningitis, pneumonia and blood poisoning, all of which can be dangerous if not treated quickly. Meningitis is an inflammation of the meninges or lining of the brain. It is a very serious condition, but if it is spotted and treated early, most children make a full recovery. The Hib vaccine gives protection against Hib meningitis, but it does not protect children against other bacterial types, such as meningococcal or pneumococcal meningitis, or viral meningitis. A baby with meningitis can become dangerously ill within hours. Early symptoms include fever, vomiting, irritability and restlessness. Refusing feeds is also common with colds and influenza. Other important signs to look for are a high-pitched moaning cry, difficulty in waking, pale or blotching skin, and red/purple spots. Common signs in older children include stiffness in the neck, severe headaches, a dislike of bright lights, confusion or drowsiness, and red/purple spots.

Polio vaccine

This vaccine protects against the disease poliomyelitis. Poliovirus is passed in the faeces of infected people and of those who have just been immunized against polio. It attacks the nervous system and may cause long-term muscle paralysis. If the chest muscles are attacked, it can be fatal. Routine immunization has meant that the natural virus no longer causes cases of polio in the UK. The vaccine is administered at 2–4 months. A booster is administered between 3 and 5 years, and another booster is given between 13 and 18 years.

MMR vaccine

This vaccine protects against measles, mumps and rubella. Measles is a very infectious viral disease. It is immediately recognizable by its characteristic rash. The infection can cause a high fever. Approximately 7% of children who contract measles are at risk of complications (e.g. chest infections, fits and brain damage). In severe cases, measles can be fatal.

Mumps, another viral infection, causes swollen glands in the face. Mumps was the most frequent cause of viral meningitis in children under 15 years before immunization was commenced. The condition can cause swelling of the gonads (testicles and ovaries) and deafness.

If a pregnant woman contracts the rubella (German measles) virus in early pregnancy, it can harm the unborn baby after birth, although the condition is usually very mild and is not likely to cause the infant any problems.

ACTIVITY

The Wakefield report of 2000 controversially raised doubts over the safety of the MMR vaccine (see Kawashima *et al.*, 2000). The researchers claimed that those children immunized with the MMR vaccine had an increased risk of developing autism later. It is generally accepted by immunology experts that the data of this report are far from being convincing, and the reader is directed to an article by Martin (2000).

BCG vaccine

The BCG (bacille Calmette-Guérin) vaccine gives protection against tuberculosis (TB). This is a bacterial infection, caused by *Mycobacterium tuberculosis*, which frequently affects the lungs. It may also affect the brain and bones. Arguably, TB no longer exists in the UK. However, there are still between 5500 and 6000 cases a year, because TB is on the increase in Africa and in some Eastern European countries.

This vaccine is administered sometimes shortly after birth but more frequently at the age of 10–14 years, when a skin test is given to see if the person already has immunity to TB. If immunity is not present, the immunization is given. A hypersensitive reaction occurs in some sensitive children resulting in abscess formation (Figure 13.28).

Hepatitis B vaccine

Several types of hepatitis exist, and they all cause inflammation of the liver (see Box 10.30, p.266). This vaccine protects against hepatitis B virus, which is passed via infected blood and may be sexually transmitted. Some people are healthy carriers of hepatitis B; if a pregnant woman is a hepatitis B carrier, she can pass it on to her child. The child may not be ill, but has a high probability of becoming a carrier and developing liver disease in later years. Because of this risk, many pregnant women are tested for hepatitis B; babies born to infected mothers will be administered a course of vaccine to prevent them contracting hepatitis B and becoming a carrier.

This has led to the removal of horse serum treatment (containing tetanus anti-toxins) in people infected with the tetanus organism.

Active artificially acquired immunity

This form of immunity involves immunization: injecting people with dead, or live but artificially weakened (attenuated), microbes as vaccines, or detoxified microbial toxins as toxoids. Vaccines and toxoids retain antigenic properties and therefore stimulate the immune response without causing disease.

Killed vaccines give protection against whooping cough, typhoid and cholera. Such administrations are given on two or three occasions, often with a booster dose after the initial programme of vaccination, because only small numbers of antigens are introduced on each occasion (see Table 13.1, p.386).

Attenuated vaccines are those in which the organism has been cultured artificially to produce a strain that no longer has any pathogenic properties. However, the organism continues to divide within the body after it has been administered, and gives rise to a full immune response, closely mimicking that followed by a natural infection. Thus, often only one administration is required to give the protection of lifelong immunity to the disease. Diseases prevented by this type of vaccine include mumps, rubella, TB and poliomyelitis.

Toxoids are preparations of bacterial endotoxins that no longer produce the disease: a chemical (e.g. formalin) is added that renders it harmless. The pathogens that cause tetanus and diphtheria both produce exotoxins, and protection is therefore achieved by the administration of toxoids.

Edward Jenner performed the first vaccination of this kind in 1796. He used the fluid extracted from cowpox blisters to confer immunity against the similar smallpox virus. Modern immunization programmes have reduced the incidence of many serious diseases, including whooping cough, TB, measles, diphtheria (see Figure 13.27), cholera, rubella, smallpox, typhoid and poliomyelitis. The success of these pro-

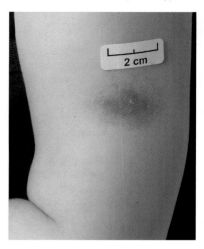

Figure 13.28 Patient exhibiting an abscess in response to the BCG. Reproduced with the kind permission of the Medical Illustration Department, Norfolk and Norwich University Hospital NHS Trust

grammes means that some diseases, such as polio, no longer occur in the UK and smallpox has been eradicated globally. In other countries where immunization is not so widely available, this is not the case. Since overseas travel is so popular now, there is a risk that diseases could be brought back into the UK and spread to individuals that have not been immunized.

Immunization can confer either lifelong immunity against infections, such as whooping cough and mumps, or short-lived immunity against certain other infections. Tetanus immunization, for example, is effective for just a number of years. Some immunity, however, may last for only a few weeks before revaccination is necessary.

The apparent loss of immunity to an infective microbe may result from contact with different microbial strains that are capable of producing the same clinical manifestations. Influenza viruses, for example, have rapid mutation rates, and even a slight mutation (i.e. change in the viral genetic make-up) produces different antigenic properties, hence we are constantly subjected to different bouts of influenza.

SUMMARY

1 The lymphatic system is associated closely with the cardiovascular system. It transports excess tissue fluid to the blood, helps defend the body against disease-causing microbes, and transports long-chain fatty acids absorbed from the gut into the blood.

2 Lymph is formed in blind-ended tubes that are closely associated with capillary networks. It then flows into lymphatic vessels that drain into the two major thoracic collecting ducts, which return lymph to blood at the junction of the subclavian and jugular veins.

3 Lymph flow is aided via the squeezing actions of surrounding skeletal muscles, low pressure in the thorax created by breathing movements and the presence of valves.

4 Any condition that interferes with the flow of lymph results in the clinical condition called oedema.

5 Lymph nodes are clinically important, as they are the production centres for lymphocytes. They also contain macrophages, and so filter foreign particles present in the lymph.

6 The spleen resembles an enlarged lymph node, hence its similar function. It also acts as a blood reservoir.

7 The body has a number of external defence mechanisms that provide formidable barriers against antigenic invasions.

8 Inside the body, the antigenic material encounters non-specific defence mechanisms (phagocytic response) and specific defence mechanisms (lymphocytic responses). The phagocytic and lymphatic responses are extremely effective in protecting the body from pathogenic activity, and at promoting recovery from infection.

9 The phagocytic response consists of inflammation and phagocytosis.

10 Monocytes give rise to phagocytic macrophages.

11 The lymphocytic response comprises cellular (T-cell) and the humoral (B-cell) immune responses. The T- and B-lymphocytes secrete cytotoxic substances and antibodies, respectively, in response to antigenic insults.

12 Stem cell lymphocytes originate in the bone marrow.

13 The thymus produces T-lymphocytes and a hormone thymosin (thymosin), which stimulates other lymphoid tissue to produce T-cells.

14 The bone marrow and other sites of the body produce B-lymphocytes.

SUMMARY

15 The memory component of the immune response ensures a quicker and boosted response following subsequent detection of an antigen, resulting in the majority of situations presenting no signs and/or symptoms of a disease should the antigen enter the body once again.

16 Immunization gives protection against a variety of infections.

17 The two principal problems associated with homeostatic failure of the lymphatic system are lymphatic obstructions and the spreading of infections.

18 Knowledge of the location of lymph nodes and the direction of lymph flow is important in predicting the source of infection and the spread of cancers.

19 Homeostatic imbalances of immune responses involving abnormal immune system responses can be categorized as being problems arising from either inadequate or excessive sensitivity. The former includes the immune deficiency diseases, which result from inadequate humoral and/or cellular immune responses. Such an imbalance may be inherited or acquired. Excessive sensitivity involves homeostatic imbalances arising from the immune mechanisms responding too well or too often. Such imbalances result in allergies, tissue rejection following transplantation, or autoimmune diseases.

REFERENCES

Charous, B.L. (2000) Update on occupational latex allergy. In: *American Academy of Allergy, Asthma and Immunology 56th AGM*. Milwaukee: American Academy of Allergy, Asthma and Immunology.

Darbyshire, J., Foulkes, M., Peto, R. *et al.* (2001) Deciphering autoimmune disease in women. *Patient Care* **34**(7): 49–59.

Haddad, M., Inch, C., Glazier, R.H. *et al.* (2001) Patient support and education for promoting adherence to highly active antiretroviral therapy for HIV/AIDS. *The Cochrane Library*. Oxford: Update Software.

Kawashima, H., Mori, T., Kashiwagi, Y. *et al.* (2000) Digestive disease. *Sciences* **45**(4): 723–9.

Kosits, C. and Callaghan, M. (2000) Rituximab: a new monoclonal antibody therapy for non-Hodgkin's lymphoma. *Oncology Nursing Forum* **27**(1): 51–9.

Martin, J. (2000) Measles, mumps and rubella. *Practice Nurse* **20**(9): 552–4.

May, D. (2000) Infection control. *Nursing Standard* **14**(28): 51–9.

McVicar, A.J. and Clancy, J. (1997) The physiological basis of fluid therapy. *Professional Nurse Supplement* **12**(8): S6–S9.

Moore, A. (2000) *Latex Allergy*. Bandolier Internet Publications.

Pace, B. (2000) JAMA patient page. Suppressing the immune system for organ transplants. *Journal of the American Medical Association* **283**(18): 2484.

Salvage. J. (2000) Now wash your hands . . . hand hygiene remains the single most important means of preventing hospital-acquired infection. *Nursing Times* **96**(43): 22.

FURTHER READING

Palmer, J. (2000) Organ transplants. *Physiotherapy Frontline* **6**(1): 16.

Peto, T. and Walker, A. (2001) Zidovudine (AZT) versus AZT plus didanosine (ddI) versus AZT plus zalcitabine (ddC) in HIV infected adults. *The Cochrane Library*. Oxford: Update Software.

THE RESPIRATORY SYSTEM

INTRODUCTION

'Respiration' is a term that refers to the utilization of oxygen by the body in the release of energy. Chapters 2 and 4 described how energy is released when chemical bonds within fuels such as glucose are broken, and is incorporated into other bonds within a chemical, adenosine triphosphate (ATP), and in that form is readily accessible to cell processes. Although some ATP is generated in cells in the absence of oxygen ('anaerobic'), most is by 'aerobic' metabolism involving oxygen. The actual oxygen requirement of individual tissues varies according to their energy needs. For example, cardiac muscle is very active and uses about 30 times as much oxygen per minute than does the relatively inactive skin. Oxygen requirements are also responsive to changing situations, for example in skeletal muscle tissue oxygen utilization may increase 15-fold during exercise.

Maintaining an adequate supply of oxygen therefore is essential to the metabolic homeostasis of cells and tissues. Tissue oxygenation occurs through four stages:

1 Oxygen is taken in from the air by blood.
2 Oxygen is carried by the blood.
3 Tissues receive adequate perfusion with blood.
4 Oxygen passes from the blood to cells.

In cells, the respiration of the main 'fuel', glucose, generates carbon dioxide. This has an important role in determining the acidity of body fluids (see Chapter 6, p.130) but in excess may cause an acidosis, a potentially dangerous situation. Excess carbon dioxide ordinarily is excreted primarily through the lungs. Lung function therefore is viewed as exchanging oxygen and carbon dioxide, and its control relates to the body's needs in this respect. Clinical terms used to identify poor control of these gases in blood and tissues are:

* *hypoxia*: a lack of oxygenation in tissues;
* *hypoxaemia*: poor oxygenation of arterial blood ('-aemia' = of blood). However, hypoxaemia will induce hypoxia and so this latter term tends to be more widely used, even if the problem stems from poor blood oxygenation;

* *hypercapnia*: excess carbon dioxide in arterial blood. The production of carbonic acid when carbon dioxide combines with water means that hypercapnia is often associated with increased acidity (acidosis);
* *hypocapnia*: deficiency of carbon dioxide in arterial blood. The lack of this important source of acidity means that hypocapnia is often associated with excessive alkalinity (alkalosis).

Carbon dioxide excretion entails more or less the opposite sequence of events from those identified above for oxygen:

1 Uptake of carbon dioxide by blood from cells.
2 Transportation of carbon dioxide by blood.
3 Transfer of carbon dioxide from blood to the air.

A common feature is ensuring that tissues are adequately perfused with blood, so that the respiratory requirements of cells are met, and this is one of the most important roles of the cardiovascular system, described in Chapter 12. The present chapter describes the other processes, that is, those involved in exchanging gases with air, in transporting them within blood, and in exchanging them at cell level.

OVERVIEW OF LUNG ANATOMY AND GENERAL PRINCIPLES OF LUNG FUNCTIONS

This section introduces the general principles of lung function; function is explained in more detail in a later section in the context of lung physiology and lung disorder. Readers should familiarize themselves with the terms frequently used in relation to lung function and respiration (Box 14.1).

The lungs are paired organs lying within the thoracic cavity (Figure 14.1). The left lung has two lobes while the right has three; the left lung is smaller than the right because of space occupied by the heart (Figure 14.2). The lungs and chest wall are lined with membranes called the visceral pleural membrane and parietal pleural membrane, respectively. The narrow cavity between these two membranes forms the fluid-filled pleural space, although the volume of fluid normally present is only of the order of 5 mL in total and so the space is extremely thin. Albeit small, the pleural space and fluid form a crucial component of the functioning of the lungs (described later).

BOX 14.1 SOME GENERAL TERMS USED IN RELATION TO THE RESPIRATORY SYSTEM

- *Respiration*: a general term relating to oxygen uptake and utilization.
- *Internal respiration*: the biochemical reactions taking place within cells that consume oxygen and produce carbon dioxide.
- *External respiration*: the processes occurring within the lungs in taking up oxygen from air and releasing carbon dioxide into it. Much of this chapter explains the processes involved in external respiration.
- *Inspiration*: the process of breathing in.
- *Expiration*: the process of breathing out.
- *Dyspnoea*: strictly speaking, this term refers to an inadequate ventilation of the lungs. It is similar therefore to the term hypoventilation (see Box 14.20, p.412) but it is more widely used in the context of difficulty in breathing (uncomfortable, laboured, even painful) since this more satisfactorily relates the problem to the patient's experience and to the nurse's observation.
- *Apnoea*: this term refers to cessation of breathing, or breathing that is ineffectual in oxygenating blood.
- *Anoxia*: not strictly related to the respiratory system *per se*, this term is used in relation to tissue oxygenation secondary to lung function. Basically it means 'no oxygenation'.
- *Asphyxia*: a physical means, such as choking, that prevents breathing from occurring, leading to anoxia.

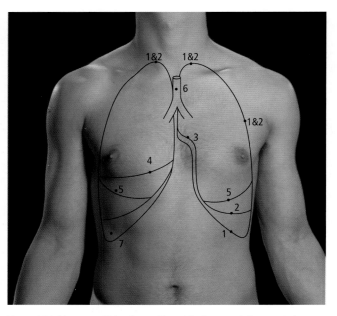

Figure 14.1 Diagram outlining the position of the lungs and pleura, anterior aspect: 1, pleural markings; 2, lung markings; 3, cardiac notch; 4, horizontal fissure; 5, oblique fissure; 6, trachea; 7, costodiaphragmatic recess. Reprinted with the kind permission of Abrahams *et al.*, from *Illustrated Clinical Anatomy*, Hodder, London.

The lungs are totally separated from the abdomen by a sheet of skeletal muscle called the diaphragm. This muscle is dome-shaped prior to lung expansion but flattens during breathing in (Figure 14.3). These actions of the diaphragm are essential to lung inflation and deflation.

Within the lungs are the airways that actually commence with the nasal cavity but extend to the minute gas-exchanging sacs, or alveoli. The general anatomy of the lung and its airways is shown in Figure 14.2. The macrostructure of the lung may be likened to that of a tree, in which the continuously dividing airways represent the branches.

The respiratory 'tree'

The airways commence with the nasal cavity, a large cavity lined with ciliated and glandular epithelium that filters and moistens the air on breathing in. The area is well supported with blood and the epithelium therefore also warms the incoming air. The efficiency of these processes is increased by the air passing over a number of projections, called conchae, that increase the cavity's surface area. The processes continue within the throat cavities, or pharynx, at the back of the mouth, which has two components: the oropharynx forms what most people would consider to be the throat itself, the nasopharynx is an extension of the throat upwards towards the nasal passages. The oropharynx opens into the oesophagus that carries food to the stomach, and the glottis, the opening to the lungs. The entrance of food into the glottis when swallowing is prevented by its closure with a small flap called the epiglottis ('epi-' = upon).

After the glottis the air enters the larynx; a structure of cartilage and ligaments that forms the 'Adam's apple'. The entire

BOX 14.2 SPUTUM

Sputum is the mucus (usually mixed with saliva from the mouth) that is removed from the airways by coughing. Mucus production is not unusual but in health it is generally of a slightly thickened consistency, and is fairly colourless.

If an infection is present* the mucus may be purulent (i.e. contains pus, the debris of dead microorganisms and body cells).The amount, colour, consistency and odour of sputum varies with different lung disorders (Johnson *et al.*, 2008).

Colour and odour are influenced by the presence of microorganisms or by the presence of blood. Infections can produce sputum of a characteristic colour. For example:

- *Streptococcus pneumoniae* produces rusty-coloured sputum;
- *Staphylococcus aureus* produces salmon-pink sputum;

- *Pseudomonas aeruginosa* causes a greenish sputum.

Consistency and volume largely depends upon the extent of infection but are also influenced by the organism present. For example, viral pneumonia produces a scanty sputum, whereas bacterial pneumonia is much more productive. Obstructive airway conditions such as chronic bronchitis may cause production of a thick, stringy mucus on coughing. Early stages of such conditions may include a non-productive cough but increased exertion with a worsening of the condition will be productive. The mucus may even contain casts of lining tissues that have been sloughed by the exertions of coughing.

*Note: some organisms are present within the mouth and so may contaminate a sputum sample that is to be analysed for its microorganisms. If of concern then a sample may be obtained direct from the trachea.

(a)

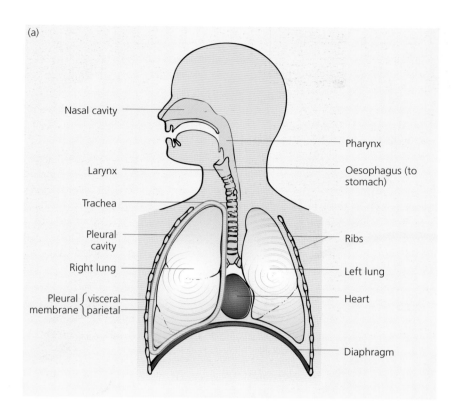

Figure 14.2 (a) Position of the lungs within the thoracic cavity. (b) The 'respiratory tree'. Pleural membranes shown on right side only

Q Which part of the 'respiratory tree' is affected by chronic bronchitis?

Q What structure maintains the patency of the trachea?

(b)

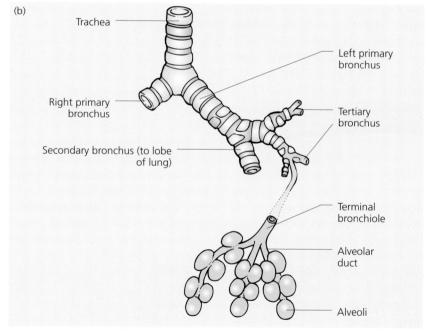

structure is supported by muscles that suspend the larynx from a small bone in the neck called the hyoid (see Figure 3.10, p.72). Within the larynx are folds of cartilage that form the 'vocal cords'. Air flowing over these causes them to vibrate and so produce sound: the voice. Their tension determines the tone or pitch of the sound and this can be altered by small muscles that pass from the cords to the cartilage of the larynx capsule. In men, actions of the sex steroid hormone testos-

terone cause elongation and thickening of the fibres during puberty and this is responsible for the larger larynx and the deeper voice tone that is produced.

From the larynx the inspired air enters the trachea, a tube of fibrous and muscular tissue some 12 cm in length and 2.5 cm in diameter, that is strengthened by 16–20 C-shaped rings of cartilage which prevent it from collapsing; the absence of carti-lage posteriorly prevents friction through rubbing with the

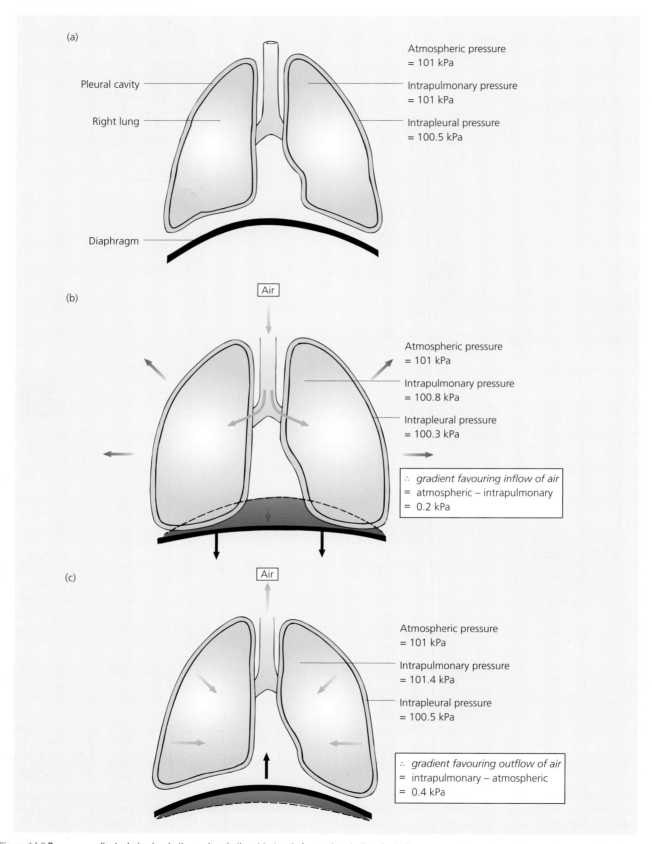

Figure 14.3 Pressure gradients during inspiration and expiration: (a) at end of normal expiration, (b) during inspiration and (c) during expiration

Q *What is the relation between alveolar pressure and atmospheric pressure (1) during inspiration and (2) at end-expiration?*

oesophagus during swallowing. The trachea is lined with a ciliated and mucus-producing epithelium: the mucus helps to moisten the airways, but also collects dusts particles and microorganisms that have been inhaled, which might be harmful should they enter the smaller airways. The particles are removed through the wafting of mucus towards the glottis by the cilia, where the mucus is swallowed and any microbes destroyed by the pH changes within the gastrointestinal tract. Coughing may also remove excess mucus, now commonly referred to as sputum, the colour and consistency of which can aid diagnosis of airway infection (Box 14.2).

The trachea divides into successively smaller airways:

- The left and right primary bronchi (singular, bronchus). The primary bronchi are generally similar in structure to the trachea, but are of smaller diameter. One primary bronchus goes to each lung.
- Secondary bronchi branch from the primary ones, and each supplies a lobe of a lung (i.e. there are three on the right side, and two on the left).
- In turn the secondary bronchi branch to form tertiary bronchi. Cartilaginous structures become less well defined in these smaller bronchi.
- Tertiary bronchi branch into numerous even smaller airways called bronchioles. Although less than 1 mm in diameter, these divide further and thus continue the extensive network of branches of the 'tree'. Bronchioles do not contain cartilage but have walls of smooth muscle.
- Bronchioles ultimately terminate in alveolar ducts that open into minute clusters of cup-shaped or globular sacs called alveoli (singular, alveolus; Figure 14.4). Each alveolus is of the order of 0.3 mm in diameter and is supported by elastic tissue. Alveoli are richly supplied with blood capillaries and the barrier formed by the capillary endothelial cells and the alveolar epithelial cells forms the surface across which gas exchange occurs between the lung and blood. Being globular and extremely numerous (approximately 300 million in total) alveoli provide a huge surface area for gas exchange between the alveoli and the blood: it has been estimated that the surface area of a pair of adult lungs is as much as 70 m².

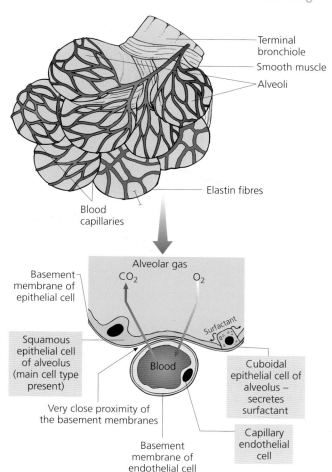

Figure 14.4 Alveoli and the alveolar–capillary membranes

Q How is gaseous exchange accomplished at the alveolar-pulmonary capillary interface?

Only the alveoli provide gas exchange surfaces within the lung. Thus, the nasal cavity, pharynx, trachea, bronchi and bronchioles do not take part in the uptake of oxygen or excretion of carbon dioxide, and are said to comprise a 'dead space'. However, these airways will be filled with air during inspiration,

---

BOX 14.3 ASPIRATION

'Aspiration' is a term used when fluids or objects are sucked into the airways during breathing in. Small particles will normally provoke a cough or sneeze reflex, the force of exhalation being sufficient to remove the objects. Fluids and larger particles are more hazardous. Aspiration of these normally does not occur because of reflex protection of the airway, for example by the closure of the epiglottis. The risk, therefore, is greatest when there is an altered state of consciousness, or when neural reflexes are depressed, for example when there is drug abuse, trauma or anaesthesia.

Medium-sized particles may lodge in the trachea or penetrate down to the primary or secondary bronchi, in which case they tend to be lodged in the right lung. This is because the left-sided positioning of the heart makes the right bronchus larger and more vertical than the left.

Such particles are difficult for the lungs to remove by a cough reflex.* Large objects may be prevented by the larynx from passage deep into the lungs (though this is not always effective). In contrast, fluids pass easily through the larynx and may pass deep into the lungs should aspiration occur, perhaps even to the terminal airways. Here they can cause serious inflammation. An example could be the aspiration of stomach acid which has refluxed out of the stomach.

*Note: Striking someone on the back or an intervention by someone standing behind the individual and squeezing up onto the individual's diaphragm (referred to as Heimlich's manoeuvre) increases the force of expiration and may be sufficient to remove the object. However, these are potentially dangerous manoeuvres and must be used with caution if trauma to tissues is to be avoided.

BOX 14.4 BRONCHIOLITIS AND BRONCHIECTASIS

Bronchiolitis is a condition in which inflammation causes obstruction of the bronchioles. It is more common in children, secondary to an upper respiratory tract infection, but can occur in adults through inhalation of toxic vapours (Bush and Thomson, 2007). Treatment is with appropriate antibiotics, anti-inflammatory steroids and chest physical therapy.

Bronchiectasis is a long-standing dilation of the bronchi. It usually occurs in conjunction with other respiratory disorders and is a consequence of long-term inflammation. The airways can become balloon-like, and heavy scarring affects smaller airways in the vicinity. Lung collapse (called atelectasis) may also occur. Blood supply to these areas may increase as part of the inflammatory response and lead to the presence of blood in sputum, which is the fluid brought up out of the lungs by coughing. This is called haemoptysis. The occurrence of scarring makes this condition difficult to treat. Antibiotics may be administered to prevent infection and physical chest therapy used to remove secretions. Bronchodilator drugs may also help improve lung ventilation.

BOX 14.5 THE RESPIRATORY SYSTEM IN CHILDREN

The respiratory system becomes functional at birth (see Box 14.21, p.412) and it should not be surprising to find that it remains functionally 'immature' for some time after birth. The lungs undergo considerable development during childhood, notably a change in size and an increase in complexity of the alveoli.

The respiratory system in infants
As might be expected, the airways differ in size and calibre when compared with older children or adults:

* The airways are shorter and narrower than in older children/adults.
* The upper airway is narrow and reduced further by the posterior displacement of the tongue (an adaptation for suckling).
* The cartilaginous rings of the trachea are less well developed, and so the trachea is more prone to collapse.
* Overall, airway resistance is some 15 times greater in infants than in adults.

The support for ventilation is also less efficient in infants:

* The chest wall is softer and more pliant and so is prone to be sucked in by the lowering of air pressure within the lungs during inspiration.
* Accessory muscles are less well formed and so breathing efforts are less sustainable.
* Alveoli are less numerous at birth (25 million alveoli compared with about 300 million at 8 years old).

The respiratory system during childhood
Development of the respiratory system during childhood is basically one of:

* Increased length of the airways, although the calibre changes little until approaching puberty.
* Increased number of alveoli (see above).

The main feature, then, in children is a respiratory 'tree' that is functionally less efficient, and one that has narrow airways. These make children especially vulnerable to conditions that increase airway resistance further, such as bronchiolitis (Box 14.4) and asthma (see Box 14.12, p.406).

---

so only a proportion of the air we breathe in actually enters the alveoli. Further, the lungs do not deflate completely when we breathe out and so the alveoli and airways are filled with gas left over from the previous breath. Thus, when we breathe in the first 'air' to enter the alveoli is that left in the airways, and so the proportion of fresh air that enters the alveoli when we inhale also has to mix with that gas. This seems inefficient but from a homeostatic point of view is very helpful as the mixing of air with alveolar gas means that the gas composition there is only slightly enriched with oxygen and depleted of carbon dioxide, and so large swings in the gas composition of blood leaving the lungs are avoided. The actual changes are described later.

General principles of lung function

At rest an adult breathes in about 500 mL of air (7–8 mL/kg body weight) with each breath. This is referred to as the tidal volume. With a normal breathing rate at rest of about 10–12 breaths/minute, this means about 5–6 L of air are breathed in (and out) each minute. This is sufficient to meet the needs of cells of the body at rest, which use about 250 mL of oxygen per minute. During exercise, however, oxygen requirements of tissues may be as high as 4 L/minute. To meet this increased demand the volume per breath and the breathing rate are both increased, with the result that the volume of air breathed is increased to perhaps 80 L/minute. Lung function, therefore,

---

BOX 14.6 THE 'RESPIRATORY QUOTIENT'

Chapter 4 described how the aerobic production of energy from glucose produces the same amount of carbon dioxide as the oxygen consumed. However, a proportion of our energy production also comes from the metabolism of fats (which produce less carbon dioxide per volume of oxygen used). The volume of carbon dioxide produced divided by the volume of oxygen used gives a parameter called the respiratory quotient. Thus,

$$\text{(Volume of } CO_2 \text{ produced)/(Volume of } O_2 \text{ consumed)} = (220 \text{ mL/min})/(250 \text{ mL/minute}) = 0.88$$

The respiratory quotient is a useful index that is sometimes used in medicine to assess which metabolic fuel predominates; for carbohydrate alone the value is 1 whereas for fats it is 0.7. The above value reflects a mixed metabolism of fats and carbohydrate

---

must be adaptive according to metabolic needs. In fact, control of lung function is such that it ensures the average gas composition of arterial blood supplying the tissues is held almost constant, even during exercise; in other words the lungs are the main effector organs that act to maintain blood gas homeostasis.

Uptake of oxygen into blood, and removal of carbon dioxide from it, takes place by simple diffusion, and so is based on the respective concentration gradients of the gases in the

BOX 14.7 GAS PRESSURES AND PRESSURE GRADIENTS

Gas molecules, such as those in air, are free to move and their random movement brings them into contact with other structures, for example with our skin. The impacts produce the gas pressure and will depend upon the density of the gas molecules and the speed at which they are moving, in other words compressing additional molecules into an enclosed chamber such as a gas cylinder will raise the gas pressure, and heating it will raise it even more as energy is passed on to the molecules and so they move more rapidly.

Gas pressures used to be measured in terms of millimetres of mercury, written as 'mmHg', in other words the height of a thin column of mercury that can be maintained by such a pressure. Modern units of measurement use the Pascal (abbreviated as Pa), where 1000 Pa (or 1 kPa) is equivalent to 7.6 mmHg. It is now unusual for the unit 'mmHg' to be used with reference to respiratory functioning, although blood pressure measurements are still referred to in these units. This inconsistency

of units used is likely to remain for some time to come, although mercury sphygmomanometers used to measure arterial blood pressure are gradually being replaced by electronic methods.

Gases move from one point to another according to pressure gradients. This principle operates even with a gas mixture, such as air. While the gas within the lung exerts an overall pressure, the movement of oxygen and carbon dioxide between blood and lung is influenced by the pressures they exert individually. The individual pressures of oxygen and carbon dioxide in the lungs are referred to as their partial pressures and are discussed in detail in a later section. For now it is important to note that the diffusion of oxygen and carbon dioxide across lung membranes will only occur if the gradient of their individual partial pressures is appropriate. Lung function is especially concerned with maintaining gradients that are conducive to adequate gas exchange.

alveoli and dissolved in blood. The air we breathe in is composed of approximately 21% oxygen and only 0.03% (physiologically, this effectively is 0) carbon dioxide. The remaining proportion (approximately 79%) is almost entirely nitrogen. Upon breathing in, the inspired air mixes with a relatively large volume of gas left in the lungs and so the 'dilutional' effect that the air has on lung gases is not pronounced. Even so, the changes in gas composition in alveoli during inspiration are sufficient to generate the necessary pressure gradients to promote oxygen diffusion into the blood and carbon dioxide from it. The volume of gas left in the lungs after breathing out is referred to as the functional residual capacity (FRC). If this is increased because of difficulties in breathing then it can have implications for the gas concentration in alveoli when we breathe in, and so is a factor to be considered in respiratory disorder (see later, p.408).

Gas composition apart, gas exchange across the alveoli will also be influenced by the barrier to diffusion that is presented by the alveolar membrane. Our lungs provide a large surface area, and as thin a barrier as possible, for adequate gas exchange to occur between blood and environment. Protection of these delicate surfaces from airborne particles is provided by:

- Filtering out particles by mucus produced by the lining of the airways (see earlier, and Box 14.2, p.399).
- Preventing dehydration by moistening the inspired air.
- Actions of the immune system. Macrophages are able to penetrate the airways, while antibody production makes it difficult for organisms to pass into the tissues (although antibodies are also responsible for hypersensitive reactions, such as asthma – readers are referred to Box 13.16, p.388).

As a final point in this overview, if a major role of the lungs is to provide adequate oxygen for tissue function elsewhere in the body, then the process would be self-defeating if the lungs themselves were to utilize much of the oxygen taken in simply to sustain the muscle activity necessary for breathing. However, the energy requirements of the lung are relatively small – during a normal resting breathing cycle the lungs and associated muscles consume less than 1% of the total uptake of oxygen. The low energy requirements are facilitated by the anatomy of the lung, described in more detail in the next section in relation to lung functioning.

DETAILS OF THE PHYSIOLOGY OF THE RESPIRATORY SYSTEM

Inspiration and expiration

Breathing movements are referred to as inspiration (breathing in) and expiration (breathing out). Inspiration requires inflation of the lungs, expiration requires deflation. Although this appears a simple process, inflation or deflation can only occur if the appropriate air pressure gradients are generated which will move gases in and out of the lungs (see Figure 14.3, p.399).

Inspiration

If we place a finger over the end of an empty syringe and try to withdraw the plunger, we can feel the suction produced inside the syringe. In other words, if the volume of a container is increased then the pressure of gas within it will decrease. Lung inflation works on this principle, and occurs because the thoracic cavity is expanded, literally sucking air into the airways down the pressure gradient that is generated. Expansion of the cavity is achieved by:

- contraction of external intercostal ('inter-' = between; '-costal' = rib) muscles, which raise the rib cage upwards and outwards;
- contraction of the muscular diaphragm, which flattens the 'dome' of this muscle sheet (Figure 14.5).

Expansion of the thoracic cavity lowers the pressure within the lung. To be precise, the expansion acts to pull the chest wall away from the lungs, but the two remain connected by the fluid of the pleural space. Thus, the chest movement lowers the pressure within the pleural fluid, which in turn 'pulls' the lung outwards and so lowers pressure within the airways. It can be seen from Figure 14.3 that the pressure gradient that is generated between

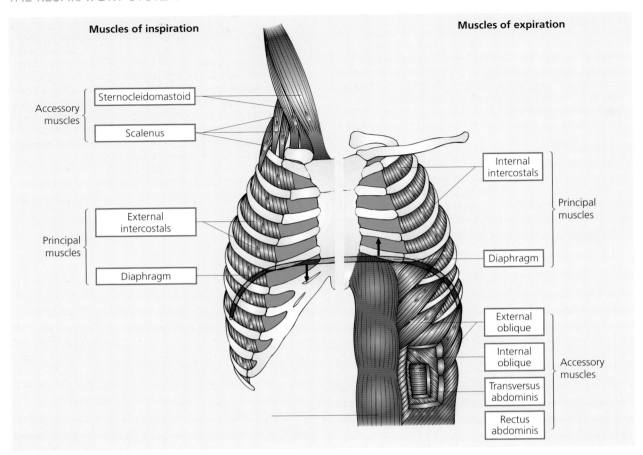

Figure 14.5 Muscles of inspiration and expiration

Q *Which are the main muscles involved in normal inspiration?*

the alveoli and air is only very slight, only 0.3 kPa (not sufficient even to generate a mild breeze in air!), yet this is sufficient to draw some 500 mL of air into the lungs (at rest). Inflation at such a small pressure gradient is indicative of the very low resistance to airflow within the lung. This may seem surprising in view of the increasingly tiny airways that make up the respiratory 'tree' but the total cross-sectional area of the airways actually increases as the airways divide simply based on the increasing number of airways present. Consequently, it is the nasal cavities and the pharynx that normally provide the main site of airway resistance. This may seem paradoxical but recall how difficult it can be to breathe easily when there is inflammation and excess mucus in the upper airways because you have a cold!

When we are at rest, contraction of the diaphragm alone may be all that is required to provide adequate ventilation of the lungs; this is called diaphragmatic breathing. The intercostal muscles become involved during even mild physical activity, while severe respiratory effort during strenuous exercise also involves 'accessory' muscles, such as the sternocleidomastoid muscle of the neck region, in order to raise the rib cage more effectively (Figure 14.5). Muscle contraction requires energy, and hence oxygen. However, the low airway resistance described above makes inflating the lungs quite effortless in

health. Extra muscle contraction in heavy exercise will of course increase the energy expended simply to maintain the appropriate level of breathing but this still represents only up to about 3% of the total oxygen consumption, and so breathing remains energy efficient. Having a low airway resistance is important; if it was high then the energy expended in muscle contraction to generate the large pressure gradients that would then be necessary to inflate the lungs would be debilitating. The fatigue observed in people who have chronic obstructive problems is an illustration of this.

Lung compliance and pulmonary fibrosis

The ease with which the lung can be inflated is referred to as lung compliance, and is a useful clinical parameter for assessing lung elasticity. It is calculated as:

Compliance = (Change in lung volume)/(Change in lung pressure)

Thus, if the lung could be inflated without causing a large increase in pressure within it (clearly beneficial in view of the small gradients normally required to maintain inflation (see above) the compliance would be high. High compliance in the lungs reflects the high elasticity of the terminal bronchioles

BOX 14.8 POSITIONING AND BREATHING MOVEMENTS

The functioning of the diaphragm is impeded if the abdominal organs are pressed against it. An upright position of the body facilitates the role of the diaphragm, and so simply sitting up a patient who has respiratory problems can make breathing much more comfortable and effective. Gravity effects may also help to reduce fluid accumulation as a consequence of pulmonary oedema (see Box 14.19, p.411).

BOX 14.9 DISTURBANCE OF THE PLEURAL SPACE: PNEUMOTHORAX AND PLEURAL EFFUSION

Pneumothorax refers to the presence of air or gas within the pleural space and arises as a consequence of ruptured pleural membranes. In open pneumothorax a penetrating wound of the chest allows air to be sucked into the pleural cavity during inspiration, which is expelled again on expiration. Lung inflation will be impaired. In tension pneumothorax air from a penetrating wound, or alveolar gas via a ruptured visceral pleura (sometimes arising spontaneously from unknown causes), enters the pleural space on inspiration but is trapped by the ruptured membrane acting as a valve. The accumulation of air/gas will cause the lung to collapse (called atelectasis) and this is life threatening.

An accumulation of fluid within the pleural cavity is referred to as pleural effusion. The extra fluid usually originates from blood vessels or lymphatics in the area and usually occurs because of high blood pressure in the pulmonary circulation (for example in congestive heart failure) or because of inflammation. Haemothorax is an accumulation of blood within the pleural cavity as a consequence of the rupture of blood vessels.

Pleural effusion compresses the lung and prevents normal inflation. The fluid usually accumulates at the base of the lung because of the effects of gravity, and may be drained by insertion of a catheter. Diagnostic methods include ultrasonography and imaging techniques (Pendharkar and Tremblay, 2007).

BOX 14.10 ORAL CARE

Oral care is an important part of health care, not least because failure to maintain oral hygiene is distressing for the patient who cannot self-care adequately. Oral hygiene also has implications for nutrition. Difficulties in inflating the lung because of increased airway resistance may cause a patient to resort to 'mouth breathing', since this circumvents the resistance provided by the nasal passages. Mouth breathing can result in drying of the oral mucosa, and tongue surface, producing considerable discomfort. Mouth care becomes very important. If oxygen therapy is involved, or even artificial ventilation, the gas is moistened to reduce the consequences for oral hydration, but even this might not be adequate to prevent drying of the oral mucosa.

BOX 14.11. EFFECTS OF REDUCED COMPLIANCE IN RESTRICTIVE LUNG DISORDERS

Conditions such as asbestosis and silicosis are those in which elastin in lungs is replaced by scar tissue; collectively this is referred to as pulmonary fibrosis. Thus, the lungs will not stretch easily on inspiration, the gas pressure inside will rapidly rise and as a consequence maintaining inspiration against such a pressure will become difficult. Restrictive disorders therefore are considered to be disorders of inspiration. Inadequate inspiration will not produce sufficient change in alveolar gas composition, leading to hypoxaemia and hypercapnia.

fibrosis and is considered as a 'restrictive' disorder, or disorder of inspiration.

Expiration

In contrast to the active, muscle-involving process of inspiration, expiration at rest is passive and utilizes the natural elasticity of the lungs and chest wall. Thus, when inspiration stops, and the inspiratory muscles relax, the lungs simply recoil like a piece of stretched elastic, and so expel the gases. No muscles are involved at rest, and this passive nature of expiration helps to keep oxygen usage to a minimum during breathing. It can only be effective, though, because the resistance to airflow is extremely low since again only a small pressure gradient is developed between the lung gases and the air outside (see Figure 14.3).

During exercise, expiratory effort can be increased through forcing gases out of the lung, rather like a pair of bellows. Thus, the lungs are compressed by contracting the internal intercostal muscles, which lower the rib cage and move it inwards, and by contracting accessory muscles such as the rectus abdominis muscle of the abdomen that help to lower the

and alveoli (see Figure 14.4), which easily stretch as the lung inflates. Poor elasticity will make the pressure within the lung rise rapidly on breathing in (Box 14.11) and so the calculated compliance value will be reduced. The difficulties with this are illustrated when we try to inflate a balloon, when generating a high pressure inside the balloon is necessary to make it begin to inflate as a consequence of the resistance of the rubber composition.

Pathologically, lungs lose compliance because the elastin proteins that are found in bronchioles and alveoli are replaced with scar tissue; collectively this is referred to as pulmonary

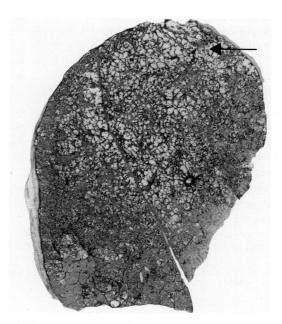

Figure 14.6 Lung with emphysema: the 'holes' (grey areas, e.g. those arrowed) are hugely distended, coalescent, alveolar spaces. Reprinted with the kind permission of Lakhani *et al.*, *Basic Pathology*. 3rd edn, Hodder, London

BOX 14.12 EFFECTS OF INCREASED AIRWAY RESISTANCE: OBSTRUCTIVE AIRWAY DISEASE

Asthma and bronchitis are common examples of disorders in which airway inflammation, excessive airway secretions, and/or constriction of bronchioles increases airway resistance.

Asthma

Asthma is a condition associated with spasmodic contraction of the bronchial smooth muscle, producing symptoms of shortness of breath (dyspnoea), cough, wheezing and, often, distress as a consequence (which exacerbates the breathing difficulty). The most common form is called atopic, or extrinsic, asthma and is a hypersensitive immune response (see Box 13.16, p.389) to environmental agents such as pollen or dust particles. This form is found mainly, but not exclusively, in children, who are more susceptible to obstructive problems because of the structure of their airways (see Box 14.5, p.402). The bronchospasm episode normally resolves in a relatively short period of time but occasionally there is a second episode several hours later. The first phase of bronchospasm is produced by histamine and parasympathetic nerve activity to the airways, whereas the second phase is a complex response to released prostaglandins, thromboxanes and leukotrienes (these are all examples of eicosanoids; see Chapter 9, p.206). Inflammatory responses are also observed, and exacerbate the increased airway resistance.

Therapy is directed at reducing airway resistance through use of bronchodilator drugs (e.g. salbutamol), or prevention by the use of drugs to impair the release of histamine or to reduce inflammation. Longer-term control is through avoidance of causative factors, if the allergen is known, and self-care has an increasingly important role for this condition (Wolf *et al.*, 2007). A poor response to bronchodilators during an asthma episode may result in a state referred to as status asthmaticus, a serious situation that will probably necessitate the use of oxygen therapy until it resolves.

Intrinsic asthma is promoted by factors such as stress or exercise and is more typically found in adults. The bronchospasm here is thought to result from an imbalance between parasympathetic nerve activity to the airways (which promotes bronchoconstriction) and sympathetic nerve activity (which promotes bronchodilation). Stress or exercise should make bronchodilation predominate but this is not the case in intrinsic asthma. Therapy is again preventative (by avoiding the causative factor), and by enhancing bronchodilation by pharmacological means.

See the case of a boy with asthma, p.659.

Bronchitis

Bronchitis is an inflammatory condition of the airways, usually as a consequence of infection or the presence of an irritant, such as cigarette smoke. Symptoms are bronchospasm and fluid/mucus secretion, and a productive cough. Airway resistance is therefore increased, which can cause mucus retention and so encourage further infections. With repeated incidences, the bronchial muscle may hypertrophy while hypersecretion of mucus may be observed, exacerbating the symptoms: a productive cough lasting for more than 3 months in a year, and occurring 2 years in succession indicates progression to chronic bronchitis.

The additional resistance has an impact on the ease of breathing in, thus increasing the inspiratory effort required, and the need for use of muscular contraction to enable normal breathing out, even at rest. Obstructive pulmonary disease, therefore, increases the energy required simply to maintain normal breathing movements. If severe, the problem is exacerbated because the extra force exerted on the airways during expiration compresses them, or moves mucus to form plugs, which increase the resistance still further, possibly even causing air trapping and overinflation of the lung. With time, the condition may also result in the loss of integrity of the airway wall, with loss of elastin and other connective tissue. The collapse of the airways on breathing out is therefore more prevalent and makes air trapping even worse, leading to the condition emphysema (Figure 14.6). The emphasis of progression on symptoms associated with difficulties in exhaling means that obstructive disorders are considered primarily to be disorders of expiration, though inspiration difficulties will also be present. Breathlessness is a very unpleasant experience for people affected in this way. Establishing a sound therapeutic relationship is essential to reduce anxiety since stress and anxiety tend to increase respiratory movements and this serves to exacerbate the feelings.

Individuals with long-standing, chronic bronchitis therefore are at risk of their condition progressing to become extremely debilitating. Bronchodilator drugs, chest physical therapy, and oxygen therapy, as required, may help to improve breathing, but the chronic state is irreversible. Prevention of progression is crucial and health education, for example reduction in smoking, is prominent in the care of this condition.

BOX 14.13 PEAK FLOW RATES

The simplest means of assessing airway resistance is to use a peak flow meter. With this, an individual is asked to inhale deeply and then to breathe out through the meter as hard as possible. The meter measures the maximum flow rate of gas through it.

Problems in making accurate peak flow measurements are:

- mouthpiece size may not be ideal for the patient;
- the patient may not be using maximal respiratory effort, or a maximal inspiration;
- values will vary between attempts. Some values therefore will be a more accurate reflection than others. It is usual to take more than one reading and record the maximum value (not the average as values are more likely to underestimate rather than overestimate airway resistance).

rib cage even more effectively (Figure 14.5). The involvement of muscles now makes expiration an active process that requires oxygen to maintain, but is essential if breathing rate and depth are to be increased during the exercise. However,

being able to move large breaths in and out of the lungs again serves to illustrate the low resistance to airflow through the airways, and in fact can be achieved consciously even at rest. Indeed, a forced expiration of a maximally inhaled breath at rest provides a useful means of clinically monitoring airway resistance since, for a given resistance, a predicted rate of gas flow should be attainable in health (see Box 14.13 and section on spirometry below).

Since peak flow rates, standardized for body size, age and gender, relate to airway resistance, then they provide an indication of any underlying change in that resistance, for example in asthma (Klements, 2001). A more accurate means of monitoring airway resistance is to use more sophisticated equipment, described later in the 'Spirometry' section (also, see Booker, 2008).

Surfactant

There is a potential danger that on expiration the walls of the alveoli may touch, adhere to each other and produce a 'friction rub'. The danger lies in the fact that alveolar membranes must be kept moist to avoid dehydration, and contact between wet surfaces produces powerful adhesion because of the phenomenon of 'surface tension'. Respiratory movements are inadequate to overcome such adhesion forces and so the collapse of alveoli in this way must be prevented. Alveoli do not, in fact, totally deflate following expiration. In addition they are also coated with a detergent-like chemical, a phospholipid called surfactant, which is secreted by epithelial cells of the alveoli (see Figure 14.4, p.401) and which acts to lower the surface tension within the alveoli, making adhesion less likely even if surfaces do touch. The role of surfactant in this respect is readily demonstrated by placing a droplet of water onto a dry piece of glass; note how it forms a globule. The surface molecules are held in place by surface tension, producing the globular shape. Add a little detergent and the drop disperses; surface tension is reduced by the detergent in much the same way as surfactant reduces it in the alveoli.

Surfactant is important throughout life and is also a crucial adaptation that enables a fetus to breathe air at birth (Box 14.14).

Pulmonary and alveolar ventilation, and dead space

The earlier 'Overview' section identified how a volume of gas remains in the lungs after breathing out and constitutes the 'dead space' provided by the major airways. This gas re-enters the alveoli during the next inspiration, closely followed by the fresh air. Thus, at the end of inspiration a portion of the inspired air will have mixed with this 'old' gas in the alveoli, but a proportion will also have filled the major airways. These parts of the respiratory tree do not exchange gases with the blood (hence the term 'dead space', or 'anatomical dead space'). Thus, for a normal adult tidal volume of 500 mL, approximately 150 mL of the inspired air will fill the dead space and only 350 mL will enter the alveoli. In some disorders non-functioning alveoli increase the volume of this dead space because their lack of contribution to gas exchange makes them an added component; they constitute a 'physiological' dead space.

The volume of air breathed into the lungs per minute is called the pulmonary ventilation rate (sometimes referred to as the 'respiratory minute volume'), while that entering the alveoli each minute is called the alveolar ventilation rate. The presence of a dead space means that it cannot be assumed that pulmonary ventilation gives a measure of the ventilation of the alveoli, yet the latter is clearly a more important parameter since this will determine the gas composition in the alveoli and hence gas exchange there. This is illustrated in Box 14.15.

Spirometry: assessment of pulmonary gas volumes and capacities

It has already been noted that the volume of air inspired per breath at rest is called the tidal volume and averages about

---

BOX 14.14 SURFACTANT AND PREMATURE BABIES

Surfactant chemicals are phospholipids, predominantly lecithin and sphingomyelin, that are secreted by cells within the alveoli.

Surfactant is not produced in quantity by the lungs until about the 34th week of fetal development, when there is a surge in production, particularly of lecithin.

Surfactant:

* enables alveoli walls to separate when an infant first inhales;
* enable alveoli walls to separate should contact occur during expiration movements.

The lack of adequate surfactant in premature babies is a major factor in their survival (Sweet *et al.*, 2007). Because of this babies born very early will be placed in an environment in which the oxygen pressure is increased. This in turn will raise the oxygen pressure in alveoli that are functioning and help to maintain oxygenation of the baby's blood until other alveoli become patent. Nevertheless, the likelihood of survival will be increased if the alveoli can be opened more effectively and researchers are developing artificial surfactants that can be administered by inhalation and will maintain alveolar patency until the intrinsic surfactant is produced in adequate quantities.

If premature delivery is anticipated then dexamethasone (a steroid) may be administered to the mother as this has been found to accelerate the production of surfactant.

Respiratory distress syndrome of the newborn (RDS) is a serious condition in premature babies which involves anatomical defects such as small alveoli and poorly developed chest structures, coupled with poor production of surfactant. Mortality rates in this condition are high.

BOX 14.15 EFFECTS OF DEAD SPACE ON ALVEOLAR VENTILATION

Consider these normal values:

Volume inspired per breath = 500 mL
Breaths per minute = 10
Pulmonary ventilation = breath volume × breathing rate = 500 mL × 10 = 5000 mL or 5.0 L/minute

Volume inspired per breath − dead space volume = 500 − 150 mL = 350 mL
Breaths per minute = 10
Alveolar ventilation = 350 mL × 10 = 3500 mL or 3.5 L/minute

Thus, alveolar ventilation at 3.5 L/minute is considerably less than the pulmonary ventilation of 5 L/minute.

Now, suppose that the volume inspired is halved (to 250 mL), but the breathing rate is doubled (to 20 breaths/minute):

Pulmonary ventilation = 250 mL × 20 = 5.0 L/minute (i.e. unchanged compared with the example above).
Alveolar ventilation = (250 − 150) × 20 = 2000 mL = 2.0 L/minute (i.e. much reduced compared with the example above).

Thus, an individual who is taking shallow, rapid breaths may seem to be achieving a reasonable lung ventilation but in fact may be experiencing a decreased alveolar ventilation, poor gas exchange, and blood gas disturbance.

The influence of dead space on alveolar ventilation has implications in diagnosis of airway problems, and for the use of mechanical ventilation therapies because the tubing used will increase the dead space. This has to be taken into account in calculating the depth and rate of ventilation, although if an endotracheal tube has been inserted into the trachea for the ventilation then this will tend also to reduce the anatomical dead space since the oral/nasal cavities are bypassed.

BOX 14.16 ASSISTED VENTILATION

Ventilation may be assisted for two main reasons:

- First, if independent breathing is not possible then artificial means of ventilation will be used.
- Second, breathing movement in respiratory disorder may not be sufficient to produce adequate alveolar ventilation, leading to oxygen lack and carbon dioxide excess. Under such circumstances oxygen therapy might be used to improve the composition of alveolar gas.

Oxygen therapy

One way to maintain adequate alveolar gas composition in respiratory disorder is to use an enriched mixture of inspired gas. Pure oxygen is toxic and produces severe inflammation of the airways. Thus the individual may be encouraged to breathe a gas mixture of air and oxygen, or perhaps a mixture of oxygen and carbon dioxide. In this way the alveolar oxygen composition can be made to be near normal even though the tidal volume is inadequate to provide normal alveolar ventilation.

The enriched gas mixture (from a gas cylinder or piped source) might be applied by free-flow through a nasal tube or through a facemask. A patient using a facemask may find it very uncomfortable, while gas pressure within the nasal tubing or facemask may also be disconcerting. It is important for carers to be aware that breathing difficulties are extremely distressing to the patient, and that both methods may add to the anxiety experienced by patients who are already feeling breathless. Feeding and speech may also be adversely affected and so adds to the frustration felt.

Artificial or mechanical ventilation

The most extreme form of assisted ventilation is that involving what was once referred to colloquially as an 'iron lung'. In this, the thorax is encased within a sealed chamber, and pressure changes within the chamber are used to produce the movements of the chest required for breathing. The method is used when paralysis of the chest arising from neck trauma or spinal cord dysfunctioning prevents the respiratory muscles from functioning.

Other methods are used to facilitate breathing by pumping air or a gas mixture into the lungs of an unconscious individual (the thorax of a conscious individual would work against the artificially induced move-

ments). The individual is connected to a ventilator by tubing, the end of which may pass into the individual's trachea. The machine pumps a preset 'tidal' volume of air/gas into the lungs at a preset rate, and so replaces the normal respiratory movements. There are a number of variations to the precise method used:

- *Continuous positive airway pressure (CPAP)*: this is maintained throughout the breathing cycle. Maintaining airway pressure ensures a positive end-expiration pressure, referred to as PEEP, and so increases the patency of alveoli and helps to prevent their collapse. It may also help to redistribute fluid into the tissue fluid space from the alveoli. There is a risk that the elevated pressure within alveoli may induce barotrauma ('baro-' = pressure) by decreasing the output from the right side of the heart and hence cardiac output from the left side. Hyperinflation also decreases the compliance of the lungs, making them harder to inflate (i.e. the work of breathing is increased), and increases the risk of pneumothorax (see Box 14.9, p.405) occurring.
- *Bi-positive airway pressure (BiPAP)*: this is a modification of CPAP in which two airway pressures are applied, with synchronization during the breathing cycle. It too ensures PEEP but it also allows a reduction in pressure during the expiration (though not sufficient to allow alveolar collapse if this is a risk) and this helps to reduce the risk of barotrauma and decreased compliance. The pressure is increased once more during inspiration, and this helps to inflate the alveoli.
- *Intermittent positive pressure ventilation (IPP)*: this method pumps air or ventilation gas into the lungs by applying a positive pressure but allows expiration to occur passively by recoil, as in normally functioning lungs. The risks of the method especially relate to the applied pressure and volume administered. If excessive then pneumothorax may occur (see Box 14.9, p.405).
- *High-frequency ventilation (HFV)*: this reduces some of the risks associated with applied pressure by administering very small volumes at high frequency. The pressure changes are not so large. The intention is to alter the composition of lung gases including those within the dead space so that small volumes can achieve the necessary 'dilutional' effect.

---

500 mL in an adult. Even at rest we can consciously increase the volume breathed in or we can also further deflate the lung, and so it is clear that the alveoli are not fully inflated after normal inspiration nor are they maximally deflated after expiration (i.e. there are inspiratory and expiratory reserve volumes; Figure 14.7). In addition the lung contains a volume of gas even after maximal expiration has occurred because deflation of the alveoli is incomplete and some gas fills the dead space; in other words there is a residual volume of gas within the lungs (of about 1.5 L in adults). Consequently, the gases within the lung into which the tidal volume air will pass when we breathe in will be the volume represented by the expiratory reserve plus the residual volume: this is an important clinical parameter called the 'functional residual capacity' – about 2.5 L in volume in an adult and approximately equal to half the maximum capacity of the lungs (called the total lung capacity). Thus the normal resting operation of the lung occurs with the lung being always about half inflated.

The importance of the FRC is illustrated by considering the consequences if it is increased. In chronic obstructive pulmonary diseases (COPDs), for example chronic bronchitis or

BOX 14.17 THE LUNG DURING PREGNANCY

The developing baby pushes up on the mother's abdominal organs, and this tends to compress the diaphragm. While this can make breathing a little uncomfortable, it also acts to reduce the volume of gas left in the lungs after expiration, and so decreases the FRC. Thus, the air breathed in has a slightly greater influence on alveolar gas composition and this in turn facilitates greater gas exchange. Alveolar ventilation is also enhanced during pregnancy through the actions of progesterone to relax the smooth muscle of the airways.

These changes are important, particularly with respect to carbon dioxide excretion, because the mother's lungs must adapt to excrete the load coming from her tissues and those of the baby. The action of progesterone to raise the sensitivity of receptors (central chemoreceptors – see later) to carbon dioxide is also important in this respect.

---

emphysema, the severity of the increased resistance prevents adequate expiration, leading to air trapping (see Box 14.12). The enlarged FRC leaves the lung overinflated and hence with a decreased inspiratory reserve. Air breathed into the enlarged FRC is then less effective at altering the gas composition and so the oxygen content of alveolar gas declines, while that of

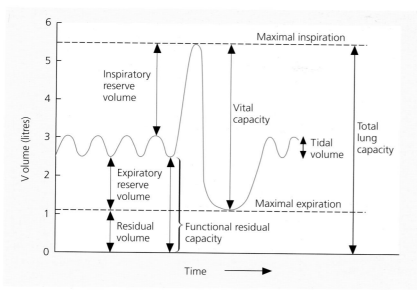

Figure 14.7 Spirometer recording (spirogram) of principal lung volumes and capacities in an adult. Note that the zero line cannot be ascertained directly (see text)

Q Define and give the average volumes in millilitres of the following: (1) tidal volume, (2) vital capacity, (3) inspiratory reserve volume and (4) residual volume.

Q Which of the lung volumes/capacities given below cannot be determined directly using a simple spirometer: (1) tidal volume, (2) vital capacity, (3) inspiratory reserve volume and (4) residual volume?

carbon dioxide increases. Similar changes occur in the blood and so these conditions can be debilitating. The problem is exacerbated because the overinflated lungs have reduced capacity to increase the breath volume during physical exertion, with the result that the individual fatigues easily (see Truesdell, 2000).

If we maximally inflate the lungs and then breathe out maximally, the volume of gas expired represents the maximum volume of gas that can possibly be expelled from the lung in a single breath (Box 14.18) and this is called the vital capacity (about 4 L in an adult). If we add the vital capacity to the residual volume (Figure 14.7) then this also gives the total lung capacity (about 5.5–6 L in an adult). The residual volume cannot be measured directly but an indirect method may be used by determining the effect of the residual gases to dilute an inert marker gas such as helium after inspiration, as this enables

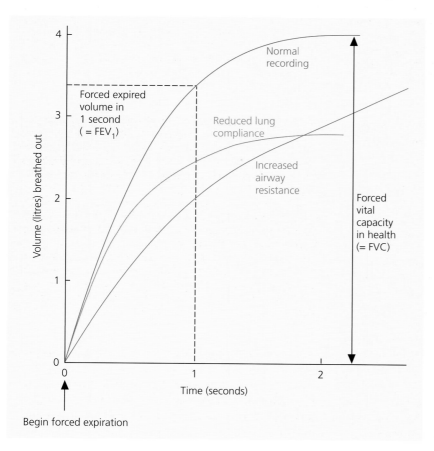

Figure 14.8 'Vitallograph' traces of vital capacity measurement to illustrate the use of forced expiratory volume in one second (FEV_1) as a diagnostic tool. Note that forced vital capacity (FVC) varies between individuals, especially in disease states. Note also the change in FEV_1 and in FVC in respiratory conditions. Values stated are examples for this illustration

Q How does long-term smoking affect the FEV_1?

BOX 14.18 USE OF SPIROMETERS TO MEASURE FORCED EXPIRATORY VOLUMES AND TO ASSESS AIRWAY RESISTANCE

It was noted in Box 14.13 how measurement of the 'peak flow rate' during expiration provides a measure of airway resistance. In performing the test the individual forcibly breathes out from maximally inflated lungs so that the vital capacity can be measured, since if someone breathes in maximally and then forcibly breathes out to completion then the entire vital capacity will be breathed out. In health, more than 80% of the vital capacity should be expelled in the first second of forcibly breathing out; the volume expired is referred to as the FEV_1 (FEV = forced expiratory volume) and the proportion it is of vital capacity as the FEV%. With increased airway resistance this proportion falls according to the severity of the condition (Figure 14.8).

Another significance of expressing the FEV_1 as a percentage (or as a ratio where 80% = 0.80) is that even if the vital capacity is severely reduced because of a restrictive condition (i.e. pulmonary fibrosis; see Box 14.11, p.405), a normal airway resistance will mean that the FEV_1 may be a normal proportion of it. Spirometry therefore provides a means of monitoring any progress in both obstructive and restrictive disorders (see also Booker, 2008).

calculation of total lung capacity. By measuring the vital capacity then it is possible to calculate the residual volume and using spirometry calculate the FRC.

Lung volumes and capacities are measured using a machine called a (re)spirometer. There are various kinds of spirometer, some of which are portable and may provide only some of the information (for example, the vital capacity may be determined using a 'Vitallograph'; Figure 14.8). Full spirometric assessment (see Figure 14.7) requires a more sophisticated spirometer, as found in lung function rooms in some larger hospitals.

Exchange of gases between alveoli and blood

Assessment of the various lung capacities and volumes provides an indication of the relationships between various airway components and lung function, and the health of the lungs. Ultimately, however, there must be gas exchange across the respiratory surface, and this is considered in this section. Oxygen and carbon dioxide move along their respective pressure gradients, and so the rate of exchange is influenced mainly by two factors:

- The thickness of the barrier formed by the alveolar membrane and the blood vessel wall (see Figure 14.4, p.401) since this influences gas diffusion for any given pressure gradient. The cells of these membranes are flattened so that the barrier is exceedingly thin (only about 0.4 μm), and so blood cells are brought into close proximity to the lung gases. The gases, however, still have to traverse the intracellular fluids of the cells which form the membranes, and across the interstitial fluid between them (although this is minimal). Much of the resistance to gas diffusion is therefore caused by fluid, and the barrier problem relates to the solubility of oxygen and carbon dioxide in water during the exchange process.

- The pressure gradient between the alveolar gas and gas dissolved in blood. The discussion prior to this point has only considered the total pressure of gases within the lung and in the air. In order to understand the exchange of individual gases within the mixture found in the lung it is important that the concept of partial pressures is understood, since it is these individual pressures that form the gradients that promote the diffusion of individual gases.

Partial pressure

As the name implies, partial pressures are those pressures generated by individual gases within a gas mixture. Each gas exerts its own pressure, determined by the relative proportions of the gases; the sum of all of the partial pressures must be equal to the total pressure of the gas mixture. For example, 21% of air is oxygen. At normal atmospheric pressure (at sea level) the total air pressure is about 101 kPa (equivalent to 760 mmHg) and so the partial pressure of oxygen will be 21% of this, which is about 21 kPa (160 mmHg). The air also contains nitrogen, carbon dioxide and small quantities of other gases. Each of these will exert its own partial pressure and the sum of these individual pressures, with oxygen, will equal 101 kPa.

The total pressure of gas in the alveoli at the end of inspiration is also 101 kPa, but analysis shows that the partial pressure of oxygen averages only 13.3 kPa (100 mmHg). This is lower than air because:

- Alveolar gas into which the air passed contains a higher proportion of carbon dioxide. The partial pressure of carbon dioxide within the alveoli averages 5.3 kPa (40 mmHg) after inspiration. It does not fall to zero, even though air is virtually free of carbon dioxide because of the large volume of gas remaining in the lungs after expiration (i.e. the FRC; see earlier).

- Alveolar gas is saturated with water vapour (which will also exert a partial pressure).

Gases simply dissolved in blood will also exert a partial pressure. The average partial pressures of alveolar gases, pulmonary arterial blood, pulmonary venous blood and air are compared in Table 14.1. Note that:

- Blood entering the lung (pulmonary artery) has a lower partial pressure of oxygen but a higher partial pressure of carbon dioxide than in the alveoli at the end of breathing in. However, when blood leaves the lungs (pulmonary venous) the gas composition has equilibrated; the partial pressure of oxygen has increased on passage through the lungs, while that of carbon dioxide has decreased. The gases therefore have exchanged with the alveoli.

- The partial pressure gradient for oxygen uptake between alveoli and pulmonary artery blood is much greater than that for carbon dioxide excretion. This is a reflection on the poor solubility of oxygen compared with carbon dioxide: a greater pressure gradient is required to 'drive' its diffusion across the alveoli–capillary membrane for a similar degree of exchange.

BOX 14.19 INFLAMMATORY LUNG CONDITIONS AND PULMONARY OEDEMA

An accumulation of fluid within the alveoli significantly increases the barrier to gas diffusion, especially so of oxygen as this gas is poorly soluble in water. Ordinarily, the alveoli are kept relatively 'dry' because the low pressure in the pulmonary capillaries is greatly exceeded by the osmotic effect of the plasma proteins in blood passing through them (refer to Chapter 6 p.124, for an explanation of capillary–tissue fluid movements).

This fluid barrier is increased if there are inflammatory exudates within the alveoli, if there is elevated blood pressure within the pulmonary circulation (pulmonary hypertension), or if there is increased permeability of capillaries within the pulmonary circulation.

Inflammation

Pneumonia describes the presence of fluid within the alveoli. Symptoms include chest pain, difficulty breathing and fatigue, together with cough (possibly with blood) and fever with chills and night sweats. It is a common cause of death in elderly people or in those with chronic or terminal illness. The fluid can be heard through a stethoscope, and there may be rales ('crackling' sounds). X-rays identify opacities within the lungs.

Pneumonia can result from infection by bacteria (e.g. *Streptococcus pneumoniae*), 'atypical' bacteria (e.g. *Mycoplasma pneumoniae*, *Legionella pneumophila*), viruses (e.g. influenza virus), fungi or chemical agents (e.g. inhalation of gastric contents – see Box 14.3, p.400).

Tuberculosis (TB) is an inflammatory condition produced by infection, most commonly by *Mycobacterium tuberculosis*. In most instances the infection remains latent and asymptomatic but when active has a high mortality rate. The organism invades macrophages within the alveoli, with the consequence that other immune system cells, especially lymphocytes, aggregate around the infected cell to form a fibrous cyst-like granuloma, or tubercle. Inside, the bacteria may die, in which case a cavity may form, or the organism remains latent (as it has been deactivated by the immune response). Symptoms of active disease are similar to those for pneumonia but as this can be a long-term condition chronic fatigue and wasting is also observed. The infection may progress beyond the airways, especially in children when it may even cause meningitis.

The BCG (bacille Calmette-Guérin) vaccination against TB has been available for over 50 years. Better, more effective vaccines are beginning to appear based on DNA recombinant technology (see Chapter 19, p.556).

Pulmonary hypertension

Pulmonary hypertension often occurs secondary to congestive heart failure. Here the failure of adequate throughput of blood in the heart (see Box 12.16, p.388) causes a 'backing up' that results in elevated pressure within the pulmonary circulation. Pulmonary arterial blood pressure ordinarily is quite low – much lower than the osmotic pressure due to plasma protein – and this helps to keep the fluid within the alveoli as little as possible (see details on capillary exchange dynamics in Chapter 6, p.124). Having little fluid present facilitates the diffusion of gases between alveoli and blood. Pulmonary hypertension disturbs that balance, as the increased blood pressure may even exceed the osmotic action of the plasma proteins, causing exudation of fluid from plasma into the alveoli.

Capillary permeability

Increased permeability of the pulmonary capillaries will lead to leakage of plasma proteins, and the formation of exudate from the capillaries. This can occur as a consequence of cardiovascular shock, or after severe trauma, and is referred to as (adult) respiratory distress syndrome (ARDS). The mechanism of ARDS remains poorly understood and mortality rates are high when it occurs.

Collectively, the occurrence of fluid within the alveoli is referred to as pulmonary oedema. If the cause is an infection then antibiotics may help but often the best means to remove accumulated fluid is debatable. Gravitational effects or diuretic drugs may be used to reduce pulmonary hypertension (but may compromise cardiac function if this is the primary disorder). Reducing inflammation is indicated where appropriate but in ARDS this is of limited benefit because of the profound changes to the structure of the barrier. Colloid infusions may be used to increase the osmotic pressure of plasma, thus withdrawing fluid from the lungs by osmosis, but they may also increase blood viscosity and impair blood flow through the lungs.

Treatment of pulmonary oedema will usually entail providing an oxygen-enriched breathing mixture, in order to raise the pressure of oxygen within the alveoli and so promote better transfer of the gas through the fluid barrier.

Table 14.1(a) Representative partial pressures of gases in air (dry), inspired air (wet) and alveolar gas after inspiration

	Air (dry) kPa	Inspired air (wet) kPa	Alveolar gas after inspiration kPa
Oxygen	21.2	19.9	13.3
Carbon dioxide	0.03	0.03	5.3
Nitrogen	79.8	77.5	76.2
Water vapour	0	6.3	6.3
Total	100.9	100.9	100.9

Atmospheric pressure is taken to be 100.9 kPa. Note how the saturation of inspired air with water vapour changes the values for other gases – the sum of the pressures must remain the same.

Table 14.1(b) Representative partial pressures and gas composition of blood entering the lungs (mixed venous blood) and leaving the lungs (pulmonary venous blood)

	PO_2 kPa	PCO_2 kPa	Volume O_2 mL/100 mL	Volume CO_2 mL/100 mL
Mixed venous blood	5.3	6.0	14	52
Pulmonary venous blood (systemic arterial blood)	13.3	5.3	19.7	48
Change	+8.0	−0.7	+5.7	−4.0

Net changes as blood passes through the lungs are shown. Note that the changes in oxygen and carbon dioxide content of blood as it passes through the lungs are produced by disproportionate changes in their partial pressures. The reason for this is that carbon dioxide is much more soluble than oxygen.

The small pressure gradient for carbon dioxide excretion is an important factor in the capacity of the lungs to regulate the gas composition of blood as it would not take much of an increase in the alveolar partial pressure of carbon dioxide to compromise excretion of the gas. In fact, the partial pressure of carbon dioxide in blood is much more important than that of oxygen in stimulating lung function changes. This is discussed later in relation to blood gas homeostasis.

LIVERPOOL JOHN MOORES UNIVERSITY
LEARNING SERVICES

BOX 14.20 PARTIAL PRESSURES AND BLOOD COMPOSITION DURING HYPERVENTILATION AND HYPOVENTILATION

Hyperventilation

In hyperventilation (Figure 14.9) the rate of alveolar ventilation is greater than appropriate for the rate of metabolism at that time, and is not a term to be used in conjunction with increased breathing in exercise since this is appropriate to the increased metabolic rate. The composition of alveolar gases alters more on inspiration, becoming much richer in oxygen (since more air is entering it) and more deficient in carbon dioxide (air is effectively 0% carbon dioxide). Hence the partial pressure of oxygen in alveoli and hence blood is increased, while that of carbon dioxide is decreased. Arterial blood is normally saturated with oxygen and so the enrichment of lung gases with oxygen has little effect. However, the carbon dioxide depletion removes the gas from blood so efficiently that arterial blood carbon dioxide content falls. This disturbance of homeostasis will produce an alkalosis but will also make cerebral blood vessels constrict (so that less carbon dioxide is washed out of the brain, thus restoring the carbon dioxide homeostasis in this tissue). This constriction will in turn impair oxygen delivery to the brain and so hyperventilating individuals will tend to feel dizzy and may even faint.

In reality, hyperventilation induced consciously is impossible to maintain in normal health since the blood gas changes will promote self-correcting responses. However, hyperventilation can be maintained in anxiety or pain. For pain this normally will require analgesia, but for anxiety the individual should be calmed and encouraged to breathe slowly and deeply. If this fails (for example in children) the individual might be encouraged to breathe in and out of a paper bag: the gas that collects in the bag will accumulate carbon dioxide and, on rebreathing, will raise alveolar and blood carbon dioxide content, hence correcting the disturbance. This in itself will improve the way that the person feels and so will have a calming effect.

Hypoventilation

In hypoventilation the rate of alveolar ventilation is inadequate for the rate of metabolism at that time. The alveolar gases become depleted in oxygen and enriched in carbon dioxide, since the volume of air entering the alveoli is insufficient to maintain the normal composition. The lower partial pressure for oxygen means that arterial blood oxygen content may decrease, and the higher partial pressure of carbon dioxide will make blood content of this gas rise.

Hypoventilation is observed in obstructive and restrictive airway disorders, or in the inhibition of breathing that is observed with brainstem trauma, drug overdose or excessive opioid analgesia.

The onset of allergy-induced hypoventilation (asthma) can be extremely rapid, and if severe can quickly produce such a profound dyspnoea as to require immediate attention. Fear and anxiety are natural in these circumstances but serve to exacerbate the problem. Oxygen therapy, reassurance and bronchodilator drugs may be used to improve ventilation, but calming reassurance is also important.

BOX 14.21 LUNG PERFUSION AND INFLATION AT BIRTH

Prior to birth the lungs are not functional as such, so much of the blood returning to the right side of the heart is shunted directly across to the left side, into the left atrium, via a perforation of the septum between the left and right atria called the foramen ovale. Of the blood that is ejected from the right ventricle towards the lungs much is shunted directly from the pulmonary arterial trunk into the aorta, via a vessel called the ductus arteriosus. Thus during fetal life, when gas exchange occurs in the placenta, the lungs receive only about 10% of the blood returning to the right side of the heart, while 90% passes into the left atrium and aorta without first passing through the lungs.

Oxygenation of the baby's tissues is promoted at birth by some precise mechanisms (it is recommended that you also refer to the structure and function of the heart of an adult in Chapter 12, p.310):

- At birth the fetal lungs are either collapsed or are partially filled with amniotic fluid, which is rapidly absorbed.
- The alveoli are inflated with air by a reflex initiation of inspiration. This occurs because respiratory centres of the brainstem (see Figure 14.1, p.418) are stimulated by the rising concentrations of carbon dioxide in the blood caused by the loss of placental gas exchange.
- Oxygen uptake across the lung raises the partial pressure of oxygen in pulmonary venous blood and this stimulates closure of the ductus arteriosus. Having closed, the ductus arteriosus will then atrophy into a ligament (the ligamentum arteriosum) during the succeeding months.

- The foramen ovale closes because more blood is arriving in the left atrium from the lungs and this produces a pressure gradient between the left and right atria that favours closure.
- The closure of the ductus arteriosus and foramen ovale ensures that all blood from the right side of the heart now perfuses the lungs.
- Pulmonary blood flow is facilitated by a decreased pulmonary vascular resistance prompted by the rising oxygenation within the lung alveoli.

Persistence of embryological features

The importance of circulatory and respiratory changes are clear:

1. A persistently low partial pressure of oxygen as a consequence of inadequate gas exchange (e.g. in infant respiratory distress syndrome) prevents adequate closure of the ductus arteriosus. Blood then flows from the aorta (in which pressure is increased at birth) into the pulmonary artery and lung, at the expense of the rest of the systemic circulation.
2. Inadequate closure of the foramen ovale means that some blood will continue to be shunted from the right to left side of the heart, without undergoing gas exchange. If severe, this will be life threatening, and even a small residual defect may become apparent years later when oxygen need increases in the growing child.

Nevertheless, the cardiovascular changes at birth are not instantaneous or complete, and it may be weeks or months before final closure of the foramen ovale or ductus arteriosus takes place.

Ventilation/perfusion ratio

At rest adults breathe in about 5 L of air per minute. The rate of blood flow through the lungs is about 5–6 L/minute at rest and so the ratio of ventilation/perfusion averages between 0.8 and 1.0. This near-matching of gas and blood movements within the lungs ensures optimal oxygenation of blood and adequate removal of carbon dioxide. However, the variation in

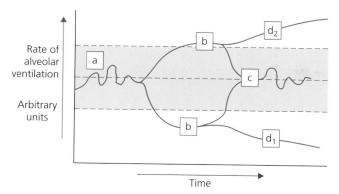

Figure 14.9 General schema for respiratory function. a, Lung ventilation operating within homeostatic range for optimal gas exchange. b, Disturbance caused by either hyperventilation or hypoventilation. c, Return to homeostatic range through monitoring of blood gas composition and pH (arterial/cerebrospinal fluid) and appropriate ventilatory changes. d_1, Imbalance owing to continued hypoventilation as a consequence of poor ventilatory response or inadequate lung function. d_2, Imbalance owing to continued hyperventilation as a consequence of poor regulatory control. [a, Represents boxes a_1–a_4 in Figure 1.7, p.11, reflecting the individual variability in the homeostatic range. The blue area represents the norm (homeostatic range) 95%]

BOX 14.22 SHUNT EFFECTS

The significance of ventilation/perfusion matching is that areas of the lung may pathologically exhibit diminished ventilation and/or perfusion and the resultant mismatch will then alter the final composition of pulmonary venous blood. Ventilation/perfusion mismatches are among the commonest causes of lung-induced oxygen deficiency in blood (hypoxaemia).

If no gas exchange occurred at all (assuming life could still survive!) then blood leaving the lungs would be depleted in oxygen and enriched in carbon dioxide: in fact it would have the same composition as mixed venous blood entering the lungs. It would be as though blood had missed the lungs completely, and the term 'shunt' was introduced as a consequence. Clearly a 100% shunt is not compatible with life but a less extensive shunt might be acknowledged in certain circumstances, for example '20% shunt' refers to a blood composition leaving the lungs that would occur if 20% of blood had not passed through it. In a newborn infant, this might actually be the case if the ductus arteriosus or foramen ovale have not closed (see Box 14.21); this literally would be an example of an anatomical shunt. With a collapsed lung blood does actually pass through the lungs but the loss of gas exchange function in those lung areas will provide a physiological shunt that may still be expressed as a 'shunt effect'. The greater the shunt effect, the greater the implication for blood leaving the lungs.

---

ventilation/perfusion ratio between regions of the lung means that regional oxygenation may be less, and carbon dioxide may be removed more or less efficiently.

Variation in the ratio arises largely because of the distribution of blood within the lungs, although it is also the case that ventilation of alveoli is uneven. Blood flow to the base of the lung is enhanced by gravity (note the anatomical position of the lung relative to the heart in Figure 14.2, p.399) whereas the perfusion of alveoli at the apex is reduced (in the upright position) since blood pressure in the pulmonary arteries is only of the order of 25/8 mmHg and this will barely maintain blood flow against gravity to the lung apex.

In this way the ventilation/perfusion ratio actually increases vertically through the lung and has an effect on the gas composition of blood leaving these areas:

- The apex of the lung is overventilated compared with the amount of blood it receives (i.e. blood is so rapidly saturated with oxygen or depleted of carbon dioxide that some of the alveolar gas is not exchanged; the extra ventilation is therefore wasted).
- The base of the lung is overperfused compared with the amount of air it receives (i.e. the alveoli are so rapidly depleted of oxygen and enriched with carbon dioxide that some of the blood does not take part in gas exchange; the extra blood perfusion is therefore wasted).

Subsequent mixing of blood from the base and apex produces the final composition found in pulmonary venous (i.e. systemic arterial) blood, averaging out the ventilation–perfusion differences across the lungs (but see Box 14.22).

Gas carriage by blood

The carriage of gases by blood, especially of oxygen, is facilitated by the pigment haemoglobin present in red blood cells.

Structure of haemoglobin

Haemoglobin begins to be synthesized in the early stages of differentiation of the red blood cell, when the cell still has a nucleus (and is called an erythroblast; see Figure 11.3, p.273). The haemoglobin will eventually fill the cell, which loses its nucleus and becomes an erythrocyte ('erythro-' = red). Haemoglobin consists of four molecules of a protein called globin, and four molecules of a pigment called haem (Figure 14.10). The globin molecules within a haemoglobin molecule are not all identical, however, because of slight differences in their amino acid composition.

Over 90% of haemoglobin of children and adults (abbreviated as HbA) contains two molecules of alpha globin and two of beta globin. In the remainder, called HbA_2, the beta-globin is replaced by delta-globin, but functionally this type of haemoglobin is similar to HbA. Changes in the proportion of HbA_2 are diagnostic, for example it is increased in the blood disorder thalassaemia.

In contrast, some two-thirds of the haemoglobin of a fetus has two alpha- and two gamma-globins in its molecule, and is referred to as HbF. This difference in the globins compared with the adult type has a significant effect on the relationship between haemoglobin and oxygen, and is an important adaptation to uterine life, as is discussed later. There is also a higher overall concentration of haemoglobin in fetuses (17 g per 100 mL compared with 12–14 g per 100 mL in adults). This will reduce to adult values within about 3 months after birth.

Haem molecules are complex structures and are an example of a group of organic chemicals called porphyrins. Each haem molecule has an iron ion at its core, and so a haemoglobin molecule contains four ions of iron, each of which can combine reversibly with an oxygen molecule (see below).

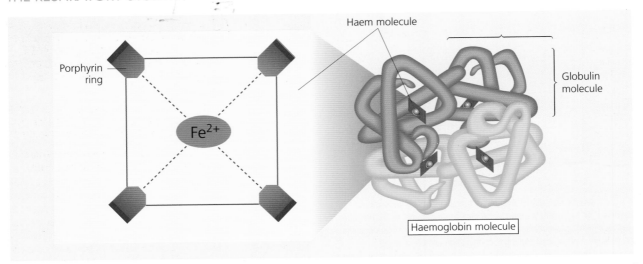

Figure 14.10 A molecule of haemoglobin, showing four molecules of globin and four molecules of haem. The haem molecule consists of a porphyrin ring surrounding an iron ion (as Fe^{2+})

Q Describe the structural relationships between the Fe^{2+}, globin and haem subunits of haemoglobin.

There are 200–300 million molecules of haemoglobin in each mature red blood cell, and this means that each 100 mL of blood contains approximately 13–15 g of haemoglobin. This amount, together with the properties of the pigment, ensure that the blood can transport adequate amounts of respiratory gases. This is particularly so for oxygen as this gas is poorly soluble in blood plasma; carbon dioxide is also carried dissolved in plasma, and also as bicarbonate ions produced by its chemical reaction with water. Haemoglobin deficiency (called anaemia), therefore, has greater implications for oxygen carriage than for the transportation of carbon dioxide.

Carriage of oxygen

Oxygen is carried mainly in association with haemoglobin. Thus:

$$Hb \quad + \quad 4O_2 \quad \leftrightarrow \quad HbO_8$$
Haemoglobin   Oxygen   Oxyhaemoglobin

When fully saturated with oxygen, haemoglobin at a concentration of 15 g per 100 mL of blood will carry about 19 mL of oxygen per 100 mL of blood. Only another 0.3 mL of the gas per 100 mL of blood will be transported dissolved in the plasma, since oxygen is poorly soluble in water. Thus, almost 99% of oxygen carried by oxygenated (arterial) blood is transported as oxyhaemoglobin, and this is a measure of the importance of having sufficient pigment. Functionally, of course, the bond between the pigment and oxygen must be reversible otherwise the gas will not be released in the tissues. It is the local partial pressure of oxygen that determines the binding:

- Within the lungs it is relatively high, so haemoglobin rapidly picks up oxygen to form oxyhaemoglobin, and blood leaves the lungs with its haemoglobin virtually saturated with oxygen. This near-saturation of haemoglobin is illustrated by the 'plateau' phase of the oxygen–haemoglobin dissociation curve (Figure 14.11a; note the graph is normally used to describe how oxygen is then unloaded from haemoglobin, hence the usual term 'dissociation curve').
- Within the tissues, oxygen is utilized and so its partial pressure is relatively low, and this causes the gas to dissociate from the haemoglobin. In Figure 14.11a note how the graph becomes very steep where the partial pressure of oxygen is low; small reductions in the pressure, for example when a muscle is exercising, will release significant amounts of the gas and so maintain tissue oxygen homeostasis.

The relationship between haemoglobin and oxygen is complex but very special: the relationship enables oxygen loading in the lungs, but unloading in the tissues. In fact, the relationship can be shifted under conditions found locally in highly active tissues so that unloading is even more efficient: an increased partial pressure of carbon dioxide, increased acidity or increased temperature, all indicative of increased metabolism, shifts the position of the dissociation curve to the right, referred to as the Bohr shift after the person who first noted it (Figure 14.11b). Thus, for a given (low) partial pressure of oxygen, more of the gas is off-loaded from the haemoglobin.

In contrast, fetal haemoglobin has a dissociation curve toward the left of that of adult haemoglobin (Figure 14.11c). This means that the pigment will have a greater saturation with oxygen for a given partial pressure. Although this may seem detrimental in terms of unloading oxygen within the fetal tissues, in fact it is an important aid in the loading of oxygen across the placenta from maternal blood that has already lost some of its oxygen.

These examples illustrate how the position of the dissociation curve in relation to partial pressures of oxygen has important physiological implications. One further example of note is the adaptation observed at high altitude, when the individ-

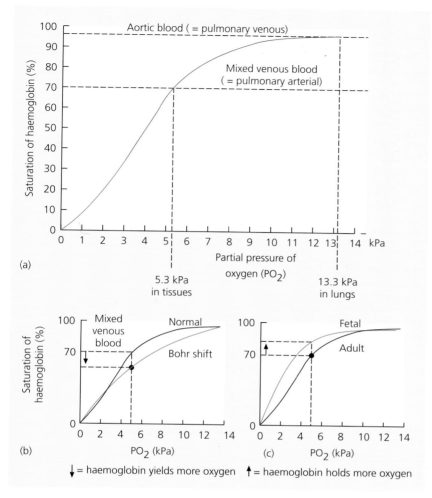

Q *Which of the following conditions in the red cell shifts the O$_2$ dissociation curve to the right: (1) rise in PCO$_2$, (2) reduction in temperature or (3) reduction in pH?*

Q *What happens to oxygen–haemoglobin formation when CO$_2$ is given off by the blood in the lungs?*

ual is exposed chronically to an atmosphere with a low partial pressure of oxygen. Under these circumstances the release of oxygen from haemoglobin is enhanced once again by a shift of the dissociation curve to the right. In this instance, the cause is a substance that becomes elevated in red blood cells, called 2,3-diphosphoglycerate (2,3DPG). As with the Bohr shift (above) this facilitates tissue oxygenation, and so is an adaptive measure that helps to maintain an adequate oxygenation of tissues even under conditions of low atmospheric partial pressure of oxygen, and so performs an important homeostatic function that enables people to live more easily at high altitude.

BOX 14.23 MEASUREMENT OF HAEMOGLOBIN SATURATION USING PULSE OXIMETRY

Pulse oximetry is widely applied as a non-invasive means of observing the oxygen saturation of blood (Vines *et al.*, 2000). Blood in the fingertips is usually observed by this method and, in the warmth, approximates to arterial blood (the fingers use little oxygen and the blood supply to them is very good when the environment is warm). The plateau phase of the oxygen–haemoglobin curve means that even a saturation of 95% (normal = 97–98%) has little meaningful consequence for oxygen carriage, and even 90% saturation represents a substantial carriage of oxygen.

Carriage of carbon dioxide

The carriage of carbon dioxide by blood is very different from that of oxygen:

BOX 14.24 CYANOSIS

Cyanosis refers to the bluish tinge of blood that is heavily deoxygenated. It occurs when there is at least 5 g of desaturated haemoglobin per 100 mL of blood and is indicative of severe oxygen deficiency of the blood. The normal concentration of haemoglobin in blood in health is about 15 g per 100 mL; anaemia would have to be very severe before someone appeared cyanotic. However, cyanosis may be apparent in the absence of severe anaemia if the blood has become heavily deoxygenated by tissues or has been very poorly oxygenated in the lungs. For example, cardiovascular shock induces 'stagnant' hypoxia in which blood flow through tissues is poor and the blood present has been almost depleted of oxygen. Poor cardiac functioning, for example congestive heart failure or pulmonary stenosis, may also cause cyanosis by impairing blood flow through the lungs.

Cyanosis can be systemic (e.g. in shock) and is readily observed by looking at the fingernails or at the gums of the person concerned, since blood circulation is superficial here. Cyanosis may also be localized as a consequence of poor local blood flow, for example in the toes in peripheral vascular disease, or in the lips on a very cold day when blood vessels are heavily constricted in the skin.

BOX 14.25 CARBON MONOXIDE POISONING

Carbon monoxide is a colourless, tasteless and odourless gas and is released in quantities into our environment as part of car emissions and from faulty gas appliances. It is highly toxic because of its high affinity for haemoglobin. The gas actually binds to the pigment more efficiently than does oxygen. However, it is not the displacement of oxygen that is the main problem. The problem is that carbon monoxide poisoning causes the pigment to hold on to its oxygen even in the tissues and so the tissues become hypoxic. This is why toxicity occurs at very low concentration of carbon monoxide.

- Carbon dioxide is a highly soluble gas yet only 7% in blood is carried simply as dissolved gas. However, this component is important because it is the dissolved gas that produces the partial pressure and so in time determines the amount of carbon dioxide carried in other forms.
- Haemoglobin transports about 23% of the carbon dioxide produced by respiring cells (after it has given up its oxygen) in the form of carbaminohaemoglobin (Figure 14.12).
- Most carbon dioxide (about 70%) is carried by blood combined with water to form bicarbonate ions. The formation of bicarbonate ions from carbon dioxide (Figure 14.12) is promoted within red blood cells by the enzyme carbonic anhydrase. Carbonic acid is initially formed and weakly dissociates into bicarbonate and hydrogen ions (see Chapter 6, p.130), thus raising their concentrations within the red blood cell. The hydrogen ions must be buffered (see Chapter 6, p.130 for explanation of buffering).
- The elevated concentration of bicarbonate ions favours their diffusion out of the blood cell and into the plasma. The disturbance in the electrical balance of plasma produced by the diffusion of bicarbonate ions out of red blood cells is corrected by the influx of chloride ions into the blood cells (hence the term 'chloride shift').

When blood reaches the lung the processes are reversed. Thus:

- Carbon dioxide gas dissolved in plasma and within blood cells diffuses down its partial pressure gradient into the alveoli, thus reducing its partial pressure in blood.
- As the partial pressure in blood decreases, carbon dioxide is released from carbaminohaemoglobin, and this too will diffuse into the alveoli.
- As carbon dioxide is removed from blood, the carbonic anhydrase enzyme in the red blood cells promotes the reformation of carbonic acid from bicarbonate and hydrogen ions, producing yet more gas for excretion (see Chapter 6, p.130 for details).
- As bicarbonate ions diffuse in, chloride ions move out of the red cells back into the plasma so that electrical balance is maintained.

At physiological values the relationship between the partial pressure of carbon dioxide and the volume of gas being carried cannot be considered to be reminiscent of the oxygen–haemoglobin dissociation curve. Rather, the relationship is virtually linear and a slight change in partial pressure of carbon dioxide in arterial blood actually represents a pronounced change in the amount of carbon dioxide, carried in its various forms. As noted earlier, it is not surprising to find that the control of lung function is very sensitive to changes in the partial pressure of carbon dioxide.

Gas exchange between blood and tissues

The exchange of gases between blood and intracellular fluid in the tissues also requires the presence of favourable pressure gradients (Figure 14.12). Notice again how a substantial gradient exists for oxygen transfer into the cells, but that for transfer of carbon dioxide out of cells into blood it is relatively small, and indicative of the 20-fold difference between the solubilities of

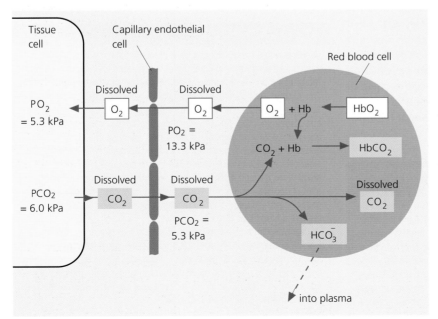

Figure 14.12 Gas exchange between blood and tissues. Partial pressure values are averages based on arterial and mixed venous blood. Note the large diffusional pressure gradient for O_2 but only a small gradient for CO_2, reflecting differences in the solubility of the two gases

Q *How does oxygen leave blood to enter tissue cells, and carbon dioxide leave tissue cells to enter blood?*

the two gases. Such a small gradient for carbon dioxide leaves little scope for adaptation to an increased partial pressure of carbon dioxide in arterial blood arising as a consequence of poor cardiac or lung function; the carbon dioxide content of intracellular fluid will rise as a consequence. This in turn will generate more carbonic acid (i.e. hydrogen ions) and eventually disturb cell homeostasis. This problem is normally avoided by the homeostatic regulation of the partial pressure of carbon dioxide in arterial blood, which facilitates removal of the gas from cells.

REGULATION OF THE RESPIRATORY SYSTEM

Breathing is largely an unconscious process closely matched to the needs of the body to maintain blood gas composition, and so facilitate tissue homeostasis through an appropriate supply of oxygen and removal of carbon dioxide. However, respiratory movements must be modifiable when we exercise, and (consciously) when we cough, or sigh, etc. Accordingly, the regulation of the respiratory system can be considered from four aspects:

- neural mechanisms that determine the actual breathing rhythm;
- influences of blood gas composition on the breathing rhythm;
- the adaptive responses to extreme situations (e.g. exercise, altitude);
- other acute responses that support respiratory mechanics (e.g. coughing).

Neural control of the respiratory rhythm

Breathing movements are largely involuntary, although they can be changed consciously, and are controlled by the rhythmical discharge of nerve impulses from 'respiratory centres'. These are located in the brainstem and impulses pass from them down the spinal cord. Some impulses are then relayed via nerves arising in the 3rd to 5th cervical segments of the cord which form the left and right phrenic nerves and innervate the diaphragm (Figure 14.13). Other impulses are relayed to nerves exiting from the 3rd to 6th thoracic segments of the cord and these form the intercostal nerves which innervate the internal and external intercostal muscles. Further spinal nerves innervate the accessory muscles of inspiration and expiration.

The respiratory centres of the brainstem are illustrated diagrammatically in Figure 14.13. Breathing movements result from an integration of nervous activity from these centres:

- *Inspiration*: this is initiated by the inspiratory centre in the medulla oblongata, following its activation by the apneustic centre, which is also in the medulla. It ceases because inputs from stretch receptors present in the lung, intercostal muscles and diaphragm (which pass to the brainstem via the vagus nerve), cause the pneumotaxic centre of the pons varolii to inhibit the apneustic centre, and hence deactivate the inspiratory centre. The role of stretch receptors is illustrated by the Hering–Breuer reflex, in which overinflation of

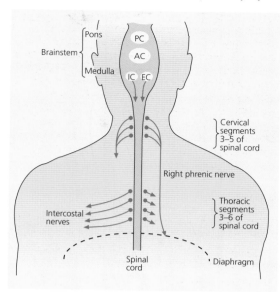

Figure 14.13 Respiratory centres and innervation of the thoracic muscles. AC, apneustic centre; EC, expiratory centre; IC, inspiratory centre; PC, pneumotaxic centre

Q *Which areas of the brain control normal quiet (i.e. diaphragmatic) breathing?*

BOX 14.26 RESPIRATORY DEPRESSION BY OPIOID ANALGESICS

When administered orally or intravenously, opioid analgesics such as morphine have their main effects on receptors located within the brainstem, where they interfere with the pain gating mechanisms (see Chapter 20, p.563). A side-effect of such drugs is to depress respiratory centre functioning and so cause dyspnoea and possibly hypoxaemia. If severe, the problem can become life threatening and an antagonistic drug (e.g. naloxone) must be administered. This is quick acting but will modulate the analgesia produced by the opioid. The problems are reduced by using intraspinal routes of administration (where spinal cord receptors are the targets) and these are increasingly popular methods.

---

the lungs causes a cessation of activity in the nerve cells that stimulate the contraction of inspiratory muscles.

- *Expiration*: in quiet breathing, expiration occurs passively by elastic recoil simply because we stop breathing in (see earlier). However, part of the apneustic centre will activate the expiratory muscles if we wish to make a more forceful expiration.

Factors that modulate respiratory rhythm: chemoreceptors

The respiratory centres also receive neural inputs from chemoreceptors that respond to changes in either blood oxygen or carbon dioxide (and acidity) content (Figure 14.14).

For oxygen, the oxyhaemoglobin curve in Figure 14.11 identifies a 'plateau' region which indicates that a change in

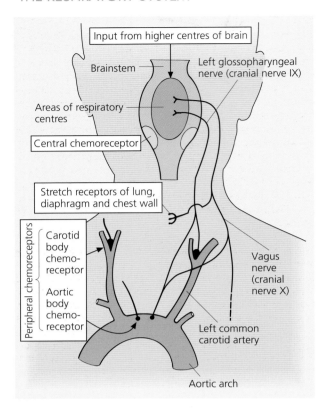

Figure 14.14 Sensory (afferent) input into respiratory centres of the brainstem

Q *Which of the factors in blood is the most important control of ventilation: PCO₂ or PO₂?*

the partial pressure of oxygen from the normal 13.3 kPa to about 10.5 kPa has little effect on the volume of oxygen carried by blood, since the haemoglobin remains well saturated with oxygen. This lower partial pressure normally still represents a reasonable pressure gradient to drive the diffusion of oxygen from blood into cells and does not provide a powerful drive to increase breathing. Consequently, there is no need for a decrease in the partial pressure of oxygen to promote increased lung ventilation, unless it falls below 10.5 kPa (i.e. when haemoglobin is less than fully saturated).

The carriage of carbon dioxide by blood was earlier identified as being very different from that of oxygen, in that it is carried in various forms. A similar proportionate increase in its partial pressure from 5.3 kPa to 6.4 kPa would represent an increase in content of about 20%, leading to a subsequent retention of the gas in the tissues and a resultant increase in the acidity of body fluids. It is therefore not surprising that the respiratory chemoreceptors are most sensitive to carbon dioxide, and even small changes in the partial pressure of carbon dioxide provide a stimulus to change lung function.

The respiratory chemoreceptors are found centrally and peripherally. Central chemoreceptors are found in the brainstem (hence the term 'central') and do not actually monitor blood gases: they monitor the acidity of the cerebrospinal fluid bathing the brain. This is separated from the circulatory sys-

tem by the 'blood–brain barrier', which is actually a secretory epithelium (the choroid plexus, see Figure 8.16b, p.181). The epithelium is impervious to hydrogen ions in the blood but is freely permeable to carbon dioxide. Thus, if the partial pressure of carbon dioxide is elevated in arterial blood the gas will diffuse into the cerebrospinal fluid, form carbonic acid and so increase the acidity of the fluid.

Central chemoreceptors do not monitor oxygen concentrations. Also, being outside the circulatory system, their responses to elevated blood carbon dioxide content will be relatively slow. They act to determine the basal respiratory rhythm needed to maintain adequate gas exchange by the lungs.

Peripheral chemoreceptors are found in the walls of the aortic arch and at the point where each of the common carotid arteries in the neck divide into their internal and external branches (an area called the carotid body). Changes in the partial pressure of carbon dioxide (and the acidity) of arterial blood stimulates these receptors and impulses are relayed to the respiratory centres of the brainstem (Figure 14.14). Peripheral chemoreceptors respond rapidly to changes in the partial pressure of carbon dioxide in arterial blood and will quickly respond to moment-by-moment changes in blood carbon dioxide content, providing a fine-tuning to the basal rhythm established by the central chemoreceptors. They also respond to a modest decrease in the oxygen content of arterial blood and are responsible for a 'hypoxic drive' (see below). It would be incorrect, however, to assume that changes in blood oxygen have only a weak involvement in the regulation of lung function. If small degrees of hypoxaemia are accompanied by an increased partial pressure of carbon dioxide, the respiratory response to the elevated carbon dioxide is potentiated as the peripheral chemoreceptors become sensitized.

Factors that modulate respiratory rhythms: adaptations to exercise and altitude

Exercise

Oxygen consumption and carbon dioxide production in strenuous exercise may each be of the order of 4 L/minute (in adults) compared with 200–250 mL/minute at rest (i.e. an increase of up to 20 times). Increased oxygen demands during exercise, and increased carbon dioxide excretion, are met by increasing the alveolar ventilation rate through increased breath volume and breathing rate. In this way as much as 100 L or more of air may be inspired per minute (compared with 5–6 L at rest).

Increased breath volume is made possible because we use the inspiratory and expiratory reserve volumes of the lungs, even to the extent of using the entire vital capacity. This results from a modification of outputs from the respiratory centres; the precise mechanism is unclear but must also include an overriding of the afferent impulses from stretch receptors within the thorax that ordinarily suppress inhalation. Efficient ventilation during exercise is also facilitated by:

* *a reduction in airway resistance*: mouth breathing is utilized, which bypasses the nasal cavity;

- *relaxation of smooth muscle in bronchioles to dilate these terminal airways*: this is induced by the actions of the sympathetic nervous system (and adrenaline/noradrenaline from the adrenal gland), which is stimulated during physical activity (see Chapter 8, p.200).

The respiratory changes compensate for the reduction in oxygen content of mixed venous blood, and elevation in carbon dioxide, that occur during exercise, and consequently the average gas composition of arterial blood does not alter, which helps to maintain cellular homeostasis. It therefore cannot be the case that the exercise-induced changes are in response to chemoreceptor activity. What promotes the increased ventilation is still unclear, but the response must result from a stimulation of receptors somewhere in the body. Suggestions include nerve impulses from muscle or joint receptors, from chemoreceptors within the pulmonary circulation (rather than aorta/carotid arteries) or from potassium-sensitive receptors, since potassium ion concentration in blood rises sharply during exercise.

Altitude

The atmospheric pressure falls on ascending from sea level, which means that the partial pressure of oxygen in the air also decreases. This in turn will lower the partial pressure of oxygen in alveolar gas and hence in arterial blood and tissues. Eventually, hypoxaemia and hypoxia results. The partial pressure of carbon dioxide will also be affected but the change is negligible since even at sea level its partial pressure in air is very close to zero, and so blood carbon dioxide remains normal. The hypoxaemia stimulates breathing but the increased ventilation will remove too much carbon dioxide from blood (i.e. it will represent a hyperventilation) and so the breathing response will quickly be reversed, leaving the individual feeling 'breathless'. Survival at altitude therefore requires adaptation to the conditions.

At this point, the reader should recall that homeostasis operates around a 'set point', in this instance the 'normal' set point for carbon dioxide in arterial blood. Over time at altitude, adaptation takes place because of changes within the brain through decreasing the buffering capacity of the cerebrospinal fluid. Thus, the acidity of the cerebrospinal fluid is held constant despite the decreased carbon dioxide content of arterial blood when the 'hypoxic drive' to breathing is operated (see Chapter 6, p.130 for a discussion of buffers). Consequently, the central chemoreceptors that determine the basal breathing rate are not stimulated to reduce the breathing response to the hypoxaemia. The reduced partial pressure of carbon dioxide in blood then becomes a new 'set point' (i.e. it is considered 'normal' and breathing rate remains elevated in response to the reduced oxygen content).

Additional adaptations to life at altitude are:

- An elevation in the 2,3DPG content of red blood cells (see earlier), which facilitates the unloading of oxygen in the tissues.
- An increased red blood cell count (hypoxaemia stimulates the release of the hormone erythropoietin, which stimulates production of red blood cells by bone marrow). The additional red cells make more haemoglobin available to carry oxygen.

BOX 14.27 VENTILATION THERAPY DURING CHRONIC OBSTRUCTIVE AIRWAY DISEASE

The text identifies a resetting of the homeostatic set point for arterial carbon dioxide on ascent to altitude, which takes several days to accomplish. With chronic obstructive pulmonary disease (COPD) the individual will undergo a similar central adaptation to modulate breathing, but this time in the opposite way so that the new set point is an elevation in arterial carbon dioxide. This occurs because the acidity of cerebrospinal fluid will be maintained as usual, despite the elevated carbon dioxide concentration in blood and cerebrospinal fluid, by buffering any change in acidity within it, and so the elevated carbon dioxide content of blood becomes a new 'set point' about which breathing movements are regulated. The adaptation is actually useful because it means that the hypoxaemia induced by inadequate lung ventilation is allowed to stimulate breathing.

Provision of oxygen therapy is not unusual in this condition but care must be taken not to remove carbon dioxide too rapidly from blood since returning the blood gas composition to its previously normal carbon dioxide content will now be interpreted paradoxically by the receptors as hypocapnia, inhibiting the respiratory drive. To reduce the hypoxaemia caused by the condition, but still leave an elevated carbon dioxide, requires the usage of only a slightly enriched oxygen mixture (perhaps 28% compared with 21% in air). In this way some hypoxaemia remains and continues to stimulate breathing, but the carbon dioxide content remains at the elevated value, now considered by the body to be normal.

- An increase in total lung capacity, which facilitates the extra ventilation required when active at altitude.

Factors that modulate respiratory rhythm: inputs from other receptors

Numerous other receptors influence respiratory movements when stimulated – some only acutely. These are chemoreceptors of the nasal mucosa, larynx and trachea that are stimulated by airborne irritants, and touch receptors of the pharynx stimulated by the presence of food particles. All produce reflex changes in respiratory movements:

- *Sneezing*: a short inspiration followed by a forced expiration with the glottis open.
- *Swallowing*: inhibits breathing movements.
- *Coughing*: short inspiration followed by a series of forced expirations against a closed glottis. Sudden opening of the glottis releases the high pressure developed in airways and carries away the irritants.
- *Hiccoughing*: spasmodic contractions of the diaphragm with the glottis closed.

The respiratory centres of the brainstem also receive impulses from higher centres of the brain. We can therefore alter breathing movements voluntarily, control expiration in singing or speech, inspire deeply with spasmodic expirations in weeping and laughing, prolong expiration in sighing, inspire deeply in yawning and produce rapid movements in fear and excitement. The functions of many of these responses are not understood.

SUMMARY

1 The carriage of oxygen (O_2) and carbon dioxide (CO_2) to and from tissues, and the exchange of these gases with air, is vital for life.

2 When a person is at rest, 5–6 L of air are taken into, and breathed out of, the lungs each minute. Exercise may increase this to 80–100 L/minute by increasing the depth of each breath and the rate of breathing. Such changes in lung ventilation ensure that the gas composition of systemic arterial blood remains almost constant.

3 The amount of energy required to maintain breathing movements is minimized by low airway resistance and a high compliance (elasticity).

4 The 'vital capacity' represents the maximum volume of gas which can be taken into the lungs, and expired from them, in a single breath. The vital capacity is used clinically to assess airway resistance and compliance.

5 Gas exchange occurs across the lung alveoli; the rest of the airway comprises a 'dead space'. This, together with the volume of gas left in the lungs after expiration, constitutes the 'functional residual capacity' or FRC. Inspired air mixes with the FRC gas and produces a slight enrichment of the oxygen content and a slight depletion of the carbon dioxide content.

6 Gases diffuse down pressure gradients. The air in the lung consists of a mixture of gases and the partial pressure exerted by each gas is physiologically more significant than the total pressure of the whole mixture. Lung ventilation ensures that the partial pressure gradients are conducive to the diffusion of oxygen into blood, and of carbon dioxide out of blood.

7 Alveolar gas composition and blood perfusion varies throughout the lungs and the partial pressures of gases in systemic arterial blood represent the mean of those in the alveoli after inspiration.

8 Oxygen is poorly soluble in water and is carried in the blood combined with the pigment haemoglobin. The oxygen is released from the pigment in tissues, where the partial pressure of O_2 is reduced by utilization of the gas. The release is facilitated by conditions associated with high rates of metabolism, such as high temperature and low pH, and this is called the Bohr shift. Fetal haemoglobin has a slightly different structure from the adult form, and this helps it to be saturated with oxygen at the partial pressures observed in the placenta.

9 Carbon dioxide is a soluble gas and is carried from tissues dissolved in blood, or in combination with water to form bicarbonate ions. Some is combined with haemoglobin. The lower partial pressure of carbon dioxide found in the lungs promotes the conversion of bicarbonate to carbon dioxide, the release of carbon dioxide from haemoglobin, and diffusion of the gas out of the blood.

10 Lung ventilation is controlled by neural activity from centres within the brainstem. The centres are modulated by neural inputs from various areas, in particular from chemoreceptors in the arterial system and in the brainstem. These especially monitor pH and so provide a means of evaluating the carbon dioxide content of blood and cerebrospinal fluid, since the gas forms carbonic acid in water. Other inputs originate from stretch receptors in the lung, from higher brain centres and from joint receptors.

11 Some homeostatic set points are altered during exercise, and following ascent to high altitude, and promote the respiratory changes observed.

REFERENCES

Booker, R. (2008) *Vital Lung Function: Your Essential Reference on Lung Function Testing*. London: Class Publishing.

Bush, A. and Thomson, A.H. (2007) Acute bronchiolitis. *British Medical Journal* **335**(7628): 1037–41.

Johnson, A.L., Hampson, D.F. and Hampson, N.B. (2008) Sputum color: potential implications for clinical practice. *Respiratory Care* **53**(4): 450–4.

Klements, E.M. (2001) Monitoring peak flow rates as a health-promoting behavior in managing and improving asthma. *Clinical Excellence for Nurse Practitioners* **24**(3): 147–51.

Pendharkar, S.R. and Tremblay, A.T. (2007) A diagnostic approach to pleural effusion: guidance on how to identify the cause. *Journal of Respiratory Diseases* (12): 565–9.

Sweet, D., Bevilacqua, G., Carnielli, V. *et al.* (2007) European consensus guidelines on the management of neonatal respiratory distress syndrome. *Journal of Perinatal Medicine* **35**(3): 175–86.

Truesdell, S. (2000) Helping patients with COPD manage episodes of acute shortage of breath. *Medical and Surgical Nursing* **9**(4): 178–82.

Vines, D.L., Shelledy, D.C. and Peters, J. (2000) Current respiratory care, part 1: oxygen therapy, oximetry, bronchial hygiene. *Journal of Critical Illness* **15**(9): 507–10.

Wolf, F.M., Guevara, J.P., Grum, C.M., Clark, N.M. and Cates, C.J. (2007) Educational interventions for asthma in children. *Cochrane Database of Systematic Reviews*, 2007 (4).

THE KIDNEYS AND URINARY TRACT

INTRODUCTION

Chapter 6 described the distribution of water within the body, and the roles of the main constituents of the intracellular and extracellular fluid compartments. In forming urine, our kidneys excrete many of the substances found in body fluids and so they are the main organs that maintain the composition of these fluids appropriate for optimal cell functioning. However, there are other functions; for example, the kidneys are the source of renin, an enzyme necessary for the production of the hormone angiotensin, which has a role in blood pressure regulation (see Figure 12.32, p.355). This chapter describes how the kidneys function and their role in homeostasis.

Urine produced by the kidneys is stored within the urinary bladder, and is eliminated from the body in a controlled process. This chapter therefore also considers the urinary tract and identifies the control of bladder emptying.

Why excrete?

Substances to be excreted fall under three categories:

1 Metabolism produces a variety of 'waste' substances that cannot be utilized and which, if allowed to accumulate, will eventually disturb the body fluid environment and hence alter cell processes.

2 The term 'waste' might also be used to describe substances produced by cells that may be important functionally but must be removed once their action is complete. Hormones, for example, must be removed from body fluids, or at least be inactivated, to stop their activities as required. Inactivation is mainly carried out in the liver but the products are usually excreted in urine.

3 In addition to products of metabolism, our body fluids are also continually influenced by substances absorbed from our diet. These may be in excess of body requirement, while some may not even be utilized at all. For example, dietary constituents such as water-soluble vitamins, minerals and water cannot be stored to any degree and therefore any excess must be removed from the body, while pigments or additives in food are frequently of no biochemical value.

Thus the solutes dissolved in our body fluids are continually being added to via metabolism or via dietary uptake, hence the need for routes for their excretion. The kidneys are often viewed as being the only organs of excretion, but there are other routes by which substances are removed from the body.

BOX 15.1 SOME DEFINITIONS: EXCRETION, SECRETION, URINATION AND DEFECATION

The following terms frequently cause confusion and are worth defining before proceeding:

• *Excretion* may be defined as the removal of substances from the body in urine, faeces, sweat and expired gases: all contain substances that have been derived from body fluids. Note that the term refers primarily to a route of removal, not a process.

• *Secretion* is a process that refers to the extrusion of substances and/or water across cell membranes. This may involve the release of substances from intracellular vesicles, as in the secretion of hormones, enzymes or neurotransmitters, or alternatively may involve the transport of substances using membrane carrier processes, for example into the forming of urine, sweat or faecal stools.

• *Urination* is the process of passing urine. Sometimes referred to as 'micturition', it relates to how the urinary bladder and the tube called the urethra facilitate the removal of urine from the body.

• *Defecation* is the process by which faeces are passed from the body. Faeces contain various substances, such as bile salts and bile pigments, which have been added from body fluids during the formation of 'stools' in the bowel, and so defecation is a route for excretion. Faecal material also includes indigestible components such as fibre that have not come into contact with intracellular metabolism and so these materials cannot be considered as excretory products.

• *Elimination* is identified as a need by models of care; it incorporates not only the biological aspects of excretion but also the psychosocial components that influence the ability of people to meet this need. The term covers both defecation and urination.

BOX 15.2 CHARACTERISTICS OF URINE

Inadequate or inappropriate kidney function will have consequences for body fluid volume and composition. Similarly, changes in hormonal functions or body fluid composition that are independent of renal pathologies will also promote a change in renal functioning. Thus, urine analysis is a valuable diagnostic procedure and health professionals should be familiar with the basic characteristics of urine.

- *Volume*: it is usual to express urine volume as a rate of production – in other words how long it has taken for the urinary bladder to accumulate the volume passed. The average rate of production in a climate such as that of the UK is 60 mL/hour but the rate will vary from about 30 mL/hour in dehydration to 800+ mL/hour in a very hydrated state. In a clinical setting, a rate of urine production of at least 30 mL/hour is looked for, but it is important to note that urine produced at this rate should be deep yellow and concentrated. If it is not, or if production is at an even lower rate, then this is a cause for concern as it may be indicative of an advanced state of renal failure. *Oliguria* is a term used to describe inadequate urinary production; *anuria* refers to little or no production at all (<100 mL/day).
- *Colour*: urine is characteristically yellow/amber in colour because of the presence of pigments, called urochromes, derived from bile pigment, and so colour will be influenced by urinary concentration (from a deep yellow to almost colourless). It may also be affected by pigments in food, for example a reddish colour after eating beetroot. Fresh urine is clear, but may sometimes be a little cloudy due to the presence of mucin secreted from the linings of the urinary tract.
- *Odour*: urine also has a characteristic odour but on standing develops an unpleasant smell of ammonia as urea (a normal constituent) within it undergoes bacterial decomposition. Urine odour may also include that produced by products in food, for example alcohol or the distinctive smell after eating asparagus.
- *Concentration*: this depends upon the state of hydration of the individual. Very low rates of urine production in dehydration are associated with high concentration, while good hydration is associated with very dilute urine. On average, urine will be quite yellow because people are usually slightly dehydrated.
- *Contents*: urine contains various solutes, especially urea and electrolytes. There should at most be only a trace of blood cells, perhaps 100 red cells/mL of urine, compared with 500 million/mL of blood. An increase in the numbers present is indicative of structural damage to the kidney or urinary tract. Similarly, urine is normally almost protein- and glucose-free compared with concentrations of about 70 g/L and 5 mmol/L, respectively, in blood plasma and an increase may again indicate underlying disease. The presence of haemoglobin (from red blood cells), protein and glucose in urine can readily be determined using a 'dip stick' method in which tabs impregnated with enzymes promote a colour formation that relates to the substance concerned. Urea and electrolytes have to be measured in a sample sent to the laboratory.
- *Acidity*: this relates to urine composition, especially of hydrogen ions and bicarbonate ions, and urine pH is readily determined using a 'dip stick' method. Normal pH range is 6.8–7.8 (i.e. slightly acidic to slightly alkaline), depending upon the acidity of blood at the time of urine formation.

In summary the routes and the substances excreted by each route are:

- *The kidneys (i.e. urine)*: metabolic products (e.g. urea, creatinine), electrolytes and water.
- *The bowel (i.e. faeces)*: bile salts, bile pigments, small amounts of electrolytes and water.
- *The lungs (i.e. expired gases)*: carbon dioxide, and water vapour.
- *The skin (i.e. sweat)*: electrolytes, water and some metabolic products (e.g. urea).

In general, the kidneys are the main routes for excretion, but in some instances, for example in the excretion of carbon dioxide and bile pigments, they play only a minor role.

Before proceeding, readers are advised to ensure that they are familiar with the material in Chapter 6, which describes the main fluids of the body and their composition, and introduces the principles of fluid homeostasis.

OVERVIEW OF THE ANATOMY AND PHYSIOLOGY OF THE KIDNEYS

General anatomy

The kidneys are paired organs situated in the superior and posterior aspects of the abdomen wall (Figure 15.1), lying outside the peritoneum on either side of the vertebral column and embedded in adipose tissue. Each weighs approximately 140 g and may be described as being bean-shaped (though some beans are kidney-shaped!) The right kidney lies a little lower than the left as it is displaced by the liver.

Each kidney receives (Figure 15.2):

- blood via a branch from the abdominal aorta, called a renal artery;
- motor nerve activity from the autonomic nervous system.

Leaving each kidney:

- is a renal vein, which drains blood directly into the inferior vena cava;
- are sensory autonomic nerves;
- is a ureter which transports urine to the urinary bladder for storage prior to urination.

Our kidneys receive a lot of blood, some 1.2 L/minute (that is, around 20% of the entire cardiac output), partly to sustain the filtration of plasma that takes place, and partly to sustain the high oxygen demands of kidney cells. Reducing renal blood flow is an important part of homeostatic responses to restore systemic arterial blood pressure when there has been a haemorrhage, or to help redirect blood to muscles during heavy exercise. It is the efferent renal nerves that produce such intense vasoconstriction. However, renal nerve activity can also be recorded under less traumatic circumstances, and has been shown to influence the urinary excretion of sodium ions as part of the mechanism of regulating blood volume. The afferent (i.e. sensory) renal nerves may provide information

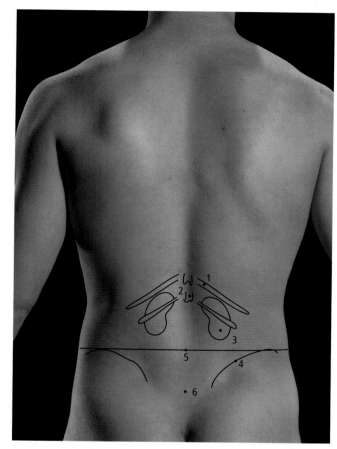

Figure 15.1 Surface anatomy of the posterior abdominal wall showing relations to the kidneys: 1, 11th rib; 2, spine T12; 3, lower pole right kidney; 4, iliac crest; 5, intercristal plane; 6, S2. Reproduced with the kind permission of Abrahams *et al.* from *Illustrated Clinical Anatomy*, Hodder, London

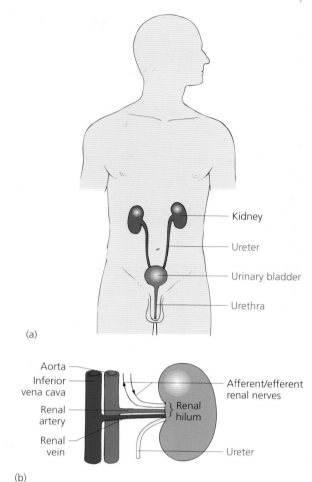

Figure 15.2 (a) Components of the urinary system. (b) Renal vessels and nerves

Q Which blood vessels bring excretory waste products to the kidney?

that enables the function of each kidney to be matched, preventing them becoming unsynchronized. Renal nerves therefore appear to have significant roles but it should be noted that transplanted kidneys (see Box 15.19, p.441) function well without them, which suggests that there may be alternative means that compensate for their actions.

A cross-section of the kidney reveals its gross anatomy (Figure 15.3):

- The outer surface is coated with a connective tissue capsule.
- Immediately under the capsule is an outer layer, or cortex, that is clearly composed of small lobules that extend into the deeper parts of the kidney. Within the cortex is found an extensive vascular system that supports the initial stage of urine formation, by a process of filtration.
- The filtrate is expressed into minute tubules, called nephrons, that eventually drain into an expanded space within the kidney, called the renal pelvis.
- Between the cortex and pelvis, the tubules pass through deeper layers of kidney tissue; this inner area is referred to as the medulla. Most tubules actually pass from the cortex into the medulla and thence back out to the cortex again, before

passing once more through the medulla and draining into the pelvis. This contorted route through these inner regions of the kidney is essential to kidney function.
- Urine drains from the renal pelvis into the ureters on the way to the urinary bladder.

The basic processes involved in urine formation

The kidney tubules (nephrons) are described in detail later but for now let us simply consider in outline the processes that take place in them that will determine the composition of urine that is finally produced (Figure 15.4).

Urine formation begins with the filtering of blood plasma as it passes through the kidneys; blood cells are retained within the circulatory system. A fluid (termed the 'filtrate') is formed that contains water and solute molecules found in plasma, other than large ones, such as proteins (though smaller proteins may gain access). The solute composition of the filtrate will therefore be, in many ways, similar to that of plasma (Table 15.1) and the process of its formation is considered in

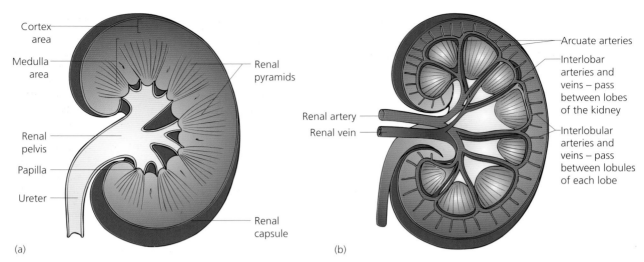

Figure 15.3 (a) General anatomy of the kidney. (b) Vasculature of the kidney

Q List the functions of the kidneys.

Q Identify the two main layers of the kidney.

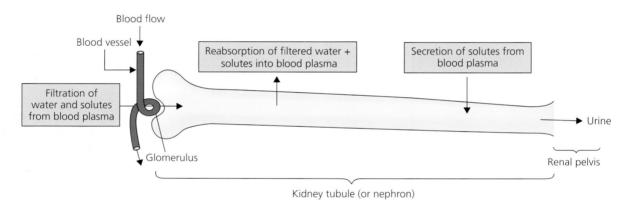

Urine volume = Volume filtered − volume reabsorbed
Solute excretion = Amount filtered − amount reabsorbed + amount secreted

Figure 15.4 Fundamental processes in the formation of urine

Q Differentiate between the following processes involved in the production of urine: (1) filtration, (2) reabsorption, and (3) secretion.

more detail when the filtering unit, called the glomerulus, is discussed later. The rate of excretion in urine of some substances, such as the metabolic waste substances urea and creatinine, is almost exclusively determined by how efficiently the kidneys are filtering. For most other substances, the composition of the filtrate is modified as it passes along the tubules by the cells that line the renal tubules.

The final urine is a complex solution of various ions and organic solutes, but not in the same proportions as they are found in plasma (Table 15.1); urine volume and solute concentration vary considerably according to our state of hydration, and because the concentrations of many solutes change independently depending upon the functioning of the renal tubules. 'Typical' values for urine must therefore be considered only as a guide. The comparison in Table 15.1 is useful, however, because it illustrates how the concentrations of many electrolytes have become enriched in urine, as also are those of

Table 15.1 Comparison of solute concentrations in plasma, the glomerular filtrate and urine

	Plasma (mmol/L)	Glomerular filtrate (mmol/L)	Urine* (mmol/L)
Sodium	140	140	200
Potassium	4	4	50
Calcium	1.3**	1.3	5
Chloride	105	113	150
Bicarbonate	25	27	2
Glucose	4	4	Trace†
Urea	4	4	250
	(g/L)	(g/L)	(g/L)
Protein	70	0.2	Trace†

*These are only representative values – concentrations vary according to conditions (see text for details).
**Represents ionized, rather than total, calcium (approximately 50% of calcium in plasma is bound to proteins).
†Presence of glucose or protein in urine warrants further laboratory tests.

Q Discuss the statement, 'the kidney is the ultimate regulator of homeostasis'.

BOX 15.3 URINE COLLECTING

Evaluating the concentration of solutes is widely applied as a clinical assessment. It is a useful parameter, especially when assessing the capacity of the kidneys to conserve water. Alternatively, the presence or absence of, say, a hormone might be looked for. Under these circumstances simply obtaining a urine sample will be adequate, perhaps after a period of 2 hours to ensure adequate volume. However, it is important to note that the concentration of a substance in urine does not necessarily reflect the actual rate of excretion, calculated as:

$$\frac{\text{(Urine concentration of the substance)} \times \text{(Urine volume)}}{\text{Collection time}}$$

In practice settings the collection time is often 12 or 24 hours since this helps to improve the accuracy of measurement and assessment, as it compensates for periods during the day when urine production might temporarily be elevated or reduced. Depending upon the setting, obtaining the urine may necessitate catheterization (for example in critical care areas or after surgery) and this involves the insertion of tubing along the urethra and into the urinary bladder (see Box 15.23, p.444). Urine is encouraged to drain into a collection bag by placing the bag low down so that gravity aids drainage. Catheter care will be important in this setting.

Alternatively, a urine sample might be taken in order to assess the presence or absence of infection. The time of collection will not be as important here, but for the clinician to be confident that the presence of infection derives from the bladder itself a mid-stream urine (abbreviated as MSU) specimen is usually taken to reduce the risk of contamination from the urethra.

nitrogenous waste, especially urea. The latter account for a considerably greater proportion of the total solute concentration in urine than in plasma, and this emphasizes the importance of urine as a route to excrete this substance.

The processes by which the composition of the filtrate is modified are referred to as 'reabsorption' and 'secretion'; body fluid composition regulation by the kidneys seems to predominantly involve appropriate modulation of reabsorptive processes and/or secretion, but not the rate of filtration:

- Reabsorption describes the movement of solutes and water out of the lumen of the kidney tubules and back into the circulatory system; the term 'absorption' infers a first-time round process of absorbing substances into the body, for example from the bowel, whereas substances being reabsorbed from the filtrate have been derived from body fluids in the first place (Figure 15.4). Some substances, such as sodium chloride, always undergo incomplete reabsorption and so they are always present in the final urine but the rate at which they are excreted will always be less than their rate of filtration from blood. Altering the rate of reabsorption is an important means by which the kidneys are able to regulate the excretion of these substances. In contrast, the reabsorption of some others, for example amino acids, glucose and small protein molecules, is almost complete; they therefore are conserved and will largely normally be absent from urine.

- With reference to kidney function, 'secretion' is used to indicate the addition of substances into the filtrate from cells lining the kidney tubules, and these secretions then become constituents of the final urine. Secretion of certain substances into the forming urine also helps the kidney regulate the rate at which they are excreted. For example, potassium filtered from plasma is almost entirely reabsorbed in the early parts of the renal tubules, and that appearing in the final urine has largely been secreted into the later parts. Altering the rate of secretion provides an important means of regulating the excretion of such substances. In this respect, one important contrast between reabsorption and secretion is that the former cannot produce a rate of excretion greater than that at which the substance was first filtered even if no

BOX 15.4 DIURESIS, ANTIDIURESIS AND NATRIURESIS

These three terms appear frequently in the medical literature in relation to urine volumes, and often confuse:

- *Diuresis*: an increased urine production. The term does not inform as to the composition of urine, which in extreme may be rich in electrolytes or may be very dilute; it simply notes the high rate of production.
- *Antidiuresis*: a fall in urine production, usually as a consequence of increased water reabsorption. Again the term does not inform on composition, although it is most widely applied to the reduction induced by antidiuretic hormone (ADH).
- *Natriuresis*: specifically refers to increased sodium excretion (natrium = sodium). This may occur in the presence or absence of pronounced changes in urine production, although urine production will normally be increased to some degree. Note though that diuretic drugs (e.g. furosemide) act by altering water reabsorption by interfering with sodium reabsorption by the kidney tubules, and in doing so promote a natriuresis as well as a diuresis (see Box 15.10, p.431).

reabsorption took place at all, but for a secreted substance more of it might be secreted into the renal tubule, if necessary, than could possibly have entered via the filtrate. This makes the excretion of substances such as potassium extremely efficient and imbalances can be reversed quickly; very appropriate considering the effects of potassium excess on the heart (see Box 6.7, p.127). Similarly, some of the organic acid products of metabolism are potentially dangerous substances and their secretion contributes to their efficient excretion.

DETAILS OF KIDNEY FUNCTIONS

Structural and functional aspects of the kidney

The previous section identified how urine composition is the net result of filtration, reabsorption and secretion processes. In order for these processes to take place, the renal tubules are subdivided into segments of different anatomical arrangement and functions: the glomerulus/Bowman's capsule, the proximal tubule, the loop of Henle, the distal tubule, and the

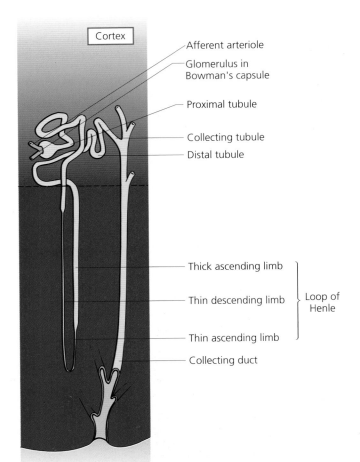

Cortex

Afferent arteriole

Glomerulus in
Bowman's capsule

Proximal tubule

Collecting tubule

Distal tubule

Thick ascending limb

Thin descending limb — Loop of Henle

Thin ascending limb

Collecting duct

Figure 15.5 Anatomical segmentation of the renal tubule

Q What is the basic structural and functional unit of the kidney?

collecting ducts (Figure 15.5). Urine collects in the renal pelvis and its passage to the bladder is completed by the ureters.

Glomerulus/Bowman's capsule

A filtrate of plasma is produced within the cortex of the kidney across microscopic filters, some 100–150 µm in diameter, called glomeruli (singular, glomerulus; Figure 15.6a), of which there are over a million in each kidney. Each glomerulus is basically a tuft of blood capillaries that provides a large surface area for filtration; the total area for both kidneys is of the order of 2 m² (about the surface of a large bath tub). The filtrate from each glomerulus is produced into individual cup-like receptacles called Bowman's capsules, from which a kidney tubule extends into the kidney mass. In some texts a single glomerulus and its Bowman's capsule may occasionally be referred to by the old name of 'Malpighian corpuscle' but this term is outdated.

The filter itself consists of two layers of cells: the cells of the wall of the glomerular capillaries and the cells of Bowman's capsule, together with the basement membranes of protein fibres which keeps the layers of cells in place. Pores through both layers, together with the matrix of the basement membranes, allow the passage of smaller solute molecules (such as electrolytes and glucose) but prevent the passage of large molecules such as plasma proteins, and of blood cells. The rate at which fluid is passed across the glomeruli into the Bowman's capsule is called the glomerular filtration rate, abbreviated as GFR. For both kidneys the total GFR in young adults is about 125 mL/minute, that is about 180 L/day or approximately 20 reasonable-sized bucketfuls per day! This is a considerable volume, equivalent to some 50 times that of the plasma from which the filtrate is derived. The potential for removing substances from blood plasma is therefore extensive. The rate at which glomerular filtrate is formed under normal circumstances is thought to be kept virtually constant (but see Box 15.6). There are two aspects to be considered in relation to this:

- How is the filtrate produced?
- Why do we filter so much?

How is the filtrate produced?

To filter such a volume requires the presence of a significant force to drive the process. This force is provided by the pressure gradient that exists across the filter, largely produced by

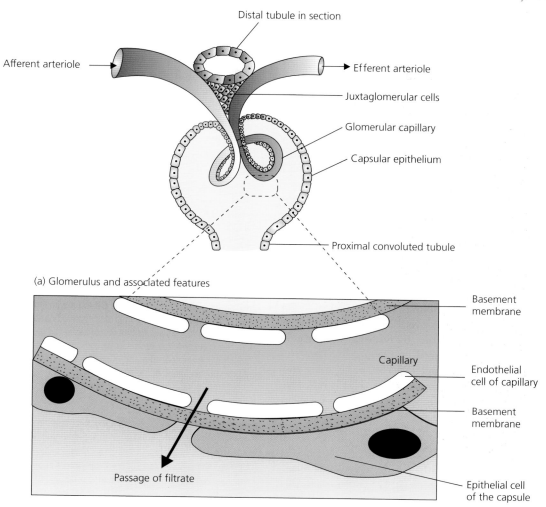

(a) Glomerulus and associated features

(b) Enlarged view to show features of the glomerular filter

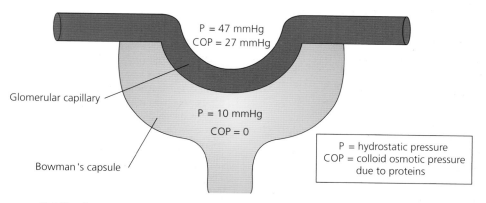

P = 47 mmHg
COP = 27 mmHg

Glomerular capillary

P = 10 mmHg

COP = 0

Bowman's capsule

P = hydrostatic pressure
COP = colloid osmotic pressure
due to proteins

Net filtration pressure = pressure favouring filtration/pressure opposing filtration
= (47–10) – (27–0)
= 37–27
= 10 mmHg i.e. positive filtration pressure

(c)

Figure 15.6 The renal glomerulus. (a) General structure. (b) Detail of the filter.
(c) Forces promoting filtration

Q Explain how the afferent arteriole is able to control the volume of blood filtered in a given time.

ACTIVITY

Compare the filtration pressure with that in a generalized capillary (see Figure 6.2, p.124).

the hydrostatic pressure of blood in the capillaries. The driving pressure is to a certain extent counteracted by the osmotic pressure generated by the plasma proteins that are retained in the glomerular capillaries (Figure 15.6c). This is similar to the situation that occurs in capillaries elsewhere, as described in Chapter 6 (p.124). However, the hydrostatic pressure in those capillaries declines along the vessel until it is exceeded by the osmotic pressure due to proteins, with the result that most of the fluid exuded out of the capillary in the early stages is now drawn back into it again. This reversal of fluid movement does not occur in the glomerulus because blood exits through another arteriole (called the efferent arteriole), a feature unique to the kidneys, which acts to maintain the hydrostatic pressure at a much higher value than in capillaries elsewhere. In addition, the constrictor activities of sympathetic nerves on the efferent arteriole helps to maintain the glomerular capillary pressure, and hence the filtration function, should blood flow to the kidney be reduced during our daily activities, for example in moderate exercise.

Producing a high volume of filtrate requires a lot of blood. Together, the two kidneys receive 1200 mL of blood per minute in an adult, of which some 700 mL will be plasma, the remaining volume being occupied by blood cells. Thus in a young adult the kidneys filter out 125/700, or approximately 20%, of the plasma flowing through them. This is called the 'filtration fraction' and is a diagnostic factor that is occasionally used in renal assessment.

Why filter so much?

As noted earlier, the average rate of urine production in a temperate climate is about 60 mL per hour (approximately 1 mL/minute). If the kidneys filter at 125 mL/minute, then about 99.9% of the filtrate must be reabsorbed to promote this rate of urine production. Even when we are very hydrated and urine production is around 1200 mL/hour (= 20 mL/minute), over 85% of the filtrate volume will still have been reabsorbed. Such levels of reabsorptive activity are extremely expensive in terms of energy usage since water reabsorption occurs by osmosis linked to the active reabsorption of solutes. In fact, the kidneys account for about 10% of the body's resting oxygen consumption, yet represent only 0.4% of body weight. This helps to explain why the kidneys receive so much blood, but it appears very wasteful of energy.

There are, however, important advantages in having such a high rate of filtration. These are:

1 The rate of excretion of substances (e.g. creatinine from muscle cells) that are not secreted or reabsorbed to any degree is entirely dependent on the rate at which it is filtered from blood plasma. Looked at in another way, a low rate of filtration would mean that any novel substances produced by metabolism, or perhaps ingested in the diet, might not be excreted efficiently unless specific transport processes to secrete them into tubule fluid were present, which is unlikely to be the case.

2 A high rate of filtration allows a high degree of flexibility in the regulation of solute excretion, particularly of sodium, and of water. This is observed in ageing kidneys which continue to excrete adequately through changing the secretion/reabsorption activities of the tubule cells as the rate of filtration declines as we grow older (Box 15.6). However, there is a limit and the kidneys may eventually exhibit a reduction in their ability to concentrate the urine as the amount of solute filtered from plasma is now insufficient to maintain the concentrating processes within the kidney (these are described later).

BOX 15.5 GLOMERULONEPHRITIS

Glomerulonephritis is an inflammation of the glomeruli commonly caused by allergic responses to toxins, by drug abuse, by 'heavy' metal poisoning (e.g. mercury) or by renal infection that has spread to the kidneys from the lower urinary tract, or perhaps elsewhere (e.g. *Streptococcus* infection of the throat; Rodríguez-Iturbe and Batsford, 2007). There may also be a genetic component in some individuals. There are many kinds of glomerulonephritis according to which cell type within the glomerulus is affected. Symptoms include excessive urinary loss of blood cells and plasma proteins, called haematuria and proteinuria, respectively, as a consequence of increased glomerular permeability. The condition can be acute or chronic and can progress to renal failure; generally speaking, the longer the duration of the proteinuria, the greater the likelihood of permanent damage.

BOX 15.6 CHANGES IN GLOMERULAR FILTRATION RATE (GFR) WITH AGE AND DURING PREGNANCY

Although the GFR of a child or adult varies little on a moment to moment basis, it does alter with age and during pregnancy.

At birth
The rate of glomerular filtration at birth is about 20% or so of the adult value (i.e. approximately 20–30 mL/minute). It reaches the adult value within about 2 years, which gives an indication of how soon renal function must mature if body fluid balance is to be maintained.

Ageing
The rate of filtration declines from about the age of 30 years and typically may be reduced by as much as 50% or more by the time the individual is 80. In health, body fluid composition is still regulated by appropriate changes in reabsorption or secretion by the tubules, and urine composition will be normal. The excretion of creatinine and urea, which is entirely dependent upon the amount filtered, may show signs of mild retention, although their production by metabolism will also reduce with age and so changes in plasma concentration will not be sufficient to be problematic.

Pregnancy
The rate of blood flow through the maternal kidneys increases by up to 50% during pregnancy. The cause of this is uncertain but it produces a substantial increase in GFR and a subsequent fall in the blood concentration of those substances that are excreted in proportion to the filtration rate, such as creatinine and urea. The improved removal of these substances presumably facilitates their transfer from the fetus across the placenta. Potentially disastrous consequences for solute and water excretion are prevented by an increased rate of absorption of most solutes by the kidney tubules. This adaptive mechanism is poorly understood.

BOX 15.7 GLOMERULAR FILTRATION RATE (GFR) IN RENAL FAILURE

In some people, the rate of decline of filtration with age is faster than that described in Box 15.6. The consequence is that eventually a rate of filtration is reached when substance excretion is compromised and, consequently, body fluid composition cannot be regulated adequately. In this instance the individual will be diagnosed as having chronic renal failure. The consequences depend upon the extent to which the GFR is reduced:

- Plasma urea and creatinine concentrations are moderately raised when GFR is about 25% of normal. This is referred to as 'renal insufficiency'.
- 'Renal failure' occurs with further reductions in GFR and is characterized by even more retention of urea and creatinine, and of other solutes, especially ions. The individual may show symptoms of fatigue, anorexia, nausea and intense itching, and the syndrome of renal failure may be referred to as uraemia. Another term that is frequently used as an alternative to uraemia is azotaemia. Strictly speaking, this term relates specifically to an observation of an increased plasma urea concentration.
- 'End stage renal failure' is when GFR is less than 10% of normal.

The consequences of renal failure upon body fluid homeostasis are described in Box 15.17, p.440.

BOX 15.8 PRESENCE OF GLUCOSE IN URINE (GLYCOSURIA)

If the glucose-transporting sites in the proximal tubule are overloaded, then glucose begins to appear in quantities in the urine (referred to as glycosuria). Overload indicates that a threshold concentration for glucose has been exceeded, such that the normal transport processes in the renal tubule are saturated. Overload can occur in two ways:

- The amount of glucose being filtered by the glomerulus is excessive. This is observed in diabetes mellitus when the raised plasma glucose concentration results in more glucose being filtered (the term 'mellitus' refers to the sweetness of the urine and dates from days when physicians would taste urine to distinguish the disorder from others. Happily, testing by 'dip sticks' has removed this necessity).
- The number of transport sites in the proximal tubule is reduced. Glomerular filtration rate is increased during pregnancy but this should not produce a significant glycosuria since transport sites in the proximal tubule should be able to cope with this excess by simply absorbing more glucose. However, there is a decrease in the number of transport sites in pregnancy and this seems to be the main cause of glycosuria when it occurs. In this instance the glycosuria is not indicative of diabetes mellitus, although this should not necessarily be ruled out. The reduction of transport sites, therefore, represents a lowering of the renal threshold for glucose.

Proximal tubule

The filtrate enters the renal tubule from Bowman's capsule, into a segment called the proximal tubule. The term 'proximal' describes its position, being close to that centralized structure. The segment of tubule has a number of characteristics:

- For most of its length it lies within the renal cortex and is referred to as the 'proximal convoluted segment' (or 'pars convoluta'), but continues as a straight section, called the 'pars recta', which takes the proximal tubule toward the medulla region. The convolutions increase its length and, therefore, the surface area available for reabsorption and secretion of substances.
- The cells have surface finger-like microvilli on their inner surface, which increases the surface area still further.
- The tubule is 'leaky' to water, and its cells are rich in transport mechanisms, which makes the absorption of solutes and the resultant osmotic movement of water very prominent here.

Consequently, about 80% of the filtrate is reabsorbed by the time it reaches the end of the proximal tubule. Some solutes, such as glucose, amino acids and small proteins, are absorbed even more efficiently, almost completely, and so the final urine is virtually free of them (but see Box 15.8); this is important if these valuable nutrients are not to be wasted. Others, for example urea or creatinine may hardly be reabsorbed at all and largely remain in the tubule fluid despite its change in volume. Other waste solutes might be secreted into the tubule fluid by the proximal tubule cells, and this promotes their excretion in urine. In general terms, the overall solute content produces an osmotic potential that is similar to that of the plasma and filtrate. In other words, the production of dilute or very concentrated urine must relate to features beyond the proximal tubule.

In diabetes mellitus (Box 15.8), one consequence of the presence of glucose in the renal tubule is that it interferes with osmosis and hence water reabsorption. This is why glycosuria is usually associated with an increased urine production rate (the term 'diabetes' is Greek for 'siphon'). Glycosuria also provides a nutrient-rich environment for bacteria, and so raises the risk of lower urinary tract infection.

Loop of Henle

Fluid leaves the proximal tubule and enters the loop of Henle (see Figure 15.5), a hairpin-like structure that carries the remnants of the filtrate deeper into the medullary region of the kidney via its descending limb and back out into the cortex again via its ascending limb. The arrangement of the two limbs act as a 'countercurrent multiplier' in that the opposite direction of flow is instrumental in the final outcome:

- In penetrating the medulla, the tubules enter a region where the tissue fluid is very concentrated – more than any other tissue in the body. As the forming urine passes down the descending limb it loses water by osmosis and, as a consequence, becomes highly concentrated.
- On passing along the ascending limb, the high concentration of solutes, especially sodium ions, now stimulates their active transport out of the tubule (hence the concentrating of tissue fluid in this region). However, this part of the tubule is much less permeable to water, and so the fluid within it becomes more and more dilute; it is frequently called the 'diluting segment'.

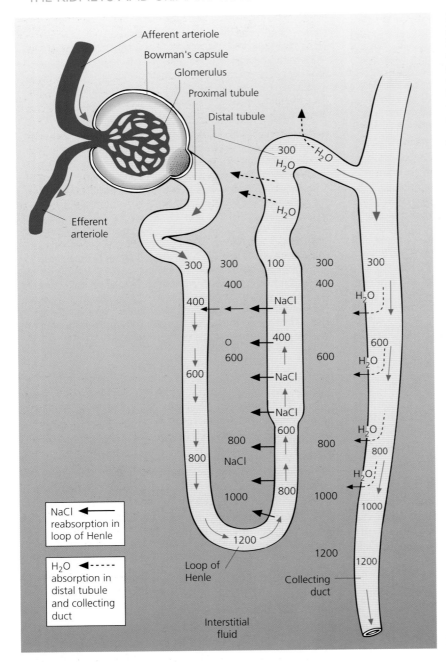

NaCl ◄────
reabsorption in
loop of Henle

H₂O ◄------
absorption in
distal tubule
and collecting
duct

Figure 15.7 The loop of Henle countercurrent multiplier mechanism in the production of a concentrated (i.e. hypertonic to plasma) urine. The numbers refer to osmotic concentration (blood plasma = 300). The arrows indicate the movement of solute (sodium chloride, NaCl; in the loop of Henle) and water (H_2O; in the distal convoluted tubule and collecting duct). The movement of water is along a concentration gradient for solute that is established between the tubule and interstitial fluid by the activities of the loop of Henle. See text for explanation. Note: the extent of reabsorption of water by the distal nephron depends on the presence of antidiuretic hormone. The fluid dilution seen as the fluid leaves the loop of Henle will continue if the hormone is absent, so that the urine will have a high volume but low concentration (i.e. the process becomes one of urine dilution, not concentration)

Q What is the role of antidiuretic hormone in water balance?

Thus, by the time fluid leaves the loop of Henle, the filtrate has become diluted (its osmotic potential is now considerably less than plasma, and the original filtrate), and lower in volume (about 85% of the filtrate has now been reabsorbed). The accumulation of solutes in the tissue fluid of the medulla is important for the role of later tubule segments.

Distal tubule

The now diluted fluid leaves the ascending limb of the loop of Henle and passes within the renal cortex into another convoluted section of tubule, which eventually joins with others to for 'collecting tubules'. The convoluted section of tubule, together with the collecting tubules, is referred to as the distal tubule. The dilution process instigated in the ascending limb of the loop of Henle continues along the distal tubule as solutes (again mainly sodium chloride) are reabsorbed in excess of water. Unlike the ascending limb, however, this is a section of tubule that has variable water permeability. If its permeability is increased, osmosis causes water to pass from the dilute tubule fluid into the cortex tissue thus concentrating what remains in the tubule; this is a site of action of antidiuretic hormone (ADH; see Figure 15.8).

Two other important processes that occur in the distal tubule are the secretion of potassium and hydrogen ions. Fluid entering the distal tubule is virtually potassium- and hydrogen-free as almost all that is filtered from plasma by the glomerulus is reabsorbed by earlier segments. Their secretion into the distal tubule is loosely in exchange for sodium ions, and is a determinant of potassium excretion and of urinary acidification.

Collecting duct

A number of collecting tubules drain within the renal cortex into a common collecting duct which descends back into the renal medulla (Figure 15.7). Solute and water reabsorption continues in this segment of tubule but the main feature is that the water permeability of the tubule wall is variable and can be controlled. Thus, promotion of water reabsorption in the distal tubule by ADH continues in the collecting ducts, but here the fluid volume can be very reduced and it is the main site where the kidney switches from producing a dilute urine to a concentrated one. Thus:

- If water permeability of the collecting ducts is low then the dilution of tubule fluid that was first initiated in the ascending limb of the loop of Henle, and which was also observed in the distal tubule, continues. The result is a dilute, almost colourless urine of relatively high volume.
- If water permeability of the collecting ducts is high then the high concentration of solute within the tissue fluid in the kidney medulla (generated by the active reabsorption occurring in the ascending limb of the loop of Henle; Figure 15.7) will promote osmosis, and hence the reabsorption of water. The result is a concentrated, deeply coloured urine in low volume.

The fluid that leaves the collecting ducts is now 'urine', and it passes into the renal pelvis, from which it drains into the ureter.

The ureters

The ureter is the muscular tube, about 25 cm long and 0.5 cm in diameter and mainly composed of smooth muscle, that connects the kidney to the urinary bladder. Urine passes along the

---

BOX 15.9 THE URINARY TRACT IN PREGNANCY

There are two main aspects here: the influence of progesterone and the compression from the growing uterus.

- *Progesterone*: the release of this hormone is greatly increased during pregnancy. One of its varied actions is relaxation of smooth muscle. In the urinary tract this results in dilation of the renal calyces, pelvises and ureters. There is a risk that peristalsis in the ureters will be less effective in transferring urine to the bladder and so retention within the kidney pelvis may occur. Accordingly, routine analysis of urine at antenatal visits will include tests for infection.
- *Compression*: the enlarged uterus presses down upon the urinary bladder reducing its capacity. Bladder tension therefore rises much more rapidly during filling, leading to increased urinary frequency.

---

ureters partly assisted by gravity and partly through peristaltic contractions.

THE KIDNEYS AND HOMEOSTATIC CONTROL OF BODY FLUID COMPOSITION AND VOLUME

Clearance

'Clearance' is a term used with reference to the extent to which the liver and/or kidneys remove a substance from blood plasma. The higher the clearance value, the more effectively has the substance been removed. Removal could be expressed in an amount per minute, but this does not tell us anything about the impact that might have on the remaining concentration in blood since we would have to know how much was being produced/added in the first place. It is more useful to express clearance as a volume of blood cleared over time. Obviously, we do not find discrete volumes of blood that have been completely cleared, while others still contain the substance, but it helps to envisage the reduction in concentration of the substance as being indicative of a volume.

'Renal clearance' can be defined as being the volume of plasma that contains the amount of a substance that is excreted

---

BOX 15.10 DIURETIC DRUGS

These drugs promote diuresis and are colloquially known as 'water tablets'.

- *Osmotic diuretics* (e.g. mannitol) interfere with the uptake of water by osmosis in the proximal tubule. They are not reabsorbed themselves and so remain in the tubule fluid, hence their effects.
- *Loop diuretics* (e.g. furosemide) are the most effective. These drugs inhibit the transport mechanism in the ascending limb of the loop of Henle and in doing so prevent the build-up of electrolytes within the surrounding tissue fluid. As a consequence the reabsorption of water by the distal nephron and collecting tubules/ducts is disrupted and large volumes of urine are produced. Electrolyte excretion will also be high, and this particularly relates to sodium chloride. Thus, loop diuretics are effective means of reducing the sodium and water content of extracellular fluid, hence their use to reduce blood volume in, for example, congestive heart failure or salt-induced hypertension. The

secretion of potassium ions by cells of the distal tubule occurs loosely in exchange for sodium ions, and is therefore promoted when sodium reabsorption is increased in this part of the tubule. The delivery of sodium to the distal nephron is increased when loop diuretics are used to reduce salt reabsorption in the loop of Henle, and stimulates sodium reabsorption and hence potassium excretion in the distal tubule. The loss of potassium ions can be such that it causes a reduction in plasma potassium concentration (hypokalaemia) and so dietary potassium supplements may be necessary in those people who take loop diuretics.

- *Distal nephron diuretics*. Thiazide diuretics act mainly on the distal tubule by reducing sodium chloride and water reabsorption there. These drugs are less effective than loop diuretics but, because they act very late in the distal nephron, do not have a major influence on potassium secretion. They are often referred to as 'potassium sparing' diuretics.

in urine per unit time. It is calculated from the timed urine volume, the urinary concentration (conc.) of the substance and its concentration in blood plasma, using the equation:

Equation 1:

Clearance of a substance (in mL/minute) =

$$\frac{\text{(Urine conc. of the substance)}}{\text{(Plasma conc. of the substance)}} \times \frac{\text{(Urine volume (mL))}}{\text{Time (minutes)}}$$

For example, let:

urine concentration of sodium	= 1.4 mmoles/mL
plasma concentration of sodium	= 0.14 mmoles/mL
urine production rate	= 1 mL/minute
Then the sodium clearance is	$\frac{1.4}{0.14} \times \frac{1}{1} = 10$ mL/minute

In other words, the rate of excretion over that period of time would remove all of the sodium from 10 mL of plasma every minute (but the kidneys receive around 700 mL of plasma per minute so this would only represent a small overall reduction in content).

Clearance values can be determined for any substance that is found in urine. For example, the method is widely applied in pharmacology to determine how efficiently a drug is removed from plasma after it has been administered, since dosages of a drug are calculated according to how long it remains at effective concentrations in blood. Thus, if its clearance rates are low then the drug may remain effective for a long period of time and so lower or more infrequent doses could be required. The pharmacologist will of course also need to know how much is removed from plasma by other routes, for example by liver clearance, but renal clearance will be an important part of the calculation.

Maintaining homeostasis

For homeostasis of body fluid composition and volume, the clearance of substances and excretion of water must be equal to the rate at which they are added to the fluids. The text so far has at times mentioned that some substances, such as urea and creatinine, are handled by the renal tubules in a different way from those such as electrolytes. In considering how balance is maintained, it is therefore convenient to consider different categories of substances separately.

Metabolic products: urea, creatinine and organic acids

The excretion of some products of metabolism, such as creatinine and urea, is largely determined by how much is filtered from the plasma, and less so by how much is reabsorbed or secreted by the tubules. The rate at which the kidneys filter is normally constant, which would suggest that the concentra-

---

BOX 15.11 USE OF RENAL CLEARANCE TO CALCULATE THE GLOMERULAR FILTRATION RATE

The filtration of plasma by glomeruli is fundamental to urine production and any clinical assessment of kidney function would be limited without knowledge of how well the kidneys were filtering. Fortunately, calculating the clearance of certain substances provides an opportunity to indirectly evaluate the rate of filtration. It involves determining the clearance of a substance that is freely filtered by the kidneys, but which is neither reabsorbed nor secreted by the renal tubule (i.e. all that is filtered actually appears in the urine). Creatinine, a waste product of creatine metabolism in muscles, is one such substance and its use to calculate glomerular filtration rate is illustrated as follows.

1 Since none of the creatinine is reabsorbed by the tubules:

Amount of creatinine filtered from plasma per minute = Amount of creatinine excreted in urine per minute

2 The amount filtered, or excreted, per minute is calculated as concentration × volume/minute (vol./min), so the equation above could also be written as:

(Plasma conc. of creatinine) × (vol. of glomerular filtrate/minute) = (Urine conc. of creatinine) × (Urine vol./minute)

3 Rearranging this equation gives:

Vol. of glomerular filtrate/minute =

$$\frac{\text{Urine conc. of creatinine}}{\text{Plasma conc. of creatinine}} \times \text{Urine vol./minute}$$

This is a form of the clearance equation given in the text, and, strictly speaking, measures the clearance rate of creatinine, which is then taken to equate with the glomerular filtration rate. The concentration of creatinine in a urine sample and plasma sample is easily measured, and the volume of urine formed per minute readily calculated from noting the time interval between emptyings of the bladder and dividing the total urine volume by the time in minutes. Thus, the glomerular filtration rate can be calculated without too much difficulty using a simple blood sample and a timed urine collection.

There has been suggestion that creatinine is not always a good 'marker' for calculating the glomerular filtration rate because at times it is actually reabsorbed to a slight degree. Other substances therefore have been used clinically to monitor the glomerular filtration rate, but they have to be administered intravenously. Inulin and ethylenediaminetetraacetic acid (EDTA) are examples of such substances. However, collecting urine normally requires a lengthy collection period, and this is highly inconvenient for patients who, for example, attend an outpatient clinic.

A less accurate way of assessing glomerular function over periods of time, but without the need for a urine sample, is simply to monitor any changes in plasma creatinine concentration. Unless someone exercises a lot, the addition of creatinine to plasma (from muscle metabolism) occurs at a fairly constant rate, and so any change in the plasma concentration over time will reflect a change in its renal clearance, and hence in the glomerular filtration rate. An actual clearance value cannot be calculated in the absence of a urine sample but if plasma creatinine concentration is measured on different occasions, any trend in changes will indicate a declining filtration rate; in this way the effect of age or chronic renal failure on glomerular filtration can be monitored.

tions of these substances in body fluids could fluctuate depending upon how much is being produced by the tissues. In practice this is generally not a major problem because any increase in their plasma concentration will simply result in more being filtered, since the amount filtered is determined by the kidneys' filtration rate and the concentration of the substance in plasma. Thus, the concentrations of these substances in extracellular fluid do not change dramatically in health unless their production is markedly increased. The process is limited, however, and regulation is not as precise as for those substances that are reabsorbed or secreted to varying degrees by the renal tubules. As a consequence changes in plasma creatinine and urea concentrations are among the first consequences of the decline in renal function that is observed with age, and likewise in kidney failure (see Box 15.17, p.440).

Urea and creatinine appear to have relatively low toxicity and only become a problem to tissues in renal failure when their concentration is excessive. Some metabolic products, known as organic acids, must be excreted much more efficiently because of the effect that acidity has on cell functions. These substances are secreted into tubule fluid, and seem to be regulated simply by the effect that a change in their concentration in blood plasma has on those transport processes. Thus an increased concentration stimulates directly the secretion of organic acid by the cells of the proximal tubule. The transport processes are sensitive and efficient, and so wide fluctuations of organic acid concentration in the extracellular fluid are prevented.

Regulation of water homeostasis and body fluid osmotic pressure

Osmotic movement of water across cell membranes ensures that the overall solute concentration (i.e. osmotic pressure; see Chapter 2, p.29) of intracellular and extracellular fluids remains in equilibrium. To maintain a constant cell volume and intracellular composition it is therefore essential that changes in the osmotic pressure of extracellular fluid are detected, so as to promote a rapid change in renal water excretion in order to restore water balance before the cells are severely compromised. The regulation of water balance is not, however, simply a question of increasing or decreasing urine volume. For example:

- Over-hydration increases extracellular fluid volume but it also dilutes it; over-hydration therefore will be more rapidly corrected by the excretion of a large volume of urine that is more dilute than plasma (i.e. by excreting water more efficiently than solutes).
- Similarly, the effects of dehydration, when plasma becomes more concentrated than normal, will be better corrected by excretion of a small volume of highly concentrated urine (i.e. by excreting solutes more efficiently than water).

The filtrate produced by the glomeruli in the first process towards forming urine has the same osmotic pressure (or potential) as the plasma from which it is derived. If urine with very different osmotic pressure is to be produced then the renal tubule must be able to separate solute and water excretion at some point along its length. As noted earlier, it is the loop of Henle and distal tubule that do this by diluting the tubule fluid, while the collecting duct has variable water permeability. It is these segments that enable us to produce urine across the range of volumes and concentrations, and hence either conserve water or excrete its excess.

Conserving water in dehydration

Dehydration raises the overall concentration (osmotic pressure) of body fluids, and this is detected by 'osmoreceptors' in the hypothalamus of the brain. These receptors are actually modified nerve cells that release ADH from their terminals within the pituitary gland (see Figure 9.5, p.214). ADH causes the collecting ducts to become more permeable to water. Recall that at this point the renal tubule contains fluid that has been considerably diluted by the actions of the ascending limb of the loop of Henle, and by the distal tubule, and that the collecting ducts run through the renal medulla where the reabsorbed solutes have collected in a high concentration. By increasing the water permeability of the collecting ducts, ADH therefore promotes the rapid uptake of water by osmosis into the renal medulla, reducing the tubule fluid volume and raising its osmotic concentration to that of the medulla. In extreme dehydration states this process may reduce urine production to just 30 mL/hour (approximately 700 mL/day), and substantially raise its concentration; osmotic 'potential' is measured in terms of osmolality (in milliosmoles (mOsm)/L; see Appendix A) and, whereas that of plasma is about 285 mOsm/L, a highly concentrated urine might be 1400 mOsm/L, about five times that of the plasma (and glomerular filtrate). In this way, solutes are being excreted more efficiently than water and so body fluid concentration will begin to decrease towards normal.

One additional component that enhances this urinary concentrating mechanism is the role of urea. When the kidneys are producing a highly concentrated urine, water reabsorption out of the collecting ducts causes a considerable increase in the concentration of urea in the tubule fluid. Urea can diffuse across the lipid membranes of the tubule cells and so its diffusion into the medulla is therefore enhanced, which adds to the solute content of the tissue fluid there and so promotes further osmotic movement of water. Urea is a product of protein metabolism, and it has been known for many years that people on a low protein intake have a reduced urinary concentrating ability.

Excreting excess water in over-hydration

The over-hydrated state dilutes body fluids and so the activity of osmoreceptors is reduced. Consequently the release of ADH decreases and the collecting ducts remain poorly permeable to water. The processes that had diluted renal tubular fluid before it reached the collecting ducts therefore enables a high-volume/low-concentration urine to be produced. Urine production can be very high, as high as 1.2 L/hour (equivalent to nearly 30 L/day, though it is unlikely that such a rate can be sustained that long). Its osmolality may be as low as 50 mOsm/L, around one-sixth that of plasma (and glomerular

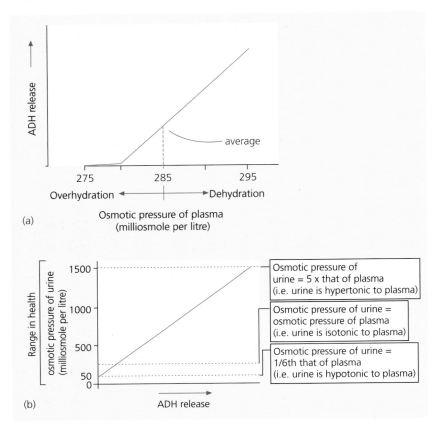

(a)

(b)

Figure 15.8 Antidiuretic hormone (ADH) and water conservation by the kidneys. Note the narrowness of the range of values for osmotic pressure of blood plasma (a) and the capacity of the kidneys to produce a very dilute or very concentrated urine, relative to plasma, according to the absence or presence of ADH (b)

Q Why do the responses have to be sensitive?

Q Why is the production of hypertonic urine when we are dehydrated so important?

filtrate). Thus, water is excreted in excess of solutes and so the concentration of body fluids begins to increase towards normal.

The mechanism of ADH release is very sensitive (Figure 15.8) but it is important to note that our need to excrete urea and electrolytes means that we must produce some urine in which these solutes are dissolved, even if we are dehydrated. Zero urine production is not an option in health. Provided that water is available to drink, the osmoreceptor–ADH–renal mechanism ensures that our water balance is maintained within the limits of ±2% of the homeostatic set point. The response is relatively quick. For example, drinking a litre of water when we are already adequately hydrated results in excretion of the excess within just 1–2 hours.

Fluid balance (homeostasis) charts

Fluid balance charts are frequently produced in clinical areas as the means of monitoring a patient's state of water homeostasis, which is influenced by water gain and also by water lost via urine and other routes. Determination of the hydration status of an individual must take these other aspects into account. A daily water balance chart for an adult in a temperate climate such as that in the UK might look like the following:

BOX 15.12 EFFECTS OF DISORDERS OF ANTIDIURETIC HORMONE (ADH) RELEASE/ACTIVITY ON KIDNEY FUNCTION

The release and action of ADH is central to the conservation of body water, and this is illustrated further by the effects of some (unusual) conditions:

The condition called syndrome of inappropriate ADH release (SIADH) induces overhydration because too much ADH is secreted relative to the state of hydration. Most commonly this is the consequence of an ADH-secreting tumour, either within the pituitary gland or more commonly at a site somewhere else within the body (referred to as 'ectopic' production of the hormone). Tumours do not exhibit the normal feedback controls on hormone release: in this instance ADH will continue to be produced even if the individual is well hydrated. The condition therefore induces a sustained dilution of body fluids, referred to as hyponatraemia (low blood sodium concentration), and cell swelling as a consequence of uptake of water through osmosis. Water intake therefore must be moderated under these circumstances.

In contrast a condition referred to as diabetes insipidus (literally translated as a 'siphoning of tasteless urine') is characterized either by a failure to release ADH or, more usually, as a failure of the kidney to respond to the hormone as a consequence of a lack of ADH receptors on collecting duct cells. In this condition, the individual will continue to produce large volumes of dilute urine, even when dehydrated, and will have a persistent thirst.

Water input (mL/day)		Water output (mL/day)	
Drink	1500	Urine	1400
Food	800	Evaporation:	
		Lungs	500
		Skin	400
Metabolic production*	200	Faeces	200
Total	**2500**		**2500**

*Mainly water produced when glucose is broken down to carbon dioxide and water during respiration.

In this illustration, most water loss is via the urine, but loss through sweat can be a very significant route during hot weather when this balance chart might look quite different. Water lost via sweat, and respiration, is termed 'insensible' loss because the volume is largely unaffected by our state of hydration (i.e. the loss does not 'make sense' when we are trying to conserve water); urinary losses, and to an extent faecal losses, are 'sensible' because they do relate to water balance.

Assessment of insensible losses, and of the volume generated by metabolism, will clearly be difficult, if not impossible, in a ward or home environment. A quick look at the balance table, however, shows that water drunk is the major component of water intake, while most water lost from the body is in urine. The role of thirst is often underplayed in biological terms, but it is actually a major part of water homeostasis and its onset should be taken seriously in patients, especially those who are particularly susceptible (Box 15.13). A reasonable estimate of fluid balance can therefore be obtained using measures of water intake and urine output, together with an estimate of insensible loss; this is the basis of ward assessment of hydration state.

Regulation of sodium homeostasis (and hence extracellular fluid volume)

The information in Table 15.1 identifies that, protein apart, blood plasma is basically a solution of sodium chloride with comparatively smaller amounts of other electrolytes and various organic substances added. This means that sodium and chloride ions are the main contributors to the osmotic potential of plasma, and of the extracellular fluid generally.

Sodium chloride is also a major salt in our foods. It is almost entirely absorbed by the small intestine and distributes throughout the extracellular fluid but is prevented from accumulating in cells by the cell membrane Na^+/K^+ exchange pump (see Chapter 2, p.30). Any increase in sodium chloride concentrations in the extracellular fluid will be detected by the osmoreceptors, referred to in relation to water balance (above), which respond if there is an increase in osmotic pressure (of plasma). This will quickly be corrected by promoting a change in water balance by the mechanism described in the previous section, that is through the release of ADH and feelings of thirst.

Consequently, any increase in sodium chloride content of extracellular fluid will promote water conservation, but the process has not been initiated by dehydration, rather it is

BOX 15.13 FLUID HOMEOSTASIS IN INFANTS AND ELDERLY PEOPLE

Box 6.1 (p.121) highlighted that infants are more susceptible to fluid imbalance partly because they have a relatively higher turnover of extracellular fluid, and because their regulatory processes are immature. The latter makes it difficult for babies to maintain fluid homeostasis if their fluid intake is inadequate, making babies more prone to dehydration. Elderly people too have a problem in maintaining fluid balance, but this time it is because ageing diminishes the production, release and actions of hormones (including antidiuretic hormone), and because dietary habits may be inadequate: dehydration therefore predominates.

BOX 15.14 EFFECTS OF SURGERY ON FLUID HOMEOSTASIS

'Nil-by-mouth' procedures will often mean that an individual is dehydrated before going into surgery (Brady *et al.*, 2007) but surgery also makes additional excretory routes significant, for example fluid loss by dehydration from internal tissues during the operative procedure, blood loss, or fluid lost through drains. Evaporative loss may also be high in the postsurgery period if the patient breathes heavily because they are in pain, or distressed or anxious. Diarrhoea, vomiting or the presence of renal complications (e.g. acute renal failure) further complicate the picture. The fluid gains that come from infusions must reflect the loss of fluid but much of the fluid loss is difficult to assess, or even estimate, and vigilance will be necessary to ensure that the infusion rate used is appropriate (see Clancy *et al.*, 2002).

caused by excessive sodium chloride. The consequence is an increase in extracellular fluid volume beyond normal. If the kidneys respond to the increased fluid volume by simply increasing water excretion, this will only cause the concentration of sodium chloride (and the osmotic pressure) of the extracellular fluid to increase again, and so once more promote water conservation. Clearly, in sodium chloride excess the sodium chloride and water must be excreted together.

Excretion of excess sodium chloride (and water)

The increase in extracellular fluid volume that occurs with sodium chloride excess is monitored, and helps provide the means of controlling sodium chloride balance. More precisely, the blood component of the extracellular fluid compartment is monitored, by receptors associated with the circulatory system. The location of all of these receptors is still debatable, though some have been found in the atria of the heart, and in the kidneys.

An increased blood volume promotes the urinary excretion of sodium chloride (and water) through the actions of hormones (Figure 15.9). Two hormones that have been implicated in the response are:

- A decreased release of aldosterone (a steroid from the adrenal gland). This hormone normally acts on the distal tubule to promote sodium chloride reabsorption, so reducing its release will increase the amount of sodium chloride in the urine. The change in hormone release is mediated by

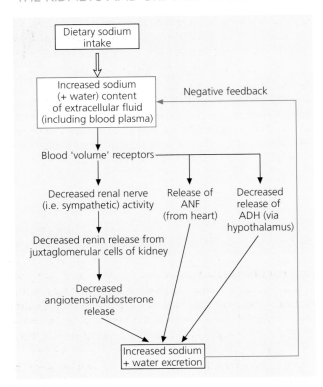

Figure 15.9 Endocrine responses to an elevated blood volume, resulting in increased sodium and water excretion. ANF, atrial natriuretic factor; ADH, antidiuretic hormone

Q How might excess sodium chloride in extracellular fluid contribute to an increased blood pressure?

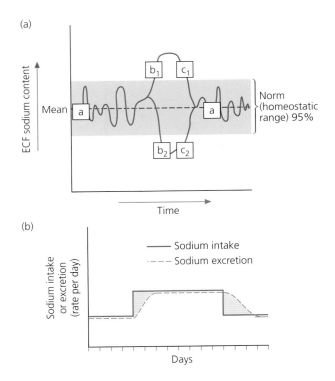

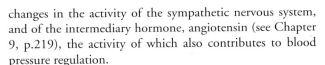

Figure 15.10 (a) The homeostatic regulation of sodium balance. a, Homeostatic range for sodium content (and volume) of extracellular fluid (ECF). b_1, Increased ECF sodium content resulting from dietary intake being in excess of excretion rate. b_2, Decreased ECF sodium content resulting from excretion rate being in excess of dietary intake. c_1, c_2, Restoration of ECF sodium content (and volume) to homeostatic norm by appropriate changes in sodium intake and sodium (and water) excretion (see Figure 15.9). (b) The delayed homeostatic response to changes in sodium intake. The delay in producing a new balance state can be seen to increase body fluid sodium content (shaded area) and volume, which increases blood volume. (a, Represents boxes a_1–a_4 in Figure 1.7, p.11, reflecting the individual variability in the homeostatic range)

changes in the activity of the sympathetic nervous system, and of the intermediary hormone, angiotensin (see Chapter 9, p.219), the activity of which also contributes to blood pressure regulation.

- A release of atrial natriuretic factor (ANF, a hormone from the cardiac atria; natriuretic = sodium-excreting). This acts by inhibiting sodium reabsorption by the collecting tubules and ducts, and its release is increased when blood volume in the heart is increased.

In addition, the decrease in sympathetic nervous activity that occurs when blood volume is expanded (necessary to prevent an increased arterial blood pressure) also reduces renal reabsorption of sodium chloride and water. The control of sodium balance is therefore multifactorial.

The renal responses to blood volume changes are relatively slow. Figure 15.10 illustrates what happens when someone is placed on a higher dietary sodium intake. The renal excretion of sodium increases gradually over a period of days during which time sodium will have accumulated (with water) in the extracellular fluid. The delay in response means that a change in sodium

balance does not produce complete correction – individuals on a high sodium intake will have a higher extracellular fluid volume (and therefore blood volume) than those on a low sodium intake. This is why there is a link between dietary sodium intake and high blood pressure (Box 15.15; see also Box 12.25, p.350).

Conserving sodium chloride (and hence water)

If the sodium chloride concentration of extracellular fluid decreases, it reduces the osmotic pressure of the fluid and this is detected by osmoreceptors and interpreted as overhydration: water is excreted, and fluid volume reduced, through inhibition of the release of ADH. The responses to a reduced sodium chloride content of extracellular fluid, and the resultant reduction in fluid volume, are largely opposite from those that promote sodium chloride excretion in excess (i.e. a stimulation of aldosterone release, and a reduction in ANF release, leading to reduced excretion of sodium chloride in urine). However, we also have a salt 'drive' when our blood volume is reduced, mediated by receptors in the hypothalamus. For example, we will tend to choose salty foods, or put more salt than usual in cooking. The presence of this 'drive' possibly reflects the

BOX 15.15 AGEING AND SODIUM BALANCE

The link between sodium chloride balance and the volume of extracellular fluid has important health implications (Chrysant, 2000). Ageing is frequently associated with an inability of the kidneys to respond adequately to hormones, or perhaps hormone secretion is diminished. Either way, the high average sodium chloride intake of people in the UK increases the risk of expanding the extracellular fluid to the extent that blood volume is sufficiently increased to cause high blood pressure (referred to as salt-induced hypertension). The common occurrence of this problem is such that there is a health education recommendation that people moderate their salt intake. General practitioners will often put people with hypertension onto diuretic therapy to increase the excretion of sodium chloride. There are other causes of hypertension but quite often this therapy will be effective.

importance of maintaining an adequate blood volume since a profound reduction in this has consequences for blood pressure control. Ordinarily, though, slight reductions in blood volume have little effect on arterial blood pressure because of the various other mechanisms that intervene to maintain blood pressure homeostasis (see Chapter 12).

Sodium balance (homeostasis) chart

In assessing sodium chloride homeostasis for clinical purposes, it is important to be aware that urine is just one route for the excretion of electrolytes, and so other routes must be taken into account. An adult's typical (UK climate) daily balance chart for sodium would look like this:

Sodium input (mmol/day)		Sodium output (mmol/day)	
Food*	200	Urine	180
		Faeces + sweat	20
Total	**200** (= approx. 9 g/day)		**200**

(Note: individual values will vary with diet.)

Urine losses of sodium predominate, and so closely relate to the sodium intake; together they provide a reasonable means of monitoring sodium balance. Note though that other routes assume greater significance if someone has diarrhoea, or if sweating rates are very high.

The sodium contents of foods can be altered if there are difficulties in excreting sodium, for example in renal failure. In contrast, saline infusions, for example after surgery, can replace or supplement dietary intake and sodium balance charts will need to take into account this new intake rate.

Regulating potassium homeostasis

The concentration gradient of potassium ions across cell membranes is the main determinant of the 'resting electrical potential' of the membrane (see Chapter 8, p.186). In nerve and muscle cells the capacity to change the electrical potential is important because it provides the means of generating the electrical currents necessary to produce the nerve impulse, and to induce muscle contraction. It is therefore essential that the resting potential (and hence potassium concentration) is maintained since any fluctuations could have dramatic effects on the sensitivity of these cell membranes to stimulation. In particular, short-term fluctuations must be avoided since the limited compensation that cells can make take some time to occur. Potassium ion concentration of blood plasma is monitored very closely, and renal responses to changes are very rapid (see section on secretion earlier), and can be extensive if necessary, and the potassium concentration is closely regulated around just 4 mmol/L (compared with 140 mmol/L for sodium).

Excretion of excess potassium

Any increase in potassium ion concentration of blood plasma is detected by receptors in the adrenal cortex, which cause the release of the hormone aldosterone. This appears to be the only

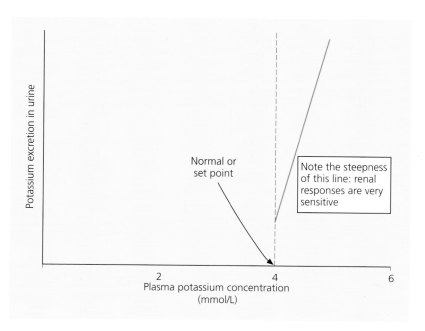

Figure 15.11 Potassium balance. The sensitivity of renal responses (and hence the narrowness of the homeostatic range) to changes in plasma potassium concentration is shown

Q *Why is it important that blood potassium concentration has a narrow homeostatic range?*

BOX 15.16 DISORDERS OF POTASSIUM REGULATION

Potassium is very abundant in foods and so disorders of potassium homeostasis are unlikely to arise from problems in obtaining it. However, inappropriate changes in renal function can induce changes in plasma potassium concentration:

- 'Loop' diuretics such as furosemide reduce sodium reabsorption in the loop of Henle and then increased delivery of sodium to the distal tubule acts to promote sodium reabsorption here, and hence potassium secretion and excretion. The rate of potassium excretion when diuretic use is high can induce hypokalaemia. Potassium supplements may be necessary to raise the intake of the electrolyte and so compensate for the losses.
- Similarly, hyperaldosteronism will also induce excessive potassium excretion. This is a condition in which the adrenal glands secrete too much of the hormone aldosterone. It can be primary (sometimes called Conn's disease), usually owing to the presence of an aldosterone-producing tumour within the gland, or secondary, as a consequence of

excessive hormones that stimulate the gland, for example angiotensin. Both forms of the disease cause a decreased plasma potassium concentration because of the actions of the excess hormone to promote potassium secretion by the distal tubule cells. Although the hormone also promotes sodium reabsorption, the occurrence of oedema as a consequence of sodium retention is unusual because the kidneys exhibit an 'escape' mechanism and compensate, and so can maintain a reasonable sodium balance. This contrast between the effects on potassium and sodium balance illustrates the multifactorial control of sodium but the unifactorial control of potassium. In secondary hyperaldosteronism caused by excessive angiotensin, hypertension may also be observed because of the actions of that hormone.

- Renal failure will prevent the normal excretion of potassium (and other ions) leading to potassium retention and hyperkalaemia ('hyper-' = greater than normal). Dietary restriction of the ion will be necessary in this instance.

---

hormone that is involved in the regulation of potassium balance. It was mentioned earlier in relation to sodium balance, and acts by stimulating sodium reabsorption by the distal tubule, but in doing so it also promotes the secretion of potassium ions into the tubule fluid. Involving secretion makes the excretory response very rapid and quickly effective (Figure 15.11), even to the extent of excreting potassium in quantities greater than those filtered from plasma in the initial stages of urine formation.

Conserving potassium

Potassium conservation follows the opposite response to that for its excretion. Thus, if potassium concentration of plasma decreases, the release of aldosterone is reduced. Sodium reabsorption by the distal tubule is therefore also reduced, leading to decreased potassium secretion into the tubule fluid (recall that most potassium in the glomerular filtrate will have been reabsorbed before the distal tubule). The impact on sodium excretion is not detrimental because sodium regulation involves other mechanisms, as outlined above.

Potassium balance (homeostasis) charts can be constructed along similar lines to those for sodium.

Regulating calcium balance

Calcium ion concentration in extracellular fluid determines the 'threshold' electrical potential at which nerve and muscle cell membranes are stimulated (see Chapter 8, p.187). About 50% of the calcium found in blood plasma is reversibly bound to plasma proteins but this component will not be physiologically active; it is the concentration (about 1.2 mmol/L) of the 50% that is free that must be closely regulated.

Unlike sodium, potassium and chloride ions, which are almost entirely absorbed from our foods and are not stored by the body, the calcium stores (as bone) are very large and only some 50% of our dietary calcium may be absorbed. The movement of calcium in and out of bone is controlled by the hor-

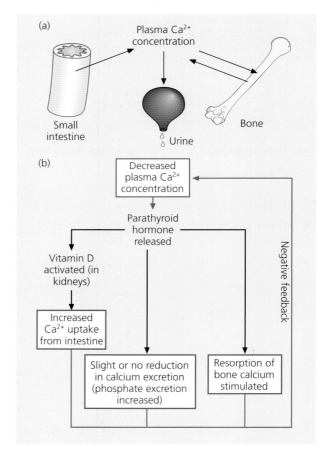

Figure 15.12 Calcium homeostasis. (a) Unabsorbed calcium in the gut and bone calcium provide a 'reservoir' that can be drawn upon if required. Note that plasma calcium concentration takes priority over bone calcium content. (b) Role of parathyroid hormone. Note that if Ca^{2+} concentration is elevated, this decreases parathyroid hormone release and so stimulates calcitonin release. Responses are therefore reversed and act to decrease calcium concentration

Q Which gland releases calcitonin?

mones (thyro-) calcitonin and parathyroid hormone, respectively, produced by the parathyroid glands.

Conserving calcium

Parathyroid hormone is released when plasma calcium ion concentration decreases, and acts to promote the release of calcium from bone (Figure 15.12). In doing so the hormone also releases phosphate ions from bone mineral. Parathyroid hormone also indirectly increases the uptake of calcium from the intestines by promoting the conversion (in the kidneys and liver) of inactive vitamin D to the active form. This is the main role of the kidney in calcium conservation since calcium excretion in urine normally is already very low, and is little changed in this process. However, phosphate excretion does increase, through the effects of parathyroid hormone to inhibit phosphate reabsorption by the proximal tubule of the kidney.

Excreting excess calcium

Calcitonin is released when plasma calcium ion concentration is increased above normal. Its main action is to promote calcium uptake into bone (for example it is used in this way in the treatment of osteitis deformans, or Paget disease), an action made more efficient because it also opposes the actions of parathyroid hormone. Calcium excretion in the urine is also increased but this is not considered the hormone's main role.

Note that changes in renal calcium excretion have only a relatively small role in the regulation of plasma calcium ion concentration; modulating uptake from the intestines and the deposition/resorption of calcium for bone are more significant processes. Dietary intake of calcium can be monitored but without knowing how much is being absorbed by the intestine, and how much is going into bone, it is difficult to construct useful balance charts.

Regulating acid–base homeostasis

Hydrogen ions are produced continually through metabolism, either directly (from protein) or indirectly (from carbon dioxide). The need to regulate body fluid pH (i.e. hydrogen ion concentration) was detailed in Chapter 6, p.128), which described how regulation is achieved by buffer chemicals that help to prevent local fluctuation in acidity within the tissues, and by hydrogen ion excretion in urine, and carbon dioxide excretion via the lungs. The main buffer chemical in plasma is bicarbonate ions, and the kidneys have a role in regulating the concentration of these ions in plasma. The regulatory process has sufficient sensitivity to ensure that moment-to-moment changes in metabolic rate produce only slight, perhaps undetectable, changes in the extracellular pH. The acidity changes become more pronounced if there is an excessive change in acid production, for example during exercise when lactic acid from muscle cells adds to the acid 'load' but even then changes are not large.

Excreting excess hydrogen ions/retaining bicarbonate ions

The regulation of pH seems largely to be governed by neural control of lung function, and by intrinsic processes within the kidneys: hormones do not appear to be specifically involved. If hydrogen ion concentration of plasma rises this stimulates the peripheral chemoreceptors and lung ventilation is increased (see Chapter 6, p.132); more carbon dioxide is exhaled than usual and this reduces the acid load produced from this source.

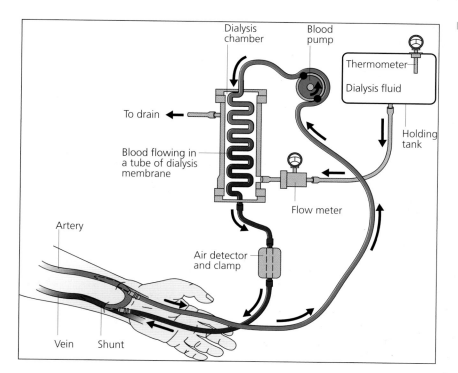

Figure 15.13 Haemodialysis (see also Box 15.18).

BOX 15.17 BODY FLUID COMPOSITION IN ACUTE RENAL FAILURE

A number of instances have been noted in this chapter in which kidney function changes that are secondary to altered function elsewhere, for example hormonal disorder, promote ill health. In such instances the removal of the primary cause should correct the altered renal function. How renal function itself relates to body fluid composition is most clearly illustrated by the consequences of acute renal failure (ARF).

ARF is linked to a number of risk factors, especially postoperatively (Kheterpal *et al.*, 2007). It is frequently observed if the kidneys have received poor supplies of blood in some lengthy surgical procedures or following severe haemorrhage. If it is caused by poor blood supply then it is referred to as having a pre-renal cause. Often the acute failure is associated with a breakdown of kidney tubule organization and function, referred to as acute tubular necrosis (ATN). The cause may be linked to the poor perfusion with blood, but sometimes the ATN arises without a pre-renal cause, for example because of sepsis or toxic chemicals. For this reason, there has been suggestion that ARF should be redefined to acute kidney injury (i.e. pre-renal cause) and acute tubular apoptosis (post-renal) (Kellum, 2008).

ARF is a condition characterized by a sudden, rapid deterioration in renal function:

* *Oliguria is observed (i.e. less than 30 mL urine/hour or less than 400 mL in 24 hours)*: the lower limit for 'normal' function relates to the ability of kidneys to conserve water when we are dehydrated. Thus urine production in ARF may be very low, but the urine will not be as concentrated as would be anticipated had the patient been very dehydrated. The patient's appearance would also not indicate dehydration of this magnitude. In some instances renal function can be so depressed as to cause anuria (0–100 mL urine in 24 hours).
* *Uraemia and uricaemia are present (raised blood urea and uric acid concentrations)*: urea and uric acid are especially dependent upon an adequate glomerular filtration for their excretion. The presence of uraemia and uricaemia is usually indicative of an inability to excrete the normal load.
* *Potassium concentration is elevated in blood plasma*: in the absence of a potassium infusion, hyperkalaemia is almost certainly caused by an inability to excrete potassium normally. Failure to maintain potassium homeostasis may cause cardiac arrhythmias and is often the cause of death in ARF.
* *Acidosis is present*: the acidosis is of 'metabolic' origin and is caused by a failure to excrete hydrogen ions. The acidosis causes breathing to be slightly elevated.

Additional imbalances produced by the renal dysfunction will be:

* Fluid overload, which is partly caused by water retention and partly by an expansion of the extracellular fluid compartment as a consequence of sodium retention. Peripheral oedema might be observed. In severe cases pulmonary oedema may occur.
* Poor appetite, nausea, and vomiting arising from the disturbed blood composition.

* Changes in mentation such as drowsiness and confusion, again as a consequence of altered blood composition.

Goals of care

It may be several hours or even several days after clinical intervention before the kidneys resume normal filtration. The reasons for the delay in recovery from ARF remain unclear, and in some people function may never be completely restored. The specific goal of care for someone in ARF is to try to normalize as far as is possible body fluid composition by managing dietary input. In this way a new homeostatic balance can be established so that 'input' once again equals 'output':

* *Restoration of fluid balance*: fluid intake is reduced, usually to 500 mL/24 hours plus a volume equal to the previous day's urine output. This is to replace the water lost through residual renal function and that lost via insensible means (lungs, skin, etc). Daily weighing is a crude means of assessing the amount of any fluid that might continue to be retained.
* *Restriction of dietary sodium intake*: this is to prevent further fluid shifts.
* *Restriction of dietary potassium intake*: ion exchange resins, such as calcium resonium, might also be administered to promote K^+ secretion into the colon. A high calorie intake is also helpful because it promotes tissue anabolism and this helps to shift more potassium into the cells.
* *Restriction of dietary protein*: this is necessary to help reduce the production of urea and other nitrogenous products and so helps to compensate for the reduced excretion of these substances.

Phases

ARF usually has three phases:

1. The oliguric phase, described above.
2. The diuretic phase. This phase follows after perhaps several days, or even several weeks, and is usually indicative that the kidneys are recovering.
3. The recovery phase. The diuresis declines and homeostasis is re-established without the need for restricted dietary inputs.

Body fluid management can still be required even when the diuretic phase commences because the kidneys are initially unable to concentrate the urine. Strict monitoring therefore is essential throughout the course of ARF. Nursing care also includes psychological support and optimum nutrition (often as total parenteral nutrition).

Approximately 60% of patients regain most or all of their renal function but it is a life-threatening condition and there is still a quite high mortality rate despite new and sophisticated technological treatment. In some individuals ARF progresses to chronic renal failure and a time may come when dialysis (or renal transplantation) will be necessary (Boxes 15.18 and 15.19).

Should the elevated acidity still persist then two processes take place as renal compensation:

* Renal tubule fluid is almost hydrogen ion-free by the time it reaches the distal tubule. Almost all that is filtered from plasma by the glomeruli is reabsorbed by the proximal tubule (even when there is increased plasma acidity) by a process that is linked to the reabsorption of bicarbonate ions.

Thus, increased plasma acidity increases the filtration of hydrogen ions by the glomeruli, which in turn stimulates hydrogen ion reabsorption by the proximal tubule. This in turn promotes bicarbonate reabsorption. The additional bicarbonate will help to maintain the buffering capacity of plasma; in chronic circumstances it may even be increased (see Chapter 6, p.132).

* Hydrogen ion secretion by the distal tubules of the kidneys

BOX 15.18 DIALYSIS

Dialysis is an artificial means of replacing kidney function, although the intermittency of its application means that the control of blood composition cannot be as precise as that normally provided by the kidneys. Dialysis is especially used in cases of renal failure when the disturbance in body fluid composition is profound. In chronic renal failure a renal transplantation would be ideal but the reality is that patients will have a prolonged spell of dialysis before a donor becomes available, if at all. Dialysis may also be used in acute renal failure, until renal function improves, or to remove poisons quickly and efficiently.

Basically there are two procedures available: haemodialysis and peritoneal dialysis.

Haemodialysis

Here blood drains from a vein, usually in the arm, and is pumped to the dialysis machine (Figure 15.13). The blood passes over a selectively permeable membrane, on the other side of which is dialysate fluid. This fluid is a carefully prepared, balanced electrolyte solution that will also permit the withdrawal of water from blood by osmosis. The blood and dialysate fluid do not mix; solute and water exchange is by diffusion alone.

Haemodialysis can maintain a patient for many years but there are psychosocial costs – the treatment is time-consuming (6–8 hours) and must be performed regularly in an appropriate clinical unit, often entailing a degree of travelling for the patient. The treatment also is not a perfect replacement for kidney functions. For example, it does not replace red blood cells, the synthesis of which is reduced in chronic renal failure

since the kidneys do not produce erythrogenin, the precursor to the hormone erythropoietin. Other complications include arteriosclerotic disease, partly because of poor calcium/phosphate control but also because uraemia is not completely removed by dialysis.

See the case of the man presenting for haemodialysis, Section VI, p.661.

Peritoneal dialysis

The principle here is to use the patient's peritoneum as the selectively permeable membrane for dialysis. Here the dialysate fluid is introduced into the peritoneal cavity at regular intervals. Exchange with blood occurs and then peritoneal fluid is slowly drained, bringing with it the 'wastes' that had accumulated from blood. The method takes longer than haemodialysis (36–48 hours) but changes blood composition much more slowly and this may be an advantage in some patients. Care must be taken to avoid the development of peritonitis (Wiggins *et al.*, 2008).

Continuous ambulatory peritoneal dialysis (CAPD) is a variant that enables patients to take an active role in their dialysis, and the treatment may take place at home. A permanent peritoneal catheter is put into place and dialysate fluid delivered from a plastic bag. After delivery the bag can be rolled up under the clothing until drainage is necessary. Several treatments a day may be performed – more than if the patient has to attend a unit – and so control of blood composition is often better. The method is clearly also less restrictive on lifestyle.

BOX 15.19 KIDNEY TRANSPLANTATION

Kidney transplantation is now a widespread intervention for failing kidneys. A single organ is usually transplanted into the groin of the individual – only one kidney is necessary for life, although it will adapt to function almost at the level of activity of two. Transplanted kidneys retain a renal artery and vein (and ureter) but will have had their nerve supplies cut.

A transplanted kidney will respond to hormones produced by the recipient and so will be able to help maintain body fluid homeostasis. Had renal nerves been central to the homeostatic mechanism then transplantation would be more problematic but fortunately hormones are the main mediators of renal functioning. The kidney does not exhibit any

deficiency in terms of water and electrolyte handling because compensatory mechanisms replace any functions of the nerves in these respects.

The transplanted kidney will not regain normal function immediately and the recipient will require monitoring for such signs. Of concern is the possibility that the individual will reject the kidney as a result of an immune response. For this reason the recipient will be given immune-suppressive drugs. Signs of rejection include malaise, elevated body temperature and reduced renal function. Alterations in blood composition may also be indicative.

---

is increased, causing an increased acidity of the urine (urine pH is normally about 6–7 but has a range of 4.5–8: i.e. acidic or alkaline according to need).

Conserving hydrogen ions/excreting excess bicarbonate ions

The secretion of hydrogen ions in the distal tubule is linked to the pH of plasma and so is decreased if plasma pH is rising. Also, fewer hydrogen ions being filtered from plasma means that less is being reabsorbed in the proximal tubule; consequently, the reabsorption of bicarbonate ions is less efficient leading to greater excretion of these ions (i.e. the urine becomes more alkaline).

THE BLADDER AND CONTROL OF MICTURITION

The urinary bladder

The bladder is a hollow organ, largely composed of smooth muscle, which lies within the pelvis between the rectum and

the symphysis pubis (Figure 15.14a,b). In women it also lies anterior to the uterus and vagina. The bladder is actually outside the peritoneal lining of the abdomen and as it inflates it extends between the peritoneum and the anterior body wall. Anatomical features are:

- The bladder wall has three layers: an outer (or serous) layer, which is an extension of the peritoneum, a middle layer of smooth muscle and an inner epithelial layer. The latter is of transitional epithelium (see Figure 2.27, p.54), which means that the cells have the capacity to stretch and so allow the bladder to fill without the epithelium rupturing. The muscle layer is itself divided into three layers: outer and inner layers of longitudinal muscle fibres and a middle layer of circular muscle. This arrangement means that contraction causes the bladder to reduce both in length and diameter, thus emptying it effectively.
- Most of the inner surface of the bladder is extremely folded. The folds, or rugae, are important because they enable the

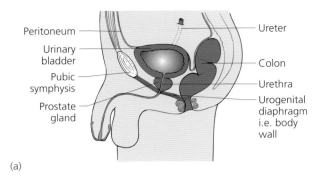

(a)

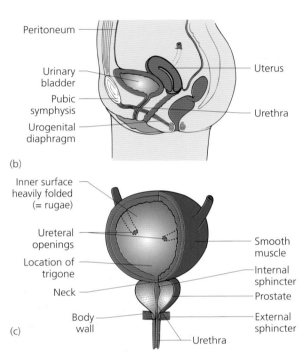

(b)

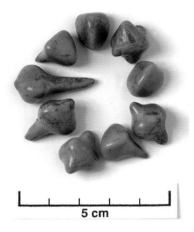

Figure 15.14 General anatomy of the urinary bladder: (a) male; (b) female; (c) detail of the male bladder

Q What is the function of the internal lining of the bladder?

Q How does the female bladder compare to that of the male?

BOX 15.20 URINARY STONES AND HYDRONEPHROSIS

Calculi (urinary stones; Figure 15.15) normally consist of calcium and uric acid (i.e. substances with a low solubility). Deposition occurs when their concentrations in urine are abnormally high, particularly if urine pH is also appropriate. They may form anywhere within the urinary tract and result in blockage of the ureter, kidney pelvis or tubules leading to urine retention, kidney distension and considerable pain. They may even form within the bladder and interfere with bladder emptying. The occurrence of stones is very painful. Stones may be removed by surgery, or may be disintegrated using ultrasound.

Obstruction of the urethra, or a ureter, or the presence of tumours within a kidney, may all cause an accumulation of urine within the renal pelvis (called hydronephrosis). The renal pelvis dilates and enlarges, and the elevated pressure may even cause a reduction in blood supply to the tissue, resulting in tissue breakdown. Treatment is aimed at removing the cause of the blockage and correcting the underlying disorder.

Figure 15.15 Urinary stones extracted from a bladder. Reproduced with the kind permission of the Medical Illustration Department, Norfolk and Norwich University Hospitals NHS Trust

bladder to fill without placing a high level of tension on the muscle wall. In contrast, the base of the bladder has a smooth triangular-shaped area, called the trigone, which lacks rugae. This area is formed between the points of entry of the ureters and the exit of the urethra (the tube to the exterior) and forms a smooth funnel-like surface that facilitates efficient bladder emptying.

- Emptying the bladder requires relaxation of two sphincters. Where the urethra leaves the bladder, the circular involuntary muscle layer is arranged so as to produce the 'internal sphincter' (Figure 15.13c), which keeps urine stored within the bladder while it is filling. The sphincter is controlled by the autonomic nervous system and we generally have little voluntary control over it. The 'external sphincter' is formed from the striated muscle of the pelvic floor (i.e. it is not anatomically a part of the bladder but it is functionally linked to it). This sphincter is under voluntary control from about 1.5–2 years of age and enables us to consciously determine when (and where!) we will urinate. The process of urination is described below.

The urethra

The urethra extends from the neck of the bladder. It opens to the exterior via the urethral meatus, or opening. No urine can enter the urethra until the internal sphincter has been relaxed. The urethra also passes through the external sphincter which unless relaxed will prevent further progress of the urine:

- In women the urethra is short, only about 4 cm long, and the meatus opens in front of the vaginal opening.
- In men the urethra is about 20 cm long and also passes through the prostate gland. Ejaculatory ducts from the testes empty into it (see Figure 18.6, p.490) and so the

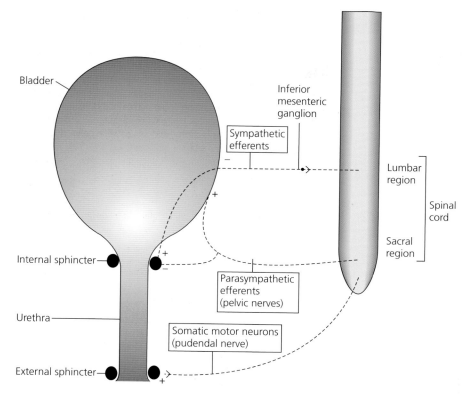

Figure 15.16 Neural control of the urinary bladder. Note that for the bladder to fill, parasympathetic efferent activity must decrease and sympathetic activity increase. For the bladder to empty, parasympathetic efferent activity must increase and sympathetic activity decrease. +, contraction when efferent nerves stimulated; −, relaxed when efferent nerves stimulated

Q Outline the neural processes involved in micturition.

male urethra performs both an excretory and a reproductive role.

Bladder emptying (urination, or micturition)

The passing of urine is referred to as micturition and results from an interplay of the autonomic nervous control of the bladder and internal sphincter, and somatic nervous control of the external sphincter:

- Contraction of the internal sphincter muscle (and external sphincter) and relaxation of the muscles of the bladder facilitates filling of the bladder.
- Relaxation of the internal sphincter (and external sphincter) and contraction of the bladder facilitates emptying.

Filling

As the bladder fills with urine, the pressure within it rises but the muscle layers actively relax through actions of the sympathetic nerves to the bladder wall (Figure 15.16). The same nerve activity causes the internal sphincter to contract. The relaxation of the bladder wall means that the pressure rises only slowly as filling continues; this allows the bladder to accommodate more urine and means that we are hardly aware of the volume present. Eventually, a point is reached when the accommodation begins to be exceeded, and so addition of further urine causes a marked rise in pressure. A sensation of a 'full bladder' is perceived that becomes more intense as the bladder continues to fill. Micturition can still be suppressed at this stage but must occur if the bladder accumulates much more (the average capacity of the bladder of an adult is about 600–700 mL of urine) when the very tense bladder wall activates pain receptors.

Emptying

The contraction of the bladder is largely a reflex response to increasing wall tension, although practice enables individuals to produce urine specimens to order. The reflex operates through sensory nerve endings in the bladder wall, which influence nerve activity from the spinal cord to the bladder

---

BOX 15.21 URINARY INCONTINENCE, FREQUENCY AND RETENTION

Urinary incontinence
Urinary incontinence is the release of small amounts of urine at a time when it should be retained in the bladder. It results from a problem of controlling micturition and has four main causes:

1. Irritation of the internal surface of the bladder by infection or the presence of precipitates will make the bladder wall 'irritable' and more prone to contract. Cystitis is an inflammation of the urinary bladder, which may cause frequent and even painful micturition.

2. Loss of muscle tone in the external sphincter is sometimes observed with age and with the stretching of the pelvic floor during childbirth, or any tissue trauma to these muscles. The shorter urethra in the female (which places the internal and external sphincters in close proximity) means that this problem is also more frequently observed

BOX 15.21 *Continued*

in women, stress incontinence is observed when an increase in abdominal pressure, perhaps through coughing or laughing, causes leakage of a small amount of urine through a weakened sphincter. Such potential for problems later in life provides a rationale for exercises to maintain the muscle tone of the pelvic floor. Immobility may also cause a loss of tone and introduce a continence problem in both sexes.

3 Spinal cord trauma often results in problems in controlling micturition since the innervation of the external sphincter exits from the lumbar/sacral regions at the lower part of the spinal cord. Cord trauma in the cervical, thoracic or upper lumbar regions may disrupt transmission from brainstem to bladder and so affect the ability to control the external sphincter.

4 Central nervous system disorder. Incontinence may be observed in dementia, probably because of a failure to promote normal conscious control of micturition.

Urinary frequency

Frequency relates to the urgency to pass urine when the urinary bladder is unfilled. Frequency may be observed as part of urinary incontinence. It might also be observed if the bladder is restricted (for example during pregnancy; see Box 15.9, p.431) or if the bladder is subjected to anxiety-induced nerve activity (in contrast some people find it difficult to void urine when they are anxious, for example in clinics, because they tense abdominal and pelvic floor muscles, and sympathetic nerve activity is increased and constricts the internal sphincter).

Urinary retention

Obstruction of the urethra will prevent adequate bladder emptying, and urinary retention. Apart from possible consequences to the kidney, this condition can also be extremely painful if severe enough to completely prevent micturition. Hyperplasia of the prostate gland is one such cause in men, where enlargement of the gland invades the area around the internal bladder sphincter. Where urinary retention is observed, a urinary catheter inserted into the bladder via the urethra will be necessary (see Box 15.23).

BOX 15.22 URINARY TRACT INFECTION

Cystitis is a term used to refer to infection of the lower urinary tract, causing irritation and soreness on passing urine. Bladder discomfort, and urinary frequency, may be observed if the infection gains access to the bladder, while the connections with the kidneys make them susceptible to infection should this 'backtrack' along the ureter to the kidney. In backtracking:

• The infection will first reach the renal pelvis, producing inflammation referred to as pyelonephritis. However, the infection is unlikely to be as localized as this and infection of renal tubules, renal interstitial space (primarily in the medulla), and the renal pelvis may be observed;

• If the infection penetrates the renal cortex then interstitial nephritis may be observed, or glomerulonephritis, which was mentioned earlier (see Box 15.5, p.428).

These conditions are not, however, caused only by infection from the urinary tract. Pre-renal causes are also possible, arising from the effects of antibody–antigen complexes secondary to infection elsewhere or from the side-effects of drugs.

These inflammatory kidney conditions are normally acute but can lead to the loss of renal tissue and scarring. Acute renal failure may ensue and may even progress to chronic renal failure.

BOX 15.23 CATHETERIZATION OF THE URETHRA

This is a technique to encourage free draining of the bladder if urinary retention is occurring. It is a useful method in the short term, for example after surgery, in which micturition is difficult, or in the long term in chronic illness where it also helps the individual maintain skin integrity and their dignity. In addition to enabling bladder emptying, a catheter also enables measurement of urine production rate, and this is very useful in assessing renal function and/or hydration states after surgery.

A 'closed-system' is used in introducing the catheter by which the catheter is initially filled with sterile saline in order to reduce the likelihood of introducing infection. Nevertheless, infection is often problematic and so catheterization should only take place when absolutely necessary, and the catheter should not remain in place longer than is necessary. Aseptic techniques are important when inserting the catheter, and when changing the urinary collection bag or cleansing the area of the urethral meatus.

Problems arising might be :

• Introduction of an infection through poor aseptic technique.
• Reflux of urine into the bladder from a poorly positioned collection bag, or during bag-changing.
• Infection with urease-producing bacteria that convert urea in urine to ammonia. This reacts with other urine constituents to produce ammonium magnesium phosphate, which can encrust the catheter causing pain on withdrawal and/or catheter obstruction, and even provide a site for microorganism growth.
• Tissue damage (and pain) during insertion of the catheter.
• Inflammation in response to the catheter composition. Solid silicone and hydrogel are usually used in catheter construction and both may promote local immune responses.

SUMMARY

1 Metabolism, and our diets, provide excesses of substances which, if retained in the body, will eventually disturb cellular and systemic functions. The main route for their excretion is via the urine.

2 Urine is initially formed in the glomeruli of the renal tubules as a filtrate of blood plasma, and at this point contains all the solutes found in plasma other than large proteins. The composition and volume of the filtrate is modified as it passes along the renal tubules, by solute reabsorption and by secretion of solutes by the tubular cells.

3 The bulk (normally >99%) of the filtrate is reabsorbed by the tubules, mostly by the proximal tubule. Separate renal handling of solute and water reabsorption by the loop of Henle, distal nephron and collecting ducts means that the final urine can be more dilute or more concentrated than plasma, with consequential effects on plasma osmotic pressure. The process is largely controlled by ADH.

4 The urinary excretion of many metabolic products, such as urea, is primarily determined by the GFR. That of electrolytes and glucose is determined by how much is reabsorbed from the filtrate or how much is secreted into it.

5 Virtually all of the glucose and amino acids filtered by the kidneys are reabsorbed and the urine is characteristically free of them.

6 Electrolyte excretion is mainly controlled by the actions of hormones on the kidneys. Homeostatic control of solute excretion is essential because of the pronounced effects that retention or excessive loss have on systemic functions. The means of detection of disturbance depends upon the physiological consequences of that disturbance, and renal responses vary accordingly.

7 Urine produced by the kidneys passes to the urinary bladder via ureters. The bladder empties to the outside via another tube, the urethra.

8 Bladder emptying is under the control of the autonomic nervous system and entails the sympathetic and parasympathetic nerves to the bladder acting antagonistically to allow relaxation of the bladder and hence its filling, and contraction for its emptying. The nerves also provide contraction or relaxation of sphincter muscles accordingly.

(Figure 15.16). The sensory fibres enter into the spinal cord in the lower (11th and 12th) lumbar segments, and when stimulated may cause an increase in parasympathetic nerve activity to the bladder. The main body of the bladder contracts, and the internal sphincter reflexly dilates. At this point relaxation of the external sphincter will allow micturition to occur. However, this is striated muscle over which we have a degree of conscious control and so we can prevent micturition unless the bladder is extremely full, and the sphincter can even be closed once micturition is in progress.

Control of the external sphincter arises through the activity of the pudendal nerve which enters/exits the lower lumbar area of the spinal cord. Sensory information regarding the tension of the bladder wall and the sphincters is relayed up the spinal cord to the sensory cortex of the brain, and final output to the external sphincter is generated from areas within the brainstem. The development of the ability to control the external sphincter takes place in young children, and is encouraged by learning through 'potty training'. The need for maturation of the brainstem areas involved means that control is not normally established until about 1.5–2 years of age.

REFERENCES

Brady, M., Kinn, S. and Stuart, P. (2007) Preoperative fasting for adults to prevent perioperative complications. In: *Cochrane Database of Systematic Reviews* (4). Oxford: Update Software.

Chrysant, G.S. (2000) High salt intake and cardiovascular disease. Is there a connection? *Nutrition* **16**(7–8): 662–4.

Clancy, J., McVicar, A. and Baird, N. (2002) Perioperative influences on water and electrolyte homeostasis. In: *Fundamentals of Homeostasis for Perioperative Practitioners*. Chapter 3. London: Routledge.

Kellum, J.A. (2008) Acute kidney injury. *Critical Care Medicine* **36**(4, Suppl.): S141–5.

Kheterpal, S., Tremper, K.K., Englesbe, M.J. *et al.* (2007) Predictors of postoperative acute renal failure after noncardiac surgery in patients with previously normal renal function. *Anesthesiology* **107**(6): 892–902.

Rodríguez-Iturbe, B. and Batsford, S. (2007) Pathogenesis of poststreptococcal glomerulonephritis a century after Clemens von Pirquet. *Kidney International* **71**(11): 1094–104.

Wiggins, K.J., Craig, J.C., Johnson, D.W. and Strippoli, G.F. (2008) Treatment for peritoneal dialysis-associated peritonitis. In: *Cochrane Database of Systematic Reviews*, 1. Oxford: Update Software.

THE SKIN

INTRODUCTION

The skin is the largest organ of the body. Its functions relate to its role in providing the main interface between the body and the external environment.

Functions of skin

Protection

Being in contact with the external environment the skin is obviously the first line of defence against potential pathogenic organisms, and to chemical agents. The structure of the skin provides a physical, impervious barrier, and the bactericidal constituents of skin secretions also provide a degree of chemical protection. Specialized skin cells called melanocytes protect against harmful ultraviolet radiation from the sun. Skin derivatives, nails and hairs, also provide a protective element.

Excretion

The skin is not an excretory organ in the sense that it has a central role in the homeostatic processes involved in body fluid regulation, although sweat composition may vary in its sodium chloride content if we are sodium deficient. However, sweat contains various other substances, including metabolic products, and the skin therefore is one route of excretion for these substances. Although normally a relatively minor route, nevertheless the amount of substance lost from the body via sweat must be considered a component of total excretion. This is particularly the case for water and electrolytes. Thus, even in cool conditions in the UK sweat accounts for almost 10% of the water output from the body, while in very hot weather sweat secretion may rise to as much as 4 L/day and far exceed the total excreted by other routes, including urine.

Prevention of tissue dehydration

The structure of the intact epidermis makes the skin impervious to water (note that sweat secretion is via ducts from sweat glands and so is a physiological process). This property of the skin is essential for our existence because it prevents evaporative water loss to the atmosphere. The importance of this role is illustrated by the effects of surgical procedures, or extensive burns, which breach the skin and expose underlying 'wet' tissues to the environment. There is extensive loss of water by evaporation, and this is a concern for care.

Support and shape

This is an obvious role of the skin. Support of the viscera is provided by muscles of the body wall but is facilitated by the tough, durable nature of the overlying skin. Muscles, skin and adipose tissues also give rise to the body shapes associated with sexual dimorphism. Being the visible aspects of the body, skin also makes clear the effects of ageing on tissues. Loss of elasticity, which will occur in other tissues and organs also, is readily apparent as the skin wrinkles with age.

Regulation of body temperature

Our bodies constantly gain heat from metabolism, and (in the UK) usually constantly lose heat to the cooler environment, though under very hot conditions the body may gain heat from the environment too. The skin therefore provides the interface for heat exchange with the environment. Maintaining an optimal temperature of the essential organs of the body is an important aspect of homeostasis, and controlling heat transfer across the skin is part of that regulatory process. The importance of skin in the regulation of body temperature is such that the topic is covered in a separate section later in this chapter.

Others

- *Energy reserves*: subcutaneous fat stores provide important energy resources for us.

BOX 16.1. ITCHING (PRURITIS)

Pruritis is caused by local irritation of the skin that stimulates nerve endings. Pruritis might result from contact of the skin with irritant agents, from inflammation or infection of the skin, or perhaps from the deposition of 'waste' substances in the skin. Deposition may arise because excretion of substances via sweat can be enhanced in renal failure. Although sweat will not compensate for body fluid disturbances in renal failure, there is an increased content of metabolic wastes in the secretion. Thus, a 'snow' of uric acid and urea may be apparent on the skin of patients, left behind when sweat evaporates. It is the deposition of crystals within the skin that causes intense itching.

- *Sensation*: the skin contains many receptors, especially temperature, pain and touch receptors, that give us information of our immediate external environment.
- *Vitamin D synthesis*: the skin provides the site of conversion of a precursor chemical to vitamin D.
- *Body odour*: normally viewed negatively because of connotation associated with bad odours (from infection of oils, etc. in sweat), normal odour is distinctive and may also be a behavioural modifier.

Some of these functions are touched upon in this chapter, and elsewhere in this book.

ANATOMY OF THE SKIN

The skin consists of two principal parts (Figure 16.1a): the inner dermis ('derm-' = layer) and the outer epidermis ('epi-'= upon). Below the dermis lies a subcutaneous layer ('sub-' = below, 'cutaneous' = of the skin; this layer may also be referred to as the 'hypodermis'), sometimes called the 'superficial fascia' since it also includes part of the connective tissue that covers muscles. Embryologically the subcutaneous layer does not develop as part of the skin, but it is functionally linked with it and so will be considered in this context.

Epidermis

The epidermis provides the immediate contact with our external environment. It therefore has adaptations to withstand the stressors we experience, most notably a multilayered structure with a tough outer layer. Nevertheless, cell attrition can be very high and the epidermis replaces itself every 35–45 days.

Cell layers

The epidermis is of the tissue type called a 'stratified squamous epithelium'. This means that it has multiple layers (strata) of simple, flattened (i.e. squamous) cells that sit, ultimately, upon a basement membrane of protein. There are various layers of cells (Figure 16.1b):

- A basal layer (stratum basale) that actually sits on the basement membrane, thus separating the epidermis from the dermis. Mitotic division by cells of the basal layer give rise to all of the other layers within the epidermis, and so it is often referred to as the 'germinal layer' of the skin. Epidermal growth factor is a peptide that has been found to promote mitosis in epithelia, including the epidermis, though its precise role in the maintenance of the skin is unclear. While some of the daughter cells produced by mitosis maintain the basal layer, others ascend toward the surface of the skin and form the following layers.
- A layer of 'prickly'-looking cells (stratum spinosum), lying above the basal layer. Within the stratum spinosum the cells become irregularly shaped and develop protuberances that cause them to appear 'prickly'. The cell extensions interlock and this is the start of the formation of a structure that will be tough and durable. Tactile nerve endings, called Merkel's discs (see Chapter 7, p.142), may also be present in this layer.

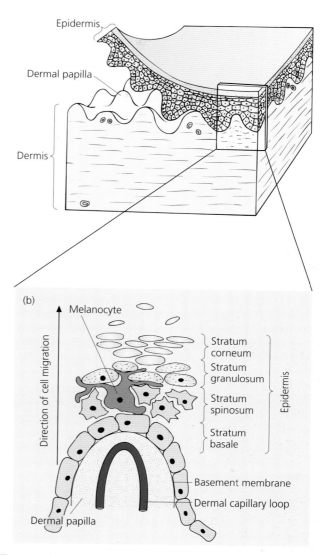

Figure 16.1 The epidermis. (a) General plan and relation to the dermis. (b) Cell layers

Q Which layer of skin is referred to as a stratified epithelium? Name the subdivisions of the layer.

Q The skin is referred to as a 'labile' tissue because of its repair capabilities. What does this mean?

- A layer of cells that contain granules (stratum granulosum), lying above the stratum spinosum. After the stratum spinosum the cells begin to flatten. They also begin to produce keratohyalin, a substance that will eventually be converted into the tough, waterproofing protein keratin. The compound is stored in the cells, hence this layer is sometimes referred to as the 'granular layer'. The nuclei of the cells within this layer begin to degenerate and consequently metabolism declines.
- A layer of tough, hardened (i.e. cornified; stratum corneum) cells, lying above the granular layer, and at the skin surface

(by this time the cells are dead). This cornified layer gives the epidermis the toughness needed to provide a barrier against external physical stresses, and environmental agents such as bacteria and chemicals. The latter include water as the epidermis is now impervious. In adults the epidermis is from 0.5 to 3 mm thick, depending upon site, and this especially relates to the thickness of the cornified layer, and hence to the physical stresses placed on that area of skin. In view of its position as the outer layer it is not surprising that cells are continuously lost from it during day-to-day living. The attrition is substantial – for example, most of the 'house dust' in bedding is composed of these cells.

- Areas of skin that are exposed to considerable frictional stress, such as the soles of the feet, have a fifth layer between the granular and cornified layers. This is a 'clear' layer (stratum lucidum) of cells: the cells produce a translucent substance that is intermediate between keratohyalin and keratin. This is called eleidin and provides a degree of frictional resistance by cushioning and absorbing shearing stresses, for example during walking.

There are no blood vessels within the epidermis itself. The demands of the cells are met by blood vessels within the dermis that extend into the vicinity of the basal layer cells.

BOX 16.2 AGEING AND THE EPIDERMIS

The thickness of the epidermis is determined by the rate of cell division in the basal layer, which must then be in balance with the rate of cell attrition from the cornified layer. One feature of ageing is that the rate of mitosis generally begins to slow down and the epidermis becomes thinner, drier and more susceptible to damage (Nazarko, 2007). In contrast, the epidermis of the soles of the feet of older people may be very tough as the cornified layer becomes even more hardened. It also shows evidence of accumulating substances that have been modified inside cells but not excreted; these are 'age pigments' and produce 'age spots'. They are indicative of changes in cell metabolism with age (see Chapter 19, p.553).

BOX 16.3 EPIDERMAL WOUND HEALING AND SKIN GRAFTING

The germinal layer of the epidermis has to be highly proliferative in order to maintain the cornified layer. Being this active means that the epithelium regenerates very quickly if damaged.

Epidermal wound healing
Wound healing was discussed in detail in Chapter 11, p.290 onwards. In that section it was noted how superficial injury is largely repaired by cell migration. In the epidermis the cell layers are all derived from the germinal layer. In other words there is no need for specific cell types to migrate from elsewhere, although lateral migration from adjoining epidermal layers may occur. Superficial wounds to the epidermis therefore heal very quickly, without a need for scarring, and tissue structure is soon reorganized and this type of wound healing is often referred to as 'invisible mend' (see Figure 11.13, p.290).

Skin grafting
This entails removal of a section of skin and its transferral to another site (Beldon, 2003). It is used when there are areas of denuded skin (e.g. burns), or where skin is inadequate to close a wound, or if skin has been removed (e.g. in excision of a tumour). Skin grafts are of three types:

- *autograft*: transplantation from that same person's skin;
- *allograft*: transplantation from one person to another;
- *xenograft*: transplantation from another species.

The graft is obtained from a suitable site using a razor or similar implement. The section of skin removed is predominantly epidermis, including some of the basal layer. Remnant germinal cells from the basal layer will re-epithelialize the donor site, although great care must be taken to ensure that the raw, exposed dermis is maintained. The graft is transferred to the graft site, which must have an adequate blood supply to support the transplanted tissue.

BOX 16.4. SKIN COLORATION

Skin colour relates to two aspects: blood passing superficially below the epidermis, and the activity of melanocytes to pigment the epidermis. The latter are described in the main text.

Skin colour produced by blood is an important indicator of well-being, and is an important aspect of healthcare assessment. In the absence of large amounts of pigment the skin is pinkish-white and its coloration is mainly determined by the visualization of blood within it:

- the skin will look flushed in hot weather when blood flow to the skin is increased;
- the skin circulation is regulated by the sympathetic nervous system, and when this is inhibited by emotional responses it may even cause 'blushing' as vessels dilate in localized areas;
- cyanosis, observed when blood is deoxygenated, can be observed through skin;
- the drainage of blood away from the skin in shock causes it to take on a greyish coloration.

BOX 16.5 SKIN TUMOURS

There are various types of skin tumour:

- *Basal cell carcinoma*: this tumour is the most common form of skin cancer and arises from granular or basal cells of the epidermis. Exposure to excessive ultraviolet light is a risk factor. The tumour has a slow growth rate and generally does not metastasize beyond skin but it can produce severe local destruction of tissue.
- *Squamous cell carcinoma*: sunlight is also an important risk factor also for this tumour. There are basically two types of tumour: the tumour may become invasive and malignant, or the tumour may be cornified, and rarely invasive or malignant, and so form a tumour '*in situ*' only.
- *Melanoma*: melanoma is the most common cancer of the skin; as its name implies it is a cancer of the pigmented melanocytes, especially occurring where the cells are aggregated in a mole. The main promoter seems to be overexposure of melanocytes to ultraviolet radiation, leading to a failure to control the cell cycle. The tumour is normally invasive and metastasizes.
- *Kaposi's sarcoma*: this is a malignancy arising from the endothelial cells that line blood vessels (in the skin). It is especially seen in immune deficiency states such as acquired immune deficiency syndrome (AIDS). The tumour can rapidly be progressive and multifocal. It normally first appears in the lower extremities but progresses to the upper body.

BOX 16.6 RADIOTHERAPY

Radiotherapy for tumours can be by internal or external means. External application exposes the skin to relatively high doses of radiation. The intention of the treatment is to disrupt the cell cycle (see Figure 2.15, p.43) of tumour cells but in doing so will also affect rapidly proliferating normal cells. These include oral, oesophageal and gastrointestinal mucosae, and the skin. Regarding the skin, local responses occur at the site of application, including reduced cell production and migration in the epidermis, skin thinning and even penetrating lesions of the epidermis and dermis (McQuestion, 2006). The skin becomes more susceptible to irritation and so patients should avoid using lotions or ointments. Skin care is therefore an important feature of care for people undergoing such treatment, and skin assessment an essential part of healthcare practice.

Melanocytes

Interspersed among cells of the basal and 'prickly' layers are cells called melanocytes, that contain the pigment melanin. Melanocytes (Figure 16.1b) have extensions that pass between cells of the other layers. When melanin production is stimulated, that released from the processes will be taken up by other epidermal cells and so will pigment most areas of skin. Skin pigmentation primarily relates to the amount of pigment present in the cells, and there is little racial difference in the actual numbers of melanocytes present. Moles (or naevi) are aggregates of melanocytes that provide a concentration of pigmented cells in one place, rather than dispersed.

Melanin is important because it is an effective filter of ultraviolet light and so protects the underlying basal layer, and the dermis, from the harmful effects of the sun. The pigment is synthesized from the amino acid tyrosine, a process that is stimulated directly by the actions of ultraviolet light, and indirectly by melanocyte-stimulating hormone (MSH, or melanotropin) released from the pituitary gland.

Albinism, which is characterized by pigment-free melanocytes and hair, occurs when a genetic deficiency prevents the synthesis of those enzymes necessary for the conversion of the amino acid tyrosine to the pigment melanin. Albinism is commonly, but not always, associated with Huntington's disease, a neurological disorder arising from an inability of cells to metabolize tyrosine appropriately. Visually, the hair is very fair, almost white, the skin is very pale and there is a deficiency of pigment in the eyes (eye colour also involves melanin). People who are albino therefore have a skin that lacks the protection normally provided by melanin against excessive ultraviolet light, and this makes skin damage, including cancers (Box 16.5), more likely if there is prolonged exposure to bright sunlight.

Other epidermal cells

Some cell types found scattered within the epidermis have the forbidding name of non-pigmented granular dendrocytes ('dendrite' = branch; the characteristics of these cells is that they are melanin-free, granulated and they have branching processes). They are cells of the immune system that at some point have migrated into the skin. They are part of the defences provided by skin, and basically remain inactive within the epidermis unless the tissue is damaged. They then interact with helper and suppressor T-lymphocytes that invade the area, in assisting immune responses (see Chapter 13, p.377).

BOX 16.7 SKIN CONDITIONS

Conditions associated with infection

- *Acne vulgaris* is an inflammation of sebaceous glands in response to bacterial infection. The problem is particularly noticeable during puberty when gland activity increases.
- *Warts* are produced by a focus of cells that have divided excessively in response to infection by a kind of virus, called a papovavirus.
- *Cold sores* are lesions produced by infection of skin with Herpes simplex virus (types 1 and 2, most commonly type 1). This virus may lie dormant for long periods, with cold sores appearing only when the virus is 'triggered'. This activation may be in response to factors such as ultraviolet light, or the release of sex steroids.
- *Chicken pox and shingles* are produced by the Varicella-zoster virus (VZV). Varicella (chicken pox) occurs as a primary infection, zoster (shingles) is usually secondary. Zoster is characterized by pain localized to a single dermatome (an area of skin supplied by branches from a single spinal nerve; see Figure 8.19, p.184), followed by vesicle eruptions. Calamine lotion or antiviral drugs offer some relief.

Inflammatory conditions

- *Acne rosacea* is an inflammatory condition of adults, but of unknown cause. It is characterized by facial erythema (red patches caused by blood vessels approaching the skin surface, a process called telangiectasis) and pustules. Hypersensitivity of the sebaceous glands may occur causing a bulbous appearance.
- *Eczema* is an inflammatory response of skin to chemical agents. The term is synonymous with dermatitis and the cause may be endogenous (e.g. in response to substances within sebum) or exogenous (e.g. allergic contact dermatitis, a type of hypersensitive immune response, or irritant dermatitis, a response that does not entail mediation by the immune system). Erythema (red patches caused by blood vessels approaching the skin surface, scaly texture and itching are usually present, and possibly oedema and crusting. Scratching exacerbates the latter and so anti-itch preparations may be used to reduce the incidence. Long-term eczema can make skin texture leathery and thickened.
- *Lupus erythematosus* (LE) is an inflammatory disease, but its causes are unclear. In discoid (cutaneous) LE the skin, especially of the face, develops lesions that contain immunoglobulin deposits (the cause of the condition is unknown but may result from sensitization to an antigen). Skin blood vessels are usually prominent producing red erythematous patches. Sensitivity to ultraviolet light is also common. Healing is frequently associated with scarring. In systemic LE many organs are affected but skin lesions and erythematous patches are again apparent, especially of the face. Photosensitivity is also present.

Inherited conditions

Psoriasis is perhaps the best-known example of an inherited skin condition, although most cases do not appear to have a familial link. Skin eruptions occur because mitotic divisions proceed too rapidly.

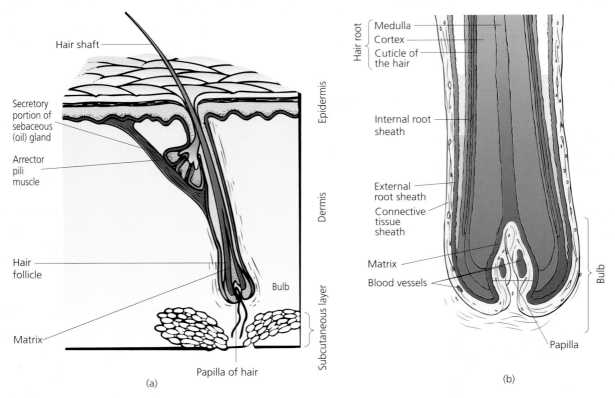

Figure 16.2 (a) Principal parts of a hair and associated structures. (b) Longitudinal section of a hair root

Q Describe the structure and functions of hair.

Q Identify the glands associated with hair.

Hair and nails: epidermally derived structures

Just glancing at Figure 16.2 gives the impression that hair is part of the dermis, and simply protrudes through the epidermis, but closer examination of the diagram shows that the base of the hair sits within a sheath made of epidermal tissue. Hair (and nails) are basically made of epidermal protein (keratin) and dead cells, and are produced by germinal cells at their base (the hair follicle and nail bed, respectively). These cells are more active than other cells of the epidermis and require a better blood supply. It therefore makes sense that the follicles and nail beds extend deeper within the skin where blood flow is adequate.

Hair

One function of hair is to protect underlying skin or structures. For example, head hair helps to prevent the heating effect of the sun on brain function, and to reduce heat loss in the cold, while eyebrows protect the eyes from direct sun and from particulate matter in the air. In some areas, notably the surface of the eyelids and in the lips, the presence of hair would affect their delicate functions and these areas are hairless. In other places the hair has become sparse (over much of the skin; thought to reduce insulation and aid heat loss), or bristly (in the ears and nose; thought to facilitate functions as filters).

However, even where hair is sparse there are touch receptors associated with hairs, and so hair also has a sensory role.

The shaft of a hair is visible externally and consists of (Figure 16.2):

- an inner structure of granulated cells and air spaces;
- a cortex of melanin-pigmented cells (with extensive air spaces in those people with white hair);
- an outer cuticular layer of heavily keratinized cells.

Note that all of these cell types are modifications of those identified above in the epidermis.

The hair root consists of the growing region of the hair and a protective sheath. The outer sheath originates from the basal and 'prickly' layers of the epidermis, while the inner sheath derives from clusters of germinative cells, called the 'matrix', which produce new hairs after old ones are shed. About 70–100 hairs are shed from the scalp each day and will be replaced by growth from the matrix. A papilla of connective tissue is present below the matrix and contains the blood vessels that supply the matrix cells. Collectively the root, matrix and papilla comprise the hair follicle (Figure 16.2). Associated with the follicles are:

- Sebaceous glands, although some are also found in hairless skin, such as the lips and eyelids. These glands secrete

BOX 16.8 HAIR LOSS AND EXCESS

Hair loss

Alopecia is the term used for hair loss. In men hair follicles on the top of the scalp may be sensitive to male sex steroids (androgens). Typically, there is loss of hair along the frontal hairline, as well as over the scalp. Alopecia may also be observed in women, but there is not usually recession from the frontal hair. Again androgens have been implicated (note that women produce male steroids from the adrenal gland – see Chapter 9, p.219) and so the occurrence is more likely postmenopausally.

Alopecia areata is rapid loss of hair from patches of scalp, usually forming rounded hairless areas. The cause is unknown but it has been linked to stressful episodes, genetic susceptibility, immune factors and metabolic disorders such as those of the thyroid. There is usually permanent regrowth of hair but this may take 1–3 months. Total hair loss can sometimes occur (called alopecia totalis), usually in young people, and regrowth is less likely in this form of alopecia.

Hair excess

Hirsutism (Figure 16.3) is excessive hair growth usually on the face and body. In men, recession of the frontal hairline is also commonly observed. The areas where the hair grows appear to be sensitive to androgens. The occurrence of hirsutism in women may be associated with excessive adrenal gland activity or underactivity of the ovaries (i.e. deficiency of oestrogens), which disturbs the normal oestrogen/androgen ratio.

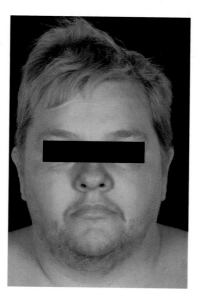

Figure 16.3 A woman with hirsutism. Reproduced with the kind permission of the Medical Illustration Department, Norfolk and Norwich University Hospitals NHS Trust

BOX 16.9 NAIL CHARACTERISTICS

- Nail formation may be influenced by infection:
  - Paronychia is an infection of the cuticle. Inflammation occurs and even abscess formation, and the shape of the nails may be affected.
  - Onychomycosis is a fungal infection of the nail plate. The nail may be raised because of deposits underneath, and is usually discoloured.
- Ageing causes the nails to become thickened and hardened. Older people who become unable to maintain the care of toenails may become disabled as a consequence. Poor-fitting shoes can exacerbate the problem.
- Nail 'colour' is also a useful observation for the health of the vascular system. For example, circulatory shock is associated with intense peripheral vasoconstriction, and so the nails lose their pink coloration. Similarly, the occurrence of a blueish tinge to the nail could indicate systemic hypoxaemia. Anaemia frequently makes the nails appear pale.
- Thin or flaking nails could reflect a poor diet: remember that the nails are primarily made of protein (keratin), and that they grow continuously from the nail root. Nails that have undergone altered rates of growth often are flecked with pale spots and patches, frequently in a lunar shape that reflects the production across the matrix at the base of the nail.

sebum, which is an oily mixture of fats, cholesterol, protein and salts, which helps to maintain the suppleness of hair and skin, and aids waterproofing of the epidermis. It also contains bactericidal chemicals. Sebum therefore helps to maintain the condition of the skin (the atmosphere is often drying) and contributes to the protective functions.

- Small arrector muscles (Figure 16.2). These are actually a part of the dermis and when stimulated cause the hairs to stand erect, a process called piloerection ('pili-' = hair). In animals this is an important thermoregulatory mechanism (see below); it also occurs during moments of anxiety and alarm (note how a cat appears to grow in size when alarmed; this is a threatening or defence response). The scarcity of body hair in humans makes these roles much less effective, although the thermoregulatory action probably contributes.

Nails

Fingernails and toenails consist of extremely hard, cornified epidermal cells. They provide protection for the tips of the fingers and toes, and aid the manipulation of small objects.

The root of the nail is hidden within the 'nail groove' at its base, and largely consists of a germinative matrix that produces the cells, which will comprise the main nail body (Figure 16.4). The proximal border of the nail and the epidermal cells of the nail groove are lined by a narrow band of epidermis called the cuticle (or eponychium). The nail body typically appears pink because the underlying epidermis is thin and so the blood vessels of the dermis are visible. The white crescent (or lunula) at the nail base is produced by the obscuring of the dermal blood by the thickened epidermal layer below this part of the nail body.

Dermis

The dermis is the subepidermal layer of the skin and is largely composed of connective tissue, including collagen and elastin fibres. These protein fibres provide the skin with durability and elasticity. The spaces between the fibres contain many of the structures associated with the skin (Figure 16.5):

- blood vessels;
- nerves;

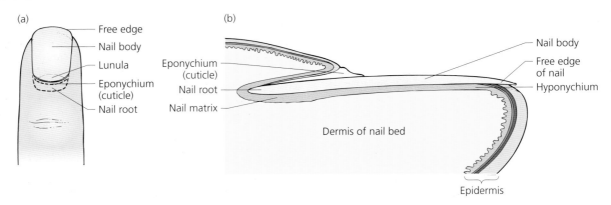

Figure 16.4 Structure of nails. (a) Fingernail viewed from above. (b) Sagittal section of fingernail and nail bed

Q Why are nails so hard?

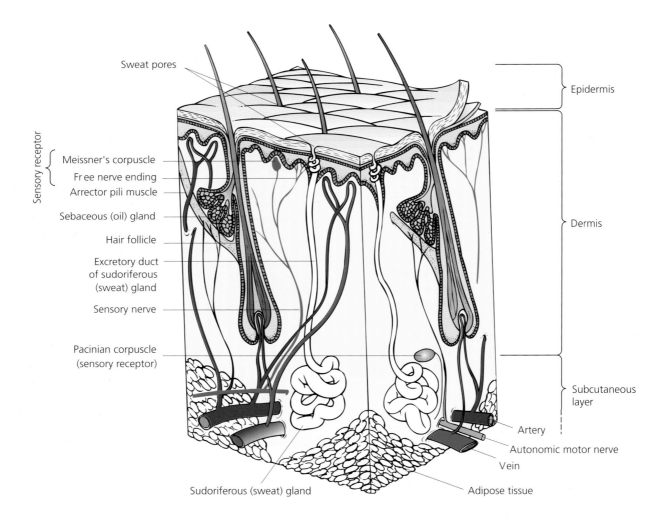

Figure 16.5 Structures of the dermis and subcutaneous layer. Note that hairs are derived epidermally and that sweat glands are actually present in the subcutaneous layer. Not shown are the collagen/elastin fibres, which form the matrix of the dermis

Q Which tissues constitute the dermis, and what are their functions?

Q List the functions of the subcutaneous adipose tissue.

BOX 16.10 LANGER'S LINES

These are not actually visible but relate to the orientation of collagen fibres within the dermis. Surgeons are aware of how the fibres are oriented in parts of the body and so will often make an incision in the axis of the fibres, rather then across them. The incision will then be stretched to reduce the need to cut further. In this way scarring is reduced, and the dermis is more likely to regain its structure afterwards.

BOX 16.11 BURNS

A classification of burns based only upon the visible extent of surface damage to the skin is now considered too simplistic. Thus, the assessment must take into account the depth of injury, if there is facial injury, if there are breathing difficulties, or if the site is prone to infection, for example in the perineal area.

Depth of injury is important because it influences the capacity for tissue regeneration (DeSanti, 2005). Thus:

- Partial thickness injury may be superficial and influence only the epidermis (also called first-degree burn) in which case healing will produce very good restoration of skin structure. Alternatively, there may be deep injury that affects some of the dermis (called second- or third-degree burn) in which case wound healing and a degree of regeneration is likely (but some scarring may occur) if the area damaged is not too extensive.
- Full thickness (or fourth-degree burn) injury includes the epidermis, dermis, and subdermal tissues such as muscle. This depth of damage will have destroyed any germinal cells and will require skin grafting.

Burns are also now classed as being major, moderate or minor: assessment includes the area of injury, site, proportion of full thickness trauma, recognition that children under 10 years have proportionately larger heads than adults (and very young children have immature immunity responses), and recognition that adults over 40 years exhibit poorer homeostatic control as a consequence of the ageing process.

Major burns are those in which:

- more than 25% of the body surface area (BSA) is damaged (more than 20% in children under 10 years and adults over 40 years) or
- more than 10% of BSA is full thickness injury, or
- the face, hands, feet, or perineal area are badly damaged, or
- there is inhalation injury, or
- there is pre-existing disease such as poor peripheral circulation.

Moderate burns are those in which:

- 15–25% of BSA is damaged (10–20% in children under 10 years and adults over 40 years), or
- less than 10% of BSA exhibits full thickness injury.

Minor burns are those in which:

- less than 15% of BSA is damaged (10% in children under 10 years and adults over 40 years), or
- less than 2% of BSA exhibits full-thickness injury.

A further complication of assessment is that electrical burns may be extensive internally, but may not be indicated by external signs.

There are a number of considerations in the intervention against burn injuries (Wiebelhaus and Hansen, 2001). In particular, wound healing must be promoted (including infection control), the flexibility of scar tissue, especially over joints, must be maintained, and fluid balance must be controlled. The effects on fluid balance arise because subepidermal 'wet' tissues are exposed leading to excessive dehydration. Inflammation of the site also leads to oedematous exudate. The latter is derived from the blood plasma and, if severe, can induce hypovolaemia and 'shock'. Intervention in this case must be aimed at preventing excessive disturbance of fluid balance and maintaining blood volume and pressure.

BOX 16.12 ULCERATION OF THE SKIN

Ulceration of the skin occurs when areas are subjected to prolonged ischaemia, leading to cell death (necrosis) and tissue atrophy. Decubitus ulcers are commonly observed in people who are immobilized, for example those people perhaps sitting for lengthy spells or confined to bed rest (and so commonly are referred to as 'bed sores'). Under such circumstances body weight acts on a point of skin, frequently the buttocks, sacrum or heels, and induces the ischaemia. The problem is exacerbated if cutaneous circulation is poor anyway, as in older people or people with diabetes mellitus. In such cases the skin may even ulcerate without the additional effect of weight.

Intervention is aimed at preventing prolonged ischaemia, and by promoting wound healing should ulceration occur. This latter process, however, can be very slow since granulation of repair tissue is itself dependent upon a reasonable blood supply to the area. The management of such wounds continues to provoke debate, especially in relation to the need to maintain hydration, nutrition and oxygenation of the wound. Interested readers are referred to Harding *et al.* (2000).

- sensory receptors (including touch and pressure receptors, thermoreceptors and pain receptors called nociceptors);
- hair follicles (though these are epidermal in origin);
- arrector muscles;
- ducts of subcutaneous glands (the glands themselves lie in the subcutaneous layer).

The upper region of the dermis has small projections called dermal papillae. These finger-like structures project into the epidermis. Such papillae contain touch-sensitive receptors (Meissner's corpuscles) and loops of blood capillaries that supply the active layers of the epidermis. These loops are vertically orientated and are visible as small pinpricks of blood when the epidermis is grazed. The papillae, which in the fingertips produce the 'fingerprints', are genetically determined and hence have a unique pattern in individuals.

Subcutaneous layer and glands

This layer consists of loose connective tissue, and adipose tissue, and attaches the dermis to the underlying tissues (Figure 16.5). The presence of relatively few collagen fibres means that:

- There is flexibility of movement of skin across the underlying tissue, and this helps to prevent shearing injuries caused by friction.
- The layer is readily distended and so it can accommodate storage of substantial amounts of fat, which provides an energy store but also a layer of insulation that reduces heat transfer from the body to environment (see later).
- From a clinical perspective, it provides an ideal site for injections, since the volume of injectate is more easily accommodated and therefore less painful.

The subcutaneous layer also contains two types of gland, the sweat (or sudoriferous) glands and the ceruminous glands (in the external ear). The ducts of these pass to the skin surface via the dermis and epidermis. Mammary glands are specialized sudoriferous glands but are not generally considered as glands of the skin; they are described in Chapter 18 (p.498).

Sweat glands

Sweat, or perspiration, is a mixture of water, salts and products of metabolism (e.g. urea, uric acid, amino acids, ammonia, lactic acid). The glands can be subdivided according to the type of sweat they produce, and therefore to their structure:

• Apocrine glands are simple tubular structures found in the skin of the armpits (axillae), pubic area, and the areolar areas of the breast. Their secretion is viscous because they contain metabolic substances such as fatty acids. These are also useful metabolic substrates for bacteria and growths of such organisms produce 'body odour'. Apocrine sweat also contains pheromones, particularly those that are sexual attractants.
• Eccrine glands are more widely distributed, though they are absent from lip margins, penis, labia minora and outer ear. They are simple, coiled tubular glands and produce a thin, watery secretion. Their main role is in temperature regulation since the evaporation of sweat from the body surface has cooling properties. The composition of eccrine sweat can be varied, however, particularly in relation to its sodium chloride content; this will occur in sodium chloride deficiency when the body is conserving this electrolyte.

Ceruminous glands

These are modified sweat glands found within the skin of the auditory canal. Their secretions are mixed with sebum (from sebaceous glands in the dermis) to form a sticky, wax-like substance called cerumen, or earwax. This provides a barrier to particulate matter and so protects the tympanic membrane. Occasionally, the secretion of cerumen may be excessive and induces conditions that promote troublesome bacterial growth. Hearing will also be impeded if excessive wax is present.

REGULATING BODY TEMPERATURE

Introduction: influence of temperature on cellular homeostasis

Metabolic reactions on the whole are more efficient if energy is put into them, and so temperatures that are suboptimal will reduce the rate of metabolism, as illustrated by the impact of hypothermia (see Box 16.15). In contrast, temperatures that are higher than optimal do not substantially raise metabolic rate, even though more energy is available to influence the process. In fact, the reverse is eventually observed. This is because the additional heat energy breaks the weak hydrogen bonds between amino acids within enzyme molecules, and this disturbs their three-dimensional shape such that they can no longer act as catalysts of chemical reactions (see Chapter 4, p.98). This is illustrated by the impact of hyperthermia (see Box 16.19, p.460). The temperature optimum is therefore a balance between the effects of heat to promote chemical reactions, and the rate at which heat denatures enzymes (Figure 16.6). The optimum temperature for most metabolic processes to occur in humans is about 37°C, but to be accurate this only applies to those tissues of the body 'core', that is, the tissues of the brain and organs of the chest and abdomen. The temperature of the 'core' is held near constant, via a homeostatic process that balances the rate of heat production by metabolism with the rate of heat transfer between the body and the external environment (i.e. across the skin and respiratory surfaces).

In contrast, the skin rarely attains a temperature of 37°C, except perhaps in very hot weather, and skin temperature can fluctuate quite considerably according to ambient conditions. The surface area of skin in an adult is some 1.8 m² and so provides the major site of heat transfer between the body and external environment. Controlling the rate of heat transfer across the skin, therefore, is an essential component of the regulatory process, hence the variability of the temperature at the skin surface. It is actually the limbs that provide the main sites for heat exchange because they have a large surface area relative to their volume, and at the kinds of ambient temperatures that we experience in the UK this usually means that the skin of the limbs is cooler than that of the chest and abdomen.

Heat balance

If the 'core' temperature of the body is to be kept constant, then the homeostatic equation must hold:

Equation 1:

$$\text{Heat gained by the body} = \text{Heat lost from the body}$$

• Heat gain is that produced by metabolism, although heat will also be gained if the environment is hotter than the body core (for example in a hot climate).
• Heat is lost from the body if the environment is cooler than the 'core' (the usual case in a temperate climate such as in the UK), or if evaporation of water can be promoted since this has a cooling effect (see below).

The physiology of temperature regulation, therefore, concerns the control of heat gain or loss, appropriate to needs. The receptors necessary to detect a change in 'core' temperature are located within the hypothalamus (see Chapter 8, p.172), and brain nuclei within this area provide the monitoring process and determine the homeostatic 'set point'. Other temperature receptors are found within the skin, but these too provide sen-

---

BOX 16.13 REMOVAL OF EXCESSIVE EAR WAX

If earwax becomes excessive then the individual may perceive a muffling of hearing in the ear, or possibly even soreness as the tympanic membrane becomes inflamed secondary to infection behind the wax.

If this is the case they may have the ears syringed to flush out the wax, possibly after a period of several days of softening the wax with a solution applied by dropper. The syringing should:

• be performed using the appropriate ear syringe (this syringe has a high degree of inertia that prevents the contents from being expelled at great pressure, with the resultant risk of damage to the tympanic membrane; it is also of high volume);
• use warmed, sterile 'normal' saline, since the temperature behind the tympanic membrane will be at 37°C;
• use a kidney dish held in place against the neck to collect the flushings.

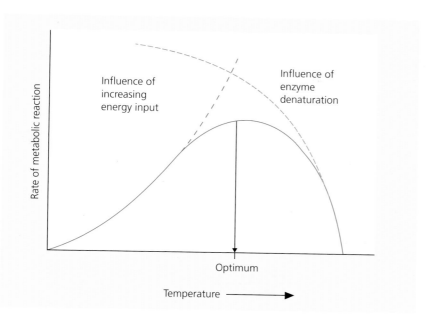

Q List four factors that determine the rate of metabolic reactions.

sory nervous input into the hypothalamic nuclei. These receptors (called Ruffini organs and Krauss end-bulbs) will detect a change in conditions at the body surface, and so homeostatic processes can be instigated even before consequential changes in 'core' temperature have occurred. Together, these central and peripheral thermoreceptors provide an efficient means of ensuring that 'core' temperature does not markedly change.

Basic principles of heat transfer

Heat is transferred to or from the environment by three main processes (Figure 16.7):

BOX 16.14 MEASURING BODY (CORE) TEMPERATURE

When body temperature is measured it is usually the core temperature that is of interest, but the core tissues themselves are internal. They can be accessed via the orifices of the body, namely the mouth, external ear and the anus, but the skin near the armpits can also give a reasonable measure of core temperature, if other routes are not possible, provided that heat is trapped in the armpit and temperature allowed to rise to that of the core tissues that lie close to the surface.

Body temperature is most often measured in a clinical setting using an electrical thermometer. This monitors the electrical resistance of a probe, which changes with its temperature, and so is very sensitive. These thermometers produce rapid readings and have good reproducibility. They also have an advantage in that unlike the traditional glass thermometers, they do not contain mercury, which is a toxic metal.

Temperatures recorded vary slightly according to site (Spitzer, 2008). For example, in adults:

- Oral temperature should be very close to 37 °C (36.9–37.1).
- Ear temperatures should be very similar to oral values, but it should be noted that values fall sharply if the thermistor is not close to the tympanum.
- Rectal temperature is usually slightly higher than the oral value, about 37.5 °C.
- Axilla (armpit) temperatures are usually slightly lower than oral values, about 36.5 °C.

- *Radiation*: any physical object at a temperature above 'absolute zero' (0 Kelvin or −273 °C) will radiate energy. The wavelength of the energy that is emitted is related to the actual temperature of the object. For example, the hot sun radiates energy at a range of wavelengths some of which constitute the 'visual' part of the light spectrum. In contrast, the radiated energy from humans is in the infrared region of the spectrum and can be visualized only by using appropriate aids. Radiated heat is normally the main way by which heat is lost or gained by the body. The rate of transfer is determined by the temperature gradient between the skin and external environment.

- *Conduction*: the direct transfer of energy between molecules that have made physical contact with each other. This will include contact between molecules within the skin and those of air or objects in contact with the skin. Once again, the rate of transfer is determined by the temperature gradient between the skin and external environment.

- *Evaporation*: converting water into vapour requires energy (584 calories/mL, or 2450 J/mL; this is called the 'latent heat of evaporation') and so the evaporation of sweat from the skin, or of water from the oral cavity and respiratory tract, are effective means of removing heat from the body.

Note that a fundamental principle that operates here is that the rate at which heat is transferred by radiation and conduction is determined by the temperature gradient that exists between the skin and external environment. Thus, heat will be lost if the skin is warmer than the surrounding environment; the greater the difference, the faster the rate of transfer. If it is cooler then heat will be gained from the environment. Note though that it is the immediate environment that is important here, that is, the environment in contact with or close to the skin surface, for example clothing or air trapped within it. Convection of air or water around the skin will introduce new

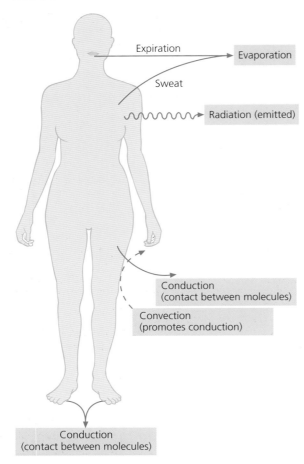

Figure 16.7 Routes of heat loss from the body. Note that heat gains by conduction and radiation will be promoted in hot environments

Q Discuss what is meant by the following terms with reference to heat transfer: (1) radiation, (2) conduction, and (3) evaporation.

environmental temperatures and therefore could promote further heat transfer across the skin. Thus convection is not of itself a route of heat transfer but it may facilitate (or even reduce) heat transfer particularly through the conduction route. This is why we feel a cooling effect from a breeze or fan.

Temperature regulation in cold climates

In cold, or just cool, environments the temperature gradient between the air and skin promotes heat loss from the body. Referring back to Equation 1, the homeostatic regulation of the 'core' temperature in cold conditions can utilize two strategies (Figures 16.8 and 16.9):

- First, the response may lower the temperature gradient between skin and air and so reduce the rate of heat loss via conduction and radiation.
- Second, the rate of metabolic heat production might be increased in order to compensate for the enhanced heat loss.

Of course, both strategies are applied but it is convenient to examine each separately.

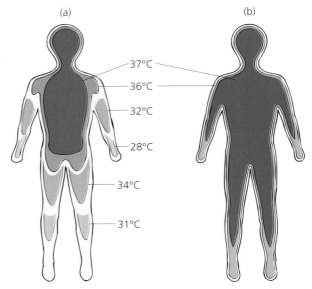

Figure 16.8 Temperature distribution in the body of a person at room temperatures of (a) 20°C and (b) 35°C. At the 20°C room temperature, the core temperature is restricted to the trunk and head. At the 35°C room temperature, a core temperature of 37°C extends almost to the surface of the body

Q Describe the homeostatic regulation of the core temperature when the body is subjected to cold environmental conditions and hot environmental conditions.

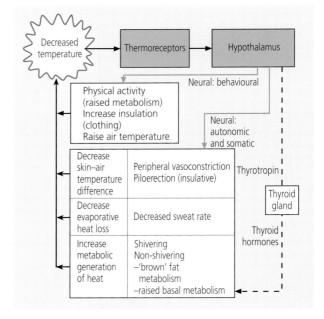

Figure 16.9 Flow chart of thermoregulatory responses to cooling. Note the range of effector mechanisms and tissues employed in the response

Decreasing the skin–air temperature gradient.

The strategies used to reduce the temperature gradient between skin and air while in a cool environment are the warming of air in contact with the skin or the reduction of the temperature of the skin itself.

Air warming

This can be widespread (e.g. by raising the central heating) or local through the warming of air close to the skin, irrespective of what the surrounding air temperature is, by externally insulating the body, or by physiologically stimulating arrector muscles of the skin that cause piloerection. Both will trap an unstirred layer of air against the skin and this will rapidly warm up because air has a low 'specific heat':

Specific heat = Heat required to raise the temperature of 1 g of substance (e.g. of air) by 1 °C.

The layer of air therefore provides us with a new skin–air interface that on warming establishes a more favourable skin–air temperature gradient. The insulative effect of the layer of warmed air is soon reduced, and rendered less effective, if air currents dislodge it, in other words by convectional currents, wind chill or fans.

A similar principle operates if the body is in water, but warming the water close to the skin requires a lot of heat since it has a high 'specific heat' and so requires a lot of energy to raise its temperature even by 1°C. This is one reason why people rapidly develop hypothermia (Box 16.15) if they fall into cold seas. However, if a thin layer of water can be confined (unstirred) at the skin surface it can form a highly effective insulation layer once it has warmed up. This is because specific heat can act to our advantage – water may require a lot of energy to warm up but it also has to lose substantial amounts to cool. Thus, once the layer is warmed it cools very slowly, especially if it is isolated from the wider environment by an insulator; this is the basis of the 'wet suit' in aqua sports.

Reducing the temperature of the skin

This is achieved by reducing the rate of blood flow to the skin, mediated by the activation of sympathetic nerves to the tissue which constrict the blood vessels. If conditions are extreme, then blood vessels in deeper subcutaneous tissues, especially in the limbs, will also be constricted. In this way the parts of the body that are at the 'core' temperature will actually contract in size (Figure 16.8) helping to ensure that absolutely vital tissues are protected. In freezing air it may be impossible for vasoconstriction to be maintained simply because of the intense cold, and the skin may then exhibit vasodilation. Although not profound, this 'flushing' is sufficient to help protect the skin from freeze damage. Thus, having 'rosy' cheeks when the weather is extremely cold does not necessarily mean that an individual is very warm; in reality they may be extremely cold.

Altering the pattern of blood flow in the limbs is another means of facilitating heat conservation. Venous blood, having cooled near the skin surface, drains into deeper veins that are in close anatomical arrangement with the arteries bringing warm blood into the limb from the 'core'. The close proximity of the vessels, and the opposite direction of blood flow between them, means that the venous blood is warmed by the arterial blood, and so returns some of the heat directly to the 'core'. This arrangement is called a 'countercurrent exchange' process.

BOX 16.15 HYPOTHERMIA

Hypothermia is a core temperature that is below normal limits. It normally arises from prolonged exposure to cold environments, but a tendency toward hypothermia is also observed in individuals with lowered metabolism because of deficient thyroid hormone secretion.

The effects of hypothermia on metabolic rate include a reduced heart rate, slowed reflexes, lethargy and poor mentation. Neurological and cardiac functions decline with progressive hypothermia, eventually leading to death. Sometimes, however, the cold produces such a profound decrease in metabolism that survival may actually be enhanced (being metabolically inactive means that cold tissues become hypoxic much more slowly). There are numerous instances of apparently 'miraculous' recoveries in people suffering prolonged cold exposure, and the principle of cooling is widely used in surgery and transplantation.

Body warming

In raising the temperature of an individual who is suffering from hypothermia it is important to raise body temperature slowly, because a sudden rise in blood temperature may promote physiological responses to cause heat loss, thus negating the improvements. Cell functions also are not very tolerant of sudden temperature changes. Blankets are ideal to prevent further heat loss, allowing heat produced by metabolism to accumulate within the body. Reflective blankets are even better because not only do they insulate and reduce conduction losses; they also reduce radiative losses by reflecting heat back onto the skin surface.

The loss of heat from skin can be reduced still further by the deposition of fat in subcutaneous tissue, since this tissue has a relatively low blood supply, and acts as an internal insulator that reduces the conduction of heat from within the body to the skin surface.

Increasing the metabolic rate

Chapter 4 described how most of the energy generated by cellular respiration is not harnessed by the cell, but is lost as heat. Raising the metabolic rate, called thermogenesis, is therefore an efficient means of generating additional heat in cold conditions. The means of generating heat can be placed into two categories: shivering (and exercise) and non-shivering thermogenesis.

Shivering

Shivering is a series of small, repeated involuntary muscular contraction–relaxation cycles, which increase the metabolic rate of the tissue. When shivering we may feel that the contraction cycles are out of control but in fact they are being coordinated by the hypothalamus, cerebral cortex and cerebellum. Shivering is extremely effective and, if severe, can double a person's total metabolic rate. It is, however, impractical as a long-term solution because it drastically impedes lifestyle, and so is best viewed as being a rapid but acute response to cold. Similarly, exercise is another excellent short-term measure to generate additional heat from muscle contraction.

Non-shivering thermogenesis

This involves an elevation of the 'basal' metabolic rate (i.e. the rate at which cells generate energy in the absence of extrinsic stimulation/physical activity). This makes it in principle a much more effective long-term adaptation to cold conditions. It is especially notable in infants in whom temperature regulatory processes are immature. 'Brown' fat is used to provide additional heat in order to compensate for the relatively high heat loss that is a consequence of having a high body surface area to volume ratio (Box 16.16). This adipose tissue is found mainly between the shoulder blades and is 'coloured' by the presence of extensive blood vessels (the more familiar 'white' fat has a poor vascularization). The tissue is supplied with sympathetic nerves and it is these that promote metabolism of the stored lipid. Little of the released energy is 'coupled' for cell metabolism (i.e. harnessed as ATP; see Figure 2.11, p.36) and so almost all of the heat is released into the blood, and is carried into the 'core'.

The capacity to generate additional heat without the inconvenience of shivering is an attractive mechanism for cold adaptation. However, adults do not have 'brown' fat reserves, and a role for non-shivering thermogenesis in adults in cold or cool climates is debatable. Some findings have implicated an increased release of thyroid hormones in the cold, which would alter basal metabolism throughout the body. This may be an important mechanism to those who live in Polar regions, but may be of too slow onset to be useful to those exposed to fluctuating temperatures during a winter season in the UK.

The 'comfort zone'

As we have seen, an air temperature that is considerably lower than that of the 'core' temperature promotes responses to conserve heat, primarily by reducing heat transfer to the environment. However, an air temperature that is similar to that of the core would also cause major difficulties. This is because heat is continually generated by metabolism and if the core temperature is to remain at 37°C then some of this heat must be lost from the body, otherwise body temperature would rise. Losing heat would be made difficult by an absence of a temperature gradient. An air temperature of around 24–25°C suffices to promote the loss of excess heat with little need to stimulate physiological mechanisms either to conserve it or promote its loss. This is termed a 'comfort zone' and provides an ideal living/working temperature, and for inactive people in hospital. There are instances, however, when a room temperature of 24–25°C can be uncomfortable, for example in certain types

of work when metabolism is much higher than usual, or in the presence of an elevated body temperature in fever, or metabolic responses to surgery or pain, or in the excessive muscle activity exhibited by people with respiratory problems.

Temperature regulation in hot climates

An air temperature above the comfort zone means that the rate of heat loss to the environment will begin to decrease, and so the balance between heat gained from metabolism and that lost from the body will be disturbed. Referring to Equation 1 from earlier, metabolic rates are little changed in hot spells, although appetite may be reduced, and so heat loss from the body must now be promoted. This will especially be the case if metabolism is increased, for example by physical activity. The strategies employed are to elevate the skin–air temperature gradient and promote sweat production. Again, both strategies will be used, but it is convenient to consider them separately.

Elevating the skin–air temperature gradient

In many ways these responses are the opposite of those described above for cold environments.

- The air temperature close to the skin may be cooled by reducing insulation (i.e. removing clothing, reducing piloerection) and by introducing air convection.
- Skin temperature is raised by vasodilation within the skin, which effectively expands the 'core' area into the periphery (see Figure 16.8). Some areas of skin such as the hands are very efficient at losing heat because they have a high surface area. A diagram of the cutaneous vasculature in these areas is shown in Figure 16.10. The feature to note is the presence of the arterial–venous 'shunt' (or anastomosis); that is, vessels that connect arterioles directly to venules thus bypassing capillaries. Dilation of these arterioles when we are hot

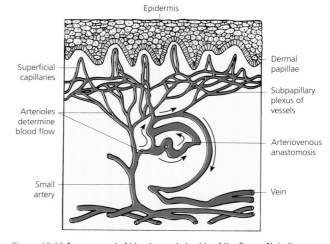

Figure 16.10 Arrangement of blood vessels in skin of the finger. Note the arterial–venous anastomosis. When patent, this will substantially increase the rate of blood flow through the skin by reducing the vascular resistance (arrows)

Q *Identify two situations when you would expect the skin vessels to vasodilate.*

BOX 16.16 TEMPERATURE REGULATION IN INFANTS

Temperature regulatory mechanisms in the neonate and infant are immature, and are compounded by the relatively large surface area to volume ratio as this favours heat loss. The surface area of the skin is the route of heat loss (in cool environments), whereas body volume influences the capacity to generate heat through metabolism. The high ratio in babies means that the newborn are very susceptible to environmental temperatures and so require a protected environment. Heat loss is partly compensated for by a metabolic rate that is relatively higher than in children and adults (non-shivering thermogenesis; see text), but hypothermia is a risk if infants are left exposed in cool environments.

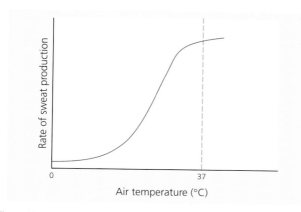

Figure 16.11 Influence of air temperature on the rate of sweat production. See also Table 16.1

Q Differentiate between apocrine and eccrine sweat glands.

Table 16.1 Relative rates of heat loss by evaporative and non-evaporative means. Note the relative importance of evaporative heat loss at high air temperatures.

Air temperature (°C)	20	25	30	35	40
Evaporative heat loss (% of total)	15	30	50	95	100
Non-evaporative (% of total)	85	70	50	5	0

Q How does evaporation help the body lose heat?

shunts blood directly into the venous system and so more blood per unit time can perfuse the skin, thus facilitating heat loss.

• The countercurrent exchange process identified earlier that helps to conserve heat in the cold would be counterproductive in warm weather, and so must be made less effective. This is achieved by directing venous blood draining the limb away from the deep veins (which lie adjacent to incoming arteries) to more superficial vessels, thus reducing the heat transfer from the arteries. This helps to explain why surface veins are more noticeable in warm weather or if someone is hot from fever or exercise.

Sweat production

As air temperature rises and begins to approach the 'core' temperature the capacity for changes in cutaneous blood flow to sustain an appropriate temperature gradient declines. Under these circumstances the evaporation of sweat from the body surface becomes the most effective means of removing heat from the body. Indeed, at very high air temperatures (>37°C), when the core–air temperature gradient is actually reversed, heat gain from the air will be promoted and so evaporation is the only physiological response available for temperature regulation (Figure 16.11 and Table 16.1). Sweating is mediated by autonomic (sympathetic) nervous activity, and secretion rates may be as high as 4 L/day. This figure is put into perspective if

BOX 16.17 PARADOXICAL SWEAT SECRETION IN SHOCK

Shock illustrates the role of the sympathetic nervous system in promoting sweat secretion, though in this condition it is normally out of context as it occurs in the absence of a need to lose heat. In circulatory shock, sympathetic activity is stimulated by the need to maintain blood pressure in the face of failing cardiovascular functioning. The symptoms of shock include a cool, pale skin as a consequence of increased peripheral resistance (see Box 12.28, p.354 and Figure 12.32, p.355) but paradoxically the individual will sweat. Clearly, the sweating is not caused by an elevated core temperature. It is in fact a secondary occurrence of the sympathetic outflow from the brain (ordinarily, such outflow would be observed in stress or exercise when losing heat by sweating would be entirely appropriate).

BOX 16.18 BODY TEMPERATURE REGULATION IN OLDER PEOPLE

Ageing reduces basal metabolic rate, decreases the effectiveness of autonomic activity to the skin, reduces the capacity to shiver (and to coordinate it) and decreases the numbers of sweat glands in skin. Physiological regulation of 'core' temperature is therefore less precise, with the result that it is more likely to move outside the homeostatic range and perhaps remain outside depending upon environmental conditions. Older people are therefore at much greater risk of hypothermia during cold spells (see Box 16.15), and hyperthermia in extremely hot weather (Box 16.19), than are younger individuals.

Major physiological effects	Thermoregulatory capabilities	°C
Death		
Proteins denature, tissue damage accelerates	Severely impaired	—44
Convulsions Cell damage	Impaired	—42
Disorientation		—40
Systems normal	Effective	—38
		—36
Disorientation	Impaired	—34
Loss of muscle control		—32
Loss of consciousness		—30
	Severely impaired	—28
Cardiac arrest		—26
Skin becomes cyanosed	Lost	—24
Death		

Figure 16.12 Normal and abnormal body temperatures, and their physiological effects

Q Why is it essential that the body has a narrow range of body (core) temperature?

Q Using information described in Chapter 22, outline how the body temperature fluctuates during a 24-hour period.

BOX 16.19 HYPERTHERMIA AND FEVER

Hyperthermia

Hyperthermia is an elevation of core temperature above normal limits. It may arise because of an inability to maintain an appropriate rate of heat loss (for example in hot climates) or because of elevated metabolism (for example transiently after heavy exercise; chronically in excessive thyroid hormone secretion states).

Neural tissues are most susceptible to a change in core temperature and nerve conduction velocity decreases at high temperatures as enzymes denature. The consequences are headache, mental confusion, delirium and lethargy (Figure 16.12). Disruption of integrative neural processes will also affect the control of other tissues already disturbed by the hyperthermia.

Fever

Hyperthermia arising from a fever (or pyrexia) is an indication that pathogenic infection has occurred. In this instance, the elevated temperature observed is actually a physiological response to the presence of substances (called pyrogens) released by the pathogens themselves, and/or by certain cells of the immune system that are activated by the infection. The pyrogens act on the hypothalamus to alter the 'set point', perhaps to 39°C or so, and hence even a 'normal' body temperature will be recognized by monitoring areas of the hypothalamus as being too low. The individual will then express feelings of being cold. Physiological mecha-

nisms such as shivering and vasoconstriction in the skin are implemented which raise 'core' temperature to the new homeostatic mean (Figure 16.13) and so the individual appears pale. In this way, core temperature rises. In clinical terms this represents a hyperthermia but note that it is physiologically induced.

As the pathogen is destroyed by immune responses, a point is reached when the amount of pyrogen released cannot sustain the new hypothalamic 'set point', and this then reverts to normal. The pyrexic temperature is now in excess of the homeostatic mean and the individual will report feeling hot. Heat loss is promoted by vasodilation in the skin, and by sweating, and so the skin will appear 'flushed' and clammy.

The advantage of such a process is that the pyrexia interferes with the metabolic enzymes of the pathogen, reducing its reproductive activities and making it more susceptible to attack by the immune system. The disadvantage is that our own metabolic processes are also affected and make us feel 'ill'. The level of hyperthermia that necessitates treatment is debatable, based on counterbalancing the impact it has on health and its impact on the pathogen. Some authorities advocate a temperature of 38°C or above, allowing a slight hyperthermia to occur. Interventions usually involve non-steroidal anti-inflammatory drugs, such as aspirin or paracetamol, since these reduce the actions of pyrogens to re-set the homeostatic set point.

See the case study of a febrile toddler, Section VI, p.664.

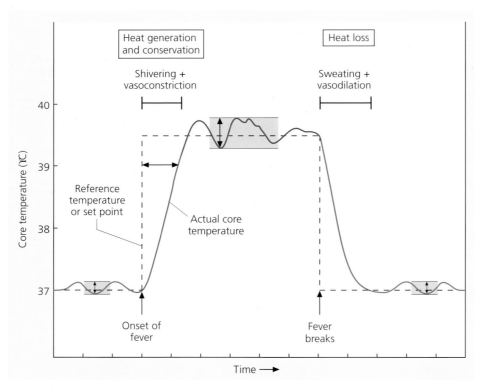

Figure 16.13 Time-course of a febrile episode. The actual body temperature lags behind the rapid shifts in set points. Note that regulation is normally maintained during the fever but that it is less precise, so temperature fluctuations are generally greater than normal

Q Describe the physiological changes associated with pyrexia (fever). See Figures 16.11 and 16.13.

Q What chemical initiates pyrexia? Refer to Chapter 13 if you have difficulty in answering this question.

one considers that the average volume of urine produced in 24 hours in a climate such as that of the UK is only about 1.5 L; the excessive loss of sweat will rapidly induce dehydration if renal compensation and thirst are ineffective.

Note, however, that sweating will only be effective at reducing body temperature if it can evaporate from the skin surface. High atmospheric humidity reduces the effect since the more

saturated with water the air becomes, the less likely it is that sweat will evaporate.

Factors that influence 'core' temperature

If the temperature regulatory mechanisms are intact then 'core' temperature is extremely well regulated with very little variation about the 'set point' of approximately 37°C, although very hot air temperature or high humidity may cause difficulties in maintaining heat loss, and may even promote a slight hyperthermia. The actual 'set point' is subject to slight variations within and between individuals and core temperature changes accordingly, although only by perhaps 0.5°C or so.

Circadian rhythmicity

Body temperature displays a 24-hour rhythmicity, linked into the day–night cycle, but which can be synchronized to match activity–rest cycles (see Figure 22.1, p.610).

Sex differences

Generally speaking, there is little difference between the core temperature of men and women. In women, however, there is a slight decrease in body temperature a few days prior to menstruation and this is maintained during the pre-ovulatory phase of the menstrual cycle. The change is less than 0.5°C (and so within the range of variation that occurs anyway) and appears to be associated with the low secretion of the hormone progesterone during this time. After ovulation body temperature rises again to 'normal'; the correlation between this rise in temperature and ovulation is useful in family planning, although the smallness of the change may make it difficult to observe.

Age

It was noted earlier how babies use non-shivering thermogenesis to elevate basal metabolism and compensate for excessive rates of heat loss. In fact the core temperature in young children (37.5–38°C) is actually higher than that found in adults.

SUMMARY

1 The skin is the largest organ of the body, the functions of which are closely associated with it being the physical barrier between the body and external environment. It is protective but also has a vital role to play in the regulation of body temperature.

2 In structure the skin consists of three layers: the epidermis, dermis and subcutaneous layers.

3 The epidermis forms the outer layer and consists of cells that eventually form the tough keratinized outer surface.

4 Nails and hair are modified epidermal structures that project into the dermis, a layer of connective tissue that contains blood vessels, neurons and various other structures.

5 The subcutaneous layer contains the sweat glands, the ducts of which project through the dermis and epidermis. Sweat performs an important role in temperature regulation but also influences fluid balance and provides a protective role.

6 Body temperature regulation is essential if the functioning of vital tissues is to be optimal, and so the temperature of the body 'core' is tightly controlled.

7 Constancy of 'core' body temperature can only be achieved if heat generation from metabolism is balanced by appropriate rates of heat loss, particularly across the skin. Changes in heat exchange with the environment are the main responses to adverse environments, but changes in the metabolic rate may also play a role, particularly in the cold.

8 The role of the skin in conserving or promoting heat loss is facilitated by its structure, by the influence of sympathetic nerves on its blood supply and by the presence of sweat glands.

9 Hyperthermia and hypothermia usually represent states in which the capacity to regulate body temperature is inadequate or has been compromised. The exception is hyperthermia produced by fever.

10 Fever is a physiological response to infection and results from a resetting of the homeostatic set point. It probably helps to reduce the metabolic activity of the invading pathogen and so reduces the rate of spread of infection.

11 Factors such as circadian rhythmicity, ageing and ovulation influence 'core' temperature.

REFERENCES

Beldon, P. (2003) Skin grafts 1: theory, procedure and management of graft sites in the community. *British Journal of Community Nursing Supplement* **8**(6): 8–18.

DeSanti, L. (2005) Pathophysiology and current management of burn injury. *Advances in Skin and Wound Care* **18**(6): 323–34.

Harding, K., Cutting, K. and Price, P. (2000) The cost-effectiveness of wound management protocols of care. *British Journal of Nursing* **9**(19, Suppl.): S6–S27.

McQuestion, M. (2006) Evidence-based skin care management in radiation therapy. *Seminars in Oncology Nursing* **22**(3): 163–73.

Nazarko, L. (2007) Maintaining the condition of ageing skin. *Nursing and Residential Care* **9**(4): 160–3.

Spitzer, O.P. (2008) Comparing tympanic temperatures in both ears to oral temperature in the critically ill adult. *Dimensions of Critical Care Nursing* **27**(1): 24–9.

Wiebelhaus, P. and Hansen S.L. (2001) What you should know about managing burn emergencies. *Nursing* **31**(1): 36–42.

CHAPTER 17

SKELETAL MUSCLES: POSTURE AND MOVEMENT

INTRODUCTION

Muscles cells are capable of changing their length and shape, and so produce movement or (as we shall see later) may actually prevent it. The changes are the result of interactions between specialized muscle proteins, present in all three types of muscle tissue found in the body – smooth, cardiac and skeletal – which all utilize a similar means of contracting, though they have different cellular anatomy, rate of contraction and control mechanisms. In addition, some other cells can become contractile by producing these proteins on occasion, for example the myofibrocytes ('myo-' = muscle) involved in drawing together surfaces of wounds during healing, and in any cells during the separation of chromosomes during cell division. However, it is skeletal muscle that is associated with the movement of the skeleton, and so it is this type of muscle that is considered in detail in this chapter.

The 'skeletomuscular system' enables us to maintain a posture against gravity, and to change posture for movement and mobility. Being mobile has a number of beneficial actions in addition to providing independence:

- It prevents loss of bone mass by helping to maintain the density of bone mineral.
- It prevents loss of muscle protein since muscle mass is influenced by the work load (see later in this chapter).
- It improves blood circulation through the limbs and so reduces the likelihood of venous thrombosis (see the case study of a woman with deep vein thrombosis, Section VI, p.651).

Chapter 3 considered the supporting role of the skeleton but also noted how movable joints within it means that maintaining a posture against gravity would not be possible without the actions of muscles to stabilize them. The muscles must also be capable of imparting movement; the control of posture and movement are part of the same mechanisms. In describing the functional anatomy of the brain, Chapter 8 also identified significant areas of the brain that are involved in the control of muscle contraction, notably the motor cortex, basal ganglia, cerebellum and parts of the brainstem. Such extensive involvement tells us that the control of posture and movement is highly coordinated and very complex. This chapter therefore considers the fundamental features of muscles, muscle cells and muscle contraction, but also provides an overview of the control of muscle contraction by involuntary (i.e. reflexes) and voluntary means.

OVERVIEW OF SKELETAL MUSCLE ANATOMY AND PHYSIOLOGY

Most skeletal muscle lies immediately below the skin; in fact there are over 600 muscles in the body (identifying individual muscles can be challenging – some suggest that there are over 800 muscles). Some are tiny, for example those muscles that move the ossicles of the middle ear, whereas others are substantial, for example the gluteus maximus of the buttock. There is no common approach to the naming of muscles, other then using 'Classical' terminology, but the nomenclature can be related to various features of the muscle, for example:

- muscle shape (e.g. the deltoid muscle of the shoulder is delta- or triangular-shaped);
- muscle size (e.g. the gluteus maximus muscle of the buttock);
- muscle location (e.g. the tibialis anterior lies in front of the tibia bone of the shin);
- muscle attachments (e.g. the sternohyoid muscle is attached to the sternum and hyoid bones);
- number of 'heads' of muscle origin (e.g. the biceps muscle of the upper arm has two 'heads'; 'cep-' = head);
- movement type (e.g. levator indicates that a muscle lifts something);
- axis of muscle fibres relative to bone (e.g. transversus).

The situation is made even more complex because frequently the nomenclature of muscles relates to more than one feature, for example:

(a)

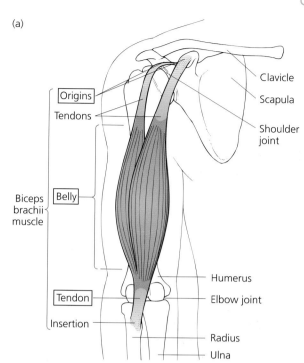

Clavicle

Scapula

Shoulder joint

Origins

Tendons

Biceps brachii muscle

Belly

Humerus

Tendon

Elbow joint

Insertion

Radius

Ulna

Figure 17.1 General appearance of muscle. (a) Muscle 'belly', insertion and origin. (b) Fascicle arrangements

Q Distinguish between the origin and insertion of a muscle.

Activity

Extend an arm and place the fingertips of your opposite hand over the biceps muscle of the upper arm. Slowly contract the biceps so that the arm bends at the elbow. It should be possible to feel the contraction occurring under the skin surface. Notice how the contraction occurs along the axis of the humerus bone of the upper arm, causing the forearm to rise in line with the upper arm. How does the arrangement of muscle fibres facilitate this?

From Figure 17.3, p.466 identify the type of lever that the elbow is classified as. How does the site of muscle attachment to the bones also help to facilitate the movement?

(b)

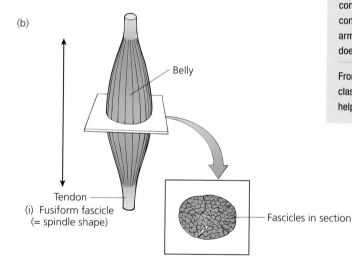

Belly

Tendon

(i) Fusiform fascicle (= spindle shape)

Fascicles in section

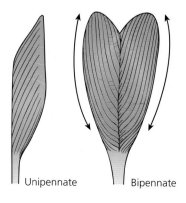

Unipennate

Bipennate

(ii) Pennate fascicle

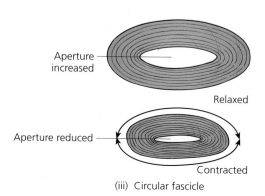

Aperture increased

Relaxed

Aperture reduced

Contracted

(iii) Circular fascicle

Levator	palpebrae	superioris
= lifter	lip	upper

(i.e. the name indicates both its position and action).

It is beyond the scope of this book to consider all muscles individually, and the interested reader is referred to the many available texts that do so. There are, however, some generic aspects of muscle structure and function that must be described if the role of muscle and process of muscle contraction is to be understood. These are muscle architecture and general anatomy, muscle histology and the mechanism of muscle contraction.

Muscle architecture and general anatomy

Generally speaking each muscle has a wide central region, or belly, and two ends which attach to other tissues, usually bone or cartilage (Figure 17.1a,b), though some muscles have more than one attachment at the same end, e.g. biceps ('bi-' = 2), quadriceps ('quad-' = 4). The connection to bone is provided by tendons (Figure 17.1a), tough cords of connective tissue that are extensions of the connective tissue of muscle and bone; the tendons therefore provide continuity between the two, and strength in that connection.

Tendons may be single or complex structures. For example:

- The 'Achilles' tendon, colloquially named after the Greek hero, is the largest single tendon in the body and attaches the large muscle of the calf (the gastrocnemius) to the heel bone (calcaneus; the technical name for the tendon is the calcaneal tendon).
- In the abdominal wall and in the palms of the hands the tendons of muscles combine to form a larger sheet-like structure called an aponeurosis.

Muscles are covered in layers of dense connective tissue, called the 'deep fascia' (there is also a superficial fascia, or subcutaneous layer, between muscle and skin; see Chapter 16, p.453). For many muscles the deep fascia acts to separate them and so enables them to function independently (Figure 17.2a). Below the deep fascia lie three distinct sheaths of connective tissue that provide support for the muscle fibres and whole muscle, and convey blood vessels, lymphatic vessels and nerves into the muscle structure. These sheaths are:

- *The epimysium ('epi-' = upon; 'myo-' = muscle)*: encloses the entire muscle.
- *The perimysium ('peri-' = surrounding)*: extends from the epimysium into the muscle itself and encloses bundles of muscle cells. The length of skeletal muscle cells means that they are often referred to as muscle 'fibres' (Figure 17.2b). Each bundle of muscle fibres is called a fascicle.
- *The endomysium ('endo-' = inner)*: which covers individual muscle fibres.

Muscle size

Muscles vary considerably in size, according to how many muscle fibres (cells) are present, the diameter of individual fibres, and the length of the muscle belly. These are all features

---

BOX 17.1 WORKLOAD AND MUSCLE MASS

The amount of work done (by a person or machine) is calculated as:

$$\text{Work} = \text{Force} \times \text{Distance}$$

As noted in the text, an athlete who regularly lifts heavy weights exhibits an adaptive change in muscle bulk, leading towards a 'Mr Universe' physique. In contrast, another athlete who regularly runs marathons may also be 'superfit' but will tend to have a very slim, wiry physique. This apparent paradox is not as contradictory as it seems. The point is that load relates to the weight or resistance encountered during the movement. For a marathon runner this simply equates to the weight of the limbs during each step, hence the very different physique from the weight lifter.

Understanding the relationship between (work) load and muscle mass also helps in recognizing why the main anti-gravity postural muscles in the body are so substantial relative to others in the body. Upon standing, such muscles must support joints against the force of gravity, and their bulk provides a reminder of how significant this force is. In particular:

- The erector spinae muscles of the back (a group of muscles with several components) have to be substantial to stabilize the back and so facilitate an erect vertebral column and head.
- The gluteus maximus of the buttock has to be substantial to stabilize the hip joint against gravity, and so facilitate an erect posture.
- The quadriceps femoris of the thigh has to be substantial to stabilize the knee joint against gravity and so facilitate leg extension.

---

related to the role of the particular muscle. For a given muscle its size is to a large extent predetermined because the length of the belly and the number of muscle fibres are a developmental feature. However, the diameter of individual muscle fibres, and hence the muscle itself, may be altered by the work performed by the muscle. Thus, regularly lifting heavy weights will stimulate protein synthesis in the biceps muscles and will in time lead to a greater muscle mass. The change in mass is an adaptation to subjecting the muscle to an increased workload as its strength correlates with its cross-sectional diameter. Conversely, someone who is immobile will have less frequent usage of muscles, with less load bearing, and the muscle protein content will fall accordingly; muscles reduce in mass, size and strength. Similar processes also operate in smooth and cardiac muscle. For example, the heart enlarges if an individual undertakes regular exercise. This influence of load on muscle mass is sometimes explained by the maxim 'use it or lose it'.

Fascicle organization

The arrangement of fascicles influences the appearance and direction of contraction of muscle (see Figure 17.1b).

The fascicles may run in parallel to the long axis of the muscle, in which case the muscle is referred to as either a 'fusiform' (spindle-shaped; the muscle has a distinct belly) or a 'strap' type. Fusiform types such as the biceps of the upper arm are generally able to generate a greater force of contraction than strap types of muscle such as the rectus abdominis muscle of the anterior abdominal wall because the muscle belly is more substantial. Note that the arrangement of fascicles will mean that the muscle fibres that make up a fascicle will also be in the

(a)

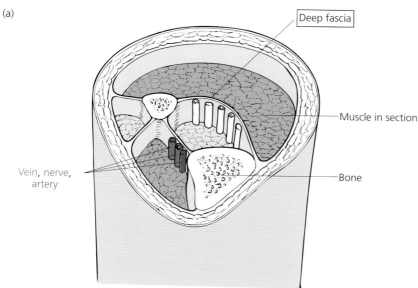

Deep fascia

Muscle in section

Bone

Vein, nerve, artery

Figure 17.2 Connective tissue sheathing of muscle. (a) Deep fascia between muscles. (b) Sheaths within a muscle

Q Name the connective tissue surrounding muscle fibres, separating them into fascicles.

(b)

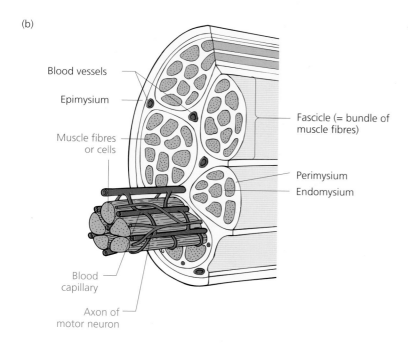

Blood vessels

Epimysium

Muscle fibres or cells

Blood capillary

Axon of motor neuron

Fascicle (= bundle of muscle fibres)

Perimysium

Endomysium

long axis of the muscle. Thus contraction will shorten the muscle along this axis.

Fascicles may be arranged obliquely to the long axis of the muscle, which gives the muscle a feather-like appearance (see Figure 17.1b). These are referred to as pennate-type muscles ('penna' = feather) and are generally stronger than strap or fusiform types. The direction of contraction will follow the fascicles and so pennate muscles will shorten in more than one axis. An example is the deltoid muscle of the shoulder, which is particularly important in maintaining the position of the shoulder girdle. The shoulder is a 'ball and socket' joint with a wide degree of possible movement and so a pennate-type muscle provides useful support here.

Fascicles may be arranged in a circular pattern around an aperture (see Figure 17.1b). Contraction of these muscles causes a change in aperture size and they are found, for example, around the mouth and form the external sphincters around the anus and urethra.

Muscle arrangement in relation to associated bones

The contraction of a skeletal muscle will usually cause a bone to move, but normally only the bone to which one end of the muscle is attached will move. This is called the 'insertion' end of the muscle; the stationary end is called the 'origin'. For example, bending the elbow involves contraction of the biceps

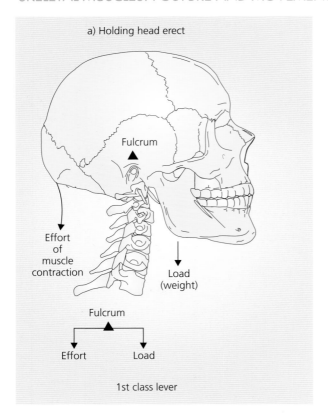

a) Holding head erect

Fulcrum

Effort of muscle contraction

Load (weight)

Fulcrum

Effort　　　Load

1st class lever

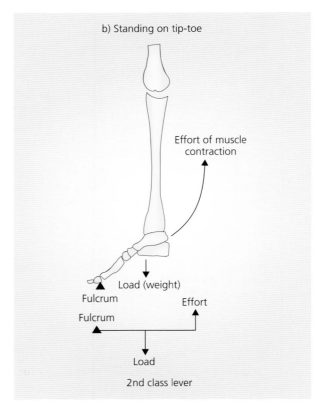

b) Standing on tip-toe

Effort of muscle contraction

Load (weight)

Fulcrum

Fulcrum

Effort

Load

2nd class lever

Figure 17.3 Skeletomuscular levers. The three classes of lever are shown. These differ in the arrangement between the pivotal point (fulcrum), the position of the load (weight) and the direction of muscle contraction (effort) that is required to move the load

Q What is the function of the following muscles: (1) an agonist (prime mover), (2) a synergist and (3) an antagonist?

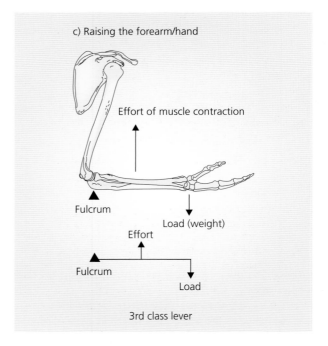

c) Raising the forearm/hand

Effort of muscle contraction

Fulcrum

Load (weight)

Effort

Fulcrum

Load

3rd class lever

muscle of the upper arm, and this has its origin in the shoulder, and its insertion in the forearm. The mode of movement varies, however, according to the particular situation and sometimes the origin end becomes the insertion end. In other words such terms are relative but are helpful when disorders of specific movements are described.

Levers

The force of contraction developed by a muscle must be sufficient to move the load placed upon it. In other words the muscle will have to work against the weight of the bone, tissues associated with the bone, body weight, or perhaps an object to be lifted. Muscle strength (and fascicle arrangement) helps provide the power required, but this is also facilitated by the position of muscle insertion relative to the joint to be controlled. Thus, skeletal muscles use a system of levers (Figure 17.3), in which the bone to be moved acts as the 'arm' of the lever, and the movement acts about the joint or fulcrum. The resistance to be overcome is the load. The arrangement of muscle, lever arm and fulcrum varies (referred to as type 1, 2 or 3 levers) but a general principle is that the further the muscle insertion is away from the fulcrum the greater the leverage will be. In this way more power can be generated when the insertion is some distance from the joint than if the same muscle was inserted close to the joint. However, the movement will be slower.

Levers enable considerable forces to be generated. Without leverage it would, for example, be difficult to stand from a squatting position unless we had a much greater muscle bulk. Levers also help us to lift considerable weights, again without the need for excessively bulky muscles.

Structure of muscle cells ('muscle fibres')

Skeletal muscle cells have numerous nuclei and this identifies that a skeletal muscle 'cell' is actually derived from a large number of cells that have fused to form a long fibre-like structure (Figure 17.4), hence the term 'muscle fibre'. Many muscle fibres are as long as the muscle itself; for example in the quadriceps femoris of the thigh the fibres extend the length of the thigh. The advantage of this differentiation is that the entire muscle fibre functions as though it is a single cell, even one as long as the thigh, and so a muscle can be induced to contract rapidly and efficiently throughout its length.

The microscopic anatomy of muscle fibres has many things in common with other cells, for example the presence of nuclei and mitochondria. However, there are features that give muscle fibres specialized functions (Figure 17.4a):

- The cell membrane is distinguished from that of other cells by being called sarcolemma ('sarco-' = flesh). This has

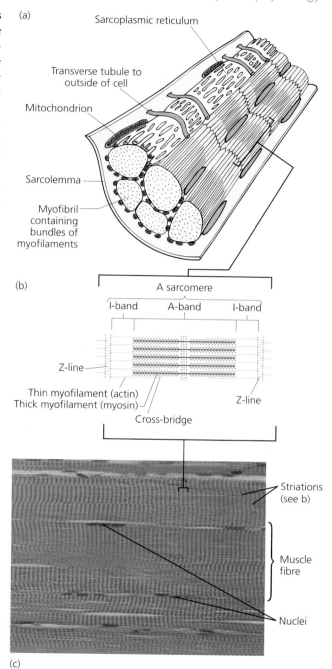

Figure 17.4 Muscle fibre histology and microfilament arrangement. (a) Intracellular features (see text for explanation). (b) Filament arrangement. I-band: striation due to actin filaments only. A-band: striation due to myosin and myosin/actin overlap. (c) Light microscopy photograph of a muscle fibre to show striations

Q Identify the scientific names of thin and thick muscle fibres.

BOX 17.2 MUSCLE STRAIN ('PULLED' OR 'TORN' MUSCLE)

A strain arises when excessive force, stretching or overuse causes microscopic tearing of muscle fibres. Treatment is as described in relation to joint sprains (see Box 3.13, p.85). Basically, a cold compress is used to reduce swelling and the muscle is immobilized as much as is practicable, using support where necessary. Use of the muscle should eventually be encouraged but return to full usage should be gradual.

The high degree of complexity of the muscle fibre, however, means that skeletal muscle is largely a 'stable' tissue in that its cells cannot divide once the fibres have formed. This means that the healing of a 'torn' muscle will include scar tissue. Being less elastic than muscle tissue (and of course non-functional), the muscle may lose some of its efficiency. There are small numbers of undifferentiated stem cells present and these can differentiate anew, but there are not enough to compensate fully if tissue damage is extensive.

Under extreme situations, when muscle damage is extensive and immobility prolonged, scar tissue may even become ossified, reducing elasticity still further. This is referred to as myositis ossificans.

numerous connections (synapses) with nerve cells, and is capable of depolarizing in a similar way to nerve cells (see Figure 8.21, p.188 for explanation of depolarization). The sarcolemma also has tubular invaginations, called transverse or T-tubules, and these are responsible for conveying the electrical signals into the cell (to the cisternae, below).

- Cytoplasm in muscle fibres is referred to as sarcoplasm, within which some organelles are modified. For example the sarcoplasmic reticulum is analogous to the endoplasmic reticulum of other cells (see Figure 2.3, p.24) but it extends into the fibre and helps to convey calcium ions, released from stores in distended areas termed cisternae, to the contractile proteins where they activate the contractile process (explained below). The calcium ions are taken up into the cisternae once again after the contraction has finished.

- The inner core of the muscle fibre is comprised of numerous minute fibre-like structures called myofibrils, which run longitudinally along the fibre, in close association with the sarcoplasmic reticulum and its cisternae. Each fibril consists of a precise arrangement of smaller, thread-like structures of protein called myofilaments (Figure 17.4a).

- Microscopically the myofilaments appear as overlapping thick and thin threads: thick ones are composed of a protein called myosin, thin ones of one called actin.

- The arrangement of mysosin and actin shown in Figure 17.4b is precise and repeats along the length of the muscle fibre in distinct functional segments; each segment of banding is called a sarcomere ('meros' = part). When viewed under the microscope a banding pattern is apparent in each sarcomere: a pale band of actin only (the so-called I-band; Figure 17.4b), and a darker band where actin and myosin overlap (the A-band). Intermediate banding occurs, for example where myosin is found alone. The arrangement makes the fibre appear to have stripes of light and dark areas and so skeletal muscle is frequently referred to as striped or striated muscle (Figure 17.4c).

DETAILS OF MUSCLE CONTRACTION

The contraction of a whole muscle necessitates the contraction of the individual muscle fibres of which it is composed. Common processes are involved in contracting the fibres, but the behaviour of the whole muscle, and the actual tension developed within it as a consequence of contraction, can vary. This section, therefore, initially considers the events that occur when a muscle fibre contracts, but continues by exploring whole muscle responses.

Contraction of an individual muscle fibre

There are two main aspects to the contraction of a muscle fibre: the stimulation of the muscle fibre by a nerve cell and the consequential events leading to the actual contraction referred to as the 'sliding filament mechanism'.

Innervation of muscle fibres

The nerve cells that cause muscle fibres to contract are collectively referred to as 'motor' neurons. The peripheral neurons for the spinal cord to the muscles are referred to as 'lower motor neurons'. Those that are present within the cord and brain, are referred to as 'upper motor neurons' and are considered later in this chapter in relation to voluntary movements. Lower motor neurons terminate at the muscle fibre in a structure referred to as the 'neuromuscular junction'.

The neuromuscular junction is actually a form of synapse, that is, the junction between two nerve cells. The synapse at the neuron–muscle fibre interface is illustrated in Figure 17.5. Its structure is somewhat different from that of a neuron–neuron synapse, detailed in Chapter 8 (see Figure 8.23, p.190), and it is called a motor end-plate to distinguish it from such synapses. However, the end-plate functions in much the same way as other synapses, and utilizes acetylcholine as the neurotransmitter chemical. Acetylcholine is released from the endings of the nerve cell by the arrival of an electrical impulse and causes a depolarization of the sarcolemma. The electrical current generated within the sarcolemma is then transmitted to the T-tubules and initiates the release of calcium ions from intracellular stores.

A muscle fibre forms numerous synapses along its length with terminals from the same nerve cell. In this way, if the nerve cell is active then impulses directed along the terminals

---

BOX 17.3 ALTERED MUSCLE FUNCTION CAUSED BY FIBRE DEFECTS

Muscle weakness caused by muscle fibre defect occurs when the fibre is deficient in protein filaments, if the sarcolemma structure prevents it from being electrically stimulated, or if there is a metabolic defect.

Protein deficiency
Protein filaments in muscle fibres are adversely affected in malnutrition and uncontrolled diabetes mellitus when the protein is utilized as an energy substrate, and in prolonged immobility when the lack of physical stress removes the need for muscles to produce a large force of contraction. Correction of muscle fibre disorder is directed at removing the underlying causes, and physiotherapy to maintain existing muscle, through the effects of loading on muscle bulk and strength (see Box 17.1, p.464).

Sarcolemma disorder
- Myotonia is a term used when the sarcolemma is over-excitable, arising from a defect that makes it difficult for the membrane to repolarize

after being stimulated. Without adequate repolarization the muscle demonstrates progressive weakness. Duchenne muscular dystrophy is a sex-linked inherited defect in the gene for a sarcolemma protein called dystrophin. The lack of dystrophin leads to eventual wastage typical of this disorder.
- Periodic paralysis is poorly understood and is characterized by intermittent episodes of muscle weakness. In some instances the problem seems to be linked to excess potassium ions in extracellular fluid (hyperkalaemia).

Metabolic deficiency
These problems are rare and include defects in the breakdown of glycogen from muscle stores (to provide glucose for respiration) or in the formation of creatine phosphate (for ATP production – see text). This group of disorders includes toxic alcohol myopathy in which cramps and severe weakness arises as a consequence of alcohol abuse.

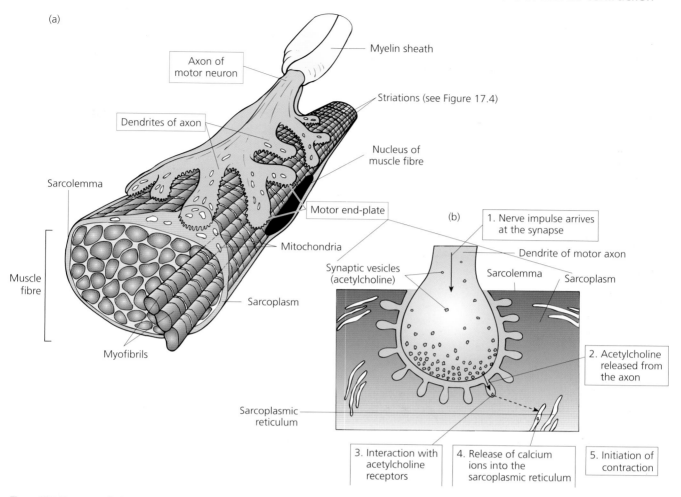

Figure 17.5 Neuromuscular junction. (a) The motor end-plate. (b) Detail of the synapse: 1–5 identify stages in stimulation of muscle contraction

Q Describe the roles of the components at a neuromuscular junction.

will stimulate the entire fibre length, thus ensuring that the whole fibre contracts simultaneously. For surgical procedures it is often useful to relax muscles before commencing the procedure, and this is achieved by blocking the actions of acetylcholine at the neuromuscular junctions, using drugs such as vecuronium or suxamethonium.

Sliding filament mechanism of muscle fibre contraction

Before commencing this section, readers should first ensure that they are familiar with muscle fibre structure, as outlined in the earlier section entitled 'Structure of muscle cells'.

The electrical activity generated at the motor end-plate (above) causes a muscle fibre to contract by initiating an interaction between the contractile proteins of the myofilaments, the myosin and actin proteins. The interaction entails a movement of the actin filaments over the myosin and the process is usually referred to as the sliding filament mechanism of muscle fibre contraction, though this is a somewhat misleading term because the filaments do not 'slide' in the conventional sense, but move via a ratchet-type of mechanism.

Figure 17.6 illustrates how the process is thought to operate:

- When electrical activity from the motor end-plate passes along the T-tubules it causes calcium ions to be released from stores within the cisternae, into the sarcoplasmic reticulum. This meshwork of microscopic tubes enables the ions to pass toward the myofilaments at the centre of the fibre.
- Proteins associated with the actin, called troponin and tropomyosin, distort and expose 'active' sites on the actin molecule that can now interact with complementary sites on the adjacent myosin filaments.
- The chemical bonds between these proteins distorts the myosin and this 'pulls' the actin filament over the myosin. The myosin sites then detach and move to the next active sites on the actin and the process is repeated. In this way the actin is pulled further along the myosin in a process analogous to a ratchet mechanism, but the whole process is very rapid and as many as 100 repeat interactions can occur per second.

BOX 17.4 ALTERED MUSCLE FUNCTION CAUSED BY PERIPHERAL NERVE DISORDER

A failure of peripheral nerves to supply muscles, or to stimulate them, will result in muscle weakness and even paralysis. For example, crushing the nerve, such as happens when an intervertebral disc has prolapsed, or if muscles of the lower back undergo spasm contractions, will affect associated muscle function and induce severe pain. There are significant disorders of lower motor neurons that affect muscle control, and they are identified below. Note though that nerve activity in motor neurones derives from the central nervous system (CNS) and there also are various disorders associated with the functioning of upper motor neurones or brain ganglia; these are considered later in Box 17.13 (p.482).

Disorder of peripheral nerves
The most prevalent peripheral neural disorder is that of peripheral neuritis, or Guillain–Barré syndrome, arising from viral infection of nerve endings. The inflammation tends to track along the nerve cells, and even into the CNS. In doing so there is ascending muscle weakness. Reflexes are absent in affected areas. As the weakness ascends it may affect respiratory function and swallowing. Corticosteroid drugs may help to reduce the inflammation but care is largely targeted at psychological support, and monitoring for signs of breathing or swallowing difficulties, and the provision of ventilation or nasogastric feeding as necessary until recovery occurs (Worsham, 2000). The individual will require rehabilitation therapy to regain mobility.

Motor neurone disease (MND) is a collection of disorders in which anterior horn cells (i.e. motor neurones) in the spinal cord and periphery are destroyed. A common disorder in adults is amyotrophic lateral scle-

rosis (ALS), in which there is a progressive and ultimately fatal degeneration (Attarian *et al.*, 2008). Muscle weakness and wasting occurs, though cramps may also be observed. The cause of ALS is not known; suggestions include damage caused by excess glutamate (an excitatory neurotransmitter in the anterior horn), autoimmunity or damage from oxidative biochemical processes within cells.

Neuromuscular junction defects
Myasthenia gravis is an autoimmune condition in which the actions of acetylcholine as a neurotransmitter is inadequate because antibodies have removed postsynaptic receptors to it. The condition normally affects extraocular muscles in its early stages, leading to difficulties in controlling eye movement and drooping eyelids (called ptosis). Facial muscles may become involved, producing a mask-like expression. Speech and swallowing difficulties are apparent if the muscles of the neck are affected. Muscle weakness throughout the body appears in later stages.

Drugs that antagonize the enzyme acetylcholine esterase (e.g. neostigmine) can help to improve muscle function since they slow the breakdown of acetylcholine by postsynaptic receptors, thus potentiating its actions on remaining receptors. Care includes monitoring for side-effects arising from drug interactions with (acetyl)cholinergic synapses elsewhere, for example abdominal cramps, diarrhoea, salivation and bronchial secretion from interactions with the parasympathetic nervous system, and irritability, headaches and insomnia from CNS actions (Cunning, 2000).

- Within a sarcomere, the ratchet-like movement of the actin myofilaments occurs towards just one end of the actin molecule, close to the middle of the sarcomere. The other ends of the actin (the I-band; see Figure 17.4b, p.467) are attached to a structure, called the Z-line, that lies transversely across the muscle fibre and marks the boundary of each sarcomere. As a consequence of the myosin–actin interaction the Z-lines at each end of the sarcomere are pulled towards each other, rather like drawing a pair of curtains, and so the sarcomere reduces in length (Figure 17.7).
- The shortening of all sarcomeres in the muscle fibre means that the entire fibre shortens.
- Contraction ends when nerve activity ceases, and calcium ions are taken up again into the cisternae. The actin then moves back to its original position; in other words the fibres (and hence muscle) relax.

Myosin also acts as an enzyme that can split adenosine triphosphate (ATP), and so cause the release of energy required for the actin–myosin interaction. The role of ATP in muscle contraction is significant because repeated interactions between actin and myosin are relatively expensive in energy terms, and so the reservoir of ATP within the fibre will rapidly be utilized. Much more must be synthesized if the contractile process is to be sustained. Muscle cells contain a substance called creatine phosphate, and the phosphate part may be removed to generate new ATP. The creatine portion is left behind and breakdown of excess creatine produces creatinine, a 'waste' substance that is excreted in urine and is an important parameter in monitoring renal efficiency (see Chapter 15, p.432).

Contraction of whole muscles

The previous section considered how nerve stimulation of a muscle fibre causes it to contract. Extrapolating from that to the behaviour of whole muscles requires further consideration as to how the whole muscle is activated, and the characteristics of that contraction.

The motor unit

It is usually the case that a single nerve cell activates more than one muscle fibre; the number of fibres innervated is called a motor unit:

- Large motor units are found in the major postural muscles, such as the quadriceps of the thighs, and make the process of developing a considerable force of contraction more efficient, otherwise an even larger number of nerve cells will be required to provide the necessary innervation of the tissue. In fact, in such muscles a single nerve cell may innervate hundreds of muscle fibres.
- Small muscles, such as the pupillary muscles inside the eye, may have fibres that are innervated by individual nerve cells. These muscles do not generate a large force of contraction, and their role requires a more subtle control than that exerted on the major postural muscles.

From a pathology viewpoint, the presence of motor units means that loss of relatively small numbers of nerve cells can result in the loss of large numbers of functional muscle fibres. Nerve cells can produce outgrowths and reinnervate nearby muscle fibres, but the resultant improvement in muscle function may only be limited.

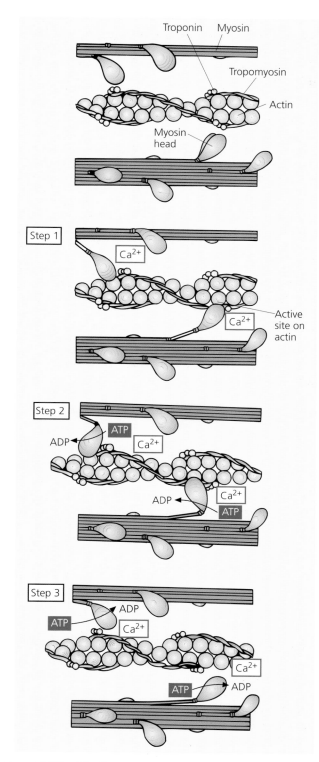

Figure 17.6 The sliding filament theory of muscle fibre contraction. Step 1, distortion of troponin–tropomyosin by calcium ions; formation of bond between myosin head and active site on actin. Step 2, splitting of adenosine triphosphate (ATP) by myosin to provide energy to move myosin–actin cross-bridges (actin is pulled along myosin), and then to break cross-bridge for new actin–myosin interaction. Step 3, movement of myosin heads to interact with next active site on actin. ADP, adenosine diphosphate

Q Describe the molecular interactions involved in muscle contraction.

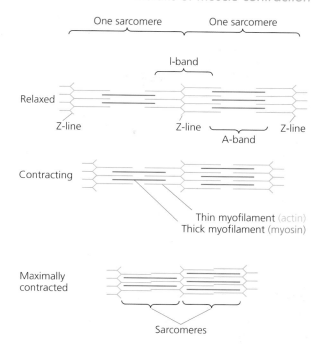

Figure 17.7 Shortening of sarcomere length during myofibril contraction. Note that myofilament lengths do not change, but the overlap between actin and myosin increases, drawing consecutive Z-lines together. Note also that the I-band striation that is reduced

Q Describe the roles of actin and myosin in shortening the sarcomere.

Twitch, treppe and tetany

Observation of the contraction of whole muscle identifies a variety of forms of contraction, depending upon the rate at which nerve stimuli arrive at the muscle:

- *Twitch*: a momentary, spasmodic contraction produced by a brief, single stimulus (Figure 17.8a). This process is essentially that described (above) when a muscle contracts on stimulation.
- *Treppe*: if a muscle is repeatedly stimulated, but is still allowed to relax between stimuli, the contraction induced by each stimulus increases in intensity to a maximum (Figure 17.8b). This principle operates when athletes 'warm up'.
- *Tetany*: if a muscle is repeatedly stimulated but is not allowed to relax fully between stimuli, the contractions induced by each stimulus are additive so that each twitch summates to produce an intense, continuous contraction called tetany (Figure 17.8c; see also Box 17.5).

Isotonic and isometric contractions

Another feature related to muscle physiology is the contrast between contraction of muscle when movement is resisted (isometric contraction), and during an actual movement (isotonic contraction).

- Isometric contraction (Figure 17.9b). In this example, the development of tension before the object can be moved occurs without moving the skeletal joint. Muscle length

BOX 17.5 MUSCLE SPASM/CRAMP AND TETANUS

The strength of contraction of a muscle will depend upon its rate of stimulation (see 'treppe' and 'tetany' in text). It will also be influenced by the local chemical environment since this will affect the sensitivity of the sarcolemma.

Spasm and cramp

The internal chemical environment is influenced by the length of time that a contracting muscle has had to spend in anaerobic conditions. Spasm and cramp occur when the excitability is increased to the point that nerve stimulation of the muscle induces a powerful contraction that is sustained, leading to hypoxia and consequently pain. Cramp is normally associated with a period of physical activity during which the muscle is subjected to a frequency of nerve stimulation that leads to tetany. Spasm is more usually associated with lower-level muscle activity and can occur, for example, simply in rising from a sitting position. Both are painful situations – nociceptors within the muscle are stimulated by the biochemical environment produced by the hypoxia and stressed muscle cells. The spasm/cramp is actually a protective device that prevents muscle damage occurring through its continued use.

Increasing blood supply to the area by the use of massage or local vasodilators will help to reverse any hypoxia, and will help to stabilize the chemical environment within the muscle. However, the sarcolemma will usually retain for a period of time a likelihood of increased sensitivity and excitability making a repeat spasm of the muscle more likely.

The threshold of stimulation required to cause the electrical changes (i.e. an action potential; see Chapter 8, p.187 for an explanation) in the sarcolemma is especially susceptible to calcium ion concentration in the extracellular fluid. Acute reductions in calcium concentration induced, for example, by hyperventilation during an anxiety 'attack' (which produces an alkalosis that facilitates the combination of calcium ions with blood proteins) may result in such a lowering of the threshold that a maximal muscle contraction is produced (i.e. tetany; see text). In alkalosis, this is often first observed as a powerful contraction of the hand, producing a movement of the thumb across the palm of the hand in a characteristic carpopedal spasm. Prior to this, an individual who has become alkalotic may report intense tingling in the fingers and hand – a prelude to muscle contraction.

Tetanus

Tetanus is a condition in which a toxin produced by infection with *Clostridium tetani* lowers the threshold for muscle excitation, making tetany likely even with very low rates of nerve stimulation (Campbell and Fallaha, 2007). For reasons that are unclear, the condition affects some muscles more markedly than others and the condition is colloquially known as 'lockjaw' because of its effects on muscles of the face. The main danger is from tetany of the muscles of the chest, since this will cause respiratory arrest. Anti-tetanus injections are available; these contain antibody to the toxin thus preventing its actions. The causal organism lives in soil and is common but vaccination programmes have made the condition rare. It is important for health carers to recognize this since anti-tetanus injections should be considered if a wound is open, and if there is no evidence that the individual has maintained a tetanus immunization.

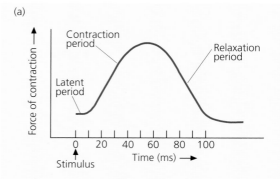

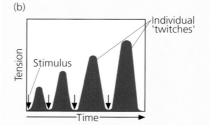

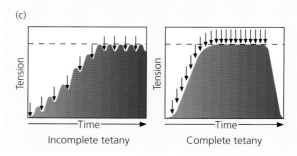

Figure 17.8 Relationship between stimulus frequency and muscle tension. (a) Twitch produced by a single stimulus. (b) Treppe produced by continued activation/relaxation. Note the increased tension with successive stimulation. (c) Tetany induced by continued activation

Q What do you understand by the term 'tetany'?

BOX 17.6 TREMORS

A tremor is a series of rapid muscle contractions that represent an oscillation in the control of tension in pairs of agonistic and antagonistic muscles (see p.477).

- *Postural or intention tremor*: many people exhibit a slight tremor, particularly if a limb is extended, and especially if being watched. The tremor probably arises from the cerebellum of the brain but is not associated with other neurological abnormalities and is not considered to relate to any underlying pathology.

- *Tremor at rest*: the tremor observed in Parkinson's disease is an example of a tremor that occurs at rest. It is produced by oscillations in the activity between the basal ganglia and cerebral cortex of the brain (see Box 17.13, p.482, and see Figure 17.16, p.481), which determine the final output to the muscles. This tremor disappears during voluntary movement, presumably because other pathways in the brain are activated that override the oscillation.

therefore remains constant despite the contraction that is occurring. The actin–myosin interaction within the muscle fibres will still be acting to move the actin myofilaments, even if they are unable to actually shorten, and this is exhibited as a rapid rise in muscle tension. The contraction is then said to be isometric ('iso-' = equal, 'metros' = length).

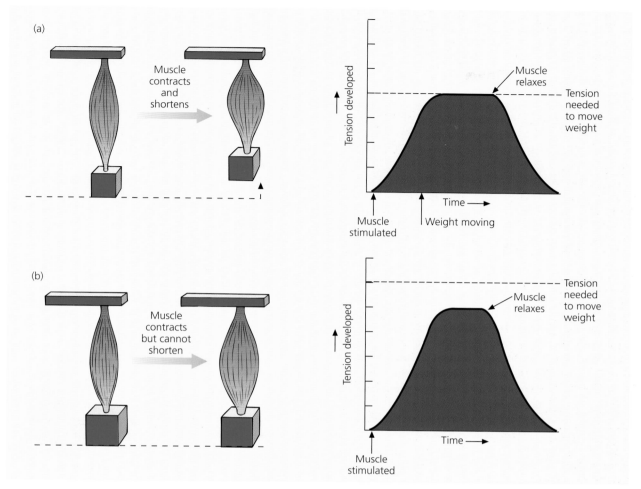

Figure 17.9 (a) Isotonic contraction. Muscle tension increases until the weight moves, and then remains constant, even though the contraction continues. (b) Isometric contraction. The weight cannot be moved: muscle tension increases during the contraction, but the muscle does not shorten

Q Define the following terms with reference to contraction of the whole muscle: (1) twitch, (2) isotonic and (3) isometric.

- Isotonic contraction (Figure 17.9a). Once the tension to move the skeletal joint has been generated then the limb begins to move, but once the object is moving further tension need not be developed. The contraction is then said to be isotonic ('isos- = equal, 'tonos' = tension). As the joint moves, the muscle shortens in length.

The two types of contraction often happen in sequence – even lifting just the weight of a limb will require a short period of isometric contraction followed by the isotonic one of the movement itself. In lifting an object, an isometric contraction is required to take the load of the limb plus the actual weight of the object, before the contraction becomes isotonic. Regular workloads of this kind trigger adaptations in which the muscle protein increases, and the cross-sectional area of the muscle is increased, thus reducing the effort to generate the required tension (see Box 17.1, p.464). The adaptation is most pronounced when frequently lifting very heavy loads. Muscle building is clearly an adaptation to the regular imposition of heavy physical loads, but there are other physiological implications to be considered (Box 17.7)

Maintaining muscle contraction: fatigue resistance

The maintenance of posture and physical activity may require muscles to maintain a degree of contraction for lengthy periods of time, for example the anti-gravity muscles (see Box 17.1, p.464). Such muscles are 'fatigue resistant' and have further adaptations to maintain the energy release required to support the contractions. In contrast, some movements involve very rapid contractions maintained for only a short period of time, for example the facial muscles, and normally are less demanding of energy supplies. Fatigue-resistant muscle fibres take longer than others to complete a cycle of muscle contraction and relaxation (although subtypes are now recognized which have intermediate rates of contraction):

- 'Slow' twitch (or type I) fibres are relatively more frequent in muscles that are unlikely to have a major role in activi-

BOX 17.7 MUSCLE BLOOD FLOW DURING ISOTONIC AND ISOMETRIC EXERCISE

The blood supply to skeletal muscles increases at, or even just prior, to producing a contraction. Once contraction begins then the chemical environment within the muscle (e.g. lowered pH, elevated potassium ions concentration in extracellular fluid and increased temperature) causes further vasodilation. These are, of course, adaptations that raise blood flow to meet the oxygen demands of the active muscle fibres.

Vasodilation is expressed during isotonic exercise. This would reduce the total peripheral resistance to blood flow within the circulatory system and cause arterial blood pressure to fall, but compensatory constriction of blood vessels elsewhere (e.g. the bowel) help to maintain the peripheral resistance. Measures of arterial blood pressure show that systolic blood pressure increases during isotonic exercise (as cardiac output has increased) but diastolic blood pressure is little changed (because the total or overall peripheral resistance is much the same as at rest).

In contrast, the tension developed during intense isometric muscle contractions tends to 'crush' blood vessels within the muscle, making the vasodilation less effective and so raising the peripheral resistance to blood flow. If the isometric phase is very pronounced then this can be sufficient to raise the diastolic blood pressure, increasing the risk of problems such as aneurysm or stroke.

Exercise and the heart

Cardiac muscle responds to increased workload if someone exercises regularly because there is an isometric contraction of the ventricles at the start of each cardiac systole, prior to the opening of the aortic and pulmonary valves; adaptation increases the heart size and this is considered beneficial as it improves the contractility of the heart and hence the volume ejected per beat. This response is considered to be one of the main benefits of regular exercise.

ties that necessitate rapid contraction/relaxation cycles. Those muscles that act to maintain posture against gravity, for example the quadriceps of the thighs, have a preponderance of slow fibres and are therefore 'slow' muscles. The muscle fibres will have an excellent blood supply, but they will also have a rich store of myoglobin, a haemoglobin-like pigment that provides a supplementary oxygen store. The fibres have the capacity to maintain ATP production by aerobic metabolism (Figure 17.10) and are therefore resistant to hypoxia and hence to fatigue. This is useful if we have to remain standing for long periods of time.

- 'Fast' twitch (type II) fibres increase in proportion in those muscles that are responsible for producing rapid movements, as in the movement of the eye or hand. Fast-type muscle fibres have lots of mitochondria but little myoglobin and so they cannot maintain contraction for long periods of time. They are not likely to predominate in the major anti-gravity muscles.

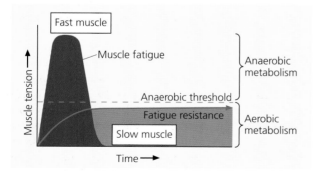

Figure 17.10 Fatigue resistance in muscles. Fast-twitch muscles rapidly exceed the anaerobic threshold during contraction. Slow-twitch muscles can maintain contraction below anaerobic threshold for long periods of time (but can also exceed threshold at times, e.g. during exercise)

Q *Distinguish between slow and fast muscle fibres. Which type of muscle would be involved in maintaining a standing posture? (see Figure 17.13, p.478)*

THE CONTROL OF POSTURE AND MOVEMENT 1: PROPRIOCEPTION, THE SENSING OF POSITION

'Posture' is the position of the body in space and includes whole-body orientation and the relative positions of body parts. The degree of tension observed in individual muscles will be appropriate for the maintenance of position of the associated joint. In this respect, this section considers (1) the kind of sensory information that is required to modulate motor nerve activity and (2) the sensory nerve pathways to the brain.

BOX 17.8 PREVENTING CONTRACTURES IN AN IMMOBILE PATIENT

A 'contracture' is a shortening of muscle in the absence of an active contractile process. It arises as a consequence of muscle spasm or weakness:

- As the result of a biochemical imbalance within the muscle fibres, for example in muscular dystrophy.
- As a result of scar contraction in a joint following joint trauma.

Prevention of contractures is important if mobility is to be retained (or restored).The aims here are to restore as much normal movement as possible, to maintain muscle strength and joint flexibility, and to facilitate muscle coordination. A range of movement exercises are employed to support joint movement through appropriate planes:

- *'Passive exercise'*: this term is a misnomer but is applied when a nurse/physiotherapist manipulates joints without assistance from the patient.
- *Active-assisted exercise*: this is performed by the patient with the assistance of the nurse/physiotherapist, and encourages normal muscle actions.
- *Active exercise*: this is performed solely by the patient. It encourages normal muscle action, and the development of muscle strength.
- *Resisted exercise*: this is active exercise performed against resistance. In doing so the isometric phase of muscle contraction (see text) is increased and this helps to increase muscle bulk and hence increase muscle power.

Sensory information: proprioreception

The brain must be 'aware' at all times of the spatial positions of the body parts, and of the orientation of the body in general, although we are not usually conscious of this information.

Two senses obviously involved are:

- *Vision*: this is clearly of use in monitoring spatial positioning, yet closing our eyes or looking away does not prevent us from being aware of our posture, the position of our hands, etc., and blind people fare as well as visually able people in this respect.
- *Mechanoreceptors of the skin*: these convey tactile information, and so inform of the contact between, say, a foot and the floor. Yet when we are, say, sitting in a chair, our brain must also be able to make a distinction between the contact of buttock with the chair and contact of the feet with the floor – the sense of touch from those areas is very similar if we are sitting on the ground. The difference seems obvious but only because we 'know' – our brain has to work it out!

Most postural information is produced by a variety of receptors collectively called proprioreceptors (or proprioceptors; 'proprio-' = position). All respond to movement but to be effective must also provide information even when the posture is unchanging, otherwise the brain will not be able to continue to identify the relative positions of parts of the body. This capacity to provide information when stationary is called a 'static' property of the receptors. In providing information about an actual movement they must also have 'dynamic' properties because they have to be capable of monitoring position change, the rate of change, the direction of change, and perhaps even any acceleratory component during the movement. The proprioceptors are the vestibular receptors, joint receptors, tendon receptors and muscle 'spindles', and are described below.

Vestibular (or equilibrium) receptors

The vestibular receptors are found within the vestibular apparatus of the inner ear (see Figure 7.2, p.142). They can generally be divided into two components: the otolithic organs, and the semicircular canals. They have in common a space that is filled with fluid (endolymph) where the receptor cells project into jelly-like structures that respond to fluid movement when the head moves and so are sometimes referred to as 'balance organs' (Box 17.9):

- The otolithic organs ('oto-' = ear, 'lith' = stone) are composed of distended structures called the utricle and saccule. Microscopically, these contain masses of small calcium carbonate crystals lying on top of a jelly-like otolithic membrane. If the position of the head alters, both the fluid and otolithic membrane moves, but the latter is more dense and so moves more slowly. The fluid movement therefore distorts the position of the crystals, and triggers the receptor cells ('hair' cells). The cells stimulate nerve endings and electrical activity is transmitted to the brain via the vestibulocochlear nerve (cranial nerve VIII). The response is relatively slow and the otoliths are largely concerned with 'static' equi-

librium, informing the brain of the position of the head relative to gravity.

- The semicircular canals are three canals in each ear, arranged at right angles to one another in three planes. At the base of each canal there is a distended region, called the ampulla, in which lies the crista, an elevated structure containing receptor cells that are inserted into the jelly-like cupula. When the head moves, the fluid currents deflect the cupula, and this activates the receptor cells. Impulses once again pass to the brain via the VIIIth cranial nerve. Comparison of the information from each of the three cristae, and each ear, gives information regarding the direction and plane of head movement, if it is rotational and how rapidly it is moving. These receptors therefore provide 'dynamic' information if the position of the head changes rapidly.

Sensory information from the vestibular apparatus of the ear passes directly to the brain: to the vestibular nuclei of the medulla, and to the cerebellum. Some information is conveyed from the medulla to the superior colliculi of the midbrain, which are areas involved in coordinating eye movement (see Chapter 7, p.153). In this way, sudden head movement detected by the vestibular receptors induces changes in eye position that help us to maintain appropriate vision. Such 'vestibular-ocular' reflexes are used in evaluating brainstem 'death' (see Box 8.9, p.178).

Joint receptors

Joint receptors are nerve endings within the cartilage and synovial capsules of joints. They respond to distortion of the joint and provide information regarding the position of the joint (a 'static' property), and the rate of change and acceleration during joint movement ('dynamic' properties). In doing so the brain can accurately determine the change in orientation of the skeleton, and can also predict where a limb will finish up after the movement is complete. Muscle contraction can therefore be modulated accordingly.

Tendon receptors (or Golgi tendon organs)

Receptors within the tendons of muscles are composed of small bundles of collagen fibres enclosed in a capsule and supplied

---

BOX 17.9 INNER EAR DISTURBANCE AND BALANCE

Disturbance of the vestibular apparatus can confuse the brain as to the position of the head, because the information does not correspond to that from the eyes. Examples of how this occurs are:

- inner ear infection, producing toxins and inflammation (thus, activation of the vestibular receptors by the infection is at odds with the actual position of the head);
- Meniere's disease, possibly occurring because of a failure to regulate blood supply to the inner ear, thus producing conflicting information as to head position;
- travel or motion sickness, including seasickness (information from the eyes and ears is unsynchronized).

In these instances the individual will usually experience nausea and may even have difficulties balancing.

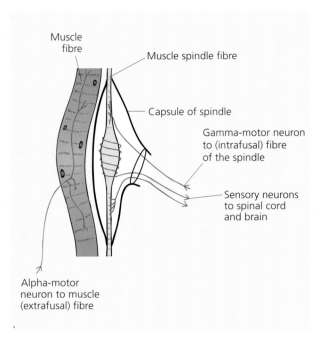

Figure 17.11 Muscle spindle fibre and its innervation

Q What information does this type of receptor provide?

tion if the tension being transmitted from the muscle to the tendons is excessive. In this way the tendons and muscles are prevented from damage, or even separation from the bone. This action is observed, for example, when muscles apparently 'give way' if the object lifted is too heavy.

Muscle spindles

Of all the proprioceptors it is the muscle spindles that are best situated to enable the brain to monitor and modulate the contraction of skeletal muscles, because the receptors are present within the muscles themselves. The spindle-shaped receptor is actually a collection of modified muscle fibres enclosed within a connective tissue capsule (Figure 17.11). The fibres are said to be 'intrafusal' ('intra-' = inside; fusiform = spindle-like), to distinguish them from the other (extrafusal) muscle fibres. The connective tissue around the spindle connects the receptor to adjacent muscle fibres, and so any stretching or shortening of the latter will also produce distortion of the spindle, and a change in intrafusal fibre length. Thus, these receptors monitor the length of the muscle spindles and hence of the muscle fibres to which the receptors are attached.

The spindle fibres have sensory nerve endings associated with them (Figure 17.11) that respond to any change in length of the intrafusal fibres, and continue to do so for a period of time after. The nerve activity conveys 'static' information regarding spindle and muscle fibre length, and 'dynamic' information regarding the rate of change of fibre length. This information is essential in involuntary muscle reflexes (below) but a critical feature of muscle spindles is that they are actually modified muscle fibres and have their own nerve supply, which

with nerve endings. The receptors are arranged in line with the muscle fibres and so provide information regarding muscle tension. However, their precise role in posture and movement is unclear. It is likely that tendon receptors provide a protective function by prompting a sudden cessation of muscle contrac-

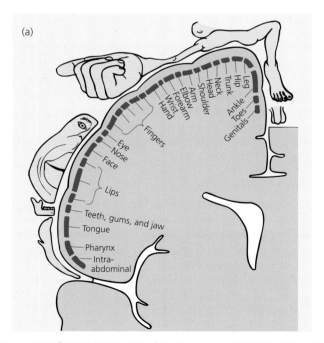

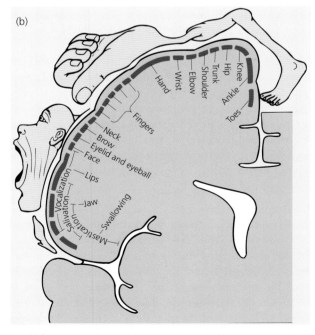

Figure 17.12 Topographical analysis of the sensory and motor areas of the cerebral cortex. (a) Somatosensory cortex, right hemisphere. (b) Motor cortex, right hemisphere

Q Identify the area associated with sending information to the jaw muscle when we are taking a meal.

means that muscle spindles also can have a role in the production of voluntary movements; this is explained later.

Sensory input to the brain

Sensory information from the proprioceptors, together with that from various mechanoreceptors in the skin, largely passes to the brain via the spinal cord, and a common feature is that these nerve pathways at some point cross over from one side of the cord to the opposite side of the brain (note also that those parts of the brain that produce motor output also cross over to control muscles on the opposite side of the body). The main neural pathways that convey this information to the brain are:

- *The posterior spinothalamic tracts (i.e. in the posterior aspect of the cord and passing to the thalamus, and thence to the cerebral cortex)*: neurons of these tracts form the 'dorsal columns' of the cord and ascend to the dorsal column nuclei of the medulla oblongata (see Figure 8.20, p.185). From here projections cross over to the other side of the medulla, pass to the thalamus via a tract called the medial lemniscus, and then they are relayed to the somatosensory cortex of the cerebrum ('somato-' = of the body). Areas of the cortex receive information from particular parts of the body (Figure 17.12a): more grey matter is devoted to the face and hands than to the entire trunk, and this relates to the complexity and volume of information from those parts.
- *The spinocerebellar tracts (i.e. from cord to cerebellum)*: these tracts ascend the lateral aspects of the cord to the medulla where they pass to the cortex of the cerebellum via tracts called the cerebellar peduncles. Many of the neurons will also have crossed over but this time within the cord.

THE CONTROL OF POSTURE AND MOVEMENT 2: MOTOR CONTROL OF MOVEMENT

'Movement' results from a change of posture and may or may not involve propulsion of the body from one point to another. It is produced by changes in the tension of muscles relative to others.

Individual muscles obviously have their own names for identification purposes. However, there also are collective terms used when describing the behaviour and relationship of muscles and muscle groups during a movement. A muscle that primarily produces a movement is called an agonist for the movement while that which opposes it is called an antagonist (note the similarity in usage of these terms in pharmacology in which agonistic drugs also promote an action and antagonistic ones prevent or reverse it; see Box 1.8, p.15). In making the movement, the antagonist clearly only opposes contraction sufficient to protect the joint involved, it will not prevent it from occurring.

The agonist muscle may act to flex (i.e. bend) the joint, or to extend it; it is therefore referred to either as a 'flexor' or 'extensor' type of muscle. Many limb movements entail both

actions, in which case a given muscle may be an agonist for one phase of the movement and an antagonist in another. For example, consider the movement of the knee joint during walking. A number of muscles in the leg are involved, but the main ones are the quadriceps femoris ('quad' because there are four parts to this muscle) of the thigh, and those that comprise the hamstring muscles at the back of the thigh (Figure 17.13). Both sets of muscles have attachments with the top of the femur or bones of the pelvis, and with the tibia of the lower leg. The quadriceps is an extensor muscle in that its contraction extends the leg; the hamstrings are flexors and cause the joint to bend during contraction. During walking the knee extensor muscles will be agonist as the leg is extended, the flexors antagonistic. When the knee is flexed, the situation is reversed. The movement therefore requires cyclical stimulation/relaxation of the muscles involved.

By altering the position of a body part, or by causing a change in body orientation, the actions of a muscle could adversely influence additional joints nearby even if they are not actually involved in the movement. For example, taking a step changes the position of the body with respect to its centre of gravity (see later) and the tendency for the body to be unbalanced is counteracted by the contraction or relaxation of muscles of the opposite leg, the back and the shoulders. Muscles that produce the stabilization are collectively referred to as synergistic muscles.

What appears as a relatively simple movement, and one that we would normally take for granted, therefore requires complex responses throughout the muscular system, and so the control of posture and movement depends upon maintaining the tension of all muscles appropriate to the desired joint position, or to the movement to be induced, and hence upon the regulation of activity of the motor nerve cells involved. That regulation is largely involuntary, but can be modulated to enable conscious, voluntary movement. This section therefore considers the control of posture by involuntary reflexes and changing posture by voluntary movements.

Control of posture by involuntary reflexes

A reflex response is extremely rapid because it involves neural pathways that remove the necessity for significant processing of information by the brain. A reflex change in muscle contraction results from a sequence of events:

- the stimulation of a sensory receptor;
- the conduction of sensory activity to the central nervous system via sensory neurons;
- the direct activation of motor neurons that promote an appropriate response.

Collectively these events are said to form a reflex arc. The fastest are 'monosynaptic' arcs, that is, one in which the sensory neuron synapses directly with the motor cell, so that is there is only one synapse en route to slow the response. The fundamental elements of a monosynaptic reflex were illustrated in Chapter 8 (Figure 8.25, p.194) in relation to a 'withdrawal' reflex in response to pain. This is a protective reflex

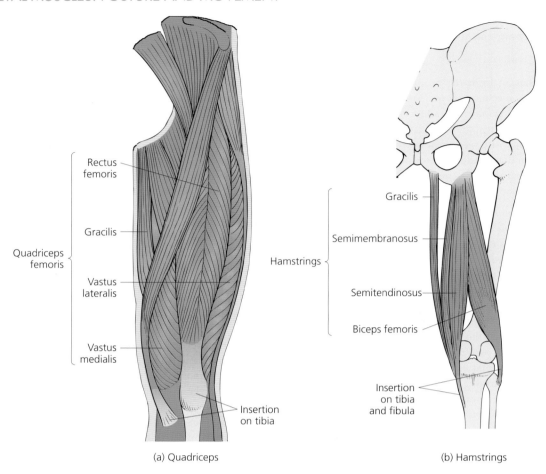

Rectus
femoris

Gracilis

Quadriceps
femoris

Vastus
lateralis

Vastus
medialis

Insertion
on tibia

(a) Quadriceps

Gracilis

Semimembranosus

Hamstrings

Semitendinosus

Biceps femoris

Insertion
on tibia
and fibula

(b) Hamstrings

Figure 17.13 Muscles controlling the knee joint. (a) Extensors, anterior view. (b) Flexors, posterior view

Q What does the difference in bulk tell you about the roles of these two muscle groups?

BOX 17.10 REFLEXES IN INFANTS

Some reflexes are apparent soon after birth, including the feeding reflex, the grasping reflex, and the 'positive supporting reaction' seen as an extension of the legs when firm contact is made on the soles of the feet. Many reflexes become modified as the baby grows. For example, while the reflex changes in position of body and limb, induced by stimulating the vestibular apparatus of the ear, must remain operative in the child and adult during involuntary head movement, it must be suppressed during voluntary movement of the head.

that entails causing a change in posture that removes the limb from the source of the pain, but it does not explain the responses of muscles elsewhere that act to stabilize the body's new position once the reflex is instigated. These further reflexes are stretch reflexes, and they play a vital day-to-day role in helping us to maintain our posture, for example in the synergistic changes observed when we take a step, noted above.

The 'knee-jerk' reflex illustrates how a stretch reflex operates. It is a rapid, reflex extension of the knee joint that involves the contraction of the quadriceps femoris muscle of the thigh. It is activated by tapping the patellar tendon, which attaches the quadriceps muscle to the tibia bone of the shin (Figure 17.14):

- Tapping the tendon stretches the muscle fibres and hence muscle spindle receptors of the quadriceps.
- The sensory nerve endings of the spindles are activated and impulses pass along the sensory neurons to the spinal cord, where they synapse directly with the motor nerve cells.
- The motor nerve cells convey impulses back to the muscle fibres of the same quadriceps muscle, causing them to contract. Simultaneously, the nerve activity to the antagonistic muscles (i.e. the hamstrings) is inhibited, which relaxes these muscles so that the movement is not impeded.

The result is that the knee is extended as a little 'kick'.

The 'knee jerk' is a demonstration of the way that spindle receptors act to keep muscle length constant. If a muscle is stretched then the subsequent contraction returns it to the original length. The 'knee jerk' is an artificial situation but the reflex it demonstrates is illustrated in the following commonplace examples:

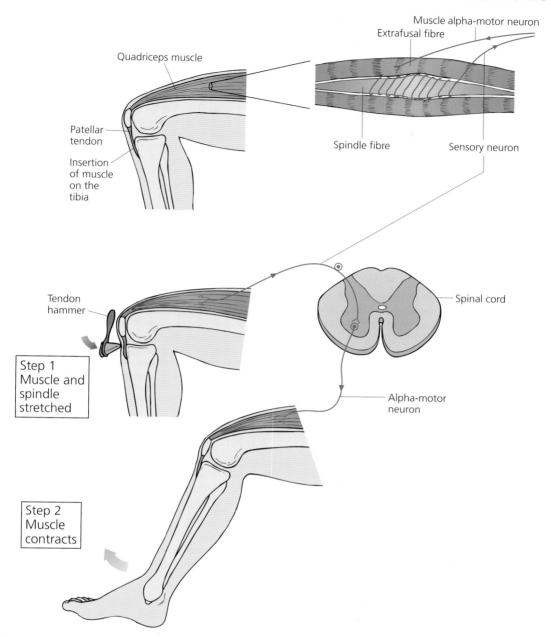

Figure 17.14 The stretch reflex, as illustrated by the knee jerk. Step 1: when a reflex hammer strikes the patellar tendon, the muscle spindle fibres stretch, resulting in a burst of activity in the afferent fibres that synapse on motor neurons inside the spinal cord. Step 2: an immediate reflexive kick is produced by the activation of motor units in the stretched muscle

Q Describe the role of muscle spindles in the reflex response.

- Upon standing, gravity acts to flex the knees, hips and intervertebral joints. The activities of the muscle spindles in the relevant extensor muscles that are stretched by these effects of gravity help to prevent us from crumpling into a heap, and so are vital if we are to maintain an upright posture unconsciously.
- Consider a situation in which an individual is bumped into by another. The unexpected and involuntary change in posture alters the length and tension of various muscles and the resultant reflexes play an important role in the quick return to stability. Other synergistic and postural muscles will also be activated because of the stimulation of other proprioceptors (e.g. the vestibular apparatus), and because of reflexes instigated by spindles within the other muscles themselves. By involving interneurons the reflex response can simultaneously promote contraction of appropriate muscles in another limb, and relaxation of antagonistic muscles. The stretch reflex thus makes a powerful contribution to the maintenance of posture.

BOX 17.11 CLINICAL USES OF THE STRETCH REFLEX (OR TENDON REFLEX)

Stimulating a stretch reflex is simple – a small tendon hammer can be used to direct an impact on various tendons of the body, especially where the tendon passes over a joint. Thus, the tendon of the quadriceps (at the knee – see text), the tendon of the biceps (at the elbow) and the tendon of the gastrocnemius (the Achilles tendon at the heel) all provide a means of testing for the presence of the reflex, and its efficiency. Such tests provide an indication of the functioning of the sensory and motor nerves to the muscle and/or spinal cord connections.

The placement of electrodes over the nerves themselves also enables a calculation of conduction velocity for the nerve pathway (from the time delay between tapping the tendon and recording the nerve activity), though this requires the use of sophisticated equipment and is not usual in general clinical practice.

BOX 17.12 SENSORIMOTOR DEVELOPMENT

Neurons are responsible for the functions we associate with the brain such as sensory processing, motor coordination, memory, reasoning, etc. For these facilities to develop in infants the process of myelination (to increase nerve cell conductivity and insulation) must progress, the cells must become more organized and intercellular communication must be established by the development and maintenance of appropriate synapses. Motor and sensory function matures earlier than 'higher' cognitive functions such as memory, reasoning and judgement. This early sensorimotor development is illustrated in:

- the production of facial expressions (here are around 20 different muscles of the face that must operate synchronously to produce an expression);
- the ability of the young child to eventually assume an upright posture, to walk, to acquire basic speech and to gain voluntary control of the urinary and anal sphincters.

The 'maturation' process of neural integration can take many years to complete (see Cech, 2002), and this is observed in the continuing development of motor skills. Gross motor control improves most rapidly and is enhanced by physical activity. It is almost complete by the end of childhood. Fine motor skills (e.g. eye/hand and arm/leg coordination) improve more slowly and development continues into the teenage years. A slight sex discrepancy is apparent, with boys developing a greater grip strength and tending toward better arm/leg coordination than girls, who exhibit better control of balance and rhythmic movement. There is a considerable overlap in the acquirement of these skills, however.

- When an object such as a ball is thrown for us to catch, or when we intend to lift an object, we unconsciously appraise the forces required, based on object size, composition, etc. An appropriate muscle tension is generated but if we have underestimated what is required, then the control of the situation could be lost. If the object was heavier than anticipated the muscles in the arm will be stretched, activating the spindles and reflexly stimulate further muscle contraction.

In all three examples the reflex response is produced independently of passing sensory information to the brain. The brain, however, must be made 'aware' of how the initiation of reflexes has altered the relative positions of parts of the body. Thus, apart from synapsing with motor neurons, the sensory neurons from the spindles will also synapse with ascending neurons within the cord that convey information to appropriate areas of the brain and so keep it 'informed'.

Changing posture by voluntary movement
Muscle spindle modulation

Voluntary movements are very distinct from reflexes. Thus, the motor nerve activity required to contract an individual muscle has not been promoted by the muscle spindle but has been generated in the brain. However, the muscle spindle still has an integral role to play because the muscle contraction will tend to passively shorten the spindles within the muscle and, from the previous discussion, the reflex response to this reduced spindle tension would be to cause muscle relaxation (to return the spindle length to that before), and so counteract the original intention. The role of spindles in the reflex maintenance of posture could therefore potentially act to restrict voluntary (conscious) movement by preventing the necessary muscular changes. A mechanism is therefore necessary to modulate the actions of spindles during voluntary movement.

It was noted earlier that the intrafusal fibres of the spindles are actually modified muscle fibres. They have their own motor nerve cells (classified as 'gamma-neurons', or 'gamma-efferents'; see Figure 17.11, p.476) and the brain may act to modulate their length independently of the rest of the muscle.

For example, they might be made to contract in time with the surrounding muscle fibres, and so not detect that the muscle has contracted. It is worth reflecting for a moment on the complexity of this process. Imagine simply taking a step forward. This entails contraction and relaxation, in the correct sequence of the agonist muscles, the opposite relaxation/contraction of the antagonistic muscles, and the contraction or relaxation of the synergistic muscles of the limb, the buttocks and the back and abdomen. In other words, every voluntary muscle movement must be accompanied by others, sometimes involving stretch reflexes, other times requiring a precise activation of specific muscles by the brain. Apart from simultaneously being capable of controlling the motor activity to each of the 600+ muscles of the body, the brain also controls the co-activation of muscle spindle fibres, if a smooth movement is to occur.

Clearly, the control of individual muscle contraction is not a 'simple' case of activating the motor nerve to it, but involves a complex integration of sensory information and the activation of appropriate motor neurons to the muscle and to the muscle spindle receptors. The brain receives a bewildering array of information regarding every aspect of posture and moment-to-moment updates on how the position of body parts and body orientation is changing. The control of posture and movement is of a complexity of the highest order; much of the brain is in fact concerned with that control. The following discussion considers motor pathways from the brain and associated brain anatomy.

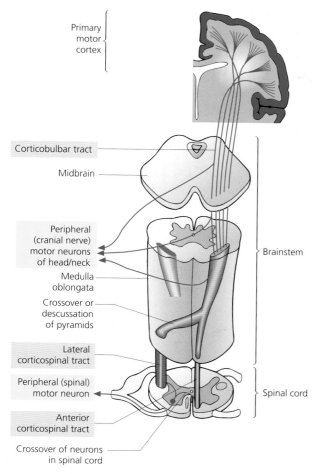

Figure 17.15 The pyramidal tracts from the motor cortex to muscles. The major tracts of neurons are identified

Q Distinguish between the pyramidal and extrapyramidal pathways.

Motor pathways from the brain, and associated brain anatomy

The mass of sensory information that is received by the brain is constantly monitored, integrated and relayed to those areas which determine the motor output from the brain. This output originates from various parts of the brain: the motor cortex, the basal ganglia and the cerebellum. Brain anatomy was described in Chapter 8, and readers are referred to that chapter for supplementary material for this subsection.

Motor cortex (and pyramidal pathways)

Much of the neural output to muscles comes from the motor cortex which lies immediately anterior to the somatosensory cortex (see Figure 8.8, p.172). Both areas of cortex can be 'mapped' to the parts of the body to which they relate (see Figure 17.12b, p.476). The complexity of controlling hand and facial movements is reflected in the disproportionate areas involved in their coordination.

Most, but not all, motor nerve activity passes out of the brain via the pyramidal pathway:

- Some passes down the spinal cord via the lateral and anterior corticospinal tracts (Figure 17.15). The lateral tracts are characterized by the crossing-over (called decussation) of the upper motor neurons within the medulla. Here these large tracts are called the 'pyramids' and so give the name to these pathways. The nerve cells continue down the cord and eventually synapse with lower motor neurons to the muscles. The anterior tract also crosses over but this time within the grey matter of the cord, where the nerve cells also synapse with lower motor neurons. Crossing over means that muscles located on one side of the body are controlled by neurons originating in the opposite side of the brain.

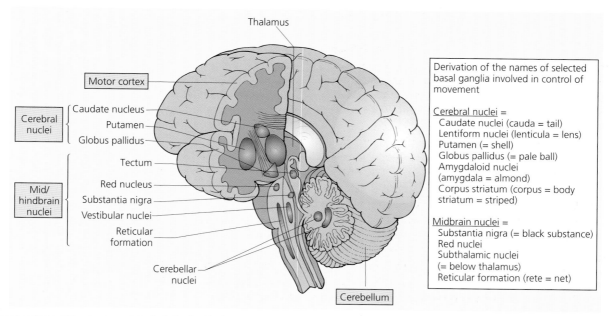

Figure 17.16 Some of the structures of the brain involved in the control of movement

Q Discuss the importance of movement and posture to health.

• Some passes to the nuclei of various cranial nerves within the brainstem, for transmission, via cranial nerves, to muscles of the face and neck. These form the corticobulbar tracts and do not project to the spinal cord, or to the pyramids, at all, but confusingly are still considered as part of the pyramidal pathways because they originate within the motor cortex of the brain.

Basal ganglia (and extrapyramidal pathways)

The basal ganglia are cerebral nuclei (i.e. of the forebrain) and some midbrain nuclei that are functionally linked to them. Their names often reflect their appearance to early anatomists, or of their position. Major ones are identified in Figure 17.16. They are involved in the subconscious production of gross intentional movement, rhythmic movements such as walking, and the positioning of the body prior to producing an intended movement. Much of the nerve activity they generate is first relayed to the motor cortex where it is modulated further before passing to the muscles via the pyramidal pathways (above). The interactions between the basal ganglia and cortex are extremely complex, involving an array of excitatory and inhibitory interconnections (see Chapter 8, p.194 for illustrations of integration).

Other neural output leaves the basal ganglia for direct transmission to muscles via the extrapyramidal pathways (i.e. those that are not part of the pyramidal pathways). They normally originate in the brainstem components of the basal ganglia and are named according to their site of origin:

BOX 17.13 ALTERED MUSCLE FUNCTION CAUSED BY CENTRAL NERVOUS SYSTEM DISORDER

Disorders of movement control arising as a consequence of changes to the central nervous system can be grouped according to cause: trauma, metabolism, imbalance of excitatory and inhibitory pathways in modulating motor nerve output, and deterioration of nerve tracts.

Trauma

Although protected by the cranium, the position of the cerebral cortex and cerebellar cortex at the surface of the brain make these structures susceptible to damage from head trauma, or from subarachnoid or subdural haemorrhage (see Chapter 8, p.178). Both cortices have central roles in the coordination of movement. The movement disorder will depend upon where the haemorrhage has occurred and its extent.

Metabolism

Deeper structures, such as the basal ganglia, are less susceptible to direct physical trauma but will be affected by localized hypoxia resulting from cerebrovascular haemorrhage (stroke), circulatory restriction (e.g. at birth, leading to cerebral palsy), or restricted respiration (e.g. asphyxia or drug-induced dyspnoea). Trauma through cerebrovascular haemorrhage affects both the basal ganglia and cortex. The outcome depends on the cerebral artery that has been affected (see Box 8.13, p.183). See also the case of a person with impaired mobility following a stroke, Section VI, p.666.

Glucose deficiency may also induce temporary disorder as energy requirements of neurons are not met. The poorly coordinated movements of someone with diabetes mellitus having a hypoglycaemic episode (and who will also be exhibiting behavioural change, such as aggression) can be mistaken as resulting from alcohol abuse.

Imbalance of excitatory and inhibitory pathways

Disturbance in the balance of excitatory : inhibitory neuronal pathways will disrupt the integration necessary to produce controlled movement:

• *Parkinson's disease:* this is of unknown pathogenesis (though several genes have been implicated) and onset peaks in the early 60s. The condition arises as a consequence of the loss of dopamine as a neurotransmitter within the pathway between the substantia nigra (a midbrain nucleus) and the corpus striatum nucleus of the cerebrum. The imbalance produced between the inhibitory neurons (that utilize dopamine) and excitatory ones (that utilize acetylcholine) results in poor coordination of motor output, leading to muscle rigidity and a tremor at rest (hypertonia; Box 17.14), and slowness of movement and occasional freezing (akinesia). The akinesia may also affect speech and swallowing. The individual may also report sudden onset of extreme fatigue. As postural muscles become involved there will be stooped posture on standing, and involuntary flexions of the head. Treatment is mainly via drugs to replace dopamine (e.g. levodopa) or anticholinergics to reduce the excitatory pathway activities (Katzenschlager *et al.*, 2002). Support and rehabilitation may be necessary to improve mobility.

• *Huntington's disease (chorea)*: this is an autosomally dominant, inherited disorder (see Chapter 19, p.547) with an onset typically of between 40 and 50 years. Neurons that utilize gamma-aminobutyric acid (GABA) as an inhibitory neurotransmitter, and are found within the pathway between the substantia nigra and other basal ganglia (the caudate and putamen nuclei) and the cerebral cortex, degenerate leading to an imbalance of pathway activities. This produces exaggerated, involuntary movements (hyperkinesia) typical of chorea: the face and arms begin the movement but eventually the whole body is affected. Cognitive problems also develop. Drugs such as tetrabenazine that prevent the release of monoamine neurotransmitter has shown some experimental promise but gene therapy possibly holds the key to future treatment of this condition (see Chapter 19, p.556).

See the case of a family with Huntington's disease, p.671.

Loss of nerve tracts

Multiple sclerosis is an immune disorder in which neurons are demyelinated, normally commencing in early adulthood. The pathogenesis is unclear but may be a response to viral infection. Plaques are produced, primarily within the white matter of the central nervous system:

• Loss of neurons in the corticospinal (pyramidal) tracts produces muscle stiffness, slowness and weakness. The lower limbs are usually more severely affected, with involvement of the bladder.

• Loss of neurons in the brainstem affects the cranial nerves, and hence produces facial/neck weakness.

• The condition may also involve other parts of the brain, for example the cerebellum and basal ganglia, producing poorly coordinated fine movement control (ataxia; Box 17.14) and even paroxysmal outbursts of abrupt movements. Sensory function may also be affected, for example of the eye. Pain is common.

Multiple sclerosis is episodic in its early phases and steroids may be helpful to reduce the rate of plaque formation. However the condition is progressive and care is supportive and rehabilitative (Barnes, 2007).

Cerebral degenerative conditions such as Alzheimer disease and Creuzfeldt–Jakob disease also produce movement problems. However, these are not normally considered to be primarily disorders of posture and movement (see Box 8.8, p.175).

BOX 17.14 SOME CLINICAL TERMS USED TO DESCRIBE DISORDERED VOLUNTARY MOVEMENTS

Clinical terminology in relation to movement and movement disorder is extensive and complex. These are some of the more common terms (others may be found in previous boxes):

- *Akinesia/bradykinesia*: a slowness of movement often reflecting a disorder of the extrapyramidal pathway.
- *Ataxia*: poor fine coordination of movement, and usually signifies a cerebellum disorder.
- *Clonus*: a form of hypertonia in which stretch reflex responses spread to other muscles. It is often seen in spasticity.
- *Dyspraxia or apraxia*: the inability to perform voluntary movements in the absence of paralysis, sensory loss, poor coordination or postural disorder. True dyspraxia arises from a failure of communication between the cerebral hemispheres.
- *Dystonia*: a condition in which damage to basal ganglia prevents the normal control of agonistic and antagonistic muscles, leading to sustained, involuntary twisting movements.
- *Hyperkinesia*: the production of abnormal involuntary movements such as spasms (paroxysmal hyperkinesia) of the face trunk and extremities (tardive hyperkinesia).
- *Hypertonia*: excessive muscle tone, noticeable when the muscle is passively stretched. It often arises as a consequence of trauma to the primary motor areas of the cerebral cortex or to spinal cord tracts (and causes uneven excessive contractions or spasticity), or as a consequence of elevated muscle spindle sensitivity (causing more even but excessive contractions or rigidity).
- *Hypokinesia*: a collective term for poor production of movement. *Paresis* is a related term used to signify weakness, whilst *paralysis* ('-plegia') signifies no movement. Hypokinesia arises through disorders associated with upper or lower motor neurons.
- *Hypotonia*: decreased muscle tone. It is characterized by little resistance to passive stretch of the muscle, indicative of depressed muscle spindle functions. This usually means poor motor output control, and so it is frequently observed as a consequence of trauma to the pyramidal tracts (e.g. spinal cord injury) or to the cerebellum (e.g. cerebrovascular accident). Milder symptoms include tiring and weakness, but the damage may even make it difficult to rise from a chair or use stairs. With time, the lack of motor output to the muscles causes the muscles to atrophy.

Lower motor neuron syndromes promote flaccid paresis or paralysis, and hyporeflexia or areflexia (i.e. depression or absence of reflexes).
Upper motor neuron syndromes promote disorders referred to as:

- *Diplegia*: the paralysis of both upper and lower extremities.
- *Hemiparesis or hemoplegia*: hypokinesia of the upper and lower extremities on one side.
- *Paraparesis or paraplegia*: weakness of the lower extremities.
- *Quadriparesis or quadriplegia*: weakness of all four extremities.

- *The rubrospinal tracts ('rubro-' = red)*: these originate from the red nuclei of the midbrain. Fibres cross over and descend in the lateral aspects of the cord.
- *The tectospinal tracts ('tectum' = roof)*: these originate from the superior colliculi of the tectum area of the midbrain, which receive input from the eyes. This tract is therefore part of the pathway that controls movement in response to visual stimuli.
- *The vestibulospinal tracts*: these derive from the vestibular nuclei of the medulla, and are influenced by input from the vestibular receptors of the inner ear.

Cerebellum

The cerebellum 'assists' the outputs from the motor cortex and basal ganglia by modulating the final neural output from the motor cortex, and hence controlling the timing and sequence of muscle contractions. The cerebellum therefore has a vital role in the precise control of fine movements necessary, for example, for writing, for buttoning clothing, for hitting a tennis ball, or simply for placing the foot during walking (i.e. without stamping!).

SUMMARY

1 The skeletomuscular system provides the support and mobility required for the performance of basic activities of living.
2 Skeletal muscles support the skeleton and provide the capacity to move joints. They are composed of bundles of muscle fibres, called fascicles, and are activated by associated motor nerves. Muscle fibres are cells that became fused together during differentiation. Each fibre acts as one cell and stimulation contracts the entire fibre.
3 Under the microscope, muscle fibres exhibit a striated pattern that repeats along the fibre. Each 'segment' is called a sarcomere, and the striations result from the arrangement of protein filaments within it.
4 Muscle fibre contraction involves an interaction between the actin and myosin protein filaments. Molecular cross-bridges between the proteins cause the actin to 'slide' over the myosin, thus pulling the ends of the sarcomere together and so shortening the fibre. The process requires the presence of calcium ions, released into the cytoplasm of the muscle fibre as a consequence of nerve stimulation.

5 The neuromuscular junction exhibits the properties of a synapse, utilizing the release of the neurotransmitter acetylcholine, which induces a change in the electrical property of the muscle fibre. Each muscle fibre within a muscle is innervated, but the numbers of fibres (called a motor unit) that are innervated by branches from a single motor neuron varies from muscle to muscle. Large postural muscles in particular have large motor units and this aids the efficiency of maintaining protracted periods of contraction.
6 Muscle fibres capable of maintaining contraction for long periods must utilize aerobic metabolism in order for them to withstand fatigue. These are called 'slow' fibres. In relative terms, 'fast' fibres produce a much faster contraction and relaxation but rapidly exceed aerobic capacity and therefore fatigue quickly.
7 The arrangement of muscles in relation to joints provides a system of levers that facilitates movement by reducing the force of contraction necessary to move the joint.

SUMMARY *Continued*

8 The degree of contraction produced by a muscle must be appropriate to the situation, and this means that all of the 600+ muscles of the body must be individually controlled. Control is provided by reflex action and by coordination of the neural output from the brain.

9 Sensory information is provided by the proprioceptors, or positional receptors. These are found in the joints, tendons of muscles, in the muscles themselves, and in the inner ear (balance or equilibrium receptors) and provide continuous information regarding the position and movement of joints, of tension in muscles, of muscle length, and of head position in relation to gravity.

10 Muscle spindle receptors are of particular importance as these not only monitor muscle length but can also act to control that length. This is possible because they consist of modified muscle fibres and can be induced to contract or relax according to the activity of their own motor innervation. Thus spindle length can be varied independently of the rest of the muscle, and in doing so can reflexly induce muscle contraction or relaxation. Muscle length, therefore, is determined by the neural activity in the motor nerve cells that innervate its fibres, and by the motor nerve cells that innervate the spindles. This dual innervation provides a high degree of control, and emphasizes the complex nature of the motor coordination provided by the brain.

11 Much of the brain is involved in receiving sensory information from around the body, and in motor control. The latter areas are the motor cortex of the cerebrum, the basal ganglia and the cerebellum of the hindbrain. Interactions between these areas occur, involving complex excitatory and inhibitory neural pathways, before the final activity is conveyed to the appropriate peripheral motor neurons.

12 Output from the motor cortex passes to the spinal cord or cranial nerves via the pyramidal pathways. That which passes directly from the basal ganglia, without first passing to the motor cortex, comprises the extrapyramidal pathways.

REFERENCES

Attarian, S., Vedel, J.P., Pouget, J. and Schmied, A. (2008) Progression of cortical and spinal dysfunctions over time in amyotrophic lateral sclerosis. *Muscle and Nerve* **37**(3): 364–75.

Barnes, F. (2007) Care of people with multiple sclerosis in the community setting. *British Journal of Community Nursing* **12**(12): 552–7.

Campbell, A. and Fallaha, D. (2007) Tetanus: pathophysiology and management. *Care of the Critically Ill* **23**(4): 100–4.

Cech, D.J. (2002) *Functional Movement Development Across the Lifespan*, 2nd edn. Philadelphia: Saunders.

Cunning, S. (2000) When the Dx is myasthenia gravis. *RN* **63**(4): 26–31.

Katzenschlager R., Sampaio C., Costa J. and Lees A. (2002) Anticholinergics for symptomatic management of Parkinson´s disease. *Cochrane Database of Systematic Reviews*, Issue 3. Art. No.: CD003735. DOI: 10.1002/14651858.CD003735.

Worsham, T.L. (2000) Easing the course of Guillain–Barré syndrome. *RN* **63**(3) 46–50.

CHAPTER 18

THE REPRODUCTIVE SYSTEMS

INTRODUCTION: RELATION OF REPRODUCTION TO HOMEOSTASIS

All organ systems of the body operate as homeostatic controls to maintain the well-being of the body, provided that the person is not genetically and/or environmentally compromised. At the cellular level of organization, reproduction may be regarded as a homeostatic process in which cells divide once they have reached their optimal size. Further growth would mean that the cell is unable to obtain sufficient levels of nutrients to sustain intercellular homeostasis, or to remove toxic chemicals, since the cell membrane (i.e. surface area) grows at a slower rate then the rest of the cell (i.e. volume) that it supports. Cell reproduction is also important to replace those in the vicinity that have become damaged or have aged. Cellular reproduction is therefore necessary to maintain the appropriate growth, development, specialization, and repair of human tissues, thus contributing to a person's well-being.

At the organism level of organization, reproduction may be regarded as a homeostatic control adapted for the survival of the species (Figure 18.1). The human reproductive system is dormant until the onset of puberty, when there seems to be a trigger that activates the genetic code responsible for the production of hormones for the initiation and continuation of this developmental stage. It is unclear what the trigger is but increased secretion of hormones from the pituitary gland is observed: one theory is that there is a maturation of the circulation between the brain and pituitary gland that facilitates the homeostatic process of regulating the gland. As we will see, the pituitary gland has a central role in determining and controlling reproductive anatomy and physiology.

Although the common purpose of both sexes is to produce offspring, their functional roles are quite different. The male role is to produce up to half a billion gametes (sperm, or spermatozoa) per day, which are then matured and activated when mixed with glandular secretions, creating a mixture called semen. This fluid leaves the male system by the process of ejaculation. The female role is to produce and mature female gametes (oocytes; i.e. immature 'eggs'), and to release (ovulate) one oocyte per month (although sometimes two oocytes are released; i.e. one from each ovary simultaneously). These gametes travel suspended in fluid to the Fallopian tubes (or oviducts) of the uterus (womb). Following sexual intercourse, the male and female gametes may fuse (in the process called

Figure 18.1 Cellular and sexual reproduction: homeostatic devices. a, Reproductive function fluctuating within its homeostatic range: on a cellular level, this reflects that cellular reproduction matches cellular loss; on an organism level, this reflects that the population size is sustainable (e.g. by its food supplies). b_1, Increased reproductive capacity: on a cellular basis, this reflects that cell reproduction is greater than cellular losses (e.g. following injury when cells are reproducing to replace lost or damaged cells), alternatively, it could indicate some underlying pathology, such as tumour growth or hypertrophied organs; on an organism basis, this reflects that the human population number has increased beyond its capabilities of maintaining such a population explosion. c_1, Homeostatic 'controls' that correct the cellular disturbance, as occurs normally during post-healing periods and when cancers are destroyed by the body's anti-cancer agents or via clinical interventions using chemotherapy, radiotherapy, surgery and/or laser therapy. Homeostatic 'controls' that correct the population explosion (e.g. limited food supplies accompanied by the survival of the fittest). c_2, Correction of underlying pathology or natural changes. d_1, An increase in cellular reproduction that is beyond control as occurs, for example, in certain cancers, or population explosion living beyond human resource level. b_2, Decreased cellular reproduction. d_2, A decreased cellular reproduction that is

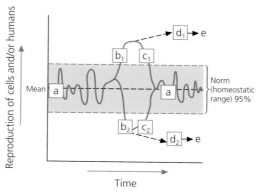

beyond control, as occurs normally with the ageing process, or abnormally in pathological wasting conditions, such as anorexia nervosa. A severe decrease in the population as occurs in natural disasters, such as war, famine, etc. e, Death at a cellular or human level. (a, Represents boxes a_1–a_4 in Figure 1.7, p.11, reflecting the individual variability in the homeostatic range) fertilization) to produce a new cell called the zygote. The zygote contains all the genetic information required to produce another human. A pregnancy is initiated if the zygote implants into the lining of the uterus. Thus, although the female and male are equal partners in the fertilization process, it is the female's uterus that provides a life-support system for the baby until birth. During this period (i.e. gestation), the female's homeostatic parameters are reset to provide a suitable environment for prebirth development and nutritional support via breast milk for the newborn until it is able to consume a mixed diet.

The intentions of this chapter are to present an overview of the anatomy and physiology of the male and female reproductive systems, and to give a detailed account of the physiological processes and hormonal mechanisms responsible for the homeostatic regulation of reproductive function. The physiology underpinning birth control will also be discussed, and boxed applications identify common male and female homeostatic imbalances, with their principles of correction identified.

OVERVIEW OF THE ANATOMY AND PHYSIOLOGY OF THE HUMAN REPRODUCTIVE SYSTEMS

The human reproductive system consists of:

- a pair of primary sex organs (gonads) that produce, store and nourish the developing sex cells (gametes). The gonads are involved in the production and initial transport of the gametes (i.e. spermatozoa and oocytes – the potential ova), and function as endocrine tissue to produce hormones that coordinate activities specific to the different sexes;
- a diverse range of other structures, such as channels (ducts) that transport gametes, accessory glands that secrete fluid into ducts, and external genitalia associated with the sexes.

The various functions of the male and female reproductive tracts are summarized in the tables accompanying Figures 18.2 and 18.3.

The male reproductive system

The male reproductive system is adapted for:

- the production of spermatozoa;
- the transportation of spermatozoa to the female reproductive tract;
- producing hormones that control the development of the secondary sexual characteristics, such as enlargement of the larynx, development of the male form, and body, pubic and facial hair.

The primary sex organs are called the testes (singular, testis). These produce the male gametes – the spermatozoa – in a process called spermatogenesis. This process is controlled by the release of a gonadotropin hormone ('-tropin' = a generic term for a hormone that acts on another endocrine gland) called follicle-stimulating hormone (FSH) from the anterior pituitary

gland (see Figure 9.5, p.214). This hormone is actually named after its role to stimulate ovarian follicles in women but it has retained its name in men. The testes store spermatozoa until they are either released from the body or broken down into their component parts and then recycled to contribute to intra-

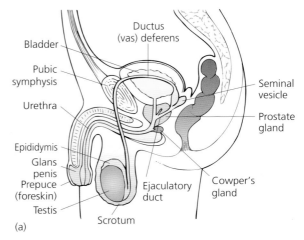

(a)

Structure	Homeostatic function
Testes	Produce sperm and sex hormone
Accessory organs	
Vas deferens, urethra	Transports sperm out of the body
Glands – seminal vesicles, prostate, Cowper's	Contribute the majority of fluid within semen
Scrotum	House the testis outside the pelvic cavity – essential for viable sperm production
Penis	Organ of copulation and excretion

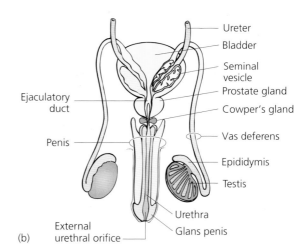

(b)

Figure 18.2 The male reproductive system: (a) sagittal view and (b) posterior view

Q Identify the accessory sex gland that contributes fructose to the seminal fluid.

Q What accessory glands contribute the majority of the seminal fluid?

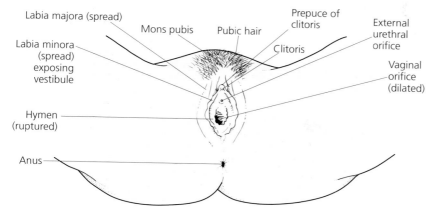

Figure 18.3 External genitalia of the female (the vulva)

Q *Name the location of the erectile tissue found in the female.*

Structure	Homeostatic function
Mons pubis	Cushions the pubic symphysis during sexual intercourse
Labia majora	Enclose and protect other external reproductive organs
Labia minora	Form margins of vestibule; protect openings of vagina and urethra
Clitoris	Gland is richly supplied with sensory nerve endings
Vestibule	Space between labia minora that includes vaginal and urethal openings
Vestibular glands	Secrete fluid that moistens and lubricates vestibule

BOX 18.1 SEXUAL DIFFERENTIATION FROM UTERUS TO PUBERTY

During embryonic development, it is the presence or absence of the male sex hormone testosterone that normally determines sexual development. Until the seventh week of gestation, the initial reproductive structures of the male and female are the same, but soon after this the gonads of a genetically male embryo begin to produce testosterone. This causes the primary male sex gonads to develop into two testes, which produce spermatozoa. The lack of testosterone, normally because the embryo is genetically female, causes the two gonads to develop into ovaries, which produce the hormone oestrogen, and will eventually produce immature oocytes.

Throughout fetal life and childhood, the testes secrete low levels of testosterone and the ovaries secrete low levels of oestrogens. Between the ages of 8 and 12 years, the gonads start to secrete more sex hormones. This triggers sexual maturation, or puberty. In girls, puberty commences at about 10 years; in boys, it begins at about 11 years. Puberty last for 2 or 3 years, and is complete when the person is capable of reproduction.

cellular homeostatic mechanisms. The testes also contain endocrine cells, which produce and secrete the male hormones (collectively called androgens), but this process is still regulated by the release of a gonadotropin, luteinizing hormone (LH; again named after its role in women), from the anterior pituitary. Testosterone is the main androgen produced by the testes.

The accessory reproductive organs consist of the scrotum, ducts, glands and penis. These protect the spermatozoa and aid their transport outside the body (Figure 18.2).

Structure of the testes

The paired oval-shaped testes originate from a location close to the developing kidneys near the posterior abdominal wall of the embryo. They develop from the embryonic tissue that also gives rise to the urinary system; indeed, the urethra of the male provides a common route for the exit of spermatozoa and urine from the body. The testes descend from the abdomen, through a channel called the inguinal canal into their sac-like scrotum to be externalized as the testicles during the seventh month of gestation, following contraction of specialized muscular tissue called the gubernaculum (Figure 18.4a). The testes are thus suspended outside the abdominal pelvic cavity. This means that their temperature is 2–3°C below the core body temperature of 37°C (see Figure 16.8, p.456). Spermatozoa development will only progress normally at this cooler temperature. The testicular venous plexus also contributes to the cooler temperature of the testes, since it coils around the testicular artery and functions to absorb heat from arterial blood, thus cooling it before it enters the testes.

Each oval-shaped testis is surrounded by the tunica albuginea, a connective tissue capsule that extends inwards, dividing it into compartmentalizing lobules. Each lobule contains one to four seminiferous tubules, which produce spermatozoa. These spermatozoa-producing factories are continuous with other tubules (the ductus efferentia, epididymis, vas deferentia and urethra) that provide the distribution route for spermatozoa exiting from the body (Figure 18.5a). A cross-section of a seminiferous tubule reveals that it contains immature spermatozoa

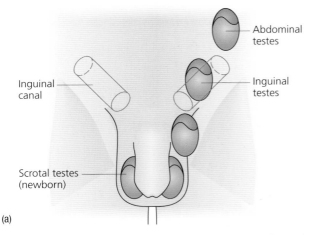

Abdominal testes

Inguinal canal

Inguinal testes

Scrotal testes (newborn)

(a)

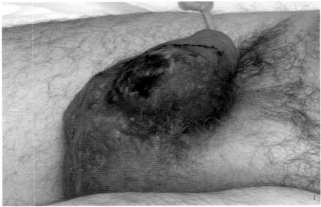

(b)

Figure 18.4 (a) Descent of the testes. (b) Patient exhibiting testicular cancer. Reproduced with the kind permission of the Medical Illustration Department, Norfolk and Norwich University Hospital NHS Trust

Q Normally, the testes descend before birth. In which homeostatic imbalance is there a failure of this descent?

Q Which hormone is responsible for the differentiation of the external genitals of the male?

cells at various stages of development. The most immature cells, called the spermatogonia, are located peripherally; the fully mature spermatozoa are located centrally within the tubule lumen. In between these two locations, the cells are of advancing maturity, and are called primary spermatocytes, secondary spermatocytes, and spermatids, respectively, i.e.:

Spermatogonia → primary spermatocytes → secondary spermatocytes → spermatids → spermatozoa

⟹ Increasing maturity of cells

Embedded between the developing spermatozoa cells are the Sertoli or sustentacular cells. Their homeostatic functions are to:

- support, nourish and protect developing spermatogenic cells;

BOX 18.2 CRYPTORCHIDISM AND TESTICULAR CANCER

Cryptorchidism is an undescended testis at birth. One or both testes may be affected. Often the testis will descend after birth. If this does not occur between 9 and 15 months a doctor will usually recommend surgery (orchiopexy) to move the testis into the scrotum, since an undescended testis increases the risk of infertility because of the higher body temperatures of the abdomen, which results in a decrease in the spermatozoa-making ability, a process that in its early stages may begin as early as 12 months of age; therefore, surgery must occur no later than the age of two.

Cryptorchidism occurs in about 5% of baby boys and 3% of premature infants (Behrman *et al.*, 2004). This condition may also cause hormonal imbalances; therefore such infants require early treatment by surgery or by testosterone injections, which stimulate the descent of the testes. If untreated, spermatogenesis is inhibited permanently and there is then a risk that an undescended testis left in the abdomen may undergo malignant changes.

Testicular cancer (Figure 18.4b) although rare is 20 times greater in people with a history of late descended or undescended testes. Most cancers arise from the spermatozoa-producing cells. Testicular tumours represent 1–2% of male malignancies, and it is the commonest cancer affecting men aged 20–24 years (Pettersson *et al.*, 2007).

Because of this risk, healthcare practitioners, such as nurses and doctors, should encourage monthly self-examination of the testes, since an alteration of or an enlarged testis, although not necessarily a malignancy, should be reported to their GP as soon as possible. Men who have not had an undescended testicle should also have medical check-ups at least once every 2 years throughout life.

As with all cancers, correction is most effective when diagnosis is made early in the development of the tumour, and necessitates removal of the cancerous tissue.

ACTIVITY

Discuss why it is important that the testes descend before birth.

- phagocytose degenerating spermatogenic cells;
- control the movement of spermatogenic cells;
- control the release of spermatozoa into the lumen of the seminiferous tubules;
- secrete chemicals that maintain testicular homeostasis; for example, the hormone inhibin depresses FSH production and hence reduces the rate of spermatogenesis, and androgen-binding protein helps prevent androgen hormones (e.g. testosterone) from going beyond their homeostatic parameters, and facilitates the actions of the androgens. These secretions provide negative feedback loops, which maintain reproductive function within its homeostatic parameters (see later, and Figure 18.14, p.505).

Accessory organs of the male reproductive system

Accessory organs of the male system comprise the duct system, various secretory glands and the penis.

After production, the spermatozoa are moved from the seminiferous tubules to the straight tubules. The latter lead to a network of ciliated ducts called the rete testis ('rete' = net), which empty into the ductus efferentia (Figure 18.5a). From

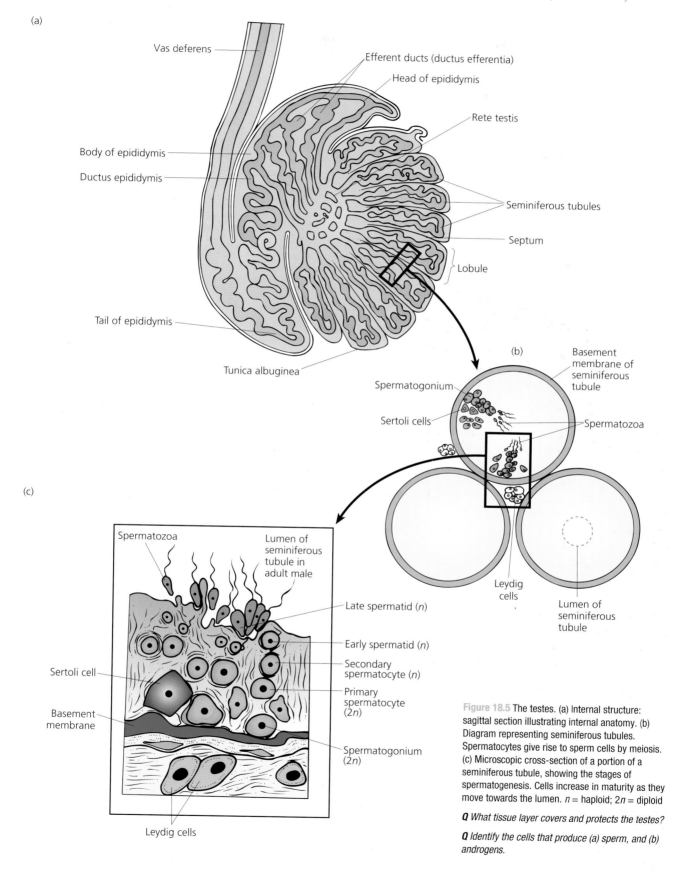

(a)

Vas deferens

Efferent ducts (ductus efferentia)

Head of epididymis

Rete testis

Body of epididymis

Ductus epididymis

Seminiferous tubules

Septum

Lobule

Tail of epididymis

Tunica albuginea

(b)

Basement membrane of seminiferous tubule

Spermatogonium

Sertoli cells

Spermatozoa

Leydig cells

Lumen of seminiferous tubule

(c)

Spermatozoa

Lumen of seminiferous tubule in adult male

Late spermatid (*n*)

Early spermatid (*n*)

Secondary spermatocyte (*n*)

Primary spermatocyte (2*n*)

Sertoli cell

Spermatogonium (2*n*)

Basement membrane

Leydig cells

Figure 18.5 The testes. (a) Internal structure: sagittal section illustrating internal anatomy. (b) Diagram representing seminiferous tubules. Spermatocytes give rise to sperm cells by meiosis. (c) Microscopic cross-section of a portion of a seminiferous tubule, showing the stages of spermatogenesis. Cells increase in maturity as they move towards the lumen. *n* = haploid; 2*n* = diploid

Q What tissue layer covers and protects the testes?

Q Identify the cells that produce (a) sperm, and (b) androgens.

here, the spermatozoa are transported through a duct system averaging 8 m in length. In order of transit, the sections of this system are called the epididymis, the vas deferens (spermatozoa tube) and the urethra (see Figure 18.2b, p.486).

The duct system

The epididymis

From the rete testis, the spermatozoa enter the head, body and then the tail of the epididymis via the ductus efferentia. It takes about 2 weeks for the spermatozoa to transit the epididymis. The homeostatic functions of this region are to:

* absorb excess fluid from the lumen, and secrete nutrients into the lumen, so as to provide a suitable environment for spermatozoa maturation. This process is referred to as 'capacitation' and is essential to ensure cell motility and fertility;
* act as a temporary storage site for spermatozoa until they are either released into the vasa deferentia when the male is sexually aroused and ejaculates, or broken down chemically, and their constituents recycled.

The vas deferens

The vas deferens (ductus deferens) is about 40–45 cm long. It begins at the epididymis and ends behind the urinary bladder, where it expands to form the ampulla region from which the ejaculatory ducts emerge. These ducts penetrate the muscular wall of the prostate gland, and upon contraction empty their contents into the urethra (see Figure 18.2b, p.486).

The urethra

The urethra extends for a distance of about 15–20 cm from the urinary bladder to the tip of the penis. This terminal portion of the male system, together with the penis, serves both the urinary and reproductive systems, as it conveys urine and semen to the exterior. Thus, these structures form a common part of the urogenital tract. Figure 18.6a shows that the urethra has three anatomical regions:

* *prostatic urethra:* passes through the prostate gland; this region conveys urine and fluid that contributes to semen;
* *membranous urethra:* a short segment that passes from the prostatic urethra to the penile urethra, and penetrates the urogenital diaphragm and the muscular floor of the pelvic cavity; this section conveys urine and fluid that contributes to semen;
* *penile urethra:* extends from the distal border of the urogenital diaphragm to the external orifice at the tip of the penis. This section conveys urine and semen (with spermatozoa).

Accessory sex glands

The accessory glands of the male reproductive tract include paired seminal vesicles, paired bulbourethral (Cowper's) glands, and a single prostate gland (see Figure 18.2, p.486). They contribute up to approximately the 95% of the fluid contained in semen (the fluid conveyed and expelled from the urethra via peristalsis during ejaculation). The seminiferous tubules and the epididymis produce secretions that contribute a small percentage to semen. Collectively, the secretions activate spermatozoa in the semen by providing nutrients for their motility, and act as a buffer mechanism, thus counteracting the acidic environments of the urethra and the female tract.

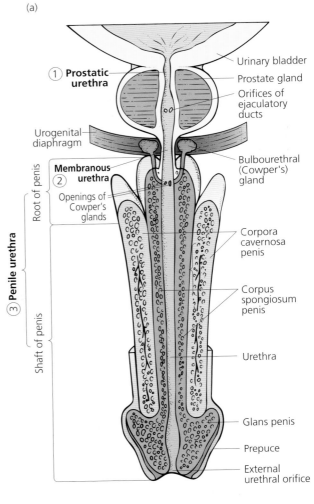

(a)

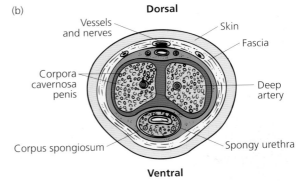

(b)

Figure 18.6 Structure of the penis: (a) longitudinal section; (b) transverse section

Q Which tissue forms the erectile tissue in the penis?

BOX 18.3 NON-SPECIFIC URETHRITIS

Typically urethritis is not normally caused by sex, but by poor hygiene or conditions, for example diabetes, that support the growth of microorganisms in the environment. The inflammation may also arise from trauma (e.g. the passage of a catheter) and chemical agents (e.g. excessive alcohol consumption).

Non-specific urethritis (NSU), however, is basically an infection of the urethra caused by a variety of organisms (although a high proportion of the infection is caused by gonorrhoea and *Chlamydia*) and therefore is usually passed on via sexual intercourse, and thus affects both sexes. In addition, bacterial agents can pass from an infected mother to infant during birth, and infect the eyes of the infant. The most important aspects of prevention of NSU are limiting the number of sexual partners and using condoms for sex. Condoms, however, do not eliminate the risk since they can split or tear, especially if not used properly.

With the infection the urethra swells and narrows, which impedes the flow of urine, and causes various symptoms (which are similar in both sexes: an increased frequency of urination, a burning sensation in urination, and there may also be a pus-containing discharge).

Complications arising from NSU are infrequent; however, for men there is a slight chance of inflamed testicles and infection of the prostate, and for both women and men there is a small risk of Reiter's syndrome – an immunological disorder associated with conjunctivitis and joint pains and/or a rash on the feet and genitals.

Although many NSU infections remain untreated, since symptoms in the male are mild and females are usually asymptomatic, the infection is easily treated with antibiotic, antiviral or antifungal medication depending on which organism is causing the problem. While taking the treatment, and until the infection has been cleared, it is best to avoid sexual contact.

The seminal vesicles

The seminal vesicles are located on the posterior wall at the base of the bladder. They secrete a viscous alkaline fluid, which accounts for approximately 60% of semen volume. This fluid contains chemicals including fructose, prostaglandins and ascorbic acid, which contribute to the life (viability) of the spermatozoa. Fructose, a sugar, provides the essential fuel necessary to initiate and maintain the beating of the spermatozoa tail (flagellum). Prostaglandins are thought to:

- decrease the viscosity of the mucus plug which guards the entrance to the uterus (i.e. the cervix) of the female, making it more passable by spermatozoa;
- stimulate anti-peristalsis, that is, contractions of the female reproductive tract away from the cervix, and so aid transportation of spermatozoa from the cervix to the site of fertilization in the Fallopian tubes;
- stimulate the release of the hormone relaxin and certain enzymes that enhance spermatozoa motility;

BOX 18.4 PROSTATISM, PROSTATIC HYPERTROPHY AND PROSTATIC CANCER

The prostate gland is susceptible to infection, enlargement and benign/malignant tumours.

Prostatism is a male urinary tract problem associated with lesions of the prostate. Symptoms include difficulty in micturition, a poor urinary stream, and urinary frequency with nocturia (micturition during the night).

Benign prostatic enlargement or hypertrophy (BPH) is a common problem: more than 50% of men in their 60s, and as many as 90% in their 80s, have some symptoms of this condition.

The prostate continues to grow during most of a man's life; however the enlargement does not usually cause problems until late in life. There are two main periods of growth: in puberty, the prostate doubles in size, and in the mid-20s the gland has a secondary surge in growth. This second growth spurt often results, years later, in BPH. Since the prostate surrounds the urethra, its enlargement can obstruct the flow of urine, resulting in secondary homeostatic imbalances of the bladder, and kidneys. It can be managed successfully with drugs (e.g. finasteride) but correction may involve partial removal of the enlarged tissue or total removal of the gland. However, if the patient cannot tolerate surgery, a permanent indwelling catheter is inserted with appropriate care, including:

- selecting the appropriate length and bore size of catheter and balloon;
- ensuring that the catheter bag is positioned lower than the bladder, that the drainage tubing is free of kinks, and that the drainage outlet is not touching any potential contaminants;
- controlling fluid intake to reduce the risk of constipation and of concentrating the urine, which can be a potential cause of bladder irritation;
- providing psychological support, since the catheter *in situ* affects body image;
- hygiene of the penile opening, or meatus, to minimize encrustation.

Although is no definite information on risk factors, the increased frequency with age has led some researchers to believe that factors related to ageing and the testes may spur the development of BPH. Men produce testosterone (see main text) from their testes, but also small amounts of oestrogen, a female hormone, from their adrenal cortex. With ageing, the blood concentration of active testosterone decreases, reducing the testosterone to oestrogen ratio, and so leaving a higher proportion of oestrogen. Studies on animals have suggested that BPH may be a result of this higher proportion of the female hormone.

See the case of a man with BPH, Section VI, p.669.

Prostatic cancer is a common and leading cause of cancer death in men. However, it rarely occurs before the age of 50 years. Genetics is a known risk factor and hence the risk is greater in a close relative, such as with a father, brother or uncle who had prostatic cancer. There also seems to be a positive correlation if several women family members have developed breast cancer, particularly if it occurs under 40 years of age, suggesting there may be a common genetic link in these cancers. A high-fat diet also seems to increase the incidence of this type of cancer.

Since testosterone stimulates an increased growth rate of the cancer, treatment may involve surgical removal of the testes, or the administration of drugs that are testosterone antagonists such as goserelin (Zoladex) and bicalutamide (Casodex). Although drug administration does not stop the cancer, it may slow growth. Radiotherapy is also an option. Palliative measures are aimed at relieving urinary bladder outlet problems, colonic obstruction (owing to compression from the tumour), spinal cord compression and pain. Treatment and prognosis depend upon the extent of the disease. There are new treatments being developed such as cryotherapy (i.e. surgery which uses liquid gas to freeze the prostate and kill cancer cells) and high-intensity, focused ultrasound (i.e. high-frequency sound waves are used to kill cancer cells.

- stimulate a chemical in semen called plasmin, which has bactericidal properties. Together with other unidentified chemicals with antibiotic properties, this may help to prevent urinary tract infections, and thus must be considered a part of the homeostatic external defence mechanisms;
- stimulate clotting factors (e.g. fibrinogen) in semen, which cause its coagulation after ejaculation, helping to retain it within the female tract;
- stimulate the enzyme fibrinolysin, which liquefies the coagulant mass about 5–20 minutes after it clots, so that the spermatozoa can swim out and begin their journey within the female tract.

Ascorbic acid in semen acts as a cofactor in some metabolic reactions within the spermatozoa's cytoplasm. This action is also promoted by the presence of prostaglandins.

The prostate

The prostate, a large gland positioned just below the bladder, secretes a thin, milky, alkaline secretion that accounts for 14–30% of semen. It contains fibrinolysin and acid phosphatase, enzymes that are important in liquefying semen and promoting maximum motility of the spermatozoa.

The bulbourethral glands

The bulbourethral (Cowper's) glands are much smaller than the prostate. They are so called because of their shape (bulbous), and because they secrete their fluid directly into the urethra. They release thick, clear, alkaline mucus just before ejaculation; this neutralizes traces of acidic urine that reside in the urethra, and lubricates the end of the penis before and during sexual intercourse. The female reproductive organs, however, provide most of the lubricating fluid for intercourse.

The penis

As has been noted, the cylindrically shaped penis is a urogenital organ. Its shape facilitates the introduction of spermatozoa into the female reproductive tract during sexual intercourse (copulation or coitus); therefore, the structure is a necessity for the perpetuation of the species. It is also the male organ of urinary excretion since it conveys urine through the urethra to the external environment.

The penis and the scrotum (testicles) constitute the male external genitalia. The penis consists of an attached root and a free body (shaft) that ends in an enlarged sensitive tip, called the glans penis, over which the skin is folded doubly to form a loosely fitted retractable case (the prepuce or foreskin) (Figure 18.6a). Internally, the penis comprises the urethra and three cylindrical masses or bodies (corpora) of spongy erectile tissue; the urethra at this point may be referred to as the spongy urethra. All three masses are enclosed by a fibrous connective tissue (fascia) and loose-fitting skin (Figure 18.6b). The two larger, uppermost cylinders form the corpora cavernosa; the

---

ACTIVITY

Describe the structure of the penis.

BOX 18.5 PARAPHIMOSIS, HYDROCOELE AND INGUINAL HERNIA

The penis may be subjected to structural abnormalities and numerous sexually transmitted infections (see Box 18.19, p.516).

- *Paraphimosis*: a condition in which the foreskin (prepuce) fits so tightly over the glans penis that it cannot retract. This can occur in catheterized patients, and results in severe discomfort. It is treated by manual reduction. Circumcision (excision or cutting of the prepuce) may be necessary once the inflammation subsides. Mild paraphimosis causes the accumulation of dirt or organic matter under the foreskin, resulting in severe infection. Severe paraphimosis can result in urinary flow obstruction; it may result in death in an infant born with the condition. After puberty, failure to achieve a penile erection occurs; although this does not affect spermatozoa production, it may cause infertility since normal intercourse may not be possible.
- *Hydrocoele*: this is an accumulation of fluid that is a common cause of scrotal swelling. Acute hydrocoele occurs in association with mumps or acute infections of the epididymis of the testes, or as a result of local trauma such as an inguinal hernia (see below). The cause of chronic hydrocoele is unknown. Treatment is only necessary if the hydrocoele compresses the testicular circulation, or if the scrotum becomes enlarged, uncomfortable or embarrassing. A surgical incision is made through the wall of the scrotum and the sac is resected or, after opening, sutured to collapse the wall. Health care involves applying an ice pack to the scrotum to reduce the oedema and bruising. A scrotal support is worn postoperatively.
- *Inguinal hernia*: this occurs because the intestines are pushed through a weakened area of the abdominal wall that separates the abdominal pelvic cavity from the scrotum. Such hernias usually occur upon lifting heavy objects, although they can also be formed congenitally. Inguinal hernias are much more common in men and femoral hernias more common in women, although they do occur in either sex. Correction involves external supports that prevent organs from protruding into the scrotum and aspiration (or drawing) of fluid, but the more serious hernias require surgical repair, thus require perioperative nursing care.

---

smaller, lower one, which contains the urethra, is the corpus spongiosum.

The male sexual act

During sexual arousal, parasympathetic nerve activity is increased causing the vascular spaces or sinuses within the spongy erectile tissue of the penis to vasodilate and become engorged with blood. The expansion compresses the veins draining the penis, so most blood flowing into it is retained. The spongy tissue is engorged with blood, enlarging the penis and causing it to become rigid. The resultant erection permits the penis to perform a penetrating role during sexual intercourse.

Ejaculation of semen is a sympathetic nerve reflex that also causes the bladder sphincter to close, and so prevents the mixing of urine and semen in the urethra (which could immobilize the spermatozoa), and prevents semen entering the bladder. Ejaculation occurs when peristaltic contractions from the testes spread to the epididymis, vas deferens and accessory glands simultaneous to the closing of the bladder sphincter. Muscles in the penis contract, and the semen is discharged.

BOX 18.6 INFERTILITY AND STERILITY IN MALES

Male infertility is the inability of the man to bring about conception, whereas male sterility is the inability to produce potent spermatozoa. However, the two terms are often used interchangeably.

Decreased production of spermatozoa (oligospermia) can result from disruption of seminiferous tubule function. The decrease may be temporary, as occurs with acute infections (the leading cause of infertility), or permanent, as occurs occasionally when a baby is born with undescended testes (cryptorchidism) or has a physical deficiency or obstruction of the reproductive ducts (the leading cause of sterility). A reduced reproductive capacity in males may also be due to factors that cause structural abnormalities of the spermatozoa. Thus, the number, motility and shape of the spermatozoa can give a hint of fertility, and are used clinically to assess the degree of infertility. Normal values are as follows:
Volume of semen ejaculated: 2–6 mL.

Spermatozoa count: 60–150 million/mL. The vast number of spermatozoa is required since only a small percentage survive and eventually reach the site of fertilization; although only one spermatozoon fertilizes an ovum, fertilization requires the combined action of large numbers to chemically break down the barrier produced by the follicular cells

surrounding the ovum. The volume and number will be progressively decreased if the man has had frequent ejaculations.
Shape: 60–80% should have the normal appearance.
Motility: 50% should be motile after incubation for 1 hour at 37°C.

Spermatozoa can be frozen and stored at −70°C; their motility and fertilizing potential reappears when thawed. This process is used when artificial insemination by husband or donor is required. It may also be used for men who are undergoing chemotherapy, since this type of treatment may cause infertility.

Undersecretion of gonadotropin-releasing hormones and gonadotropins (follicle-stimulating hormone and luteinizing hormone) can lead to sterility in either sex, since functional gametes will not be produced. The depression of hypothalamic secretion of gonadotropin-releasing hormones may be a consequence of dietary disturbances, distress or anaemia. In males, fatigue, alcohol abuse and emotional factors are more common causes of impotency (i.e. inability to perform sexual intercourse). High testicular temperatures decrease spermatozoa production and thus are also associated with sterility. Pituitary, gonad and adrenal gland tumours may also cause infertility by secreting abnormal types and amounts of gonadotropin or sex hormones.

The penile flaccid state returns when the arteries constrict and pressure on the veins is relieved.

ACTIVITY

Read the article by Meston and Frolich (2000), which describes how Viagra works.

The female reproductive system

The female reproductive system is adapted for:

* oogenesis (i.e. the production of oocytes/ova);
* receiving spermatozoa;
* providing a suitable environment for fertilization and for prebirth development (see Figure 19.4, p.526);
* producing hormones that control the development of secondary sexual characteristics, such as pubic hair, and the provision of the feminine form.

The female reproductive system, therefore, has a greater variety of tasks than the male system, which is involved only in spermatozoa production and ejaculation. This is reflected in the greater complexity of the female reproductive organs.

The primary female sex organs are the paired ovaries. The accessory reproductive organs consist of the uterine (Fallopian) tubes, the uterus (womb), the vagina, and the external genitalia that comprise the vulva (Figure 18.7a). In addition, the mammary glands have a significant role in female reproduction (see later).

Ovaries

The paired ovaries are structures about twice the size of almond nuts. One lies on each side of the pelvic cavity. Their position is supported by ovarian ligaments, which anchor them medially to the uterus, suspensory ligaments, which anchor them laterally to the pelvic wall, and broad ligaments, which anchor them to the posterior wall of the pelvis (Figure 18.7b).

Each ovary contains a hilus, or site where nerves, blood, and lymphatic vessels enter/exit. Just as the testes are adapted for spermatozoa and hormonal production in the male, the ovaries are adapted for the production of oocytes (cells that develop into mature ova following fertilization) and hormones (progesterone, oestrogens and relaxin). Therefore, they contain germ cells, distributed as a germinal epithelium found as a surface layer of cuboidal cells in the outer cortex of this organ (Figure 18.8) and glandular cells. Other structures include the tunica albuginea, that is, a capsule of connective tissue immediately encloses the general epithelium, and a stroma, a region of connective tissue deep to the tunica albuginea in the outer cortical and inner medullary regions.

The cortical region of the ovary contains the ovarian follicles. As the menstrual cycle proceeds, the follicles progressively change their structure, as follows:

1 In the early stages of the menstrual cycle, primary follicles consist of a couple of external layers of epithelial cells and a primary oocyte. The inner layers comprise the granulosa cells.
2 Secondary follicles develop fluid-filled spaces around the granulosa cells. The spaces unite to form a central fluid-filled cavity or antrum.
3 A Graafian follicle is observed just before the release of the oocyte at ovulation. This is the most mature stage of follicular development. The oocyte is now referred to as a secondary oocyte.
4 A glandular tissue, the corpus luteum (= 'yellow body'), may develop after ovulation. This consists of the Graafian follicle minus its secondary oocyte and encasing granulosa cells. The

(a)

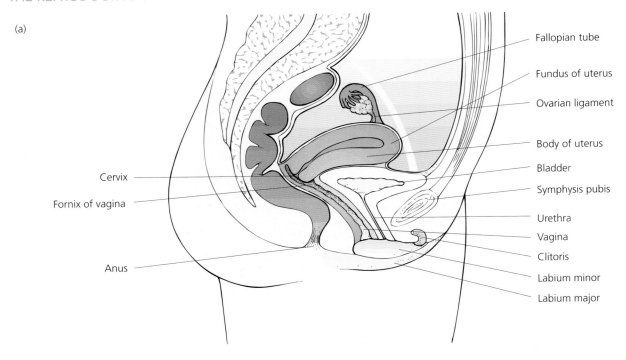

(b)

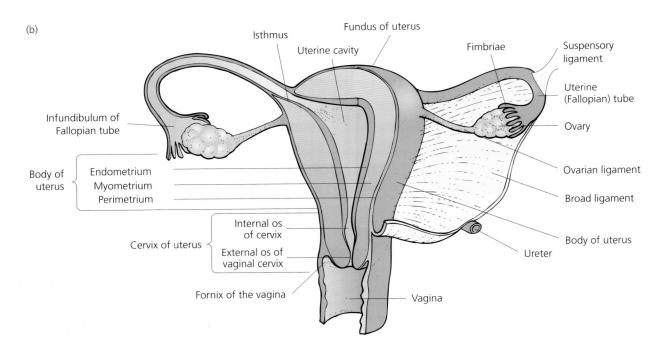

Figure 18.7 The female reproductive system: (a) sagittal section; (b) frontal section

corpus luteum degenerates into the corpus albicans (= 'white body'), unless fertilization takes place, in which case it is retained for a while as the corpus luteum of pregnancy (see later).

Like the testes, the ovaries originate from embryonic tissue close to the posterior abdominal wall near the developing kidneys. During development, they descend to locations just below the pelvic brim, where they remain attached to the lateral pelvic wall.

ACTIVITY

Identify and describe the structure of the primary sex organs of the female, and state the equivalent in the male.

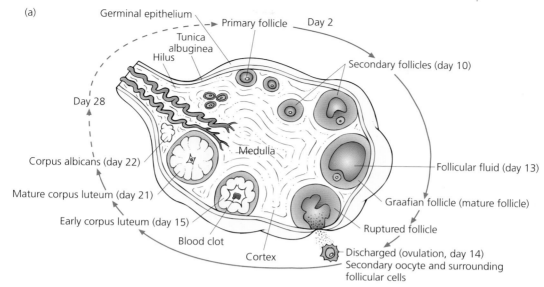

(a)

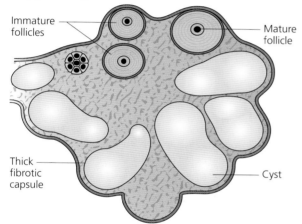

(b) Polycystic ovary

Figure 18.8 (a) An ovary. Approximate times in parentheses are for an average menstrual cycle of 28 days. (b) Polycystic ovarian syndrome

Q What structures in the ovary contain endocrine tissue, and what hormones do they secrete?

The uterine or Fallopian tubes

The two Fallopian tubes (oviducts, or uterine tubes) transport the secondary oocyte to the uterus, during which time it may be fertilized. The oviducts are attached to the uterus at its superior outer angles, which lie in the upper margins of the broad ligaments. Each tube is about 10 cm long and has three distinct regions:

* *isthmus*: the narrow, thick-walled portion that joins the uterus;
* *ampulla*: the intermediate, dilated portion that makes up about two-thirds of the tube's length;
* *infundibulum*: the funnel-shaped, terminal component that opens into the peritoneal cavity surrounding the ovary. The opening has a fringe of finger-like projections, called the fimbriae (Figure 18.9).

The wall of the Fallopian tube consists of three layers:

* *internal mucosa*: has a ciliated surface adapted to aid the movement of the oocyte and to provide it with nutritional support. This layer is in direct contact with the peritoneum of the pelvic cavity, and is continuous with the cavity of the uterus, and hence with the vagina;
* *muscularis layer*: the middle region comprising inner circular, and outer longitudinal, muscle sublayers responsible for the peristaltic movements that move the oocyte towards the uterus;
* *serosa*: an outer serous connective tissue membrane.

Approximately once a month, a secondary oocyte ruptures from the surface of the ovary near the infundibular region of the Fallopian tube in a process called ovulation. The oocyte is swept into the tube by suction pressure generated by the ciliated epithelium of the infundibulum. It is then propelled along the Fallopian tube by ciliary action, supplemented by peristaltic contractions of the muscularis layer. Fertilization

BOX 18.7 OVARIAN CYSTS AND POLYCYSTIC OVARY SYNDROME

Ovarian cysts (fluid-filled sacs) are normally benign (non-cancerous), rarely become dangerous and frequently disappear within a few months of their emergence. However, some are cancerous, or may become cancerous over time. There are several types of ovarian cysts but for the purpose of this text only two of the more common subtypes of cysts are noted: follicular and corpus luteum cysts. The cyst develops when there is a 'functional' fault with ovulation: follicular cysts develop from a follicle that fails to rupture completely and corpus luteum cysts develop from the corpus luteum if it fails to degenerate (Figure 18.8a).

Ovarian cysts vary in size from less than the size of a baked bean to the size of a tennis ball. Follicular cysts may grow to about 5 cm across, whereas the corpus luteum cyst can grow slightly larger.

Women who have endometriosis (see Box 18.8, p.497) may develop one or more cysts on their ovaries. The cysts are blood filled and the 'old' blood within them looks like chocolate and hence these cysts are sometimes called 'chocolate cysts'.

Most ovarian cysts cause no symptoms. However, a minority of cysts cause the following problems:

- Constant or intermittent pain in the lower abdomen, particularly on sexual intercourse.
- Irregular, or heavy or lighter periods.
- A cyst may burst causing a sudden severe pain in the lower abdomen.

- Large cysts can cause the abdominal swelling, and/or press on nearby organs, such as the bladder, which may cause urinary symptoms.
- Some cysts have a risk of becoming cancerous.

Since the majority of ovarian cysts cause no symptoms, many cysts are diagnosed by chance, for example by a routine examination. An ultrasound scan confirms diagnosis. Treatment depends on various factors such as age, childbearing status, the appearance and size of the cyst and presenting symptoms. Usually, if the ultrasound confirms a small functional cyst (common in premenopausal women) the specialist will request a repeat ultrasound in a month or so, and since most cysts disappear on their own over a few weeks then no further action may be needed. However, removal of the ovarian cyst may be advised if the patient presents with symptoms, or the cyst is potentially cancerous or at risk of becoming cancerous. Removal of some smaller cysts may be via laparoscopic surgery ('keyhole' surgery), while others require a more traditional style operation. In some cases, the ovary and sometimes other nearby structures (e.g. uterus) may also be removed.

Polycystic ovary syndrome (PCOS)
'Polycystic' means 'many cysts' in the ovary (Figure 18.8b). These cysts develop because of a problem with ovulation caused by a hormone imbalance. However, the exact cause is not clear, and glandular cells within the cysts themselves cause further hormone imbalance: this syndrome is associated with period problems, reduced fertility, hair growth, obesity and acne.

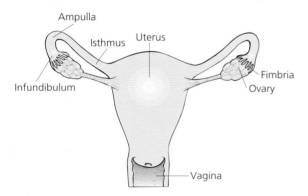

Organ	Homeostatic function
Ovary	Production of egg cells and female sex hormones
Fallopian tube	Conveys egg cell toward uterus; site of fertilization; conveys developing embryo to uterus
Uterus	Protects and sustains life of embryo during pregnancy
Vagina	Conveys uterine secretions to outside of body; receives erect penis during sexual intercourse; transports fetus during birth process

Figure 18.9 The Fallopian tubes, uterus and vagina

usually occurs in the ampulla of the uterine tube, though it can take place even in the uterus. At this point, if the oocyte is fertilized by a spermatozoon then it completes its development to become an ovum, and then by fusing with the spermatozoon nucleus forms a new cell, called a zygote. Fertilization may occur at any time up to 24 hours after ovulation. The resultant zygote divides by mitosis, producing a specialized structure, the early embryo called a blastocyst, which descends into the uterus over the next few days. If unfertilized, the secondary oocyte disintegrates, and the remains leave the female tract.

ACTIVITY

See p.592 for the details of fertilization. Describe the path taken by the spermatozoon and secondary oocyte from their respective reproductive systems, clearly identifying how the gametes are moved along the Fallopian tubes.

The uterus

The uterus is located between the bladder and rectum, and is the site of menstruation (if fertilization has not occurred), or of embryo implantation, embryo–fetal development and labour. A woman who has never been pregnant has an inverted pear-shaped uterus that is about 7 cm and 5 cm at its widest and narrowest parts, respectively (Figure 18.9). Anatomically, the uterus is divided into an expanded superior body called the fundus, a constricted isthmus, and a narrow neck region called the cervix, which opens into the vagina at its external orifice, the cervical os (see Figure 18.7b). The cervix can be felt

BOX 18.8 PELVIC INFLAMMATORY DISEASE

Pelvic inflammatory disease (PID) is a collective term used to include any extensive bacterial infection of the pelvic organs, especially the uterus, Fallopian tubes or ovaries. The external opening of the female tract makes this area susceptible to infection by pathogens (e.g. gonococcal bacteria). Spreading of inflammation is also common. Salpingitis (inflammation of the Fallopian tubes), for example, spreads readily and causes peritonitis (inflammation of the peritoneum), a potentially serious problem.

The infection causing PID may spread to other tissues, including the blood, where it may cause septic shock and death. The infection may be very distressing for the patient. The hospitalized patient is maintained on bed rest. Local warmth may be applied to the abdomen to provide comfort externally. Healthcare professionals provide support in explaining how PID occurs and how it can be controlled (see Best, 2000).

Early treatment with antibiotics (tetracycline or penicillin) is essential to stop the PID spreading. To prevent recurrence, sexual partners must also be treated with antibiotic combinations (Stones and Mountfield, 2001).

Endometriosis may also be a cause of PID, though it is a benign condition and not an infection. Endometriosis is the presence of functional endometrial tissue outside the uterus. The displaced tissue can occur in many different locations, although it is most often found in or on pelvic and abdominal organs. The tissues develop and regress cyclically, influenced by the normal hormonal events of the menstrual cycle; symptoms include premenstrual pain or unusual menstrual pain (dysmenorrhoea) caused by the displaced tissue being shed during menstruation (see Box 18.15, p.510).

BOX 18.9 CERVICAL CANCER

Cervical cancer is a relatively common disorder that kills about 2000 women in the UK each year (Shepherd *et al.*, 2001). The condition begins with cervical dysplasia (i.e. an abnormal change in the shape, growth and number of cervical cells). If the dysplasia is minimal, cells may regress to normal, but if severe it may progress to cancer. As with other malignant cancers studies have demonstrated that cervical cancer is a disease with multifactorial causes. However, unlike the majority of other cancers, cervical cancer has been shown to have a central causal agent, Human papillomavirus (HPV) infection, whose involvement in the risk of the cancer is much greater than that of any other recognized risk factors.

In some studies the prevalence of HPV DNA in cervical tumours has been greater than 90% (Franco *et al.*, 2001). This raises the possibility one day of prevention in most instances with a vaccine.

Depending on the progression of the disease, cervical cancer may be detected in its early stages by a 'Pap' (Papanicolaou) smear and regular cervical screening is widely promoted. Treatment of precancerous or early cancerous tissue may consist of tissue removal by cutting out (excising) the lesions, by hysterectomy (removal of the uterus or womb), and/or by radiotherapy, chemotherapy and laser therapy to destroy discrete areas of tissue.

readily by inserting a finger into the vagina; it feels like the tip of the nose. The space within the uterus is called the uterine cavity. Three pairs of suspensory ligaments stabilize the position of the uterus and limit its range of movement.

Histologically, the uterine wall can be divided into three main layers:

- an inner endometrium;
- a muscular myometrium;
- an outer serosa or perimetrium.

ACTIVITY

The suffix '-metr-' means uterus. Can you remember the meanings of the following prefixes: 'endo-', 'myo-' and 'peri-'?

The endometrium will receive the implanted embryo should fertilization take place, and it undergoes cyclical development in the menstrual cycle to ensure that it can perform this role. It is a mucous membrane that consists of three distinct layers:

- *stratum compactum*: a compact surface layer of ciliated epithelium;
- *stratum spongiosum*: a spongy middle layer of loose connective tissue;
- *stratum basale*: a dense inner layer attached to the underlying myometrium.

The superficial functional zone of the endometrium (layers 1 and 2, sometimes collectively referred to as the stratum functionalis) nourishes the developing embryo, and is maintained by high levels of the sex hormones oestrogens and progesterone. It is sloughed off following birth (or during menstruation if fertilization has been unsuccessful) in response to falling levels of those hormones.

The thick myometrium layer forms the bulk of the uterine wall, and its thicker upper fundic and thinner lower cervical regions are good examples of structural adaptations to function: to expel a fetus, the fundic region contracts more forcibly than its cervical counterpart, dilating the cervix to encourage childbirth. The myometrium also has three layers of involuntary muscle fibres that extend in all directions, giving the uterus great strength while ensuring even constriction across the organ during birth.

The uterine cavity is directed downwards and opens at the cervical canal at the internal os. The lower region of the cervical canal (or external os) opens into the vagina.

The vagina

The vagina is a thin-walled, muscular, tubular organ located between the urinary bladder and the rectum. It extends from the cervix to the external genitalia. On average, it is about 7–9 cm long. The fornix – the region where the vagina attaches itself to the cervix – is an important anatomical landmark for the positioning of the contraceptive diaphragm (see Figure

18.17, p.513). The vagina is a distensible organ that serves as a passageway for menstrual flow and for childbirth, hence it is often called the birth canal. It is the receptacle for the penis (and semen) during sexual intercourse; thus its wall is composed mainly of involuntary smooth muscle, and its folded lining is lubricated with mucus to aid its role during intercourse. The vaginal secretions are acidic (pH 3.5–4.0) and provide a hostile, protective environment against microbial growth, but will also be hostile to spermatozoa. The alkaline semen acts to neutralize this acidity to ensure survival of spermatozoa. However, this is only partly successful, since most spermatozoa die because of the effects of the acidic pH on their enzymes before the neutralizing process is effective.

The external genitalia

The external genitalia (vulva) lie immediately external to the vagina. The vulva is comprises a number of components: the mons pubis, labia majora (labia = lips), labia minora and the components of the vestibule and the clitoris (see Figure 18.3, p.487).

The mons pubis is an elevated, rounded fatty-tissue area that cushions the underlying bony pubic symphysis during sexual intercourse. During puberty, it becomes surrounded by pubic hair. From the mons pubis, two elongated pigmented fatty folds of skin, called the labia majora (the developmental homologue of the male scrotum), extend downwards, enclosing and protecting other external genitalia. On the outside, these folds contain numerous hairs, sweat and sebaceous glands; inside, there are two delicate hair-free skin folds, the labia minora. These contain sebum-producing cells and function to protect the opening of the urethra and vagina. They also enclose the vestibule, which comprises:

- the hymen, a folded mucous membrane that partly closes the vaginal orifice;
- the vaginal orifice;
- the external urethral orifice;
- the opening of the mucus-secreting paraurethral (Skene's) glands (the homologue of the male prostate gland);
- the mucus-secreting greater vestibular (Bartholin's) glands (the homologue of the male bulbourethral glands).

The role of the mucous glands is to lubricate the area, thereby facilitating intercourse.

The clitoris

The clitoris looks small externally, but it is much larger than it appears because much of it is internal. This organ is composed of two layers of erectile tissue (corpora cavernosa), and it is the homologue of the male glans penis. The junction of the labia minora folds forms its hood, a layer of skin called the prepuce or foreskin. The clitoris is richly innervated with sensory nerve endings; therefore, like the penis, it is capable of enlargement upon tactile stimulation; this contributes to female sexual arousal.

The perineum

The perineum is a diamond-shaped, muscular region found in both sexes between the external genitalia and the anus.

BOX 18.10 EPISIOTOMY

Clinically the perineum is of importance to females because of the danger of it being torn during childbirth. To avoid this, an incision (called an episiotomy) may be made in the perineal skin and underlying tissues just before delivery. After delivery, the incision is sutured to promote healing and prevent later vaginal prolapse (i.e. its downward displacement). The perineum is extensively innervated, so the laceration is likely to be very painful. Sitting, defecation and the establishment of breast-feeding may therefore all become more difficult. Aperient and high-fibre diets are encouraged to prevent constipation. Scrupulous hygiene is also required to avoid infection. Pelvic floor exercises are encouraged soon after delivery to improve blood flow to the area, which minimizes infection risk, maximizes the healing process and increases the tone of any muscle affected by the incision.

ACTIVITY

Draw and label the male and female reproductive tracts.

The female sexual act

The phases of female sexual arousal resemble those of the male (i.e. involving erection, lubrication and orgasm). During arousal, parasympathetic activation leads to the erectile tissue of the clitoris and other parts of the female genitalia becoming engorged with blood. Parasympathetic impulses also cause mucus secretion and hence the lubrication of the vagina, which facilitates intercourse. During intercourse, rhythmical contractions of the clitoris and vaginal walls produce stimulation that eventually leads to orgasm. Female orgasm is accompanied by peristaltic contractions of the uterine walls, vaginal walls and the perineum muscles. The pleasurable sensation experienced with the contractions is analogous to that produced by male ejaculation.

The mammary glands

The mammary glands are accessory organs of the reproductive system present in both sexes.

The mammary glands are modified sweat (sudoriferous) glands, and they are actually a part of the skin. The breast extends from the second to the sixth rib, and from the sternum

---

BOX 18.11 DEVELOPMENT OF THE MAMMARY GLANDS

When a child approaches puberty, the primary sex glands remain underdeveloped, but in girls a surge of ovarian hormones (oestrogens and progesterone) stimulates further development of the mammary glands. In boys, secretion of female sex hormones from the adrenal gland (see Chapter 9, pp.218–20) may also cause the breasts to appear enlarged, because of the accumulation of fatty tissue. During puberty, some males experience gynaecomastia, a condition in which the breasts enlarge temporally as a result of this hormonal imbalance.

A woman's breasts only become biologically functional following pregnancy, since their role is to produce and secrete milk in order to provide a source of nourishment to the newborn. The size of the breast is determined by the amount of fat surrounding this glandular tissue, and is not related to its functional capacity.

(a)

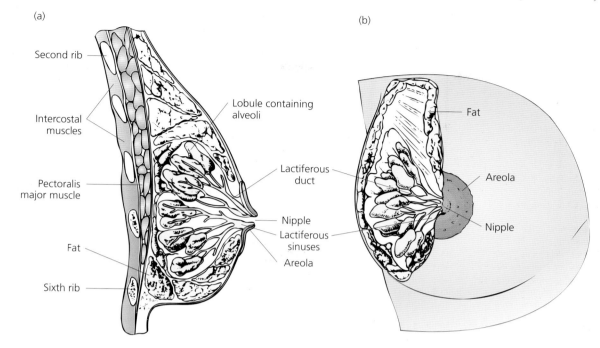

Second rib

Intercostal muscles

Pectoralis major muscle

Fat

Sixth rib

Lobule containing alveoli

Lactiferous duct

Nipple

Lactiferous sinuses

Areola

(b)

Fat

Areola

Nipple

Figure 18.10 The anatomy of the mammary glands: (a) sagittal section; (b) anterior view (partially sectioned); (c) hormonal control of lactation. PRF – Prolactin-releasing factor.

Q Identify the roles of the female hormones involved in development of the breast during pregnancy and lactation.

BOX 18.12 AREOLA: A MARKER OF FIRST PREGNANCY

In Caucasians the areola changes colour from delicate pink to brown early in the first pregnancy, a fact that can be useful in identifying a first pregnancy. Although it never returns to its original colour, the colour intensity decreases after lactation has ceased. In darker-skinned women, there is no noticeable colour change.

(c)

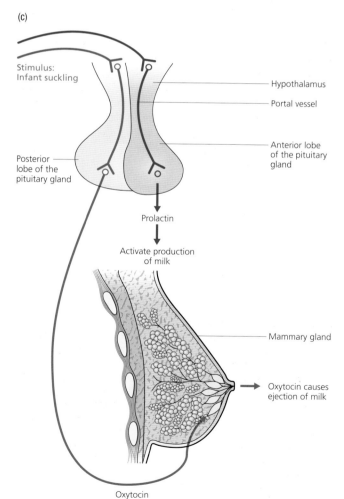

Stimulus: Infant suckling

Hypothalamus

Portal vessel

Anterior lobe of the pituitary gland

Posterior lobe of the pituitary gland

Prolactin

Activate production of milk

Mammary gland

Oxytocin causes ejection of milk

Oxytocin

to the armpits (axillae). It overlies, and is connected to, the pectoralis major muscles (Figure 18.10). Slightly below the centre of each breast is a ring of pigmented skin, the areola, which surrounds a central protruding nipple. Large areolar sebaceous glands give this region a slightly bumpy appearance; these glands secrete sebum to lubricate the areola and nipple during breast-feeding. Exposure to cold, tactile or sexual stimuli stimulates the smooth muscle fibres in the areola, causing the nipple to become erect.

Internally, each breast consists of 15–25 irregularly shaped lobes radiating around the nipple, each of which is separated from the others by a wall of connective tissue that forms the suspensory ligaments of the breast. In each lobe, smaller lobules called alveoli (see Figure 14.2b, p.399, lung alveoli, for structural comparison) are present in which are found the milk-secreting cells. During lactation, milk is passed from the alveoli to the lactiferous ducts. These enlarge to form the lactiferous sinuses just before their openings on the surface of the nipple. The milk accumulates in the sinuses during 'nursing'.

BOX 18.13 FIBROCYSTIC DISEASE AND MALIGNANCIES OF THE BREAST

Fibrocystic disease of the breast is the most common cause of breast lumps in women. One or more cysts (fluid-containing sacs), and thickening of the alveoli, occur. The condition is common in women aged 30–50 years, and is possibly caused by an excess of oestrogens or a deficiency of progesterone in the postovulatory phase of the menstrual cycle. The condition usually causes one or both breasts to become lumpy, swollen and tender a week before menstruation.

Malignancies of the reproductive tract and related organs, especially the breast, account for the majority of cancer cases amongst women. Figures from breast cancer statistics website (http://www.cancerresearchuk.org/) in February 2007 reveal that:

* Breast cancer is now the most common cancer in the UK.
* Each year more than 44 000 women are diagnosed with breast cancer, that's more than 100 women a day.
* Each year around 300 men are diagnosed with breast cancer.
* Breast cancer survival rates have been improving for more than 20 years. In the 1970s around 5 out of 10 breast cancer patients survived beyond 5 years. In 2006 it was 8 out of 10.
* Each year in the UK more than 12 000 women and around 100 men die from breast cancer.

In 1998, genes (e.g. *BRCA1* on chromosome 17; *BRCA2* on chromosome 13) responsible for a small number of inherited breast cancers were identified. Mammary cancers often spread (metastasize; see Figure 2.17a, p.46) to the ovaries, producing ovarian cancers. Breast cancer has one of the highest fatality (death) rates of all cancers affecting women. It often goes undiscovered, since its associated pain becomes evident only when the cancer is quite advanced. The incidence of breast cancer is age-related; approximately 1 in 19 000 women will develop breast cancer at the age of 25, 1 in 2500 by the age of 30 and 1 in 50 by the age of 50. Breast cancer can also occur in men, it accounts for 1% of male cancers, and the age at which it peaks is 60–69 years of age. Corrective measures for breast cancers depend on the size and type of cancer, but usually involve a combination of:

* *Surgical approaches*: lumpectomies and mastectomies ('-ectomy' = cutting out). The axillary nymph nodes may be removed if metastasis is suspected and this may lead to lymphoedema of the arm (see Figure 2.17d, p.46). The operation obviously has implications for body image, sexuality, self-esteem and relationships.
* *Radiotherapy*: the use of X-ray radiation to kill cancer cells prior to metastasis.
* *Chemotherapy*: this prevents cancer cells from replicating (see p.32). In breast cancer this may also involve administration of oestrogen-antagonists such as tamoxifen and raloxifene since some cancers are oestrogen dependent. Before the menopause, the ovaries may also be removed to reduce oestrogen secretions; postmenopausally, the steroid aminoglutethimide may be given, which inhibits the conversion of androgens into oestrogens.
* *Combined therapies*: radiotherapy and chemotherapy, radiotherapy and surgery, or chemotherapy and surgery.
* *Immunotherapy (pharmacogenomics)*: this is a new and expanding field of pharmacological research based upon the knowledge base of genetics. Researchers predict that in the future it will be possible to administer drugs that are tailor-made to the individual's causal factors, such as drugs designed to inactivate oncoreceptors (such as oestrogen receptors), inactivate oncogenes (such as *BRAC1* and *BRAC2*), competitively inhibit cancer enzymes or provide suboptimal conditions for cancer enzymes (hence slowing the progression of the cancer) or competitively inhibit cancer metabolic endproducts (see Figure 2.9, p.33). This new and exciting area is not without its critics, and it may be currently 'over-hyped' according to a report in 2007 from the Royal Society, the UK's National Academy of Science, which stated that this area of research is still 10–15 years away from living up to its promise in clinical practice, largely owing to shortages of researchers and lack of international coordination. Conversely, a group of researchers from the University of Nottingham in 2007 stated that the impact of pharmacogenomics on clinical medicine is going to be felt more quickly since they have pharmacological tests in progress and predict that there will be new tests in oncology at least over the next 5 years.

The healthcare professional's role in planning and implementing care will include the reduction of emotional stress, fear and anxiety, since the patient's problems may include the fear of coping with the diagnosis, the treatment, its side-effects and prognosis, and the impact of surgery and therapies on body image.

See the case study on a woman with breast cancer, Section VI, p.630.

In non-pregnant, non-nursing women, the breasts and the duct system are underdeveloped. The homeostatic control of breast development, from puberty onwards, and especially during pregnancy and for a short time after delivery (lactation), involves the female sex hormones: oestrogens stimulate the development of the duct system and progesterone stimulates the development of the alveolar regions. Initiation and maintenance of lactation involves two further hormones, prolactin and oxytocin, released from the pituitary gland, which stimulate milk production and control milk let-down, respectively (Figure 18.10c).

ACTIVITY

Describe the structure of the mammary glands, and identify gender-specific differences.

REPRODUCTIVE PHYSIOLOGY

Gametogenesis

Gametogenesis is a general term that refers to the production of the sex cells, or gametes, by the gonads. Spermatogenesis and oogenesis are the specific terms for the production of spermatozoa by the testes and oocytes by the ovaries, respectively. Gametogenesis involves both mitotic and meiotic divisions of cells. You should therefore review the mechanism of cell division discussed in Chapters 2 and 9, since it is our intention at this point only to review of a few key concepts.

Humans reproduce sexually by producing germinal cells by mitosis and the gametes by meiosis, a reduction division that ensures that the chromosome number in the gametes is halved to 23 (the haploid number). The fusion of male and female gametes at fertilization then produces a zygote containing 23 pairs of chromosomes (i.e. 46, which is the diploid number),

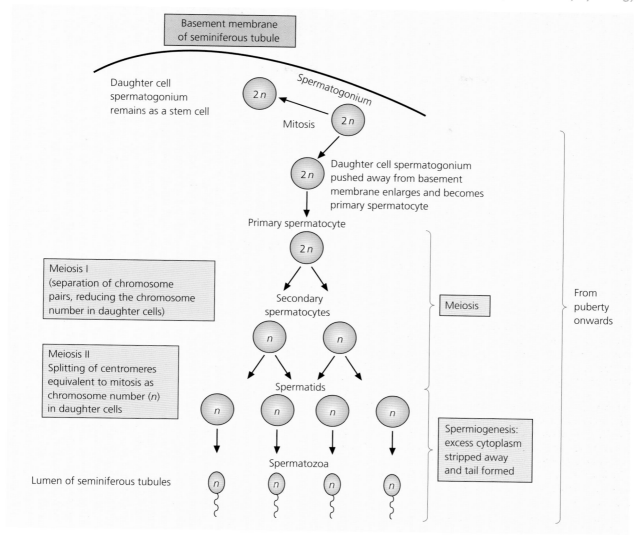

Figure 18.11 Flow chart of events of spermatogenesis. 2*n* = diploid; *n* = haploid

Q What do the terms 'diploid' and 'haploid' mean?

one partner of each pair from the spermatozoon cell and one from the ovum. The zygote divides by duplication division – mitosis – to ensure that cells derived from it all contain the diploid number of chromosomes. Consequently, just before this cell division, the zygote and subsequent daughter cells must duplicate their DNA so a copy can be passed into each new resultant cell.

Spermatogenesis

Spermatogenesis ('-genesis' = creation) is the sequence of events that occurs in the seminiferous tubules of the testis and leads to the formation of spermatozoa. As discussed previously, histological investigation of the seminiferous tubules reveals that the majority of the cells comprising the tubule walls are at various stages of cell division (see Figure 18.5c, p.507). These cells, collectively called spermatogenic (spermatozoa-forming) cells, develop into mature spermatozoa via a number of cell

divisions and transformations that involve mitosis, meiosis and a development process called spermiogenesis.

Mitotic division of spermatogonia

The undifferentiated spermatogenic cells in direct contact with the germinal epithelium of the testis are called the spermatogonia. These stem cells divide continuously by mitosis until puberty; consequently, all of the spermatogenic cells in a young male are undifferentiated spermatogonia, and each contains 23 pairs (i.e. diploid number) of chromosomes, the usual number for human cells. During early adolescence, certain hormones (the gonadotropins and steroidal androgens) stimulate mitotic divisions of the spermatogonia giving rise to daughter cells, some of which provide a reserve supply of spermatogonia (i.e. the germ cell line), while others migrate towards the lumen of the tubule, where they enlarge and become primary spermatocytes. The latter are destined to become mature spermatozoa via the processes of meiosis and spermiogenesis (Figure 18.11).

Meiotic division of spermatocytes

Meiosis involves two successive divisions (Figure 18.11) that reduces the 23 pairs of chromosomes to just 23 in total. During the first meiotic division, the chromosome pairs of the primary spermatocytes separate so that each forms two haploid secondary spermatocytes; at this point each chromosome still comprises its two copies of DNA, or chromatids. Each secondary spermatocyte in turn gives rise to two spermatids via the second meiotic division, which separates the two chromatids (i.e. meiosis generates four new cells from each primary spermatocyte, each with 23 molecules of DNA).

Spermiogenesis

Spermiogenesis is the final stage of spermatogenesis, in which the spermatids differentiate into mature spermatozoa. This transformation involves streamlining the non-motile spermatid by shedding most of its superfluous cytoplasmic 'baggage' and providing a tail (see 'The structure of spermatozoa', below).

Each day, spermatogenesis produces several thousand spermatozoa. Subsequent to their production, they migrate to the epididymis of the testis for storage. Over the next 18 hours to 10 days, they undergo further maturation, a process called capacitation. After this, the spermatozoa are either expelled via ejaculation or broken down chemically and their constituents recycled. Capacitated spermatozoa are also stored in the vas deferens where they can retain their fertility for up to several months. Once ejaculated, however, they have a life expectancy of about 48 hours within the woman's reproductive tract.

ACTIVITY

Write brief notes on the distinguishing features of meiosis and mitosis.

The structure of spermatozoa

The mature spermatozoon is a tiny (approximately 60 μm long) tadpole-shaped structure consisting of three distinct regions: a flattened head, a cylindrical body or midpiece, and an elongated tail (Figure 18.12). The head is composed primarily of a nucleus, which contains 23 densely packed chromosomes. Its anterior tip forms the acrosomal cap, which contains hydrolytic enzymes (e.g. hyaluronidase) with roles in fertilization. A very short neck attaches the head to the midpiece. The latter contains a central filamentous core with a large number of mitochondria arranged in a spiral. These organelles provide energy (ATP) for the contraction of protein filaments in the tail; the resultant propulsive forces move the spermatozoa at a rate of 1–4 mm/minute.

A mature spermatozoon lacks many of the usual cell organelles, including endoplasmic reticulum, Golgi complex, lysosomes and cytoplasmic inclusions. It also does not contain glycogen or other energy reserves, so it must absorb nutrients, primarily fructose, from the surrounding seminal fluid.

Oogenesis

The female homologue of spermatogenesis is called oogenesis. As discussed previously, spermatozoa production in males

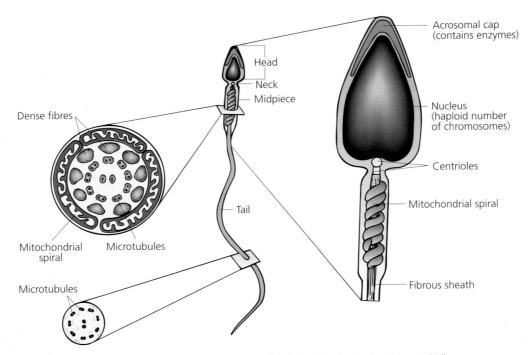

Figure 18.12 Schematic diagram of a sperm cell, showing its internal structure and parts, including the head, midpiece and tail

Q Which organelle would be highly represented in the acrosomal cap of the sperm?

Q Which sugar is used to give the sperm energy to 'swim' to the site of fertilization?

development can be found on pp.522–33 and summarized in Figure 19.4, p.526.

BOX 18.14 SPERMATOGENESIS AND AGE

Spermatogenesis occurs from puberty and throughout life. However, with advancing years, there is a decline in spermatozoa production since there is a significant atrophy of the testes with depletion of the germinal and Sertoli cells. Sertoli cells are essential for spermatogenesis, since they facilitate the progression of germ cells to spermatozoa by controlling the environment milieu within the seminiferous tubules.

Hormonal regulation of gametogenesis in the male

The production of spermatozoa clearly does not require the refinement that is associated with ova production. Nevertheless, the control of spermatogenesis has two important aspects: development of spermatozoa from spermatogonium cells must be stimulated, and the spermatozoa must undergo a 'maturation' process, without which they are incapable of independent life and functionality.

Spermatogenesis is controlled by the interplay between the male sex steroid hormone, testosterone, and gonadotropin hormones, a relationship sometimes called the hypothalamic–pituitary–testicular axis. Another gonad hormone, inhibin, may also be involved.

Clusters of interstitial cells between the seminiferous tubules, called cells of Leydig, secrete testosterone in response to the gonadotropin LH from the anterior pituitary gland (Figure 18.14). Testosterone is essential for the growth and maintenance of the testes, and for the maturation or capacitation of spermatozoa in the epididymis. The gonadotropin FSH and to some degree LH, stimulates Sertoli (sustentacular) cells in the testis. These cells lie among the developing spermatogonia, and secrete nutritive substances and chemicals that promote spermatozoan development. For example, an androgen-binding protein is released, which facilitates the binding of testosterone to spermatogenic cells. In this way, FSH helps to make the spermatogenic cells receptive to the stimulatory effects of testosterone.

The whole process of spermatogenesis, therefore, depends on the presence of appropriate concentrations of the pituitary gonadotropins and the male sex steroid. The release of these hormones is kept in check by negative feedback. Thus, as testosterone is released beyond its homeostatic range, it inhibits the release of LH and FSH by acting on the hypothalamus to suppress the secretion of the gonadotropin-releasing hormone (GnRH) that in turn is required to stimulate secretion of the gonadotropins by the anterior pituitary gland (Figure 18.14). As LH release declines, the secretion of testosterone will consequently be reduced. Testosterone already present in the blood is metabolized, the concentration of the hormone decreases, and inhibition by negative feedback becomes less effective. Consequently, when the blood concentration of this steroid is below its homeostatic range, LH release increases again, and so on.

A second control component is also present, in that the Sertoli cells exert a degree of control on the rate of spermatogenesis. These cells release another hormone, called inhibin (a peptide), when the spermatozoa count goes beyond its upper homeostatic limit. Inhibin directly inhibits the release of FSH from the pituitary, and probably also inhibits the hypothalamic secretion of GnRH. When the spermatozoa count falls below its lower homeostatic limit (around 20 million/mL of semen), inhibin secretion is prevented and the rate of spermatogenesis is stimulated again.

begins at puberty and generally continues throughout life. Gamete production in the female, however, is quite different: the first meiotic division of the undifferentiated oogonium, which produces the primary oocytes, begins before birth but the second meiotic division to produce the ovum does not take place until after the secondary oocyte has been fertilized.

Figure 18.13 illustrates how the fetal oogonia, which are diploid at this stage, multiply rapidly by mitosis to produce a reserve of germ cells. Subsequently, oogonia enter a growth phase; gradually, early or primordial ovarian follicles appear and the oogonia are transformed into primary oocytes, surrounded by a single layer of flattened follicle cells called the corona radiata. Many primordial follicles deteriorate before birth; those remaining occupy the cortical region of the immature ovary. By birth, a girl's life supply of primary oocytes is approximately 750 000 cells. These cells are 'stalled' in the early stages of the first meiotic division, and will not complete meiosis and produce functional gametes until stimulated to do so by hormonal changes following puberty.

Once the menstrual cycle is established, a small number (i.e. about 500 cells) of the primary oocytes begin their growth and developmental cycles each month. Thus, as in the male, nature has provided a generous supply of sex cells. However, the primary oocytes are not replaced and so total numbers continuously decline, although there is easily sufficient for a lifetime). Only one of these oocytes per month (or perhaps one from each ovary) completes the first meiotic division, which ends when two haploid daughter cells, called a secondary oocyte and the first polar body, are produced. The secondary oocyte only undergoes the second meiotic division following fertilization by a spermatozoon cell; this division produces a haploid ovum and the second polar body. The first polar body may or may not divide again.

The ovum, then, is only one of the daughter cells produced from the primary oocyte. The polar bodies are often referred to as the 'nuclear dustbins', since their DNA is destroyed. The mature ovum occurs only as a brief stage of oogenesis, as the haploid nuclei of the ovum and spermatozoon soon combine (now called a zygote) to restore the normal diploid number of chromosomes. Details of conception, and embryonic and fetal

ACTIVITY

Distinguish between the following developing cells: primary oocytes, secondary oocytes, polar bodies, ova and zygotes.

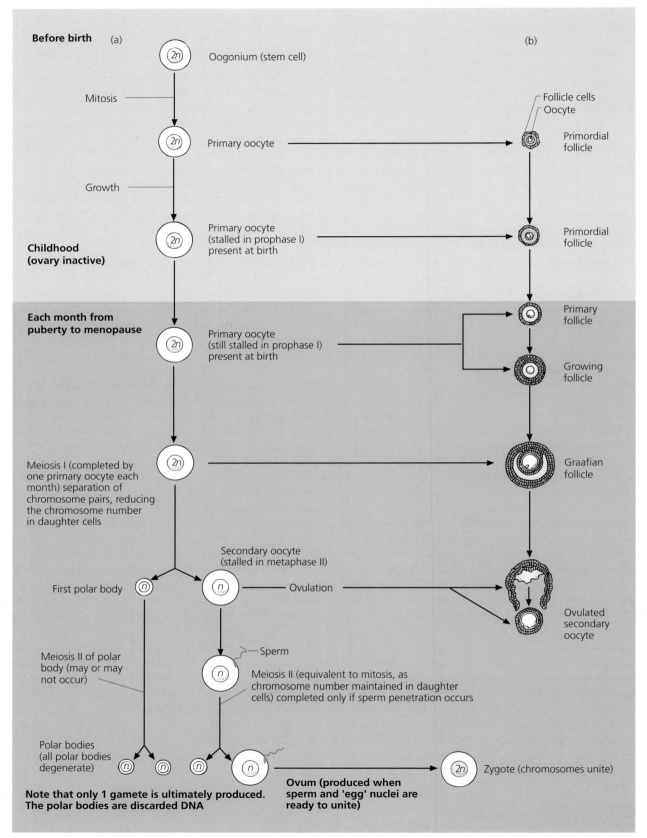

Figure 18.13 (a) Flow chart of events of oogenesis: $2n$ = diploid; n = haploid. (b) Follicle development in the ovary

Q *How does the age of the primary spermatocyte in the male compare with the age of a primary oocyte in a female?*

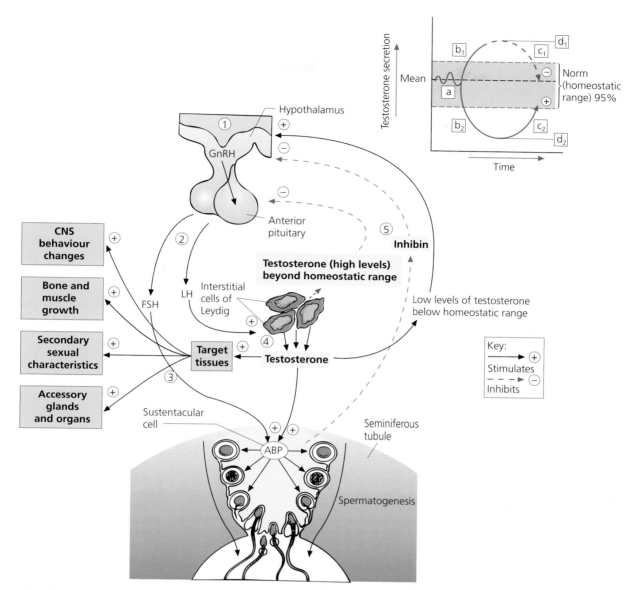

Figure 18.14 Hormonal regulation of testicular function by the hypothalamic–pituitary–testicular axis. 1, The hypothalamus releases gonadotropin-releasing hormone (GnRH). 2, GnRH stimulates the anterior pituitary to release the gonadotropins follicle-stimulating hormone (FSH) and luteinizing hormone (LH). 3, FSH acts on the sustentacular cells, causing them to release androgen-binding protein (ABP). 4, LH acts on the interstitial (Leydig) cells, stimulating their release of testosterone. ABP binding of testosterone then enhances spermatogenesis. 5, Rising levels of testosterone and inhibin exert feedback inhibition on the hypothalamus and pituitary. Inset: a, testosterone fluctuating within its homeostatic parameters; b_1, hypersecretion of testosterone; c_1, correction of imbalance via natural negative feedback (e.g. inhibin) or via clinical removal of the underlying pathology causing the imbalance (e.g. removal of testicular cancer, see Figure 18.4b, p.488); d_1, irreversible clinical hypersecretion (e.g. hypothalamic and pituitary tumours); b_2, hyposecretion of testosterone; c_2, correction of imbalance via natural negative feedback stimulated by LH; d_2, irreversible genetic disorders that result in low levels of testosterone. CNS, central nervous system. (a, Represents boxes a_1–a_4 in Figure 1.7, p.11, reflecting the individual variability in the homeostatic range)

Q Which pituitary hormone stimulates the secretion of the male hormone testosterone?

Q Which male hormones inhibit secretion of FSH and LH by the anterior pituitary gland?

Q What do the acronynms FSH and LH mean?

Spermatogenesis is thus controlled by tight negative feedback loops (Figure 18.14) involving the following hormones:

- *gonadotropin-releasing hormones from the hypothalamus*: these stimulate the release of gonadotropins from the pituitary;

- *pituitary gonadotropins (FSH and LH)*: these stimulate spermatogenesis and the secretion of testosterone and inhibin;
- *testicular hormones (testosterone and inhibin)*: these exert negative feedback controls on the secretion of hypothalamic releasing hormones and the pituitary gonadotropins.

The names of the gonadotropins are derived from their functions in the female, but the hormones are chemically identical in both sexes. In males, LH is sometimes called interstitial cell-stimulation hormone (ICSH), in recognition of its role in promoting testosterone secretion from the interstitial cells of the testes.

Testosterone exerts a number of actions in addition to the capacitation of spermatozoa, including:

* promoting the descent of the testes in the fetus towards the end of the gestation period;
* regulating the development of the male accessory sex organs;
* controlling the development and maintenance of the secondary sexual characteristics, such as the growth of facial, axillary and pubic hair, enlargement of the larynx and provision of masculine muscular development;
* being partly responsible for promoting a number of behavioural characteristics associated with adolescence.

Removal of the testes does not usually lead to a loss of secondary sexual characteristics, however, since there is an increased output of androgen steroids from the adrenal gland (cortex). The testes also produce female sex hormones, but their function in males is unclear.

Table 18.1 summarizes the major male reproductive hormones.

Hormonal regulation of the female reproductive cycle

Changes occur periodically in the female between the onset of menses (the menarche) and its cessation (menopause or climacteric). Menstruation is the visible external sign that cyclical changes to the endometrium are occurring, and hence cyclical release of the ovarian sex hormones is taking place. This section discusses the hormonal regulation of the menstrual and ovarian cycles.

The menstrual cycle involves cyclical changes within the endometrium and mammary glands in a non-pregnant woman in response to changing levels of ovarian hormones (Figure 18.15). Each month, the endometrium is prepared to receive a fertilized ovum. The development of this lining is essential for embryonic and fetal development during the period of pregnancy (gestation). If fertilization does not occur, part of the endometrium is shed as the menstrual flow (menses).

The ovarian cycle involves changes that occur in the ovaries during the menstrual cycle. These include the maturation of a secondary oocyte, its release at ovulation, and the development and degeneration of the corpus luteum (Figure 18.15). The hormonal control of the events of both cycles is influenced by hormones of the hypothalamic–pituitary–ovarian axis: the gonadotropin-releasing hormones from the hypothalamus, the gonadotropin hormones (LH and FSH) from the anterior pituitary, and the steroidal oestrogens and progestins from the ovary (Figure 18.16).

The complete menstrual cycle becomes established with the eventual onset of ovulation. The menstrual cycle, therefore, is a sequence of changes to the reproductive tract of a non-pregnant

---

Table 18.1 Major reproductive hormones

Hormone	Functions	Source
Male		
GnRH	Controls pituitary secretion of FSH and LH	Hypothalamus
FSH	Increases testosterone production, aids sperm maturation	Pituitary gland Controlled by hypothalamus
LH	Stimulates testosterone secretion	Pituitary gland Controlled by hypothalamus
Testosterone	Increases sperm production, stimulates development of male primary and secondary sex characteristics, inhibits LH secretion	Leydig cells in testes (controlled by LH)
Female		
GnRH	Controls pituitary secretion of FSH and LH	Hypothalamus
FSH	Causes immature oocyte and follicle to develop, increases oestrogen secretion	Pituitary gland (controlled by hypothalamus)
LH	Stimulates further development of oocyte and follicle, stimulates ovulation, increases progesterone secretion	Pituitary gland (controlled by hypothalamus)
Oestrogen	Stimulates thickening of uterine wall, stimulates oocyte maturation, stimulates development of female sex characteristics, stimulates lactiferous ducts of the mammary glands, inhibits FSH secretion, increases LH secretion prior to ovulation	Ovarian follicle, corpus luteum (controlled by FSH)
Progesterone	Stimulates thickening of uterine wall, stimulates formation of alveolar regions of the mammary glands	Corpus luteum (controlled by LH)
hCG	Prevents corpus luteum from disintegrating, stimulates oestrogen and progesterone secretion from corpus luteum	Embryonic membranes, placenta
Prostaglandin	Initiates parturition (labour)	Endometrium
Relaxin	Relaxes symphysis pubis and dilates uterine and cervix	Corpus luteum
Prolactin	Promotes milk production by mammary glands after childbirth	Pituitary gland (controlled by hypothalamus)
Oxytocin	Stimulates uterine contractions during labour, induces mammary glands to eject milk after childbirth	Pituitary gland (controlled by hypothalamus)

FSH, follicle-stimulating hormone; GnRH, gonadotropin-releasing hormone; hCG, human chorionic gonadotropin; LH, luteinizing hormone.

Q Do the gonadotropins derive their name from their functions in the male or female?

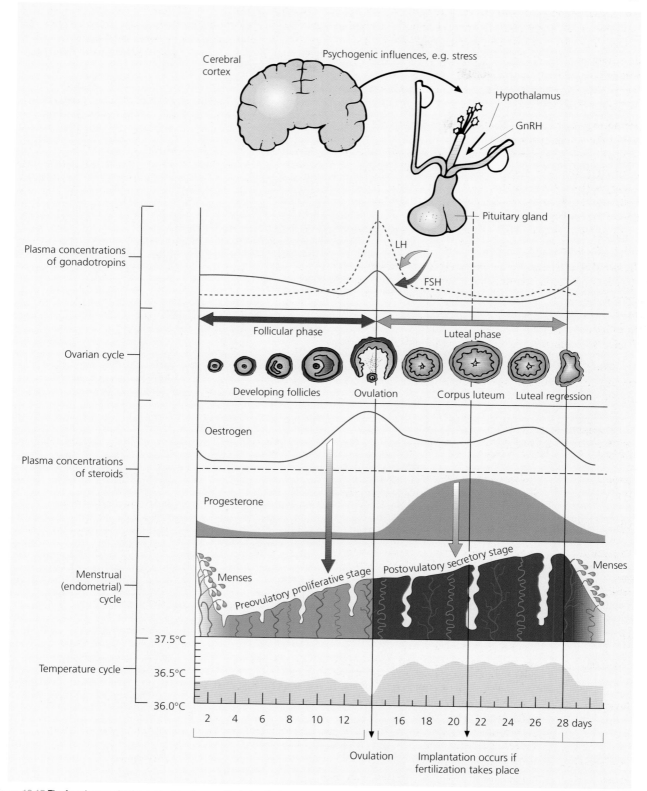

Figure 18.15 The female reproductive cycle. The diagram illustrates the interrelationship of cerebral, hypothalamic, pituitary, ovarian and uterine functions throughout a usual 28-day cycle. Note that the luteinizing hormone (LH) surge causes ovulation. The low levels of steroids initiate menstruation. FSH, follicle-stimulating hormone; GnRH, gonadotropin-releasing hormone

Q *Which hormones are responsible for regulating the preovulatory, ovulatory and postovulatory phases of the menstrual cycle?*

Q *Which hormones are responsible for regulating the growth of the corpus luteum and the surge of LH mid-cycle?*

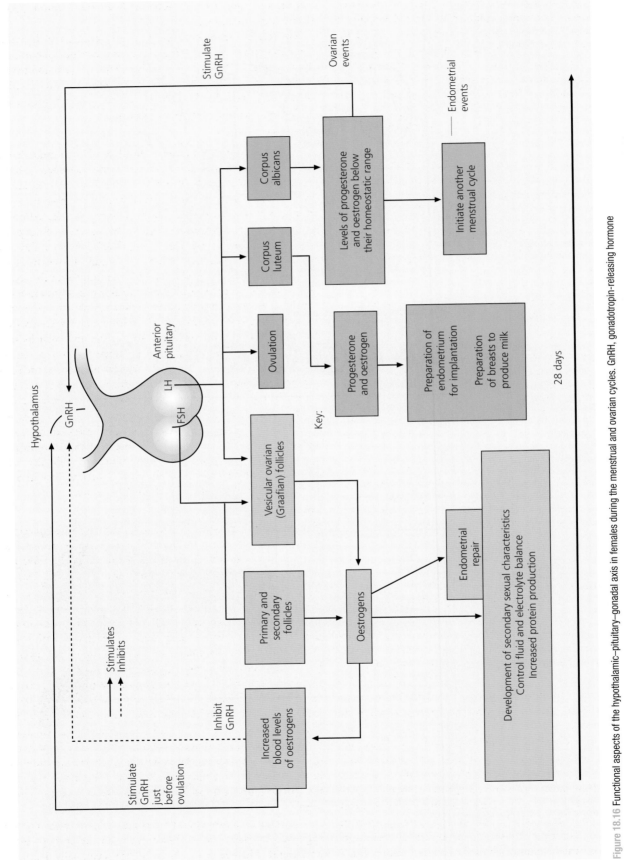

Figure 18.16 Functional aspects of the hypothalamic–pituitary–gonadal axis in females during the menstrual and ovarian cycles. GnRH, gonadotropin-releasing hormone

Q *Using your knowledge of the hypothalamic–pituitary–gonad axis, suggest potential sites of endocrine tumours that may give rise to female pseudohermaphroditism (see Chapter 9 for help).*

woman, and is controlled by interplay of the ovarian steroids and gonadotropin hormones. From a functional viewpoint, the uterus is anatomically most suited to carry just one developing fetus, although multiple births are not uncommon. The cycle normally promotes the release of a single secondary oocyte from an ovary; this becomes a mature ovum if it is fertilized. The product of fertilization (the zygote) develops into the early embryo, which must implant in the endometrium for a pregnancy to occur. The hormones involved in controlling these events, therefore, must:

* promote the development of a new endometrium;
* promote ovulation at a time when the endometrium is sufficiently developed for implantation to occur;
* promote further nutritive development of the endometrium, and prevent its shedding, in order to support the early embryo should implantation occur;
* cause the endometrium to be shed if conception does not take place (why it is shed is subject to debate but menstruation is observed in all mammals and so is taken to be of biological importance; perhaps it prevents an accumulation, over time, of harmful agents that could affect embryo development).

The processes involved are illustrated in Figure 18.15. The menstrual cycle typically has a duration of 28 days, although there is individual variation and it is subject to many environmental influences. Conventionally, timing begins at the onset of menstrual bleeding, when the endometrium that developed in the previous cycle begins to be shed; this typically lasts for about 5 days. During this time (and just before it), the release of ovarian steroids is diminished; it is the lack of these that causes the endometrium to be shed. In addition, as ovarian steroid release is reduced, the negative feedback they exert on the anterior pituitary weakens, and increasing amounts of gonadotropins are secreted, stimulating development of the next cycle.

Preovulation

The preovulatory phase of the menstrual cycle involves the maturation of a (normally) single ovarian follicle and growth of a new uterine endometrium. The gonadotropins FSH and LH are released concurrently. As its name implies, FSH promotes the development of ovarian follicles, which basically consist of an immature oocyte surrounded by a mass of follicle cells. Perhaps 20 or so of these primary follicles will be stimulated in this way, but normally one is more advanced than the others. As the follicles develop, the gonadotropins stimulate the follicular cells to secrete oestrogens, which then feed back and inhibit gonadotropin release by the pituitary. Thus, further development for most of the follicles (now called secondary follicles) is retarded, and they atrophy and die. The most advanced follicle, however, somehow becomes independent of the need for FSH by this stage, and so continues to grow as follicular cells proliferate. In addition to regulating this part of the cycle, the oestrogens released by the follicles also promote the growth of a new endometrium, i.e. a new stratum func-

tionalis (functional layer) develops from the stratum basalis (basal or germinating layer).

The role of the follicular oestrogens is reflected in the name sometimes given to this part of the cycle – the follicular or proliferative phase (although 'preovulatory phase' is a better term).

Note that 'oestrogens' is a collective term used to describe six different steroids. The three most abundant oestrogens are 17-beta-oestradiol, oestrone and oestriol.

Ovulation

Ovulation requires the transient release of LH in a surge that is sufficient to prompt the shedding of the secondary oocyte from the mature Graafian follicle. Ovulation occurs at about 14 days into the cycle, but again timing is variable between individuals. As Figure 18.15 shows, oestrogens released up to about 11–12 days powerfully inhibit the secretion of the pituitary gonadotropins via negative feedback. By an unknown mechanism, this negative (inhibitory) feedback switches to a positive (stimulatory) feedback, with the result that the secretion of pituitary stores of LH (and FSH) is strongly stimulated by the presence of high concentrations of oestrogens in the blood. The resulting surge of LH release triggers events that cause the mature ovarian follicle to rupture and shed its secondary oocyte. This action can be detected as a very slight, sudden increase in body temperature – an indicator of the timing of ovulation. The positive feedback influence on LH release is transient and soon reverses to negative feedback.

Oestrogen secretion by the remnant follicle decreases slightly once the secondary oocyte has been released, but soon picks up again. The release of LH before ovulation also triggers the further proliferation and development of follicular cells within the follicle; these form the corpus luteum. The importance of LH in this respect is reflected in its name.

Postovulation

The postovulatory phase is marked by the continued development of the endometrium under the influence of progestins, principally progesterone, from the remnants of the Graafian follicle (the corpus luteum). The corpus luteum secretes increasing quantities of both oestrogens and progesterone. Up to this point, progesterone release from the ovary has been only slight. The significance of its release after ovulation is that it promotes the secretory activity of glands within the endometrium, the vascularization of the superficial layer of the endometrium, and glycogen storage within the endometrium cells. These actions prepare the endometrium to receive the embryo, should the secondary oocyte be fertilized. The activities peak about 1 week after ovulation, which is about the time an embryo could be expected to arrive in the uterus after passage along the Fallopian tube. The importance of the corpus luteum and progesterone is reflected in the alternative names for this phase of the cycle – the luteal or secretory phase (although 'postovulatory phase' is a more correct term).

The release of progesterone has an additive effect on the negative feedback actions of oestrogens on the anterior pituitary gland. The release of LH (and FSH) eventually decreases

BOX 18.15 PREMENSTRUAL SYNDROME, OVULATORY PAINS AND DYSMENORRHOEA

Premenstrual syndrome

Premenstrual syndrome (PMS) is also known as premenstrual tension (PMT) but increased tension may not be the only symptom. The woman may have one or two symptoms, or have several. The most common are reported to be:

- *'Psychological' symptoms*: tension, low mood, loss of confidence, feelings of aggression or anger, irritability, tiredness, anxiety, feeling emotional. There may also be a change in the sleep pattern, sexual feelings and appetite. Relationships may become strained because of these symptoms.
- *'Physical' symptoms*: breast swelling and/or pain, swelling of the feet or hands, weight gain, abdominal bloating and headaches. Patients with epilepsy, asthma, migraine or cold sores may find that these conditions become worse prior to the commencement of bleeding.

Although PMS is a term notably reserved for the severe physical and emotional distress that can accompany the premenstrual phase of the menstrual cycle, it sometimes overlaps with menstruation.

About five in 100 women in the UK have what has been described as 'true' PMS. This is where the symptoms disrupt their day-to-day functioning, and quality of life. Sometimes it is difficult to distinguish that the symptoms are caused by PMS, or if they are attributed to other conditions such as anxiety or depression. It is when the symptoms occur, not just their nature, which indicates PMS. Therefore:

- Symptoms are initiated some time following ovulation. Symptoms may occur for just a few days prior to bleeding (i.e. a period), although some women have symptoms for 2 weeks or so leading up to a period. Usually, symptoms progressively get worse as the period approaches.
- Symptoms disappear a few days following the commencement of a period.
- Symptoms that occur all of the time are not caused by PMS.

The causes of PMS remain unclear. However, it is now generally accepted that it is not caused by a hormone imbalance (i.e. too much oestrogen or too little progesterone). Currently, it is thought that women with this condition are hypersensitive to the normal level of progesterone secreted following ovulation. This over-sensitivity to progesterone seems to lead to a decrease in the level of a brain neurotransmitter called serotonin. This may lead to some of the symptoms of PMS, and may explain why medicines that increase the serotonin level are sometimes successful in its treatment (see below). Other potential links to PMS are inadequate levels of the neurotransmitter dopamine, vitamin B_6 deficiency, hypoglycaemia and the water retention that accompanies high levels of steroid release through an overlap with the actions of the salt-retaining steroid, aldosterone.

The treatment of PMS is a changing area as research continues to clarify which treatments actually work and tries to find better treatments. Currently treatments focus on relieving the symptoms of PMS, which include oedema, breast swelling, abdominal distension, backache, constipation, fatigue, depression and anxiety. The following gives a brief description of some suggested treatment options.

Non-prescription therapies include:

- *Vitamin B_6 (pyridoxine)*: despite this being a treatment for PMS, which has been used for many years, there is only limited research evidence that it works.
- *Vitex agnus-castus (Chaste Tree) fruit extract*: it is claimed that this extract may increase levels of brain neurotransmitters such as serotonin and dopamine.

Prescription therapies include:

- *SSRI medicines (selective serotonin re-uptake inhibitors)*: these antidepressant drugs increase the concentration of serotonin in the brain and are usually prescribed to treat severe PMS even when the woman

has not been diagnosed as being depressed.

- *The contraceptive pill*: in theory, preventing ovulation should help PMS, since ovulation and the subsequent secretion of progesterone into the bloodstream postovulation seems to activate symptoms of this syndrome. Despite this, most contraceptives do not help with PMS since their content of progestogen hormones have similar action to progesterone. However, a pill called Yasmin contains a progestogen (called drospirenone) that does not seem to have the drawbacks of other progestogens and the early indications of clinical studies acknowledge that this may be a good treatment for PMS.
- *Other ways of inhibiting ovulation*: in addition to progesterone-based 'pills', there are alternative way to ways to prevent ovulation.
  - Oestrogen administration. However, to protect the uterus progestogen is also administered, since there is an increased risk of developing cancer of the uterus if oestrogen alone is administered. To prevent any rise in blood progesterone an intrauterine contraceptive system (IUS) may be inserted. These devices release a small amount of progestogen into the uterus, and a minimal amount into blood thereby protecting against symptoms of progesterone excess.
  - Some medicines prevent ovulation, for example GnRH analogues (e.g. buserelin and triptorelin). These have been reported to work well, but reports of side-effects may limit their usefulness in treating PMS.
  - Surgery. Removal of both ovaries (oophorectomy, see later) prevents ovulation, and obviously cures PMS. Surgery, however, is only considered in exceptionally severe cases of PMS where other treatments have not helped.

For women sufferers with one or two physical symptoms, treatments are aimed at the specific physical symptom. For example anti-inflammatory painkillers may help if painful symptoms develop, and diuretics can help reduce fluid retention and bloating. However, it is generally reported that these treatments are unlikely to alleviate psychological symptoms (that is, unless the physical symptom is causing or enhancing the psychological symptoms, such as anxiety, etc.).

Other potential treatments that are currently attracting media attention in the treatment of PMS include St John's Wort (a plant extract) and bright-light therapy. The herbal extract (St John's Wort) is commonly used as a means to self-treat depression, while bright-light therapy has been successful in the treatment of seasonal affective disorder (SAD). How these therapies may help in PMS is unknown and therefore more research (in particular 'controlled trials') is needed to confirm if they are useful remedies for most women with PMS.

Ovulatory pains

Ovulatory pains may be caused if pain-producing chemicals released from the ruptured follicle irritate the peritoneum, causing sharp pain in the lower abdomen.

Dysmenorrhoea

Dysmenorrhoea refers to painful menstruation. It can be classified as primary or secondary dysmenorrhoea.

Primary dysmenorrhoea occurs in the absence of associated pelvic pathology, and is thought to be caused by an excessive secretion of certain uterine prostaglandins, since these chemicals cause painful spasms of the uterine muscle. Vasopressin (antidiuretic hormone, ADH), which stimulates myometrial activity and leukotrienes, and thus increases smooth muscle activity, has also been indicated in the aetiology of dysmenorrhoea. Prostaglandin synthesis inhibitors, such as aspirin and ibuprofen, are sometimes used to relieve the symptoms. Oral contraceptives that inhibit uterine contractions may also be administered.

Secondary dysmenorrhoea can be due to a narrowing (stenosis) of the cervix or to various inflammatory conditions. Correction involves treating the underlying pathology.

BOX 18.16 PSEUDOHERMAPHRODITISM

The phenotypic sex of the newborn depends upon hormonal cues received by tissues during development (i.e. it is not dependent entirely on the genetic sex of the individual – although the two are usually associated). Pseudohermaphroditism is a condition in which a person's genetic and anatomical sexes differ. Although such cases are relatively infrequent, the most common cause of female pseudohermaphroditism is adrenal genital syndrome (adrenal hypertrophy), in which an excessive secretion of androgens exists. This can occur in the female fetus or in the mature woman; in the latter case, the androgens gradually transform the woman's appearance into a male form. An absence of menstruation (amenorrhoea) occurs, causing sterility. Other causes of female pseudohermaphroditism include androgen drug abuse, pregnant females exposed to androgen drugs, maternal pituitary and/or adrenal endocrine tumours, and the genetic condition known as XY females in which the usual genetic stimulation of testosterone produc-

tion does not take place and so the gonads develop as ovaries (see earlier).

Male pseudohermaphroditism occurs in response to an undersecretion of androgens. A common cause is testicular feminization syndrome. This homeostatic imbalance involves a defect in the cellular receptors that respond to androgens. Consequently, embryonic and adult tissues cannot respond to the existing normal levels of these male hormones, and the person develops and remains physically female. However, the menstrual cycle does not appear (amenorrhoea), the uterus is absent and the vagina ends in a blind pocket. The genetic condition known as XX males also exists (the genes responsible for testosterone production in an XY embryo are actually on the X chromosome, and in this instance are inappropriately active).

Correction involves hormonal therapy and surgery to produce a sexually functioning male or female.

to levels at which the hormone is incapable of maintaining the corpus luteum. If pregnancy has not occurred, this degenerates into the corpus albicans and secretion of oestrogens and progesterone subsequently declines sharply. Consequently, the endometrium cannot be sustained and it is shed – and so the next menses begins. As ovarian steroid release diminishes, the negative feedback signal is reduced and secretion of gonadotropins increases again: further ovarian follicles begin to develop, and a new cycle is initiated.

Should the secondary oocyte be fertilized, and the early embryo implants in the endometrium, then the release of the ovarian steroids increases and initiates the maternal physiological changes associated with pregnancy. In this case, the functional integrity of the corpus luteum must be maintained for a few weeks in the absence of adequate LH. A hormone called human chorionic gonadotropin (hCG), which is released from the implanted embryo, brings this about. By the time secretion of hCG has diminished, the developing placenta will also be secreting steroids (oestrogens and progestogens) at a rate appropriate to maintain the pregnancy.

In addition to maintaining the endometrium, progesterone and oestrogens also prepare the mammary glands for lactation. Relaxin, a hormone secreted by the placenta towards the end of pregnancy, relaxes the pelvic ligaments and the pubic symphysis to aid the dilation of the uterine cervix to facilitate delivery. Pregnancy, therefore, is an altered state of health in which the homeostatic set points are reset.

The female gonadal steroids clearly have potent physiological actions, and their release cannot continue unregulated. The secretion of gonadotropins and steroids therefore fluctuates with time, and utilizes negative feedback to establish a physiologically appropriate range of values. The onset of menopause is signalled by the climacteric, when the release of steroids is insufficient to maintain the usual menstrual cycles, which therefore become less frequent. The climacteric typically begins between the ages of 40 and 50 years, and occurs because of a failure of the ovary to respond to the pituitary gonadotropin hormones. The details of menopause are discussed in Box 18.18, p.515.

Table 18.1 (p.506) summarizes the major female reproductive hormones.

ACTIVITY

Discuss the similarities and differences between the timing of oogenesis and spermatogenesis.

PHYSIOLOGY OF BIRTH CONTROL

Most adults, whether for physiological, logistic, financial and/or emotional reasons, practise some form of birth control during their reproductive years. Methods of birth control in the extreme case include the removal of the gonads and the uterus, but more usual methods are sterilization and mechanical and chemical contraception. Although research is making progress in its search for a male chemical contraceptive, so far the burden of birth control lies predominantly with women, since the complexity of the reproductive biology of women provides more target points for contraceptive development, especially chemical contraception, and so most methods are directed at women (Figure 18.17). All methods are used to avoid unwanted pregnancies, and each has potential risks and benefits, which must be analysed carefully on an individual basis. Interested readers should read other texts to consider the pros and cons of such methods, as we provide only a brief overview here.

Surgical methods

The surgical removal of the testes (castration), the ovaries (oophorectomy) and the uterus (hysterectomy) are all absolute and irreversible methods, and are performed only if the organs are diseased. The removal of the gonads (testes and ovaries) has adverse effects because of their important endocrine roles. Premenopausal women undergoing a hysterectomy do not experience an artificial menopause straight away, since the ovaries are not removed. However, if an oophorectomy is performed at the same time, then the artificial menopause will be

BOX 18.17 INFERTILITY AND STERILITY IN WOMEN

Homeostatic imbalances associated with infertility or sterility are common, and most are attributed to problems with the female reproductive system. Natural female fertility seems to decline quite rapidly after the age of 35 years but this is just an average and the actual point of decline for any individual may vary significantly.

An infertile woman has a low ability to produce functional oocytes/ova and/or support a developing embryo/fetus. Physiological (functional) infertility and sterility have multifactorial aetiologies. Sexually transmitted diseases, for example, may damage reproductive structures, and thus abolish the reproductive capacity. In addition, developmental structural abnormalities of the reproductive system (e.g. endometriosis, polycystic ovarian syndrome – see Box 18.7, p.496) and physiological problems (e.g. pituitary infarction – Sheehan's disease) affecting hormonal and neural regulation of reproductive function can cause sterility (i.e. an inability to become pregnant) (see Figure 18.18).

Menstruation reflects the health of the endocrine glands that control the process, and imbalances of the female reproductive system frequently involve menstrual/ovarian disorders. These may occur at the level of the hypothalamus and/or anterior pituitary gland and/or the ovary. For example, hypothalamic and pituitary tumours can cause a displacement or destruction of normal hypothalamic/pituitary tissue, which results in an undersecretion of gonadotropin-releasing hormones and gonadotropins [follicle-stimulating hormone (FSH) and luteinizing hormone (LH)], respectively that can lead to sterility, since functional gametes will not be produced. An undersecretion of oestrogens by the ovaries has a similar effect, and may be a consequence of dietary disturbances, distress or anaemia can cause amenorrhoea.

Other factors that can cause amenorrhoea include:

- *Abnormal ovarian and uterine development*: polycystic ovarian syndrome (see Box 18.7, p.496) is usually, but not always, associated with obesity, and fatty (sclerocystic) ovaries fail to ovulate. Structural deformity of the uterus (e.g. bicornuate uterus) may be more likely to cause recurrent abortion from failure to conceive, while significant distortion of the uterine cavity by fibroids can prevent implantation and hence affect fertility.
- *Infection causing damage to the Fallopian tubes*: anyone investigated for infertility should be tested for *Chlamydia* infection as sexually transmitted diseases, especially *Chlamydia* and gonorrhoea, are a common cause of infertility. Illegal, medical or spontaneous abortion can also lead to infection of retained products of conception. Postpartum infection can also affect fertility. Infection may be less direct and spread from areas such as the appendix, even without overt peritonitis. Infection can also damage the uterus – the presence of adhesions in the uterus and cervix is called Asherman's syndrome.
- *Endocrine disorders*: for example hyperprolactinaemia.
- *Chromosomal disorders*: for example Turner syndrome (see Figure 19.19a, p.543).
- *Nutritional disorders*: anorexia and obesity.
- *Other diseases*: systemic disease is particularly associated with the hypothalamic–pituitary axis, and may include causative autoimmune disease (e.g. rheumatoid disease). Chronic renal failure and poorly controlled diabetes mellitus have been associated with impaired fertility.
- *Medication*: phenothiazines and metoclopramide cause hyperprolactinaemia which impairs fertility. Non-steroidal anti-inflammatory drugs can impair the rupture of ovarian follicles to release an oocyte. Chemotherapeutic agents, such as those used to treat childhood leukaemia, may result in subsequent sterility. Surgery and radiotherapy may also be relevant if they involved the pelvic region. Some illicit drugs have adverse effects on fertility for example, cocaine is linked to tubal infertility and cannabis with impaired ovulation.
- *Athletic amenorrhoea*: this is related to excessive training and not being underweight is uncommon.
- *Smoking cigarettes*: this also impairs fertility.
- *Excessive alcohol consumption*: this also impairs fertility.

Correction involves treating the underlying disorder or condition. The use of fertility drugs involves stimulating the hypothalamic–pituitary–ovarian axis. Clomiphene, for example (usually administered with human chorionic gonadotropin), is thought to block oestrogen receptors in the hypothalamus. Consequently, the levels of FSH and LH are raised (since the negative feedback mechanism is inhibited) to induce follicular development and ovulation, though multiple ovulations (super-ovulation) sometimes occur, resulting in multiple pregnancies. Gonadotropin administration has also proved successful as a fertility treatment. However, the administration of gonadotropin-releasing hormone has so far proved ineffective in fertility treatment.

---

experienced soon after the operation. After a simple hysterectomy, pregnancy is, of course, impossible and menstruation will cease. However, a woman's femininity or enjoyment of sex should not be altered.

In contrast, sterilization in either sex denies the provision of functional gametes for fertilization, but maintains the endocrine function of the gonads. One means of male sterilization is a vasectomy, in which segments of the vas deferens are removed or destroyed by heat (a process called cauterization), thus making it impossible for spermatozoa to pass from the epididymis to the distal portions of the male reproductive tract. The cut (cauterized) ends do not reconnect (though there have been celebrated cases when this appears to have happened), and scarring eventually forms a permanent seal; if this happens then the vasectomy is irreversible, making the method unsuitable for men who still plan to have children but want to select the time. However, vasectomies can be reversed in a modified procedure that involves simply blocking the cut ends of the vas deferens with silicone plugs, which can later be removed.

Vasectomies do not impair normal sexual function, since the epididymal and testicular secretions account for only about 5% of semen. Spermatozoa continue to develop as normal in the epididymis until they are broken down chemically and recycled, and some may still be found for a while within the vas deferens stores: men therefore may remain fertile for up to 8 weeks after their vasectomy. The duration of fertility depends upon the frequency of ejaculation since this depletes the stores. During this period, there is obviously a need for extra contraceptive methods. The man is usually required to go back to the clinic twice with a specimen of his ejaculate to check for the absence of spermatozoa before an assurance of sterility can be given.

Female sterilization is generally achieved by ligating the Fallopian tube, which prevents the secondary oocyte and spermatozoa meeting. The procedure may be reversed, although

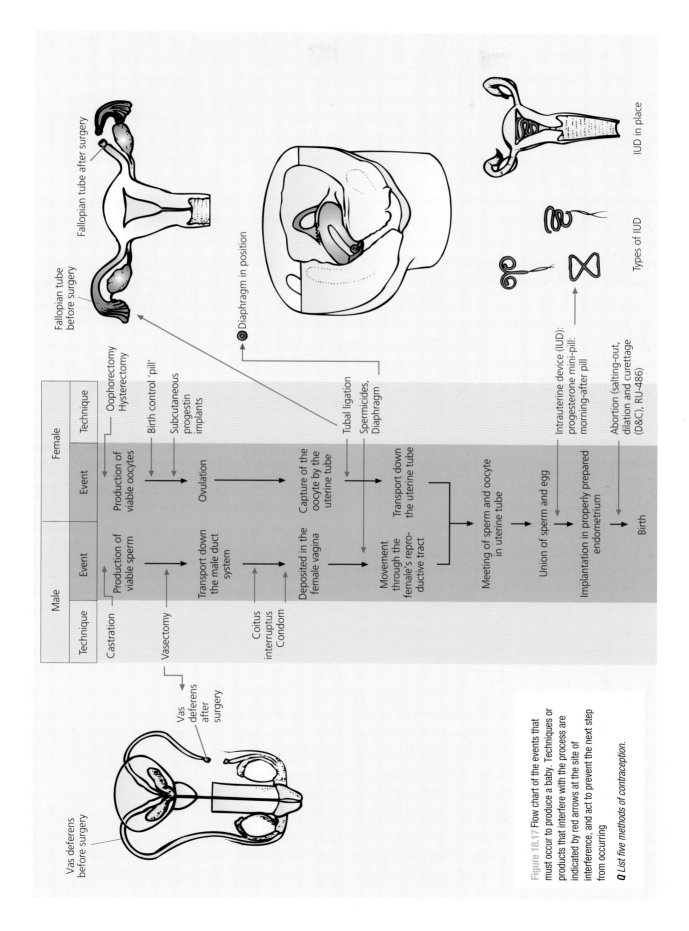

Male					Female	
Technique	Event				Event	Technique
Castration	Production of viable sperm				Production of viable oocytes	Oophorectomy Hysterectomy
Vasectomy	Transport down the male duct system				Ovulation	Birth control 'pill' / Subcutaneous progestin implants
Coitus interruptus / Condom	Deposited in the female vagina				Capture of the oocyte by the uterine tube	Tubal ligation
	Movement through the female's reproductive tract				Transport down the uterine tube	Spermicides, Diaphragm
					Meeting of sperm and oocyte in uterine tube	
					Union of sperm and egg	Intrauterine device (IUD): progesterone mini-pill; morning-after pill
					Implantation in properly prepared endometrium	Abortion (salting-out, dilation and curettage (D&C), RU-486)
					Birth	

Vas deferens before surgery

Vas deferens after surgery

Fallopian tube before surgery

Fallopian tube after surgery

Diaphragm in position

Types of IUD

IUD in place

Figure 18.17 Flow chart of the events that must occur to produce a baby. Techniques or products that interfere with the process are indicated by red arrows at the site of interference, and act to prevent the next step from occurring

Q List five methods of contraception.

this cannot be guaranteed. There is no impairment of sexual performance or enjoyment.

Natural and mechanical methods

Natural and mechanical contraceptive methods prevent fertilization without altering fertility. Natural methods include:

- *coitus interruptus*: involves the withdrawal of the penis just before ejaculation. The voluntary control of ejaculation, however, is never assured, since involuntary premature ejaculations are quite common;
- *rhythm or fertility awareness methods*: these take advantage of the fact that a secondary oocyte is fertilizable for a period of only about 3 days during each menstrual cycle; the couple therefore avoids intercourse during this fertile period. The period is recognized by noting changes in the consistency of vaginal mucus, since the mucus changes from a sticky to a clear and stringy consistency during the fertile period, and by noting body temperature, since this rises slightly (by about 0.2–0.4°F or 0.1–0.2°C after ovulation (see Figure 18.15, p.507).

The effectiveness of these techniques is limited, since few women have perfectly regular cycles, and some women occasionally ovulate during the so-called safe period of menstruation and so may become pregnant very soon after menstruation has ended.

Mechanical (barrier) methods of contraception include:

- *the condom*: prevents the deposition of spermatozoa in the vagina. This method has become the most common form of birth control in recent years, as it also reduces the incidence of sexually transmitted diseases;
- *the diaphragm*: stops spermatozoa from passing into the cervix;
- *the intrauterine device (IUD)*: thought to change the uterine lining so that it produces a substance that destroys either the spermatozoa, thus preventing fertilization, or the products of the fertilized ovum by preventing implantation. The use of IUDs is not as widespread as other barrier methods, since they have been associated with pelvic inflammatory diseases, uterine perforations and infertility.

Chemical methods

Chemical methods of contraception include spermicidal agents (foams, creams, jellies and suppositories) that kill spermatozoa, and oral contraceptives based on reproductive hormones. Oral contraceptives inhibit ovulation by activating the negative feedback inhibition of the menstrual cycle. Many contraceptive pills are now available, and they are in widespread use. However, the high-oestrogen pill initially introduced has been associated with serious health risks, including cancer and heart disease, and withdrawn, while the 'mini-pill', or progesterone-only pill, has proven to be less effective in preventing pregnancy, as the negative feedback response is weaker than that of oestrogens. The hormone does promote the formation of a mucus plug in the cervix, but this is not a perfect

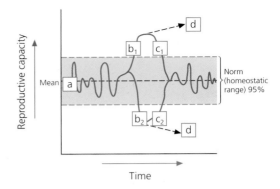

Figure 18.18 Reproductive capacity, a homeostatic function. a, Reproductive capacity fluctuating within its homeostatic range. This corresponds to the acquisition of 'normal' requirements for gametogenesis and the absence of factors (e.g. emotional) that may diminish the desire to have sexual intercourse. b_1, Increased fertility, which accompanies increased spermatogenesis (high sperm counts) or increased monthly ovulations. The latter can occur naturally, as in the case of non-identical twinning, or artificially, as a result of the *in vitro* fertilization (IVF) programme, producing 'super-ovulation'. b_2, Decreased fertility, as occurs: (1) temporarily in females accompanying distress or anaemia, in males accompanying high testicular temperatures, fatigue or increased alcohol intakes and in both sexes, accompanying malnutrition, fever, radiation, infection (e.g. sexually transmitted diseases, STDs); (2) permanently, such as a result developmental structural abnormalities (e.g. male and female hermaphroditism and cryptorchidism) and physiological, neural and hormonal mechanisms (e.g. hyposecretion of the gonadotropins). c_1, Contraception (either reversible or irreversible) encouraged to decrease the number of conceptions and potential offspring. c_2, Correction of the underlying pathology (e.g. surgical removal of tumours, surgical correction of hermaphroditism, hormone administration in hyposecretion imbalances). d, Irreversibility of homeostatic imbalance as occurs with certain cancers. (a, Represents boxes a_1–a_4 in Figure 1.7, p.11, reflecting the individual variability in the homeostatic range)

Q Describe the major male and female homeostatic imbalances mentioned in this chapter that may be associated with infertility and sterility.

barrier to spermatozoa. The most commonly used chemical method is the combination pill, which contains both progesterone and oestrogens (with the former in higher concentrations). The combined effect of these hormones is to decrease the secretion of gonadotropins by inhibiting the secretion of hypothalamic GnRH. Accordingly, the levels of gonadotropins (FSH and LH) are not adequate to initiate follicular maturation or to induce ovulation, and the absence of the secondary oocyte means that pregnancy cannot occur.

Contraceptive pills are administered in a cyclical fashion, beginning 5 days after the start of the menses and continuing over the next 3 weeks. Placebo pills, or no pills, are taken in the fourth week of the cycle to promote shedding of the endometrium that will have developed in response to the steroids in the pill. Despite its popularity, the use of the oral contraceptive pill is not without potential risks. Approximately 40–45% of women taking it experience side-effects ranging from minor problems, such as nausea, weight gain, irregular periods and amenorrhoea, to life-threatening conditions, such as thrombosis (and its associated risks of heart attacks or strokes), liver tumours and gall bladder diseases. A major side-effect of the contraceptive pill reported by

BOX 18.18 MENOPAUSE AND HORMONE REPLACEMENT THERAPY

The menopause is a normal developmental event in all women and is defined as the last menstrual period. However, it is frequently referred to as the 'change of life' since most people view the menopause as the time of life, perhaps a number of years, leading up to, and following the last period. The average age of occurrence of the menopause in the UK is 51 years.

Menopause may be asymptomatic but it is common for one or more symptoms to exist which result from a low level of oestrogen secretion. Symptoms are classified as short-term and long-term.

Short-term symptoms:

- *Hot flushes*: these occur in the majority of women and the number and frequency varies. They occur infrequently in some women to approximately 20 times per day in others. Hot flushes last a few minutes and cause flushing of the face, neck and chest. Some women become giddy, faint, or feel weak or sick during a flush. Flushing commences just prior to the menopause, and normally continues for a couple of years.
- *Sweats*: these can coincide with hot flushes, and can occur on their own, usually in bed at night.
- *Other symptoms*: headaches, palpitations, tiredness, difficulty sleeping, depression, increased irritability and anxiety, aches and pains and loss of libido.

Long-term changes and problems:

- *Skin and hair*: collagen production in the skin is decreased, hence the skin becomes thinner, drier and itchy.
- *Genital area*: decreased oestrogen causes the tissues in and around the vagina and the vulva to become thinner and drier. Therefore, the vagina may shrink a little, and expand less easily during sex and this may result in some pain upon sexual intercourse.

Osteoporosis following the menopause

Women lose bone material faster than men especially following menopause because of their decreasing levels of oestrogen (this female hormone is protective against bone loss). Many studies have shown that by the age of 75 years some women have lost approximately one-third of their bone material and as a result these women become more susceptible to bone fractures. However, not all women develop osteoporosis following menopause. Osteoporosis is like most diseases (i.e. its occurrence results from nature–nurture interactions) and therefore it is more likely to develop if one or more 'risk factors' exists:

- a strong family history of osteoporosis;
- commenced menopause before the age of 45 years;
- body mass index (BMI) of 19 (i.e. woman is very underweight);
- smoking;
- history of a previous bone fracture following an insignificant fall;
- periods stopped for approximately 12 months or more prior to the menopause;
- history, or currently taking a steroid medicine for 3 months or more (a side-effect of steroids is to promote bone loss);
- deficiency in calcium and/or vitamin D;
- sedentary lifestyle, or has never taken exercise;
- presence of medical conditions that can affect the bones such as, primary hyperthyroidism, Cushing's disease, and other conditions which result in poor mobility.

ACTIVITY

Using information from Chapter 1, p.17 Identify the genetic and environmental components associated with the risk factors above.

Hormone replacement therapy

Technically, hormone replacement therapy (HRT) relates to replacement of any hormone that is lacking, but it is more widely used in the context of the menopause. It may be prescribed for women during or after menopause to relieve the symptoms caused by the decreasing levels of oestrogens. All types of HRT contain an oestrogen hormone. Oestrogen may be administered orally, intravenously, as transdermal patches, or as implanted pellets. If the major symptoms are vaginal, then a topical oestrogen cream is often applied. The oestrogen in HRT is usually combined with a progestogen hormone.

The side-effects of taking HRT are not serious. In the first few weeks some women may develop slight nausea, or breast discomfort or leg cramps; some have more headaches, while others may experience dry eyes.

Evidence from research has shown that within the first year or so of starting HRT there is a small increased risk of developing and intravascular thrombosis which can cause deep vein thrombosis (DVT) and the clot may travel to the lung (increasing the risk of pulmonary embolism) or the heart (increasing the risk of myocardial infarction) or the brain (increasing the risk of cerebrovascular accident) (see Figures 12.13b, p.324 and 12.7c, p.313). Studies have shown there is also a small increased risk of developing cancers of the breast, the uterus (womb), the ovary and gut, and of developing dementia. Therefore, it is recommended that women on HRT undergo regular check-ups for cervical smears, blood pressure and weight recordings because of these associated risks.

As always, the benefits have to be balanced against the risks in each individual.

---

many women is loss of libido. Refinement of pill composition and health checks have now made major problems rare, although women who combine this form of contraceptive with smoking and/or other risk factors associated with heart attacks and strokes are obviously increasing their chances of developing these conditions.

Norplant, launched in 1993, is a revolutionary contraceptive for women. The method involves administering a potent synthetic progesterone-related hormone (levonorgestrel) via six flexible tubes, each about the size of a matchstick, inserted under the skin of the upper arm. Norplant has a 98.5% reliability (second only to the combined contraceptive pill). It provides reversible protection for up to 5 years, after which the capsules have to be removed and replaced with new ones if contraception is still required. Norplant operates by:

- preventing 50% of ovulations (i.e. negative feedback suppression of LH/FSH release is incomplete);
- thickening the cervical mucus, so spermatozoa cannot swim through;
- slowing down the transport of the successfully ovulated secondary oocytes, so that fertilization becomes less likely;
- thinning the endometrial lining, so that the fertilized ovum cannot develop.

As discussed previously, the secretion of FSH by the pituitary is also inhibited by another gonadal hormone, inhibin

BOX 18.19 SEXUALLY TRANSMITTED DISEASES

Sexually transmitted diseases (STDs) are infectious, and spread via direct sexual contact. They include the traditionally known bacterial venereal diseases syphilis and gonorrhoea, previously the most common STDs. During the 1980s, these were superseded by human immuno-deficiency virus (HIV) infections and consequently acquired immune deficiency syndrome (AIDS). One method of transmitting HIV is during sexual contact.

The use of condoms provides a physical barrier to prevent the spread of STDs. The use of condoms has been strongly advised since the discovery of HIV infection and the fatal outcome of AIDS. HIV and its progression into AIDS are discussed further in Box 13.16, p.388 and in the case study of a young man with symptomatic HIV/AIDS, Section VI, p.656.

Syphilis

Syphilis is caused by the bacterium *Treponema pallidum*, acquired through sexual contact or via placental transmission. Confirmed cases of syphilis have increased in the last few years in men who have sex with men. Infected fetuses are usually stillborn or die shortly after birth. Sexually transmitted syphilis can affect any system of the body, as the bacteria easily penetrate intact mucosal membranes and skin abrasions, from where they then have easy access to local lymphatics and the circulation (see Figures 13.4a, p.367). Within a few hours of exposure, a body-wide infection is in progress. If the disease is untreated, it advances through primary, secondary, latent and, sometimes, tertiary stages.

During the primary stage, an open sore (chancre) occurs at the point of contact. In men, this is typically the penis, and thus is easily identifiable. In women, however, vaginal or cervix lesions are often undetected. The lesion persists for 1 week or more, in which time it ulcerates, becomes crusty, heals spontaneously and disappears. Approximately 6–24 weeks later, symptoms such as a rash, fever and aching joints and muscles indicate the secondary stage. The symptoms then disappear, and the disease ceases to be infectious. During this symptomless latent stage, the bacteria may invade body organs; the signs of organ degeneration (such as brain changes) mark the appearance of the tertiary stage. The antibiotic penicillin interferes with the ability of dividing bacteria to produce new cell walls, and is still the treatment of choice for all stages of syphilis.

Gonorrhoea

Gonorrhoea is caused by the bacterium *Neisseria gonorrhoeae*. This STD affects primarily the mucous membranes of the urogenital tract, rectum and, occasionally, the eyes, throat and lower intestines. Transmission is by direct contact, usually sexual, although bacteria can be transmitted to the eyes of the newborn through the cervix. Administration of 1% silver nitrate solution to the baby's eyes prevents infection. Symptoms vary depending on the sex of person. Most infected women experience few symptoms, and medical treatment is not sought. Consequently, these carriers may spread the infection. The most common symptom in men is urethritis, accompanied by painful urination and pus discharge from the penis. If untreated, gonorrhoea in men can lead to urethral constriction and inflammation of the entire duct system; in females it may lead to sterility. Correction involves antibiotic therapy (e.g. procaine penicillin), although strains are becoming increasingly resistant to these antibiotics, and gonorrhoea is becoming increasingly prevalent. New cases reported to genitourinary medicine clinics have been decreasing in line with the Department of Health '1992 Health of the Nation' projection.

Genital herpes

Many people are unaware that they suffer from genital herpes. Herpes simplex virus (HSV) type II is the most reported organism responsible for most herpes infections below the waist, including genital blisters on the prepuce and glans penis in men, and the vulva and sometimes the vagina in women, however HSV type I can also cause genital herpes. Type I is responsible for the majority of infections above the waist (e.g. cold sores).

The painful lesions of the reproductive organs observed in genital herpes are usually more of a nuisance than a threat to life. If a pregnant woman suffers symptoms at the time of birth, a Caesarean section is strongly advised to prevent complications in the newborn, since congenital herpes can cause severe malformations. Unlike syphilis and gonorrhoea, genital herpes is viral; the virus remains inside the body, and the person may suffer recurrent symptoms several times a year. Sexual abstinence for the duration of HSV 'eruption' will not prevent transmission as asymptomatic shedding of the virus is now well documented and prior to an eruption they will be shedding the virus.

Treatment involves management of the symptoms via the administration of antiviral agents (e.g. aciclovir), analgesia and saline compresses.

(see Figure 18.14, p.505). Inhibin appears to have a more limited range of physiological actions and so may eventually prove to be an ideal contraceptive for both women and men.

Abortion

Abortion is the expulsion of the products of conception from the uterus. There are many forms of abortion, but they can be classified broadly as spontaneous (naturally occurring) and induced (intentionally performed).

Induced abortions are used in various circumstances, including as a form of contraception when the birth control methods discussed above have not been practised or have failed, although this is highly controversial. Procedures include vacuum aspiration (suction), surgical evacuation (scraping) and the induction of uterine contractions by use of saline solution or drugs. The last method interferes with the hormonal actions necessary to maintain pregnancy. For example, RU-486 (mifepristone) acts by blocking the quieting effects of progesterone on the uterus. It is taken in the first 7 weeks of pregnancy in conjunction with prostaglandins to induce uterine contractions and a miscarriage. The drug has a 96–98% success rate. Similarly, anti-hCG vaccine inhibits the actions of chorionic gonadotropin, and therefore stimulates menstrual flow instead of maintaining pregnancy.

SUMMARY

1 Sex cells, or gametes, are reproduced by: (i) mitosis, a duplication division that occurs in all body (somatic) cells and ensures that the diploid number of chromosomes is sustained, so that homeostatic functions can proceed within their normal parameters; and (ii) meiosis, a reduction division that occurs in the gonads and ensures that gametes have the haploid number of chromosomes, so that the diploid number (essential for normal embryonic/fetal development) is restored at fertilization.

2 Reproductive organs have specialized exocrine tissues adapted to produce, maintain and transport gametes, and endocrine tissue adapted to produce steroidal hormones.

3 Primary sex organs include the male testes and the female ovaries. These organs produce spermatozoa (a process called spermatogenesis), secondary oocytes (oogenesis), and sex hormones. Accessory organs include the internal and external reproductive organs.

4 At puberty, hypothalamic GnRH stimulates the production and secretion of gonadotropins (FSH and LH) by the pituitary gland. These hormones are important in gametogenesis and in the production of the male sex hormones (androgens) and female sex hormones (oestrogens and progestogens, mainly progesterone).

5 In males, mature spermatozoa are produced in the seminiferous tubules and collect in the epididymis, where they are stored until they are broken down chemically and recycled or released into the vas deferens upon ejaculation. The vas continues as the urethra at the base of the bladder; this latter part provides the exit route for both spermatozoa and urine at the tip of the penis.

6 The seminal vesicles, prostate and Cowper's glands (and, to a small extent, the seminiferous tubules and the epididymis) add secretions to the spermatozoa cells and produce the semen.

7 Testes descend via the inguinal canal into the scrotal sacs before birth. Cryptorchidism is an imbalance that reflects undescended testes. Inguinal hernia is a dropping of a portion of the intestines into the inguinal canal.

8 The penis is the male copulatory organ with specialized tissue (corpora cavernosa and corpus spongiosum) that becomes engorged with blood when sexually aroused, producing a rigid and erect structure necessary for the insertion into the vagina during sexual intercourse.

9 In the female, gametes are produced and matured in ovarian follicles at puberty under the hormonal influence of pituitary FSH. Adequate FSH release signals the onset of menarche (the first menstrual flow).

10 The mature (Graafian) follicle releases the secondary oocyte (and some of its surrounding follicular cells) at ovulation. These cells are taken to the uterus via the Fallopian tubes. The trigger to ovulation is an LH surge from the pituitary gland caused by a transient positive (stimulatory) feedback mechanism produced by oestrogen, the release of which is relatively high at this point within the menstrual cycle.

11 LH converts the follicle cells remaining in the ovary after ovulation into the corpus luteum, a body that secretes steroid hormones (progesterone and oestrogens). These hormones suppress FSH and LH release by negative feedback, in order to prevent further follicular development, and to promote further development of the endometrium.

12 The uterine cycle (average 28 days) begins with menstruation (up to the fifth day). Following this, steroids (from the preovulatory follicles and the postovulatory corpus luteum) prepare the uterus for implantation of the fertilized ovum. If fertilization does not occur, the corpus luteum becomes the corpus albicans, which then degenerates and is recycled. Consequently, steroid secretion from the ovary decreases, removing their inhibitory action over the gonadotropins; their subsequent release is associated with the next menstrual cycle.

13 The vagina is the female copulatory organ. The hymen guards its entrance in virgins. Bartholin's glandular tissue secretes a lubricant in anticipation of, and during, sexual intercourse. The external genitalia of the vulva are comprised of the mons pubis, labia majora, labia minora, clitoris and vestibule.

14 During sexual arousal, the engorgement of blood in the clitoris causes its erection.

15 Fertilization occurs high in the Fallopian tubes. The fusion of spermatozoa and ovum nuclei produce the diploid zygote.

16 Contraceptive methods are designed to prevent gamete formation or prevent the spermatozoa reaching the secondary oocyte. Methods are classified as being natural, mechanical and chemical.

17 Homeostatic imbalances of male and female reproductive tracts are divided into anatomical and physiological abnormalities, both of which may be responsible for infertility or sterility in either sex.

REFERENCES

Best, K. (2000) How to minimize PID risks. *Network* **20**(1): 7–11.

Behrman, R.E., Kliegman, R.M. Jenson, H.B. and Stanton, B.F. (2004) Disorders and anomalies of the scrotal contents. In: *Nelson Textbook of Pediatrics*, 17th edn. Philadelphia: Saunders, 245–50.

Franco, L., Duarte-Franco, D. and Ferenczy, A. (2004) Cervical cancer: epidemiology, prevention and the role of human papillomavirus infection. *Canadian Medical Association Journal* **164**(7): 1017–25.

Meston, C.M. and Frolich, P.F. (2000) The neurobiology of sexual function. *Archives of General Psychiatry* **57**: 1012–30.

Pettersson, A., Richiardi, L., Nordenskjold, A., Kaijser, M., and Akre, O. (2007) Age at surgery for undescended testis and risk of testicular cancer. *New England Journal of Medicine* **356**(18): 1835–41.

Shepherd, J., Weston, R., Peersman, G. and Napuli, I.Z. (2001) Interventions for encouraging sexual lifestyles and behaviours intended to prevent cervical cancer. *The Cochrane Library*, Issue 1. Oxford: Update Software.

Stones, R.W. and Mountfield, J. (2001) Interventions for treating chronic pelvic pain in women. *The Cochrane Library*, Issue 1. Oxford: Update Software.

FURTHER READING

Aiken, C. (2000) The impact of the cyclical symptoms of PMS. *Practice Nurse* **19**(4): 148, 150–2.

American Urological Association (2003) Guideline on the management of benign prostatic hyperplasia: Chapter 1: Diagnosis and treatment recommendations. *Journal of Urology* **170**(2 Pt 1): 530–7.

Bailey, K. (2000) The nurse's role in promoting breast cancer. *Nursing Standard* **14**(30): 34–6.

Bhasin, S. (2007) Approach to the infertile man. *Journal of Clinical Endocrinology and Metabolism* **92**(6): 1995–2004.

Barnard, N.D., Scialli, A.R., Hurlock, D. and Berton, P. (2000) Diet and sex-hormone binding globulin, dysmenorrhea, and premenstrual symptoms. *Obstetrics and Gynecology* **95**(2): 245–50.

Challen, V. (1998) Prostatic cancer screening – does it fulfil the criteria for medical screening? *Radiography* **4**(2): 115–20.

Cook, N. (2000) Clinical: health promotion. Testicular cancer: testicular self-examination and screening. *British Journal of Nursing* **9**(6): 338–43.

Crayford, T.J.B., Campbell, S., Bourne, T.H., Rawson, H.J. and Collins, W.P. (2000) Benign ovarian cysts and ovarian cancer: a cohort study with implications for screening. *Lancet* **355**(9209): 1060–3.

Frye, G.M. and Silverman, S.D. (2000) Women's health. Is it premenstrual syndrome? Keys to focused diagnosis, therapies for multiple symptoms (fifth in a series). *Postgraduate Medicine* **107**(5): 151–9.

Goswami, D. and Conway, G.S. (2005) Premature ovarian failure. *Human Reproduction Update* **11**(4): 391–410.

Lutchman Singh, K., Davies, M. and Chatterjee, R. (2005) Fertility in female cancer survivors: pathophysiology, preservation and the role of ovarian reserve testing. *Human Reproduction Update* **11**(1): 69–89.

Trinder, J. and Cahill, D.J. (2002) Endometriosis and infertility: the debate continues. *Human Fertilization* **5**(1 Suppl.): S21–7.

USEFUL WEBSITES

http://www.cancer.gov/cancertopics/factsheet/Detection/PSA.

http://www.prostate-research.org.uk

http://www.prostate-cancer.org.uk

http://www.pms.org.uk

http://health.yahoo.com/sexualhealth-causes?pd=healthwise

INFLUENCES ON HOMEOSTASIS

CHAPTER 19

GENES IN EMBRYO DEVELOPMENT AND AGEING

INTRODUCTION

The human body is composed of billions of cells, each specialized for its role. Specialization largely occurs during the differentiation of cells in the embryo, and is primarily controlled by the genetic information encoded within the cell, but is modified by environmental stimuli. Differentiation is a complex and incompletely understood process but can be envisaged as resulting in the generation of cells of distinct structure and activity. Proteins are crucial in this, particularly the activities of enzymes, which must be present at the appropriate time.

The molecular shape of a protein (and hence the specificity of enzyme action; see Chapter 4, pp.98–9) results from variations in the number of amino acids present, the types of amino acids present and the sequencing of those amino acids. Here lies the importance of the genetic code within the cell's nucleus since cells construct proteins according to the 'blueprint' encapsulated within DNA. The process of protein synthesis is summarized in Figure 2.14 (p.41) and readers should familiarize themselves with this process, and the nature of the genetic code, before continuing with this chapter.

Chromosomes

The majority of genes in a cell are located on chromosomes ('chromo-' = colour, 'soma' = body), which are the molecules of DNA within the cell. There are 46 molecules of DNA within a human body cell (not a sex cell) and hence there are 46 chromosomes. The 46 chromosomes are comprised of 23 pairs because one member of each pair was inherited from each parent, and then copied into each new cell. In sex cells there are just 23 chromosomes, that is, just one member of each chromosome pair.

The chromosomal make-up of a cell is called its karyotype. Karyotyping is useful because it identifies if there is a chromosomal defect (i.e. too many or too few, or perhaps fragmented chromosomes). It does not, however, give information about the specific genetic make-up of a cell, called the genome, since this relates to the actual genes within the chromosomes. Chromosomes differ in size and according to their broad role within the body. Two of the chromosomes are called sex chromosomes because they are involved in the development of the sexual characteristics of the fetus (but with some involvement in other functions). The remaining 44 are called autosomes (Figure 19.1) and are mostly concerned with the non-sexual functioning of the body. The autosomes are numbered according to their size: pair 1 is the largest, pair 22 the smallest.

Most of the chromosomes are indistinguishable between men and women. The exception is the pair of sex chromosomes. In women, the sex karyotype is referred to as XX, because there are two X chromosomes. In men, there is only one X chromosome; the other member of the pair is considerably smaller and is called the Y chromosome (i.e. the male karyotype is XY). This difference has implications for the inheritance of certain disorders as some are linked to these particular chromosomes, and the disorder typically is observed in men. Both autosomal and sex-liked inheritance are considered later in this chapter.

Are genetic disorders inherited or acquired?

The activities of genes are evident throughout life, and science increasingly is identifying genetic causes of ill health. A number of inherited disorders are recognized (approximately 3000, mostly rare though) and many readers will have heard of the commoner ones such as cystic fibrosis and Duchenne muscular dystrophy. One feature of inherited disorders is that they are usually present from birth, although some inherited genes may only become problematic later in childhood, or even adulthood, because gene expression may be 'masked' for a while. However, recent advances are now beginning to identify how genetic disturbances can also be acquired during life. Thus disorders such as cancer and heart disease are now known to have genetic components that become problematic because

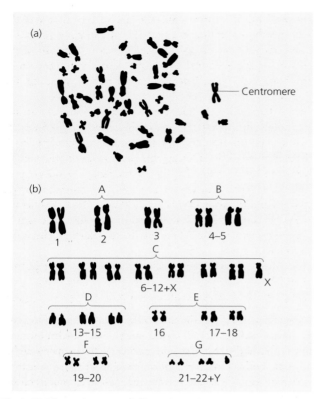

Figure 19.1 Human karyotype. (a) Chromosomes from a normal human cell. (b) Karyotyping of chromosomes from a male

Q *How does the female karyotype differ from that of the male?*

at the birth of an affected child. Counselling may then be initiated should the parents plan further pregnancies.

Genetic counsellors are members of a healthcare team with specific background in medical genetics. They offer advice and support to patients and families who have members with genetic diseases and to families who may be at risk for a multiplicity of inherited disorders. The counsellors identify families at risk, investigate the problem that exists in the family, resolve information as regards the condition, scrutinize inheritance patterns and risks of reappearance, and inform the family of all the available options. The role of a genetic counsellor seems certain to expand in the near future. This is because the 'new' genetics, which is a product of the Human Genome Project (explained later) is going to have a major impact on understanding the nature of health and ill health with new screening mechanisms, new health education measures, gene therapies and new pharmaceuticals that will affect us all.

This chapter ends with an exploration of the directions and prospects of recent research in this area, but to set the scene much of the earlier sections address the fundamentals of genetics, including main stages in tissue specialization during embryo development, the inheritance of characteristics, and how acquired gene changes seem to be an important factor in the declining function that is associated with ageing.

EMBRYO DEVELOPMENT AND THE ROLE OF GENES AS MEDIATORS OF TISSUE DIFFERENTIATION

This section outlines the processes of moving from a fertilized ovum to a formed fetus. Critical steps that are actioned by genes during differentiation and lead to tissue specialization are highlighted. It should be noted, however, that while recent research has identified some of the genes that are essential in these processes (called 'homeobox' genes), other crucial genes remain to be identified. The normality of these genes (and others) and of their expression is vital to the whole process.

Stages of embryo development

It is convenient to consider the milestones of tissue differentiation in two substages: that of the early embryo prior to implantation in the uterus and that of the later embryo after implantation.

Differentiation of the early embryo

Fertilization and formation of the zygote

A later section identifies that the cell division process referred to as meiosis generates four 'daughter' cells from the original germinative cell, each with reduced numbers of chromosomes. Producing four cells from one is advantageous in men as this helps the testes to generate lots of gametes (i.e. spermatozoa). In women, it is usual to produce just one gamete (ovum), which means that three of the daughter cells cannot develop. In the first instance, ovulation releases from the ovarian follicle a secondary oocyte and a nucleus (rather than a whole cell)

the genetic code is altered during life. Acquired genetic changes are also evident in the ageing process, for example raising the risk of onset of Alzheimer disease and diabetes mellitus Type II. Yet even with the consequences of acquired changes, it is clear that some people inherit certain genes that give them a greater likelihood (i.e. a susceptibility) of developing the changes.

In relation to ill health, therefore, two significant aspects are:

- the genes which we inherit that either influence embryo development or give a propensity to later acquired conditions, and
- the genetic changes that we acquire during the lifespan.

The likelihood of genetic disorder in offspring has traditionally been established by pedigree analysis of family history. Thus familial incidences of a disorder, going back through a number of generations, can identify the presence of an affected gene within the family line. Such analyses, however, can only highlight the possibility that an individual is a carrier of the affected gene, and similarly if his/her partner might also be a carrier. It is also the case that family histories are incomplete, or only extend back one or two generations, and so people are often unaware of any inherited disorders within the family line. Thus, a couple often only become aware that they are carriers

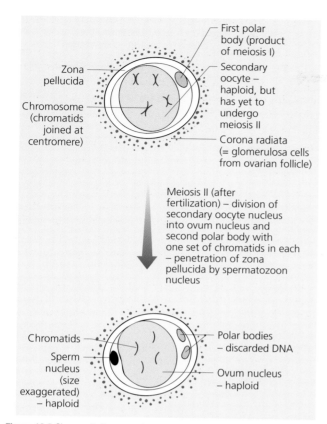

Figure 19.2 Changes in the secondary oocyte at fertilization. For clarity, only four chromosomes are shown. The ovum and sperm nuclei soon fuse, and the polar bodies degenerate

Q When does a secondary oocyte become an ovum, and an ovum a zygote?

called the first polar body (Figure 19.2; see also Figure 18.13, p.504). The secondary oocyte is the cell that will form the ovum, while the polar body plays no further role and disintegrates. This is the first part of the cell division process; the polar body is the first daughter cell to be discarded.

When released the oocyte is surrounded by a protective layer of glycoprotein called the zona pellucida, and a cloud of granulated cells called the corona radiata (from the ovarian follicle). These layers help to protect the oocyte as it passes along the Fallopian tube (oviduct); at this point the oocyte is very vulnerable and its well-being will be affected by any adverse changes in the fluid composition within the tube.

Fertilization normally takes place within the Fallopian tube:

- Of the millions of spermatozoa ejaculated during intercourse only a few hundred will arrive in the vicinity of the oocyte, and only one will penetrate and fertilize it. To do this a spermatozoon must penetrate the protective layers of the zona pellucida and cumulus oophorus. This is achieved by spermatozoa in the vicinity of the oocyte secreting enzymes collectively called acrosin, which change the properties of the matrix and makes passage of the spermatozoa easier.
- Once a single spermatozoon has penetrated the oocyte the sperm nucleus initiates further enzyme activity (the cortical

reaction) but this time within the oocyte. The nature of the cell membrane of the oocyte, and of the zona pellucida, alters and prevents access of further sperm. The tail of the sperm separates from it during fertilization and only the head (i.e. nucleus) of the sperm actually penetrates the oocyte.

- For a short while the nuclei of the spermatozoon and the oocyte remain separate; the oocyte is around 30–50 times the diameter of the nucleus of the spermatozoon, and so can readily accommodate it. During this period the oocyte nucleus begins to complete its division by meiosis. The oocyte produces two more daughter nuclei: these are called the ovum nucleus and the second polar body (Figure 19.2). As before, the polar body nucleus disintegrates leaving only the ovum.
- The spermatozoon nucleus swells to produce the male pronucleus.
- The nucleus of the ovum swells to form the female pronucleus.
- The pronuclei fuse i.e. fertilization occurs. This is the zygote.

It is of note that only the nucleus of the spermatozoon takes part in fertilization. Consequently, all inclusions in embryo/fetal cells other than the nucleus will have been exclusively derived from those of the ovum; thus the small quantity of extranuclear DNA that we all carry within our mitochondria (see later) is derived from our mother, grandmother, and so on. Such conservation of DNA from the maternal line has provided science with the opportunity to study lineages, including population and ethnic groups that may have dispersed thousands of years ago.

The morula

Cell division begins immediately after the ovum and spermatozoon nuclei have fused. The cells divide approximately every 12 hours, eventually producing a ball of 64 cells. This stage is called the morula (= mulberry; the appearance is likened to this fruit – Figure 19.3). There is no increase in overall size, however, as the cells (which therefore must decrease in individual size) remain encapsulated within the zona pellucida that was present when the oocyte was shed from the ovary. This coat continues to provide protection for the morula as it is wafted along in fluid within the Fallopian tube, to the body of the uterus over a period of a few days.

The cells within the morula appear very simplistic. While some genes are undoubtedly active within the cells, a cell can actually be removed at a point of morula development without affecting the future development of the embryo; this has to be done around the 8- to 12-cell stage since by the time there are 16 cells or more present each cell will have become compacted within the confines of the zona pellucida and removal of a cell will in all likelihood cause others to be damaged. The cells, therefore, do not yet have a predetermined 'destiny': the developmental genes have still to be activated.

The blastocyst

By the time the morula reaches the uterus it has become transformed:

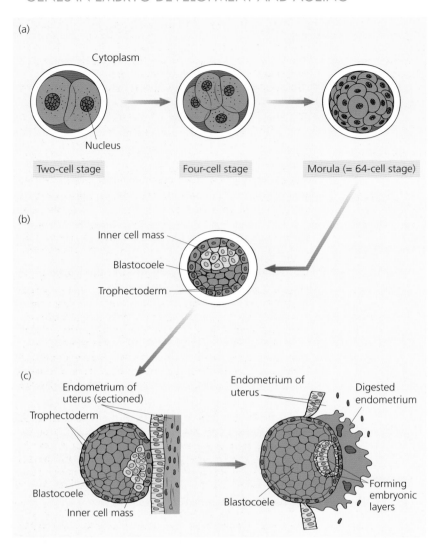

Figure 19.3 Preimplantation development. (a) Cleavage stage. Development of the morula from the zygote. (b) The blastocyst (in section). (c) Implantation

Q Discuss the events leading to the formation of the zygote.

Q Distinguish between the morula and blastocyst stages of development.

BOX 19.1 TWINS AND TRIPLETS

Should twinning take place it usually occurs at or soon after fertilization:

- If two ova (i.e. from two oocytes released at ovulation) are independently fertilized then dizygotic (two zygotes), or fraternal, twins may result. Another term is non-identical twins. Each embryo will be genetically distinct and will develop independently.
- Monozygotic (one zygote) twins develop when the zygote divides into two and each new part develops into a separate embryo. Monozygotic twins are therefore genetically identical. Each embryo develops inde-

pendently but if twinning occurs some time after fertilization then the pair may only partially separate, producing conjoined twins. The timing of twinning also has implications for development of the embryonic membranes.

- Triplets can be monozygotic (i.e. all three embryos are genetically identical and derived from a single zygote), dizygotic (i.e. where one of two fraternal zygotes divides again to form identical twins), or trizygotic (i.e. all three embryos develop from separate zygotes).

- Some cells have migrated to the outer surface, leaving a fluid-filled cavity called the blastocoele ('-coele' = space or compartment). The cell layer is called the trophectoderm ('troph-' =' nutrition, ectoderm = outer layer), and individual cells are referred to as trophoblasts. Note though that the trophectoderm bears no relation to the embryonic ectoderm mentioned later. The two terms are confusing but a general rule is that any reference to tissues in a fetus, infant, child or

adult as being 'ectodermal' in origin will usually be referring to the ectoderm, not the trophectoderm. Cells derived from the latter will eventually be incorporated into one of the membranes that surround the embryo (the chorion) and the placenta.

- A small cluster of cells, called the inner cell mass, will have collected at one side of the cavity. These cells are destined to become the embryo (and may be referred to as 'embryoblasts').

BOX 19.2 SCREENING METHODS 1: PREIMPLANTATION DIAGNOSIS

Preimplantation diagnosis (PreGD) involves taking biopsies for genetic testing. Samples are obtained from oocytes or cleaving embryos following *in vitro* fertilization (IVF). Only embryos without chromosomal or genetic disorders are made available for replacement in the uterus. However, PreGD is not a novel approach – it has been used since 1968 in animal husbandry for routinely determining the sex of an animal. Human research into this type of genetic diagnosis has been going on since 1992, but it is only relatively recently that it has been developed for the prevention of genetic disease in humans as an alternative to post-implantation testing (these tests are described in Box 19.6, p.593) or actual terminations.

A PreGD can take place at various stages in the early embryo: it is an *in vitro* technique (i.e. takes place outside the body), entailing the development of early embryos from aspirated oocytes. The ovaries are first stimulated by administration of exogenous gonadotropins, such as follicle stimulating hormone (FSH) and luteinizing hormone (LH) (see Figure 18.15, p.507), to boost events of the ovarian cycle. The events are monitored by pelvic ultrasound, and many ovarian follicles are recruited. The number, size and maturation of oocytes are hormonally controlled, and approximately 34–38 hours following the initiation of the events the oocytes are collected using aspiration of the follicular fluid, guided by transvaginal ultrasound. The oocytes are then added to a culture medium and either:

- left overnight with semen to fertilize (= *in vitro* fertilization, IVF), or
- immediately inseminated by intracytoplasmic sperm injection (ICSI). Only one spermatozoon is transferred; ICSI is therefore analogous to the normal fertilization process.

The latter is the preferred procedure when the potential father has a low spermatozoa count or quality, or for mothers with poor fertilization success. The following day 'embryos' are examined for the presence of the two pronuclei, which indicates normal fertilization (see text for explanation). In IVF, those embryos without two pronuclei are transferred back to the culture medium to allow more time for fertilization.

- *Polar body stage biopsy*: 14–20 hours following normal fertilization the first/second polar bodies (see Figure 19.2) are aspirated from the zygote. Their sampling poses no detrimental affects to embryo development. The major advantage of polar body samples is that they contain identical genetic material from the mother and so may be expressing early functional changes. However, polar bodies comprise solely maternal DNA and so a major disadvantage is that testing is only

beneficial at detecting 'maternal syndromes', for example monosomies, trisomies and altered genes in the maternal line (see later). It cannot reveal inheritance from the spermatozoon.

- *Cleavage stage biopsy* (Figure 19.3): biopsy sampling soon after the zygote has begun to divide (i.e. at the 2- to 4-cell stage) is unsuccessful as there is a removal of a large mass of embryo which is damaging to any further developmental potential. Sampling at the 8- to 12-cell stage (3 days) is mostly successful because removal of a cell is a less significant proportion of the total. The advantage of such early sampling is that the cells taken at this stage have the ability to develop into any stem cell type; they have yet to exhibit a 'destiny'. The cells removed are examined and embryos considered suitable are allowed to continue to develop to the early blastocyst stage and are then transferred to the uterus (on days 4 or 5). Biopsy at the 16-cell stage of the morula is not possible because cells become joined together via tight junctions in the process called 'compaction'.

- *Blastocyst biopsy*: the major drawback with both polar body and cleavage stage sampling is that only a small amount of genetic material is accessible, which can make it imprecise and unpredictable in genetic diagnosis. Biopsies at the blastocyst stage eliminate some of these problems as the embryo can comprise 300 or more cells so more cells can be removed without apparent detrimental effect. Blastocyst biopsy involves removing the more accessible trophoectodermal cells (see Figure 19.3); another advantage here is that those blastocyst cells are not the precursors of the eventual embryo itself.

The use of PreGD is extremely important since it prevents unwanted psychophysiological trauma imposed on a potential mum (and significant others) carrying an unborn child which is destined for prenatal death or a child with gross congenital malformations that will result in early neonatal death. PreGD is also a useful tool for those couples who do not have the reproductive capacity to produce offspring, since it increases the success of IVF.

To date, the majority of the research has been focused on identifying known genes, or in measuring enzyme activity in embryonic cells, for conditions characterized by an excess or absence (or reduction) of specific enzyme. As a result of the completion of the Human Genome Project in 2004, geneticists today, and in the future, are now focusing their attention on specific genes known to cause disease, and genes that make people susceptible to disease.

The developmental significance of these changes is that cells have now shown a degree of identity. This stage of development is called a blastocyst ('blast-' = a simple, as-yet unspecialized cell, '-cyst' = fluid-filled mass; Figure 19.3) and provides the earliest evidence of functional specialization resulting from selective gene activation/deactivation.

Two or three days after arrival within the uterus (i.e. around the sixth day after fertilization) the blastocyst orientates itself so that the inner cell mass is adjacent to the surface of the endometrium, usually in the upper areas of the uterus. It then 'hatches' from the zona pellucida and adheres to the endometrium.

At this point the cells that form the (outer) trophectoderm layer begin to secrete enzymes which digest the immediate endometrial cells, and so initiate implantation (Figure 19.3).

The trophectoderm itself has undergone a number of changes by this time (see below) but the involvement in the outer cells in obtaining nutrients for the embryo is reflected in the name often given to them: trophoblasts. Implantation is completed by about the day 11 after fertilization.

The following describes the critical stages of implantation:

- The blastocyst becomes positioned adjacent to the endometrium.
- Genes are activated that cause the blastocyst to secrete chemicals that remove barrier proteins from the surface of endometrial cells, which then in turn secrete proteins that adhere the blastocyst to the endometrium.
- Upon adhesion, the trophoblast cells of the blastocyst differentiate into two layers. The outer layer in contact with the

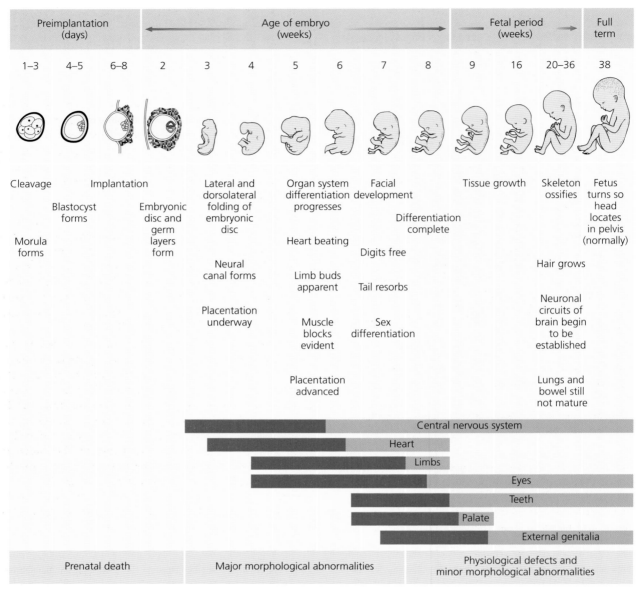

Figure 19.4 Embryo/fetal development. Chronology of tissue differentiation. Horizontal bars at the bottom of the figure provide examples of developmental susceptibility to teratogenic agents

Q Distinguish between the embryo and fetal stages of development.

Q Discuss the role of genes and the environment in the initiation of each stage of human development.

endometrium begins to fuse into a syncytium, that is, a mass without distinguishable cell boundaries, and so the cells of this layer are referred to as syncytiotrophoblasts. Cells of the inner layer retain their individual structure and are distinguished by referring to them as cytotrophoblasts ('cyte-' = cell); their role at this point is to maintain the syncytium. The two layers invade the underlying connective tissue layer of the endometrium, called the stroma. In doing so they trigger the decidual reaction by which the stromal cells become swollen with high-energy glycogen and lipid stores to form a distinct region called the decidua. Continued invasion by

the blastocyst releases nutrients from the decidual cells and fuels the continual outgrowing of the trophoblasts.

- Invasion of the decidua causes fluid-filled spaces, or lacunae, to appear. These will have an important role in placentation as the finger-like villi of the placenta will grow into them, but at this stage the spaces are blocked and so prevent maternal blood filling them (which would expose the embryo to the mother's immune system).
- The site where the blastocyst entered the endometrium is plugged, initially by a blood clot and then by the epithelium which quickly regenerates over the area.

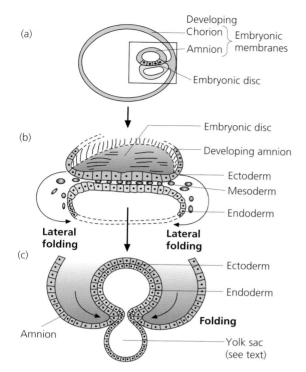

(a) Developing Chorion / Amnion } Embryonic membranes
Embryonic disc

(b) Embryonic disc
Developing amnion
Ectoderm
Mesoderm
Endoderm
Lateral folding **Lateral folding**

(c) Ectoderm
Endoderm
Folding
Amnion
Yolk sac (see text)

Figure 19.5 The embryonic germ layers and differentiation of the neural canal. (a,b) The embryonic disc. (c) Folding to internalize the endoderm (mesoderm not shown)

Q Name the three germ layers. To what organs do the layers give rise (use Table 19.1 if you have difficulty in answering this question)?

The interactions between blastocyst and endometrium are therefore complex, requiring an integration of gene activation in both tissues. Failure of blastocysts to implant is a significant factor in conception problems, especially with *in vitro* techniques. It will be some time before the contribution of the chemicals involved is fully understood but, interestingly, scientists working to improve the success of *in vitro* fertilization methods suspect that chromosomal abnormalities might be involved when implantation fails.

Differentiation of the later embryo

For clarity, development after implantation can be divided into the differentiation of the inner cell mass into the embryo/fetus, and the development of the extra-embryonic membranes. Concurrent with these developments are the formation of the placenta and umbilical cord. The chronology of tissue differentiation is briefly described in this section, but is detailed in Figure 19.4.

The inner cell mass

The inner cell mass of the implanted blastocyst first becomes organized into a flat structure called the embryonic disc. This disc of cells then undergoes gastrulation, that is, it becomes stratified into three distinct layers of cells called the ectoderm, mesoderm and endoderm ('derm' = layer, 'ecto-' = outer; 'meso-' = middle, 'endo-' = inner). The embryo is about 14–18 days old at this stage (postfertilization).

Once formed, this gastrula begins to fold by the curling over of the ectoderm, with the result that the endoderm and mesoderm form concentric tube-like layers within it (Figures 19.5 and 19.6). In this way, a two-dimensional structure is transformed into a three-dimensional one, while the names of the layers now reflect their final position within the developing embryo. Clearly, further gene activity has been initiated to produce such changes. The phase should not be underestimated in the development of a new human being since this seemingly simple act lays down the basic body plan: if one imagines a cross-section through the adult abdomen it can be clearly envisaged which tissues the cell layers are destined to develop into (Table 19.1):

Table 19.1 Structures produced by the three primary germ layers

Endoderm	Mesoderm	Ectoderm
Epithelium of digestive tract (except the oral cavity and anal canal) and its associated glands	All skeletal, most smooth and all cardiac muscle	Nervous tissue
	Cartilage, bone and other connective tissues	Epidermis of skin
Epithelium of urinary bladder, gall bladder and liver	Blood, bone marrow and lymphoid tissue	Hair follicles, arrector pili muscles, nails, and epithelia of sebaceous and sudoriferous glands
	Endothelium of blood vessels and lymphatics	
Epithelium of pharynx, external auditory tube, tonsils, larynx and airways of the lungs	Dermis of skin	Lens, cornea and optic nerve of eye, and internal eye muscles
	Fibrous and vascular coats of eye	Inner and outer ear
Epithelium of thyroid, parathyroid, pancreas and thymus glands	Middle ear	Neuroepithelium of sense organs
Epithelium of prostate and bulbourethral glands, vagina, vestibule, urethra and associated glands	Epithelium of kidneys and ureters	Epithelium of oral and nasal cavities, paranasal sinuses, salivary glands and anal canal
	Epithelium of adrenal cortex	
	Epithelium of gonads and genital ducts	Epithelium of pineal gland, pituitary gland and adrenal medulla

Q What do the prefixes 'endo-', 'meso-' and 'ecto-' mean?

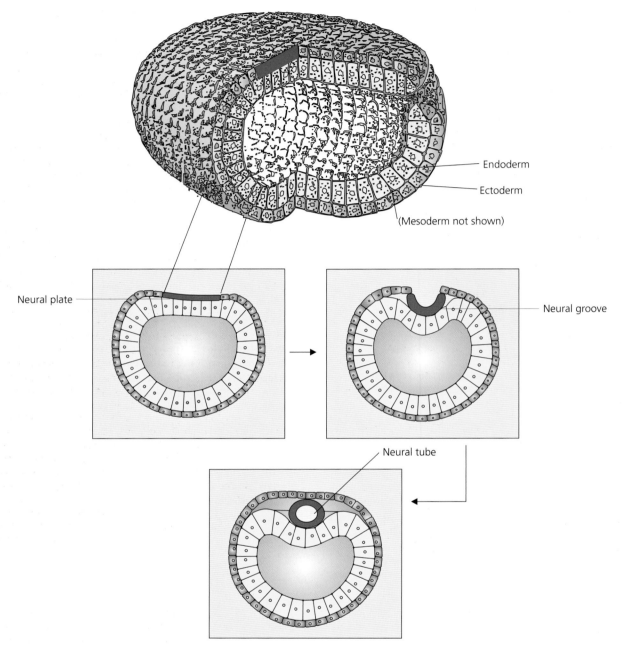

Figure 19.6 The first (visible) signs of organ development in the embryo: formation of the neural tube

Q From which embryonic germ layer is the neural tube derived?

- the gut and associated structures are derived from the endodermal tube;
- the epidermis of the skin and nervous system is formed from the embryonic ectoderm;
- the skeleton, skeletal muscle layers, most viscera and blood are structures found between the skin and gut and are derived from the mesoderm;
- the perforation at each end of the tube-like structure eventually become the mouth and anus, and so the ends of the tube are set to become the 'head' and 'tail' end respectively.

The embryo still has some way to go before these organ systems have differentiated.

Morphogenesis

The emphasis of the discussion so far has been the role of genes at the cellular level: their role in determining cell function and appearance. 'Morphogenesis' is a term used to describe the development of tissues and organs, and their place within the body ('morph-' = shape, form; '-genesis' = creation). Over 80 years ago, Spemann and Mangold demonstrated the central

BOX 19.3 ABNORMALITIES OF EARLY DEVELOPMENT

The following provides some examples of conditions that illustrate how congenital disorders can have a profound effect on the neural and cardiovascular systems.

Abnormalities of neural development

- *Spina bifida*: an incomplete closure of the neural arch of one or more vertebrae. In its most severe form a fluid-filled sac (called a myelomeningocoele) protrudes through to the skin, usually in the lumbar region. This thin protection afforded to underlying spinal neurons is usually inadequate, leading to infection, damage and resultant paralysis. Spina bifida is a congenital condition but its incidence has decreased dramatically in recent years since it was recognized that folic acid deficiency was a major contributing factor (Wald, 1991). Supplementation of this vitamin in the mother's diet early in pregnancy is now recommended to reduce the risk of the embryo developing this neural tube defect.
- *Microcephaly*: an abnormal smallness of the head in relation to the rest of the body, caused because the brain does not develop fully.
- *Hydrocephalus*: this occurs when there is an interference in the circulation of cerebrospinal fluid within the brain. It produces a raised pressure of the cerebrospinal fluid that acts to compress neural tissue. Such cranial hypertension may be observed at any life stage, e.g. as a consequence of head trauma, but in infants it often arises because there is poor connection between the ventricles (these spaces form the fluid which then drains to other spaces around the brain and spinal cord; see Chapter 8, p.180). Hydrocephalus in infants normally induces an enlargement of the head because the sutures of the skull are not closed. The rise in intracranial pressure presents itself by drowsiness and vomiting, and neurological dysfunction.
- *Cri du chat syndrome*: a congenital condition caused by absence of one of the arms of chromosome number 5. The widespread loss of genes that this produces causes profound abnormalities, both physical and mental. The name refers to a cat-like cry in infancy.

Abnormalities of cardiac development

Readers may find it helpful to review Box 14.21, p.412, before reading this section.

- *Transposition of the great vessels*: as the heart develops in the embryo, a large artery normally divides into the two vessels that form the aorta and pulmonary trunk artery. The aorta normally drains the left ventricle and the pulmonary trunk the right ventricle. If the insertion of the vessels into these chambers is reversed, then the aorta will take deoxygenated blood from the right ventricle and direct it to the body tissues, bypassing the lungs (for arrangement of the adult circulation, see Chapter 12). In contrast, the pulmonary vessel will now direct oxygenated blood arriving from the lungs back to the lungs. In other words, there will be a complete separation of the pulmonary and systemic circulations. This is clearly not viable for life and babies born with this problem will usually be reliant on the small amount of blood mixing that occurs through fetal features: the foramen ovale between the atria, and the ductus arteriosus between the aorta and pulmonary trunk artery, that allows blood to largely bypass the developing lungs in the fetus. These features disappear soon after birth, so corrective surgery will be necessary very early on.
- *Valve stenosis*: failure to form the cardiac valves may produce stenosis (i.e. the cusps of the valves thicken and fail to function appropriately). This has consequences for the passage of blood through the heart, and hence its output, and may promote excessive pressure in the heart chamber preceding the valve causing the chamber to hypertrophy and eventually fail to empty normally.
- *Persistent foramen ovale*: this was noted above as a feature of the fetal circulation. The foramen is located in the wall between the atria and normally closes at or soon after birth, as lung circulation improves. If it does not close, then some blood will pass from the left atrium to the right (pressure changes in the left atrium at birth promote this reversal in blood flow) during the cardiac cycle, leading to a reduced cardiac output. While not, perhaps, having immediate consequences for the infant, it may influence growth during childhood.
- *Septal defects*: the foramen ovale is a normal embryological feature. Septal defects relate to abnormal openings, usually in the septum between the two ventricles. They occur because the septum ends have failed to fuse as they grow towards each other during the development of the heart chambers. A ventricular septum defect will result in blood passing from the left ventricle to the right during systole, since the pressure is higher than that in the right. Cardiac output will decrease, and there will be excessive volume in the right ventricle. This may cause excessive growth of this chamber, and may also have long-term consequences by causing right heart failure, resulting in pulmonary oedema.

---

role of genes in this process too when they reported that transplanting cells from specific points within a single embryo of a newt to another position on a recipient embryo could produce two (joined) newt embryos (De Robertis, 2006). In other words, the transplanted cells were capable of determining body axis, and of inducing precise morphogenesis in tissues adjacent to the transplant site. There is likely to be more than one cluster of such cells, referred to as 'organizers', and they have since been identified in embryos of all animal groups. In these cells, gene 'families', such as those called HOX and PAX, appear to become active and promote the production of enzymes that stimulate differentiation in surrounding tissues by interacting with the genes and gene products of those cells. Some genes have been shown to have a widespread involvement, for example the 'Hedgehog' gene and its subtypes appear to have involvement in the morphogenesis of many organs, from intestines to the brain.

Collectively, the gene products that promote morphogenesis are known as morphogens. Among those best studied are 'transcription factors' that interact with the DNA of cells to trigger certain genes to become active and hence govern the cell's structure and hence how the cell looks and functions. Morphogens secreted from within a restricted area of tissue will spread away from that source; cells close to the source are therefore subjected to a high concentration, whereas those a distance away receive a lower concentration as the substance dissipates. It is this concentration gradient that seems to influence how cells respond to the morphogen. The process is clearly very complex and highly coordinated. Readers are referred to technical reviews for more detail, for example Tabata and Takei (2004).

The first signs of a specific organ being formed is the appearance of a raised neural plate of cells in the ectoderm surface. This collection of cells then becomes a neural groove and thence a neural tube (Figure 19.6); this hollow structure is eventually reflected in the cerebral ventricles and spinal canal of the central nervous system. The nervous system must begin to develop early, partly because of its ultimate complexity and partly because of its role in coordinating fetal tissue functions. Similarly, further gene activation will ensure that the heart and circulation also develop early since it is this system that must ensure adequate delivery of nutrients and oxygen to tissues in order to support the rapid growth that is taking place. The early development of the nervous and circulatory system, and the need for continued development throughout the embryo/fetal period, makes these systems especially susceptible to developmental disorder (see Box 19.3 and Figure 19.4, p.526).

Thus, within just 3 weeks of fertilization gene activities have established the general plan of the body, and specific tissues and organs have begun to develop. Tissue differentiation continues during the following weeks, and the embryo becomes increasingly humanoid in shape (see Figure 19.4, p.526). The final process is that of sex determination, which occurs from about the seventh week and is mostly complete by the end of the eighth week (see below). All organs therefore are basically defined by the end of 8 weeks of embryonic development, although their functions may be only rudimentary, and so this early period is when the embryo is particularly susceptible to environmental agents (mutagens and teratogens; see later) that could cause errors in gene expression. It is also a period when the mother may not even be aware that she is pregnant.

The embryo is now considered to be a fetus. Further development of the fetus primarily entails growth and the functional maturation of the organs laid down during the embryonic period. This does not mean that the fetus is now no longer susceptible to abnormalities of development but the risk declines.

Sex differentiation

There are a number of congenital disorders of sex development (discussed later) and it is worthwhile noting here how sex differentiation occurs.

Tissue that can form both male and female gonads develops at the same site within the abdomen of the embryo; these are, of course, non-functional and it would be incorrect to consider that the embryo is hermaphrodite, that is, with both male and

---

BOX 19.4 RESEARCH ON HUMAN EMBRYOS

Excess embryos produced using *in vitro* fertilization techniques (see Box 19.2, p.525) are frozen in case of later need/opportunities: these embryos also provide a focus for new research directions should they be made available for research purposes.

At the time of writing, 'hot' topics on the research front are:

- *Research on embryo development*: the UK Human Fertilization and Embryology Act (1990) currently permits research on embryos up to 14 days (postfertilization) age, around the time when the embryonic disc has formed. However, there is increasing pressure to permit embryos to develop further so that more complex genetic interactions might be studied, and the Act is under review.
- *Exploitation of embryonic stem cells (i.e. those that have not differentiated into specific cell types)*: these cells are of interest to medicine because understanding developmental genes means that there is potential to artificially transform stem cells into specific cell types for transplantation into disease-affected children or adults. Embryonic stem cells are especially attractive because they are completely undifferentiated and therefore are 'pluripotent'; that is; they may potentially be directed to form almost any tissue required. Cord blood is one source of stem cells, but embryos cultivated for the purpose could also potentially provide a rich source.
- *Exploitation of embryos for cloning (i.e. production of identical genetic copies)*: a clone is produced by extracting the nucleus from an adult's body cell, injecting it into a secondary oocyte from which the nucleus has been removed – referred to as somatic cell nuclear transfer (SCNT) – and activating the newly constructed cell to develop into an embryo. Allowing complete development is referred to as reproductive cloning and currently is banned in humans in the UK. However, early embryos potentially may also be used to yield stem cells that are genetically identical to the nuclear donor and so could be triggered to produce tissue cells that are less likely to be rejected if the actual recipient was the nuclear donor. This is referred to as therapeutic cloning.
- *Embryo selection*: the analysis of chromosomal number and size/shape (karyotyping) has long been applied in practice using embryo/fetal cells obtained from pregnant women via amniocentesis or chorionic villus sampling (see Box 19.6). The identification of specific genes on chromosomes (genotyping) is a relatively new technology that is not yet widely available but seems likely to become more so. Both methods can also be used to screen early, preimplantation embryos since extracting a cell from the morula stage (see Box 19.2, p.525) does not have a consequence for its further development. Preimplantation genetic diagnosis has implications for embryo selection where parents are known to be carriers of a particular gene, but potentially also could identify genes that are increasingly recognized to have an impact on health later in life, or even those that could predict more innocuous features such as eye colour.
- *Genetic engineering*: this is the technology by which 'normal' genes can be implanted into another cell and hence restore those activities that had been deficient, for example through inheritance of a recessive genetic disorder (normal genes are dominant to these; the terms recessive and dominant are explained later). One technical problem is ensuring that implanted genes are present in all cells, but there is potential to achieve this by engineering sex cells prior to fertilization. Such engineering of embryos is not allowed in the UK.

There are rigorous legislative measures that govern embryo research in the UK. These are overseen by the Human Fertilization and Embryology Authority (HFEA), introduced in 1991, which regulates and inspects UK clinics providing *in vitro* fertilization, donor insemination or storage of ova, spermatozoa or embryos, and licences all human embryo research in the UK (see http://www.hfea.gov.uk/cps/rde/xchg/hfea). The potential of technologies for medical advancement across the human lifespan continues to put pressure on the HFEA to grant limited, special permissions. For example in 2004 a group of British scientists were granted a licence to clone human embryos, while another was granted permission in 2006 to screen embryos for those genes that may lead to certain cancers in middle age.

Not surprisingly, such technologies have introduced intense moral and ethical debate as to whether science should exploit embryos in these ways, and if it should then how might the technologies be best applied and abuse avoided.

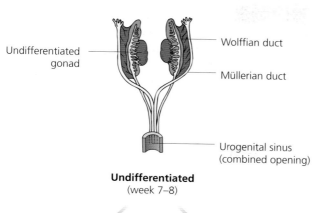

female gonads. Rather, the embryo has bi-potential in that it may become male or female. Associated with the undifferentiated gonadal tissue are two sets of ducts, called the Wolffian and Müllerian ducts (Figure 19.7; named after the people who first identified them). If a Y chromosome is present then male sex determination is triggered by activation for a short period of time of genes on this chromosome. These in turn stimulate certain genes on the X chromosome, which act to promote the differentiation of the gonadal tissue into testes, which then begin to produce the male sex steroid hormone testosterone and a peptide hormone called Müllerian inhibiting substance (MIS). These hormones promote the appropriate duct system:

- Testosterone stimulates the differentiation of the Wolffian ducts into the vas deferens and associated structures of the male reproductive tract, and external genitalia develop accordingly.
- MIS causes the Müllerian ducts to degenerate.

In the absence of a Y chromosome the early gonadal tissue will not be activated to produce testosterone and so the Wolffian ducts regress and atrophy. Similarly, MIS is not produced and so the Müllerian ducts persist and develop into the Fallopian tubes and uterus of the female tract. The undifferentiated gonads develop as ovaries, and so the embryo becomes female.

BOX 19.5 BIRTH WEIGHT

Various factors such as race and gestational age affect birth weights, and there are accepted 'norms'. The term 'weight-for-gestational age' is usually applied. Body weights outside the normal range are frequently the result of altered gene expression rather than a consequence of changes to the genes themselves.

- *Excessive weight-for-gestational age*: excessive stimulation of fetal growth produces birth weights in excess of the norms. Thus, maternal diabetes mellitus induces increased insulin release in the fetus, with subsequent deposition of food stores. Excessive birth weight has obvious implications for labour, for example cephalo-pelvic disproportion (CPD) or obstructed labour.

- *Low weight-for-gestational age*: low birth weights reflect either inadequate placental blood flow, which restricts nutrient supply to the fetus (e.g. the effects of nicotine from smoking) or depressed metabolism (e.g. in the fetal alcohol syndrome, and possibly from carbon monoxide in cigarette smoke).

- *Very low weight-for-age*: these babies are more susceptible to neonatal difficulties (Agustines *et al.*, 2000). Recent studies have also suggested that there may be a link between low birth weight and increased risk of ill health later in life, and this suggests that tissue development as well as growth might have been adversely affected (e.g. Zwicker and Harris, 2008).

In rare cases, the activities of the Y chromosome cannot be (fully) expressed and so the baby develops as a female with no, or at most only rudimentary, testes. This situation may arise because the Y chromosome fails to activate the appropriate genes on the X chromosome. Alternatively, it may be that the early gonadal tissue fails to secrete adequate testosterone, or perhaps the male reproductive tract tissue fails to develop adequately under the effects of the testosterone. The situation introduces a potential dilemma in that genetically the individual is XY (i.e. male) but phenotypically they are female.

Extra-embryonic membranes

Screening programmes for embryological abnormalities can be implemented quite early (11–16 weeks) in pregnancy. The methods basically entail obtaining samples of fetal tissue so that chromosomal and biochemical analyses can be performed. Information is provided in Box 19.6 but to understand how tissue can be sampled it is important to first consider the development of the membranes that support and provide for the growing embryo/fetus.

There are four membranes that develop from embryological tissue:

- The *chorion* partly develops from the trophectoderm of the blastocyst and it eventually increases in size until it lines the uterine cavity. Parts of the chorion will be incorporated into the placenta. The remaining three membranes develop as outgrowths of cell layers of the actual embryo.

- The *amnion* develops from ectoderm of the embryonic disc and distends, as the gastrula folds, to encompass the entire developing embryo (see Figures 19.5, p.527 and 19.8). It secretes amniotic fluid (the 'waters'), which provides support for the growing fetus, helps to maintain a constant temperature and acts as a shock absorber during maternal movement. The fluid is also swallowed by the fetus and a dilute urine excreted into it, and this facilitates the functional development of the gut and kidneys. Its volume at term is 1–1.5 L, and the amnion will have grown outwards to meet the chorion and so also lines the uterine cavity.

- The *yolk sac* grows from the endoderm but also incorporates migrated mesodermal cells. It projects into the fluid-filled cavity enclosed by the growing chorion and helps in the nutrition of the embryo (Figure 19.8). Blood vessels develop from the mesodermal cells, which are also responsible for early synthesis of red blood cells. The sac therefore has an important role in the early processes of embryo development, but then becomes incorporated into the developing 'body stalk' that attaches the embryo to the developing placenta, which takes over the nutritive role and so the sac is no longer required. Blood vessels develop from mesoderm within the 'body stalk', which is destined to become the umbilical cord.

- The *allantois* is another endodermal sac. It originates close to the base of the yolk sac (Figure 19.8) and contains mesodermal cells. Blood vessels that develop from these cells also help to establish the vascularization of the chorion/placenta. The membrane is eventually incorporated into the umbilical cord although a part of it is incorporated into the growing fetal bladder.

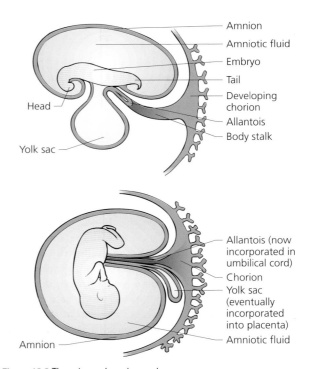

Figure 19.8 The extra-embryonic membranes

Q What is the purpose of amniotic fluid?

BOX 19.6 SCREENING METHODS 2: POSTIMPLANTATION DIAGNOSIS

Screening for inherited problems in the developing fetus is by two main approaches: fetal testing and maternal testing.

Fetal testing

Fetal testing falls under two broad categories: examination of fetal cells, and imaging of the fetus. Cell sampling enables examination of fetal tissue for chromosomal abnormalities: cells are obtained by amniocentesis and chorionic villus sampling (Figure 19.9). Other testing methods are less invasive, using ultrasound and chemical screening.

- *Amniocentesis*: for women who may be 'at risk' of chromosomal abnormalities, samples of about 20 mL of amniotic fluid are aspirated following a transabdominal insertion of a needle from week 15 of gestation. The fluid contains cells of the amnion membrane and also cells (hence their chromosomes) shed from the fetus. The fluid itself is also of value in screening; for example, alphafetoprotein (AFP) or the enzyme acetylcholinesterase may be measured, and these are elevated in various abnormalities of development, especially neural tube defects. The risk of spontaneous abortion via amniocentesis is about 1 in 100 (Alfirevic *et al.*, 2007).
- *Chorionic villus sampling (or placental biopsy)*: this is a diagnostic test that can be performed from 10 weeks onwards (i.e. when the chorion is well developed). It entails taking a sample from the chorion at the edge of the placenta, using a hollow needle and suction. This membrane originated from the embryological cells that formed the outer layer of the blastocyst stage of development. The risk of spontaneous abortion via the process of a placental biopsy is approximately 2–3 in 100 (Alfirevic *et al.*, 2007).
- *Ultrasound*: since the early 1990s imaging via ultrasound technology and other diagnostic procedures following implantation of the embryo has evolved to allow sonographers and clinicians to build a more complete representation of the developing fetus and is beginning to supersede cell sampling as a screening tool. For example, detailed ultrasound scanning of the spine is now possible, and has largely superseded the chemical screening method. Other measurements are utilized as indicators of development, such as the thickness of the nuchal (neck) fold of the fetus and the biparietal diameter of the fetal skull.

A fairly novel procedure called the nuchal translucency test may be used to evaluate the fluid at the back of the baby's neck. Results from this test can be highly indicative as the test picks up approximately 75% of fetuses with trisomy 21 (Down syndrome; Said and Malone, 2008). It is predicted that in the near future this test will routinely be offered to women at 11–14 weeks of pregnancy.

Maternal testing

The risk of miscarriage as a consequence of fetal testing through amniocentesis or chorionic villus sampling makes maternal testing an attractive alternative. This entails assessing chemical markers in maternal blood samples:

- For example, AFP that is released from the fetus into the amniotic fluid enters the mother's circulation. Its secretion is increased if there is incomplete neural tube closure in the embryo, so raised concentrations in the maternal blood may be indicative of such a defect.
- In contrast, the maternal serum AFP concentration may be reduced if the baby has Down syndrome. The test is not conclusive, however, and other tests are required to raise confidence in the assessment.

The level of confidence of diagnosis is increased by the concomitant presence of a lower-than-normal concentration of unconjugated oestriol and a higher-than-normal concentration of human chorionic gonadotropin (hCG). Together with the AFP test, these tests constitute the 'Barts' triple test', which is commonly applied as a diagnostic aid during pregnancy in women at risk. However, the level of confidence provided by this test is still not especially high – of the order of 70% (Harrison and Goldie, 2006) – and false positive and false negative results are possible. The triple test may therefore be combined with other parameters, such as another protein called inhibin A (to produce a 'quadruple test') or, increasingly, with fetal data obtained by imaging (see above) in order to raise the level of diagnostic confidence still further.

The chorion and amnion are the most developed of these membranes. Together, they are the membranes that 'burst' in the first stage of labour, while the 'waters' are predominantly amniotic fluid released from the cavity.

Genetic and environmental factors in congenital disorders

Congenital disorders are present at birth and are caused by errors of development or function. It is usually the case that they have an impact on health and they arise from:

- *Dysplasia*: the failure of differentiation of tissue in the early embryo, which usually has genetic cause.
- *Defect*: this is failure of further development of tissue and may have a genetic cause or may arise through the influence of environmental factors (e.g. drug abuse by the mother).
- *Deformation*: this is an altered tissue size or shape arising as a consequence of the effects of physical forces on tissue growth, for example the poor brain growth in a fetus with hydrocephalus (excessive cerebrospinal fluid which compresses the brain tissue against the bones of the skull).

Tissue differentiation and development therefore largely depends upon two factors: the expression of genes and the actual genetic complement of the embryo. Note, however, that the majority of instances of congenital abnormality have no known attributable cause. In other words this is an area that is still poorly understood (but see later).

Gene expression

Agents that prevent cell differentiation and/or morphogenesis induce physical problems in the newborn, and are referred to collectively as teratogens; these include 'mutagens' that alter genetic structure but also include those agents that alter the expression of genes and the actions of morphogens.

There is a tendency to look upon teratogens as being agents that are introduced in some form into the embryo/fetus. Various agents are known to influence tissue differentiation and include toxins produced by certain bacteria that increase the risk of congenital problems, and numerous chemicals that are relatively harmless to the mother but influence embryo/fetal cells. Some examples are given in Table 19.2.

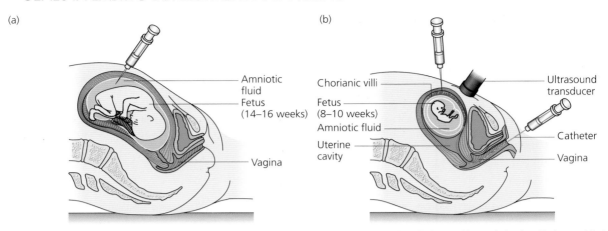

Figure 19.9 Postimplantation diagnostic investigations: (a) amniocentesis, (b) chorionic villus sampling. Redrawn with permission from Tortura and Grabowski. *Principles of Anatomy and Physiology*. (1999) John Wiley and Sons

Table 19.2 Selected teratogenic influences on embryo/fetal development. It should be noted that these influences raise the risk; the occurrence of problems is not certain, or even likely in many instances

Teratogenic influence	Possible effects on fetus or newborn
Drugs taken by mother	
Androgens	Masculinization of fetus
Anaesthetics	Depression of fetus, asphyxia
Antihistamines	Abortion, malformations
Aspirin	Persistent truncus arteriosus, abnormal heart
Diuretics	Polycystic kidney disease
Heroin and morphine	Convulsions, tremor, neonatal death
Insulin shock	Fetal death
LSD (lysergide; lysergic acid diethylamide)	Chromosomal anomalies, deformity
Nicotine (from smoking)	Stunting, accelerated heart beat, premature birth, organ congestion, fits and convulsions
Oestrogens	Malformations, hyperactivity of fetal adrenal glands
Streptomycin	Damage to auditory nerve
Thalidomide	Hearing loss, abnormal appendages, death
Maternal infection	
Chicken pox or shingles	Chicken pox or shingles, abortion, stillbirth
Syphilis	Miscarriage
Cytomegalovirus (salivary gland virus)	Small head, inflammation and hardening of brain and retina, deafness, poor mental development, enlargement of spleen and liver, anaemia, giant cells in urine from kidneys
Hepatitis	Hepatitis
Herpes simplex	Generalized herpes, inflammation of brain, cyanosis, jaundice, fever, respiratory and circulatory collapse, death
Mumps	Fetal death, endocardial fibroelastosis, anomalies
Pneumonia	Abortion in early pregnancy
Poliomyelitis	Spinal or bulbar poliomyelitis, acute poliomyelitis of newborn
Rubella (German measles)	Anomalies, haemorrhage, enlargement of spleen and liver, inflammation of brain, liver, and lungs, cataracts, small brain, deafness, various mental deficiencies, death
Scarlet fever	Abortion in early pregnancy
Smallpox	Abortion, stillbirth, smallpox
Syphilis	Stillbirth, premature birth, syphilis
Toxoplasmosis (protozoan parasite infection)	Small eyes and head, learning disabilities, cerebral oedema (encephalitis), heart damage, fetal death
Tuberculosis	Fetal death, lowered resistance to tuberculosis
Typhoid fever	Abortion in early pregnancy

Q Differentiate between mutagens and teratogens.

Q Using this table and Figure 19.3, identify the critical periods of gestation in which administering the drug thalidomide to a pregnant woman would cause (1) major changes in limb formation, (2) minor changes in limb formation, and (3) no changes to limb formation.

It is also the case, however, that a deficiency of essential substances may also be teratogenic. For example, studies (see Box 19.3) have shown that the incidence of spina bifida can be dramatically reduced by ensuring that the maternal diet contains adequate folate, a vitamin of the B group. Folate (folic acid) has a particular role in maintaining neural functions and it should not, perhaps, be surprising that it has a profound role in neural development. Retrospect is much easier than foresight, however, and the protective effects of folate have only recently been recognized.

Genetic complement

Genetic change can occur while the embryo is *in utero*, either spontaneously or because of an extrinsic agent (e.g. radiation) that acts as a mutagen. In most instances, however, the genetic complement of an embryo is determined by the genes inherited from the spermatozoon and oocyte at fertilization and so disordered development arises when inherited, mutated genes are expressed, or when genes are in excess or absent because of chromosomal defects.

Inheritance is a large topic and to appreciate how those genes inherited may or may not affect development it is necessary to explore it in detail. The next section therefore considers the many aspects of inheritance.

THE FUNDAMENTALS OF INHERITANCE: GENES, ALLELES AND CELL DIVISION

Terminology

Like all branches of biology, genetics has its specific terminology. First, then, some general definitions:

- Collectively the entire gene composition of the DNA of an individual is called the *genome*. Thus, a genome provides the full genetic 'blueprint' of an individual.
- The genes of an individual are largely responsible for observable or measurable characteristics called the *phenotypes* of that individual. Such characteristics are normally expressed as physical ones, but, as outlined in Chapter 2, the activities of genes are observed at the biochemical level of cell activity. The term 'phenotype' therefore could be applied to characteristics ranging from a particular enzyme, to cell organelles, to tissue types, to organ function, to external features of the individual. Some characteristics are produced by a single gene while others involve several genes.
- It is the gene or genes responsible for a given phenotype that comprise the *genotype* for that characteristic.

The occurrence of chromosomes in pairs, one set inherited from each parent, has major implications because each set of 23 chromosomes within a cell will contain the 'blueprint' for an individual. Thus, each chromosome within a pair will usually carry genes for the same characteristics, and so there is normally a duplication of genes – if a chromosome contains genes inherited from the mother that provide the code for, say, eye colour then there will be a complementary set of genes on the

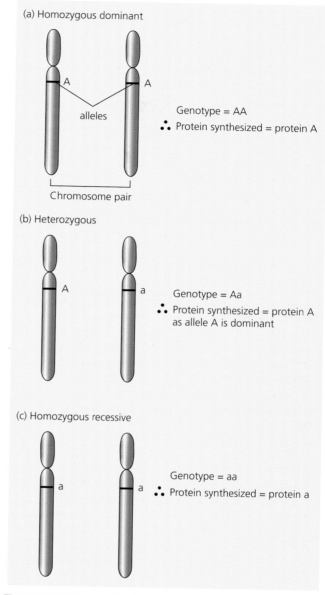

(a) Homozygous dominant

alleles

Chromosome pair

Genotype = AA
∴ Protein synthesized = protein A

(b) Heterozygous

Genotype = Aa
∴ Protein synthesized = protein A as allele A is dominant

(c) Homozygous recessive

Genotype = aa
∴ Protein synthesized = protein a

Figure 19.10 Genotypes and protein synthesis for a gene A found on a (hypothetical) chromosome. (a) Homozygous dominant: genotype is AA; therefore protein synthesis is protein A. (b) Heterozygous: genotype is Aa; therefore protein synthesis is protein A. (c) Homozygous recessive: genotype is aa; therefore protein synthesis is protein a

***Q** Define the terms 'homozygous' and 'heterozygous'.*

other member of the chromosome pair that was inherited from the father. Thus, most phenotypes of an individual reflect the net effects of pairs of genes and the genotype will be written to reflect this (e.g. for a gene we could call 'A' the genotype might be written as 'AA'). Pairs of chromosomes are said to be homologous chromosomes ('homo-' = same) in recognition that each member of the pair will carry genes that are complementary for the same characteristics.

Being aware of this is important because although a pair of genes may be responsible for a single, given characteristic they may not necessarily have precisely the same genetic coding, either to each other or to those of another individual (Figure 19.10). If this variation in the actual genetic code is expressed as a gene product, then it may introduce some variation into the characteristic it produces, a concept that is fundamental to evolution theory, since that variation may confer an advantage to the individual concerned. Since the pair of genes may not be identical, the two forms are called allelomorphs or *alleles* for short. As a general rule, if reference is made to a gene for a particular characteristic (e.g. 'the gene for cystic fibrosis') this will normally refer to the allele that is mainly responsible for that characteristic.

If a pair of alleles have identical genetic coding then either will cause the cell to produce the same protein (Figure 19.10). Accordingly the individual is said to be homozygous for the characteristic that is produced. If the two alleles are slightly different from one another then they could cause the cell to produce slightly different proteins; the individual is said to be heterozygous ('hetero-' = different) for that characteristic. Having heterozygous genotypes has significant implications in the inheritance of characteristics, as is explained later.

Although alleles can vary, many are actually going to be identical in everyone because they code for essential processes that operate in us all. For example, the ability of cells to generate ATP from glucose will involve much the same genetic code in all individuals otherwise the vital enzymes could not be synthesized and life would not be possible. Nevertheless, the difference in appearance of people is a clear indication of how variable some alleles may be. In health care the tendency is to only consider those gene mutations that cause ill health through disruption of normal embryo development. This forms the focus of the chapter, and instances are cited below, but it is also important to recognize that gene variation can be a positive influence as it may enable adaptation to a changing environment; for example it is clear that some individuals have an inborn resistance to infection with human immuno-deficiency virus (HIV) infection. It could be argued that such genes are essential for human survival since it is hard to imagine the environment will ever stop changing and presenting new challenges to the continuation of the human species.

Alleles and cell function

How can one allele have a different genetic code from its counterpart? The answer is that the allele has undergone a change to the genetic code either as a result of deletions or substitutions of the chemical bases that comprise the code, or from a rearrangement of their order within the DNA molecule (Figure 19.11). This is what is meant by 'gene mutation', and it can occur spontaneously or result from the actions of certain environmental agents, such as radiation, toxins or viruses. The consequence of mutation is that the changed protein that is now the gene product might have novel effects on the cell, or alternatively the absence of the 'normal' protein may itself affect cell function (Figure 19.12). Thus, in the heterozygous state, there is a question as to which allele will be responsible for determining the phenotype.

(a) Consider this sentence:

THE OLD CAT WAS TOO FAT

This is an understandable sentence. By analogy, if this was genetic code, its translation would be acceptable to a cell.

Rearranging the words:

THE FAT CAT WAS TOO OLD

In this genetic code, the translation would still be acceptable, but the meaning of the original sentence (by analogy a protein synthesized by the cell) has been lost. The function associated with that sentence is no longer available, but has been replaced with the new one, which may or may not be to a cell's advantage, or may even be a disadvantage.

Alternatively:

THE OLD CAT WAS TOO FTA

The original meaning has been lost, and been replaced with a nonsensical sentence. By analogy, this new code (i.e. protein) will not have any action in the cell.

(b) Using this principle to illustrate gene mutation, the following is a piece of genetic code:

GCA ACC CAG CUU CAC UCA UCC GGC ACG

In the next sequence, a gene mutation called a substitution has occurred, in which a base at one point in the original has been changed into another:

GCA A**A**C CAG CUU CAC UCA UCC GGC ACG

In the next sequence, a gene mutation called an insertion has occurred in the original, in which an extra base has been inserted into the sequence:

GCA ACC **G**CA GCU UCA CUC AUC CGG CAC G..

Compare these to the original above. Which of the two mutations is likely to be most effective as far as changing cell function is concerned? To answer this, you might want to refer to Table 2.3 (p.41) and 'translate' these codes into a sequence of amino acids.

Figure 19.11 Gene mutation. The base sequence (i.e. genetic code) of DNA is 'read' in groups of three bases; each group of three bases represents an amino acid. In this way, a cell constructs a protein of a specific amino acid sequence (see Chapter 2). (a) Genetic code in the form of a simple English sentence highlights the principle of gene mutation. (b) An example of gene mutation by substitution or insertion of a base (i.e. a 'letter' in the three-letter word).

Dominant and recessive alleles

It is likely that we all have mutated alleles that if expressed are capable of producing disordered functioning. So why are the dysfunctional changes not always observed? The explanation is that the alleles are usually paired with a 'normal' counterpart that exerts dominance over the mutated one, which is then said to be recessive. The cell therefore synthesizes the 'normal' protein, and the altered allele is ineffective. In writing the genotype it is usual to show the dominant allele as a capital letter and the recessive one as a lower case letter (e.g. 'Aa'; see Figure 19.10). Of course, if both alleles are of the recessive mutation (e.g. genotype 'aa') there is no 'normal' form to dominate cell function and so the recessive alleles can express themselves. Most genetic disorders involve a recessive allele and so we

(a)

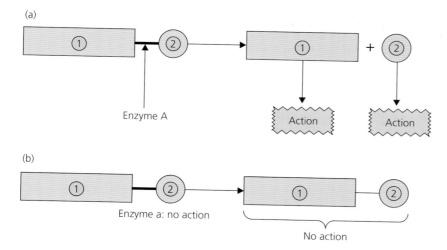

(b)

(c)

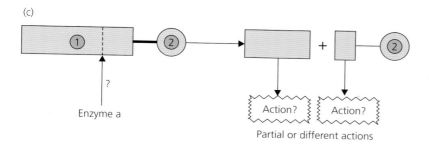

Fig. 19.12 Schematic representation of consequences of gene mutation. (a) Action of enzyme A to catalyse production of chemicals 1 and 2. (b) Gene mutation (homozygous recessive) induces production of enzyme a. Chemicals 1 and 2 are not produced, and the cell loses the actions associated with them. (c) Gene mutation (homozygous recessive) induces production of enzyme a, which, although unable to produce chemicals 1 and 2, catalyses the original molecule into two similar molecules. These may have a partial action similar to that of chemicals 1 and 2, or may have different actions in a cell

Q Why are some mutations lethal?

would have to inherit both recessive copies of the allele if the condition is to be expressed.

The expression of a gene is referred to as 'penetrance'; dominant alleles have better penetrance than recessive ones. How one allele assumes dominance over another is still poorly understood, but it is clear that occasionally penetrance of a dominant gene is incomplete, in which case if both dominant and recessive alleles are present then both are active to some extent, for example in the sickle cell trait (see Box 19.13, p.548). In some instances mutated alleles may even be dominant to the 'normal' form, in which case having just one copy of it will alter cell or tissue functioning, for example in retinoblastoma (also Box 19.13).

When mutated alleles are expressed, the consequences for the individual's well-being will depend upon the extent of their influences on cell and tissue functioning:

- The characteristic produced may not markedly be altered because many other genes also have an influence on it; that is, it is a 'polygenic' phenotype (below).
- The changes induced may be benign (Box 19.7).
- Some genes are vital to basic cell processes. Thus, a single mutated gene may give rise to serious inherited conditions, for example cystic fibrosis.

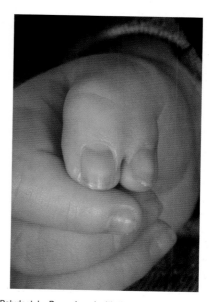

Figure 19.13 Polydactyly. Reproduced with the kind permission of the Medical Illustration Department, Norfolk and Norwich University Hospital NHS Trust

BOX 19.7 BENIGN GENE MUTATIONS

The consequences of altered genes do not have to be detrimental to health (for example see Figure 19.13).

For example, try to roll your tongue lengthways. If you can do this then you have inherited two copies of a recessive gene. Similarly, is your ear lobe rounded or does it taper to the side of the neck? This too relates to inheritance of a gene mutation.

Other examples are even more readily apparent; the breadth of variation between physical appearances results from 'gene mixing' but basically entails the inheritance and expression of various genes that will differ between people because of genetic variation.

Multifactorial, or polygenic, phenotypes

Many phenotypes represent complex integrated functions and result from the net effect of the activities of a number of genes, rather than a single one, which are not necessarily all found on the same chromosome. The net appearance of such polygenic phenotypes will depend upon how many of the alleles of the functional group are mutated and expressed: the more variations present, or the more 'crucial' the genes that are affected, the greater the likelihood of an altered phenotype. This has become an important principle in understanding susceptibility to 'adult-onset' disorders such as cancer, diabetes mellitus, coronary heart disease, and Alzheimer disease.

The net expression of the numerous alleles is additive. For example, skin pigmentation results from the expression of several genes but as an illustration we could consider just two (i.e. two pairs of alleles). The inheritance is summarized in Figure 19.14. If both pairs are homozygous for the recessive alleles then skin colour is 'white'. If both are homozygous for the dominant form, which increases the amount of the melanin pigment present, then skin colour is 'black'. However, if one gene pair is heterozygous and the other homozygous, then an intermediate skin colour will be produced.

Lethal alleles

Occasionally (thankfully rarely) a mutation of an allele can occur that has such a drastic influence on tissue functions that life is impossible. Such alleles are called lethal alleles and they may be dominant or recessive in nature. One protection we have against such mutations is the presence in DNA of numerous 'back-up' copies of some of the most vital genes.

Gene transmission during cell division
Forming the chromosomes

Cell division is concerned with the production of new cells. In doing so the DNA in a cell must be assorted so that the new 'daughter' cells contain the appropriate amount and the correct genetic code. Cell division forms only a part of a cell's life cycle (see Figure 2.15, p.43), and during much of the time that a cell is actively performing its functional role the DNA forms an almost amorphous mass within the nucleus. In order for the cell to manipulate the DNA during cell division this must first

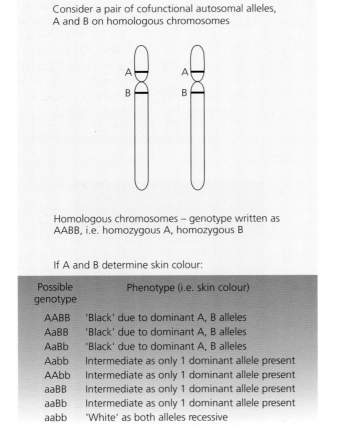

Consider a pair of cofunctional autosomal alleles, A and B on homologous chromosomes

Homologous chromosomes – genotype written as AABB, i.e. homozygous A, homozygous B

If A and B determine skin colour:

Possible genotype	Phenotype (i.e. skin colour)
AABB	'Black' due to dominant A, B alleles
AaBB	'Black' due to dominant A, B alleles
AaBb	'Black' due to dominant A, B alleles
Aabb	Intermediate as only 1 dominant allele present
AAbb	Intermediate as only 1 dominant allele present
aaBB	Intermediate as only 1 dominant allele present
aaBb	Intermediate as only 1 dominant allele present
aabb	'White' as both alleles recessive

Figure 19.14 Effect of allelic variation on a phenotype determined by more than one gene

Q Define the term 'allele'.

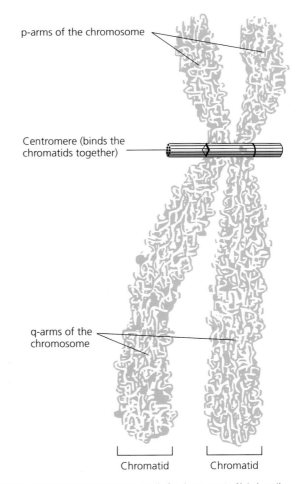

Figure 19.15 Drawing to show the detail of a chromosome. Note how the structure has a coiled appearance. A chromosome is comprised of two (identical) DNA molecules, each forming one chromatid

p-arms of the chromosome

Centromere (binds the chromatids together)

q-arms of the chromosome

Chromatid   Chromatid

BOX 19.8 THE HUMAN GENOME PROJECT

The entire collection of genes within an individual's body cell is called the genome and will comprise those genes for the various characteristics of that individual. The ability of science to identify genetic coding wherever it lies within a chromosome has made possible the identification of the genetic coding of the entire human genome. Much of the human genome (95%) is considered to be 'junk' DNA – functionless leftovers from the evolutionary process – but within the genome will be the genetic coding of the genes that make up the remaining 5%.

The Human Genome Project commenced in the late 1980s as a collaborative venture between various countries. Publication of the draft genome was in 2001, with revisions in 2003, but the final version was not released until 2004. Thus, the complete human 'blueprint' has been identified:

- The human genome contains 3.2 billion nucleotide bases (A, T, C and G; see Figure 2.13, p.40).
- 99.9% of bases are exactly the same in all people (i.e. human variation arises from differences in just 0.1% of the bases).
- The average gene comprises 3000 bases. However, sizes vary a great deal, the biggest human gene (to date), called dystrophin, has 2.4 million bases.
- The total number of human genes is estimated to be around 25 000.
- The functions are unknown for over 50% of genes discovered.

- Chromosome 1 has the most genes (2968) and the Y chromosome has the fewest (231).
- Geneticists have isolated about 1.4 million sites where single-base DNA differences (in scientific terms, single nucleotide polymorphisms or SNPs) occur in humans; these are sites of variation, possibly disease.
- The ratio of spermatozoon and oocyte mutations is 2:1.

The five questions to be answered at the time of writing are:

1 How does the relatively small number of genes enable the synthesis of the vast array (100 000–150 000) of proteins found in the human body?
2 Exactly where are the genes within the genome? Many have been identified but have yet to be linked to a given characteristic.
3 Now genes are being identified; what are their roles in health and ill health?
4 Can a commercial company claim ownership of genes that their laboratories have identified and/or classified? This argument places business and scientists in academia in opposition and is still under discussion at the time of writing.
5 How can healthcare intervention resolve genetic disorders? (but see 'Gene transmission during cell division', p.538).

---

be packaged into units that can be easily moved around the cell. An analogy would be trying to assort 46 strands of wool that are tangled together within a ball (viz. strands of DNA within the cell nucleus): assortment is much easier if the strands have first formed 46 individual small balls (the DNA molecule coils around and folds in on itself, and so becomes shorter and fatter). It is these small packages of DNA that are the chromosomes, mentioned earlier, and so these become visible under a microscope only when cells are undergoing cell division.

To form the chromosome:

- The DNA molecule duplicates; this is necessary because a fundamental aspect of cell division is that new cells will each require a faithful copy of the original DNA.
- The duplicated DNA takes on a characteristic shape (Figure 19.15), with each half of the chromosome comprising a single molecule of DNA, and being joined together near the central point (a structure called a centromere). Each half of the chromosome is referred to as a chromatid. The centromere is not exactly at the mid-point and so the two 'arms' of each chromatid are not equal in length: the shorter one is referred to as the p-arm, the longer one as the q-arm. Reference to the p- or q-arm is used when a gene location on a chromosome is identified (Figure 19.15).

The process of duplicating DNA is obviously crucial in forming the chromosome. The structure of DNA was described in Chapter 2 (see Figure 2.13, p.40), but it is important to remember that it basically consists of two strands of structural molecules and pairs of molecules, called nucleotide bases, that connect the two strands together rather like the rungs of a ladder. If a molecule of DNA is 'unzipped' (via the

actions of certain enzymes) to expose the constituent bases of each strand, it is a relatively straightforward process for a new set of complementary bases to combine with those that have been exposed (see Figure 2.16, p.44). New strands complete the process and as a result two molecules of DNA, identical to the original, will have been produced. Complementary pairing of bases ensures that the process of attaching new bases is not random and so the new DNA molecules, and hence the genetic code contained within it, is conserved.

Cell division by mitosis

Mitosis is fundamental to tissue growth, and to cell replacement. The general process is relatively simple:

1 As a cell prepares to divide, its chromosomes are formed, each being composed of the two duplicates of DNA, or chromatids, as explained above.
2 The membrane around the nucleus breaks down, and the chromosomes align within the cytoplasm across the centre of the cell (Figure 19.16).
3 The chromosomes are held in place by the attachment of their centromeres to an array of protein fibres called a spindle. This latter is produced by small organelles called centrioles that are found in all cells but which only produce this spindle when the cell is dividing. The spindle fibres are secured at opposite ends, or poles, of the cell.
4 The pair of chromatids that make up each chromosome separate, and the spindle fibres draw them to the opposite poles of the cell (Figure 19.16). Thus, 46 chromatids will accumulate at each pole of the cell. In this way, each pole will have 46 molecules of DNA of identical structure to the 46 DNA molecules of the original cell.

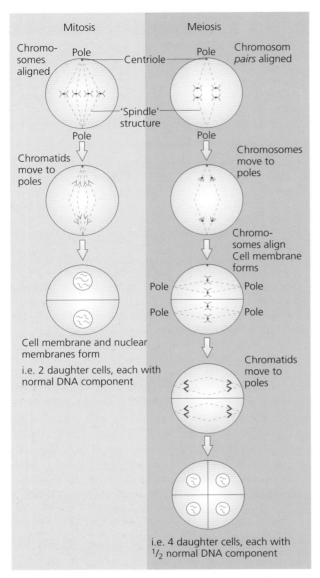

Figure 19.16 Comparison of chromosomal behaviour in mitosis and meiosis. Both processes are shown at the metaphase stage to begin with (i.e. chromosomes are aligned across the middle of the cell)

Q Identify the area within women and men where meiosis takes place.

That is not to say that they will always retain those same functions; for example one daughter cell may simply replace the original while the other transforms into another cell type. This happens when germinative cells divide, for example in the production of spermatocytes, or epidermal skin cells.

Cell division by meiosis

Meiosis is the form of cell division that occurs during the production of sex cells, or gametes, a process summarized in Figures 18.11, p.501, and 18.13, p.504 (see also Figure 19.2, p.523). Mitosis would not be appropriate for this because it would produce spermatozoa or ova with a cell's usual 46 molecules of DNA, and fertilization would then produce a zygote with 92 (i.e. 46 + 46) molecules of DNA, and hence an embryo with this number in its cells. In the succeeding generation this would become 184, and so on. Clearly, the 46 molecules of DNA must be reduced to 23 in the ovum and spermatozoon so that the usual 46 will be restored in the zygote. This is why cell division by meiosis is sometimes referred to as 'reduction division'.

The reduction in chromosome number is through a carefully regulated process. An important principle operates here and was noted earlier: meiosis involves the separation of the members of the chromosome pairs to leave just one member of each pair within the gamete (Figure 19.16):

1 Like mitosis, meiosis commences with duplication of the germ cell's DNA to form the chromosomes.
2 The nuclear membrane then breaks down, and the chromosomes align themselves at the centre of the cell and attach to the spindle by their centromeres. At this point meiosis and mitosis begin to differ.
3 In meiosis the chromosomes actually align in their pairs. The two chromosomes in each pair are bound together for a while by proteins, during which time they may exchange genetic material: the significance of this mixing is explained later in relation to the inheritance of genes.
4 The next stage is for the binding proteins to break, and for the pairs of chromosomes to separate, pulled apart by the spindle fibres. In this way, entire chromosomes pass along the spindle fibres, with members of each pair moving to opposite poles of the cell. The chromosome pairs have thus been separated and there will be just one copy of each pair at each pole of the cell (Figure 19.16).
5 An intervening cell membrane forms. At this point the original cell is said to have completed the first part of meiosis, referred to as 'meiosis I'. Each chromosome still has the characteristic shape since they are still composed of their chromatids.
6 Each 'group' of chromosomes then becomes attached to new spindles (Figure 19.16) and the chromatids immediately separate, in a process analogous to mitosis division.
7 The chromatids pass to the poles of the newly formed cells.
8 New nuclear membranes and further intervening cell membranes form. The second part of meiosis, 'meiosis II', has now been completed.

5 A nuclear membrane forms around each cluster of chromatids, and an intervening cell membrane develops between the two new nuclei. Thus two 'daughter' cells have been produced from the single 'parent' cell, and each will be genetically identical to it. The term 'diploid' is used to indicate that the cells have the usual complement of chromosomes.

Each stage of mitosis has a characteristic name (see p.42) but such names can serve to confuse readers unfamiliar with the process: it is more important for practitioners to understand the significance of the behaviour of the chromosomes during cell division. Thus, mitosis provides new cells with a genetic 'blueprint' that is identical to the original and so the new cells should have the same structure and functions as the original.

BOX 19.9 CLONING

This term refers to a technique by which individual organisms are produced that have an identical genetic make-up to that of another living (or dead) organism. The method entails removing the nucleus from an oocyte, and then taking the nucleus of a cell from, perhaps, an adult animal (the donor of the oocyte or another one) and transferring it into the enucleated oocyte. This newly constituted cell is then transferred to a uterus where, if successful, it will implant and form a new individual genetically identical to the donor of the nucleus. From a purely scientific perspective, demonstrating that cloning is possible highlights that the activation of development genes is feasible even in DNA taken from an adult cell, but the success of cloning experiments has also raised serious ethical and moral issues (Elsner, 2006).

The technique has only recently been performed successfully. 'Dolly' the sheep is credited with being the first cloned animal (in 1996) but the method has been extended to other animals, and in late 1999 to humans (although human embryos produced in this way were destroyed after a few days). On the positive side, the method is considered to have potential beneficial applications in agriculture and in the development of tissue for transplantation (see Box 19.4, p.530). On the negative side, there is concern that there is enormous potential for abuse, for example by enabling an individual to clone him or herself either while still alive or after death.

9 As a result four 'daughter' cells have been formed from the original parent cell (mitosis only produces two), but each has only 23 molecules of DNA; they are referred to as being haploid.

Each stage of the meiosis process has a characteristic name but once again it is the behaviour of the chromosomes that is important here. Whereas mitosis conserves genetic information in the new cells, the separation of the pairs of chromosomes during meiosis means that gametes contain only half of the total genetic make-up of the parent cells.

Thus, when a zygote is formed at fertilization, half of the genetic material of the resultant embryo will be of maternal origin (from the ovum) and the other half paternal (from the spermatozoon). This genetic mixing has important implications for the inheritance of characteristics and of congenital disorder, as we shall see in a later section.

Meiosis and inheritance

If meiosis occurs normally then sex cells will be formed with half the usual number of chromosomes. Since we all inherit half of our DNA from one parent and half from another then logic suggests that it ought to be possible for someone to inherit a set of chromosomes from say their mother which are identical in genetic code to the set that she inherited from her mother, and so on. While we all know people who look very similar to a parent or even a grandparent, they are never identical. This is because meiosis also promotes gene mixing, which is achieved in three ways: (1) segregation of alleles, (2) independent assortment of alleles and (3) crossover of alleles between chromosomes.

Segregation of alleles

This has been the focus of much of the discussion on inheritance so far. Remember, when the homologous chromosome

pairs separate during meiosis in the formation of the gametes, the process also separates (or 'segregates') the pairs of alleles on those chromosomes. This means that for a given gene an individual will only inherit one allele from each parent, thus raising the likelihood of a different pairing in the offspring. For example, it raises the possibility that a recessive allele will be paired with another recessive allele from the other parent. If this happens then the recessive alleles will be operative in the offspring.

Independent assortment of alleles

It was noted earlier how characteristics often result from the expression of several genes. It is likely that the genes that make up this 'group' are located on more than one pair of chromosomes. For these alleles the inheritance of the characteristic will also therefore depend upon which members of the chromosome pairs passes into the gamete. This in turn depends upon how the different chromosomes assort themselves when they line up during meiosis – a process that appears to be random.

Figure 19.17 illustrates a possible arrangement of three pairs of homologous chromosomes during meiosis. Note how the combination of alleles passed into the gametes varies depending upon how these chromosomes are assorted before they separate. In this way meiosis once again ensures that alleles are mixed in the next generation.

Translocation (or crossing-over) of alleles

When a pair of homologous chromosomes align prior to their separation during the first stage of meiosis they are briefly

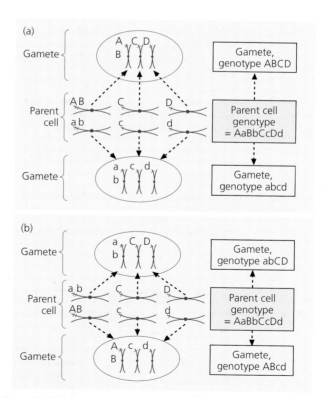

Figure 19.17 Two examples of the effects of independent assortment of three chromosome pairs on the genotypes of gametes produced by meiosis. The genotype of the parent cell is the same in each case

bound together by proteins. At this point some of the DNA may be exchanged between the chromosomes, taking with it the constituent alleles (Figure 19.18). This is called 'crossing over' or, more technically, 'translocation' and causes the composition of the chromosomes concerned to be altered. If a num-

ber of alleles on a single chromosome contribute to a particular phenotype then translocation mixes these and can potentially alter the phenotype. As a point of interest, the enzymes that facilitate this exchange of DNA are used by scientists to 'clip out' or 'paste in' pieces of DNA in genetic engineering.

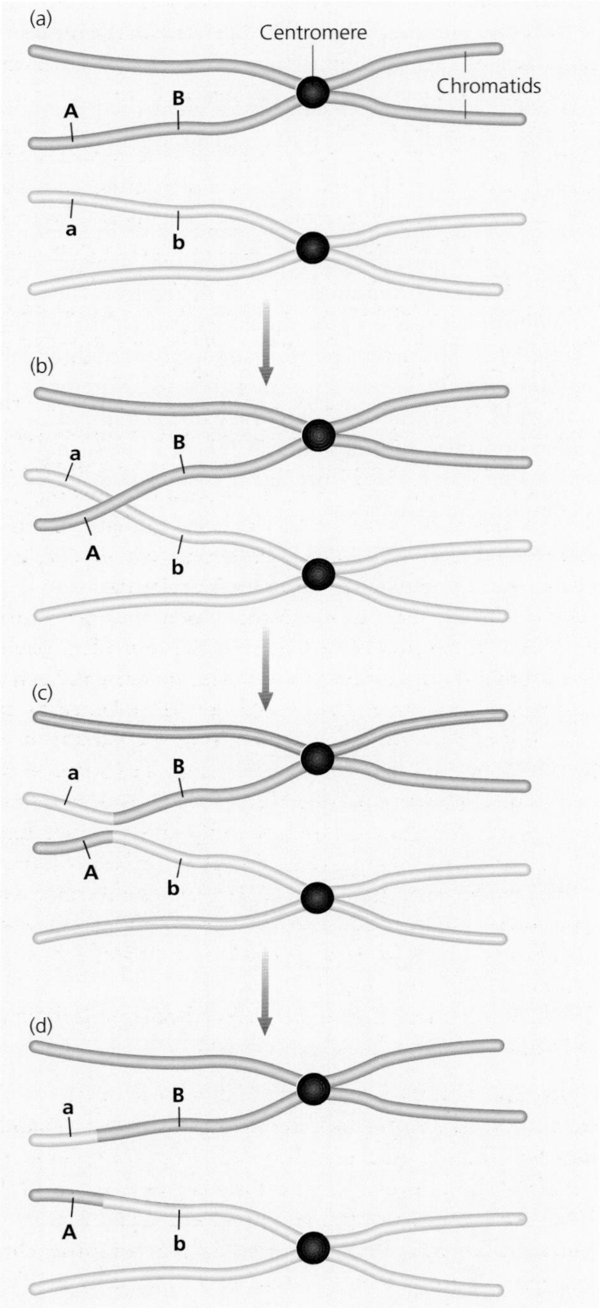

Figure 19.18 Allelic mixing produced by exchange of DNA (crossover) between chromosomal pairs during meiosis. (a) Chromosome pair aligns at metaphase stage of meiosis. (b) Arms of the two chromosomes interact. (c) Crossover of DNA from one chromosome to another complete chromosome. (d) Chromosome pair ready to separate during the next stage of meiosis. Note the different allelic pairing on each chromosome, compared with (a)

Q What is crossover?

PRINCIPLES OF THE INHERITANCE OF CHARACTERISTICS

The previous section explains how the separation of chromosomes during the production of sex cells by meiosis ensures that there is a mixing of genes in the next generation. Since most genes comprise two alleles, and these may be identical (referred to as a 'homozygous genotype') or differ slightly ('heterozygous genotype'), the characteristics inherited by succeeding generations will depend upon whether dominant or recessive alleles have been inherited. In order to understand how such inheritances occur, it is necessary to consider some of the general principles involved.

Gregor Mendel (1822–1884) was the first person to record how characteristics can arise in offspring even though they are not apparent in the parents (the term 'recessive' was not used in his time). Mendel went on to identify many of the features of the inheritance of characteristics but was restricted by the lack of knowledge at the time regarding DNA, chromosomes, etc. However, his contribution is recorded in posterity and the general principles of inheritance are referred to as 'Mendelian'.

Mendelian principles and the inheritance of genetic disorder

Most DNA is found within the cell nucleus (nuclear or chromosomal DNA) but small amounts also occur outside the nucleus, in the mitochondria (mitochondrial DNA). Inherited disorders caused by changes of mutations in mitochondrial DNA are rare, but acquired changes to these genes are of interest in relation to free-radical theories of ageing (see later).

The great majority of disorders that have been linked to genetic changes are caused by altered chromosomal DNA. The inheritance of altered phenotypes, especially in relation to disorder, can be considered from the perspective of chromosome number or size, and the inheritance of altered genotypes of single genes or multiple genes.

Chromosome number or size

Non-dysjunction

As we have seen, cells other than the gametes normally contain two copies of each autosome and two sex chromosomes. The inheritance of a numerical disturbance would arise:

- if a chromosome pair failed to separate at meiosis when the gametes were formed; or
- if the chromatids of a chromosome in the second stage of meiosis failed to separate.

Failure of separation is referred to as non-dysjunction (Figure 19.19). Whichever stage of meiosis it occurs in, non-dysjunction will result in a gamete that contains two of the same molecule of DNA (i.e. chromosome). If this gamete contributes to fertilization, then the resultant zygote will have three of the chromosome, referred to as trisomy: two copies will have been inherited from the gamete with non-dysjunction, and one as normal from the other. If non-dysjunction leaves both copies of a chromosome in one cell, then it follows that there will also be a cell formed that lacks the chromosome. If that gamete takes part in fertilization then the resultant zygote will have just one copy of the chromosome, referred to as monosomy: the one copy will have been inherited from one partner as normal, the other gamete will not have a copy owing to non-dysjunction.

Trisomies and monosomies mean that an embryo has, respectively, either a great excess of alleles or only one set of alleles associated with the chromosome. The imbalance seems

to be particularly detrimental to development if the chromosome is one of the autosomes, especially for monosomies, but babies with trisomies 13, 18 and 21 do occur (Box 19.10). Both trisomies and monosomies are observed for the sex chromosomes (Figure 19.19).

Non-dysjunction can occur in the formation of either spermatozoa or oocytes, but most often arises during the formation of the oocyte. The reason for this is that meiosis commences in women around the time that they are born, and the further development of the oocytes is suspended until they are reactivated after puberty. The stage at which development is suspended is when the homologous pairs of chromosomes have aligned in meiosis I; this is the point at which chromosomes are bound together and so they remain bound in oocytes for many years. Failure to break the bonds relates to maternal age, presumably because of ageing of the primary oocytes in the ovary. For example, the incidence of trisomy 21 in Down syndrome is about 1 in 700–1000 births overall, but if the mother is over 35 years old then the risk is 3 in 1000 (Bittles *et al.*, 2007)

Occasionally non-dysjunction can occur twice during a single meiotic division. If this occurs then a pair of chromosomes remain together after meiosis I, and one or both chromosomes pass intact (i.e. with both of their chromatids) into the new cells after meiosis II. This can lead to gametes that have up to four copies of a chromosome. Such excessive copies are only viable in relation to sex chromosomes (Box 19.10).

Mosaicism is a very unusual form of non-dysjunction that results in a proportion of cells within the individual having chromosomal abnormalities while the rest are normal. Such an occurrence within the embryo could not be explained by the inheritance of an extra chromosome from the parents, as all cells would be expected to have the same karyotype as the zygote. The condition arises because of incomplete separation of chromatids during mitosis of cells in the embryo itself, especially in the early stages of tissue differentiation. It is a form of non-dysjunction that may produce developmental abnormalities but these cannot be considered inherited (though they will be 'congenital' since this term covers both inherited influences and those that occur *in utero*).

In relation to mosaicism in Down syndrome, non-dysjunction in mitosis means that some cells will:

- contain the normal complement of chromosome 21;
- contain the whole of a chromosome 21 (i.e. two chromatids) together with the usual one chromatid from the other member of the chromosome pair (i.e. three copies, not two) of the DNA molecule that comprises chromosome pair 21;
- contain one copy of the DNA molecule that comprises chromosome 21, rather than the usual two (these cells are likely to be dysfunctional and not proliferate).

Once non-dysjunction has occurred, the numeric disturbance in the affected cells continues into later cell populations as the embryo grows; more cells will have the trisomy, hence the symptoms of Down syndrome.

Approximately 1% of cases of Down syndrome arise through mosaicism (i.e. many cells are trisomic for chromosome 21)

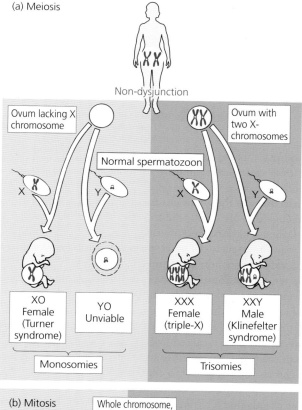

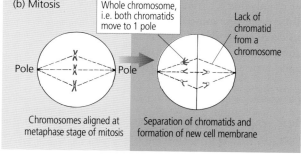

Figure 19.19 Non-dysjunction of (a) sex chromosomes during meiosis and (b) chromatids during mitosis

Q What is Down syndrome?

BOX 19.10 INHERITED TRISOMIES AND MONOSOMIES

Trisomy and polysomy of the sex chromosomes

Klinefelter syndrome is observed in males, in whom there is an extra X chromosome (i.e. these individuals are XXY). The consequence is that the testes are small and androgen secretion is low. Spermatozoa may be absent, though some people with the syndrome have fathered children (note that the presence of the Y chromosome makes these people male). Cognitive functions may be affected but only slightly at most (Porche, 2007).

Trisomy of the X chromosome is called triple X syndrome and is also frequently found within a population, but individuals usually do not have distinctive phenotypic characteristics. In the absence of a Y chromosome, triple-X individuals are always female. Although some of these women have menstrual difficulties, many are fertile.

Non-dysjunction during both meiosis I and meiosis II may also lead to the inheritance of multiple sex chromosomes (i.e. polysomy). Even the pentasomy, XXXXX, has been observed, though the consequences are more severe than for trisomy and it is associated with learning disabilities.

Trisomy of the autosomes

Trisomy of chromosome 21 is the only viable autosomal trisomy, although even with this form the majority of fetuses do not go to term. Trisomy 21 is usually referred to by its clinical name of Down syndrome (after the clinician who first described it). Others are known (e.g. Patau syndrome, 3×13, and Edward syndrome, 3×18) but these babies are so profoundly affected that the pregnancy rarely goes to term and when

infants are born their period of survival is usually very short.

Trisomy 21 produces a number of developmental anomalies:

- learning disability, which may be profound but varies between individuals because the trisomy may only be partial (see below);
- distinctive facial characteristics, especially of the forehead and eyes;
- an open mouth with a protruding tongue;
- cardiovascular anomalies, especially of heart structure;
- a third fontanelle of the skull;
- a single palmar crease.

Not all cases of Down syndrome represent complete trisomy 21, although about 95% do. Partial trisomy 21 is possible and is observed in about 3–4% of cases. The remaining cases occur through 'mosaicism' involving chromosome 21.

Monosomy

Cells usually require at least two copies of each chromosome and so monosomic fetuses might not be expected to be viable. The exception is of the X chromosome (Turner syndrome) in which individuals are XO. About 98% of such fetuses spontaneously abort and the 2% born are female as no Y chromosome is present. Development of the gonads, and body growth, are slowed, and there may be a range of systemic problems (Doswell et al., 2006).

Should a zygote inherit just a Y chromosome (i.e. YO) it will not develop. Apparently at least one copy of an X chromosome is a minimum requirement.

---

while other cells are derived from embryonic cells that divided normally and therefore have the usual two copies. Clearly, the consequences for development will depend upon the extent of the mosaicism, and this relates to the period of embryo/fetal development when the non-dysjunction occurred. If it occurred early in development then most cells in the later embryo will be trisomic, if later in development then many of the cells and tissues will have a normal chromosome number.

Chromosomal fragmentation (errors of translocation)

It was noted earlier how chromosomes swap sections when the homologous pairs are lined up at the start of meiosis (illustrated in Figure 19.18). Fragmentation occurs when this process is disrupted, with sections of chromosome not being swapped in the conventional way. Thus, a fragment can become attached to the other member of the pair without any exchange occurring, or perhaps to a different chromosome entirely. As the chromosomes segregate during meiosis, this means that a cell may be produced that contains a chromosome plus the extra fragment, or one with the shortened chromosome that 'lost' the fragment. The chromosome with the additional fragment will therefore contain some duplicated alleles, while the shortened one is now deficient in alleles. The effects on the health of the infant will depend upon the additional alleles gained or lost.

Down syndrome may occur through fragmentation that results in translocation of a fragment of chromosome 21. Approximately 3–4% of cases arise because a piece of chromosome 21 breaks off during the crossing-over stage of meiosis and translocates to become attached to another chromosome, often

number 14. The zygote then may inherit a copy of chromosome 21 from each parent, and the additional fragment attached to another chromosome. This results in a 'partial trisomy' 21, and causes many of the symptoms associated with Down syndrome, although they are usually milder than the full trisomy.

Losing a section of chromosome may not be so detrimental as in most instances the other member of the pair that is inherited will have its normal complement of alleles. In the case of the sex chromosomes, however, the X chromosome contains alleles that, in males, will be the only copies present.

Fragile X syndrome results from fragmentation of the X chromosome and is a frequent cause of learning disability. In this case the error is caused by a 'fragile' section of DNA which tends to break during meiosis with the result that a whole piece of chromosome is lost. As a consequence, any resultant zygote will be deficient in the alleles on the lost fragment. The presence of only one X chromosome in boys means that the effects will be more pronounced than in girls and this condition is considered to be sex-linked. The cause of the breakage of the chromosome is not fully understood but there is evidence for a 'fragile' gene at the location of the break.

Inheritance of altered genotypes 1: single gene disorders

When genes are altered (mutated) their products may no longer perform a normal cellular function, and a disorder may occur. Single-gene disorders are triggered by alterations in the nucleotide base sequence of one gene. Advocates of the operon theory of gene expression and non-expression may argue that there are no single-gene disorders, since the operon involves

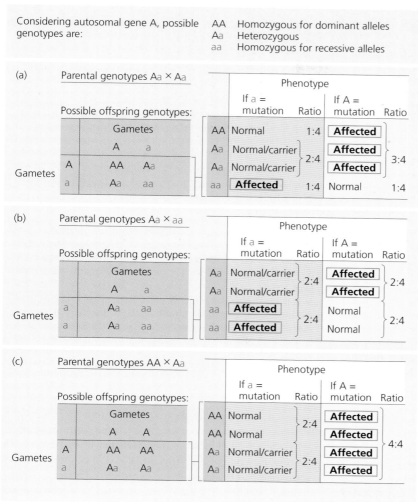

Considering autosomal gene A, possible genotypes are:

AA	Homozygous for dominant alleles
Aa	Heterozygous
aa	Homozygous for recessive alleles

Figure 19.20 Autosomal inheritance: influence of parental genotype on the phenotype of offspring. In each case the phenotype outcome is shown if the recessive allele a or the dominant allele A is a gene mutation that potentially could induce change

Q What would be the genotypes and phenotypes of offspring with the following genetic crosses of parental ABO blood groupings: (1) AO × BO; (2) AA × OB; (3) AB × AB?

three genes: operator, structural and repressor genes (see Figure 2.19, p.49). Therefore, a mutation in one, two or all three genes may result in a disorder previously thought of as a single-gene mutation. Nevertheless, at the present time some disorders are specifically linked to one (structural) gene.

The likelihood of progeny inheriting single-gene problems depends upon whether the alleles concerned are recessive or dominant, or if they are found on the autosomes or sex chromosomes.

Autosomal recessive inheritance

We have seen how meiosis separates homologous chromosomes and in doing so separates the gene alleles. If the individual is heterozygous for a given pair of alleles (e.g. one 'normal' dominant, one altered recessive), then half of the gametes formed will contain the 'normal' allele and half the recessive form. Should his/her partner also be heterozygous it can be seen that there is a one in four statistical likelihood that a zygote formed will be homozygous for the recessive allele (Figure 19.20).

In contrast, there is no possibility of a recessive, homozygous genotype when one parent is heterozygous and the other is homozygous for the 'normal' (i.e. dominant) alleles, as the

child will inherit at least one 'normal' allele. There is, however, a one in two chance that the child will be heterozygous (Figure 19.20). In this case, any disorder associated with the recessive allele will 'skip' that generation but there remains the possibility that the homozygous form will appear in the following one. For this reason the heterozygous individual is frequently referred to as a *carrier* of the recessive allele (or condition).

There are many examples of recessive disorder that result from just a single gene change. Those genes responsible for some of the commoner disorders have now been identified, and the impact on cell processes studied. The commoner disorders are included in Box 19.11.

Sex-linked recessive inheritance

Some disorders appear predominantly in males because the genes involved are found on the X chromosome. An important factor is the discrepancy between the sizes of the X and Y chromosomes as this has important implications for gene mutations on the X chromosome. The relatively small size of the Y chromosome means that most alleles on the X chromosome do not have counterparts on the Y (additionally, the Y chromosome appears to be functionally 'quiet' after birth). In females, with

BOX 19.11 AUTOSOMAL RECESSIVE CONDITIONS

Cystic fibrosis

This is the commonest inherited condition in the UK, and is characterized by the secretion of viscous mucus in the lungs and gastrointestinal tract, that may obstruct airways and the pancreatic duct. The disorder actually arises because of a problem in chloride transport, and hence water movement, across the cell membranes of mucosal cells as a consequence of a failure of the recessive gene to cause the synthesis of the appropriate protein. The gene is found on chromosome 7. Care is aimed at removing secretions (using physiotherapy) and preventing infection in the obstructed tissues (Baker and Denyes, 2008). Severe pancreatic obstruction may compromise digestion, and pancreatic enzymes or simple foodstuffs may then have to be administered directly into the small intestine.

Phenylketonuria (PKU)

This condition is characterized by an accumulation of the essential amino acid phenylalanine in tissues. The amino acid is obtained from dietary protein and some is converted in the liver to tyrosine which is used by the body for many reactions for example to synthesize proteins, the pigment melanin and catecholamine hormones. Tyrosine synthesis is catalysed by the enzyme phenylalanine hydroxylase and it is the absence of this enzyme that promotes the disorder. Young children in particular are at risk of the consequences of this problem (phenylalanine accumulation interferes with brain uptake of other amino acids, and so slows brain development) but the condition is controllable by reducing the dietary intake as compensation for the decreased utilization (Weetch

and MacDonald, 2006). Analysis of a blood sample (the neonatal screening test, previously called the Guthrie test) will clearly show if excessive phenylalanine is present. The gene for this condition is found on chromosome 12.

Familial hyperlipidaemia (or hypercholesterolaemia)

In this condition there is an excessively high lipid concentration in the blood, which promotes the development of atheromatous deposits in vessels (see Figure 12.13, p.324). The elevated lipid results from a problem in the uptake mechanism by which cholesterol is taken into liver cells. The gene for this condition is found on chromosome 19. Care is aimed at education to encourage the individual to have a low (saturated) fat diet, and to use cholesterol-lowering drugs.

Tay–Sachs disease

In this condition, an altered gene on chromosome 15 means that nerve cells cannot produce the enzyme hexosaminidase A. This enzyme degrades fatty substances called gangliosides (another term for the disorder is gangliosidosis). These are important but harmful if allowed to accumulate. Consequently, the disorder is characterized by profound neurological and neuromuscular problems: blindness, deafness, dementia, muscle paralysis and seizures. The condition is normally fatal before the age of 4 years. The incidence of Tay–Sachs disease is particularly high among people of Eastern European and Askhenazi Jewish descent (Weinstein, 2007). Patients and carriers of Tay–Sachs disease can be identified by a simple blood test that measures beta-hexosaminidase A activity.

two X chromosomes, the expression of a recessive allele on these will only be observed if both have a copy of it, much as is the case for recessive alleles on the autosomes (above). In males, however, a recessive allele on the X chromosome will often be expressed because there is no 'normal' allele on the Y chromosome to dominate it (Figure 19.21). This is not to say that such conditions are necessarily always restricted to boys. The issue is the likelihood of girls inheriting two recessive forms of an allele.

For example, red–green colour deficiency arises because of a gene mutation on the X chromosome and so colour deficiency is more likely to be found in boys than girls. However, it does not affect 'survivability' and there are many girls who also are

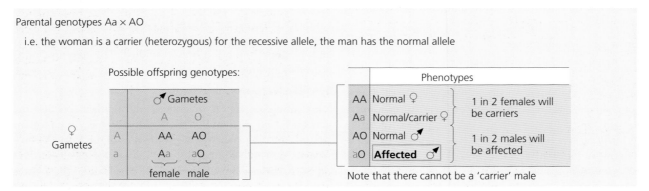

Figure 19.21 Sex-linked inheritance

Q *Describe what is meant by sex-linked inheritance.*

BOX 19.12 SEX-LINKED RECESSIVE CONDITIONS

Duchenne muscular dystrophy

This condition is characterized by loss of the muscle protein dystrophin, which has a role in the maintenance of the cell membrane, or sarcolemma (Emery, 2006). Loss of the protein results in progressive wastage of muscle. The example of inheritance given in Figure 19.21 is the most likely pattern of inheritance for this condition. This is because a woman who had the condition would have to be homozygous for the gene and so would have to have inherited an affected X chromosome from her father (who would have had this progressive condition himself and so would be unlikely to have children). Thus, a woman might have one copy and so be a carrier of the muscular dystrophy allele but is unlikely to have two copies and hence have the condition. Nevertheless, a handful of cases of women with Duchenne muscular dystrophy are known world-wide.

Haemophilia A

This condition results from a loss of the liver enzyme necessary for the synthesis of clotting factor VIII. The condition has been known for many years to be primarily a condition of boys, although a few incidences in girls have been documented. Unlike Duchenne muscular dystrophy, haemophilia is now controllable (through administration of extrinsic factor VIII) and so does not now place a reproductive restriction on the inherited genotype (but see Petersen, 2006). Thus it should be feasible for the man with haemophilia to father a daughter who, if she also inherited an affected X chromosome from her carrier mother, would be homozygous for the condition. The sex-linkage of this condition there-

fore seems likely to be weaker than it is for Duchenne muscular dystrophy. However, the mutated allele has a low frequency within the population; this means that the partner of the father is unlikely to be carrying the gene and so the condition remains predominantly a problem in males.

Severe combined immune deficiency syndrome

Severe combined immune deficiency syndrome (SCID) is a recessive disorder in which there is a deficiency of proteins involved in the interactions between interleukins and lymphocytes in the immune system. These interactions entail a combination of interleukin (IL) with a cell-surface receptor, and the triggering of intracellular events (second messengers; see Chapter 9, p.208). A SCID arises if there is gene mutation leading to deficiency at any of the critical steps in this pathway, and so the pattern of inheritance of SCID is irregular. The sex-linked form, X-SCID, is the best known in which the IL-2 receptor gene on the X chromosome is mutated. Another form involves mutation to the Janus kinase 3 gene, responsible for the production of one of the second messenger proteins, but this gene is autosomal and so the form is not sex-linked. The consequence of SCID is that there is a defective, often deficient, population of T-lymphocytes (see Figure 13.18, p.384), and sometimes of B-lymphocytes, leading to a severely compromised immune system. It is often colloquially referred to as 'Boy in the Bubble' disease after a highly-publicized case in the 1970s when a child was physically isolated from his environment, but died as a teenager when that protection was removed.

colour deficient. In contrast, some sex-linked disorders present such severe problems that a boy with the condition is reproductively restricted; however, modern medicine and clinical support means that these conditions are frequently now survivable into adulthood and there is an increasing possibility of a daughter inheriting two copies of the allele (Box 19.12).

Autosomal dominant inheritance

An altered allele will occasionally (rarely) behave in a dominant fashion. This means that the influences of that allele will be observed even in the heterozygous condition because the 'normal' allele will now be recessive to it. Thus:

* with two heterozygous parents there is a three in four, or 75% chance that the offspring will have the phenotype associated with the allele because of a two in four chance that the offspring will be heterozygous, and a one in four chance that a child will be homozygous for the dominant allele (see Figure 19.20);
* if only one parent is heterozygous, and the other is homozygous for the 'normal' (now recessive) allele, then there is still a 50% chance that the dominant phenotype will be inherited (Figure 19.20);
* if a parent is homozygous for that gene then all children will inherit the phenotype.

The dominant allele therefore has a high inheritance/penetrance. Conditions associated with it might be expected to be apparent from birth, and place a reproductive restriction on the affected person, but this is not necessarily the

case as some genes seem to be screened in a way that remains unclear, and become apparent much later in life. Examples of autosomal dominant conditions are given in Box 19.13.

Inheritance of altered genotypes 2: multifactorial disorders

Multifactorial disorders arise via a combination of environmental factors and mutations of a number of genes. Polygenic characteristics are produced by the actions of several genes located on one or more chromosomes; the genes involved for a character may be referred to as the haplotype for the characteristic. When several genes are involved pronounced changes in cell function will arise only if a 'vital' gene within the sequence is altered, or if a number of the genes within the group are altered by environmental factors during the individual's lifespan. Although the number of genes involved makes inheritance or susceptibility to a disorder unpredictable, some genes in a functional group appear to be more critical than others and so disorders (e.g. some cancers, heart disease, Alzheimer disease, insulin-independent diabetes mellitus) can sometimes exhibit a weak familial link (Box 19.14).

Introduction to population genetics

The above sections consider the likelihood of gene mutations carried by the parents being inherited by their offspring. The chances of the affected gene being present in both parents will relate to the frequency of the gene within the population since this influences the chance of someone meeting another carrier. The alleles present within a population comprise the *gene pool*

BOX 19.13 AUTOSOMAL DOMINANT CONDITIONS

Retinoblastoma

This condition is a rare eye tumour that originates in the retina of one or both eyes (Rao *et al.*, 2008). In approximately half of cases the condition is acquired in the early years, but it can also be expressed as an inherited condition. The reason for this variation is that the gene is one that can exhibit incomplete penetrance (i.e. for some reason in some instances the dominant gene is not expressed; the mechanism is unclear). The gene is located on chromosome 13.

Huntington's disease (or Huntington's chorea)

This is a neurological disorder but its expression typically does not occur until well into adulthood (on average 40–50 years of age) and so an individual may be totally unaware of its inheritance until long after they have had children of their own. The condition is characterized by a deficiency of the neurotransmitter gamma-aminobutyric acid (GABA) from neurological areas involved in the control of movement (see Box 17.13, p.482). Why there should be a delay in expression of the disorder is unclear. The gene is found on chromosome 4.

See the case of a family with Huntington's disease, Section VI, p.671.

Incomplete dominance

Sickle cell anaemia is the commonest form of sickle cell disease, in which 'sickle-shaped' red blood cells are a feature (other forms are sickle haemoglobin C disease, sickle beta-plus thalassaemia, and sickle beta-zero thalassaemia). This condition arises because a gene mutation on chromosome 11 means that one of the polypeptide chains in a haemoglobin molecule contains a single amino acid substitution (forming haemoglobin S), when compared with 'normal' haemoglobin (haemoglobin A). This small change alters the properties of the pigment, causing it to distort after releasing oxygen and so produce the sickling of the erythrocyte. The cell membrane is more fragile in the sickled state, resulting in haemolysis. The red cell therefore has a much-shortened lifespan (16 days compared with 120 days) and so anaemia is present.

It is observed in the homozygous condition, where both sickle cell alleles are present. In this way, it behaves in much the same way as the usual recessive inheritance. However, blood samples from heterozygous individuals (i.e. just one sickle cell allele present, the other 'normal') will also show numbers of sickled erythrocytes, in addition to normal ones, as both 'normal' and 'sickle' alleles are expressed. Thus, this condition represents an example of one produced by alleles that exhibit 'incomplete dominance', or 'incomplete penetrance' of the dominant allele. Symptoms may be present but the degree of sickling in the heterozygous state is usually insufficient for them to be very severe, and so the condition is referred to as *sickle cell trait*.

BOX 19.14 CANCER: AN EXAMPLE OF A POLYGENIC CONDITION

Colorectal cancer is an example of an inherited predisposition. In this condition familial linkage is recognized, but is lower than might be anticipated from Mendelian principles. The cancer exhibits a benign precancerous phase as polyps within the colon or rectum; the presence of polyps shows a much higher genetic concordance (the gene for familial polyposis coli is found on chromosome 5). As with other cancers, it is currently thought that the polyps arise because of inherited alleles or the occurrence of mutation through the actions of 'initator' factors, and progress to cancerous lesions because of further mutations to genes by 'promotor' factors (further genes involved in the genesis of colorectal cancer have been identified on chromosomes 5, 12, 17 and 18; Takayama *et al.*, 2006). This multiple 'hit' approach to gene mutation means that lifestyle factors are likely to figure prominently in the genesis of cancer (and disorders of other polygenic characteristics such as heart disease, diabetes mellitus, etc.) and research is targeting the genes involved in an attempt to understand the factors concerned, and to raise the possibility of new therapeutic approaches.

BOX 19.15 'NATURAL SELECTION' AND ALLELE FREQUENCY IN THE GENE POOL

'Natural selection' (see text) might be expected to reduce the incidence of severe genetic disorders, and this undoubtedly is a factor in the rarity of most such conditions. Exceptions are the high frequency of the allele for sickle cell anaemia in Afro-Caribbean cultures, and of the allele for cystic fibrosis alleles in Caucasian cultures (Streetly *et al.*, 2008). The implication of these two examples is that 'natural selection' has actually favoured the occurrence of the allele within the population, even though having two copies produces the inherited disorder, because having one copy conveys a survival advantage.

An individual who has just one copy of the sickle cell allele has a degree of protection against malaria because the parasite finds it difficult to live inside the red blood cells. The individual may experience mild symptoms of sickle cell anaemia but the protection against malaria is thought to be so advantageous to survival in some parts of the world that 'natural selection' increased the frequency of the allele in the population.

An advantage to the frequency of the cystic fibrosis allele is less clear. The same ion transport mechanism is affected in both cystic fibrosis and cholera and so perhaps it was advantageous to be a carrier of the allele when cholera was once rife. The link is tenuous, however, and remains to be determined.

and the frequency of a gene within this is determined by various factors: natural selection, inbreeding, population drift and spontaneous or acquired mutations.

Natural selection

'Gene mixing' during meiosis and reproduction produces offspring with genotypes that will differ from those of the parents. This variation may prove beneficial for those individuals who have a particular gene change when compared with other people who live in the same environment, and so over many generations the success of such offspring could be expected to increase the incidence of the advantageous alleles. Similarly, any gene mutation that is detrimental to life should tend to reduce in frequency in the gene pool. This is the basis of the proposals forwarded by Charles Darwin in the nineteenth century in his 'theory of evolution'. Darwin called the process 'natural selection' (Box 19.15).

For many conditions, however, medical advances in recent years have ensured survival at least until adulthood and, to some degree, have negated selection processes.

Inbreeding

Inbreeding within a family line increases the likelihood that both parents are carriers of a particular allele. This, for example, is why the incidence of haemophilia A in the royal line traced back to Queen Victoria is much greater than that of the population as a whole. The effect is not simply confined to inbreeding between close relatives: if a population is small and stable with little immigration or emigration then the likelihood increases of people being related, perhaps from several generations earlier. This is a factor in the incidence of clusters of inherited conditions in some districts, when compared with national figures.

Population drift

The immigration or emigration of individuals into or out of a population will, respectively, add to or remove genes from that population. The process can alter the incidence of a particular gene mutation within a gene pool and may even result in the introduction of novel mutations. We see this in the physical characteristics of people in parts of the world where cultures have integrated. In another example, Huntington's disease appears to have been introduced into North America by European settlers.

Spontaneous or acquired mutation

Cells can often self-repair any alterations to the genetic code that have occurred spontaneously, but some of these may persist and therefore be inherited. This means that inherited conditions are unlikely to be eradicated from a population as new mutations will continuously occur within the gene pool. The cause of 'spontaneous' mutation is unclear. Cosmic radiation is one factor but it may be that there are other as yet unidentified environmental factors. The acquisition of gene mutations produced by environmental factors may also help to explain the occurrence of local clusters of disorders; for example it has been suggested that leukaemia can be induced by radon gas emission from granite rocks.

GENES AND AGEING

This chapter has provided an overview, with examples, of why genes and their actions are so important to cell activity and health. The focus has very much been that of genes and basic tissue functions, in particular to explain the occurrence of congenital disorder. The following section of this chapter considers how the acquisition of gene changes are also involved in ageing and conditions associated with increasing age.

Ageing and declining homeostatic efficiency (senescence)

The functions of individual organs and tissues in healthy individuals are at a premium during the mid-to-late years of our twenties, when the conditions necessary for 'normal' cell function are optimally maintained, via finely controlled and efficient homeostatic processes. Adaptive mechanisms are also in place and so the capacity to change organ function to perform exercise will also be at a peak. The integrated, homeostatic efficiency of the adult means that the individual is considered as having a maximal functional capacity.

Ageing *per se* does not necessarily mean a complete loss of homeostatic control, but the effectiveness of that control in response to physical challenge declines (Figure 19.22). Problems become apparent at all stages of the control process. Thus, receptor density decreases and the threshold rises at which stimulation occurs (i.e. a greater change in a parameter is required to stimulate a response). The afferent and efferent signalling becomes less precise because hormone release or neural function declines. Further loss of efficiency occurs because the effector tissues respond more slowly because of age-related changes in the cells of tissues (e.g. tissue atrophy,

Table 19.3 Selected age-related changes in homeostatic parameters and systemic functions

System	Change and/or consequence	
Nervous	Loss of neurons, myelin, neurotransmitter, synaptic receptors (e.g. memory loss, reduced reflexes, reduced postural control)	
Senses	Decreased receptor density/sensitivity, decreased accommodating ability of eye lens, decreased blood flow to cochlea (e.g. loss of hearing, visual acuity, taste)	
Endocrine	Decreased synthesis/release/actions of hormones (poor regulation of parameters, e.g. blood glucose)	
Cardiovascular	Effects of autonomic inadequacy, atherosclerosis, and reduced peripheral circulation (e.g. hypotension, hypertension, coronary heart disease, ulceration)	
Skeletal	Decreased bone density (e.g. osteoporosis), decreased vertebral column length (i.e. decreased height), fissures of joint cartilage (e.g. osteoarthrosis)	
Gastrointestinal tract	Effects of autonomic inadequacy (e.g. decreased motility, decreased secretions)	
Lungs	Loss of elastin (reduced vital capacity)	
Kidneys	Loss of nephrons (decreased glomerular filtration rate)	
Immune system	Decreased immunity, increased autoimmunity	

Q Why are the above changes associated with ageing?

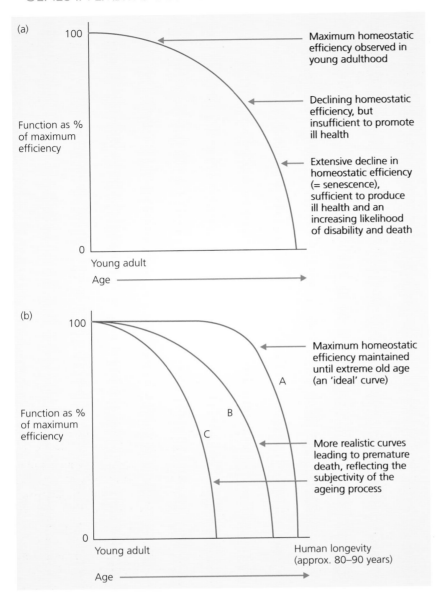

Figure 19.22 Survival curves. (a) Survival during ageing is depicted in terms of the failing capacity with age to maintain homeostasis. (b) Different-shaped curves indicate relative differences in the consequences of ageing. Curve A indicates maximal survival of a population (i.e. health maintained to maximal longevity). Curve B indicates a situation much as today. Curve C indicates a situation more representative of the early twentieth century when average lifespan was much shorter than it is today

disruption of cell architecture, loss of membrane receptors, decreased contractility of muscle cells and decreased secretory activity of glandular cells; Table 19.3). The picture is one of increasingly profound alterations in cell functions (Figure 19.23).

Functional decline generally commences after about the late twenties, and leads to an increased susceptibility to disease and an increased probability of death (collectively referred to as senescent changes). The considerable physiological 'reserve' that people possess means that functional decline causes little serious hardship for many people until the 'reserve' is significantly reduced. Thus, a capacity to compete in physical events may be diminished by early middle age but day-to-day functioning is generally adequate. For most people, therefore, senescence does not produce notable physical difficulties until the late adulthood/elderly years (and even then many do not

experience major difficulties). With improvements in the treatment of infectious disease, and a growing understanding of the nature of many inherited disorders, it is these senescent processes that are increasingly viewed as the major challenge to health in the developed world.

Humans have a finite lifespan and the effects of age *per se* on the functioning of physiological systems exhibit many similarities between individuals. However, the rate at which function declines with time varies considerably. Reasons for this are not entirely understood, and the completion of the Human Genome Project (see Box 19.8, p.539) is expected to provide opportunity for further research into the genetic components. There is also an association of certain disorders of, for example, the circulatory system, the digestive and respiratory tracts and the skeletomuscular system with environmental influences such as diet, employment and lifestyle, and such extrinsic links

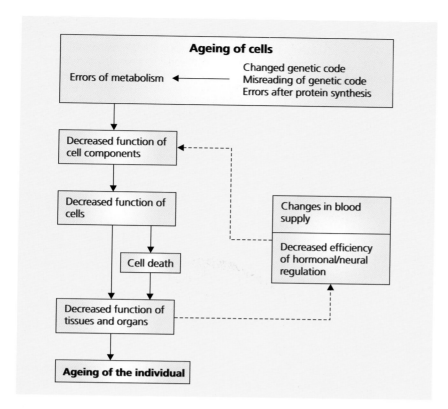

Figure 19.23 Cellular ageing and ageing of the individual. Note the role of genes/gene expression within cells (see also Figure 19.24), and the positive feedback effect of deterioration in circulatory, hormonal and neural functioning

have prompted vigorous health education and promotion programmes in recent years. As the genome is increasingly better understood it is likely that new health education recommendations will evolve that will reduce the risk of accumulating genetic changes that might also lead to ill health (see 'Multifactorial, or polygenic, phenotypes', p.538, and Box 19.14). In other words, senescence may not be considered inevitable, or at least its progress might be slowed. Various theories have been proposed during the last 50 years to explain physiological decline during adulthood.

Theories of biological ageing

Traditionally, ageing has been viewed as a process of 'wear and tear'. In other words as we age our tissues begin to 'wear out'. The loss of teeth might be fitted into this theory because any wear is not repaired as it is accrued. However, major changes such as the gradual deterioration of skeletal joints cannot be considered in the same light since these are dynamic tissues that are repaired through life. 'Wear and tear' therefore reflects a declining ability of the tissues to carry out this maintenance. Theories of ageing therefore seek to explain this declining capacity, and how the rate of decline seems to be variable between people.

Programme theories

Some researchers have looked for evidence of the presence of a 'central clock', or controlling tissue, which might be responsible for triggering ageing. For example, the thymus gland involutes toward the end of adolescence and then atrophies. The incidence of autoimmune disorders also increases with age and

this, together with thymus changes, could implicate the immune system as an ageing 'clock'. It is also feasible, however, that autoimmune responses are a consequence and not a cause of the ageing process. Other research has centred on the pineal gland. This gland produces melatonin (involved in circadian rhythmicity – see Figure 22.6, p.615) and calcifies during adulthood, hence its putative link with ageing. Interestingly melatonin is a potent anti-oxidant and so may provide a degree of protection against cellular changes with age (see 'free radical' theory, below) and its secretion is decreased with age. The possibility of a central clock mechanism cannot be entirely discounted but most age research today focuses on processes that are occurring within individual cells.

In the 1960s Hayflick and coworkers demonstrated that cultured human cells could only undergo about 50 cell divisions before the culture declined and died (Hayflick and Moorhead, 1961), and that this was independent of factors such as nutrient supply. Findings that the maximum possible divisions (called the 'Hayflick limit') is considerably reduced in cultured cells from individuals with inherited forms of accelerated ageing (called progeria; e.g. Hutchinson–Gilford syndrome), and in normally aged individuals, strongly suggest that ageing is an intracellular phenomenon. Although unrepresentative of cells that do not undergo cell division through life, the 'Hayflick number' is considered by most researchers to reflect the ageing process (Box 19.16). Recent studies therefore have tended to concentrate on cellular processes and ageing. Theories in this respect have also been around for a long time, but have gained credence.

BOX 19.16 TELOMERES

These are pieces of DNA found at the tips of the chromosomes. The integrity of these stretches is maintained through the activity of an enzyme called telomerase. The 'Hayflick limit' to cell division is related to the loss of telomere length, caused by declining activity of telomerase. These are interesting findings because the process provides insight into the declining ability of cells to divide as we age (Goyns and Lavery, 2000). Finding a means of manipulating telomerase is an avenue of current research into the biology of ageing.

Of further interest is the way in which cancer cells are able to maintain telomerase and their telomere length. In doing so they are able to 'escape' the 'Hayflick limit' and so become 'immortal' (Ju and Rudolph, 2006). Preventing cancer cells from behaving this way is another area of research activity.

BOX 19.17 LONGEVITY OR SENESCENCE?

'Longevity' is a term used in connection with the maximal lifespan of a specie. In humans this is of the order of 90 years or so (longevity does not equate with statistics of average life expectancy); some people do live longer than this but they are exceptional. Longevity varies between species and undoubtedly has a genetic basis. Indeed, some of the genes involved have now been identified, leading to speculation that gene manipulation might in the future extend human longevity to 120 years or even more.

'Senescence' covers the processes of chronic decline in biological function that contributes to species longevity but also determines the individual's actual lifespan. It is these processes that social change and medical science has influenced during the last 150 years (see Figure 19.22) but has led to concerns of demographic change in which the numbers of elderly people in the population are increasing. The problem is largely one of dependency – if senescence can be better understood so that late adulthood is still a period of health and/or economic activity then the demographic change becomes less of a concern. Extending human longevity, therefore, may not be desirable unless the rate of senescence can be reduced. This means understanding more of the cellular mechanisms of ageing, but also of the environmental factors that contribute to functional decline.

The 'programme theory of ageing' suggests that there are specific genes that promote metabolic decline once they are activated or deactivated. These act as a genetic 'clock' and could help to explain the widely different lifespans of different animal species. The inherited syndromes of accelerated ageing (e.g. the progeria Werner syndrome involving a gene on chromosome 8) provide strong evidence for the presence of such genes. In addition, molecular biologists have identified genes that may be activated during the normal ageing process. The role of 'ageing genes' is debatable, however, and some researchers consider that such genes probably determine the maximal longevity of species but there are other mechanisms that promote senescence, the rate of which varies considerably between individuals (Box 19.17). For example, breeding experiments in animals, such as roundworms, flies and mice, have identified that continually selecting for long-lived individuals can increase the longevity of the laboratory population, perhaps by 50%. Senescence is seen as a different process, and many studies suggest that cumulative disturbances of enzymatic processes in cells are involved.

Damage or error theories

These theories suggest that senescence is the consequence of an accumulation by cells of metabolic disturbances, or their consequences in cells. Indeed, senescence is sometimes explained in terms of a 'disposable soma', that is, genes and hence cell functions are maintained during the peak reproductive years but then errors are then 'allowed' to accumulate and so cell functions begin to decline. In their proposals many overlap with genetic ideas, although they do not propose a 'programme' theory as such. Metabolic disturbances may result from cumulative genetic mutation, or the activation of 'ageing' genes or errors in protein synthesis (Figure 19.24).

Genetic influences

The 'somatic mutation theory of ageing' suggests that DNA mutations accumulate throughout life, with consequences for cell functions. There is a degree of evidence for this but the extent of nuclear DNA mutation that has been observed is probably insufficient to account for the extent and range of functional disturbances associated with ageing.

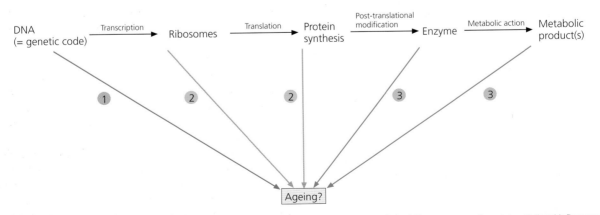

Figure 19.24 Putative effects of ageing on metabolism. 1, genetic influences; 2, effects on transcription/translation processes; 3, post-translational influences

Q What effect does ageing have on metabolism?

Recent studies have extended this theory by showing that mitochondrial DNA and mitochondrial membranes are damaged during life. Mitochondrial DNA is extranuclear DNA, which contains only a small number of genes that are particularly involved in controlling mitochondrial function. Mutation of these genes will have consequences for cellular respiratory processes and evidence indicates that oxidative metabolism does indeed decline with age (Trifunovic and Larsson, 2008).

Superoxidant chemicals, called 'free radicals', have been implicated as the cause of mitochondrial damage. These are produced by normal respiratory reactions but are so reactive that they are rapidly catabolized. Although existing only transiently, their continued production means that they are always present, albeit in small quantities, and will exert some activities. The 'free-radical theory' (proposed by Harman, 1956) is not new, but recent advances in the study of molecular biology have only recently made it possible to investigate its implications. This is now the major theory in the biology of ageing (Barja, 2007).

Transcriptional/translational errors in protein synthesis

The 'error catastrophe theory' (Orgel, 1963) proposes that errors in transcribing the genetic code, or in ribosomal translation of that code, results in the loss of vital enzymes, or perhaps the production of novel ones. This theory is supported by findings that substances do indeed accumulate in cells with age, for example lipofuscin (age pigment) is observable as brown patches in the skin. Lipofuscin does not appear to be detrimental to cell function, but it is possible that other accumulations may be. The theory is 'catastrophic' as it implies that the loss of enzymes, or the production of novel substances, could disturb the activities of other enzymatic processes, which in turn causes further disruption, and so on.

Recent studies have found that there is indeed an accumulation of aberrant proteins during ageing, for example proteins that have been glycated (collectively called Maillard products). Glycation is the spontaneous, but inappropriate, combination of glucose with proteins and occurs as a consequence of the continuous presence of glucose within the cell. It is distinct from the process by which certain proteins are metabolically combined with glucose to produce glycoproteins that are vital for cell function. Glycated enzymes will not be effective. The theory suggests that the resultant accumulation of Maillard products disturbs cell function. Readers interested in this topic might like to consult Bengmark (2006) for further information.

The 'cross-linkage theory' (Bjorksten, 1968) proposes that proteins synthesized by cells increasingly link together during life, with resultant disruption of protein structure and function. For example, the loss of intermolecular cross-linkage of collagen is largely responsible for the loss of tissue elasticity, including skin wrinkling. This too might be considered as aberrant protein and the older we are the greater will be their accumulation.

A unified theory?

In terms of their basic proposals, the theories that suggest post-translational changes in proteins are responsible for senescence overlap with theories of genetic mutation and transcriptional/translational errors. A growing view is that age-related changes in cell functions arise through an integration of effects arising from increasing amounts of inactive proteins, a rise in the functional half-life of proteins, increased damage to mitochondria and a drop in energy generation per mitochondrion.

When does ageing begin?

Metabolic theories of ageing imply an accumulation of errors in cell functioning, and this could mean that the ageing process is initiated much earlier in life, perhaps even before birth. The emphasis currently placed on preconceptual and antenatal care might support this notion. For many people, however, biological ageing is synonymous with physiological decline during adulthood. The involution of the thymus gland in late adolescence, and the possibility that 'ageing genes' are activated at some time during the life cycle, could support the triggering of ageing as an event in early/middle adulthood.

In functional terms, the years between conception and adolescence mark a period of increasing physiological efficiency, and this also argues against the view that age-related cellular homeostasis decline occurs throughout life. It could, of course, be that the dynamic changes induced by developmental responses, prompted by altered genetic activity and resultant hormonal changes, exceed any negative effects of the ageing process.

Clearly, this is an area of debate but is one that is important in the context of producing health promotion and health education programmes, for example in the possible use of anti-oxidant vitamin supplements to counteract oxidative damage by free-radical activity (Foksinski *et al.*, 2007).

IMPLICATIONS OF ADVANCES IN GENETICS FOR HEALTH CARE

Genetic disorders have proved extremely resistant to curative methods. Therapies have generally been directed at the maintenance of health for as long as possible, rather than cure. However, large leaps in the identification of genes, and understanding as to how they operate, have been made during the last 20 years as part of the Human Genome Project and related research. Recent advances in molecular biology have also furthered knowledge and understanding of genetic disease and advances in the treatment of such disorders are on the horizon. New therapies including gene therapy and pharmaceutical preparations that will modulate gene actions or actions of gene products are beginning to appear or enter trials. Alongside these developments are studies that are increasing the understanding of how environmental factors influence gene and gene expression.

It is likely that in the future an individual's medical records will contain their total genome as well as a personalized list of single base-pair variations that can be used to precisely predict their reaction to certain drugs and environmental stressors. This will allow individualized treatments and hence new successful treatments. Medically, it will be possible to gauge a person's susceptibility to specific homeostatic imbalances (diseases), which will then give the person the opportunity to alter their lifestyle so as to decrease the probability of developing such imbalances or to be treated with preventive or disease-delaying drugs.

In other words, advances in gene technologies and in understanding how genes work seem likely to have a major impact on future health and healthcare delivery, not to mention on social factors (e.g. issues surrounding genetically modified foods, and even the use of gene scanning for approval for life insurance policies). While some of this may sound futuristic an important message here is that the genetic revolution is happening now; the future is on the horizon. This section outlines some of the processes that will underpin future health developments based on genes and their activities.

Genetic screening

Gene tests (see Table 19.4) are the modern and most complex of the methods used to test for genetic diseases. They involve direct examination of the DNA. Other genetic tests include tests for gene products (enzymes). Genetic tests are increasingly used for:

- preimplantation genetic diagnosis (of embryos generated by *in vitro* techniques);
- prenatal diagnostic testing;
- newborn screening;
- screening of adults for recessive alleles;
- presymptomatic testing for predicting adult onset of inherited disorders such as Huntington's disease;
- confirmational diagnosis of a symptomatic individual;
- forensic/identity testing.

As noted earlier (see Box 19.6, p.533), application of amniocentesis and chorionic villus sampling to identify fetuses at risk is not new. The focus has mainly been on karyotyping, with more recent introduction of maternal testing for blood-borne markers of congenital disorder. This situation is changing rapidly as techniques are now available that can identify the presence of certain mutated genes in cells, although this might only be looked for if there is a known risk. The screening of early embryos is possible *in vitro* because cells can be removed from embryological stages without affecting later development of that embryo (see Box 19.2, p.525). Chromosomal and gene analysis of the extracted cell can then identify which embryos will be affected; unaffected embryos might then be chosen for implantation. This technique has already been applied in a number of cases of single-gene disorders when the parents are known carriers of the allele, for example cystic fibrosis.

Neonatal genetic testing for monogenic diseases will probably become the norm. Some of the ambiguity of early embryonic

Table 19.4 Examples of common DNA tests

Test names, ABBREVIATION	Description of the diseases or symptoms
Alpha-1-antitrypsin deficiency, AAT	Emphysema and liver disease
Amyotrophic lateral sclerosis, ALS	Lou Gehrig's disease; progressive motor function loss leading to paralysis and death
Alzheimer disease*, APOE	Late-onset variety of senile dementia
Gaucher disease, GD	Enlarged liver and spleen, bone degeneration
Inherited breast and ovarian cancer*, BRCA 1 and 2	Early-onset tumours of breasts and ovaries
Hereditary nonpolyposis colon cancer* , CA	Early-onset tumours of colon and sometimes other organs
Congenital adrenal hyperplasia, CAH	Hormone deficiency; ambiguous genitalia and male pseudohermaphroditism
Cystic fibrosis, CF	Disease of lung and pancreas resulting in thick mucous accumulations and chronic infections
Duchenne muscular dystrophy/Becker muscular dystrophy, DMD	Severe to mild muscle wasting, deterioration, weakness
Dystonia, DYT	Muscle rigidity, repetitive twisting movements
Fanconi anaemia, group C, FA	Anaemia, leukaemia, skeletal deformities
Factor V-Leiden, FVL	Blood-clotting disorder
Fragile X syndrome, FRAX	Leading cause of inherited learning disability
Haemophilia A and B, HEMA and HEMB	Bleeding disorders
Hereditary haemochromatosis, HFE	Excess iron storage disorder
Huntington's disease (HD	Usually midlife onset; progressive, lethal, degenerative neurological disease
Myotonic dystrophy, MD	Progressive muscle weakness; most common form of adult muscular dystrophy
Neurofibromatosis type 1, NF1	Multiple benign nervous system tumors that can be disfiguring; cancers
Phenylketonuria, PKU	Progressive learning disability due to missing enzyme; correctable by diet
Adult polycystic kidney disease, APKD	Kidney failure and liver disease
Prader Willi/Angelman syndromes, PW/A	Decreased motor skills, cognitive impairment, early death
Sickle cell disease, SS	Blood cell disorder; chronic pain and infections
Spinal muscular atrophy, SMA	Severe, progressive muscle-wasting disorder in children
Thalassemias, THAL	Anaemias – reduced red blood cell levels
Tay–Sachs disease, TS	Fatal neurological disease of early childhood; seizures, paralysis

* Susceptibility tests, provide only an estimated risk for acquiring the disease.

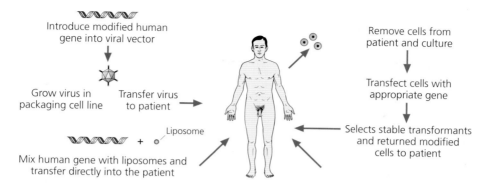

Figure 19.25 **Gene and cell therapies.**

health and illness developmental processes will be known as scientists will know the timing of human gene expression.

In adults gene screening techniques could also identify their carriage of alleles (perhaps because of family history) that might be inherited in their future children. Also, the risk of developing a polygenic condition later in life might be estimated since the genetic predisposition can be assessed. This could provide a means of enabling people to predict risk; for example, a gene scan might one day enable assessment of the risk of someone developing insulin-dependent diabetes mellitus (most of the group of genes involved are now known, although their functional significance is not). The advantage is that if there are any environmental risk factors in the progression from predisposition to the actual condition then these could perhaps be minimized or avoided. However, gene tests provide only a statistical probability for acquiring the disease: some individuals who carry a disease-associated genetic mutation certainly do not develop the disease. Geneticists consider that these mutations may cooperate together with one another and/or with unknown mutations and/or with environmental stressors to cause disease. Nevertheless, if there is access to the information then this could have implications if the individual wishes to obtain life insurance, or perhaps even long-term employment. Individuals also may not wish to be aware of the propensity, or perhaps may not be able to afford a scan.

The advancement of gene profiling of individuals will be more clear-cut, and profiling increasingly will be used in cases of determining paternity and in criminology in identifying criminals, victims of criminal injustice and proving mistaken identities.

There are important moral and ethical questions to be asked but these situations are increasingly possible, and likely. Gene analysis may seem extraordinarily 'high-tech' but the cost of gene analyses is falling rapidly as technology improves and there has even been speculation that self-testing might be a possibility in the near future.

Functional genomics

The Human Genome Project already is having an impact on identifying genes connected with disease. A number of genes (and their base sequences) have been identified, positioned and associated with specific diseases, examples of which are provided in this chapter. The location of these genes offers precise targets for the development of useful new therapies.

The possession of an individual's base sequence, it is predicted, will permit a novel approach to genetic research. Prior to the publication of the human genome geneticists studied one or a few genes at a time; now, however, geneticists are armed with whole-genome sequences, so they can tackle questions much more systematically. For example, for a breast tumour, geneticists can study all the genes in a genome, or how blocks of numerous genes and their enzymes cooperate with each other interdependently to control the chemistry of life.

The volume of genomic data increases almost daily, so the test in the future will be to determine how genes and enzymes cooperate with each other and with the environment to create the complicated homeodynamic mechanisms with human beings throughout their lifespan. Scientists have predicted that systematic studies of functional genomics (i.e. transcriptomics, proteomics, structural genomics, new experimental methodologies and comparative genomics) will be the attention of biological research in this century and onwards:

- Transcriptomics involves the scrutiny of messenger RNAs, produced when genes are active, and will identify when, where and under what conditions genes are turned 'on' and 'off'.
- Proteomics involves the study of gene products (i.e. enzyme production, structure and function). These studies will provide more information as to what is happening in the cell than gene-expression studies. This has applications for drug design.
- Structural genomics research entails producing three-dimensional structures of one (or more enzymes) from each enzyme family, thereby presenting clues to function and to targets for drug design.
- Experimental methodologies can now evaluate the tasks of genes and the enzymes they encode through 'knockout studies' to inactivate genes and so analyse alterations to metabolism that could reveal gene functions. Several animal 'knockout' models, especially strains of mice, are now available to scientists.

BOX 19.18 GENE THERAPY METHODS

Most studies involve inserting a 'normal' gene into the genome to replace a defective disease-causing gene. A vector (i.e. a carrier molecule) is used to transport the therapeutic gene to the patient's specific target cells (Advani *et al.*, 2007). At present, the most frequent vector is a virus that has been genetically modified to transport normal human genes. Viruses encapsulate and carry genes to human target cells in a pathogenic manner (see Chapter 13, p.362). Scientists use this knowledge to manipulate the virus genome to remove disease-causing genes and insert normal (or therapeutic) genes. A patient's target cells (e.g. liver cells) are infected with the viral vector. The vector then transports its genetic material (plus the therapeutic human gene) into the target cell. The production of a normal functional enzyme from the therapeutic gene restores the cell to a normal state.

Viral vectors

- *Retroviruses*: the nuclear material of this type of virus is in the form of RNA, which has to be copied to make DNA via the process of reverse transcription (the virus has an enzyme called reverse transcriptase for this purpose). The new double-stranded DNA is then inserted into the chromosomes of host cells. Attenuated viruses will not be able to manufacture new viral RNA but the DNA will be engineered to include human genes.
- *Adenoviruses (e.g. common cold virus)*: the nuclear material of this type of virus is in the form of double-stranded DNA. Such a genome cause respiratory, intestinal and eye infections in humans and so the modified viruses provide potential vectors for delivering engineered DNA into these tissues.

- *Herpes simplex viruses*: the nuclear material of this class of virus (e.g. Herpes simplex virus type 1 is a common human pathogen that causes cold sores) is in the form of double-stranded DNA. They infect various tissues, for example nerve cells, and could be vectors for engineered DNA in these tissues.

Non-viral vectors

An alternative technique involves the creation of liposomes. These comprise a synthetic lipid sphere with an aqueous core (which carries the therapeutic genes). The lipophilic nature of the liposomes allows the passage through the lipid component of the cell membrane of the target cell.

Therapeutic genes may also enter target cells by chemically connecting the DNA to a molecule that will attach to specialized cell receptors. The DNA–receptor complex enters the target cell via the process of phagocytosis (see Figure 13.10, p.378). This delivery method is less effective than other options.

Synthetic chromosomes

Scientists are experimenting with introducing an engineered 47th man-made human chromosome into target cells. The theory is that this chromosome would reside independently alongside the other 46 chromosomes without affecting their workings. The advantages of carrying large quantities of therapeutic genes may protect the individual from multiple diseases. The dilemma with this potential method is the complexity in transporting such mass amounts of genetic material to the nucleus of a host's target cells.

- Comparative genomics consist of comparing the genes of humans with those of other organisms, so as to understand further how human gene organic base sequences influence function.

Genetic engineering and gene therapies

Genetic engineering utilizes 'recombinant DNA technology' that was developed during the 1970s and 1980s as a means of producing large quantities of a particular gene or gene product so that sufficient of it was available for research purposes. It involves either:

- incorporating a fragment of DNA into a host cell (usually a bacterium) which, by multiple cell division, then produces multiple copies of the DNA fragment and its genes which can then be extracted; or
- utilizing the enzyme DNA polymerase to directly produce multiple copies of the DNA fragment.

Modern genetic engineering has extended these techniques to the incorporation of DNA fragments into cells of higher, more complex organisms including humans, with the intention of altering cell functioning.

Gene transplantation (called transgenics) first involves incorporating a piece of DNA that contains the required allele into a vector such as a modified virus or a microscopic lipid droplet (called a liposome), and allowing the vector to penetrate the target cells (Box 19.18).

The DNA becomes incorporated into the genome of the recipient cell. If the transplanted allele is a dominant form, then this will influence cell function. To be effective in correcting an established disorder, a normal allele must be transplanted into the majority of the affected cells in extensive, already differentiated, tissues. One way is to transplant the gene into stem, or germinative, cells from which new tissue cells will be derived; another is to use a method which provides access to large areas of tissue, using perhaps viruses that specifically infect those tissues. The expansion of technologies to facilitate this application can be seen in the increasing developments of genetically modified foods. Clinically, the method has been used, with apparent success, to treat leukaemia in young babies and attempts are currently being made to introduce sufficient genes to produce significant health improvements in people with conditions such as cystic fibrosis. Transgenics therefore is an exciting development, which for the first time could aid the prevention or correction of genetic disorders.

The transplantation of genes into embryos involves much the same techniques and so is technologically feasible. The manipulation of genes within embryos is restricted and such work has been confined to animal studies. It understandably raises concern regarding the legal and ethical position of embryo manipulation and the prevention of abuse of these techniques to enable parents to select 'desirable' characteristics for their offspring.

'Designer' drugs

Explorations into the function of each gene will offer information on how faulty genes are involved in causing disease. Consequently, commercialism is moving away from diagnos-

BOX 19.19 STEM CELLS

Gene therapy has potential for the development of transplantation tissue from stem cells. These are cells found in most, if not all, tissues even in adults and are undifferentiated, or only partially differentiated cells that might be triggered to develop further and differentiate into cells of a particular tissue type. This may occur within a damaged tissue, and recent research has begun to identify the chemical factors produced by tissues that trigger this, and which also might be used by medicine to manipulate the differentiation. This, coupled with cloning techniques, raises the possibility of producing large numbers of activated stem cells *in vitro* for transplanta-

tion, for example into neural tissue. Such cells could regenerate new tissue in disorders such as Parkinson's disease or where there has been tissue trauma.

Large numbers of stem cells are required to raise the confidence of success and the level of functional improvement should the transplantation be accepted. Young cells (i.e. embryological cells) are likely to be most effective. These two aspects have led to suggestions that the government allow the cultivation of early human embryos to provide the stem cells. This is clearly an emotive area and one that is fraught with moral and ethical issues (Harris, 2004).

---

tics and toward developing a pioneering generation of therapeutics founded on genes.

'Pharmacogenomics' is the study of how a patient's genome affects their reaction to drugs (Court, 2007). New medicines derived from a rational and logical approach to the use of gene sequence and enzyme structure and functioning is replacing the traditional trial-and-error means. Drugs targeted to specific places in the body provide the assurance of having fewer side-effects than many of today's medicines. For example, some areas of cancer research are currently investigating this approach by using antibody–drug complexes to target abnormal antigens on tumour cells, or by using drugs that will act to modify or replace the actions of those altered proteins involved in the cell cycle.

It is predicted that in the future doctors will be able to test genetic profiles against classes of drugs available, for maximum potential benefit for the individual. Matching drugs to the individual and adapting them to each person's genome will be a significant advance towards individualizing care.

Cloning

Boxes 19.4, p.530 and 19.9, p.541 identified some of the issues in relation to cloning. One major potential benefit is the use of such techniques to produce tissue for transplantation. If (when?) developmental genes can be modulated then cloning techniques could generate tissues that have been triggered to form specific cell types for implantation into recipients. In this way, functioning tissues could be transplanted to replace dysfunctional ones, leading to new repair technologies in disorders such as Parkinson's disease that as yet have no known cure (Box 19.19).

Genetic fingerprinting

The ability of scientists to replicate a DNA sample many times over, and hence to determine the genetic coding of the sample, has enabled the analysis of minute traces of DNA. This has facilitated crime investigations (hence the term 'DNA fingerprinting') and the identification of related species of plant or animal (both extant and extinct!). In addition, the human genome contains within it sequences that mutate little and which will be almost constant between closely related individuals. The family link can also be assessed by comparing mitochondrial DNA (i.e. DNA found within the cell mitochondria rather than in the nucleus). This DNA is only inherited through the female line as the mitochondria of spermatozoa are jettisoned with the tail at fertilization.

SUMMARY

1 Genes are sections of DNA and a sequence of constituent bases that provides the information necessary for a cell to synthesize a specific polypeptide, and hence determine that cell's characteristics.

2 The DNA of a cell is packaged prior to cell division as chromosomes. There are 23 pairs of chromosomes in each body cell (i.e. 23 chromosomes inherited from each parent). There is thus a duplication of genes (except on the sex chromosomes of males where the Y chromosome is considerably smaller than the X chromosome). Each member of a pair of genes is called an allele. The pairs of alleles separate in meiosis during the formation of the gametes, however, and the alleles on either chromosome can potentially be inherited by offspring.

3 Fertilization of an oocyte by a spermatozoon produces a zygote which undergoes a number of changes prior to implantation into the uterus. Selective gene activation is first apparent in the blastocyst phase. Tissue differentiation continues and increases in complexity following implantation. Differentiation is further evidence of selective gene activation and most tissues are basically formed by weeks 7–8 after fertilization. The embryo is now considered to be a fetus.

4 Fetal development is primarily one of growth and functional maturation. Nutrient exchange with the mother is facilitated by the development of the placenta, although this also has numerous other functions.

5 Embryo differentiation and fetal development are influenced by the gene mix that has been inherited from the parents, and by environmental factors that affect uterine environment and/or maternal well-being.

6 Mutation, or alteration, of the genetic code in one of a pair of alleles is possible, in which case the person is said to be heterozygous. Such a mutation may be of no consequence if the mutated allele is recessive to the normal dominant one on the homologous chromosome, since the normal protein associated with the gene will be synthesized. If the mutation is dominant, however, then the cell will synthesize the protein determined by that allele, with possible damaging effects.

7 Although recessive alleles may remain 'hidden' in heterozygous individuals, there is always a possibility that a child may inherit copies of the allele from each parent. With no dominant counterpart to sup-

SUMMARY

press it, the mutated allele will now contribute to protein synthesis and cell function. The potential effects of losing a normal protein, or of producing the novel protein, can be devastating and is the basis of most recognized genetic diseases.

8 Mutated alleles on the X chromosome are unlikely to have corresponding alleles on the smaller Y chromosome. Thus male offspring will always be affected even if the mutation is recessive to the normal form. This means that males cannot be 'carriers' of a recessive allele in the usual sense and some disorders typically are observed more frequently in boys than girls.

9 Characteristics produced by the net effects of multiple genes are less sensitive to the effects of mutation of an individual allele within the group, but the more mutations that are inherited the greater the likelihood will be that mutation of the remainder of the 'group' will occur during life. Thus a susceptibility to a disorder can be inherited, with consequences later in life.

10 Functional changes during adulthood are mainly those of declining homeostatic efficiency, with an increasing susceptibility to ill health.

11 Theories abound as to how the ageing process affects tissues, and most focus on interference with the synthesis of functional proteins, especially enzymes. Recent advances have pinpointed specific

metabolic effects, primarily in relation to cell respiration, but the influence of extrinsic factors on the ageing process is still unclear.

12 Pedigree analysis can identify people at risk of genetic disorder and so pregnancies can be avoided (depriving a couple of children) or couples prepared for the outcome. Traditional therapies for inherited disorder have been aimed at maintaining as high a standard of life as possible – cures have not been possible. Alternatively, affected fetuses may be aborted. The development of *in vitro* fertilization techniques, coupled with recent advances in the identification of mutated genes, has meant that the implantation of embryos known to be lacking certain mutations is possible, and will result in an unaffected child.

13 Identification of the human genome has accelerated the understanding of what genes do, and how their expression is controlled. It is opening up new, radical possibilities for diagnosis, embryo selection, and evaluating health risks. Advances in genetic engineering are beginning to make the treatment of certain genetic disorders appear possible, and such genetic therapies could represent a major breakthrough in medicine. However, gene therapy and related genetic technologies evoke powerful moral and ethical debate, the outcomes of which have many ethical–moral issues that are still to be resolved.

REFERENCES

Advani, S.J., Weichselbaum, R.R. and Chmura, S.J. (2007) Enhancing radiotherapy with genetically engineered viruses. *Journal of Clinical Oncology* **25**(26): 4090–5.

Agustines, L.A., Lin, Y.G., Rumney, P.J. *et al.* (2000) Outcomes of extremely low weight infants between 500 and 750 g. *American Journal of Obstetrics and Gynaecology* **182**(5), 1113–16.

Alfirevic, Z., Sundberg, K. and Brigham S. (2007) Amniocentesis and chorionic villus sampling for prenatal diagnosis. *Cochrane Database of Systematic Reviews* Issue 3, CD003252. Oxford: Update Software.

Baker, L.K. and Denyes, M.J. (2008) Predictors of self-care in adolescents with cystic fibrosis: a test of Orem's theories of self-care and self-care deficit. *Journal of Pediatric Nursing* **23**(1): 37–48.

Barja, G. (2007) Mitochondrial oxygen consumption and reactive oxygen species production are independently modulated: implications for aging studies. *Rejuvenation Research* **10**(2): 215–24.

Bengmark, S. (2006) Impact of nutrition on ageing and disease. *Current Opinion in Clinical Nutrition and Metabolic Care* **9**(1): 2–7.

Bittles, A.H., Bower, C., Hussain, R. and Glasson, E.J. (2007) The four ages of Down syndrome. *European Journal of Public Health* **17**(2): 221–5.

Bjorksten, J. (1968) The cross-linkage theory of aging. *Journal of the American Geriatric Society* **16**: 408–27.

Bortolotti, L. and Harris, J. (2006) Embryos and eagles: symbolic value in research and reproduction. *Cambridge Quarterly of Healthcare Ethics* **15**(1): 22–34.

Court, M.H. (2007) A pharmacogenomics primer. *Journal of Clinical Pharmacology* **47**(9): 1087–1103.

De Robertis, E. (2006) Spemann's organizer and self-regulation in amphibian embryos. *Nature Reviews Molecular Cell Biology* **7**: 296–302.

Doswell, B,H., Visootsak, J., Brady, A.N. and Graham J.M. Jr (2006) Turner syndrome: an update and review for the primary pediatrician. *Clinical Pediatrics* **45**(4): 301–13.

Elsner, D. (2006) Just another reproductive technology? The ethics of human reproductive cloning as an experimental medical procedure. *Journal of Medical Ethics* **32**(10): 596–600.

Emery, A.E.H. (2006) *Muscular Dystrophy*, 3rd edn. Oxford: Oxford University Press.

Foksinski, M., Gackowski, D., Rozalski, R. *et al.* (2007) Effects of basal level of antioxidants on oxidative DNA damage in humans. *European Journal of Nutrition* **46**(3): 174–80.

Goyns, M.H. and Lavery, W.L. (2000) Telomerase and mammalian ageing: a critical appraisal. *Mechanisms of Ageing and Development* **114**(2), 69–77.

Harman, D. (1956) Aging: a theory based on free-radical and radiation chemistry. *Journal of Gerontology* **11**, 298–300.

Harris, J. (2004) *On Cloning*. London: Routledge.

Harrison, G. and Goldie, D. (2006) Second-trimester Down's syndrome serum screening: double, triple or quadruple marker testing? *Annals of Clinical Biochemistry* **43**(Part 1): 67–72.

Hayflick, L. and Moorhead, P.S. (1961) The serial subcultivation of human cell strains. *Experimental Cell Research* **25**, 585–621.

Ju, Z. and Rudolph, K.L. (2006) Telomeres and telomerase in cancer stem cells. *European Journal of Cancer* **42**(9): 1197–203.

Orgel, L.E. (1963) The maintenance of accuracy of protein synthesis and its relevance too aging. *Proceedings of the National Academy of Sciences, USA* **49**: 5117–21.

Petersen, A. (2006) The best experts: The narratives of those who have a genetic condition. *Social Science and Medicine* **63**(1): 32–42.

Porche, D.J. (2007) Klinefelter syndrome. *Journal for Nurse Practitioners* **3**(7): 443–4.

Rao, A., Rothman, J. and Nichols, K.E. (2008) Genetic testing and tumor surveillance for children with cancer predisposition syndromes. *Current Opinion in Pediatrics* **20**(1): 1–7.

Said, S. and Malone, F.D. (2008) The use of nuchal translucency in contemporary obstetric practice. *Obstetrics and Gynecology* **51**(1): 37–47.

Streetly, A., Clarke, M., Downing, M. *et al.* (2008) Implementation of the newborn screening programme for sickle cell disease in England: results for 2003–2005. *Journal of Medical Screening* **15**(1): 9–13.

Tabata, T. and Takei, Y. (2004) Morphogens, their identification and regulation. *Development* **131**(4): 703–12.

Takayama, T., Miyanishi, K., Hayashi, T., Sato, Y. and Niitsu, Y. (2006) Colorectal cancer: genetics of development and metastasis. *Journal of Gastroenterology* **41**(3): 185–92.

Trifunovic, A. and Larsson, N.G. (2008) Mitochondrial dysfunction as a cause of ageing. *Journal of Internal Medicine* **263**(2): 167–78.

Wald, N. (1991) Prevention of neural tube defects: results of the Medical Research Council Vitamin Study. *Lancet* **338**(8760): 131–7.

Weetch, E. and MacDonald, A. (2006) The determination of phenylalanine content of foods suitable for phenylketonuria. *Journal of Human Nutrition and Dietetics* **19**(3): 229–36.

Weinstein, L.B. (2007) Selected genetic disorders affecting Ashkenazi Jewish families. *Family and Community Health* **30**(1): 50–62.

Zwicker, J.G. and Harris, S.R. (2008) Quality of life of formerly preterm and very low birth weight infants from preschool age to adulthood: a systematic review. *Pediatrics* **121**(2): e366–76.

CHAPTER 20

PAIN

INTRODUCTION

Most people think they know what pain is, yet from a scientific point of view, much still has to be discovered. It is difficult for researchers to agree upon a definition, and further difficulties arise in developing a suitable theory to account for all the different observations that have been made (Melzack and Wall, 1965, 1996). A person's personality, culture, mood and social influence have all been suggested by many studies to affect the perception and expression of pain. Although pain perception can be considered to be a 'sense', to understand how pain can be subjective needs more discussion than was possible when the senses were described in Chapter 7.

This chapter begins with a definition of pain. It then investigates the functions of pain, and the types of pain a person may perceive. The neurophysiology associated with Melzack and Wall's gate control theory of pain perception will also be discussed. An integrated scientific perspective using the nature–nurture interactions as a template will be used to understand the gate control theory. This involves linking the socio-psychology with the neurophysiology associated with pain perception. Various assessment tools will be also reviewed, and those factors that must be taken into consideration during objective assessment of pain will be discussed. The principles of the gate control theory will be used to explain the site of action of pharmacological and non-pharmacological agents commonly used by healthcare professionals.

Definition of pain

The word 'pain' is derived from the Greek word 'poine' for 'penalty', and thus suggests the concept of punishment and retribution. Any credible definition must include the subjective nature of pain, as emphasized by McCaffery's (1983) famous definition that 'Pain is whatever the experiencing person says it is, existing whenever he says it does'.

Pain thresholds

Pain threshold refers to the level of stimulation at which the person just begins to perceive pain. There is considerable debate over the existence of an absolute pain threshold for each individual, since the threshold is affected by socio-psychological and 'physical' factors, such as anxiety, hospitalization, age and experience. Thus, individual thresholds fluctuate within the individual, as well as being personal to individuals within the population. Some of the factors that account for this subjectivity are highlighted later in the chapter. Thresholds can be divided into those of:

- pain perception, when the perception of stimuli (e.g. temperature change or pressure) reaches a level when the person begins to feel pain for the first time;
- severe pain – the point when the pain becomes unbearable for the person if stimulus strength is increased further. This is sometimes referred to as pain tolerance.

In general, studies have shown little difference between the values obtained for pain perception thresholds across different social and ethnic groups, whereas values for the severe pain threshold differ markedly, and this may be explained by cultural and psychophysiological variations.

Functions of pain

Pain has survival and protective values. For example, the pain sensation that occurs before serious injury, such as when a person picks up a hot object, produces immediate withdrawals in order to prevent further damage. Subsequently, through conditioned learning and socialization, the person avoids future injurious objects.

Pain associated with injuries may be considered a homeostatic disturbance, since damaged cells are involved in the release of pain-producing substances. Injuries set limits on activity by enforcing inactivity and rest, which itself aids faster recovery. In this sense, rest and inactivity could be considered as crude homeostatic adaptive mechanisms. Injury pain therefore serves useful purposes. However, on occasions, long-lasting pain may be considered a homeostatic imbalance (i.e. since it is continual and persistent) that seems to have no useful value (e.g. some amputees suffer excruciating phantom limb pain for years and sometimes for life; Ehde *et al.*, 2000).

ACTIVITY

Discuss what you understand by the statement that 'pain is a homeo-static imbalance'.

Varieties of pain

Classifying the type of pain aids the selection of appropriate assessment tools and therapies to suit the individual needs of the patient. Clinically, pain is classified as acute or chronic.

Acute pain

Acute pain is usually (and should be) dealt with adequately, and is relatively short lived: a beginning and an end are often identifiable. It is viewed positively as a warning signal, which draws attention to injury or illness, and is experienced by everyone at some stage in their lives. Acute pain can range from a relatively minor acute pain, such as toothache, to a relatively major pain, such as postoperative pain. The characteristics of acute pain are usually those associated with tissue damage and anxiety-led features exhibited in the psychophysiological 'fight, flight and fright' reactions (see Figure 21.6, p.598). Accompanying these reactions is a preoccupation with the cause of the pain and its consequences.

Chronic pain

In contrast to acute pain, chronic (intractable) pain has no biological value. It is disabling and is easily recognizable, but it is poorly understood. The pain overwhelms the patient, and is often associated with anxiety, depression and insomnia.

A qualitative difference between acute and chronic pain exists since it affects the person differently, whether psychologically, physiologically, emotionally or spiritually. It is impossi-

ACTIVITY

Read the articles by Fitzsimons *et al.* (2000), and Chen and Chang (2000).

ble to predict when chronic pain will end; it often gets worse rather than better, it is poorly controlled and therapies are generally ineffective (Cunningham, 2000). Examples include arthritic and cancer pains. Chronic pain can be so terrible and detrimental to one's life that some people would rather die than continue living with it.

ACTIVITY

Distinguish between acute and chronic pains.

Pain perception: an overview

Pain perception involves five components (Figure 20.1):

- *Specialized pain receptors*: it is unclear what constitutes a pain receptor (nociceptor). Some nociceptors are probably free nerve endings, which are only sensitive to chemicals (e.g. bradykinin, lactic acid, prostaglandins) perhaps released from damaged cells in the vicinity. These are classified as a type of chemoreceptor. Other nociceptors are complex encapsulated structures sensitive to pronounced mechanical deformation (e.g. stretching, crushing, tearing, cutting) and extreme temperature change (e.g. scalding, burning and freezing). These are classified as types of mechanoreceptors and thermoreceptors, respectively. Some nociceptors respond to only one type of stimulus, while others are capable of responding to chemical, mechanical and thermal stimuli; these are known as polymodal nociceptors. Nociceptors are attached to distal ends of primary afferent pain fibres. Various aspects of the anatomy of pain pathways are recognized:
- *Primary afferent pain fibres*: these are sensory fibres that transmit the pain message as an electrical impulse towards the central nervous system. Other primary afferents function to inhibit the passage of pain impulses (covered later).
- *Ascending nociceptive nerve fibre tracts*: these are stimulated by a pain neurotransmitter released from the primary afferent pain fibres at synapses throughout the dorsal horn of grey matter in the spinal cord (and certain brain sites, e.g. thalamus). They conduct the pain impulse to the higher pain centres of the brain (i.e. within the cerebral cortex).
- *Higher pain centres of the brain*: these interpret the electrochemical impulses conducted in pain fibres, originally derived from the noxious stimuli, as a perception of pain.
- *Descending nerve fibre tracts*: the descending nerve fibres conduct impulses from the brain to the spinal cord. These are involved in modulating the perception of pain by influencing neural transmission in the ascending tracts.

Once pain has been perceived, the individual responds in a variety of ways which is personal to them. Responses to pain

BOX 20.1 PERIOPERATIVE ACUTE PAIN

Surgical nurses and other allied healthcare practitioners are certain to encounter patients in pain during the perioperative period. In acute situations, the surgical patient is often admitted in pain; postoperative pain is also a normal occurrence of surgery itself, and a considerable number of patients discharged from hospital are in pain (Clancy *et al.*, 2002). Perhaps the problem of inadequate pain control may be enhanced further, since there are increasing numbers of patients undergoing day-case or short-stay surgery. Thus, there is a need for better education of hospital staff in postoperative pain control (Redwood, 2000). In support of this, we would argue that surgical nurses (and all healthcare practitioners) must have a sound knowledge of the neurophysiology associated with the subjective nature of this experience, since this would be helpful in the understanding of:

- the different types of pain expressed by the surgical patient;
- the variation that exists between patients in their expression of differing pain intensities, and duration and qualities of pain;
- the site of action of pharmacological and non-pharmacological methods of pain control.

Such an understanding is paramount in assisting the decision-making processes that underpin effective individualized perioperative pain management.

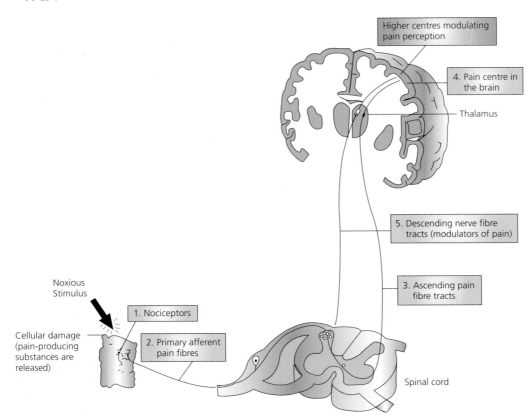

Figure 20.1 The sensory components involved in pain perception

Q What is the relative distribution of sodium and potassium ions on either side of the cell membrane of neurons/muscle cells required to establish the resting membrane potential? What movement of these ions is necessary to produce the (1) depolarized, (2) repolarized and (3) hyperpolarized phases of the action potential?

are categorized as either behavioural or physical, manifested by sympathetic activity. The former responses include vocal responses (e.g. moaning,), verbal statements (e.g. 'Ouch, that hurts'), facial expression (e.g. grimacing), restricting movement and/or adopting a guarding behaviour ('protective rigidity'). Sympathetic responses include nausea, vomiting, gastric stasis, decreased gut motility, and impaired renal activity.

NEUROPHYSIOLOGY OF PAIN PERCEPTION

In order to generate pain, there is usually cellular damage. This may arise as a result of a surgical incision, traumatic injury, tumours compressing surrounding soft tissues, myocardial infarction, etc. Tissue damage promotes the appearance of the classic signs of inflammation (see Figure 11.16, p.293). Accompanying inflammation are a variety of chemicals secreted from nerve endings, blood vessels, phagocytes, lymphocytes and tissues cells as a number of homeostatic reflexes go into operation to promote the healing of the damaged tissue (Clancy and McVicar, 1997). These chemicals are responsible for promoting the familiar localized signs (swelling/oedema, redness/erythema, heat/vasodilation, and pain) of the inflammatory process. This chapter is concerned only with the chemicals that induce pain and those that enhance responses to painful stimuli.

Pain-producing substances

Pain-producing substances released from damaged tissue include histamine, prostaglandins and kinin-like compounds, such as bradykinin. These substances combine with receptor binding sites on nociceptors, the initiators of the neural transmission associated with the perception of pain. In order to initiate a neural impulse, the interaction between pain-producing substances and nociceptors must reach the level of stimulation required to activate the nociceptor (i.e. generate an action potential; see Chapter 8, pp.186–9); in most circumstances this level seems to equate to a person's pain perception threshold. The brain interprets the intensity of pain according to the number of pain impulses it receives within a set period of time: the more impulses it receives, the greater the intensity of the pain (Figure 20.2).

Prostaglandins are among the most important initiators of pain. These chemicals are synthesized from an essential fatty acid, arachidonic acid, aided by the enzyme prostaglandin synthetase. Prostaglandins sensitize nociceptors, thereby enhancing the effects of other pain-producing substances. Accordingly, these chemicals may be considered the most important pain-producing substances in the human body (Clancy and McVicar, 2002; Clancy *et al.*, 2002). They also enhance pain fibre response to non-noxious stimuli in polymodal nociceptors. Kinins (e.g. bradykinin) sensitize polymodal nociceptors to heat and mechanical stimuli.

The secretion of histamine from certain white blood cells (basophils or mast cells) is instigated by a number of chemical mediators, including interleukin 1 and nerve growth factor, released in the vicinity of damaged tissue. At low concentrations, histamine stimulates sensory neurons to produce an itching sensation; at high concentrations, it evokes a painful sensation.

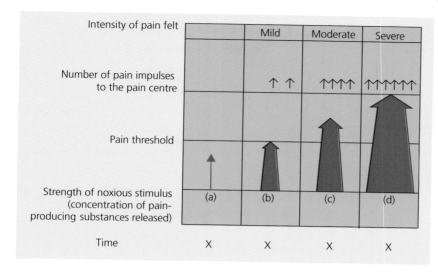

Figure 20.2 Pain threshold and the intensity of pain perception. (a) Minimal tissue damage, threshold not met, no pain impulse, no pain felt. (b) More tissue damage, threshold reached, few pain impulses sent to the pain centre, 'mild' pain felt. (c) Further tissue damage, threshold superseded, more pain impulses sent to the pain centre, 'moderate' pain felt. (d) Severe tissue damage, threshold superseded further, many more pain impulses sent to the pain centre, 'severe' pain felt

Q Using the text and this figure, distinguish between the following: (1) pain perception threshold, (2) severe pain threshold, and (3) pain tolerance.

Nociceptors (free nerve endings) are located extensively in the dermal layer of the skin (see Figure 16.5, p.452), periosteum (layer of fibrous tissue surrounding bones), articular surfaces of joints, walls of arteries and the dura mater (outer membrane covering of the spinal cord and brain). Deeper tissues, particularly the walls of the internal organs (collectively called viscera) are supplied less extensively. Cutaneous pain receptors have a relatively high threshold. Thus, a strong stimulus is required to generate an electrical signal that initiates the train of events resulting in pain perception.

ACTIVITY

List the pain-producing substances released from cells following injury.

Anatomical location of nociceptors

Nociceptors are located at the distal end of afferent pain neurons. These neurons are of two particular types (the classification of neurons can be found in Table 8.3, p.189): small-diameter, myelinated A-delta fibres and smaller, unmyelinated C fibres. These are classified as the 'fast' and 'slow' pain fibres, respectively, since faster transmission is associated with thicker fibres and the presence of a myelin sheath. The A-delta fibres conduct impulses at a speed of 5–25 m/second; C fibres conduct messages at 0.5–2 m/second. To put these into context, an A-delta fibre could potentially conduct an impulse from a toe-end receptor to the brain (say, approx 2 m in an adult) in 0.1–0.4 seconds but that in a C fibre would require 1–2 seconds. This difference in speed has implications for quickness of response, for example in a withdrawal reflex (see Box 20.2 and Chapter 8, p.193). Nociceptors for fast pain fibres are located only in the skin and mucous membranes; nociceptors for slow pain fibres are found in the skin and most other body tissues, except the brain's nervous tissue, which is insensitive to pain.

The gate control theory

Melzack and Wall in 1965 proposed a gating mechanism within the dorsal horn of grey matter of the spinal cord. These gates were the layer of cells called the substantia gelatinosa, through which sensory (afferent) pain impulses have to pass before they are relayed to, and perceived in, the pain centre(s) of the brain. It is now generally accepted that every neuron is a

---

BOX 20.2 SHARP AND DULL PAINS AND REFLEXES: AIDS TO DIAGNOSING

If the patient describes their pain as sharp and prickling, this informs the healthcare practitioner that the pain fibres involved are mainly of the A-delta type. This type of pain can be located precisely by the patient, because A-delta fibre nociceptors send pain signals along discrete pathways to the somatosensory cortex of the brain, which enables the pain to be established to within a few centimetres of the source (Bennett, 2000).

Fast pain is often accompanied by withdrawal reflexes, activated via flexor motor neurons in the anterior horns of the spinal cord that activate the effector organ, usually a muscle, to instigate a protective withdrawal contraction in an attempt to avoid any further damage (Bennett, 2000; see Figures 8.18, p.184 and 8.25, p.193). This reflex exhibits itself when a person stands on a sharp object or touches a hot surface. To the trained practitioner, protective withdrawal reflexes may be used to establish the origin of the damage, and thus may be considered an aid to diagnosis. For example, when a patient instinctively covers the right lower quadrant of the abdomen or the left side of the chest, the practitioner may suspect the pain/damage is of appendix or cardiac origin, respectively. This knowledge, together with other signs and symptoms, may aid a diagnosis of appendicitis and angina, respectively.

If the assessment indicates that the pain is characteristically dull, burning, troublesome, aching, poorly localized, of persistent nature, and is somatic in origin, it informs the practitioner that the pain fibres involved are C-type fibres. Torrance and Serginson (1997) proposed that the immediate pain of a surgical incision is mediated by A-delta fibres, but within a few seconds, the pain becomes more widespread because of C-fibre activation.

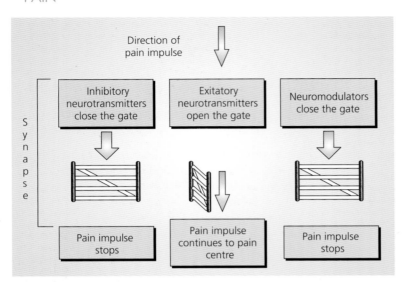

Figure 20.3 The chemicals involved in opening and closing the gateway of pain

Q Name the pain-producing substances mentioned in this chapter.

'gate'. The gates are symbolic of synapses between afferent neurons and various ascending and descending tract neurons. The gate control theory suggests that information can pass through when the gate is 'open' but not when the gate is 'closed'. The opening of the gate is caused by the release at the synapse of an excitatory neurotransmitter (called substance P). The closing of the gate is brought about by the release of inhibitory neurotransmitters and neuromodulators (Figure 20.3).

ACTIVITY

Before continuing, review the relevant sections in Chapter 8 for a discussion on excitatory and inhibitory neurotransmitters involved in synaptic conduction (see also Figure 8.24, p.192). It will help your understanding if you also look at Figures 20.3 and 20.4 while reading the following section.

The gating mechanism depends upon two modifying factors:

• the balance of activity of primary afferent (sensory) neurons;
• the modulatory control of pain provided by descending fibres from the brain's higher centres.

Primary afferent fibre input

The afferent neurons, which provide input to the gate, are:

• *the nociceptors of A-delta and C pain fibres*: these neurons release substance P, an excitatory neurotransmitter, at synapses (i.e. 'gates') within the central nervous system;
• *the mechanoreceptors containing thick myelinated faster-transmitting A-beta neurons*: these fibres release inhibitory neurotransmitters (e.g. serotonin) at synapses within the central nervous system. They do not themselves convey pain information but are modulators of the pain afferent neurons.

BOX 20.3 REDUCING THE PAIN ASSOCIATED WITH INJECTION

Before giving an injection, some healthcare practitioners pinch the area to be injected. This activates mechanoreceptor and their faster-transmitting A-beta fibre input to the gate, thereby closing it and inhibiting the slower pain signals induced by the penetrating needle.

ACTIVITY

Using Figure 8.22 and Table 8.3, p.189, review the conduction properties of myelinated A-delta and A-beta fibres (i.e. saltatory transmission) and unmyelinated C fibres (i.e. local circuitry, non-saltatory transmission).

If the dominant input to the gate is via the faster-transmitting A-beta fibres, then the gate will close due to the release and action of the inhibitory neurotransmitters.

There are many possible modes of action of these inhibitory neurotransmitters (Clancy and McVicar, 2002; Clancy *et al.*, 2002), either by acting presynaptically (i.e. before the release of substance P) or postsynaptically (i.e. after the release of substance P). These are summarized in Figure 20.4.

Inhibitory neurotransmitters may be operative presynaptically via a number of possible mechanisms:

• repressing the gene activity necessary for the enzyme synthesis involved in substance P production. This seems an unlikely mechanism in acute pain as it assumes that substance P is produced upon stimulation, whereas presynaptic neurons typically store neurotransmitter in vesicles (see Figure 8.24, p.192);
• blocking the 'active site' of the enzyme, thus inhibiting the production of substance P. Again, unlikely in acute pain;
• destroying the presynaptic fibres stores of substance P;
• preventing substance P release by decreasing the presynaptic membrane permeability to electrolytes or substance P itself, or by inducing its hyperpolarization of the presynaptic

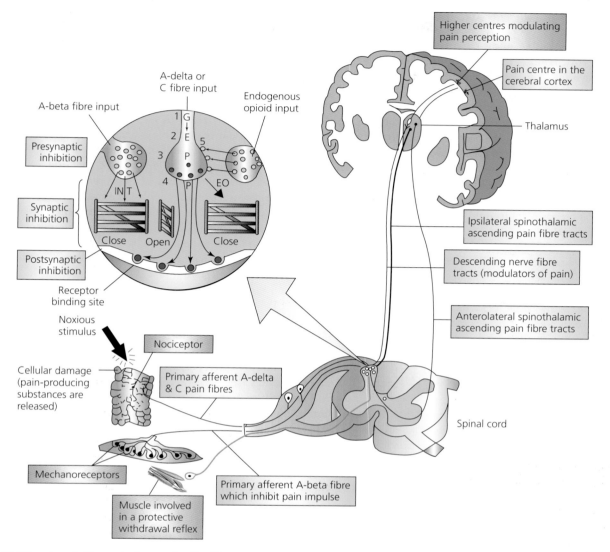

Figure 20.4 The gate control theory of pain perception. Possible sites of action of inhibitory neurotransmitters (INTs) and endogenous opiates (EOs – neuromodulators). Presynaptic inhibition: 1, INTs repress the gene necessary for the synthesis of enzyme for substance P (P); 2, INTs block enzyme activity, thus inhibiting the production of substance P; 3, INTs destroy vacuolated substance P; 4,5, INTs and EOs prevent substance P release by decreasing the presynaptic membrane permeability. Synaptic inhibition: INTs destroy substance P within the synapse. Postsynaptic inhibition: INTs compete for substance P receptor-binding sites. PPS, pain-producing substances. E, enzyme; G, gene

Q Outline the principles behind the gate control theory of pain perception, using the following terms: pain-producing substances, inhibitory neurotransmitters, excitatory neurotransmitters, neuromodulators, nociceptors, endogenous opiates, A-delta pain fibres, C pain fibres, A-beta fibres, threshold, afferent input, descending fibres, pain centre, higher cortical centres, kinins, prostaglandins, endorphins, and enkephalins.

Q Differentiate between the following: (1) nociceptor and polymodal nociceptors, and (2) inhibitory neurotransmitters and excitatory neurotransmitters.

membrane, thus making it more difficult for impulses to conducted.

Inhibitory neurotransmitters may be operative synaptically by:

- destroying substance P within the synapse (although this seems unlikely);
- competing for substance P's receptor binding sites on the postsynaptic membrane, hence inhibiting the impulse from travelling in postsynaptic pain fibres.

In contrast, if the dominant input to the gate is from the afferent A-delta and/or C pain fibres, the gate may be open (see later section on additional influences from descending modulator control), owing to the release and the postsynaptic action of the excitatory neurotransmitter substance P (Figure 20.4). The pain impulse normally passes from the dorsal horn of the grey matter in ascending pathways, which, in the main, cross to the opposite side of the spinal cord before relaying upwards to the thalamus of the brain. These pathways are logically called the anterolateral spinothalamic ascending pain tracts.

Some ascending pain fibre tracts (referred to as ipsilateral spinothalamic tracts; 'ipsi-' = same) relay upwards to the thalamus, while remaining on the same side of the cord.

Most A-delta fibres terminate in the thalamus, where they synapse with further neurons that transmit the signals to other basal areas of the brain and to the somatosensory cortex. Up to one-quarter of the C pain fibres terminate in the thalamus; the rest terminate in three distinct areas of the brainstem. Specific pain centre(s) have not yet been located. Melzack and Wall (1996) stated that the cerebral cortex may not contain specific pain centres, and may just process the information it receives before transmitting it deeper into the brain tissue. It is generally believed that pain is perceived via activity in the midbrain, but the appreciation of its unpleasant qualities depends on the cerebral cortex.

In some ways the passage of sensory impulses from nociceptors to the brain is analogous to the general pattern of afferent pathways of the senses (see Chapter 7, p.143). However, as we have seen, transmission of pain can be modulated within the ascending pathway by mechanoreceptor inputs. It is also important to note that pain perception will also only occur if there is no or insufficient interference via descending fibre input to the gate from higher centres of the brain.

Descending modulator control from higher centres of the brain

The gate theory proposes that even if A-delta and C fibre input into the central nervous system dominates over the mechanoreceptor A-beta fibre input, the pain gate may still be closed. This is because areas of the brainstem, such as the reticular formation, raphe nuclei, trigeminal nuclei and vestibular nuclei, together with various nuclei of the hypothalamus and cerebral cortex, can modify the gating process via descending neural mechanisms (Figure 20.5). These are termed pain inhibitory complexes where the interaction takes place in the dorsal horns of the spinal cord (Bennett, 2000). The neurons of descending fibres release a variety of endogenous opioids (i.e. opium or morphine-like in action but not extracted or derived from opium extract; e.g. endorphins, enkephalins, dynorphins). These neuromodulators bind to receptor sites on the presynaptic membrane of the pain fibres, and 'close the gate' by inhibiting the release of the pain neurotransmitter, substance P (Figure 20.4). Because of their function, these opioids have been referred to as the body's own natural painkillers (Clancy and McVicar, 2002). Morphine and related opioid analgesics, and opiates such as heroin (note: opioid and opiate are often used interchangeably but technically an opiate is a chemical extracted or derived from opium. Thus, heroin and morphine are true opiates but synthetic analgesics based on morphine are not), also act on the opioid receptor sites, hence their effectiveness in pain management. The distribution of opioid-binding sites has been found to be uneven, with the highest concentration in the limbic system, thalamus, hypothalamus, midbrain and spinal cord, suggesting that these are important locations of pain gates.

The reticular formation projections from the brainstem exert a powerful inhibitory control over the spinal gating mechanism. These projections are also influenced via somatic (body) input, and input from auditory and visual centres. In addition, cortical projections, particularly from the frontal cortex (this area subserves cognitive processes, such as past experience), also pass to the reticular formation to mediate the control over the spinal gating mechanism. Cognitive processes can also influence gating mechanisms directly via their large fast-conducting corticospinal (pyramidal) fibre tracts (Figure 20.5). Melzack and Wall (1965) proposed the idea of a 'central trigger' that activates particular brain processes, such as past experience and memories. Psychological processes have an extremely important role in pain perception, and research has shown that factors such as anxiety and helplessness can intensify the pain experienced. Thus, interventions that reduce anxiety or helplessness can reduce the pain experienced and enhance coping.

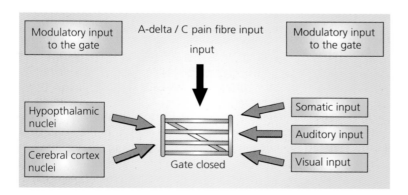

Figure 20.5 Higher centre descending fibres modulating control of pain. This shows that the higher centre input to the gate dominates over the pain fibre input so pain is not felt; however, this is not always the case

Q Name the endogenous opiates mentioned in this chapter.

ACTIVITY

Review your notes and reflect on your learning. Use Figure 20.4 and the interim summary below to revise your understanding of the operational workings of the gate control theory of pain perception.

Interim summary

If the combined effect of pain modifiers (i.e. inhibitory neuro-transmitters and endogenous neuromodulators) does not exceed the pain fibre input to the gate, then the gate is opened, and afferent pain neurons transmit their activity via the antero-lateral spinothalamic tracts from the spinal cord to the thalamus. Within the thalamus, they synapse with other neurons, which transmit the impulses to the pain centre(s) of the brain (wherever they are!). Therefore, it follows that the 'closing of the gate' is the basis of pain relief and is thus achieved via the inhibition of:

- the synthesis and/or the secretion of pain-producing substances;
- nociceptor activation;
- the electrical events associated with depolarization of pain fibre membranes;
- the synthesis or release or the actions of substance P.

In short, for the person to perceive pain, the afferent pain fibre input to the gate must dominate. To provide analgesic relief, this domination must be removed via increasing the mechanoreceptors afferent input and/or the descending neuron input to the gate. The concept of individualized pain relief is therefore based on knowledge of the patient's background, the progress of the illness, the type and magnitude of the injury (e.g. surgical procedure employed), the area undergoing damage, and the durability/delicateness of the surrounding tissues. These are all relevant factors that need to be considered if peri-operative pain management is going to be successful.

The subjectivity of pain

Pain is a subjective experience, since each individual has a unique personal range of anatomical, physiological, social and psychological identities. These identities, using the nature–nurture interactions template, can be applied to the gate control theory to help explain the subjective nature of pain perception. The concept of individualized pain relief is also perhaps based upon this template to the gate theory.

Anatomical subjectivity

The size and shape of the human body is controlled genetically and modified by environmental factors (e.g. diet, exercise, occupation, predisposing illness, etc.). Thus, a tremendous variation in human body shapes and sizes exists (see the case study on obesity in Section VI, p.636), and so it follows that the number and distribution of nociceptors and their pain fibres, together with inhibitory afferent fibres and neural modulatory descending fibres varies enormously between individuals. This could be expected to produce regional variations of anatomical subjectivity in sensitivity and, or desensitivity (or resistance) to noxious stimuli.

Biochemical and physiological subjectivity

Individuals have different production capacities of the bio-chemicals involved in the pain pathway. A person's active genome is responsible for the production of physiologically active enzymes necessary for the biochemical synthesis of pain-producing substances, substance P, inhibitory endogenous opioids and inhibitory neurotransmitters. From an evolutionary perspective the genome has been shown to change by the action of the five forces of evolution (i.e. mutation, random genetic drift, natural selection, population mating and culture) so it is possible that the genes responsible for the synthesis of pain-producing substances and/or substance P are changed (i.e. mutated) or repressed (switched off), and/or that the nociceptors become desensitized to pain-producing substances, and so perhaps these people then would experience tissue injury without perceiving pain, or less pain. Alternatively, some people may not report pain, despite tissue damage, if the genes necessary for the production of the endogenous opioids or inhibitory neurotransmitters are repeatedly expressed, since their high levels would close the gate. Conversely, high levels of pain-producing substances (including substance P), or low levels of endogenous opioids and/or inhibitory neurotransmitters as a consequence of gene activity or inactivity, respectively, would lead to pain hypersensitivity. Congenital disorders of pain perception exist; some people are born insensitive to pain, while others feel pain without any detectable injury (Melzack and Wall, 1996).

Generally, though, studies suggest that the strength of stimulus required to activate nociceptors does not vary enormously between people; variation relates to pain perception and, especially, to pain tolerance.

ACTIVITY

Review your understanding of the operon theory in Chapter 2, p.47.

Sociological subjectivity

Social factors affect psychophysiological functioning of the human body (interactionist theory – see Chapter 1, p.16) and therefore may be responsible indirectly for either opening or closing the pain gate. Social factors influence the development of the brain; these higher cortical centres may conceivably influence the physiological, neuronal and synaptic activity of the gate by influencing the descending control.

Anxiety is a state that may be determined genetically and/or socialized environmentally. It is well documented in the healthcare literature that an elevated anxiety level is associated with an increased pain perception and reduced tolerance, and vice versa. Consequently, a role of the healthcare practitioner is to reduce a patient's anxiety in order to potentially decrease or abolish their pain. The gate control theory would attribute this

BOX 20.4 CARE AND ANXIETY

Usually, the patient's anxiety level is heightened with admission to hospital, the thought of the impending diagnostic procedures and, if applicable, surgery itself. As noted, anxiety influences pain and so these features influence the person's perception of pain, and are often associated with pre-hospitalization sleep loss (Desjardins, 2000). This has implications for pain assessment since it may not represent a reasonable baseline for subsequent times. Healthcare practitioners should aim to reduce the patient's anxiety before attempting to 'quantify' the pain that the patient perceives. Perhaps, then, an appropriate healthcare action might be just to empathize and support the patient in pain, since this physical assurance perhaps can have analgesic qualities.

increased anxiety to a reduced levels of endogenous opioid and/or an increased level of substance P. Some advocates of the descending fibre control theory state that decreased endogenous opioid is the most likely scenario. However, the authors of this text suggest that it is not quite as straightforward as this. Some studies have shown anxiety to be associated with a temporary increase in endogenous opioids. Obviously, we are not advocating that health carers should raise a patient's anxiety, since for the majority of the time, depressed endogenous opioid release is the norm.

Cultural differences in the perception of pain are observed, and therefore need to be taken into consideration when assessing pain. This could suggest that past socializing experiences and individual conditioning have important influences on the subjective elements of pain. Socialization determines psychological behaviour, which could conceivably affect the output of endogenous opioids.

The importance or meaning of a situation can affect one's perception of pain (Box 20.6).

BOX 20.5 CARING FOR ALL CULTURES

Healthcare curricula should be dynamic in meeting the demands of today's multicultural societies. Practitioners should be concerned with management of pain by using constant patient monitoring, and according to the patient's perception of their pain. Professionals should be familiar with cultural differences when reducing the patient's anxiety before assessing the appropriate care to be implemented.

BOX 20.6 THE PROCESS OF HOSPITALIZATION MAY EVEN REDUCE PAIN

In general, studies reflect that pain perception is affected by the process of hospitalization. That is, before hospital admission the pain to the patient seemed almost unbearable, whereas following admission, interviews indicate that the pain has lessened or even gone. Perhaps the fear of a serious diagnosis results in a surge of endogenous opioid gene activity! If this is the case, then it demonstrates how environmental factors, such as the clinical setting, presence of doctors and other healthcare practitioners, and unfamiliar and possibly high-technology equipment, may influence gene activity and subsequent opioid release, thus reducing or abolishing the pain and reducing the need for painkillers (Clancy and McVicar, 2002).

ACTIVITY

What do you understand by the following statement: 'Pain is a subjective experience depending on an individual's characteristics'? Think about your answer using the nature–nurture template described in this book.

Pain management: a gate control perspective

The different characteristics associated with acute, chronic benign, chronic malignant, phantom, bone and muscle pains necessitate different therapeutic approaches emphasizing the subjectivity of pain management. Perhaps it could be argued that nurses and other allied healthcare professionals adopt a psychological approach in assisting the patient to understand and to cope with their pain, while doctors are more concerned with the physiological role of diagnosing pain and instigating treatment. However, a considerable degree of overlap exists, depending on the philosophy of the hospital staff, a factor itself that demonstrates subjectivity. We would argue that all healthcare practitioners who care for patients in pain must have a sound knowledge of the neurophysiology associated with this subjective experience, since such an understanding is paramount in assisting the decision-making process underpinning effective individualized pain management.

You are advised to refamiliarize yourself with the content of the previous pages before continuing. In theory, pain can be prevented or relieved by pharmacologically blocking the initiation and/or the transmission of nerve impulses anywhere from the site of damage to the pain centres in the brain. In practice, this is so (Figure 20.6). Thus, the inhibition or modulation of:

- the stimulatory effects of pain-producing substances and the blockade of the nociceptive binding sites can be achieved pharmacologically with local mild oral analgesics;
- the electrical transmission along afferent pain fibres can be achieved via the administration of local anaesthetics;
- the secretion of the pain neurotransmitter, substance P, through synapses ('gates') can be achieved by the administration of opioid analgesics.

Non-pharmacological approaches are also available for pain management and basically operate via increasing the patient's production of endogenous inhibitory neurotransmitters and neuromodulators (Figure 20.6, pathways D and E).

A review of the specific analgesic qualities of pharmacological and non-pharmacological agents now follows. However, before this discussion, it must be stressed that good verbal and non-verbal rapports with the patient (if conscious) are essential aspects of caring, so that the patient feels confident in the practitioner's ability to reduce or abolish their pain. Perhaps this works on a placebo basis – that is, working by increasing the body's natural opioids. (A placebo is any inactive substance resembling medicine given during controlled experiments or to satisfy a patient.)

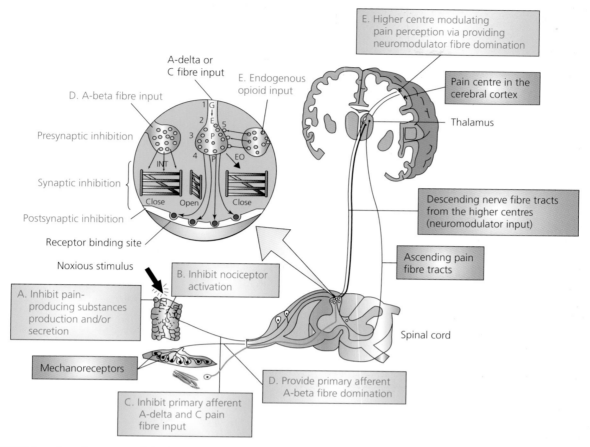

Figure 20.6 Perioperative pain management. A gate control perspective. Analgesia action is provided by: Box A, inhibiting the production and/or secretion of pain-producing substances; Box B, inhibiting nociceptor activation; Box C, inhibiting afferent pain fibre input; Box D, replacing afferent pain fibre input domination by promoting mechanoreceptors afferent fibre input; Box E, replacing afferent pain fibre input domination by promoting neuromodulator descending fibre input domination. E, enzyme; EO, endogenous opiates; G, gene; INT, inhibitory neurotransmitters; P. substance P

PHARMACOLOGICAL PAIN MANAGEMENT

The use of analgesic drugs is the mainstay of immediate pain management. The important aspects of pharmacological therapies are to provide the patient with sufficient pain relief to allow rest, relaxation, pain-free sleep and mobilization, and to avoid the toxic effects of the drugs and the occurrence of breakthrough of pain (Zeppetella *et al.*, 2000). The administration of regular, adequate doses will prevent the latter (Figure 20.7a). If breakthrough pain occurs, higher dosages may be deemed necessary by the healthcare practitioner, rendering the possibility of the appearance of drug toxicity (Figure 20.7b).

Analgesic drug administration can be via a variety of routes, namely oral, sublingual, rectal, inhalation, intramuscular, intravenous, subcutaneous, transdermal, spinal and epidural. Intravenous drugs may also be administered using patient-controlled administration systems.

Pain may be controlled using non-opioid and/or opioid analgesics. If pain persists, then the principles of the 'analgesic staircase' are employed in an attempt to improve pain control (Figure 20.8). The choice of drug depends on:

- the location, type and severity of pain experienced. In general, non-opioid simple analgesics are given to relieve mild to moderate pain. Non-steroidal anti-inflammatory drugs (NSAIDs) are used for generalized pains or local inflammation. Some weak opioids are used to relieve mild to moderate pain, and others are used to relieve moderate to severe somatic pain. Stronger opioids are used for severe somatic pain;
- the pharmacological mode and site of action;
- the potential toxic effects.

Non-opioid analgesics

The non-opioids that are used frequently in clinical pain management are paracetamol and the NSAIDs – diclofenac, ketoprofen, naproxen and ibuprofen (administered for mild to moderate pain relief) and ketorolac (administered for moderate to severe pain relief). Intravenous infusion of diclofenac is also used to prevent the occurrence of postoperative pain (Omoigui, 2005).

Since NSAIDs do not have the side-effects of opioid drugs (e.g. respiratory depression, inhibition of gastrointestinal motility), they are useful alternatives in the management of

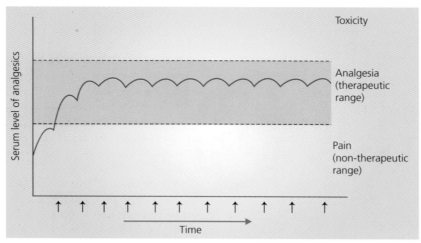

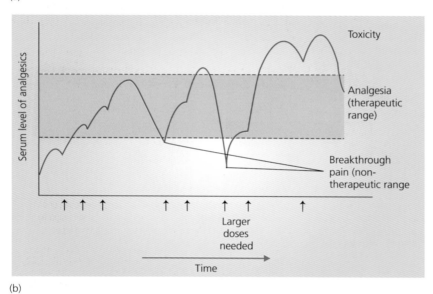

Figure 20.7 (a) Drug administration in successful analgesia. Regular, adequate doses of analgesia are required to alleviate pain. (b) Drug administration in breakthrough pain. Analgesics given at irregular intervals may result in breakthrough pain. Higher doses may then be deemed necessary, rendering the possibility of drug toxicity

Q How is breakthrough pain prevented?

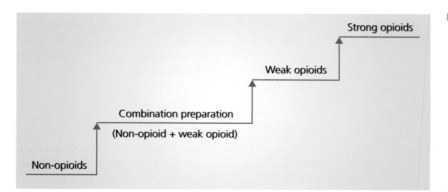

Figure 20.8 Pharmacodynamics (see text for details)

postoperative pain, although they may be inadequate for relief of severe pain as they do not act on the pain gates within the neurotransmission pathways.

Analgesically, some non-opioids act outside the central nervous system in the periphery at the site of injury. For exam-ple, paracetamol (e.g. Panadol) inhibits the formation of prostaglandins by inhibiting the enzyme prostaglandin syn-thetase (see Figure 20.6, pathway A). Aspirin and ibuprofen (a NSAID) are also inhibitors of the enzymes under the umbrella term of prostaglandin synthetase.

ACTIVITY

Refer to Chapter 4, pp.97–9 for a discussion of the lock and key theory of enzymatic action and competitive inhibition of enzyme activity.

Diclofenac and aspirin are thought to inhibit prostaglandin secretion from cells in the damaged area. Ibuprofen, ketoprofen and naproxen (and aspirin) provide analgesic relief by inhibiting the secretion of other chemical initiators (e.g. bradykinin, histamine) of pain (Omoigui, 2005).

Opioid analgesics

Narcotics or weaker substitutes are classified as opioids because of their chemical resemblance to the body's endogenous neuromodulator opioids (i.e. the endorphins, enkephalins and dynorphins). Thus, their analgesic sites of action are the specialized opioid receptors located on the presynaptic membrane of the afferent pain fibres (see Figure 20.6, pathway E). Aspirin also operates centrally on these opioid receptor sites, thus inhibiting pain transmission (Omoigui, 2005).

Opioids provide analgesic relief by:

* depressing the transmission of pain at the spinal cord level in the dorsal horn region;
* stimulating activity in descending inhibitory pathways in the brainstem;
* exerting mood-elevating effects, acting through the limbic system;
* allaying anxiety.

Weak opioid analgesics

The weak opioid analgesics frequently used for the treatment of mild to moderate pain are mainly based on codeine and include codeine phosphate, co-dydramol, co-proxamol and co-codamol. These opioids are classified as narcotic agonists (i.e. their analgesic site of action is at the endogenous opioid receptor-binding site, although their binding/activation of the receptors is less effective than for strong opioids such as morphine). Codeine phosphate is often used in combination with non-narcotic analgesics, such as paracetamol, for symptomatic treatment of mild to moderate pain.

Potent narcotic opioid analgesics

Potent opioid narcotics are the most effective analgesics. These drugs are particularly suitable for treating moderate to severe pain of somatic origin. The most commonly ones used in the UK are morphine, diamorphine, fentanyl, hydromorphone, oxycodone and methadone.

Important pharmacological factors that inform the choice of drug are (1) its pharmacodynamics, (2) the best route of delivery and (3) the adverse effects of the drug.

Pharmacodynamics

This section should be read in association with Figure 20.9. Pharmacodynamics involves the efficacy and potency of the drug. 'Efficacy' is the extent to which a drug has the desired effects, in this instance analgesia. Opioid analgesics are especially effective because they act to modulate neural synapses within the sensory pathway (Clancy & McVicar 1998; Davies & McVicar 2000b). They do this by acting as agonists of receptors to the intrinsic analgesic opioids (i.e. by inhibiting substance P release; see Figure 20.6, pathway E). There are a number of types of receptor to these substances (see 'Adverse reactions' below) and the most effective opioid drugs exhibit a high activation of the type referred to as the **mu** (μ) receptor. Since all of the strong opioids are highly agonistic of the **mu** receptor, they have comparable efficacies.

'Potency' relates to the dose of drug that is required to provide the desired effect. With similar efficacies it might be anticipated that drug doses of strong opioids would also be similar, but this is not the case. This is because the 'bioavailability' of the drugs varies depending upon how the drug is released after swallowing, how it is absorbed across the lining of the tract, and how easily it is distributed to the target tissue including across the blood–brain barrier.

Potency is especially important when considering an oral route of administration. Table 20.1 illustrates how bioavailability and potency varies between the strong oral analgesics,

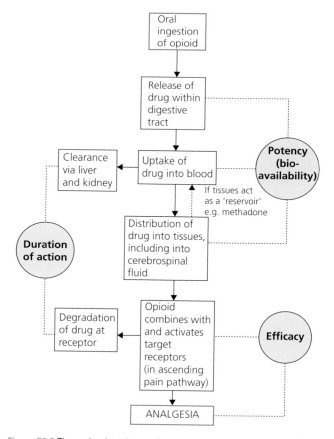

Figure 20.9 The analgesic staircase. This pathway may be used in order to reduce or abolish a patient's pain. If the pain is not removed using non-opioids (e.g. paracetamol), then a combined preparation may be given (e.g. paracetamol plus codeine phosphate). If the pain is still not removed, then weak opioids are given. If pain persists, then a strong opioid is given (Davies and McVicar, 2000b)

Table 20.1 Potency, plasma half-life and duration of action of commonly used strong opioid analgesic drugs. Potency is expressed as a comparison with oral morphine (potency ratio = 1). Data are adapted from Twycross *et al.* (1998)

Analgesic	Potency ratio (relative to morphine)	Oral bioavailability (% of dose)	Time of onset of analgesia after oral administration	Plasma 'half-life'	Duration of action
Morphine	1	18–68%	20–30 minutes	1.5–2 hours	3–6 hours
Hydromorphone	7.5	37–62%	20–30 minutes	2–3 hours	4–5 hours
Oxycodone	1.5–2	70%	20–30 minutes	3–4 hours	4–6 hours
Methadone	5–10	40–100%	30 minutes	8–75 hours*	8–24 hours
Fentanyl	150	Not taken orally	Not taken orally	24 hours*	72 hours**

*Form a reservoir within tissues. See text for details.

**Continuous delivery via skin patch over 72 hours.

but note that the time of onset of analgesia is very similar. This is because the dosage given can compensate for variation in potency.

Duration of action

Once a drug has entered body fluids it will begin to be cleared from blood via the liver and kidneys. Generally speaking, the faster the clearance then the sooner the concentration of the drug in blood will fall below a therapeutic value, leading to breakthrough pain (see Figure 20.7b). Clearance rates may be indicated as the plasma 'half-life' of the drug (i.e. the time required for the concentration of drug in blood plasma to decrease by 50%), but 'duration of action' is a more useful clinical parameter since this can be used when planning therapy. The duration of action of morphine, hydromorphone and oxycodone are broadly similar (Table 20.1) and this reflects their similar rates of clearance.

Methadone and fentanyl have much longer 'half-lives' (Table 20.1) because they form a reservoir in tissues and so clearance is apparently slower. Thus, methadone is more soluble in lipids and distributes more readily throughout the body (it also binds to plasma proteins and so is less easily cleared), while fentanyl is delivered via a skin patch (see 'trans-dermal diffusion', below) and forms a reservoir in the skin. The subsequent extended duration of action of these drugs complicates any titration of analgesia, or conversion to alternative analgesic. The problem is not insurmountable but it does mean that the drugs may not be a first-line choice unless they convey additional benefits:

* Methadone interacts with other types of opioid and non-opioid receptors found within the pain pathway and so has a slightly broader spectrum of action than morphine. Consequently it can be useful if there is hyperexcitability to morphine, or in neuropathic pain that is poorly responsive to morphine (Twycross *et al.*, 1998).
* Fentanyl has less severe adverse reactions than morphine, and its administration via skin patches is easier than infusing diamorphine, and is more convenient for patients (see below).

Route of delivery

Analgesics may be administered via a variety of routes (Table 20.2):

* oral
* injection
* infusion

Table 20.2 Rationale for choice of analgesic drug for administration by injection, via transoral mucosa, or rectally. See text for discussion of other routes: oral administration, infusion and transdermal diffusion

Route	Advantages	Disadvantages
Injection	Excellent bioavailability, very rapid onset of analgesia. Morphine, diamorphine and methadone are all available as injectate Diamorphine is highly soluble so can be injected in relatively small volume	Intravenous injection is likely to precipitate excessive response unless given slowly. Intramuscular (IM) or subcutaneous (subcut) injection preferable Most opioids have low solubility so injectate volume is relatively high. IM or subcut injection likely to be painful
Transoral mucosal	Good bioavailability, rapid onset of analgesia. Only available currently as fentanyl 'lozenge on a stick'	Necessitates retention of drug within the oral cavity so generally not feasible for most opioids. Recent tests of fentanyl have shown rapid onset of analgesia, and good potency
Per rectum	Good bioavailability, rapid onset of analgesia. Oxycodone and morphine are both available in suppository form	The discomfort of this method makes usage in palliative care unlikely

Table 20.3 Comparison of continuous delivery of analgesic via subcutaneous diamorphine and fentanyl skin patch. Data are taken from the text, and adapted from Twycross *et al.* (1998)

	Diamorphine infusion	Fentanyl patch
Efficacy	Good	Good
Time of onset of analgesia	Rapid (10–30 minutes)	Slow (24–48 hours) on first application of patch
Plasma 'half-life'	Short (3 minutes)	Long (17–24 hours)
Titration	Rapid onset and short 'half-life' make titration relatively straightforward	Titration made more difficult by slow onset and long 'half-life'
Conversion	Rapid onset and short 'half-life' make conversion relatively straightforward	Conversion made more difficult by slow onset and long 'half-life'
Adverse reactions	Pronounced in some patients	Often less severe than diamorphine
Cost	Relatively low cost on a per dose basis, but dependent on equipment and professional support so hidden costs	More expensive than diamorphine on a per dose basis but not dependent upon equipment and patches can be self-applied

- transdermal diffusion (via a skin patch)
- transoral mucosal
- Per rectum.

The oral route of administration (for example tablets, solutions or suspensions) is the most common route for administering opioids, apart from fentanyl (but see 'Transoral mucosal'; Table 20.2). The delay to onset of analgesia is 20–30 minutes, but dosage varies between the drugs because of different potencies.

Oral medication as a route for delivery has a significant disadvantage in that blood concentration exhibits fluctuations between doses, and these may be quite sharp. Modified release preparations help to reduce this variability. These preparations maintain blood concentration better because they are formulated in such a way that the release of the drug is controlled, thus reducing the frequency of taking medication.

Deterioration in the condition of a patient, perhaps complicated by dehydration and difficulties in swallowing, may make compliance with oral medication difficult and so continuous administration becomes a better means of maintaining a therapeutic concentration of an analgesic in body fluids. Two methods are used: infusion or transdermal diffusion.

The high solubility of some drugs (for example, dimorphine) make them more suitable for subcutaneous infusion, thus reducing the risks associated with long-term intravenous delivery (discomfort, infection and phlebitis). Direct application into body fluids means that the time of onset is rapid. This, together with a very short (a few minutes) plasma 'half-life', means that titration/conversion can be made readily and effectively.

Transdermal delivery involves applying an easy patch that contains a concentration of drug sufficient to promote its diffusion into and across the skin. This is therefore conceptually similar to subcutaneous infusion, but without the need for an access point or syringe driver. Fentanyl is the only opioid currently available for use in patches. Using skin patches to deliver the drug introduces a number of issues (Table 20.3):

- *Does the patch/drug cause irritation of the skin?* Skin tolerance to fentanyl is good but as an additional precaution it is usual for the patch to be applied to a clean, healthy area of hair-free skin, and to rotate sites for replacement patches to reduce the likelihood of sensitivity developing.
- *Is the rate of diffusion near constant?* Fentanyl is lipid soluble and so readily crosses skin. Uptake of the drug from a patch will be influenced by the rate of blood supply to the skin (i.e. increased if the skin is warmed using a heat pad or if there is fever, and decreased in older people). The patches contain sufficient drug for 72 hours of sustained delivery.
- *On applying a patch for the first time how long does it take for analgesia to be effective?* Blood concentration rises with time. There is a degree of subjectivity but generally, studies using fentanyl patches suggest it takes about 24 hours for a significant decrease in pain to occur and up to up to 48 hours for full analgesia. During this initial phase it is likely to be necessary to provide supplemental analgesic. For example if conversion from morphine to fentanyl is required then morphine can be continued for 12 hours while fentanyl concentrations rise in blood, and any breakthrough pain after this is readily controlled by oral medication (Mitten, 2000).
- *Upon removing the patch, how long is the duration of action?* Fentanyl is metabolized quite quickly. However, the drug continues to be released from a reservoir that forms within the skin and so the plasma 'half-life' is of the order of 17–24 hours (Twycross *et al.* 1998; Fallon, 2000). This makes titration and conversion more difficult when compared with diamorphine infusion. Nevertheless, if breakthrough pain does occur it can readily be controlled by administering a short-acting opioid.

Adverse reactions

The analgesic qualities and side-effects of opioids are a result of the opioid system being comprised of four distinct types of receptors: mu (μ), kappa (κ), delta (δ) and sigma (σ). There are two types of mu receptor: mu-1 and mu-2. Both mu and kappa receptors are believed to mediate analgesia, while delta and sigma mediate the side-effects of respiratory depression, nausea, vomiting and constipation. The distribution of receptors varies; for example mu receptors are found in highest density in the brainstem, and kappa receptors are mainly located in the spinal cord. Thus, exogenous opioid stimulation of kappa receptors results in spinal analgesia, respiratory depressions and sedation. Opioid stimulation of sigma receptors results in dysphoria, depression, hallucinations and vasomotor stimulation. Delta receptors are only stimulated by endogenous opioids. The opioids have different affinities for these receptors (e.g. morphine's affinity for mu receptors is 100 times greater than its affinity for kappa receptors). Hence the frequency and severity of these reactions varies: constipation, drowsiness and nausea are the most common. If a patient finds that morphine-induced reactions are intolerable, it is common policy for a different opioid to be administered. This will be one that induces less severe reactions, usually fentanyl, oxycodone or hydromorphone (Fallon, 2000).

All narcotics produce powerful depression of the respiratory centres in the brain, and acute poisoning is always associated with slow, inadequate respiration, which can endanger the life of these patients (naloxone, an opioid antagonist is administered to reverse respiratory depression). All the drugs of this type are liable to induce nausea and vomiting because they have a stimulant action on the vomiting centre in the brain postoperatively; this may necessitate giving anti-emetics (e.g. metoclopramide or cyclizine) at the same time. Many of them produce characteristic stimulation of the parasympathetic nervous system, which results in constipation (Joint Formulary Committee, 2007).

The dangers (particularly of respiratory depression) of the opioids have stimulated research into discovering analgesic compounds that minimize this side-effect. A number of such compounds exist, e.g. codeine phosphate and dihydrocodeine (DF118) are weak analgesics but are very good cough suppressants. They are, however, constipating.

Rationale for selecting the first-line analgesic

The main consideration in choosing an analgesic is the need to manage pain effectively. Morphine is globally the most commonly recommended first-line strong opioid (World Health Organization, 1996); the drug is successful in controlling about 80% of cancer pain (Twycross *et al.*, 1998). However, it is clear that other effective opioids are available, and this raises the question as to what other factors govern choice.

In relation to oral medication, the slow clearance rate of methadone (Table 20.1) would be problematic from the point of view of titration or conversion, and the availability of suitable alternatives makes it unlikely that it would normally be chosen as a first-line analgesic. This argument does not hold for hydromorphone or oxycodone. These drugs also seem to produce fewer or less severe adverse reactions than does morphine and, being more potent, might therefore be expected to be first-line analgesics rather than a second-line alternative. However, adverse reactions to morphine are not usually intolerable, and largely can be controlled, and so in many instances these drugs do not provide significant additional benefits. Cost effectiveness (and drug availability in some countries) then becomes an important factor and oral preparations of morphine are considerably cheaper than both hydromorphone and oxycodone (*British National Formulary*; Joint Formulary Committee, 2007).

When it is required, the continuous delivery of analgesic is usually achieved either by subcutaneous infusion of diamorphine or by transdermal fentanyl. A summary comparison of these drugs is provided in Table 20.3. Diamorphine and fentanyl are equally efficacious, but the side-effects of fentanyl are tolerated in a higher proportion of patients. However, the patch delivery method for fentanyl produces a delayed time of onset from first application, and extended plasma 'half-life' that introduces considerations regarding titration or conversion. These characteristics have consequential implications for breakthrough pain, though maintaining adequate analgesia is readily achieved using morphine/diamorphine or the fentanyl 'lollipop', although the latter is being phased out in some UK Regional Health Authorities (see Table 20.2). The need to manage pain effectively therefore does not exclude the use of fentanyl patches if continuous opioid delivery is required.

Once again, a further influencing factor will be cost. Fentanyl patches are more expensive than diamorphine infusion (*British National Formulary*; Joint Formulary Committee, 2007). However, using diamorphine might have greater indirect costs, notably the provision of a syringe driver and the resultant input of nursing care/time. Therefore, real cost difference between the two drugs may be less than it at first appears.

Fentanyl is as clinically effective as other opioids, but it is less invasive than subcutaneous diamorphine, and has fewer or

---

BOX 20.7 PALLIATIVE CARE PATIENT/CARER EXPERIENCE

Before reading this section please refer to Figure 1.8c, p.14, and its associated text.

Chronic pain is a complex phenomenon that affects quality of life. Its qualities can be hard to describe and perception of it is not always proportional to the stimulus (Clancy and McVicar, 2002). Successful management therefore requires a thorough 'holistic' assessment including the patients' perception of the pain experience and its effect upon their quality of life (Davies and McVicar, 2000a). Chronic pain also affects those close to the patient and therefore assessment and management ought to include them.

The core standard for palliative care relating to effectiveness states that all patients have their symptoms managed to a degree that is acceptable to them, and achievable by multiprofessional healthcare team intervention with current palliative care knowledge. When one considers the above evidence, there is little to choose between the opioids in terms of clinical effectiveness, but the side-effects and method of administration may be considerations for individual preferences. The aim of pain control is the optimal dose with the fewest side-effects, but when embracing patient choice this becomes the most acceptable side-effects.

Titration

A wide range of analgesics are available to manage chronic pain. Titration is commonly practised in palliative cancer care, in which the type of opioid drug is altered, and dosages are increased if necessary, until pain management is effective (Mercadante, 2007).

BOX 20.8 PATIENT-CONTROLLED ANALGESIA

Patient-controlled analgesia (PCA) is an essential part of the healthcare professional's role in ensuring patient compliance. It allows patients to give themselves their own analgesia by activating a syringe pump or driver and provides a flexible form of pain control. Studies generally acknowledge that the more the patient feels in control of their own pain management, the lower the requirement for analgesia (Parsons, 2000). Other reported advantages of PCA include:

- its apparent safe method of analgesic delivery;
- it bypasses the delays and deficiencies of the more conventional intra-muscular injection method;
- it reduces anxiety. However, we would dispute this generalization, since not all patients feel comfortable being in control of their own analgesic relief. Reassurance may be required that the patient will not become addicted or overdose themselves.

more acceptable side-effects. Consequently, it may be preferable to patients with difficulty taking oral medication (Radbruch *et al.*, 2000). Indeed the survey of Thomason *et al.* (1998) concluded that the most frequently reported barrier to effective pain control was patients forgetting to take their medication (up to one-third of patients), while 18% of patients also stated that unwanted side-effects were a barrier to taking medication. Thus by providing 3 days worth of analgesia, fentanyl could have a niche in relation to patient compliance and more acceptable side-effects (patient choice and quality of life).

Fentanyl therefore, would seem to be one drug that could have significant benefit for patients receiving palliative care, and conforms to Summary Points 3–5 drawn from the discussion so far. In relation to cost effectiveness, however, fentanyl appears to be more expensive than the other opioids. This brings us back to the question of patient choice being limited by cost; in other words the principles of palliative care may be at odds with health economics.

Local analgesics (local anaesthetics)

Local analgesics such as lidocaine provide regional anaesthesia by stabilizing afferent pain fibre membranes, by maintaining the activity of the Na^+/K^+ ATPase pump and thus inhibiting the ionic fluxes required for the initiation and conduction of electrical impulses (see Figure 8.21, p.188). In short, they cause a reversible block to conduction along the pain afferent nerve fibres (see Figure 20.6, p.569, pathway C).

ACTIVITY

Review Figure 8.21, p.188 and its associated text in Chapter 8, and reflect on your understanding of the activity/inactivity of the Na^+/K^+ ATPase pump during a resting membrane potential and an action potential.

The local anaesthetics used vary widely in their potency, toxicity, length of effects, solubility, stability and ability to permeate mucous membranes. These variations determine their suitability of administration route, e.g. infiltration, plexus,

topical (surface), epidural or spinal block (Omoigui, 2005). Epidural analgesia is commonly used during surgery, often combined with general anaesthesia, because of its protective effects against the stress response of surgery. It is often used when good postoperative pain control is essential, such as in aortic aneurysms or major bowel surgery (*British National Formulary*; Joint Formulary Committee, 2007).

It is common practice to give several drugs with different actions to produce a state of surgical anaesthesia with a minimal risk of toxic side-effects. An intravenous anaesthetic is usually administered for induction, followed by maintenance with inhalation anaesthetics, perhaps supplemented by other drugs administered intravenously. Specific drugs are used to produce muscle relaxation. For certain procedures, controlled hypotension may be required, thus labetalol may be used. Beta-blockers may be used to control arrhythmia during anaesthesia. Glyceryl trinitrate is used to control hypertension, particularly postoperatively.

Local anaesthetics that are used frequently include bupivacaine, chloroprocaine, etidocaine, lidocaine and procaine. Lidocaine is the most widely used anaesthetic drug. It acts more rapidly and is more stable than other local anaesthetics. The duration of block (with adrenaline) is about 1.5 hours.

Bupivacaine's onset of action is fairly rapid, and the duration of anaesthesia is significantly longer than with any other commonly used local anaesthetic, which is a great advantage of this local anaesthetic. It is often used in lumbar epidural blockade. Epidural administration provides long-acting neural blockade. Transmission is blocked at the nerve root and dorsal root ganglia. Bupivacaine is the principle drug for spinal anaesthesia in the UK (*British National Formulary*; Joint Formulary Committee, 2007).

Intravenous administrations of chloroprocaine may also produce central analgesia perhaps owing to inhibition of substance P secretion from afferent C pain fibres, and central sympathetic blockade with a decrease in pain-induced reflex vasoconstriction.

Procaine has a similar potency value to lidocaine, but has a shorter duration of effect. It is now seldom used. Etidocaine provides a significant motor blockade and abdominal muscle relaxation when used for peridural analgesia.

NON-PHARMACOLOGICAL TECHNIQUES OF PAIN MANAGEMENT

Non-pharmacological techniques are frequently more within the direct control of the healthcare practitioner. They may be used in isolation or combination with medically prescribed analgesics, and may be used as a useful adjunct to analgesia in the immediate postoperative period in lessening the side-effects of drugs (Torrance and Serginson, 1997).

A variety of non-pharmacological approaches to pain management exist. These can be grouped as:

- Therapies that provide inhibitory neurotransmitter domination, including touch, and transcutaneous nerve stimulation (see Figure 20.6, p.569, pathway D).

- Therapies that provide neuromodulator domination, including giving information and verbal support to the patient, and the therapies of relaxation, distraction, imagery, biofeedback and neurosurgery (see Figure 20.6, p. 569, pathway E).

While some of this fall naturally to the role of the nurse, others require specialized therapists.

The next sections discuss these methods in more detail.

> **ACTIVITY**
>
> Review Figures 20.3–20.6, pp.564–9 to gain maximum benefit from the following discussion.

Therapies that provide inhibitory neurotransmitter domination

Transcutaneous electrical nerve stimulation

The technique in administering transcutaneous electrical nerve stimulation (TENS) requires very little training. It involves the electrical stimulation of the nervous system using a pulse generator, an amplifier and a system of electrodes (Figure 20.10). The mode of action is controversial. Gadsby and Flowerdew (2001) suggest that TENS stimulates the release of endogenous neuromodulator opioids, while Melzack and Wall (1996) suggest that it provides continuous analgesic relief by ensuring the domination of A-beta afferent fibre input to the pain gates, and thus reduces the need for narcotics. The place of TENS in today's management of postoperative pain is in doubt: some health authorities have abandoned its use since it has been tried and found to be ineffective in many cases.

Touch

Touch therapies include massage, aromatherapy, acupressure and reflexology. Their analgesic qualities stem from encouraging domination of the A-beta afferent fibre (with the mechanoreceptors at their distal ends) input to the pain gates. It may even simply involve holding a patient's hand, or lightly stroking the patient's forehead or forearm.

Reflexology – the art of foot and hand massage – brings relief from some stress while encouraging the homeostatic reflexes associated with wound healing (Clancy and McVicar, 1997). Aromatherapy is the use of essential oils that have been extracted from plants to treat problems such as dyspepsia, nausea or flatulence; the oils may be used as relaxing agents (Torrance and Serginson, 1997).

Touch therapies are designed to comfort and relax patients, and thus promote pain relief perhaps by enhancing the release of endogenous opioids. Touch promotes hypothalamic stimulation of the parasympathetic nervous system; used correctly, it can also relieve anxiety and reassure the patient that someone cares and understands (Torrance and Serginson, 1997). One must be careful with this therapy, however, as the practitioner may invade the patient's 'personal space', which may elevate anxiety levels, thus emphasizing therapeutic subjectivity

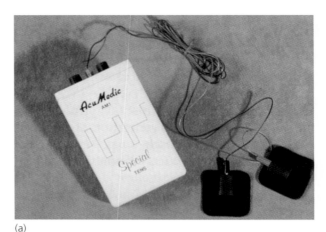

(a)

(b)

Figure 20.10 (a) Transcutaneous electrical nerve stimulation (TENS) machine with electrodes attached (photograph kindly supplied by the Acumedic Centre, London). (b) Electrode placement for brachial plexus lesion: A, complete anaesthesia below the elbow and pain in the whole hand; B, complete anaesthesia below the elbow and pain in the little and ring fingers; C, complete anaesthesia below the shoulder

Q How does the application of TENS relieve pain?

(Clancy and McVicar, 2002). There is general belief that TENS and touch therapies (e.g. Bowen therapy) provide dual analgesic relief through stimulating inhibitory neurotransmitter input and endogenous neuromodulator input to the pain gates (see Figure 20.6, p.569, pathways D and E).

Therapies that provide neuromodulator domination

The actions of neuromodulators such as endorphins on descending fibre input to the pain gates forms the psychophysiological basis of auditory and visual distraction and diversion therapies, hypnosis, biofeedback, counselling and placebo (Melzack and Wall, 1996).

Information and verbal support

Melzack and Wall (1996) stated that anxiety could produce a physiological response similar to acute pain. Thus, the criteria that should be part of any pain management plan are based on establishing a good patient–nurse (healthcare practitioner) relationship, so as to reduce the patient's anxiety and fears regarding:

- their impending stay in hospital;
- progression of their disease state;
- different pain relief techniques;
- potential complications.

The authors emphasize, however, that this information is to be provided in a manner that the patient can understand, so as to individualize care.

Anxiety promotes behavioural responses, including muscle spasms and increased sympathetic activity. The former response compromises blood flow to tissues, causing ischaemia, thus increasing pain perception via the release of pain-producing substances, such as lactic acid (a byproduct of anaerobic metabolism). The latter response can lead to pulmonary problems, increased cardiovascular work, altered muscle metabolism, increased oxygen consumption, and even death. Such behavioural responses can be minimized by the nurse and other healthcare practitioners by using appropriate communications skills to reduce the patient's anxiety and pain (Torrance and Serginson, 1997). Perhaps, then, an appropriate nursing action might be just to empathize, sit and support the patient in pain, since this physical assurance may have analgesic qualities (Clancy and McVicar, 2002). This is because of the pain–anxiety linkage. Perhaps nursing care should aim to reduce the patient's anxiety levels before attempting to quantify the pain that the patient perceives.

The reassurance and communication skills used by healthcare practitioners during the patient's stay in hospital probably enhance the neuromodulatory descending fibre input to the pain gates.

Relaxation, distraction and imagery techniques

Relaxation is thought to remove or reduce pain by allaying a patient's anxiety. Relaxation and distraction techniques may act on both the higher centres involved in pain perception and the pain gating mechanism (see Figure 20.6, p.569).

Distraction draws attention away from the pain, focusing it to a pleasant sensory stimulus. The use of appropriate music can help the patient to relax, and simple deep breathing exercises enhance this effect (Biley, 2000; McCaffery and Good, 2000). It could be argued, however, that the music must be pleasing to the patient to be beneficial, otherwise it may be a source of irritation, raising anxiety levels and thus the patient's perception of pain.

Imagery involves the patient focusing on a situation that is completely incompatible with pain. It may include one or a combination of all senses, incorporating a pleasurable sensation. This ranges from a simple sensation, such as getting the

ACTIVITY

Read the articles by Szirony (2000), Johnson (2000), Reilly (2000), Schofield and Davis (2000) and Cosentino (2000).

patient to describe a favourite pastime, to a complex mental visualization, which involves deep concentration on detailed tasks. Imagery promotes relaxation, which in turn alleviates or eliminates anxiety (Ackerman and Turkiski, 2000). The effectiveness of this therapy depends on the image used and the imagery ability of the individual patient.

Neurosurgery

Neurosurgery is concerned with sectioning nerves, or deleting nerve tracts, within the afferent pain pathways. However, neurosurgeons have now abandoned the use of such techniques in favour of non-destructive methods, such as devices that electrically stimulate nerves, the spinal cord, and discrete but accessible areas of the brain.

According to Melzack and Wall (1996), neurosurgery is regarded as being fully justified to improve the quality of life of patients who have a limited time to live (e.g. in the later stages of terminal cancer as a short-term analgesic control). However, long-term analgesia is rarely achieved and this method may be associated with additional unpleasant sensations. For example, surgical section of peripheral nerves permanently disturbs 'normal' input patterning, but may also produce 'abnormal' inputs from scar tissue.

Interim summary

Many pain therapies exist, and numerous texts are available for further details. The aetiology and management of perioperative pain is varied and sometimes complex. Management of pain requires adequate planning and skill on the part of the healthcare team in terms of both assessment and implementation of care. Therapies used fall into two categories: pharmacological and non-pharmacological. Analgesic drugs have actions that can be related directly to the neurophysiology of pain, especially in relation to the gating mechanisms put forward by Melzack and Wall in 1965. The decision-making processes currently consider morphine to be the first-choice oral analgesic and diamorphine as the first choice for infusion. It is clear though that alternatives with a more convenient means of administration, or fewer/less severe side-effects, may well be more popular with patients under certain circumstances. In the interest of patient choice, patients ought to be informed of the advantages and disadvantages of the various drugs as applicable to themselves, though the reality is that there often are other considerations that apply, for example economics.

Non-pharmacological therapies have actions that remain debatable, although many can be related to the known neurophysiology, for example on neural processing of information in the cerebral cortex (perhaps by imagery or distraction) and psychological impacts on descending pathways (perhaps by relaxation or biofeedback). These alternative or complementary therapies provide potentially useful additional methods for pain relief (and so may be referred to in the literature as 'adjuvants'), and can reduce the amount of analgesia used. The use of such methods emphasizes how psychosocial aspects can influence physiological processes and serves to highlight the subjective nature of pain. Therefore, any approach employed is effective only if it is adapted to the patient's individual needs. If the patient is dissatisfied, then care must be reassessed and be

---

ACTIVITY

To test your understanding of the site of action of various analgesia interventions, study and complete Table 20.4.

Table 20.4 The site of action of pharmacological and non-pharmacological analgesics. Essentially, successful pain management blocks the electrochemical impulses of the pain pathway at different locations en route to the brain's pain centre. Using this information, place a tick in the appropriate boxes of this table to show the proposed operational activity of the listed therapeutic interventions. Note that there may be more than one tick required for each intervention

Therapeutic interventions	Site of action						
	A	B	C	D	E	F	G
Non-opioid analgesics							
Paracetamol							
Diclofenac							
Ketoprofen							
Ketorolac							
Ibuprofen							
Naproxen							
Local anaesthetics							
Lignocaine							
Chloroprocaine							
Bupivacaine							
Etidocaine							
Procaine							
Weak opioid analgesics							
Codeine phosphate							
Co-dyaramol							
Co-proxamol							
Co-codamol							
Narcotic opioid analgesics							
Morphine							
Diamorphine							
Alfentanil							
Fentanyl							
Pethidine							
Distraction and relaxation therapies							
Transcutaneous nerve stimulation							
Verbal support							
Imagery							
Touch therapies							

A, inhibits prostaglandin synthetase; B, inhibits secretion of prostaglandin; C, inhibits secretion of bradykinin and histamine; D, activates the sodium/potassium ATPase pump; E, dominates the A-beta fibre input to the pain gates; F, blocks the secretion of substance P; G, dominates the descending neuromodulator fibre input to the pain gates.

---

adapted to ensure that the patient's comfort is achieved as soon as possible.

The complexity of pain demands a multifaceted and multidisciplinary approach if the patient is to achieve effective pain relief. A prerequisite to good patient care is that the practitioner actually believes the patient. Unless this happens, one cannot get much further with pain assessment, and consequently its management. We suggest that a good understanding of the individualistic nature of the patient's pain, underpinned by a sound knowledge of the neurophysiology of pain, is essential before practitioners attempt to plan and rationalize a patient's care.

ASSESSMENT OF PAIN

Pain and health care are linked inextricably, because assessment and management of the pain process is one of the most common roles of the health carer. The measurement of pain, however, is a contentious and controversial issue with debate

---

BOX 20.9 PAIN RELIEF DURING CHILDBIRTH

A broad spectrum of analgesics is used in maternity care during both normal childbirth and operative procedures. All methods of pain relief offered should provide the optimum level of pain relief without compromising the health of the woman or fetus.

Woman today are turning increasingly to non-drug forms of pain relief for labour and childbirth, including relaxation techniques, breathing exercises to cope with the waves of labour pains, the adoption of positions that maximize comfort, aromatherapy, acupuncture, reflexology and transcutaneous electrical nerve stimulation. None of these techniques, if administered by appropriately qualified professionals, has an effect on the fetus.

Hospitals now offer routine administration of Entonox (50% oxygen, 50% nitrous oxide) via a facemask or mouthpiece. This method is very popular, as it is controlled by the woman and has the added benefit of aiding fetal oxygenation.

Also available is the narcotic pethidine, a powerful opioid analgesic with sedative and anti-spasmodic effects. The dosage ranges from 50 to 200 mg, and may be prescribed and administered by a midwife for a woman in labour. Unfortunately, pethidine is not strong enough to completely remove labour pain, but it does enable most women to cope with it. There are a number of side-effects, including nausea and vomiting (for which an anti-emetic is provided), loss of self-control and reduction in blood pressure. A concern is that the drug passes through the placental barrier and affects the fetus: if the baby is delivered within 2–3 hours of administration, pethidine may cause drowsiness and delay in the onset of respiration or respiratory depression, requiring the antagonist naloxone hydrochloride 0.01 mg/kg to reverse the effects.

Regional epidural analgesia is now available in most maternity units; this is performed by an experienced anaesthetist. Improvements in local anaesthetics have improved the effects of the block provided, and women are now more able to move freely after administration; a 'mobile epidural' allows the woman to bear weight and even to walk/mobilize. An epidural may be topped up with stronger anaesthetics in cases where operative vaginal or abdominal delivery is required.

In the event of elective or emergency Caesarean section, spinal (subarachnoid) analgesia is used, in which local anaesthetic is introduced into the subarachnoid space between L2 and L5 (see Figure 8.4, p.166) Spinal analgesia has a rapid effect, and is quicker to perform than an epidural. Postoperative pain management is usually in the form of narcotics, with epidural top-up from narcotics or bupivacaine.

from two schools of thought. One school of thought believes that pain measurement is necessary and feasible. Certainly, communication is an essential step towards measurement and relief of pain. Therefore, problems in communication and poor understanding of the complexity of pain can result in its poor management. However, it must be stated that the ward environment influences the success of communication. For example, critical care patients are often vulnerable to communication barriers, such as the presence of highly technical equipment and the sight of other critically ill patients. Technical equipment may increase or decrease anxiety levels, since its presence may or may not aid the patient's understanding of their condition or alleviate the fear of the unknown. The presence of other critically ill patients also may or may not increase anxiety, according to individual experience.

A second school of thought believes that pain experiences can never be measured because of the subjective nature of pain. In support of this, there are numerous pain assessment studies, which have demonstrated that nurses (and doctors, pharmacists and paramedics) tend to underestimate the patient's pain, and that if assessment of pain is judged simply on a patient's behaviour (such as restlessness, groaning or grimacing), it can be misleading. In addition, classical signs such as an increased heart rate and lowered blood pressure may also be absent in some patients experiencing pain, thus exposing the dangers of using generalizations.

Both schools of thought emphasize that there is no easy way of understanding what a patient is suffering, or of conveying information from one person to another, although doctors, nurses and other healthcare practitioners need to do so.

In short, many factors affect pain assessment, and these are often interrelated. They all stem from the complex nature of pain, and one cannot expect a certain stimulus to produce a predictable outcome, as other factors may intervene. Melzack and Wall (1996), who stated that pain could not be measured directly so one cannot be sure how much pain someone is suffering, support this. It could also be argued, however, that accurate pain assessment and measurement are essential if the sufferer is to obtain appropriate and successful pain relief.

Clinicians treating patients need to know how the pain changes throughout the day, the descriptive quality of pain and whether there are any aggravating or relieving factors. Such information will perhaps make clinical diagnosis more accurate and allow easier evaluation of treatments.

An individualized approach to the assessment and control of pain is the obvious solution. This is easier said than done, because in order to assess pain, one must take into account individuality with respect to those who have the pain (patients) and those who are trying to assess it (practitioners).

Patient factors

Patient factors affect the patient's expression of pain, rather than the amount of pain perceived; consequently, assessment must also be affected. This is complicated further by the fact that patients have difficulty in describing the pain and in expressing its location.

Cultural backgrounds

Different cultures have different socialization attitudes and behaviours, thus the cultural background of the patient may be responsible for some aspects of inadequate pain assessment and management. It is important to recognize how cultural bias can influence patient care.

Personality typing

Anxiety is heightened by hospitalization and surgery, and therefore exacerbates the patient's interpretation of pain. Personality and anxiety can be interrelated; this is supported by the historical findings of Friedman and Rosenmann, who, in 1974, correlated personality types A, B and C with the incidence of anxiety-provoked myocardial infarctions.

Social class

Social class is an instrumental factor in pain assessment. If the health carer's and patient's social classes are comparable, then more sympathy and better management of pain ensues. Patients from higher social classes are usually more effective in expressing their pain, and thus are more likely to receive better pain management. Language, therefore, is another significant factor, and impairment of communication (e.g. impaired hearing or sight or foreign languages) makes pain assessment, and hence management, more difficult (Melzack and Wall, 1996).

Past experience

The patient's past experiences are significant, since attitudes to pain and suffering are, in part, socially learned responses and hence affect one's judgement of pain and what the pain means to the patient. For example, a layperson having an electrocardiogram (ECG) for the first time may suffer psychosomatic pain if the practitioner does not clarify that the electrodes do not produce painful electric currents when they are applied to the chest and limbs. However, on subsequent visits, when the person has had time to reflect on the method, socially learned responses result in the individual not experiencing psychosomatic pain.

Location of the pain

The location of the pain is important, since some areas of the body are more acceptable discussion topics than others. For example, rectal pain may be an 'unacceptable' topic for discussion and needs to be assessed differently from pain associated with a sore finger.

Gender differences

Gender differences need to be taken into consideration when assessing a patient's pain, since in Westernized societies males tend to be socialized into being courageous, and females into expressing their emotions. McCaffery and Ferrel (1992) demonstrated that generally there are differences in how a nurse thinks men and women respond to pain. They observed that, of 362 nurses, approximately one-third argued that there were gender differences in pain expression. Regarding the

BOX 20.10 PRACTITIONER FACTORS IN THE ASSESSMENT OF PAIN

The factors that affect the patient's experience and interpretation of pain are equally likely to affect that of the practitioner, since individual differences are evident according to nature–nurture interactions. In addition, a number of other factors are important. Some authorities believe that training has placed the responsibility of pain control with the doctors; consequently, nurses are unaware of their importance in pain control. Nursing and other healthcare training affects attitudes to painkillers, and misplaced concerns, such as opioid analgesic addiction and dependency, may cause the nurse to give less than the prescribed analgesia, both in terms of frequency and amount (Bell, 2000). Therefore, more realistic training in pharmacology would help reduce such fears and benefit patient care.

The practitioner has to infer the amount of pain and suffering a patient is experiencing, since it cannot be assessed directly. Although complex, it is our view that knowledge of the nature–nurture interactions associated with the subjective nature of pain is therefore essential to improving the practitioner's assessment and management of pain. The nurse's or health carer's own beliefs and values might influence their assessment of pain, and they must be aware of this in order to be objective.

Pain relief may be affected further by busy ward routines, staff shortages and frequent staff changes, all of which increase the difficulties in establishing a good practitioner–patient relationship. Frequent patient changeover in a ward also affects patient–patient relationships, which can affect the expression of pain by the patient. Thus, ward policy may influence assessment, and hence pain management. Current cost-cutting changes to the skill mix in nursing may well compound the problem.

It will always be difficult to assess adequately an individual's perception of pain, because of the complexity in understanding subjectivity. The concept of 'holistic' care attempts to close this gap and minimize the differences between practitioner and patient assessments. Superficially, pain assessment seems easy, and healthcare practitioners may underestimate the difficulties associated with pain perception/assessment. Some tools seek to provide the breadth of information that would help in assessment, for example the McGill–Melzack pain questionnaire, but the necessary communication skills need time and training to develop, and may cause inaccuracies in assessment (Davies and McVicar, 2000a): some patients assume that the practitioner knows when they are in pain, and some nurses assume that patients will report their pain. It is not surprising that the pain then goes unchecked, and is controlled inadequately. Thus, there needs to be a good working relationship between the patient and the practitioner in which both parties must have mutual trust in each another.

patient's pain tolerance, approximately 50% of the nurses thought that females tolerated pain better than males, while only 15% thought men had a better tolerance. Pain and distress trends seemed to be reversed: 41% believed men showed greater distress when in pain, while only 18% believed women exhibited more distress. Fifty-three per cent, compared with 27%, believed that men rather than women were likely to under-report their pain. However, the practitioner must not sexually stereotype the relationship, since this would not be treating the patient as an individual.

Interim summary

The experience of pain is so complex, being influenced by many variables (subjective to the patient and practitioner), that

the practitioner may or may not be able to predict them. It must be stressed, however, that at all times it is important not to stereotype the factors mentioned above. For example, when caring for patients from different cultures, the practitioner must be aware not only that cultural differences exist in pain expression, but also that individual differences occur within each culture. That is, if the practitioner expects a Caucasian patient to be stoic and they are not, then there may be a danger that they could be labelled as attention-seeking or even malingering. Thus, it is still the patient who is the only one who knows how much pain he or she has. The patient must be involved, whenever possible, in any assessment of pain. An individualized approach in assessing and controlling pain is the obvious solution. To conclude, nurses and other healthcare practitioners who operate on the basis of stereotyping (cultural, gender, social class, etc.) are in danger of ignoring the individuality of pain perception, and consequently pain assessment and management become unsatisfactory.

The clinical measurement of pain

An accurate assessment of pain is essential for adequate therapy. The subjective nature of pain, both in the sufferer and in the observations made by the health practitioner, makes assessment difficult. This section highlights the strengths and shortcomings of frequently used clinical assessment methods.

Measurements of pain involve informal and formal observations. The informal observations are made when the patient is unaware that he or she is being assessed, as this is when the most natural reactions occur. These involve monitoring facial expression, difficulties in performing physical movement, and mood. Formal observations encourage a more accurate assessment, and are important in providing continuity of care. They stress the objective measurements performed by doctors, nurses, midwives and other healthcare practitioners and are based on the patient's experiences and comments, and the observer's own experience of pain and/or traditional/cultural beliefs about pain and the level to be expressed in a given illness, etc. Verbal report is of obvious significance: we hope this chapter has supported that, owing to nature–nurture interactions, pain occurs when the patient says it does.

A 'word' scale could be used in the clinical measurement of pain, but these are open to distortion and observer bias. More attention is thus currently being paid to pain involving the patient's own estimate of pain as a basis for treatment. Such measures include the scales and charts detailed below. The article by Stephenson and Herman (2000) compares different pain scales.

Simple verbal rating scales

For example: No pain, Mild pain, Moderate pain, Severe pain, Unbearable pain.

Verbal rating scales (descriptive scale) are crude, and give only a rough approximation of the pain experienced. In addition, individuals cannot be compared readily. Although these scales are easy to use, they can have a limited usefulness in that there may be:

- misinterpretation of words by the patient/practitioner;
- a limit to the number of words one uses;
- different assumptions made by the practitioner or patient that the intervals between the words are of equal value.

Descriptive scales also are too complicated for use in acute pain.

Visual analogue scale

Visual analogue scales (VASs), also known as graphic rating scales, have been used in an attempt to overcome the problem of expressing 'pain language'.

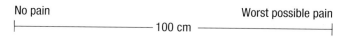

The patient marks the line, and this represents the level of pain at that moment. The distance of the mark from the left end is measured and is called the 'pain score'. This may be repeated several times each day to form the basis of a pain profile for the patient. This type of scale avoids the use of gradation, reduces the misinterpretation of language, is user friendly, and may be modified to assess pain relief by having 'no pain relief' and 'complete pain relief' at opposite ends of the scale.

Shortcomings of the scale are that it is an abstract concept that can be difficult to understand, most answers cluster around the extremes of the scale with little use of the midpoints, and the relevance to patients experiencing acute pain is questionable.

Both the verbal and visual scales view pain one-dimensionally, since they do not take into account other variables that may have an impact on the amount of pain experienced.

Numerical scales

Numerical scales use a continuum comprising a numerical rating scale of either 0–10 or 0–100, with 0 signifying no pain and 10 or 100 signifying unbearable pain. These scales allow greater sensitivity and avoid misinterpretation of the meanings of words. Such scales are used commonly in assessing pain associated with acute myocardial infarction patients, relating pain scores with morphine requirements.

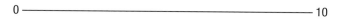

The pain thermometer

The pain thermometer ('painmeter'), designed by the Burford Nursing Development Unit at Oxford, UK (Figure 20.11), acts as a visual aid for the patient to describe their pain experience. It has been used extensively in the care of older people, because patients find it easy to understand. The practitioner and the patient decide how often the painmeter is to be used, and analgesia can be administered accordingly. Although limited in range, it may be helpful in assisting the healthcare practitioner to improve the control of pain relief.

The London Hospital pain observation chart

The London Hospital pain chart (Figure 20.12) improves communication between the practitioner and the patient by making

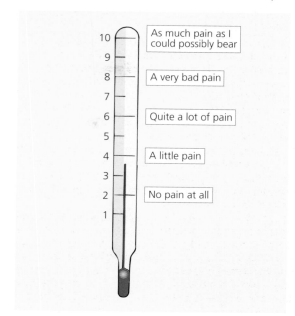

Figure 20.11 The pain thermometer

the recording of pain more systematic. It makes the information that is useful when making decisions about the management of pain readily available in one place. The chart focuses attention on the mechanisms of different pains by recording each site of pain separately, and is a means of communication to be used with the patient, not on the patient. Occasionally, the patient keeps one chart and the staff keeps another.

The McGill–Melzack pain questionnaire

Rather than viewing pain as a specific sensory experience, this questionnaire attempts to measure pain on a broader level by categorizing it into dimensions of pain experience: the sensory, affective and evaluative levels (Figure 20.13). From the list presented, the patient selects the words that best describe their pain; from these measurements, the pain is assessed quantifiably and quantitatively (the higher the total score, the greater the pain).

The questionnaire is used frequently in clinical practice, mainly for work in pain clinics with chronic pain sufferers. However, difficulties arise in the interpretation of the words into the dimension of pain experienced, and it appears difficult to adapt its bulky format to the acute pain setting. Possibly, the questionnaire benefits from being used with other assessment tools, and is in need of some refinement before it can become widely applicable.

Home diaries

Home diaries are useful in combining measurements with the patient's description of the pain (Figure 20.14). These include how the pain changes with respect to time, the precipitating factors of pain, and the success of the analgesic method used to alleviate the pain.

This chart records where a patient's pain is and how bad it is, by the nurse asking the patient at regular intervals. If analgesics are being given regularly, make an observation with each dose and another half-way between each dose. If analgesics are given only 'as required', observe two-hourly. When the observations are stable and the patient is comfortable, any regular time interval between observations may be chosen.

To use this chart, ask the patient to mark all his or her pains on the body diagram below. Label each site of pain with a letter (i.e. A, B, C, etc).

Then, at each observation time, ask the patient to assess:

1. The pain in each separate site since the last observation.
   Use the scale above the body diagram, and enter the number or letter in the appropriate column.

2. The pain overall since the last observation. Use the same scale and enter in column marked overall.

Next, record what has been done to relieve pain. In particular:

3. Note any analgesic given since the last observation, stating name, dose, route and time given.

4. Tick any other nursing care or action taken to ease pain.

Finally note any comment on pain from patient or nurse (use the back of the chart as well, if necessary) and initial the record.

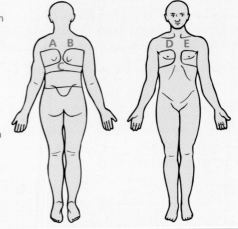

Date _____ Sheet number _____ Patient identification label

Time	Pain rating By sites									Measures to relieve pain (specify where starred)							Comments from patients and/or staff	Initials
	A	B	C	D	E	F	G	H	Overall	Analgesic given (Name, dose, route, time)	Lifting	Turning	Massage	Distracting activities	Position change*	Additional aids*	Other*		

The complete Pain Observation Chart.
Adapted from the London Hospital Pain Observation Chart

Figure 20.12 The London Hospital pain observation chart. Reproduced, with permission, from Latham, J. (1989) *Pain Control*, Austen Cornish.

Q What are the advantages of this assessment tool over the pain thermometer?

Figure 20.13 The McGill–Melzack pain questionnaire

1	8	16
Flickering	Tingling	Annoying
Quivering	Itchy	Troublesome
Pulsing	Smarting	Miserable
Throbbing	Stinging	Intense
Beating	**9**	Unbearable
Pounding	Dull	**17**
2	Sore	Spreading
Jumping	Hurting	Radiating
Flashing	Aching	Penetrating
Shooting	Heavy	Piercing
3	**10**	**18**
Pricking	Tender	Tight
Boring	Taut	Numb
Drilling	Rasping	Drawing
Stabbing	Splitting	Squeezing
Lancinating	**11**	Tearing
4	Tiring	**19**
Sharp	Exhausting	Cool
Cutting	**12**	Cold
Lacerating	Sickening	Freezing
5	Suffocating	**20**
Pinching	**13**	Nagging
Pressing	Fearful	Nauseating
Gnawing	Frightful	Agonizing
Cramping	Terrifying	Dreadful
Crushing	**14**	Torturing
6	Punishing	**PPI**
Tugging	Gruelling	0 No pain
Pulling	Cruel	1 Mild
Wrenching	Vicious	2 Discomforting
7	Killing	3 Distressing
Hot	**15**	4 Horrible
Burning	Wretched	5 Excruciating
Scalding	Binding	
Searing		Constant
		Periodic
		Brief

This questionnaire enables researchers to compare to some extent people's level of pain. Each descriptive word carries its own score – the lower down in its group, the higher its value. The sum of the scores gives what is termed a person's 'pain rating index' – in other words, their overall pain intensity. The final 'present pain intensity' (PPI) section gives an idea of the pain level at the moment the questionnaire is completed.

Indirect clinical measures of pain

Such techniques depend on the effect that pain has on bodily functions, or on the amount of analgesia required to bring pain relief. Specific measures have been developed for use in specific clinical environments, for example the following questions could be used in the coronary care setting:

1 How do you feel? Describe the sensation.
2 Where does it hurt?
3 Does the sensation travel anywhere?
4 Did anything trigger it off?
5 How long has it lasted?
6 Has anything made it worse or better?
7 Are there any other relevant signs or symptoms?

This has the advantage of being a quick procedure with the questions overlapping each other in the scope of the answers, and allowing a place for physical signs and symptoms that may be relevant. The disadvantages of the method are that the replies cannot be standardized, and the assessment is still subject to the practitioner's interpretation of the patient's reply.

Interim summary

The use of pain assessment tools has been shown to improve pain control and aid care. The tools, however, are still not in common practice. Introducing a pain system of measurement would improve the practitioner's awareness of pain, which would inevitably result in improved patient care. However, the tool that is chosen depends on the type of pain, the clinical setting, and the patient group, among other factors. Measurement tools are essential to avoid possible difficulties in practitioner–patient communication, and therefore to avoid unnecessary patient suffering. However, it could be argued that the assessment of pain barely considers the patient's social,

	Notes of any different pain, symptom or problem, and any unusual activity or exercise during each day	Any other comments
Day 1		
Day 2		
Day 3		
Day 4		
Day 5		
Day 6		
Day 7		

LHMC

HOME DIARY

NAME.................................
DATE STARTED ....

How to fill in the home diary

1 *Sleep:* In this column, fill in hours slept, then ring word that best describes how much your pain disturbed your rest.
2 *Pain:* In the column for each part of the day, write the number of doses of painkiller (tablets, spoonfuls) taken. Then choose the best word to describe your pain for that part of the day. Put in the chart the *pain number* next to the word you chose.
3 On the back of the diary, make a note of any different pains, symptoms or problems, and note any unusual activities or exercise that day.
4 Add any other comments of your own.

Excruciating	5
Very severe	4
Severe	3
Moderate	2
Just noticeable	1
No pain at all	0

	Sleep	Morning (to 12 noon)	Afternoon (noon to 4 pm)	Early evening (4 – 8 pm)	Late evening (from 8 pm)
Day 1	Hours of sleep / Pain disturbed sleep never/a bit/often/a lot	No. of painkillers / Pain number	No. of painkillers / Pain number	No. of painkillers / Pain number	No. of painkillers / Pain number
Day 2	Hours of sleep / Pain disturbed sleep never/a bit/often/a lot	No. of painkillers / Pain number	No. of painkillers / Pain number	No. of painkillers / Pain number	No. of painkillers / Pain number
Day 3	Hours of sleep / Pain disturbed sleep never/a bit/often/a lot	No. of painkillers / Pain number	No. of painkillers / Pain number	No. of painkillers / Pain number	No. of painkillers / Pain number
Day 4	Hours of sleep / Pain disturbed sleep never/a bit/often/a lot	No. of painkillers / Pain number	No. of painkillers / Pain number	No. of painkillers / Pain number	No. of painkillers / Pain number
Day 5	Hours of sleep / Pain disturbed sleep never/a bit/often/a lot	No. of painkillers / Pain number	No. of painkillers / Pain number	No. of painkillers / Pain number	No. of painkillers / Pain number
Day 6	Hours of sleep / Pain disturbed sleep never/a bit/often/a lot	No. of painkillers / Pain number	No. of painkillers / Pain number	No. of painkillers / Pain number	No. of painkillers / Pain number
Day 7	Hours of sleep / Pain disturbed sleep never/a bit/often/a lot	No. of painkillers / Pain number	No. of painkillers / Pain number	No. of painkillers / Pain number	No. of painkillers / Pain number

Figure 20.14 Home diary. Reproduced with permission from Lady Hayden Medical College

psychological and neurophysiological factors, all of which must be considered if assessment is to be accurate. The development of appropriate assessment tools specific to certain clinical settings must be considered of vital importance in the practitioner's bid to improve the quality of patient care.

ACTIVITY

What factors should be taken into consideration when assessing pain? List the clinical tools used to assess pain, and comment on the usefulness and drawbacks of the tools mentioned in this chapter.

SUMMARY

1 Melzack and Wall's gate control theory of pain perception is a credible model that explains pain perception and control.

2 Pain perception is dependent on the balance of afferent neuron input to the gating mechanisms, and, the descending neuron input to the gating mechanisms. If the afferent pain fibre input dominates, the gate is 'open' and one perceives pain. If the mechanoreceptor's afferent input and/or the descending neuron input dominate, then the gate is 'closed' and pain is not perceived.

3 Pain is a subjective experience that depends on the nature–nurture interactions that determine the characteristics of the individual. Subjectivity is determined by the individual's unique blend of genes and his/her unique environmental experiences.

4 The subjective nature of pain has wide implications for assessing, evaluating, planning and monitoring the care of people in pain. Thus, the complexity of pain states demands a multifaceted and multidisciplinary approach if the patient is to achieve effective pain relief.

5 Pain relief is by pharmacological and non-pharmacological techniques. If pain persists the principles of the analgesic staircase are employed to reduce or abolish it.

6 Common non-opioids include paracetamol and non-steroidal antiinflammatories – NSAIDs. These block pain in the periphery at the site of damage.

7 Common oral opioids include weak ones (e.g. codeine phosphate, co-proxamol and co-codamol) and strong ones (e.g. morphine).

8 Non-pharmacological techniques for pain control include transcutaneous nerve stimulation, relaxation, distraction and imagery techniques.

9 Healthcare professionals have a duty to ensure that the patient voice is heard. This will require patient education, and empowerment and advocacy in order to support patient autonomy and choice.

10 Assessment of pain is multifactorial. It is affected by factors attributed to the patient, the practitioner, ward policy and hospital environments, and it must be questioned whether it can really be assessed adequately.

11 Pain assessment tools, it could be argued, are of limited use in measuring pain. Their usefulness is largely in monitoring the effectiveness/appropriateness of the analgesic method used, and the effectiveness of the practitioner in managing the patient's pain.

12 A prerequisite to good patient care is that the practitioner actually believes the patient. Unless this happens one cannot get much further with pain assessment, and consequently its management. We suggest that a good understanding of the individualistic nature of the patient's pain is essential before practitioners attempt to plan and rationalize a patient's care.

13 Biomedical and physiological research have provided great understanding of some dimensions associated with pain, and psychological research has increased knowledge of the relationships between stress, anxiety and pain. Psychometric studies have generated various methods of measuring pain. However, because of the complexity of the phenomenon we call 'pain', there are many unanswered questions; continued research into the interrelations of these disciplines is the only way forward to unfold some of these mysteries.

REFERENCES

Ackerman, C.J. and Turkiski, B. (2000) Using guided imagery to reduce pain and anxiety. *Home Healthcare Nurse* **18**(8): 524–30.

Bell, F. (2000) A review of the literature on the attitudes of nurses to acute pain management. *Journal of Orthopaedic Nursing* **4**(2): 64–70.

Bennett, G.J. (2000) Update on the neurophysiology of pain transmission and modulation: focus on the NMDA-receptor and NMDA-receptor antagonists: evolving role in analgesia. Proceedings of a meeting sponsored by Algos Pharmaceutical Corporation, New York City. *Journal of Pain and Symptom Management* **19**(1S Suppl.): S2–6.

Biley, F.C. (2000) The effects on patient well-being of music listening as a nursing intervention: a review of the literature. *Journal of Clinical Nursing* **7**(5): 668–77.

Chen, B. and Chang, M. (2000) Anxiety and depression in Taiwanese cancer patients with and without pain. *Journal of Advanced Nursing* **32**(4): 944–51.

Clancy, J. and McVicar, A.J. (1997) Wound healing: a series of homeostatic responses. *British Journal of Theatre Nursing* **7**(4): 25–33.

Clancy, J. and McVicar, A.J. (1998) Neurophysiology of pain. *British Journal of Theatre Nursing* **7**(10): 15–24.

Clancy, J. and McVicar, A.J. (2002) *Physiology and Anatomy. A Homeostatic Approach*, 2nd edn. London: Arnold.

Clancy, J. McVicar, A.J. and Baird, N. (2002) *Perioperative Practice. Fundamentals of Homeostasis*. London: Routledge.

Cosentino, B.W. (2000) Guided visualization and imagery for chronic pain. *Nursing Spectrum (New York/New Jersey Metro edn)* **12A**(10): 8–9.

Cunningham, M. (2000) Chronic pain: potential sequel of cancer and cancer treatment (reprinted with permission from Mary Cunningham, MS, RN, AOCN). *Missouri Nurse* **69**(6): 8–9.

Davies, J. and McVicar, A. (2000a) Issues in effective pain control 1: assessment and education. *International Journal of Palliative Nursing* **6**(2), 58–66.

Davies, J. and McVicar, A. (2000b) Issues in effective pain control 2: from assessment to management. *International Journal of Palliative Nursing* **6**(4), 162–9.

Desjardins, P.J. (2000) Patient pain and anxiety: the medical and psychological challenges facing oral and maxillofacial surgery. *Journal of Oral and Maxillofacial Surgery* **58**(10 Suppl. 2): 1–3.

Ehde, D.M., Czerniecki, J.M., Smith, D.G. *et al.* (2000) Chronic phantom sensations, phantom pain, residual limb pain, and other regional pain after lower limb amputation. *Archives of Physical Medicine and Rehabilitation* **81**(8): 1039–44.

Fallon, M. (2000). Rationale for using alternative drugs to morphine. *Palliative Care Today* **9**(1), 10–15.

Fitzsimons, D., Parahoo, K. and Stringer, M. (2000) Waiting for coronary artery bypass surgery: a qualitative analysis. *Journal of Advanced Nursing* **32**(5): 1243–52.

Friedman, H. and Rosenmann, R.H. (1974) *Type A Behaviour and Your Heart*. London: Wildwood.

Gadsby, J.G. and Flowerdew, M.W. (2001) Transcutaneous electrical nerve stimulation and acupuncture-like transcutaneous electrical nerve stimulation for chronic low back pain. *The Cochrane Library*. Oxford: Update Software.

Johnson, M.I. (2000) The clinical effectiveness of TENS in pain management. *Critical Reviews in Physical and Rehabilitation Medicine* **12**(2): 131–49.

Joint Formulary Committee (2007) *British National Formulary*. London: British Medical Association and Royal Pharmaceutical Society for Great Britain.

McCaffery, M. (1983) *Nursing the Patient in Pain*. London: Harper Row.

McCaffery, M. and Ferrell, B.R. (1992) Does the gender gap affect your pain control? *Nursing* **22**(8): 48–51.

McCaffrey, R.G. and Good, M. (2000) The lived experience of listening to music while recovering from surgery. *Journal of Holistic Nursing* **18**(4): 378–90.

Melzack, R. and Wall, P.D. (1965) Pain mechanisms: a new theory. *Science* **150**: 971–9.

Melzack, R. and Wall, P.D. (1996) *The Challenge of Pain*, updated 2nd edn. London: Penguin.

Mercadante, S. (2007) Opioid titration in cancer pain: a critical review. *European Journal of Pain* **11**(8): 823–30.

Mitten, T. (2000). Introduction to pain control. In: Cooper, J (ed.) *Stepping into Palliative Care. A Handbook for Community Professionals*. Chapter 1. Abingdon: Radcliffe Medical Press, 4–43.

Omoigui, S. (2005) *The Pain Drugs Handbook*. London: Mosby.

Parsons, G. (2000) Patient controlled analgesia was more effective than nurse controlled analgesia after cardiac surgery. *Evidence-Based Nursing* **3**(2): 53.

Radbruch, L., Sabatowski, R., Lowick, G. *et al.* (2000) Constipation and the use of laxatives: a comparison between transdermal fentanyl and oral morphine. *Palliative Medicine* **14**(2), 111–19.

Redwood, S. (2000) Clinical. Improving pain management: breaking down the invisible barrier. *British Journal of Nursing* **9**(19): 2067–72.

Reilly, M.P. (2000) Clinical applications of acupuncture in anesthesia practice. *CRNA – the Clinical Forum for Nurse Anesthetists* **11**(4): 173–9.

Schofield, P. and Davis, B. (2000) Sensory stimulation (snoezelen) versus relaxation: a potential strategy for the management of chronic pain. *Disability and Rehabilitation* **22**(15): 675–82.

Stephenson, N.L. and Herman, J. (2000) Research brief. Pain measurement: a comparison using horizontal and vertical analogue scales. *Applied Nursing Research* **13**(3): 157–8.

Szirony, G.M. (2000) A psychophysiological view of pain: mind–body interaction in the rehabilitation of injury and illness. *Work: a Journal of Prevention, Assessment and Rehabilitation* **15**(1): 55–60.

Thomason, T.E., McCune J.S., Bernard S.A. *et al.* (1998) Cancer pain survey: patient-centred issues in control. *Journal of Pain and Symptom Management* **15**(5): 275–84.

Torrance, C. and Serginson, E. (1997) *Surgical Nursing*. London: Baillière Tindall.

Twycross, R., Willcock, A. and Thorp, S. (1998) *Palliative Care Formulary*. Abingdon: Radcliffe Medical Press Ltd.

World Health Organization (1996) *Cancer Pain Relief and Palliative Care*. Report of a WHO expert committee. Technical Report Series 804. Geneva: WHO.

Zeppetella, G., O'Doherty, C.A. and Collins, S. (2000) Prevalence and characteristics of breakthrough pain in cancer patients admitted to a hospice. *Journal of Pain and Symptom Management* **20**(2): 87–92.

STRESS

INTRODUCTION

Stress is an inextricable part of life, and according to the physiologist Selye (1976), 'it is essentially reflected by the rate of all the wear and tear caused by life'. Stress is evident to most people, since it manifests itself with obvious, often visible physiological and psychological responses (Table 21.1). Responses to particular stressful situations are highly personal; hence there is a strong subjective element. An understanding of stress has contributed considerably to the present understanding of health and illness. The existence of a link between stress and illness has grown to near-acceptance in the scientific world.

According to Clancy and McVicar (1998a), few people now doubt that 'physiological' and 'psychological factors' play an important role in 'mental' and 'physical' illness.

The multidefinitional aspects of stress will be explored briefly in this chapter, taking the view that stress is a psychophysiological response (since mind–body interactions are inseparable) instigated by environmental stressors. Thus, 'nature–nurture' interactions will be the main focus in describing the personal nature of stressor perception, the stress response and coping methods. Stress-related illnesses will also be discussed with this nature–nurture template in mind. The stress models used in reviewing this subjectivity are the transactional theory of Cox

Table 21.1 Some psychophysiological indicators of the stress response

Physical indicators	Behavioural indicators	Emotional indicators
▲ High blood pressure	● Poor work performance	● Emotional outbursts/crying
● Increased heart rate	● Accidents at work and home	● Irritability with people
● Increased respiratory rate	● Overindulgence in smoking, alcohol and	▲ Depression
▲ Increased muscle tension	drugs	● Tendency to blame others
▲ Increased restlessness	● Loss of interest	● Hostile and insulting behaviour
▲ Upset stomach	● Daydreaming	● Tiredness
● Sweaty palms	● Diminished attention to detail	● Anxiety
● Loss of appetite	● Forgetfulness	
▲ Indigestion or heartburn	● Mental blocking	
● Change in sleep patterns	▲ Social isolation	
▲ Tension headaches	▲ Marital and family breakdowns	
▲ Cold hands and feet		
▲ Nausea		
▲ Nail biting		
▲ Constipation or diarrhoea		
▲ Backache		

Note: The above are termed psychophysiological indicators because physical, behavioural and emotional indicators are inseparable, being both cause and effect, i.e.

Physical ⟷ Behavioural
Emotional

• Usually short-term effects. ▲ Usually long-term effects.

Q Distinguish between exogenous and endogenous stressors.

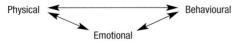
LIVERPOOL JOHN MOORES UNIVERSITY
LEARNING SERVICES

BOX 21.1 HEALTHCARE PRACTITIONERS NEED TO UNDERSTAND STRESS

It is essential that health carers have a clear understanding of the subjectivity of stress perception in everyday life, in relation to illness, and in the process of diagnosis, prognosis and hospitalization. Because of their contact with patients, their relatives and loved ones, healthcare practitioners are in an ideal position to take action to prevent unnecessary stress and to minimize or alleviate prolonged stress. Health carers with this insight will be able to cope effectively with their own stress, that of their peers, colleagues, patients and their relatives (see Box 21.4, p.594).

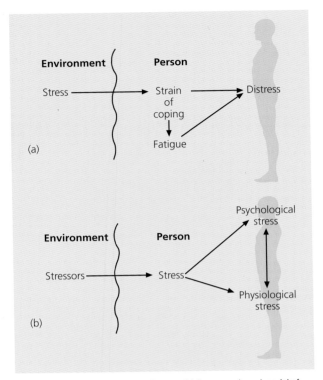

Figure 21.1 (a) Layperson's model of stress. (b) Response-based model of stress

Q Differentiate between stressors and stress.

and McKay (1976), a physiological theory called the general adaptation syndrome (GAS) described by Selye (1956), and a modified GAS or psychophysiological model put forward by Selye and Lazarus (1966, cited in Selye, 1976).

Definitions of stress

Various attempts have been made to find a suitable definition of stress; the following text explores this and the conclusion is that stress has different connotations for different people.

Stimulus-based definition

A layperson often views stress as an environmental incident (stimulus) that causes strain within the body in the form of fatigue and/or distress (Figure 21.1a). These environmental stresses for the person normally are major events or situations and could be, for example, a situation or conditions at work, the formalities of a divorce process, the death of a loved one, unemployment, repossession of the house, the highly technical equipment used in the intensive-care setting, the dentist, lifestyle problems created after being diagnosed human immunodeficiency virus (HIV) positive, etc.

Such stimulus-based definitions are incomplete, since any situation may or may not be stressful, depending on the individual and the meaning of the situation for that person.

Response-based definition

Although there is no generally accepted definition of 'a state of stress' in biological or social systems, biologists and behavioural scientists continue to use the term. Biologists and medical scientists tend to be concerned with the sources of stress that are concrete and observable, and can otherwise be considered as 'causes' of illness and injury. The response-based definition views stress as a person's bodily physiological and/or psychological responses to environmental stressors. What is not explained satisfactorily is the uniqueness of the perception of stressors to individuals, and the personal responses. Presumably, this is because the complexity of humans makes it impossible to comprehend fully the interrelationships of psychological and physiological (mind–body) processes that arise owing to environmental influences. Thus, environmental stresses are recognized as stressors to the biomedical scientist, and it is the accumulation of these that produces stress within the body, identified as physiological stress or psychological stress. However, as stated above these disciplines are inseparable from one another (Figure 21.1b) and from the environment (see systems theory, Figure 1.11, p.19). For example, in anxiety provoked by an environmental threat one may become consciously aware of a faster and more powerful heartbeat (a so-called physiological stress response), which in turn may increase the person's perception of their anxiety state (a so-called psychological stress response). However, because of their interdependency of mind–body interaction we prefer to consider anxiety as a psychophysiological bodily state induced by environmental stressors.

Social and behavioural scientists tend to be concerned with sources of stress that represent information arising from outside the person, and responses are mediated by higher centres of the brain. It is clear that such psychological stresses can lead to alterations of internal functions, even at the biochemical level, and that these are potential causes of disease. Equally, psychological responses are a consequence of biochemical (enzymatic) changes induced by gene expression (see Chapter 1, p.17–20). These are interdependent on other mechanisms, including environmental stressors, which ultimately are of a sociocultural origin. In other words, the sources of stress are environmental/social stressors outside (exogenous) and/or inside (endogenous) the body that may produce a psychophysiological stress response.

Selye (1956) defined stress as 'the non-specific response of the body and that freedom from stress is death'. This definition views stress as being the non-specific (i.e. common) result

Table 21.2 Psychological and physiological indicators of eustress and distress*

	Eustress	Distress	Severe distress
Psychological	Fear/excitement Increased level of arousal, and mental acuity	Unease Apprehension Sadness Depression Pessimism Listlessness Lack of self-esteem Negative attitudes Short temper Fatigue Poor sleep	Burnout: emotional exhaustion depersonalization and disengagement decreased personal accomplishment
Physiological**	Autonomic arousal Increased arterial blood pressure Increased heart rate Quicker reaction times Release of metabolic hormones especially cortisol Increased metabolic rate Mobilization of glucose, fatty acids, amino acids	Increased smoking/alcohol consumption Persistently elevated arterial blood pressure Indigestion Constipation or diarrhoea Weight gain or loss	Clinical hypertension Coronary heart disease Gastric disorders Menstrual problems in women Increased asthma attacks in sufferers
Impact on the individual	*Adaptive:* Increased alertness Attention focused on the situation Individual more responsive to changing situations Fight, flight and fright preparation for activity: 'Energised'	Variable between individuals, but usually *maladaptive*	Variable between individuals but usually *severely maladaptive*, possibly life-threatening***

* The evidence that both cognitive and physiological responses occur simultaneously is debatable, except in extremely distressful situations, but it is convenient to consider cognitive and physical responses separately. See Sarafino (2002) for further information.
** Physiological responses based on the general adaptation syndrome (Selye, 1976).
***The health impact may be compounded in nurses by health-risk behaviours, for example excessive smoking and alcohol abuse (Plant *et al.*, 1992).

Q List some potential eustressors associated with the occupation of nursing.

of any mental or somatic demand placed upon the body. That is, stress is the response to a 'threat' (i.e. a change in the environment), and its integrity is based on evaluating the information received.

A generally accepted historical definition of stress is 'a state which arises from an actual or perceived demand–capability imbalance in the organism's vital adjustment actions which is partially manifested by a non-specific response' (Lazarus and Folkman, 1984). Thus, although historically stress has been viewed in terms of separate physiological, psychological and sociological (environmental) phenomena, the authors' view is that theorists integrate the disciplines in order to appreciate the subjective nature of stress; thus any suitable definition should encompass this integration. For example:

• Using the concept of homeodynamism, expressed in Box 1.7, p.15 an adapted Lazarus–Folkman definition would be that perceptional stress is a psychophysiological homeostatic adaptation (of increased sympathetic activity and stress hormones) arising when there is an actual and/or perceived demand–capability mismatch between the individual and his or her environment (namely, a homeostatic disturbance), thus facilitating coping and restoring homeostasis.

• Following on from this, psychophysiological homeostatic

imbalances would arise when there is a temporary actual and/or perceived demand–capability mismatch that cannot be managed adequately, and is becoming more severe. Finally, psychophysiological homeostatic imbalances (e.g. hyperplasia of endocrine organs producing stress hormones) arise when there is a long-lasting or permanent actual and/or perceived demand–capability mismatch. These imbalances (i.e. signs and symptoms of stress) lead to the label of stress-related illness. In other words, what was referred to briefly in the introduction as the interactionist or transactional model of stress.

Stress is generally thought of, and expressed, in a negative sense, with a view that stress is potentially harmful when the stress threshold is reached or superseded. The threshold is the minimum cumulative stressor value necessary to evoke a stress response in an individual. However, as Selye (1976) stated, stress can also be related to positive and pleasurable experiences, for example the stress associated with competitive sport, with reviving an unconscious patient, with meeting a deadline, etc. He referred to this type of stress as 'the ecstasy of fulfilment' or the 'spice of life' that contributes to the wear and tear of life. Thus, stress can be associated with both positive and negative experiences. Selye referred to 'eustress' and 'distress' to distinguish between the two.

Eustress and distress

Eustressors lead to the experience of eustress. Accompanying eustress is a sense of 'psychological' and 'physiological' alertness whereby the person feels energized and hence the response is viewed as part of 'well-being' (see Table 21.2, eustress column).

Distressors are extreme, long-lasting or unusual stressors which produce distress (i.e. the negative or 'unhealthy' stress response; see Table 21.2, distress column). If homeostasis is restored, it is at a cost to the body (i.e. the person's resistance to stress is reduced). If homeostatic mechanisms are not re-established, then homeostatic imbalances (see Table 21.2, distress column) persist leading to a label of a stress-related illness (see Table 21.2, severe distress column) or even death may result.

Eustress triggers homeostatic mechanisms to remove, adapt or cope with the initiating stressor(s) and so restore homeostasis, but it is time-dependent, so if the homeostatic mechanisms are unsuccessful then eustress is transformed into distress.

Figure 21.2 illustrates homeostasis as a dynamic concept in which the individual may or may not be consciously aware of the impact of stressors. Essentially:

- The individual always experiences 'stress' since we continually react to our environment. In most instances, the stress levels are within the homeostatic range (Figure 21.2, label a); this equates to Selye's statement that 'freedom from stress is death'. We consider that this stress is when an individual's 'stress' threshold has not been met, and therefore, while the person may be responding, they are not consciously aware of the body's response to the stressors. Stress hormones in the blood are close to their basal level.

- In order for the individual to become consciously aware, the stress level must change to the extent that it is now outside the homeostatic range (i.e. threshold is reached or superseded). The person now consciously experiences eustress or distress. Eustress is when the person is homeostatically adapting psychophysiologically to the environmental cumulative stressors (i.e. a rise in stress hormones in the blood, and behavioural responses, are considered normal and acceptable). Distress is experienced when the individual is undergoing a greater level of psychophysiological homeostatic disturbance (Table 21.2, distress column) and return to homeostatic control is more difficult, though possible. If, however, distress, prolonged, or added to by other distressors, the disturbance becomes more severe (i.e. positive feedback), resulting in an imbalance and/or stress-related illnesses (Table 21.2, distress and severe distress columns) if there is a failure of the individual's coping mechanisms. The main focus of this chapter is this maladaptive stress, since it is this form of stress that produces most distress and disease.

One important aspect of this dynamic concept is that eustress may transform into distress in some circumstances. An example of the transition of eustress into distress can be found in competitive sports, such as boxing. At the commencement of a fight, a boxer usually believes he is going to beat his oppo-

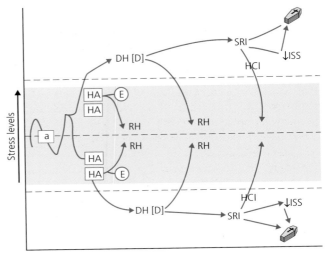

Figure 21.2 Perceptional stress: a homoeostatic adaptation and/or a homeostatic disturbance, and/or an homeostatic imbalance. a, Subconscious ('resting metabolism') stress levels: an expected/natural rise in sympathetic nervous stimulus and stress hormones accompanying an environmental 'threat'. These changes are when the homeostatic parameters moved upwards so as to adapt to the stressor (i.e. 'metabolism is more active; see Figure 1.7, p.14 and associated text), but the individual is still unaware of it (= HA) and/or the stress threshold has been reached or superseded and the individual consciously experiences 'eustress' (= HA-E; see Table 21.2, Eustress column). The eustressed individual in time either re-establishes homeostasis (RH) or if prolonged, the eustress is transformed into distress (= DH, disturbed homeostasis; see Table 21.2, Distress column). The distressed individual in time either re-establishes homeostasis (RH), or if prolonged, or if additional stressors come into play the individual experiences severe stress (see Table 21.2, Severe distress column) and a stress-related illness (SRI) results. HCI, healthcare intervention re-establishes the homeostatic status for the patient (RH), or decreases signs and symptoms without establishing the homeostatic status (= ↓SS) to a state that the individual can tolerate and/or intervention fails completely resulting in death ⚰. [a, Represents boxes a₁–a₄ in Figure 1.7, p.11, reflecting the individual variability in the homeostatic range. The blue area represents the norm (homeostatic range) 95%]

Q Define the concept of stress threshold.

nent, and so experiences eustressful responses on the first bell. The perception extends until the boxer gets tired or is hurt; then he doubts winning, and eustress is transformed into distress. Similarly, a patient's optimism that their health deficit will be managed can change to distress if intervention fails or is only partially successful.

ACTIVITY

Identify three situations you may come across in your day-to-day health care of a patient when a eustressful experience is transformed into a distressful one, and vice versa.

Interim summary

Stress is the psychophysiological response (i.e. perceived as adaptive eustress and maladaptive distress) of the body to environmental (exogenous and endogenous) stimuli called stressors (eustressors or distressors). The perceptions of stressors differ quantitatively and qualitatively between individuals, as do the stress thresholds. Psychophysiological responses to stressors are also subjective, since individuals experience either eustress or distress, depending upon their perception of the demands made by the stressors, and their capacity to meet those demands. In addition, as Table 21.1 demonstrates, there is a range of physical, emotional and behavioural indicators that occur when people are stressed (the main emphasis is on indicators when one is distressed), and it is unlikely that two people will display the same indicators. The psychophysiological response is also time dependent. For example, eustress may be transformed into distress, and perceptions of the response vary daily, and even within the same day, since humans are social beings who display circadian rhythmicity of body functioning and hence have a variable stress threshold.

The individual nature of the psychophysiological stress response can be explained using the nature–nurture interaction template:

Genotype ⟶ Phenotype
(determines free running   (circadian
endogenous rhythms)   parameters)
Environment
(exogenous modulators)

The unique genotype that a person possesses partly determines the measurable psychophysiological indicators (phenotypes) of the stress response. Genes are expressed or suppressed when the necessary environmental factors (stressors) prevail. For example, crying (a phenotype) in response to a situation is a common indicator of a psychophysiological stress response. This act is labelled an emotion, and as such is usually dealt with in the realms of psychological teaching. It must be remembered, however, that psychological perception of environmental stressors is a consequence of physiological processes (nerve impulses), so giving credibility to the interactionist or transactional model of stress. Thus, crying is a result of excessive tear production and secretion. Tears are chemicals, and are the end-product of chemical reactions produced as a result of gene expression, which will be influenced by the dominant environmental stressor within the cumulative stressors one perceives at that point in time. Crying can be a distressful or eustressful response, depending on how the individual perceives the major contributory stressor(s) (i.e. as joyful or unhappy events).

This concept underpins notions of subjectivity of stress perception and responses, considered in the next section.

THE SUBJECTIVITY OF STRESS

Humans react to stress in different ways because of the different societies they live in, the way they live their lives within that society, the type and dynamic fluctuations of societal stressors, and genetic variation. Subjectivity (or individualism) exists as a result of factors that influence expression of an individual's unique genotype, together with how the individual perceives and reacts to the environment in which they live. This explains why identical twins can differ in personality and health. Although developed from the same zygote, their biochemistry will not be completely identical because there will be

some genetic uniqueness since some genetic mutations are likely to occur during intrauterine development (see pp.536–7) and with age (see pp.549–53), and their family experiences may vary; although parents like to think that they treat their children the same, in reality they often do not. Different experiences for twins even occur in the womb, depending on how the mother is living her life in different gestatory periods; even the position and the degree of placentation influences development.

Before we become aware of the bodily stress response, the cumulative stressors one perceives at that point must have reached or superseded the stress threshold. As noted, the perception of stressors, and the stress threshold, are dynamic and subjective, fluctuating with night–day activities (broadly defined as circadian rhythms, and covered in detail in Chapter 22) in the individual and between individuals as they proceed through the developmental stages of life. For example, consider the fondness for loud music by some young people; while this may be included in your own list of distressors now, it may not have always been so.

The subjectivity of stressors

People are constantly exposed to potential stressors, but may not be consciously aware of their existence. Stressors are classified as being social, physical, psychological, environmental and developmental.

Social stressors

Social readjustment rating scale

An historical publication by Holmes and Rahe (1967) identified 43 common stressful life events by examining the case his-

Table 21.3(a)   The Holmes and Rahe social readjustment rating scale

Event	Life crisis score (points)
Death of spouse	100
Divorce	73
Marital separation	65
Personal injury or illness	53
Marriage	50
Pregnancy	40
Sexual problems	39
Change in responsibilities at work	29
Outstanding personal achievement	28
Trouble with the boss	23
Change in working hours or conditions	20
Change in social activity	18
Vacation	13
Christmas	12

Q What are the main criticisms of this scale?

Table 21.3(b)   Magnitude of life crisis

Magnitude of life crisis	Life change unit score
Mild	150–199
Moderate	200–299
Severe	300+

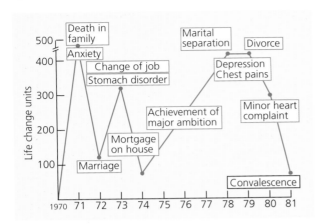

Figure 21.3 How stress affects your health. Life change units used from Holmes and Rahe's social readjustment rating scale (see also Table 21.4)

tories of about 5000 people and identifying the life events that regularly preceded the onset of illness (Table 21.3a). Holmes and Rahe argued that there is an increase in the incidence of stress-related illnesses following stressful life events because of

the extent of coping activities such 'adaptive' changes require. 'Negative' and 'positive' perceived events, such as divorce and marriage, respectively, are stressful since they necessitate adjustments by the person to a new lifestyle. Using their rating scale, the person reports any change in lifestyle, and each change is assigned a life change unit (LCU) score; a total LCU score is then calculated. Holmes and Rahe ranked people as experiencing mild, moderate or severe stress (according to their LCU score; Table 21.3b).

Life events operate as stressors to the extent that they tax or exceed the adaptive resources of the person. They may be divided into major and minor. The former include events such as divorce, unemployment, serious illness and death of a loved one; the latter include daily stressors such as noise, job dissatisfaction and enjoyment.

Daily hassles of life

In 1981, Kanner *et al.* developed the 'Daily Hassles Scale', comprising 117 items that people may find frustrating or irritating, such as silly practical mistakes, losing one's purse, or having an argument with a loved one or workmate (revised in 1985 by Lazarus *et al.*). Participants of the study were required

---

BOX 21.2 SOCIAL READJUSTMENT RATING SCALE: ANY USE IN CLINICAL PRACTICE?

In support of such rating scales, it is possible to trace retrospectively from a patient's medical notes documented life events over a period of time preceding a stress-related illness. Figure 21.3, for example, highlights some common and most dominant (with regard to the life change unit, LCU, score) stressors a person who has had a coronary might perceive during a 10-year period.

The stressor scales are clinically useful in identifying potential distressors, so that the person can avoid them or learn how to cope with them, and in emphasizing the cumulative effects of multiple stressors in a person's life that cause the resultant signs of distress. However, theoretical and methodological weaknesses include:

- Some individuals undergo considerable life event changes without experiencing illness of any kind. Even Holmes and Rahe (1967) stated that 20% of scores bordering severe stress levels (LCU = 300) are not associated with a stress-related illness. Thus, individual differences in the ability to cope with stressful life events are overlooked.
- Attempts to quantify stressors in numerical order are crude and unscientific, since individuals rank life events differently according to their own perceptions. Thus, the transactional model of stress gives no consideration to the subjective appraisal of potential stressful situations. For example, when caring for a spouse during the terminal stage of cancer, death may not be the highest-ranked distressor in that person's life (at that particular moment in time), but it will depend on a number of factors, such as age, length and happiness of the relationship. Death of the partner may even bring relief to some, as it does not prolong the agony associated with seeing a loved one waste away.
- Some items appear ambiguous and vague (e.g. change in responsibilities at work).
- Self-reported stressful life events may also be unreliable because this depends on an individual's ability to recall accurate perceptions. A person's state of mind is influential (e.g. a patient who is unwell may dwell on and over-report negative events and under-report positive events).
- The meaning of specific events also changes with time, changing social, political and economic climates, and because one's perception

changes with experience. Adult emotional distress relies upon personality characteristics formed early in life, but primary, secondary and tertiary socialization must also be taken into account. These include current experiences that take place with continuing changes (stressors) in one's life. Values, beliefs, ideologies, interactional patterns, interests and activities – indeed the entire range of dispositions and behaviours – are subject to modification as one proceeds through life. While exposure to stressful situations varies with the social circumstances of people, it is also true that identical circumstances have different effects on individuals within the group, depending on the social contexts. For example, retirement may be eustressful to a person that has an unstimulating job, or in a culture, such as Japan, that values its elders. Alternatively, retirement may lead to chronic distress and consequently depression in a person who thoroughly enjoyed their work and now does not have enough to occupy their mind, or in a culture, such as Britain, that views elderly people negatively. Societies influence individual change and adaptation. They are sources of hardship and challenges and, by providing contexts that give meaning to the consequences of these hardships, help people fend off the harmful emotional distress that may otherwise result. The strain among people of different ages is especially relevant to developmental concerns. They can be summarized simply because of their uniqueness to particular individuals, whether it is work related or the strains associated with being single, married or divorced. Temperamentally, however, everyone is different. Thus, how we respond to stressors is subjective. Personality, it could be argued, is largely determined socially, since the family is important in providing mental stability or instability in developing our attitudes to eustress/distress. The way in which we face a crisis or disaster is learned from those around us in our youth.

- The scales focus only on distressful events and omit eustressful experiences.

This variation demonstrates that subjectivity exists even in the perception of stress. We would argue that this is caused by differences in the adaptability of individuals to cope with stressors.

to distinguish which hassles they had come across during the preceding month and then rate each entry on a three-point scale to indicate how severe the hassle had been during that period. Lazarus and Folkman (1984) stated that 'daily hassles are experiences and conditions of daily living that have been appraised as salient and harmful to the person's wellbeing.' Lazarus is working within a transactional model of stress where stress is influenced by a person's appraisal of a situation and their perceived ability to cope with it.

When quantifying stress within this conceptual framework, subjective elements such as personal beliefs and appraisal have to be included, since the perception of stress is more important than the event itself. These workers argued that the influence of hassles might be reduced by 'uplifts' (i.e. desirable experiences, such as feeling healthy or working well with your colleagues). They then developed a 135-item Uplifts Scale. This scale was administered alongside the Hassles Scale, and the strength of uplift was also rated on a three-point scale.

Major life events and daily hassles are almost certainly connected. For example, a major life event such as the death of a spouse may create a number of more minor hassles, such as sorting out financial arrangements, being a one-parent family, sorting out childcare facilities, and so on.

Further research is clearly needed to explore the complex relationship between major life events, minor frequent irritations and the onset of illness, especially since individual variation has been reported in the way people react.

Physical stressors

Physical distressors involve overexertion as well as bodily change, which may affect one's mood. They result from malnutrition, hormonal/biochemical imbalances, illnesses, injuries caused, for example, by too much activity and strain on the skeletomuscular system, or from drug and alcohol abuse. An example of physical eustress is when exercise increases one's perception of fitness level.

Psychological stressors

Psychological stressors include innate and socialized 'fears' and 'fantasies' that, if provoked, will produce either distressed (anxiety) or eustressed responses.

Environmental stressors

Environmental stressors include:

- Societal pressures, such as overcrowding, antisocial behaviour, conforming to societal norms and values, and parental wishes.
- Work distressors associated with imposed conditions, such as levels of noise, glare, or restricted movement, 'work overload' in terms of too much work (quantitative overload) or too difficult work (qualitative overload) and, conversely, quantitative and qualitative 'underload'. Conditions of employment, such as low pay, low status, shift work, staff shortages and lack of resources are also included. Relationships at work are also important, and poor commu-

---

BOX 21.3 POSTPARTUM BLUES

The 'stress' following birth is well documented (Evans *et al.*, 2001; Glover, 2001; Heron *et al.*, 2004). Nolan (2002) identified that between 50% and 80% of all the mothers experienced 'postpartum blues'. The onset of 'blues' usually occurs within the first 3–5 days after delivery and normally lasts for 2 weeks. 'The blues' are described as rapid mood fluctuations, where for no specific reason tears may follow elation. Although distressing for some women, these emotional mood swings usually resolve independently after a few days, but approximately one out of every five women will go on to develop postpartum depression which is a more severe and longer-lasting disorder that occurs in 13–15% of mothers (Nolan, 2002). The women experience psychological problems for several months – sometimes years – following birth. Women who experience postnatal depression are at increased risk of further depression particularly after subsequent births.

The most serious form of postnatal depression is puerperal psychosis, which is rare and affects two or three in 1000 women (Nolan, 2002). Symptoms include depression, mania, delusions and delirium, which resemble schizophrenia. The main concern is that the woman may be at risk of unintentionally harming herself or her baby as a result of her symptoms. The onset is sudden, and urgent treatment is required, usually in a psychiatric mother-and-baby unit on an inpatient basis. The disorder has an excellent prognosis, with a 2- to 3-month recovery period in most cases.

Although traditionally maternal depression has only been recognized after the birth of the baby, Hammond and Crozier (2007) identify antenatal depression of the precursor to postnatal depression.

---

nication channels within these may be a source of distress. A lack of understanding of social support and accountability levels, and other aspects, including career and promotion prospects, may all result in frustrations and distress, which may be associated with high absenteeism and work-related illnesses, and can result in the individual leaving that employment.

- Organizational stressors, such as work policy and procedures, could be restrictive and hence become distressful. Conversely, they may be viewed as being helpful in the day-to-day management of an individual's workload, and hence are potentially eustressful. Lack of positive feedback on performance or acceptance of new ideas could be perceived as a source of frustration and distress.
- The individual's organizational role could be a source of irritation (e.g. there may be a lack of defined authority, or no definite role specification). Interdepartmental conflicts with superiors or with colleagues/staff may occur. Difficulty in delegation, lack of involvement in decision making and lack of training for management, etc. are also perceived as sources of distress.
- Work–home interactions: two broad categories of stress for the person in work are occupational and private (domestic/personal). Stress, whether eustress or distress, in one part of life tends to spill over into other areas. Home and work conflicts may also arise with women's 'double shifts'. Their domestic labour, childcare, caring for dependants, etc. results in a lack of time for their choice of employment. Colleagues or spouse may relate this to the lack of recognition at work (Box 21.4).

BOX 21.4 THE STRESS OF THE HEALTHCARE PROFESSIONS

Assessing stress is very difficult in an occupation as diverse as health care, and to cover the stress associated with all health carers is outside the scope of this text. This section will review the implications of the subjective aspects of stress perception for nurses as a professional group most likely to report very high levels of workplace stress (Smith *et al.*, 2000).

Assessment of stress is further complicated because the term 'stress' is often used too simplistically. 'Stress' therefore should be viewed as a continuum along which an individual may pass, from no perception to feelings of eustress, to those of mild/moderate distress, to those of severe distress. Indicators of distress are recognized (see Tables 21.1, p.587 and 21.2, p.589), but those of mild/moderate distress may not be observed collectively, or may have differing degrees of severity, and so symptoms at this level of distress are likely to vary between individuals. In contrast, severe and prolonged distress culminates in more consistently observed symptoms of emotional 'burnout' and serious physiological disturbance.

It is the transition to severe distress that is likely to be most detrimental for nurses, and is closely linked to staff absenteeism, poor staff retention, and ill health (McGowan 2001; Shader *et al.* 2001). If severe distress is to be prevented then it is important to understand what factors promote the transition. Nursing provides a wide range of potential workplace stressors.

Since the transition from eustress to distress will depend upon the individual's own stress perceptions, it follows that variability between individuals in the identification of workplace stressors might be expected. In addition, temporal changes in the sources of stress might also be anticipated since working conditions are not static.

A systematic review from the literature 1985–2003 of Adult and Child care nursing by McVicar in 2003 identified six main themes for the sources of workplace distress (Table 21.4). The review indicated that most sources of stress (that is, workload, leadership/management issues, professional conflict and emotional demands of caring) have been identified consistently by nurses for many years. Perhaps this should not be surprising as they relate to the main generic characteristics of practice.

Hillhouse and Adler (1997) suggest that it is the actual characteristics of the work environment, and workload, rather than any differences in practice requirements that are important in evaluating sources of stress. However, McVicar also stated a small number of studies suggest that, while overall reported stress levels may be similar, the actual ranking of sources of stress may vary according to practice area. Foxall *et al.* (1990) found that nurses working in intensive care ranked coping with 'death and dying' more highly as a source of distress than did nurses from medical–surgical care, who ranked workload and staffing issues higher. More such comparative studies are required but from the few studies reviewed by McVicar (2003) it would appear to be important that the National Health Service (NHS) should consider that the needs of nurses could differ between practice areas.

Stordeur *et al.* (2001) ranked stressors in order of severity of impact, the main ones being:

- high workload;
- conflict with other nurses/physicians;
- experiencing a lack of clarity about tasks/goals;
- a head nurse who closely monitors the performance of staff in order to detect mistakes and to take corrective action.

Healy and McKay (2000) also found workload to be most significantly correlated with mood disturbance. However, Payne (2001) did not find a significant relationship between workload and burnout, although levels of burnout in her study were lower than in related studies. The reasons for this variation are unclear, but seem likely to include differences of stress 'hardiness' (Simoni and Paterson, 1997), of coping mechanisms (Payne, 2001), of age and experience (McNeese-Smith, 2000) or of the level of social support in the workplace (Healy and McKay, 2000).

Inter- and intra-professional conflict continues to be an important source of stress for nurses. Interprofessional conflict, particularly between nurses and physicians, appears to be more of a problem (Bratt *et al.*, 2000). The *'Working Well'* survey for the Royal College of Nursing found that 30% of nurses on long-term sick leave reported harassment and intimidation arising from sex/gender, age, race, sexuality or personal clashes, as the main cause of their absence.

Demerouti *et al.* (2000) and McGowan (2001) identified lack of reward and shift working as major sources of distress, but these did not appear as significant stressors in earlier studies. In contrast, the emotional aspect of caring does not appear as frequently in the recent literature as a source of distress as it did in earlier studies. The emotional costs of providing care are unlikely to have reduced, and so it is possible that the increased significance of sources such as reward have assumed a greater significance for nurses. If this were so then it would suggest that the problem is becoming one of growing dissatisfaction among nurses with the terms and conditions of their employment, rather than nursing *per se*.

Demerouti *et al.* (2000) also sought to distinguish between those factors that were most likely to result in emotional exhaustion and (job) disengagement, the two main components of burnout arising as a consequence of severe distress (see Table 21.2, p.589). They found that job demands (workload, time pressure and demanding contacts with patients) were most associated with emotional exhaustion, whereas job resources (lack of participation in decision making, lack of reward) were most associated with disengagement from work. These findings extend understanding by distinguishing between the type of impact that major stressors may have, but in terms of their general meaning are in broad agreement with those of Stordeur *et al.* (2001) noted above. However, data from these two studies also identify that there are limitations to such attempts to rank or categorize stressors. Thus, while Stordeur *et al.* (2001) identify 'workload' as the most frequently reported stressor, even this had a relatively low contribution (22%) to the variance in emotional exhaustion identified in that study. Similarly, although the impact of those combinations of stressors that contributed to exhaustion and disengagement was much higher, 55% and 66% respectively (Demerouti *et al.* 2000), the data still suggest that perceptions vary considerably even between nurses working in the same area.

In his review of the literature McVicar (2003) stated that it is too simplistic to suggest that any one, two or even three sources of distress are the causal factors for all nurses, or to consider that the transition of an individual nurse from mild to severe distress can be predicted reliably at present. He concluded that the progression along the continuum from no conscious perception of stress to eustress to distress is subjective, depending upon the relationship between the individual and their environment. Thus, while there is recognition that workload, leadership style, professional relationships, and emotional demands are the most frequently reported major factors that cause workplace distress for staff, it is clear that the impact of these sources varies considerably. There are differences in the perceptions of nurses from different workplaces, and even between individuals in the same workplace. The workplace is also not static: lack of reward and complications of shift working have also been identified recently as further significant sources of distress for nurses.

The implications for the impact of organizational interventions to reduce stress in nursing is outside the scope of this text, but is discussed in detail in the review by McVicar (2003) and is covered in various Departmental of Health reports (see further reading).

BOX 21.4 *Continued*

McVicar (2003) also concluded that initiatives introduced by the NHS to address the problem of stress in nursing have the potential to go some way towards improving the situation, but there is a need for more comparative studies to help to clarify how interventions might be directed at specific clinical areas. Improvements are most likely in leadership/management styles and interprofessional conflict but the issues of workload (i.e. staffing levels), emotional labour, pay and shift work are likely to remain a problem, at least for the foreseeable future. Inadequate pay is increasingly a source of distress, exacerbated by high workload and by falling levels of staffing. The government and NHS are seeking to improve the situation but, while initiatives will help, it is questionable that they will remove the problem.

Table 21.4 Major workplace stressors that impact on work satisfaction for staff nurses*

Stressor	References: 1985–1997	References: 1998–April 2003
Workload/inadequate staff cover/ time pressure	Hipwell *et al.* (1989) Baglioni *et al.* (1990) Foxall *et al.* (1990) Lees and Ellis (1990) Tyler and Ellison (1994) Tyler and Cushway (1995) Hillhouse and Adler (1997)	Healy and McKay (1999) Demerouti *et al.* (2000) McGowan (2001) Stordeur *et al.* (2001)
Relationship with other clinical staff	Foxall *et al.* (1990) Lees and Ellis (1990) Tyler and Ellison (1994) Hillhouse and Adler (1997)	Hope *et al.* (1998) Healy and McKay (1999) Bratt *et al.* (2000) Stordeur *et al.* (2001)
Leadership and management style/ poor locus of control/ poor group cohesion/ lack of adequate supervisory support	Constable and Russell (1986) Lucas *et al.* (1993) Tyler and Ellison (1994) Leveck and Jones (1996) Morrison *et al.* (1997)	Bratt *et al.* (2000) Demerouti *et al.* (2000) Schmitz *et al.* (2000) McGowan (2001) Shader *et al.* (2001) Stordeur *et al.* (2001)
Coping with emotional needs of patients and their families/poor patient diagnosis/death and dying	Hare *et al.* (1988) Hipwell *et al.* (1989) Foxall *et al.* (1990) Lees and Ellis (1990) Tyler and Ellison (1994)	Bratt *et al.* (2000)
Shift working		Demerouti *et al.* (2000) Healy and McKay (2000)
Lack of reward		Demerouti *et al.* (2000) McGowan (2001)

*Those stressors that relate to the same theme are collated, and presented pre- and post-1997, that is before and after recent policy changes in the workplace (Department of Health, 1999, 2002a,b,c, 2003). The stressors are not listed in order of importance.

Physical eustress could be the perception of enjoyment one feels on a long-earned holiday or break from the distressors of work.

See also Box 21.5 for a discussion of burnout and disease of adaptation

Developmental stressors

In an attempt to make sense of the 'meaning of life', science has always tried to classify objects, living matter, etc. Human development is no exception: various stages of development have been attributed labels, so we can distinguish one developmental stage from another in order to aid advances in specialist knowledge in these areas. Thus, we have (arguably) the 'beginnings of life' stage, known as the zygote. This stage progresses into the morula, the blastocyst, the embryo, the fetus (see Figure 19.4, p.526), the neonate, the infant, the child, the pubertal adolescent, the adult, the stage we equate with old age, retirement and beyond, and finally the terminal stage of 'death', which, according to Selye, is when we are finally free from stress!

Each stage is identifiable from the others by differential psychophysiological phenotypes (i.e. measurable characteristics). For example, the emotional and physical characteristics of the adolescent and adult are obviously different. Each psychophysiological phenotype arises through enzymatically controlled reactions, through a combination of gene expression and modification by environmental factors (including stressors), and the timing of exposure to such stressors influence this gene expression, and so are responsible for the range of onset of developmental stages. For example, the onset of puberty is between 10 and 12 years for girls and between 12 and 14 years for boys; this results from the production of adequate quantities of the male and female steroid hormones, which promote the development of the secondary sexual characteristics. Genes must be expressed for this hormone synthesis to cause puberty. Most people have the genetic potential for puberty, and the age range of the onset demonstrates subjectivity of gene expression instigated by environmental triggers of puberty. Perhaps premature or delayed onset may be a result of premature or delayed exposure to those environmental factors necessary for gene expression.

Therefore, psychophysiological subjectivity exists across the lifespan. Society, which provides the environmental triggers, therefore also has positive and negative effects on development.

ACTIVITY

List the potential social, physical, psychological, developmental and environmental distressors that a healthcare practitioner may encounter with (1) his/her patients, and (2) the occupational hazards of nursing.

Interim summary

So far, this discussion has focused on the subjectivity of how people perceive stressors. The cumulative effect on an individual of such stressors (social, developmental, physical, environmental and psychological) also demonstrates individuality. Thus, stressors may or may not be perceived consciously as such by different individuals, because no two people are alike.

It is also unlikely that any two people will experience identical stressors. Furthermore, the perceived stressors must reach or supersede the stress threshold of the individual. Stress thresholds are dynamic and are not fixed entities. They are subjective to individuals, according to the individual's resistance to stressors, their available coping mechanisms or 'adaptation energy', and to the stress-related conditions they have experienced throughout their lives.

Subjectivity is based upon the nature–nurture interactions of at least five factors:

1 The person's genotype.
2 The person's upbringing.
3 The person's environment.
4 The person's personality (which depends on factors 1 and 2).
5 Circadian rhythm fluctuations (e.g. people who are 'moody' first thing in the morning).

Once the cumulative effect of the stressors has reached or superseded the stress threshold, then individuality of the psychophysiological bodily response is observed, and the person experiences either distress or eustress, depending on the cognitive interpretation of the 'stressors'.

THE SUBJECTIVITY OF STRESS RESPONSES

Historically, many models of stress have been put forward; this section will now consider only the well established ones.

Transactional model of stress

Cox and McKay in 1976 described the stress response as occurring when there is a mismatch between the perceived environmental demands and the person's perceived capabilities (Figure 21.4a). An important aspect of this model is that it is the individual's perception of demands (and not actual demands) placed upon them that may produce the stress response. That is, if the person's perception of demands exceeds their perceived capabilities to cope with them, then too much stress (hyperstress) becomes apparent. Conversely, if perceived capabilities of coping exceed the perceived demands, then too little stress (hypostress) is evident. When capabilities and demands are matched, then, the authors of this text consider that the individual is experiencing eustress. It follows then, that coping (or adapting) to situations of hyperstress or hypostress involve changing one's perceptions of demands according to one's capabilities and vice versa (Figure 21.4b). Yerkes-Dodson in 1982 (Dodson, 1982) stated that optimum stress provides maximum performance, and from this one may then potentially experience eustress. Stress levels below or above these optima result in deteriorating performance and can be a potential source of distress (Figure 21.5).

ACTIVITY

'Stress is a subjective perception.' Discuss this statement using the principles of Cox and McKay's transactional model of stress.

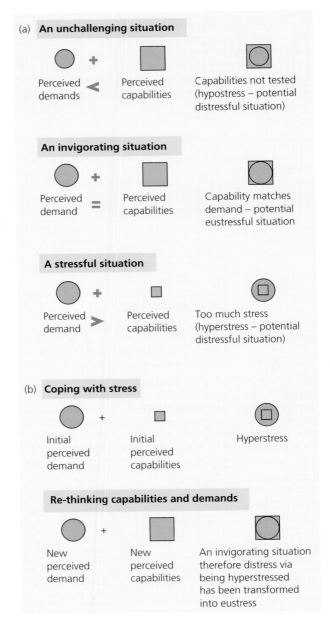

Figure 21.4 (a) Cox and McKay's transactional model of stress. (b) Coping with stress

Q *Distinguish between perceived demands and perceived capability.*

See the case studies of occupational hyperstress and hypostress, Section VI, p.675.

The general adaptation syndrome

The demand–capability model can be linked with the earlier work of Selye (1956), who described the GAS. This model attempts to explain the physiological responses to stress. Selye labelled the response as a non-specific (i.e. stereotypic) response – 'the sick syndrome' – as he realized that patients with a variety of diseases had similar signs and symptoms, including weight loss, appetite loss, decreased muscular

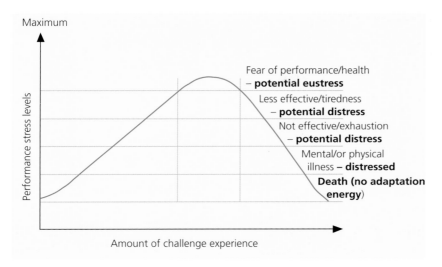

strength, and no ambition. His animal studies demonstrated that three changes occurred during exposure to continued or extreme stress:

1 The adrenal cortex enlarged (or hypertrophies), and therefore becomes hypersecretive.
2 The thymus gland, spleen and lymph nodes decreased in size (or atrophy).
3 Bleeding ulcers appeared in the gastrointestinal tract.

Selye argued that a variety of dissimilar situations, such as arousal, grief, pain, fear, unexpected success and loss of blood, are all capable of producing similar physiological stress responses. Thus, although people may face quite different stressors, in some respects their bodies respond in a stereotypical pattern. According to Selye, this involved identical biochemical changes that enabled them to cope with any type of increased demand on the body. Thus, Selye believed that stress was the non-specific adaptive response of the body to any demand placed upon it. Later, he argued that stress, whether pleasurable (eustress) or threatening (distress), produced physiological changes to restore homeostasis, which was disrupted by the stressors. Selye also suggested that continued exposure to stressors results in three distinct phases of alarm, resistance (or adaptation) and exhaustion.

The alarm stage

Alarm is predominantly initiated and controlled by the sympathetic nervous system, and affects organs such as the brain, heart and skeletal muscles (Figure 21.6). These initial effects are prolonged by the simultaneous sympathetic input to the adrenal medulla, which causes the release of the catecholamine hormones adrenaline and noradrenaline. These hormones function at the sympathetic neuromuscular and neurosecretory effector sites. Selye viewed this response as being anticipatory of a threat, and the necessity of taking action. The alarm stage is equivalent to Cannon's (1935) famous 'fright, fight, flight' statement when describing the effects of adrenaline and noradrenaline. The authors of this text consider the effects of

this stage as being normal homeostatic adaptations operating, hopefully, to enable the individual to cope with, or adapt to, the dominant stressor(s), which had resulted in the person reaching the stress threshold. If the adaptations are successful, or the dominant stressor is perceived to have fallen below threshold level, then visceral organ functions return to their 'normal' homeostatic ranges or baselines (e.g. heart rate returns to resting level, etc). However, if the stressors remain at or above threshold level, and/or additional stressors occur, then Selye argued that the individual goes into the second stage of resistance or dies. Progression through the GAS depends on the person's perception of the intensity and duration of the demand.

ACTIVITY

List the four most common signs of the alarm stage that you have experienced in patients who are undergoing admissions to your ward. Compare these with the actions of the sympathetic nervous system outlined in Table 8.6, p.200.

Resistance or adaptation stage

The resistance stage is controlled predominantly by the hormones of stress and is therefore mediated by the hypothalamus, which provides the main mind–body functional link (see Figures 9.5, p.214 and 9.12, p.219). In the context of this text, such events are still regarded as homeostatic adaptations (i.e. normal adaptive responses to a changed situation). This stage is maintained largely by the hormone cortisol, the main glucocorticoid hormone produced by the cortex of the adrenal glands. Growth hormone is also released from the pituitary gland; the actions of cortisol and growth hormone are highlighted in Figures 21.6 and 21.8. Note in particular the actions of the two hormones to mobilize metabolic fuels. Cortisol is sometimes referred to as the 'hormone of stress', since people who are unable to produce it in sufficient quantities adapt very poorly to stressful situations.

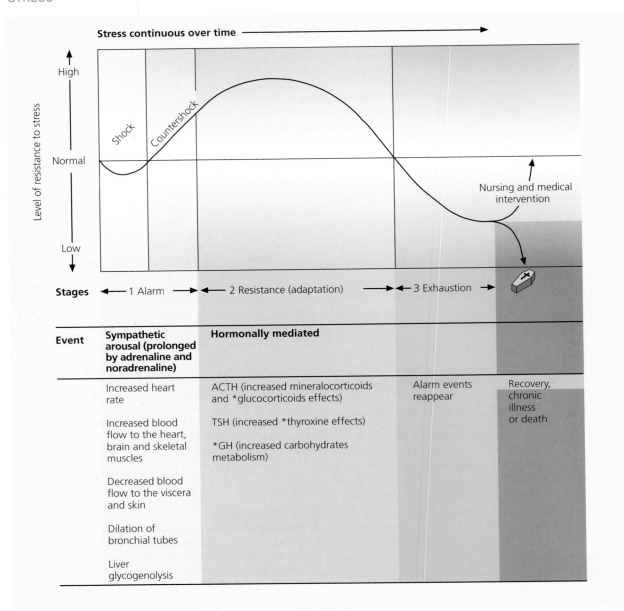

Figure 21.6 Selye's general adaptation syndrome. ACTH, adrenocorticotropic hormone; GH, growth hormone; TSH, thyroid-stimulating hormone; *, increased glucose availability for catabolism (possibly provides a source of adaptation energy)

Q Describe the events associated with the triphasic stages of the general adaptation syndrome.

The alarm and resistance phases facilitate our ability to cope with stressors. In other words, although it may seem that neural and hormonal homeostasis in these phases has failed, the responses do promote the conditions necessary for survival and so are examples of homeostatic adaptation rather than homeostatic imbalance.

The majority of hormones released are hyperglycaemic agents (i.e. chemicals that raise the blood sugar levels) and as such provide cells with energy to cope with the effects of the stressors. Selye (1956) referred to the concept of 'adaptation energy'. He stated that our amount of adaptation energy might be compared with our inherited bank account, determined by

our individualistic genotype, from which we can make withdrawals, but into which we apparently cannot make deposits. 'Adaptation energy' is conceptual, not a measurable entity, though advances in stem cell research might influence such statements. However, according to Selye, stressors cause wear and tear, leaving some irreversible 'scars' (or costs), which accumulate and contribute to the signs of ageing (see Table 19.3, p.549 and Figure 19.23, p.551). If this is the case, then adaptation energy should be used wisely rather than squandered. It is still not understood what is lost, except that it is unlikely to be simply the product of calorific energy (i.e. ATP). If there is no adaptation (or resistance), or if attempts to reduce

BOX 21.5 BURNOUT AND DISEASE OF ADAPTATION

Burnout

To burn out is 'to fail, wear out or become exhausted by making excessive demands on energy, strength or resources'. Some of the signs of burnout include feelings of exhaustion and fatigue, not being able to shake off a cold, feeling worn out, frequent headaches and gastrointestinal tract disturbances, loss of weight and depression. Burnout is sometime viewed as progressive stress and can be divided into five stages:

1 *Honeymoon stage*: idealistic enthusiasm is demonstrated by a high degree of personal motivation to achieve goals (some of which may be unrealistic). This is sometimes referred to as the 'honeymoon period' for example within a new job and it may last up to a year. However, in theory if the patterns of coping are positive, adaptive, then an individual can stay in the honeymoon period almost indefinitely.

2 *Balancing stage*: the individual realizes that some days are better than others regarding how well they are handling the 'stress' for example of the job. An awareness of a notable increase in the following is indicative of this stage:

   (i) Job dissatisfaction.

   (ii) Motivation declines progressively and outside interests begin to take precedence over work.

   (iii) Working inefficiency and losing things; the goals become unrealistic and unachievable.

   (iv) Fatigue; personal energy levels begin to fade.

   (v) Sleep disturbances.

3 *Chronic stage*: chronic symptoms appear marked by intensification some of the factors in stage 2; for example, chronic exhaustion, anger, depression and physical illness may result.

4 *Crisis stage*: the symptoms of stage 3 become critical. The individual obsesses about frustrations, such as at work, and develops escapism activities (including eating, smoking, drinking, watching TV). Pessimism and self-doubt dominate thinking.

5 *Enmeshment stage*: the symptoms of burnout are so embedded that they are likely to be labelled as having some significant physical or emotional problem, and are likely to be considered a burnout case.

Managers and nurses and other healthcare practitioners should be aware of these stages, since the teaching of stress management will reduce the risk of burnout.

ACTIVITY

Examine your own behaviour and that of colleagues for signs of burnout.

Diseases of adaptation

In the context of this book, 'diseases of adaptation' occur when stress is maladapted and therefore it is when clinical intervention is required to restore the person's homeostatic mechanisms. First, there is a need to assess or identify the major stressors associated with the illness. Care must then be planned and implemented so as to minimize, remove or treat these stressors. For example, bacterial infection or perhaps social problems would be treated with antibiotics or controlled by teaching stress management techniques, respectively.

Only the most severe stress leads rapidly to the exhaustion stage and maybe death. Most physical and/or psychological exertion, infection and other stressors act upon us for a limited period and produce changes corresponding only to the first and second stages. Thus, throughout life, we go through these first two stages many times in order to adapt to all the demands within our environment.

The triphasic nature of the GAS indicates that the body's adaptation energy is finite, since continuous distress eventually produces exhaustion, and the person succumbs to a stress-related condition. The type and severity of these conditions reflect, yet again, subjective elements. Selye (1976) classified GAS responses as 'synotoxic' and 'catatoxic reactions of the body's defence against potential internal and/or external aggressors (stressors)'. Synotoxic reactions help us put up with the aggressor, whereas catatoxic reactions help us to destroy it. Synotoxic stimuli act as tissue 'tranquillizers', permitting a peaceful coexistence with the aggressors, whereas catatoxic agents mainly involve the induction of destructive enzymes, which generate an attack on the pathogen, usually by accelerating its metabolic degradation.

Corticoids are among the most effective synotoxic hormones. This hormonal group inhibits inflammation and promotes other defence mechanisms, such as transplant rejection. The main purpose of inflammation is to prevent irritants from entering the circulation by localizing them. However, once the foreign agent is rendered harmless, the suppression of inflammation becomes advantageous. Clinically, anti-inflammatory corticoids are given in such cases, and have proven to be effective in treating diseases in which the major complaint is inflammation of the eyes, joints or respiratory passageways.

Alternatively, when the aggressor is dangerous, the defence reaction should be increased above the normal level. This is achieved by catatoxic substances, such as antibodies, lysozymes and pain-producing substances, which carry messages to fight the 'invaders' (stressors) even more actively than normal.

The major physiological responses of the body to excessive stress are vascular in some form, usually compromising blood supply at some point. The body may overcome this by neural/endocrine changes that re-establish vascular homeostasis. This response is potentially life saving in acute situations, but if stressors are prolonged or intense, it can lead to organ system failure, resulting, for example, in cardiovascular and gastrointestinal disease. The interdependency of organ systems and their component parts means that if one system is affected, then others will also be affected (see Chapter 1, p.8–10).

A good example of this is in maturity-onset diabetes mellitus, which demonstrates that a failure at cellular level results in multiple organ system failure. This condition is exacerbated by the prolonged effects of carbohydrate-rich (distressor) diets, which promote hyperglycaemia (= excessively high glucose concentration in blood) as the insulin target receptor sites become 'desensitized' to the hormone insulin. The hyperglycaemia (now a distressor) must be corrected. Glucose is excreted in the urine (glycosuria), which helps to moderate the hyperglycaemia, but there are no endogenous agents, other than insulin, that will reverse it. In addition, diabetes is also associated with fat breakdown, which produces hyperlipidaemia (another distressor) with an atherosclerotic effect. Atherosclerosis is another distressor in diabetes; it diminishes the functions of the blood vessels of multiple organs, and partly explains why a diabetic person's eyes, heart, blood pressure and kidneys may all be affected. Although diabetic people exhibit the same biochemical and response mechanisms, the degree of change is individual, so the organs that are affected, and how much they are affected, varies. Perhaps the host of factors that form the basis of nature–nurture interaction subjectivity also explains this variation.

A severely stressed person also presents a clinical picture that results from the cumulative effects of various stress hormones. For example, hypertension could result from the vasoconstrictory actions of adrenaline, noradrenaline and angiotensin II, or the circulatory volume-expanding effects of aldosterone and antidiuretic hormone, or from an increased cardiac output caused by adrenaline and noradrenaline (see Figure 12.29a, p.349, and associated text). Adrenaline and noradrenaline may also cause tachycardia, hyperventilation, bowel dysfunction, and other fight, flight and fright responses (alarm reactions). Again, however, there is individual variability.

the cumulative effects of the stressors below threshold level are unsuccessful, then, Selye argued, we would go into the final stage of exhaustion.

Exhaustion

In exhaustion, the signs of the alarm stage reappear. This is an indication that the body's homeostatic adaptive processes have failed since the body's adaptive responses have not been sufficient and so have made necessary further activation of catacholamines. Consequently stress-related illnesses appear (Box 21.5; Selye called these 'diseases of adaptation') or death results.

Analysis of the general adaptation syndrome

Although on the whole we agree with Selye's ideas, looking at Table 21.1 we could argue that stressed people do not have consistent (non-specific) physiological, behavioural and emotional response indicators. In addition, when stressed, individuality is again observed according to whether the person perceives the stress response as distress or eustress, and whether the person is consciously aware of this stress response.

The pituitary–adrenocortical activity in response to stress is also not as broad and consistent as Selye suggested. He found that some physically harmful stressors, such as fasting, did not increase corticosteroid levels when the stressors were weak. However, when fasting was strengthened by psychological factors (e.g. an unhealthy desire to be thin), the non-specific response occurred. Thus, it is only demands that tax the person's capabilities that are stressful (i.e. those that reach or exceed the person's stress threshold). The extent of the stress response depends on the individual's evaluation of the consequences of unfulfilled demands. The stress response is not stereotypical, and stress is not manifested as a single syndrome, such as the GAS. Multiple factors governed by situational and individualistic variables are involved.

The disadvantages of Selye's GAS are that it fails to clarify what conditions cause stress or what constitutes a demanding stressor capable of initiating it, and it does not take into account situational and individualistic variables involved in the activation of this stress response. Consequently, it really describes a theory of adaptation to stress rather than a stress theory.

Selye's work, however, can be defended easily using the stress threshold concept. If stressor strength is below threshold level ('subconscious' stress), then the reactions of the GAS do not appear; it is only when the threshold is met or superseded that the reactions of the GAS come into operation.

Cognitive models of stress

The influence of Lazarus (1966) marked a change in the stress research field, which previously had been dominated by Selye. Lazarus identified three important aspects of stress:

1. Stress is determined by the perception of a stressful situation rather than by the situation itself.
2. Individuals differ in their reactivity to stress.
3. The extent of stress depends partly on the capabilities of the individual to cope.

ACTIVITY

Identify clinical situations in which healthcare professionals use perception of control, predicting the outcome and past experiences to minimize distress in patients.

Therefore, according to Lazarus (1966), 'Stress occurs when there are demands on the person which tax or exceed his adaptive resources'. This definition emphasizes the role of cognitive appraisal in relation to a demand–capability imbalance. Factors important in the perception of environmental stressors involve:

- *perception of control*: if one is not in control then distress is more likely;

ACTIVITY

'Stress is a subjective phenomenon.' Discuss this statement in relation to the individualistic nature of the following: (1) stressors; (2) stress threshold; (3) stress response; and (4) stress-related illnesses. Suggest why it is difficult to measure or assess subjective experiences such as stress.

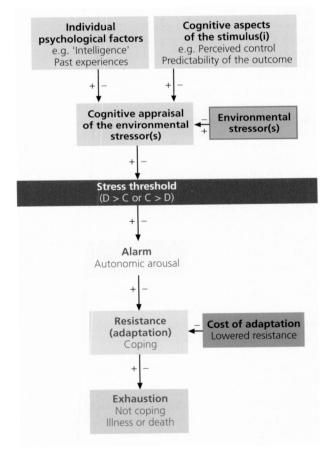

Figure 21.7 Psychophysiological model of stress. C, capabilities; D, demands; +, continue; −, remove

Q Stress is said to be a psychophysiological bodily response arising through environmental stressors. What do you understand by this statement?

BOX 21.6 STRESS REDUCTION: A CLINICAL PERSPECTIVE

Scientific breakthroughs include the use of tranquillizers in combating 'mental' illnesses, and the use of anti-ulcer drugs. However, most of these agents are directed not against stress, but against some of its manifestations and therefore do not enable people to manage the cause of their problem. Many authorities are therefore critical of a reliance on 'medical' solutions, and increasing attention is given to psychological and behavioural techniques that anyone can use to avoid producing the

stress response. There are various approaches that are beyond the remit of this book, but enabling people to reappraise their situation through cognitive behavioural therapy is a popular one, coupled with measures to improve day-to-day coping, for example relaxation techniques such as transcendental meditation, which should be given the respect they deserve as they do work on some of those people who try them.

- *predictability of the outcome*: if one cannot predict the outcome, then distress is more likely;
- *past experiences*: if one has no past experience with potential distressors, then one is more likely to experience distress until a coping strategy can be developed.

In contrast to Selye's biological theory, the emphasis of 'psychological' stress is on the input side, in particular on the kind of situation and the individual interaction that evokes a stress state. Both approaches are complementary. Lazarus's psychological theory outlines the conditions that determine the evocation of stress, while Selye's physiological theory describes its form (Figure 21.7). This integrated approach provides Selye's formulations with the breadth needed to encompass the stress of living.

The psychological effects of stress are subjective and multiple. They may result in depression, lack of personal accomplishment, avoidance of decisions, depersonalization or a feeling of emotional emptiness. The effects of these stressors can result in a shift from a positive to a negative view, which can lead to an uncaring disposition. Absenteeism, guilt, error

---

BOX 21.7 THE METABOLIC STRESS RESPONSE TO SURGERY

Surgical trauma promotes metabolic responses, which can be divided into various phases. Following surgery, the patient rapidly enters the 'ebb' phase, in which there is reduced metabolism and the concentration of metabolic fuels within the blood increases. This phase is usually quite short, and may start before injury owing to responses associated with the 'alarm' phase of stress responses, as identified by Selye. After several hours, the patient enters the 'flow' phase, which is characterized by tissue catabolism and an increased metabolic rate: these responses may be substantial, especially after severe trauma. In the longer term, anabolic phases can also be identified, during which the metabolic status of the patient returns to normal. This box is concerned largely with the flow phase, since this phase covers the immediate week or so after surgery, and it is within this period that the major adaptive responses for recovery are observed.

Although the GAS can be criticized for various reasons (see earlier), the hormonal responses it describes are identifiable in the patient undergoing physical trauma, such as surgery. They illustrate the adaptive aspects of such responses and so, in this context, stress responses would be eustressful if the patient recovered from surgery, but could potentially be distressful if the hormonal responses were excessive or persistent. The principles of the GAS therefore provide a useful means of introducing these responses, but you should bear in mind that the hormonal changes it describes largely occur simultaneously following injury (Clancy and McVicar, 1998b).

Stress response in the postoperative period
The metabolic changes that are promoted in the alarm and resistance phases equate with the injury (i.e. ebb and flow) phase of surgical recovery. This section looks at how these responses enable the individual to cope with, and recover from, surgical stress.

The activity of the sympathetic nervous system, adrenaline and cortisol during the ebb phase stimulate breakdown of glycogen (glycogenolysis) and fat (lipolysis), and hence promote the mobilization of glucose and fatty acids. However, sympathetic activity to the pancreas inhibits insulin secretion, while growth hormone released from the pituitary gland reduces the capacity of cells to take up glucose (i.e. insulin resistance is promoted): the mobilization of glucose, coupled with an inhibited insulin release and elevated insulin resistance, leads to high blood sugar

concentration (hyperglycaemia). This favours the functioning of insulin-independent tissues, especially the brain, while tissues that are insulin sensitive, such as liver, adipocytes and skeletal muscle, will become more dependent on the generation of energy from fatty acids, thus resulting in the consequential accumulation of ketone bodies.

Despite these changes, basal metabolism does not increase overall during the ebb phase; in fact, it often decreases, suggesting that there are additional biochemical adaptations. However, the ebb phase is usually quite short, and the patient soon enters the flow phase, when the metabolic responses facilitate an increased metabolic rate.

ACTIVITY

Remind yourself of what the term 'basal metabolic rate' means, and its significance to clinical practice, and identify the factors that might influence it during the postoperative period.

As the flow phase becomes established, fatty acid metabolism will still be the most important energy store for the body as a whole, although glucose supply to insulin-independent tissues continues to be supported by hyperglycaemia. The latter is maintained by further glucose synthesis prompted by the actions of cortisol to induce protein breakdown and the release of amino acids. Protein catabolism also results in the increased synthesis and excretion of urea (a 'waste' product of amino acid metabolism). Protein synthesis is also decreased, exacerbating the reduction in protein. Muscle provides the main source of protein in the body, but the increased protein catabolism may also decrease the concentration of some plasma proteins, although fibrinogen and those involved in immunity may even increase, perhaps as haemostatic and anti-infection mechanisms. The flow phase responses are summarized in Figure 21.8.

The elevated metabolism observed during the flow phase causes an increase in body temperature, an elevation in heart rate (to promote effective circulation), and an elevation in lung ventilation (to promote oxygen uptake and carbon dioxide excretion). The significance of increased mobilization of metabolic fuels is that cell division and tissue growth and repair are facilitated. A further action of an elevated release of cortisol is to reduce immune responses. Although at first this might

BOX 21.7 *Continued*

seem detrimental to recovery from surgery, the response is probably important later in the flow phase when the persistence of inflammation and fibrosis will hinder wound healing. The anti-inflammatory actions of steroids are well known and they are used widely in clinical practice; the effects of cortisol released during stress are also of interest to researchers studying incidences of infection following lifestyle stress. Chronic use of steroids also has depressive actions on the immune system.

ACTIVITY

Using Chapter 9, pp.218–19 review how the control of cortisol is normally controlled. Using Figure 21.6, p.598, and associated text identify the site of action of non-steroidal anti-inflammatory drugs (NSAIDs) in the pain pathway.

Circulatory responses
The cardiovascular actions of sympathetic nerves, backed up by catecholamines, represent part of the stress response to surgery. They are worth reviewing here because they reinforce the advantages that stress responses facilitate during and after trauma. The roles of sympathetic activation can be related to the circulation and to haemostasis.

A significant loss of blood during surgery could be expected to stimulate sympathetic nerve activity, and to promote the release of vasoactive hormones (especially adrenaline, vasopressin and angiotensin II), but there is an additional aspect. Contact with, and manipulation of, internal organs is a very powerful stimulus for the release of the hormones, regardless of fluid loss. In a 'natural' sense, such contact would represent a severe trauma that would ordinarily be expected to induce haemorrhage, so the alarm response can also be viewed as being anticipatory of hypovolaemia. This helps to explain why abdominal and thoracic surgery is a particularly powerful stimulus for hormone release.

Surgery is a controlled trauma, in that blood loss is minimized. With limited blood loss, a powerful release of vasoactive hormones might be expected to elevate arterial blood pressure, but their actions are offset against the effects of anaesthetics, some of which depress the brainstem control of the autonomic nervous system, hence causing a decline in sympathetic output to the heart and blood vessels. However, the release of vasoactive hormones in the alarm phase will actually help to control arterial blood pressure in the presence of anaesthesia. The permissive actions of cortisol on the catecholamines provide additional support following trauma.

Further actions of adrenaline, vasopressin and angiotensin II include the promotion of blood clotting (adrenaline) and the initiation of water and electrolyte conservation (all three hormones, but especially vasopressin and angiotensin). These actions again are of obvious benefit should blood loss have occurred, but they will also have implications for the patient's water balance in the postsurgical period (Clancy and McVicar, 1997a).

ACTIVITY

Using Chapter 20, p.578 review the actions of local anaesthetics on the sodium/potassium ATPase pump in inhibiting the pain stimuli.

Implications of metabolic responses to surgery
The metabolic responses to surgery represent a resetting of homeostatic range, and hence homeostatic means, and so promote the functional changes necessary for recovery. As such, according to stress and homeostatic theories, they are homeostatically adaptive, eustressful mecha-

nisms that promote the health of the patient. The release of the hormones supporting the changes declines gradually as the flow phase progresses, so homeostatic ranges and means eventually return to their normal homeostatic parameters. However, there is a metabolic 'cost' of the flow phase, particularly in relation to protein synthesis: the catabolism of muscle proteins produced by growth hormone and cortisol during the flow phase induces a loss of muscle tissue. The resultant increase in urea production from amino acid metabolism promotes a negative nitrogen balance, since urea has incorporated into it the nitrogen found in amino acid molecules. Persistence of protein depletion may hinder long-term wound healing and has implications for the general welfare of the patient.

Selye's general adaptation syndrome would relate these implications to a transition from resistance into exhaustion and distress (i.e. the metabolic cost of recovery places the patient at risk of ill health). Wound healing can be enhanced, and protein depletion reduced, by ensuring that the patient has adequate protein nutrition during the flow phase. The amino acids arginine and glutamine are especially important in this respect, as they stimulate collagen production, fibroblast activity and immune functions, all of which are central to the wound healing process (Clancy and McVicar, 1997b). A good-quality diet should be available to patients, although commercially available supplements may also be used, and will help to minimize protein depletion before the patient enters the anabolic phase of recovery.

Diabetes mellitus and surgery
The discussion so far has centred on the responses of patients that do not have an underlying metabolic problem on admission for surgery (although malnourishment, particularly dehydration, is not rare in the surgical patient because of presurgical 'nil-by-mouth' procedures and hormonal responses). Patients with diabetes are faced with additional hazards, which are related to chronic complications of the disorder (e.g. nephropathy, angiopathy and neuropathy) and that result from the imposition of metabolic responses to surgery upon the person's disturbed metabolism. Under these circumstances, responses that are ordinarily adaptive can become maladaptive, and so have immediate implications for health.

ACTIVITY

How might the presence of nephropathy, angiopathy and neuropathy in the patient with diabetes affect processes involved in wound healing?

In diabetes, the shortage of insulin or the presence of insulin resistance intensifies the metabolic response to surgery. The risks associated with this are:

- enhanced hyperglycaemia, with the associated risk of coma. Polyuria and polydipsia would also be expected;
- increased fatty acid mobilization and ketone body formation, to the extent that the risk of ketoacidosis is increased.

Such risks mean that monitoring blood glucose concentration accurately, and paying particular attention to maintaining the patient's metabolic control, will be important aspects for perioperative care of people with diabetes mellitus.

ACTIVITY

Review your understanding of the two main types of diabetes mellitus, and consider how metabolic control might be achieved with each type after surgery.

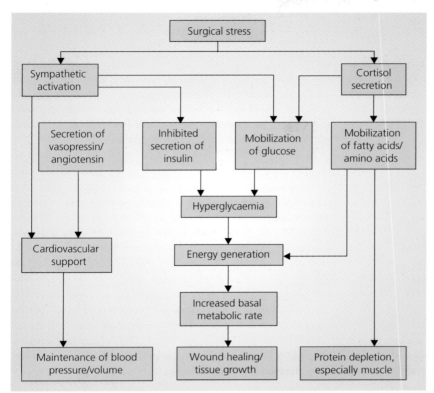

Figure 21.8 Summary of the main events in the flow phase of recovery from surgery. Note how the net effect of the responses is generally one of facilitating recovery, apart from the metabolic 'cost' of protein depletion

and helplessness can follow. Such signs are often described in the context of 'disengagement' and (eventually) 'burnout'.

COPING MECHANISMS AND FEATURES OF FAILURE

Stress management attempts to reduce or prevent distress and its harmful effects. There are three classes of management:

- change one's environment and/or lifestyle;
- change one's personality and/or one's perceptions;
- change the biological response to stress.

In general, the term 'coping' is usually reserved for behavioural (psychological) responses, and 'adaptation' is applied to the physiological responses. Thus, as stress is viewed by the authors as a psychophysiological bodily response, then we prefer the use of the term 'adaptive coping', as stress-management techniques are employed to alleviate the negative consequences of the whole-body stress response. It is obviously outside the scope of this chapter to describe stress-management techniques in any detail; however, some methods are illustrated in Table 21.5, and the principles behind them are explained in the sec-

tion on 'Principles of coping'. The important point to note is that the usefulness of each technique is subject to an individual's beliefs, and that these beliefs are time-dependent and dynamic.

Principles of coping

Everyone possesses strategies or defence mechanisms that they often do not recognize they have used, including:

- *denial:* for example, a practitioner who refuses to concede the existence of stress (the nurse who continues to work against all odds);
- *escape:* for example, taking time out to avoid stressful encounters or avoiding the demands of the job to concentrate on trivial tasks;
- *displacement:* transferring feelings or blame from one person to another, often easier scapegoat;
- *intellectualization:* distancing oneself from the person or situation causing stress.

An awareness of these mechanisms allows one to observe signs of stress in oneself and in others.

This section is concerned with how people generally cope

Table 21.5 Some stress management techniques

Environmental/lifestyle	Personality/perception	Biological response
Time management	Assertiveness training	Progressive relaxation
Proper nutrition	Thought stopping	Relaxation response
Exercise	Refuting irrational ideas	Meditation
Finding alternatives to frustrated goals, e.g. stopping smoking or drinking.	Stress inoculation modifying type A behaviour	Breathing exercises, biofeedback autogenics

with stress using cognitive appraisal of distressors, but does not discuss individual coping strategies. This book has demonstrated that stressors are necessary to perform the 'characteristics of life', and that it is how a person copes or fails to adapt to distressors that is important in determining whether he or she succumbs to stress-related conditions, or progresses through developmental stages of the lifespan.

Cognitive coping

A cognitive approach to coping involves transferring distress into eustress, or removing distressors to below the stress threshold level by reducing perceived or actual demands on the body. The success of coping methods is subjective, since individuals differ in respect of their cognitive and behavioural efforts to manage, reduce or tolerate the internal and external demands of the person–environment transactions. Success is also time dependent, since individuals have circadian rhythm fluctuations (see Chapter 22, p.609–11) that influence cognitive and behavioural appraisals and responses.

It is generally accepted that a mismatch between perceived demands and capabilities produces a source of distress, so it is important that the person copes or adapts to these distressors in order to prevent the occurrence of stress-related illness. The term 'coping', like 'stress', has acquired many meanings. It may refer to efforts to master conditions of harm or threat of challenge, when a routine or automatic response is not readily available. Here, environmental demands must be met with new behavioural solutions, or old ones must be adapted to meet the current stress. There are two sources of coping: problem-focused (essentially how to reduce or remove the source of distress) and emotion-focused coping (changing the cognitive appraisal of the stressor and capacity to deal with it) (Figures 21.4b, p.596 and 21.7, p.600). For example, in trying to understand this entire book you may be struggling because there aspects that you feel you need to understand but others that are of less significance. But how do you determine what is of significance? What do you need to understand from the breadth of material within the book that would help you to gain a better understanding of those relevant aspects? How can you apply the learning from your professional experience?

Another method of cognitive coping could involve 'moulding' one's personality into a less distressed or even a eustressful personality. For example, personality type A is often described as being hard-driving, hasty, hostile, hurried, agitated, impatient, irritable, frequently a poor listener, rushed, overcompetitive and overambitious. People who have few of these characteristics are referred to as personality type B, being calm and content, easy-going personalities, good listeners, not easily irritated, patient and unhurried. Type A personalities often claim that they 'thrive on stress' (perhaps they are addicted to adrenaline and noradrenaline, which are released in the stress response alarm and exhaustion stages). Excessive, frequent and prolonged release of these catecholamines is thought to increase one's susceptibility to stress-related conditions, such as heart disease, hypertension, migraines and ulcers. However,

not all type A personalities succumb to the ill effects of stress. Perhaps if a type A person consciously recognizes what is happening, they can actually become more resistant to stress (i.e. he or she becomes type C, sometimes referred to as type H or hardy personality). These people now look upon situations as challenges rather than threats, and convert the distressful life events of type A into opportunities or possibilities (eustressful life events) for personal growth and benefit (i.e. they have rethought their demands and capabilities).

In order to be 'stress-wise', it is important, therefore, to identify type behaviour in ourselves by recognizing attitudes and expectations that engage us in a constant struggle to gain control over our environment. For example, when a type A personality perceives emotional threats or challenges, the stress response is triggered automatically, even when there is no real danger (e.g. when waiting in a traffic jam, queuing in the bank, etc.). As a result, much unnecessary 'stress' (and loss of adaptation energy) is created, which keeps the person frequently outside the normal range of the stress balance and in the distressed area. The difficulty is in appraising our behaviour and altering our responses to stressors. Lazarus (1966) put forward a stress appraisal model based on coping with mental illnesses. According to Lazarus, primary appraisal of the initiating situation involved three possibilities:

1 A stressor is considered irrelevant.
2 A stressor is seen as being positive with respect to well-being, having positive and pleasant emotions.
3 The stressors are regarded as damaging and threatening, with negative emotions such as anxiety.

These three possibilities can therefore be equated to being unconsciously aware of the psychophysiological indicators of the stress response, eustress and distress. The outcome of these possibilities determines the emotions experienced. This experience promotes the necessary action to be taken, and results in

---

ACTIVITY

Describe a cognitive coping strategy used on your ward that reduces distress in patients.

BOX 21.8 TYPE A PERSONALITY NURSES

According to Howells-Johnson (1998), there is an increased prevalence of type A behaviour among nurses. Whether a type A person becomes a nurse, or whether nursing changes people into type A personalities, is difficult to assess.

Ask yourself these questions. How often as a nurse do you:

- engage in races against the clock trying to squeeze more and more patient care into each shift?
- perform two or more jobs at any one time?
- view peers as competitors?
- interpret an offer of help as a slur on your competence?
- work double shifts, denying time for restful periods?

BOX 21.9 COPING FAILURE: PSEUDO-ORGANIC AND ORGANIC DISEASE

Pseudo-organic disease

Some people with coping failure present symptoms that suggest the presence of an organic disease (e.g. pseudo-angina), which upon consultation and examination show no evidence of the actual disorder. Frequently, such patients are treated with mild analgesics; if these prove ineffective, then more powerful analgesics may be administered. The patient may be very anxious and complain that it is the pain that is the stressor, and that this is causing a lack of sleep. Consequently, the patient may be prescribed antidepressants; after taking a few months to recover, the patient then rarely complains of the 'angina' again. It may be speculated that the reason for an increased pain perception is that there is a decrease in arousal levels in the depressed state. That is, the depression is a failure of adaptation, and is a sign that may be attributed to the exhaustion stage of the general adaptation syndrome, when the levels of endogenous painkillers such as endorphins might be expected to be low. Guillemin was awarded the Nobel Prize in 1977 for discovering endorphins, which have anti-stress effects by acting as painkillers. They may be among the first mediators in the alarm stress response.

Organic disease

There are possibly two pathways in which stress is related to the onset of disease. First, stress may have direct psychophysiological effects that affect health via disturbed homeostatic controls within cells influenced by the neuroendocrine responses to stress. Second, stress may lead to health-impairing habits (e.g. smoking and alcohol abuse) and altered behaviours (e.g. biting nails). These are referred to as palliative coping methods.

These two pathways explain the relationship between stress and the onset of disease. For example, hormonal changes and immune system decline are thought to reduce the host's resistance, thereby increasing the risk of disease. Once an illness occurs, then one may be subjected to illness behaviour, which influences the course of the disease, and so would form a third pathway. For example, in the case of bereavement, a clear link exists between the increased incidence of mortality and an increased likelihood of illness among widows and widowers who have suffered a recent bereavement of their spouse. One may argue that the evidence is suggestive but not conclusive. However, what is important is that the dominant stressor (death of the spouse) demonstrates individuality with respect to the differing illnesses acquired, and even death in those who seem unable to cope with the bereavement. As far as cardiovascular diseases are concerned, there are a number of well-designed retrospective studies that provide evidence in favour of the hypothesis that factors such as personality type may be important in the aetiology of disease.

Some may question whether ischaemic heart disease is a disease of stress. In a 'biological' sense it is; however, since 90% of myocardial infarctions are caused by atherosclerosis, a contributory factor (stressor) to this process is a constant and heavy intake of saturated fat as a source of 'stress' for the person. In this case, the liver responds to the hyperlipidaemia by synthesizing large amounts of cholesterol from circulatory fats. As time passes, more and more cholesterol is deposited in blood vessels, including the coronary arteries, which may be sufficient to restrict blood flow to the organs they supply. At first, this may be transient or partial (e.g. at times of high oxygen demand, angina pectoris may be induced), and later, total and permanent (e.g. in myocardial infarction). The stress response observed will vary according to the nature–nurture interaction subjectivity associated with the resultant ischaemic pain (see Chapter 1, pp.16–17 and the case study of a woman with myocardial infarction, Section VI, p.654). Myocardial oxygen demands are not within the affected person's capabilities, but the degree of angina or the extent of the myocardial infarction emphasizes the subjectivity of this process. Following the classic formulation of Selye, people with ischaemic heart disease either adapt partially (angina) or do not adapt at all (myocardial infarction).

In our opinion, diseases are not caused solely by one predisposing factor (stressor), but result from the cumulative affects of multiple stressors. Using the example above, the stressors include all the risk factors associated with cardiovascular disease. These can generally be classified as being:

- within the body (e.g. a genetic predisposition – endogenous stressor – to hypercholesterolaemia). A gene on chromosome 19 was identified in 1992 that predisposes the individual to a myocardial infarction;
- outside the body (e.g. cigarette smoking, high dietary fat and distressful life events – exogenous stressors, all of which are hypercholesterolaemic agents). This again demonstrates stressor subjectivity with relation to an individual's exposure to such a diverse range of stressors.

It is the cumulative effect of all coronary risk factors that is responsible for the resultant cardiac problem. The common view of stress is that it results from difficulties associated with lifestyle and professional or personal relationships. The authors of this text consider, however, that every illness can be viewed ultimately as a stress-related illness, whereby the individual's homeostatic controls have failed to cope with the disturbance, then the imbalances (i.e. the signs and symptoms that contribute to the label of the stress-related illness), or when the 'adaptation energy' has been depleted. This applies regardless of whether it is:

- a commonly referred to stress-related condition, such as coronary heart disease or an infection. Then, all the risk factors could be referred to as stressors, which may be linked to environmental influences on gene expression;
- a serious condition not commonly labelled as being stress related, such as acquired immune deficiency syndrome (AIDS). The stressors associated with AIDS are human immunodeficiency virus and the pathogenic stressors of the opportunistic infections that have led to the person being diagnosed with AIDS. Perhaps the disease can be regarded as a phenomenon that occurs when an agent or condition threatens to destroy the dynamic state (i.e. homeostatic mechanisms) upon which the integrity of the organism depends, and the manifestations of disease appear to be, in large measure, manifestations of the organism's efforts to adapt to and contain threats to its integrity. In this sense, all diseases are, to some extent, disorders of adaptation, as Selye suggested in 1956.

---

a secondary appraisal that involves planning and evaluating possible coping methods:

- to change the stressors or situation;
- to modify the meaning of the situation;
- to regulate the experienced emotions.

In other words, distress may be transferred into eustress, the person may flee the situation, one's perceptions of demands and capabilities may be altered or distressful emotions may be minimized.

ACTIVITY

What do you understand by the statement, 'all illnesses are stress related'?

SUMMARY

1 Short-term stress manifests itself via certain psychophysiological homeostatic adaptive bodily responses, whereas prolonged stress results in homeostatic disturbances/imbalances and stress-related illness.

2 Stress is perceived only when the cumulative effects of stressors reach or supersede the stress threshold, which varies between individuals and within the individual with time, since it may be influenced by circadian fluctuations and as the individual goes through the different developmental stages.

3 Stress is perceived as either eustress or distress. The former is regarded as a healthy bodily response, the latter an unhealthy response.

4 A person's perception of stressors, stress thresholds, resistance or adaptation to stress, coping strategies, the stress-related illnesses experienced and their eventual outcome are all subjective.

5 The basis of subjectivity depends on an individual's unique genotype (i.e. nature) and the individual's unique environmental perceptions (nurture) they are exposed to throughout their lives.

6 Although the GAS has been criticized, it is accepted as a description of the physiological responses observed when the body is subjected to stress. Stress induces changes that involve the sympathetic nervous system and various hormones and, superficially, would appear to represent a significant failure of the homeostatic process. However, as this book has illustrated, homeostasis is not about constancy or balance, but is about the provision of optimal conditions. Thus, physiological processes in general have to be adaptable. Stress responses help to maintain the circulatory system and facilitate wound healing,

and so should be viewed as being of benefit (i.e. eustressful) to the recovery, for example, from trauma and surgery. However, they are influenced by factors such as sensitivity and an altered metabolic baseline; under these circumstances, optimal conditions may not prevail, or the adaptive responses themselves promote a metabolic 'deficit', so the responses become distressful with consequences for general well-being and recovery. Nutritional support and the use of fluid therapies are therefore important considerations in the postoperative care of the surgical patient, especially if there is a pre-existing metabolic disturbance, such as diabetes mellitus. In this case, even normal adaptive responses can be distressful.

7 Integration of sociology, psychology and physiology is required to investigate stress from a nature–nurture perspective. This would involve focusing attention on the multiple cumulative stressors that are responsible for each stress-related condition, since it is the author's opinion that all diseases are a result of cumulative stressors (including physical, psychological, environmental, social and developmental). Some disorders are easily identifiable, while others are difficult to pinpoint.

8 Since stress is acquired via nature–nurture interactions, it follows that stress management must involve a multidimensional approach based on nature–nurture interactions. Organizations and individuals must work together for their mutual self-interests. It is important for everyone to become educated in this area of research, in order to identify distress in oneself and then to take appropriate action via individualized coping methods so as to transfer distress into eustress, or to remove or adapt to distressors. It may be a matter of life and death – yours!

REFERENCES

Baglioni Jr, A.J., Cooper, C.L. and Hingley, P. (1990) Job stress, mental health and job satisfaction among UK senior nurses. *Stress Medicine* **6**: 9–20.

Bratt, M.M., Broome, M., Kelber, S. and Lostocco, L. (2000) Influence of stress and nursing leadership on job satisfaction of paediatric intensive care unit nurses. *American Journal of Critical Care* **9**(5): 307–17.

Cannon, W.B. (1935) Stresses and strains of homeostasis. *American Journal of Medical Sciences* **189**: 1–10.

Clancy, J. and McVicar, A.J. (1997a) Homeostasis – the key concept to physiological control: perioperative influences on water and electrolyte homeostasis. *British Journal of Theatre Nursing* **7**(8): 27–32.

Clancy J. and McVicar, A.J. (1997b) Homeostasis – the key concept to physiological control: wound healing – a series of homeostatic responses. *British Journal of Theatre Nursing* **7**(4): 25–34.

Clancy, J. and McVicar, A.J. (1998a) Homeostasis and nature–nurture interactions: a framework for integrating the life sciences. In: Hinchliff, S.M., Norman, S.E. and Schober, J.E. (eds) *Nursing Practice and Health*, 3rd edn. London: Arnold.

Clancy, J. and McVicar, A.J. (1998b) The metabolic response to surgery. *British Journal of Theatre Nursing* **8**(3): 12–18.

Constable, J.F. and Russell, D.W. (1986) The effect of social support and the work environment upon burnout among nurses. *Journal of Human Stress* **12**: 20–6.

Cox, T. and McKay, C.J. (1976) *Psychological model of occupational stress*. Paper presented to the Medical Research Council Meeting – Mental Health in Industry. London: MRC.

Demerouti, E., Bakker, A., Nachreiner, F. and Schaufeli, W.B. (2000) A model of burnout and life satisfaction amongst nurses. *Journal of Advanced Nursing* **32**(2): 454–64.

Department of Health (1999) *Agenda for Change – Modernising the NHS Pay System*. London: Department of Health.

Department of Health (2002a) *Human Resources and the NHS Plan: a Consultation Document*. London: Department of Health.

Department of Health (2000b) *Code of Conduct for NHS Managers*. London: Department of Health.

Department of Health (2000c) *Working Together – Learning Together. A Framework for Lifelong Learning for the NHS*. London: Department of Health.

Department of Health (2003) *The NHS Plan – a Progress Report*. London: Department of Health.

Dodson, C.R. (1982) *Stress. The Hidden Adversary*. Lancaster: MTP Press, 29–30.

Evans, J., Heron, J., Frankcomb, H., Oke, S. and Golding, J. (2001) Cohort study of depressed mood during pregnancy and after childbirth. *British Medical Journal* **323**: 257–60.

Foxall, M.J., Zimmerman, L., Standley, R. and Bene, B. (1990) A comparison of frequency and sources of nursing job stress perceived by intensive care, hospice and medical-surgical nurses. *Journal of Advanced Nursing* **15**: 577–84.

Glover, V. (2001) *Antenatal and Postnatal Mood: the Effects on The Foetus and Child, Postnatal and Maternal Mental Health: a Public Priority*. London: 'Community Practitioners' and 'Health Visitors' Association.

Hammond, S. and Crozier, K. (2007) Gloomy anticipation. *Midwives* **10**(40): 164–6.

Hare, J., Pratt, C.C. and Andrews, D. (1988) Predictors of burnout in professional and paraprofessional nurses working in hospitals and nursing homes. *International Journal of Nursing Studies* **25**: 105–15.

Healy, C. and McKay, M.F. (1999) Identifying sources of stress and job satisfaction in the nursing environment. *Australian Journal of Advanced Nursing* **17**(2): 30–5.

Healy, C. and McKay, M.F. (2000) Nursing stress: the effect of coping strategies and job satisfaction in a sample of Australian nurses. *Journal of Advanced Nursing* **31**(3): 681–8.

Heron, J., O'Connor, T.G., Evans, J., Golding, J., Glover, G., APLSPAC Study Team (2004) The course of anxiety and depression through pregnancy and the postpartum in a community sample. *Journal of Affective Disorders* **80**: 65–73.

Hillhouse, J.J. and Adler, C.M. (1997) Investigating stress effect patterns in hospital staff nurses: result of cluster analysis. *Social Science and Medicine* **45**(12), 1781–8.

Hipwell, A.E., Tyler, P.A. and Wilson, C.M. (1989) Sources of stress and dissatisfaction among nurses in four hospital environments. *British Journal of Medical Psychology* **62**(1): 71–9.

Holmes, T.H. and Rahe, R.H. (1967) The social adjustment rating scale. *Journal of Psychosomatic Research* **11**: 213–18.

Hope, A., Kelleher, C.C. and O'Connor, M. (1998) Lifestyle practices and the health promoting environment of hospital nurses. *Journal of Advanced Nursing* **28**(2): 438–47.

Howells-Johnson, J. (1998) Manifestations and management of stress in healthcare workers. *British Journal of Nursing* **8**(3): 25–30.

Lazarus, R.S. (1966) *Psychological Stress and the Coping Process*. New York: McGraw Hill.

Lazarus, R.S. and Folkman, S. (1984) *Stress, Appraisal and Coping*. New York: Springer.

Lazarus, R.S., DeLongis, A., Folkman, S. and Gruen, R. (1985) Stress and adaptational outcomes: the problem of confounded measures. *American Psychologist* **40**: 770–9.

Lees, S. and Ellis, N. (1990) The design of a stress-management programme for nursing personnel. *Journal of Advanced Nursing* **15**(8): 946–61.

Leveck, M.L. and Jones, C.B. (1996) The nursing practice environment, staff retention and quality of care. *Research in Nursing and Health* **19**: 331–43.

Lucas, M.D., Atwood, J.R. and Hagaman, R. (1993) Replication and validation of anticipated turnover model for urban registered nurses. *Nursing Research* **42**(1), 29–35.

McGowan, B. (2001) Self-reported stress and its effects on nurses. *Nursing Standard* **15**(42): 33–8.

McNeese-Smith, D. (2000) Job stages of entry, mastery and disengagement among nurses. *Journal of Nursing Administration* **30**(3): 140–7.

McVicar, A. (2003) Workplace stress in nursing: a literature review. *Journal of Advanced Nursing* **44**(6): 1–10.

Morrison, R.S., Jones, L. and Fuller, B. (1997) The relation between leadership style and empowerment on job satisfaction of nurses. *Journal of Nursing Administration* **27**(5): 27–4.

Nolan, P.A. (2002) *Data on Postpartum Mood Disorders. A Report to The Rhode Island General Assembly*. Providence: Rhode Island Department of Health.

Plant, M.L., Plant, M.A. and Foster, J. (1992) Stress, alcohol, tobacco and illicit drug use amongst nurses: a Scottish study. *Journal of Advanced Nursing* **17**, 1056–67.

Payne, N. (2001) Occupational stressors and coping as determinants of burnout in female hospice nurses. *Journal of Advanced Nursing* **33**(3), 396–405.

Sarafino, E.P. (2002) Chapter 3 in *Health Psychology. Biopsychosocial Interactions*, 4th edn. New York: John Wiley & Sons, 70–96.

Schmitz, N., Neumann, W. and Opperman, R. (2000) Stress, burnout and locus of control in German nurses. *International Journal of Nursing Studies* **37**(2): 95–9.

Selye, H. (1956) The general adaptation syndrome and diseases of adaptation. *Journal of Clinical Endocrinology* **6**: 117–18.

Selye, H. (1976) *The Stress of Life*. New York: McGraw-Hill.

Shader, K., Broome, M.E., West, M.E. and Nash, M. (2001) Factors influencing satisfaction and anticipated turnover for nurses in an academic medical center. *Journal of Nursing Administration* **31**(4): 210–16.

Simoni, P.S. and Paterson, J.J. (1997) Hardiness, coping, and burnout in the nursing workplace. *Journal of Professional Nursing* **13**(3): 178–85.

Smith, A., Brice, C., Collins, A., Mathews, V. and McNamara, R. (2000) *The Scale of Occupational Stress: a Further Analysis of the Input Of Demographic Factors and Type of Job*. Norwich: HSE Books, HMSO.

Stordeur, S., D'Hoore, W. and Vandenberghe, C. (2001) Leadership, organizational stress and emotional exhaustion among hospital nursing staff. *Journal of Advanced Nursing* **35**(4), 533–42.

Tyler, P.A. and Cushway, D. (1995) Stress in nurses: the effects of coping and social support. *Stress Medicine* **11**: 243–51.

Tyler, P.A. and Ellison, R.N. (1994) Sources of stress and psychological well-being in high-dependency nursing. *Journal of Advanced Nursing* **19**: 469–76.

FURTHER READING

Department of Health (2002) *Human Resources and the NHS Plan: a Consultation Document*. London: Department of Health.

Department of Health (2002) *Code of Conduct for NHS Managers*. London: Department of Health.

Department of Health (2002) *Working Together – Learning Together. A Framework For Lifelong Learning for the NHS*. London: Department of Health.

Department of Health (2003) *The NHS Plan – a Progress Report*. London: Department of Health.

Jones, M.C. and Johnston, D.W. (2000) A critical review of the relationship between perception of the work environment, coping and mental health in trained nurses and patient outcomes. *Clinical Effectiveness in Nursing* **4**(2): 74–85.

For more information about stress at work, please visit the Centers for Disease Control and Prevention (CDC) website:

National Institute for Occupational Safety and Health (NIOSH) Safety and Health Topic: Stress at Work:
http://www.cdc.gov/niosh/topics/stress/

NIOSH Publication Nos. 99–101: STRESS ... At Work:
http://www.cdc.gov/niosh/stresswk.html

NIOSH Publication Nos. 2003–114d: Working With Stress (Video):
http://www.cdc.gov/niosh/docs/video/stress1.html

NIOSH Publication Nos. 2003–114d:
http://www.cdc.gov/niosh/video/stressdvd1002.html

CHAPTER 22

CIRCADIAN RHYTHMS

INTRODUCTION: RELATION OF RHYTHMS TO HUMANS

The term 'circadian' stems from the Latin words 'circa' meaning 'about', and 'dies' meaning 'day'. A rhythm refers to a sequence of events that repeat themselves through time in the same order and at the same interval. Thus, human circadian rhythms refer to the physiological, biochemical and behavioural (or psychological) events that are repeated in the body every 24 hours. Some human rhythms, however, are persistent and are of shorter duration (i.e. not circadian). For example, the adult heart rate, with approximately 70 beats/minute. For historical interest, Luce (1977) reported that it was Ogle in 1866 who first identified human circadian rhythm (of body temperature) and Simpson and Galbraith in 1906 who established that the monkey's temperature rhythm was harmonized (or synchronized) according to the light and dark cycle. Most human studies came much later. In 1959, Halberg stated that physical, psychological and biochemical parameters are intrinsic to individuals with a day and night periodicity of 20–30 hours (i.e. the intrinsic rhythm must be entrained to one of 24-hour periodicity).

Rhythms, though not necessarily circadian, are associated with all forms of life. Since organisms are a part of the physical environment they live in, they are responsive to natural rhythmical changes within that environment.

Circannual rhythms are of a yearly periodicity and are very important in plant and animal species as they determine breeding and hibernation seasons. Humans are not obviously a rhythmic or cyclical species, as they have no breeding season, migration, hibernation, etc. Thus, it is debatable whether these long-cycle rhythms are present in humans, although they may be responsible for mood swings at certain times of the year. That is, some people feel good and are at their happiest during the spring and summer months, which may explain in part why suicide rates are at their lowest at this time of the year. In contrast, some people feel low and depressed in winter months with atypical features of increased appetite (this corresponds with seasonal affective disorder, SAD – see Box 22.5, p.616), which may be linked to the higher suicide rates during this time of the year. The mood swings may be related to the amount of natural daylight, since light is arguably one of the most important environmental stimuli that control human rhythms.

ACTIVITY

Distinguish between circadian, circannual and persistent rhythms.

CIRCADIAN RHYTHM PATTERNS

It is obviously outside the scope of this book to discuss 'psychological' circadian rhythms; these will be omitted owing to the nature of this textbook. Biochemical rhythms will be limited to just a few common examples associated with physiological rhythms. The reader should be aware, however, that these three parameters of bodily function are inseparable and are interdependent entities (see Chapter 1, pp.16–17). Although physiological rhythms such as body temperature will be described, the reader should bear in mind that heat is produced as a consequence of metabolic reactions that are ultimately dependent on cellular respiration (see Figure 2.11, p.36). In addition, physiological parameters can be influenced by one's psychological functions (or vice versa); for example, the majority of 'psychological' performance indicators peaks are associated with peak in body temperature. The purpose of this chapter is to emphasize that if we were to 'look inside' our bodies, we would see a number of repetitive psychophysiological patterns. Thus, some cells would be more active in the morning when the body is in its awake state, while others will be more pronounced at night when we are asleep. These 'normal' patterns become disturbed in illness, or when we change our natural timing of sleep–wake patterns, such as in staying up late at weekends, admission to hospital, doing shift work or travelling across different time zones.

Technical advances now mean that non-invasive assessment of physiological variables can be performed, and that measurements can be made on very small samples of fluids, including plasma, urine and saliva. Thus, sequential measurements can be carried out during the circadian period. These non-invasive procedures, together with questionnaires and interviews are the basis of much of the circadian rhythm research of today.

Body temperature

The circadian rhythm of body temperature does not vary markedly in 'normal' healthy people (although the timing of peaks and troughs can differ slightly between people), and thus is one of the most reliable indicators of 'time' inside the body. Body temperature is an indicator of the level of a person's metabolism: an increased body temperature is associated with a high rate of metabolism, which necessitates quicker heart and respiratory rates in order to deliver more nutrients and oxygen to the active cells. A high rate of metabolism requires more energy (as ATP) to drive the metabolic reactions (see overview section in Chapter 2, p.22). Consequently, the metabolic pathways of cellular respiration are faster, with the result that more heat energy is produced, thus increasing the body temperature. The potential of a metabolic acidosis also arises (Clancy and McVicar, 2007a,b).

Figure 22.1 illustrates the expected circadian rhythmicity of oral temperature. The pattern of change is:

1 A steep rise in the morning, becoming maximal during late morning (or early afternoon in some people).
2 A slight decline from the maximum, followed by a return to the maximum or a value close to it later in the afternoon; this is called the 'post-lunch dip' (PLD).
3 A decline in the afternoon or early evening, continuing through the night.
4 The lowest point (or nadir) in the early hours of the morning.

One would expect such rhythmicity, since the increase in body temperature, hence metabolism, begins just before awakening, preparing the body for the waking process and subsequent events. The rise continues during the morning and early afternoon, which are the times when we require a higher rate of metabolism to deal with daily activities. The fall-off during late afternoon and the declining levels in the evening are a consequence of our activities slowing down and getting ready for sleep. Upon sleeping, such parameters are at their lowest (body temperature falls at night by about 0.5°C, which represents a considerable change in metabolic activity), since a function of sleep is to replenish energy levels in preparation for the following daily activities. The temperature reflects changes in secretion of thyroxine and cortisol, since these hormones control the metabolic rate during the 24-hour period. Only people who are very sick, such as those with cancer, fevers (pyrexia – see Figure 16.13, p.460) or severe infections such as encephalitis, show distortions of this rhythm.

Body temperature is actually related more closely to changes in skin temperature than it is to metabolism. Constriction of superficial skin (cutaneous) blood vessels reduces heat loss, and so promotes a rise in body temperature. The change in skin temperature occurs before the body temperature is elevated, so body core temperature changes seem also to be a consequence of rhythmic vasomotor changes in the skin vessels, in addition to a change in metabolic rate (see Figure 16.9, p.456).

ACTIVITY

Explain why an increased metabolism is associated with an increased body temperature and why body temperature increases with increased cellular respiration?

The diurnal rhythm of task performance and arousal seem to parallel that of body temperature. The most consistent improvement in task efficiency occurs during the first 3 hours, when the temperature rise is most noticeable. On a general note, peak performance corresponds to the peak temperature and arousal levels, occurring between midday and 6 p.m., which is also the period of quickest reaction times and best psychomotor coordination. The poorest performance coincides with the intervals of lowest temperature and arousal; this is between 3 a.m. and 6 a.m. This is generally referred to as the 'dead spot', and its occurrence is not surprising since there is a natural urge to sleep between 2 a.m. and 7 a.m.

Subjectivity of circadian rhythmicity

The timing or duration of maximum temperature and PLDs may vary between people, but the rhythmicity tends to be consistent in the same individual as long as they remain healthy. 'Morning larks' in whom temperature shows a faster rise and peaks earlier in the morning (i.e. the peak in Figure 22.1 would move to the left), claim that they perform physical and mental tasks better in the morning. In 'night owls' (i.e. people who claim that they are more alert at night) the day temperature rises more slowly and peaks later (i.e. the peak in Figure 22.1 moves to the right). The steepness of the rise, the timing and duration of the peaks of temperatures (morning and evening people), PLD variations, the steepness of the decline, dead spot times, etc., all demonstrate that there is subjectivity of circadian rhythmicity within the population.

The PLD phenomenon has not been explained satisfactorily, as it occurs irrespective of whether we have lunch or not. The PLD does not affect one's performance during this period simply because an increased proportion of the cardiac output is

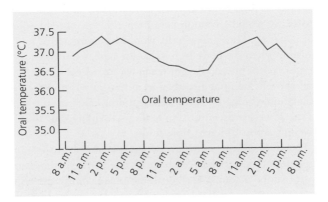

Figure 22.1 Oral temperature over 36 hours

Q Differentiate between the 'normal' circadian patterns of body temperature experienced by 'morning' and 'evening' people.

diverted to the gastrointestinal tract, since there are no corresponding post-breakfast or post-dinner dips! However, if one becomes consciously aware of the slight 'lull' in performance, one may arrange to perform automatic tasks in this period. The small rhythmical change in body temperature is also not so large that motivation cannot compensate for it. Therefore, performance is not greatly affected in someone who enjoys his or her job for example.

Other functions of the body have a reverse or an intermediate rhythmicity to that of temperature. For example, growth hormone release and the concentrations of some electrolytes in body fluids tend to have their maximal value nocturnally. Growth hormone secretion rises at night probably to divert the body's energy (ATP) stores to growth, repair and regeneration of body tissues (see Figure 11.11, p.287), since during the day ATP utilization is spread among many different metabolic reactions associated with physical and mental tasks.

ACTIVITY

Describe the 'normal' circadian pattern of body temperature, and relate it to performance of physical and mental tasks and arousal levels during a 24-hour period.

Urination

Figure 22.2 demonstrates a rhythm in urinary excretion, which involves the production of a large volume of urine in the morning and midday and lower volumes at night. The urinary circadian rhythm may result from the influence of bodily rhythms in parameters such as glomerular filtration rate (GFR), tubular reabsorption, or antidiuretic hormone (ADH) secretion, or from fluid intake. The rise in urine flow is dependent on the switchover from dark to light. A decreased recognition of light cues in older adults and people who are blind, therefore, may result in abnormal rhythms.

Urinary excretory products, for example sodium (Na^+) and potassium (K^+), demonstrate separate activities (Figure 22.3). Generally, for a person who goes to bed at 11 p.m. and rises at 7 a.m., most potassium excretion would be between 10.30

BOX 22.1 URINATION AND THE OLDER ADULT

Circadian rhythmicity of urine production, especially being lowest during the night, aids sleep. Disturbances of the rhythmicity in older people can result in them producing more urine at night than during the day. This can lead to social problems, such as insomnia (inability to fall asleep), nocturia (urination at night) and nocturnal (night-time) wandering, and the appearance of these problems could be labelled incorrectly as 'confusional behaviour' by the health carer. However, any resultant sedation may well make the problems worse.

---

a.m. and 2.30 p.m. Variations in these are explained by individual differences in diets and routines.

Blood components

Figure 22.4 illustrates individual variation with reference to the timing of peaks and nadirs (i.e. lowest point), and the duration of troughs and plateaux of the concentrations of certain plasma components. The rhythms of iron, phosphate and corticosteroid hormones demonstrate considerable consistency, and thus can be of practical importance. For example, corticosteroids are released from the adrenal gland in a series of discrete episodes, including an increase in release early in the morning, and a declining frequency as the day proceeds, although throughout this broad pattern there is a series of small, sharp peaks. Figure 22.5 illustrates a typical circadian pattern in a 'normal' healthy subject. A steep rise from low nocturnal values to a maximum about 1 hours before waking is observed, and the peak is just before the end of the dark phase at a time when we are usually awakening. Perhaps this may promote central nervous system arousal, which causes waking up. Many of us may be aware of this, since it is reflected by us sometimes waking to switch the alarm off before it has been activated. Corticosteroids are also important metabolic hormones, and their release would be appropriate for the move in metabolism that occurs at this time.

Rhythm synchronization

At rest, the basic inborn (innate) sleep–wake rhythm is generally longer than 24 hours; therefore circadian (24-hour) periodicity is dependent on:

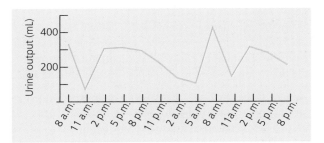

Figure 22.2 Urine output over 36 hours

Q How is the urinary output circadian pattern associated with the sleep–wake cycle?

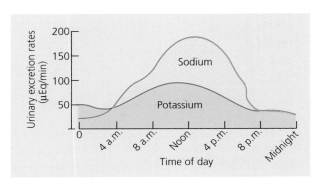

Figure 22.3 Urinary excretion of potassium (K^+) and sodium (Na^+)

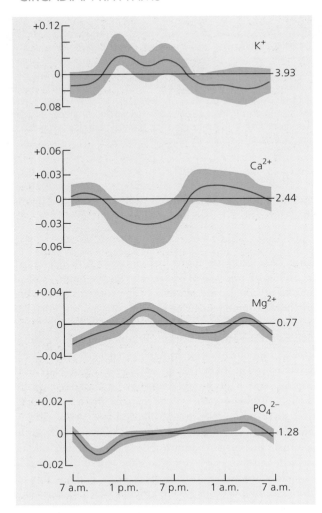

Figure 22.4 Mean diurnal cycles of plasma concentrations of potassium (K^+), calcium (Ca^{2+}), magnesium (Mg^{2+}) and phosphate (PO_4^{2-}). Shaded areas indicate the subjectivity of individual circadian parameters

Q Discuss what circadian pattern variation or subjectivity means.

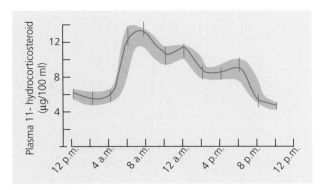

Figure 22.5 Circadian rhythm of plasma 11-hydrocorticosteroid concentrations. The shaded area represents subjectivity in the population studied

Q Describe the 'normal' circadian pattern of hydrocorticosteroid, and relate it to performance of physical and mental tasks and arousal levels during a 24-hour period.

BOX 22.2 CLINICAL IMPORTANCE OF CIRCADIAN RHYTHMS (CHRONOBIOLOGY)

Recognizing the occurrence of time in the body (chronobiology) is of clinical importance. Pathology, haematology and clinical biochemistry reports indicate the upper and lower normal values, which are associated with 'health' and the homeostatic ranges that have been referred to frequently throughout this book (and itemized in Appendix B). These take into account circadian variation. The authors would advocate that the sampling of blood, and urine, etc., should, ideally, coincide with the patient's mean values (since *ad hoc* sampling could be measuring the patient's peaks and troughs for a parameter), so the daily comparative sampling (and assessment) becomes more accurate and is therefore of greater value if it is performed at the same time of the day.

Clinical chronobiology investigates circadian influences on human disorders, for example their incidence, the variation in severity of signs and symptoms over the circadian 24-hour (or other) period, the response of patients to exploratory/diagnostic procedures and the effect on the individual of clinical treatments. The signs and symptoms of long-standing or chronic diseases (e.g. coronary heart disease, arthritis, asthma, epilepsy), for example, frequently display circadian, seasonal and (in women) menstrual patterns. The life-threatening events of myocardial and cerebral infarction also exhibit predictable-in-time patterns over the circadian period and the time of year. For example, the neural outputs from the respiration and cardiac control centres of the brainstem are at their lowest in the middle of the night and the subsequent higher blood carbon dioxide and lower oxygen means the person may become quite hypoxic. Consequently, the individual's life functions are at their lowest; therefore it is not surprising that most deaths occur in this 'critical period'.

Admission to hospital routine and the phenomenon of the 'white coat syndrome' (an anxiety response to seeing a doctor!) influence blood pressure assessment, spirometric evaluation, and many more assessments (see Boxes 22.7, p.622 and 22.9, p.624). Bodily rhythms also affect the pharmacokinetics and dynamics of medications (see Box 22.8, p.623). Healthcare professionals should also be careful in monitoring their own health, because shift work causes circadian disturbances and in the long term can result in shift-related illness (see Box 22.6, p.620 and section 'Circadian rhythm desynchronization: homeostatic disturbances – imbalances/disorders').

- environmental cues, such as the night–day cues. The removal of such cues, as observed in studies in which participants have been confined in underground caves produces non-circadian (or 'free-running') sleep–wake cycles with a periodicity range of 16–50 hours. The huge range demonstrates the individual's variation in control over the sleep–wake 'activity' cycles;
- levels of circulating compounds, which influence the sleep–wake cycle. For example, waking may be associated with the stimulatory effects of corticosteroid hormones on the brainstem, including the respiratory and cardiac areas.

When all the rhythms are following their expected patterns then the body is said to be in a state of internal synchronization. It is now considered unusual to find a 'physiological' variable without a rhythm. The authors suggest that since mind–body functions are interdependent, this synchronization can be achieved only by integrating psychophysiological rhythms and observing how the environment affects each

BOX 22.3 POOR SLEEPERS

Body temperature curves strongly suggest that poor sleepers might be out of synchrony with the 24-hour day. Their temperature declines less when compared with good sleepers, and is still declining when they rise in the morning. Poor sleepers may wish that they could go to bed later and rise later than is socially convenient, because the body time may lag behind the clock time (i.e. showing a longer period than 24 hours). These free-running periods are common in response to distress, and may help to explain the insomnia that accompanies many illnesses, particularly in people with mental health problems. Thus, during this free-running period, the individual is performing their waking tasks with a 'sleeping' body, and subsequently may develop psychosomatic and emotional symptoms as a result of this imbalance or desynchronization.

rhythm. In this way, nature–nurture interactions become instrumental in our understanding of circadian rhythms and individual variations in circadian patterns. An understanding of such integration would enhance the understanding of illnesses and how, for example, hospitalization affects patients.

ACTIVITY

How is the body temperature circadian pattern associated with the sleep–wake cycle?

Control of circadian rhythms

It is generally accepted that circadian rhythms result from two interacting processes: a genetic (nature or endogenous) basis of control, and entrainment (environmental or exogenous) mechanisms to keep these rhythms 'on track' (i.e. circadian). In the elderly the endogenous and exogenous processes are affected, and as a consequence of, for example, no job stressors, a disruption in sleep and daytime functioning may occur in this group (see Boxes 22.1, p.611, 22.5, p.616, 22.8, p.623 and 22.9, p.624).

As noted, endogenous rhythms are 'free-running' (i.e. shorter or longer than 24 hours), being modified exogenously to give 24-hour rhythmicity; this is the process of entrainment or synchronization. These modifying exogenous cues (called 'zeitgebers' – 'time givers' – or synchronizers') include light/dark, clocks, radio, television and a regular lifestyle involving work, leisure and mealtimes.

Rhythms vary in the relative influence of their endogenous and exogenous components. For example, body temperature has a large endogenous component, which is why its circadian variation is minimal, but the release of some hormones has a large exogenous component (e.g. adrenaline surges occur whenever the individual is stressed and may be time-linked depending upon the source of stress).

ACTIVITY

Using Figure 21.6, p.598, list other hormones that are released in the adaptation stage of the Selye's general adaptation syndrome.

BOX 22.4 THE HUMAN GENOME PROJECT TO IDENTIFY CIRCADIAN GENES?

One of the objectives of the Human Genome Project was to identify the endogenous location(s) of circadian rhythms in humans (see Box 19.1, p.524). For example, the genetic basis (i.e. a gene called *hPer2*) of a rare syndrome (called familial advanced sleep-phase syndrome) in which individuals have a 'fast' biological clock, which prompts them to awaken each morning and fall asleep each evening several hours earlier than normal. In-depth DNA nucleotide sequence studies of the gene in the affected family members exposed a single substitution mutation of a single amino acid (i.e. serine to glycine) in the associated protein. Many within the older adult population have similar kinds of problems whereas many adolescents have the opposite problem (called delayed sleep-phase syndrome), which in affected individuals prevents them from getting to sleep at a reasonable time.

One dilemma with distinguishing a familial circadian syndrome is that there are widespread normal variations in sleep patterns. There are some people referred to as 'morning larks' and others as 'night owls', whereas the majority of people fall somewhere between. These variations are complex, involving contributions from numerous genes (polygenic), and various environmental factors.

A thorough understanding of the molecular basis for the human circadian clock might suggest future therapies. That is, the gene and the enzyme produced by any mutated gene potentially could be targeted (see Figure 2.9, p.33) to adjust the disrupted sleep patterns of these early risers, and others, including the 'night owl' adolescents, the older adults who exhibit polycyclic sleep (see Box 22.9, p.624), those facing jet lag or shift work, which disrupts their circadian rhythms, and for conditions such as sleep deficit disorders (e.g. insomnia, seasonal affective disorder) and depression.

Light and dark cues are generally considered to be the most important exogenous cues to which species synchronize their bodily rhythms. In humans, the importance of light as an exogenous zeitgeber is supported by isolation studies, studies involving blind people and studies of Inuit peoples living above the Arctic Circle.

Isolation studies

Mills (1973) studied a young man who wore a wristwatch throughout a 3-month stay in a cave. Although the subject resolved to sustain a 24-hour routine, Mills demonstrated that the subject got out of bed later, slept when tired, and generally lived on an activity–rest cycle that was longer than 24 hours. In other words, free-running rhythms were exhibited because of the removal of exogenous cues. Other studies have demonstrated sleep–wake (endogenous) rhythms to be of a greater periodicity than 24 hours, although the range documented for this cycle has been between 16- and 50-hourly rhythms. The difference in the free-running periods demonstrates individual variation in the control of the sleep–wake cycle. Subjectivity is not surprising, as each individual has their own unique blend of genes and their unique interpretation of environmental cues. Although the environment is controlled to a certain extent in isolation studies by the removal of exogenous cues, the authors would argue that it is not possible to control the individual's perceptions of that removal.

In contrast to the sleep–wake cycle, rhythms such as body temperature are controlled more genetically and are less dependent on environmental modification, as they exhibit a 25-hour rhythmicity in isolation studies. Thus there are two classes of circadian oscillations:

1. Poorly entrained and easily modified patterns (e.g. sleep–wake cycle).
2. Strongly sustained rhythms (e.g. body temperature, hormone secretion, and urine excretion).

Studies involving people who are blind

The endogenous control and exogenous modification of circadian rhythms is evident in studies involving people that are born totally blind. These people still exhibit rhythmicity, although the rhythms are a little disorganized and low in amplitude; consequently, these are often referred to as 'flattened' rhythms. The majority of people who are blind have rhythms that are 'free-running' and consequently the condition is linked with periodic insomnia and daytime sleepiness. Despite this, they still show some degree of periodicity that approximates to about 25 hours. Perhaps this rhythmicity is brought about by people who are blind putting a greater emphasis (compared with sighted people) on exogenous cues, such as televisions and clocks, in order to entrain their rhythmicity. These changes have also been demonstrated in older adults who have a decreased sensitivity to light (see Boxes 22.1, p.611, 22.5, p.616, 22.8, p.623 and 22.9, p.624). Since some studies have shown that the administration of melatonin can entrain circadian rhythms in blind people who have free-running rhythms, perhaps melatonin administration may benefit the older adults (Box 22.5).

Studies involving Inuit peoples

The Inuit year includes 6 months of continuous light and 6 months of continuous dark (twilight) and are therefore devoid of night–day exogenous cues, and so their rhythms are free running. Interestingly, short-duration studies have, to date, demonstrated no adverse effects of this, so it could be questioned as to why we have circadian rhythms. However, researchers involved in longitudinal studies may identify adverse effects – only time will tell.

Whether or not light is the most important zeitgeber in humans remains unresolved. What is certain is that human circadian rhythms are a result of the cumulative zeitgebers, such as choice of mealtimes, sleep times, time to be sociable, lifestyle, etc., that enable us to cooperate as a social group. Thus, cultural differences, and differences within the same culture, produce individual variation.

ACTIVITY

What is the German equivalent name for synchronizers?

Location of circadian control

The occurrence of free-running rhythms in the absence of synchronizers supports an innate location of rhythm generation.

Early suggestions of a 'biological clock' within the hypothalamus were put forward as the 'inherited clock theory'. That is, the rhythm may be 'born, not made'. In 1994, the so-called 'clock' gene on chromosome 5 was identified; whether this is activated only in the hypothalamic cells remains to be seen.

There is almost certainly more than one clock, and perhaps they all operate at once. These may, however, be controlled or synchronized to a 24-hour rhythm by a 'master' clock. The clocks may be the homeostatic control centres of the brain, such as the medullary cardiac, respiratory and vasomotor centres, which in turn would be responsible for free-running patterns. Considerable research has sought to establish the location(s) of the clock(s) and the neuroendocrine communicating channels between them. The suprachiasmatic nuclei (SCN) of the hypothalamus (i.e. a group of neurons about 3 cm behind the eyes) have been strongly advocated as being the link between the clocks, and hence could be the 'master' clock. This is a plausible theory, since the hypothalamus is the centre of many activities that control the activity of the rest of the body, probably via its neuroendocrine activity; it also controls satiety, hunger and temperature. In addition, if the hypothalamus is the master clock, then damage to the SCN (e.g. compression by expanding pituitary tumours) should mean that the ability to express any overt circadian rhythms is destroyed. There is also substantial evidence that suggests that damage to the hypothalamic temperature control area (as occurs when one is subjected to recurrent fever) results in other interrelated bodily rhythms being affected (e.g. those of heart rate and respiratory rates). The circadian rhythms that become desynchronized presumably would depend on which area of the hypothalamus is damaged.

The pineal gland (located centrally in the brain; see Figure 9.3, p.212) has also been suggested to be the 'master' clock, since it is an important link between light and dark reception and central nervous system function. However, a direct anatomical retinohypothalamic link has been found which terminates in the hypothalamic SCN. This is connected by a neural pathway to the pineal gland and could support the notion that the hypothalamus is the master gland; it may also explain why light is such an important exogenous cue (Figure 22.6).

In this way, light incident on the retina will inhibit the pineal gland output of melatonin (Figure 22.6a). Melatonin secretion is 20 times greater in the dark than during the light phase (Figure 22.6.b). The function of melatonin that has received most research attention is its role in the induction of sleep; however, many other roles have been cited such as its ability to increase endocrine secretions from the pituitary gland, gonads and adrenal glands. Furthermore, homeostatic deficits in melatonin secretion have been linked with several diseases (e.g. cardiovascular disease, severe immunodeficiency syndromes, diabetes mellitus and Alzheimer disease), hence it may have a role to play in preventing these diseases; biomedical research is seeking to conclusively demonstrate these links. Early research studies suggest a potential adjuvant therapeutic role for melatonin administration in cancer therapy.

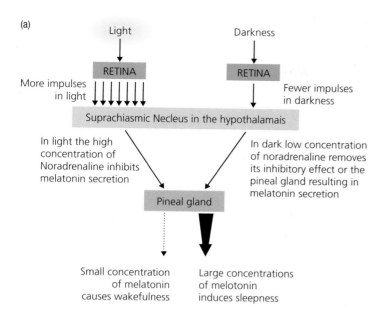

(a)

Figure 22.6 (a) Melatonin secretion during the day and night. (b) Melatonin secretion during the night is 20 times that of daytime secretion

Q *'Circadian rhythms are controlled endogenously and modified exogenously.'* What do you understand by this statement?

The fact is that we still do not know where the clock is, or even if there are many clocks controlled by a 'master' clock. Although the inherited clock theory receives most support, other theories do exist. For example, the basis of the 'imprint theory' is that initially an animal is arrhythmic (without rhythms), and it then learns from environmental conditions and parental behaviour what 24 hours constitutes. This theory does not receive much support, as some rhythms appear during uterine development. It cannot be demonstrated, however, that these rhythms are inherent in the fetus or result from changes in the mother, but it is likely that the fetus does respond to maternal rhythms, and that we are born with some form of rhythmicity. Neonatal rhythms are low in amplitude (flattened). As the body adapts to the light–dark activity, the rhythm becomes more mature, and eventually full maturity is developed in a light and dark environment. The rate of maturation varies between individuals with respect to the different rhythms. For example, the sleep–wake cycle must develop before there is a capability to entrain to light–dark cues. At approximately 20 weeks of age, some infants begin to synchronize with parents, but in others it takes more time (up to a few years) before synchronization is fully mature. Bladder control at night, which normally occurs within 2 years, can take up to several years; this late control is thought to be a result of a lack of light and dark modification of endogenous control of urine volume early on in the developmental processes. Further support comes from studies of children in nurseries in which artificial light predominates, which is thought to delay bladder control in some children. Other evidence includes studies involving babies who are jaundiced at birth; these babies are put into high-intensity light to reduce the jaundice, but the light prolongs the time for maturation of circadian rhythms.

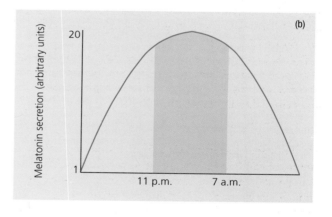

ACTIVITY

Suggest why older adults are more reliant upon exogenous time-givers for circadian rhythmicity. Discuss the suggested roles of the hypothalamus and the pineal gland in the entrainment of circadian rhythms.

ROLE OF CIRCADIAN RHYTHMS IN HOMEOSTASIS

Cells are the 'basic units of life', and therefore must ultimately control each circadian rhythm, and hence homeostatic function, via:

Genotype   ⟶   Phenotype
(determines free-running   ↑   (circadian parameters)
endogenous rhythms)

Environment
(exogenous modulators)

BOX 22.5 MELATONIN IN THE OLDER ADULT AND MELATONIN ADMINISTRATION

Melatonin in the older adult

Melatonin secretion in some older adults appears to be elevated during daylight because they have a reduced sensitivity to light/dark as a result of:

- the eye becoming opaque (e.g. in glaucoma), which therefore limits the amount of light penetrating the eye;
- the retina–hypothalamic–pineal neural pathways having a diminished function, owing to decreased neural conduction and synaptic functioning as a consequence of the ageing process;
- calcification of the pineal gland, which inhibits its secretory function.

Consequently, the older adult potentially has disturbed endogenous circadian rhythms (whether the hypothalamus or the pineal gland is the master gland) and so have to rely more on exogenous (social) synchronizers such as the arrival of the milkman, timing of favourite TV and radio programmes, etc., to help give them 24-hour rhythmicity.

Melatonin administration

Currently available as a dietary supplement melatonin is publicized as being a potential weapon against sleep deficit illnesses associated with insomnia, seasonal affective disorder, depression, jet lag, ageing and shift-related sleep disturbances (see Box 22.6, p.620). Melatonin secretion has been found to entrain the sleep part of circadian rhythms and as such, is not unreasonable to support since the research states it can be administered to successfully treat jet lag, delayed sleep-phase syndrome, and sleep disorders in the blind and in some neurologically impaired children. However because of its hypnotic effect, only extremely low dosages of melatonin should be taken, since it can even cause insomnia, particularly in the older adult (and other disorders stated above). The dose–effect relationship is perhaps why melatonin cannot be bought over the counter in the UK. However, it can be purchased overseas or is available on the Internet; if it is used then it should be done so with caution. Melatonin secretion is decreased by alcohol and caffeine (found in tea and coffee) so if melatonin is taken to solve minor sleep disturbances the authors would advocate first to avoid caffeine-loaded products after 6 p.m. to see if this on its own solves the sleep disturbance.

Phenotypes include all the measurable circadian parameters within the body: body temperature, levels of biochemicals such as neurotransmitters (e.g. acetylcholine, adrenaline), hormones (e.g. growth hormone, insulin), chemicals such as glucose, amino acids and electrolytes, and others such as pain-producing substances (e.g. kinins, prostaglandins), and pain-relieving substances (e.g. endorphins, enkephalins). Owing to the interdependency of mind–body functions, factors such as mood, sleep and cognition all have circadian phenotypes.

All circadian parameters are influenced by cellular metabolism and thus ultimately are mediated enzymatically. The production of enzymes is determined genetically (endogenously) and influenced environmentally (exogenously) by social modulators. For example, noise disturbances (exogenous modulator) may lead to less sleep because 'stress' hormones are increased, which affects the activity–rest (wake–sleep) cycle, which in turn can alter neural metabolism and affect one's mood. So is it the genetic, biochemical, physiological and psychological homeosta-

tic disturbances that affect circadian rhythmicity, or is it circadian rhythm disturbances from exogenous changes that lead to psychophysiological disturbances? Your guess is as good as ours!

Circadian rhythm desynchronization: homeostatic disturbances – imbalances/disorders

It can be argued that health occurs only when the body has normal synchronized psychophysiological circadian rhythms. Once these rhythms are acquired, then their disturbance or desynchronization must be caused by unnatural or 'abnormal' exogenous cues, such as shift work, travelling across time

ACTIVITY

Look up the World Health Organization definition of 'health'. How do circadian rhythms link with this definition?

zones, illness, staying up late at weekends or hospitalization. These cues can modify the expression of a person's genotype to produce psychophysiological circadian imbalances by changing the body's pronounced daily rhythms of eating, sleeping, body temperature, performance, etc. This disturbance requires the body to resynchronize, or re-establish homeostasis; otherwise, if desynchronization is chronically imposed, it can be detrimental to health, producing circadian imbalances (signs and symptoms), which lead to an illness – a clinical label! Such disturbances are referred to as 'phase shifts', because rhythms persist but the peaks and nadirs occur at times out of phase with periods of activity and inactivity (Figure 22.7).

The following sections discuss the consequences of such phase shifts as experienced by shift workers and by patients through their illness and hospital admission.

Shift work

Health consequences of shift work

A significant percentage of the working populations of industrialized countries are shift workers. Continuous shift work is necessary for a variety of reasons:

- *Economic gains*: shift work is a high priority for the country's gross national profit.
- *Technological reasons*: some industries, such as petroleum and steel, need to operate on a 24-hour basis.
- *Human services*: the population requires public services throughout 24 hours for security (police, military, etc.) and health reasons (healthcare workers).
- *Economic necessity for the workers*: shift work brings financial bonuses that may be needed in order to maintain standards of living. Workers may have to choose between shift work and redundancy.

Shifts produce a chronic alteration in environmental time (i.e. exogenous cues) (Figure 22.8). As a result, shift work has important implications for both the personal well-being of the

Figure 22.7 Circadian rhythms: a homeostatic function. a, Homeostasis = synchronized psychophysiological circadian rhythmicity = health. The range is dynamic, reflecting individual variation of parameter rhythmicity within the population based on the individual's unique genotype and perceptions of environmental cues. b, Disturbed homeostasis = desynchronized psychophysiological 'circadian' rhythms = phase shifts caused by: (i) extreme, unusual or abnormal exogenous cues (stressors, zeitgebers, etc.), such as shift work, travelling across time zones, potential pathogens and hospitalization; and (ii) a deviation in genotypes (e.g. congenital malformation, cancer, etc.). c, Homeostatic control systems re-establishing the balance = circadian rhythm resynchronization, as occurs following the removal of extreme, unusual or abnormal exogenous cues, such as shift work patterns, ceasing chronic travelling across time zones, the body's successful defence against potential pathogens and community care. d, Homeostatic imbalances as a result of control failure = free-running psychophysiological rhythms = ill health/illness. e, Clinical intervention (e.g. health education, community care, etc.). f, Untreatable clinical imbalances (e.g. terminal illness). (a, Represents boxes a_1–a_4 in Figure 1.7, p.11, reflecting the individual variability in the homeostatic range)

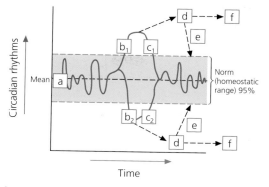

Q Describe why illness and hospitalization are said to cause circadian rhythm desynchronization.

Q Give an example of a rhythm that has a strong endogenous component, and a rhythm that is easily disrupted by exogenous cues.

workers and the safety of the general public, both in and out of the work place.

Research has identified many potential problems for the long-term shift worker. 'Social' problems may exist as a result of a lack of qualitative and quantitative time spent with family and friends, and a lack of regular leisure time. Perhaps this may explain in part the high divorce rate seen in shift workers. These social stressors can lead to a sense of isolation and helplessness in the shift worker, which have been linked by research to an increased incidence of psychophysiological imbalances/disorders including:

- neurosis;
- depression;
- some cases of schizophrenia;
- disorganized and poor eating patterns, which lead to a significantly higher incidence of gastrointestinal tract disorders. Common complaints are peptic and duodenal ulcers. An increased incidence of gastroduodenitis and other gastrointestinally associated problems, such as anorexia and constipation, are also common. It is possible that shifts promote the eating of more 'junk food', and increased caffeine consumption and smoking, which are all responsible for, or contribute to, the bowel (and other) disorders;
- disorganized sleep patterns: some workers have difficulty falling asleep because their sleep–wake pattern is affected. This is not surprising, because in night workers, the cycle of sleep and wakefulness is reversed completely and is initially at odds with other rhythms. Sleep disturbances are more common in the evening shift, while fatigue is associated with the night shift because day sleep is shorter. On average, night workers get 1.5 hours less sleep than day workers (i.e. 6 hours versus 7.5 hours). The quality of sleep is reduced, even when daily noises are absent, and rapid eye movement (REM; see Chapter 8, p.195) sleep is of low amplitude. There is also less REM sleep, and sleep is of shorter periods. Changing sleep patterns can have dramatic effects: sleep is one of the most important circadian rhythms, and its desyn-

chronization has multiple effects on other circadian rhythms. Sleep disturbance may also be a contributing factor to the higher consumption of alcohol, cigarettes, sleeping pills and tranquillizers in shift workers. Performance is affected because night workers are working when bodily rhythms are geared up to sleep, and they sleep when the rhythms are geared for activity. For example, low levels of corticosteroids and adrenaline at night when night workers must function at their best cause them to be less efficient, and vice versa. It is not surprising, therefore, that sleep is of a poor quality and quantity.

- cardiovascular problems: shift work is associated with an increased risk of myocardial infarction (MI) when the shift pattern lasts between 11 and 15 years, although the incidence appears to decrease if the shift is continued for more than 20 years. A greater incidence of hypercholesterolaemia occurs in shift workers, the link possibly being that 90% of MIs are a result of atherosclerosis;
- nervousness, tension and fatigue.

Shifts and work performance

The imbalances listed above (which may be considered as distressors) and any resultant disorders are likely to affect work performance. Research has demonstrated that generally accidents in factories and cars are greater at 1 a.m., and most industrial accidents occur between 2 a.m. and 4 a.m. Sweden's meter readers recorded most errors at night, and telephone operators identified 3 a.m. to 4 a.m. as their 'dead spot', since more errors were recorded. Research involving doctors and other healthcare practitioners on night shifts demonstrate similar findings. In addition, impaired retention, decreased factual recall, poorer manual dexterity, slow information processing, slow problem solving, increased anxiety, hyperirritability, less social interaction, depersonalization and divorce problems are also frequently quoted as homeostatic disturbances/imbalances as a result of shift work. These disturbances/imbalances, if prolonged, may cause stress-related disorders, such as ulcers,

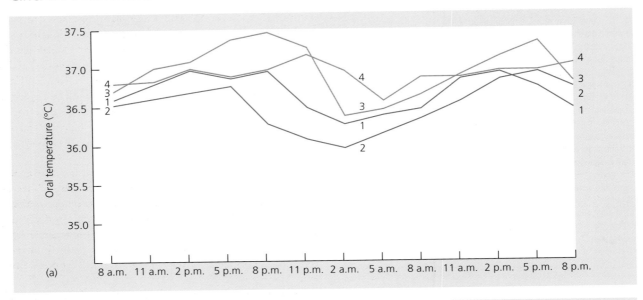

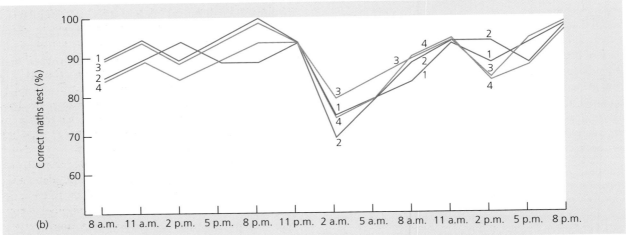

Figure 22.8 (a) Relationship between oral temperature and time over 36 hours. (b) Relationship between mathematical testing efficiency (%) and time over 36 hours. (c) Times of peak temperature values in non-shift workers and shift workers over a 7-day period. (d) Times of peak performance levels in mathematical testing between non-shift workers and shift workers over a 7-day period. 1 and 2, control subjects (non-shift workers); 3 and 4, experimental subjects (shift workers before commencing the shift; Clancy and McVicar, 1995)

Q Suggest why shift work researchers use the phrase 'maladaptation syndrome'.

hypertension, cardiac complaints, depression, neurosis, and possibly even an increase in suicidal tendencies.

Night shifts, in particular, are associated with a high rate of absenteeism because of reported 'stress-related' conditions. The question is whether these conditions are caused by the night work itself or are a consequence of the person's daily activities. Whichever is the case, we can safely say that night work is less efficient from the employers' and less healthy from the employees' points of view.

Afternoon (late) shifts are the most popular among shift workers, followed by morning (early) shifts, and then nights. Factors contributing to the popularity of late shifts are the lesser effects on social life, less susceptibility to digestive disorders and less fatigue.

The scheduling of shifts is often cited most often as a reason for resignation for nursing staff; it is now identified as a significant workplace stressor by nurses (McVicar, 2003). The authors hypothesize that this could also be the main reason in other health carers. Thus, we can only assume that financial gain, job security and devotion to patients are a few reasons why they remain.

The authors advocate longitudinal research into any health impacts of the effects of the 12-hour shift system since this scheduling is gaining popularity within the workforce (see Box 22.6), and as a workforce we must have evidence whether this pattern of shift scheduling enhances or alleviates some of the well-known problems associated with the shifts mentioned above.

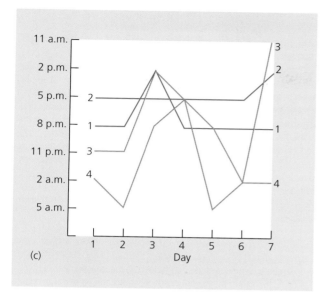

(c)

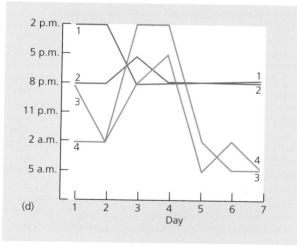

(d)

'Adaptation' to shift work

Adaptation is a problem, since it takes several days to completely readjust to just a 1-hour phase shift. It is not surprising that when a person works on night shift, their entire body enters a state of transition for many days. Although the individual responds by 'resetting' or synchronizing sleep and activity cycles, the problem is that our numerous rhythms do not reset at once. Blood pressure takes about 2 days to adapt, but body temperature takes more than 5 days, in response to a 1-hour time change in shifts; other rhythms (e.g. serum potassium) may take up to 2 weeks to reset to a new schedule of sleep and rest.

The 'perceived adaptability' of some individuals suggests that some feel more comfortable doing shift work than others.

Despite this perception there is a positive correlation between shift workers and disorders indicating the reality is shift workers do not actually adapt, even though they think they do! Research has also identified a significant increase in road traffic accidents in the week after a change of the shift work, and suggests that this may be caused by the rhythms still being desynchronized. The nature of this transitional vulnerability arising through phase shifting, perhaps owing to a desynchronization of internal rhythms, remains one of the interesting questions of work–rest scheduling.

Longitudinal studies, which investigate the desynchronizing effects on the human lifespan, are not forthcoming. However, we would suggest that the cumulative effects of shift-induced disturbances/imbalances (stressors) would result in decreasing one's adaptation resistance to stress at a greater rate in shift workers. Also, a removal of shift work may actually decrease or diminish the stressors associated with the shift worker's situation.

Shifts probably affect people differently, since an individual's tolerance varies depending on their genotype and their perceived environmental (socializing) experiences. In addition, the rate and direction of shift change varies as a result of social, societal, organizational and public requirements, which is very important in one's perception of adaptation. The problem is that the individual may think that they are in control (and hence 'adapted'), but most people are unaware of the damaging effects of shift work on their bodies and their relationships. This was supported by the Rhone Valley survey of 1000 industrial workers, 45% of whom could not adjust to a 7-day shift rotation and 34% could not adjust to a 2-day rotation. Thus, 55% and 66%, respectively, thought they were adapted (Luce 1977). Interestingly, body temperature did not adapt in either group. The phrase 'shift maladaptation syndrome' is used in shift work research since it describes a condition that affects people who cannot adapt to shifts.

Body temperature is often used as an index of adaptation as it is normally the most consistent rhythm; in shift work involving consecutive night work for periods of 1–3 weeks, a phase shifting of the minimal body temperature will be observed. The temperature will shift to a point within the new sleeping period after 7+ days of night shift (i.e. adaptation has occurred).

Plasma potassium (K^+) concentration can also be used, as it is a good indicator of how quickly a person is adjusting to phase shifts and living to non-circadian schedules. For a reversal of the patterns, the shift worker must work 14 nights to achieve adaptation, i.e. 14 consecutive nights before the K^+ concentrations have been inverted from their daily pattern of change.

Hence the night shifts of approximately 3–5 nights' duration will demonstrate that some rhythmic patterns will be adapted and others will not. For example, blood pressure will be adapted to the night shift, since it takes 1–2 days to adapt, body temperature takes a week to adapt, and therefore body temperature (and performance) will not be adapted within this period. Because of the body's attempt to resynchronize during

BOX 22.6 SHIFT WORK IN HEALTH CARE

Shifts are classified according to the number of hours worked. Historically, 8 hours constitutes a shift, and in order to provide 24-hour coverage shifts are split into mornings ('earlies'), afternoons ('lates') and nights. The scheduling of shifts in health care depends on regional and hospital policies. Historically, weekly work patterns of some healthcare practitioners (e.g. nurses, midwives, paramedics, operating departmental practitioners) are either two shifts (earlies and lates) in association with permanent nights, or three shifts (mornings, e.g. 7 a.m. to 3 p.m.; afternoons, e.g. 2 p.m. to 10 p.m.; and nights, e.g. 9.30 p.m. to 7.30 a.m.). The latter pattern is described as rotational, as workers rotate their shifts between afternoons, nights and earlies. Health authorities state that the reasons for rotational shift work in their health carers were that:

- slow rotation results in slow adaptation, so efficiency of work declines for up to 1 week. Thus, in a month of shifts there will be three efficient weeks and one inefficient week. However, improved safety measures for these healthcare workers and the patient are needed at lower efficiency levels, and, as mentioned in the text, the health carer's body clocks are tending to revert back to their normal circadian patterns during the days off. In the author's opinion, three efficient weeks is a misconception;
- rapid rotation (the majority of nursing and midwifery shifts) produces very little adaptation of circadian rhythms, and workers just feel tired and fatigued. It is generally considered that rapidly rotating shifts do not affect efficiency, but substantive longitudinal data is lacking, and is required to look at the cumulative effects of rapidly rotating shifts on the well-being of the health carer, and on efficiency levels, which are going to affect the well-being of the patients.

Some health authorities have implemented a 12-hour shift and these are becoming popular in the UK. In particular, the implementation of the 12-hour shift system is becoming fashionable in human-led services (police, fire brigade and healthcare professions) and businesses in the UK. One reason for its popularity is that the day-on, day-off pattern and the on-shift coverage is relatively easy to understand. However, like any shift pattern, the 12-hour shift has advantages and disadvantages relative to alternative shorter shift patterns. The advantages commonly quoted when compared with shorter shifts (i.e. 10-hour and 8-hour) are for the same hours worked each year, the 12-hour shift worker works

fewer days, and therefore will have more days and more weekends off and more holidays. Minimizing the number of shifts makes the planning of social and family events much easier. Most studies conclude that the change from 8-hour to 12-hour shifts was in fact positive in other respects such as increased satisfaction with sleep, alertness, health, perceived accident risk, and work performance (tasks based on reaction times), while recovery time following night work also reduced.

The frequently mentioned disadvantages are that the 12-hour days are long, and can be tiring, with employees increasingly distracted from duties towards the end of the shift. Twelve-hour shifts may also have an adverse impact on shift worker lifestyles, on their actual work days and their days off. In summary, before the 12-hour system becomes more widespread data from longitudinal studies need to answer the following questions:

- *Can the shift worker work more consecutive hours without any adverse impact on productivity, quality and health and safety?* To date researchers commonly state that as long as the total number of hours remains the same, the majority of occupations can be performed just as well on short and long shift patterns. However, jobs which focus on tedious detail tasks are best kept to shorter shifts, unless the workers change duties from time to time to keep themselves alert.
- *Does long-standing exposure to damaging environmental conditions increase the risk of shift-work related illnesses?* There is an abundance of evidence to support that an 8-hour exposure to extreme temperatures, noisy machinery, antigenic insults and hard mental or physical work can seriously damage the health of some workers. The authors therefore would hypothesize that a 12-hour shift may simply be too much to endure and will have an obvious knock-on effect on individual's health and rates of absenteeism. Advocates of the 12-hour system dispute this because there are more days off to recover.
- *What do the workers want?* While longer shifts are appealing nationwide (for the advantages above) they are not the first choice of all workers, so to enforce them on every employee takes away personal choice, which may have a knock-on effect on the health of some individuals. Longitudinal data is needed on the potential health effects of those that self-selected a 12-hour shift, so ideally the workers can make an informed decision of which shift pattern to choose.

---

rest days, following the shift, there can be no shift pattern with totally synchronized circadian rhythms, with the exception of the 'normal' synchronized daily shift, i.e. approximately between 8 a.m. and 6 p.m.

Hypothetically, an ideal shift pattern would be one that takes into account the adaptation of all the rhythms. Thus, since 14 nights are necessary for adaptations of some rhythms, such as K^+ ions, then one would have to be constantly at work, as days off would result in the individual trying to resynchronize to the 'normal' circadian pattern. Even constant working (without time off) would not help, however, since the worker would become easily fatigued and exhausted, which consequently would enhance the likelihood of illness (which itself also desynchronizes rhythms) and absenteeism. During absence from work, the person would then revert back to the 'innate' rhythms associated with a daily work routine.

Three major strategies have been used to address the well-documented evidence of problems of adaptation to rotational shifts:

1 Schedule workers on straight shifts without rotation. The problem would be staffing the night shift, since research data suggests that this is the least popular choice of the workforce.
2 Use a rapid rotation of shifts in order to escape the consequences of partial resynchronization of some rhythms. The problem is that some circadian rhythms will still be affected; this is reflected by reports that rapid rotation is associated with the worker reporting increased tiredness and fatigue.
3 Select people who seem to have the best tolerance to shift work or have abnormal sleeping rhythms (i.e. those with rhythms of low amplitude). This does not include people who think they are adapted to shift work, since data suggests

the perception of adaptation is not actually reflected in the biochemistry of their body.

In summary, shift work will always be a necessity because of the importance to the country's economy of providing a 24-hour service. This will become more of a problem to health as more and more of the world becomes industrialized, and so trends to run continuous around-the-clock operations increase. Since it is the authors' view that no shift can provide totally synchronized circadian rhythms (except 'normal' day work), then one must seek compensatory behaviours to reduce the desynchronizing effect of shift work. Such interventions include napping and exercise.

Napping

Napping can be used as a sleep supplement. For many years, Japanese companies have offered their workers rest rooms for this 'activity' during their shifts. They believe that this results in decreased fatigue and reinstated arousal, which increases the performance of their workforce. This idea has been implemented informally in many 24-hour healthcare environments, whereby night workers are often given the opportunity to have a 'cat-nap' during their shift. However, to the individual napper, this can reduce the quality and duration of the subsequent night's sleep, and research has shown that naps need to be controlled with reference to the individual's shift pattern if the person is to benefit. For example, if the next main sleep is on the following night, it is better not to take a nap in order to ensure that the sleep is of good, restorable quality. However, if the following night is a working night, then an afternoon nap is advisable to reduce the inevitable fatigue that accompanies night work.

Exercise

Regular, moderate exercise increases one's fitness and, as a result, decreases skeletomuscular signs of fatigue. There is also an increased alertness. Perhaps exercise increases resynchronization efficiency, resulting in quicker adaptation rates.

ACTIVITY

Suggest what interventionary schemes may be used to compensate for desynchronized rhythms associated with shift work.

Interim summary

Further research is needed in this area to minimize the disadvantageous effects of shift work. This is being addressed in some countries, where chronobiological departments have been developed to study circadian rhythms in an attempt to improve schedules. Chronobiologists (scientists who study time; 'chrono-' = time) believe that the best shift is the one that takes account of the natural circadian patterns. They also believe that night workers are able to accommodate their sleep disruption more satisfactorily if they go to sleep as soon as they finish their night shift, rather than staying up for a few hours following their night shift and going to sleep before normal sleep time. These scientists have demonstrated that improved shift change patterns are those that rotate clockwise (i.e. mornings to afternoons to evening, and back to morning). In most shifts, this is usually at a frequency of 1 or 2 days, but if this period is extended, then it also improves circadian effects. Rotational shift patterns are a source of debate, as rhythms are constantly being disrupted and adaptation depends on the speed of rotation. The time interval between each shift in a slow rotation is generally only long enough for the rhythms to adapt partially; this partial resynchronization is potentially harmful to rhythms that do not adapt fully. Rapid rotation avoids the problems of continued partial resynchronization, and so is considered more satisfactory. The major problems associated with rapid rotation are the greater disruptions they cause to domestic and social life, which is why many people prefer slow rotation. With regard to rapid rotation, it is not known what cumulative effects will result over a long period of time. Some companies in Germany provide optional medical check-ups for their employees, and special hospital admission arrangements for them to normalize their desynchronized rhythms in an attempt to avoid long-term problems. Organizations in the UK offer employers' advice on the problems associated with shift work.

In the context of the dynamic model of homeostasis presented in this book, the rhythmic changes in physiological and biochemical parameters provide the optimal internal conditions for external expression of behaviours and activities, the latter especially linked to the daytime. An effective change to night-time activity with shift working largely becomes possible because exogenous cues establish the phases of change and so many rhythms can be resynchronized to meet the new activity–sleep schedule, thus adapting to a new homeostatic set point. However, this resetting takes time, and not all rhythms can be reset, and so there are 'costs'.

ACTIVITY

Distinguish between the following terms: synchronization, desynchronization and resynchronization.

Travelling across time zones

When crossing time zones, a person becomes desynchronized as the body time is not in phase with the external cues. Body temperature adjustment times vary from 5 to 21 days according to different studies, demonstrating individual variation. This is hardly surprising when we consider that if we fly west from the UK to the USA, there is a time difference of between 5 and 8 hours (east and west coasts, respectively). Thus, the phases of Americans are approximately 5–8 hours behind, and consequently the peaks and troughs of their body chemistry occurs earlier than those of Europeans (Figure 22.9). People

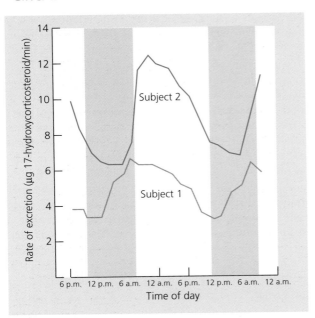

Figure 22.9 Excretion rates of 17-hydroxycorticosteroids in adults at different times of the day. Subject 1, Americans; Subject 2, Europeans

Q Describe why travelling across different time zones is said to cause circadian rhythm desynchronization.

find it hard to adjust, and most (if not all) travellers are aware of the fatigue associated with 'jet lag'. Furthermore, continued exposure to this causes the 'jet syndrome', with symptoms of general malaise, sleep disruptions, feelings of disorientation,

headaches, burning or unfocused eyes, gastrointestinal tract problems, sweating and shortness of breath. These are similar problems to those experienced by shift workers. Research has demonstrated that the life expectancy of persistent flyers is reduced by 10%; however, this is not irreversible, and the symptoms disappear with time when persistent flyers stop flying.

The components responsible for travel fatigue are:

- *external desynchronization*: the weak time cues on arrival lead to slow adjustment;
- *internal desynchronization*: leads to a decrease in psychomotor skills.

When we invert our sleep pattern by east–west travel, or vice versa, we expose our bodies to potential pathogens, viruses and infection during the very phase when production of antibodies is at its lowest. Perhaps this may account for the high incidences of colds and infections that many travellers, students studying for exams and people doing shift work experience.

The hormone melatonin is sold over the counter in some countries as an aid to decrease the incidence of jet lag, and to aid quicker recovery in sufferers of jet lag (see Figure 22.6, p.615). The UK is still awaiting clinical evidence on the reliability and validity of exogenous melatonin administration (see Box 22.5, p.616). However advocates of melatonin administration argue that its benefits support the evidence that the light and dark cycle is one of the most important circadian rhythms, and so altering the light–dark schedule on long-distance flights, or the use of artificial light aids, are some of the methods promoted to ameliorate jet lag.

BOX 22.7 CIRCADIAN RHYTHMS, ILLNESS AND HOSPITALIZATION

All illnesses are associated with desynchronized circadian rhythms. The rhythms that are most disturbed depend on the illness. For example, feverish illness produces pronounced desynchronized body temperature rhythms (and associated rhythms, e.g. heart, respiratory and metabolic rates). Some illnesses produce specific changes in normal circadian rhythms. For example, variations and desynchronized patterns of blood glucose occur in people with diabetes. Patients with liver disease show urination and temperature peaks at night instead of in the morning.

It is feasible that desynchronization of circadian rhythms could eventually explain recurrent symptoms; perhaps all illnesses need to be studied for disturbed circadian rhythms so as to contribute to the understanding of the associated signs and symptoms. Constant exposure to distressors (in this case desynchronized rhythms = homeostatic imbalances) leads to a deterioration of the adaptive system, and consequently one succumbs to an illness (stress-related illness). It is possible, perhaps, that this deterioration may even be caused by one or more circadian rhythm(s) moving out of phase.

Observations of circadian patterns have demonstrated that there are times in the day–night cycle that correlate with specific illnesses. For example:

- The peak frequency for the onset of myocardial infarctions is between 8 a.m. and 10 a.m.

- Peripheral circulation in the arms and legs reaches a low point between midnight and 4 a.m. Tissues receive less oxygen during this period, and therefore it is not surprising that some people with peripheral arterial disease are awakened with acute pain from their sleep at this time.
- There appears to be a peak time for births. Most labours begin around midnight, and births are more frequent in the early hours of the morning. Induced births, however, are opposite to natural labour, since from an economic point more staff are available during the day. Interestingly, the number of stillbirths follows the induced curves, and it is tempting to speculate, therefore, that the timing of the induction may be a contributory factor to the number of stillbirths, since it is not the natural time for delivery.
- Deaths are more likely to occur at night, but this is not surprising, since metabolism is at its lowest and so we are more at risk.

Hospitalization
Exogenous cues ('zeitgebers') are markedly altered by hospitalization.

As mentioned previously, illnesses will already have induced desynchronized circadian rhythms, and these may be disturbed further by hospitalization, and other unaffected rhythms may become desynchronized upon admission to hospital, since exogenous synchronizers are replaced partly by those cues determined by the ward policy and new environ-

BOX 22.7 *Continued*

ment. In addition, admission can potentially produce a greater desynchronization in people (e.g. people who are blind and older adults) who have a greater dependency upon set exogenous cues for their circadian rhythmicity. Furthermore, not only are older adults desynchronized to a greater extent following hospital admission, but they also find it more difficult to adapt to the imposed hospital zeitgebers.

All patients upon admission lose some of their exogenous synchronizers. Some wards still wake their 'older adult' patients during the night to commode, which further disrupts the sleep–wake and associated rhythms; the nurse may report this as confusion. However, the authors would argue that any person may appear temporarily confused and distressed when awakened at these times, especially if they are awakened when in stage IV (deep) sleep. When labelled confused there is a risk that the patient may be sedated, thus disrupting the sleep–wake and associated circadian rhythms further. Awakening policies are not restricted to 'care-of-the-elderly' wards, since research has shown that many patients also have disrupted during sleep through the activities of hospital staff, and by noises and lights on surrounding the ward.

The hospitalized patient, whether old or not, has many additional routines or zeitgebers. For example, the last drug round perhaps is at 10 p.m., with lights out soon after this. The patient may be awakened at 6.30 a.m. to 7 a.m., and there are specific meal times (breakfast at 8.30 a.m., lunch at midday and dinner at 5.30 p.m.). Patients must also adapt to the presence of complicated and unfamiliar machinery in a specialized ward (e.g. intensive care units). During this period of adaptation, the patient may appear to be confused. Increasing social interaction may be

the way to reduce or remove this confusion. Historically, research has highlighted the importance of face-to-face therapy, at the patient's level of understanding, since a potential desynchronizer to patients comes from poor communication between nurses and other healthcare practitioners.

The removal of wall-to-wall seating, which is still found in many hospital rest rooms, may improve social contact and so help remove the appearance of 'confusion' in patients and abolish unnecessary sedation. Perhaps it may also decrease the amplitude of circadian rhythm disturbances and reduce the adaptation period, thus improving the quality of care.

The study of circadian rhythms may aid the assessment of the individual needs of patients. Forcing patients particularly older adult patients, and infants or young children, into a rigidly conforming pattern of care is not only going to potentially make them worse, but may also make them confused and disoriented, thus increasing the level of dependency on the nurse and other healthcare practitioners. Conversely, it could be argued that rhythmicity might be promoted by adopting a highly regularized living routine, even if different from the one followed previously, since some improvement is noted in some older adult patients following an initial post-admission period of confusion. Perhaps this may be due in part to mundane routine rather than medical intervention. It remains controversial whether imposing environmental rhythms that do not coincide with a patient's own internal rhythms fosters well-being.

See the case study of a man with learning disabilities leaving a long-stay institution, Section VI, p.678.

BOX 22.8 CIRCADIAN RHYTHMS AND VULNERABILITY TO DRUGS

Although the application of circadian rhythms to pharmacology is a relatively new area of research there is much evidence over the last 20 years to suggest that a lower pharmacological tolerance exists at night; thus if the same dosages are given at night then they have greater pharmacological effects. For example, the cardiac stimulant digitalis is 40 times more effective at night than during the day, but ward policy in some areas of the UK is to administer digitalis in the morning. This is 'normal' practice with drugs that are administered once daily, and depressed tolerance levels are not, on the whole, taken into account for drugs that are needed two, three or four times a day, as the same dosage is given at night as during the day.

Drug tolerance depends on the absorption rates of drugs, their distribution rates, their metabolism by the liver, and their excretory rates (for example, see the discussion on opioid analgesics in Chapter 20, pp.568–9). All of these are depressed at night. Drug tolerance variation is even more pronounced in the older adult, since absorption rates are potentially much slower. However, the main problem is that this group of the population are more likely to be affected by drug combinations since many are taking several drugs. Thus, there is an increased drug distribution, resulting in a longer half-life of the drugs. This also arises because these adults have lower plasma albumin (which binds to certain drugs) concentrations, leaving more 'free' drug, so there is increased pharmacological activity.

There is also a decreased activity of drug-metabolizing enzymes in the livers of older people. Depressed drug metabolism may also be caused by a decrease in hepatic blood flow, therefore reduced dosages are required and dosage intervals need to be less frequent. Kidney

clearance of drugs by this group of people is also reduced, which also supports the need for decreased dosages and less frequent intervals. A misunderstanding of drug dosages and drug intervals could conceivably lead to further desynchronization of circadian rhythms and, as a result, hospitalization (it is increasingly recognized that a proportion of hospital admissions are due solely or partly to adverse drug reactions). Older patients seem to be a particularly vulnerable group. Adverse drug reactions in them stem from the fact that high proportions are taking some form of drug medication, and many are taking several drugs. Many older people are given repeat prescriptions without regular medical check-ups. As a result, older people may exhibit drug-induced symptoms. For example, overindulgence in laxatives (drugs to counteract constipation) has been demonstrated to have a strong link with the incidence of colonic cancers. It must also be remembered that sedatives and opiates also alter a patient's perception and ability to respond to environmental cues, and use of these classes of drugs is common in older people.

Major goals of clinical chronobiology are chronotherapeutics (i.e. drugs formulated to administer varying dosages at different times over the 24-hour period), the optimization of pharmacotherapies (i.e. taking into consideration rhythm-dependencies in the workings and dynamics of medications), plus predictable-in-time variability in the manifestation and severity of human disease. Chronotherapies need to positively correlate with biological need. In theory this could improve efficacy. In effect, this is working in some clinical areas; for example, chronotherapy for cardiovascular disease is now routinely applied in the form of the evening administration for lipid-lowering medications.

BOX 22.9 IMPLICATIONS FOR CARE

There is a need for the healthcare professions to be aware that patients' circadian rhythms, and their disturbances, as rhythm desynchronization (= homeostatic imbalances) is an important diagnostic tool because these may be signs and symptoms of clinical labels. For example, a continued increase in plasma calcium ion concentration beyond its normal circadian parameters could represent a gradual decalcification of bone, which is known to accompany continuous recumbency, and a fall in blood nitrogen is typical of the effects of starvation. Deviation in patterns can be indicative of disturbed homeostatic functions; for example in Addison's disease and Cushing's syndrome, the normal variation in cortisol release is largely or entirely absent. In Addison's disease, cortisol concentrations are lower, but may not be any lower than is observed in unaffected people at night. Conversely, with Cushing's syndrome, elevated cortisol levels may be no higher than those shown in a healthy individual first thing in the morning. Diagnosis would therefore be aided by taking a morning and evening serum sample. If only single samples are permitted by hospital policy, then a morning sample would be better to detect Addison's disease and an evening sample would be better to detect Cushing's syndrome. The timing of samples, however, is complicated if the patient is a shift worker, as there is no guarantee of their 'adapted' rhythmicity. In addition, the patient's nationality and frequency of overseas travel may have to be taken into consideration when assessing the patient (e.g. baseline observations) otherwise missed diagnoses may occur. For example, a resynchronizing American visitor or a recent visitor to the USA would have rhythms 5–8 hours (depending on which coast they came from) ahead of Europeans (Figure 22.9). All these variations demonstrate the importance of individualized care for patients.

Where possible circadian rhythms should be applied routinely to all aspects of care. The following should become a matter of routine in order to improve the quality of care administered:

- Clinical staff could investigate optimal times (i.e. increased responsiveness) for chemotherapeutic administration, especially for medications that commonly cause allergic responses. Allergy testing should be investigated in the evening, when allergic responses are at their highest.
- Clinical staff could investigate optimal times for laboratory specimens. Variations in the peaks of leucocyte counts, electrolyte concentrations, haematocrit, blood gas composition, temperature, urinary output, etc. all exist, so it makes the common practice for collection of samples questionable. The 'typical' sample should be collected closest to the mean for that person, rather than at the time when it would be at its highest or lowest values. In addition, daily comparative sampling will be of maximal value only if it is performed at the same time of day every time to take into account circadian fluctuations. At present, samples are usually drawn at 6 a.m., when some of the rhythmic values are at their minimum, so that they are ready for when the physician arrives at the unit. If regular samples (e.g. every 4 hours) were taken, then a circadian pattern for the patient could be plotted after a few days (a process called 'circadian mapping'). Once established, circadian patterns can be used to avoid:
  - reactionary responses (e.g. decreased urinary output at night should not be controlled diuretically);
  - increased stressors or exercise at the patient's lowest resource point (e.g. the lowest pain response is between midnight and 4 a.m., so intravenous catheterization and other painful procedures could be started early in the rest cycle in order to minimize the pain response). The optimal time for treatment and surgery scheduling is thought to be in the early morning hours when the patient's metabolism is low, despite the practitioner's metabolism also being low and consequently risking error and accident. Also, care may be improved by monitoring patients closely at more susceptible times.

For example, exaggerated bronchoconstrictory rhythm occurs in people with asthma at about 6 a.m., and special alertness is required at this time.

- A knowledge of circadian patterns can be of value from a health-education point of view, since the body temperature peak is associated with a better performance in relation to both teaching (practitioner) and learning (patient). We would argue that the most important teaching time ideally would coincide with the patient's peak temperatures, in order to gain maximum benefit from the teaching. However, body temperature cannot always be used as a reliable indicator of the person's performance, since illness and hospital admission may be associated with rhythm desynchronization in the patient.
- Research needs to investigate the circadian timing of 'stress-related' events, in order to avoid 'stressors', which can potentially affect the circadian rhythms of the patient.
- One could minimize circadian problems for patients by maintaining the patient's natural social synchronizers (e.g. emphasizing community care, particularly for the older person). Night admission wards could be introduced to cater for insomniacs, people who are nocturnally disturbed, and people who are frightened of being alone at night. In addition to providing an extra element of care, this would also remove the 'burden' from families who obviously have their sleep patterns disturbed by the nocturnal activities within their homes.

The patient is in a period of desynchronization and/or resynchronization because of the illness itself, the admission process, and the stressors associated with being a patient. Therefore, care should support previous circadian rhythms where possible, and should not be associated with ward conformity. For example, sleep is usually influenced by social and occupational pressure, and removal of these pressures (e.g. with retirement or hospital admission) may result in a 'polycyclic' sleep pattern (i.e. 'cat-naps' during the day). Napping reduces the quality and quantity of night-time sleeping. We would argue that the best treatment would be to detect the stressors (e.g. boredom) that cause the naps, and remove (e.g. increase social interaction) or replace (e.g. face-to-face therapy) them, thus benefiting the patient by reducing medication and giving a sense of time.

If polycyclic sleep is evident on the wards, then one must question whether it is imposed or if it is a normal routine for the patient. The nurse must try to remove it only if it is not the patient's normal routine, since a disturbed rest–activity cycle can lead to desynchronization of other rhythms. Providing a stimulating environment specific to each patient can prevent it. If polycyclic sleep is a normal occurrence for the patient, then we would argue that this should be encouraged in hospitals.

Patients are often overloaded with many additional stressors, and other healthcare practitioners should minimize these potential desynchronizers by various means. Interviews should be conducted as a series of short meetings rather than one long-winded interview, in order to develop a care plan. This should be by the same nurse if possible. The interviews should coincide with the patient's most receptive time, borne out by the body temperature peak. The patient should be involved in the decision-making process. Also, subsequent to discussions with the nurse, the patient should be allowed to 'sleep on it' before coming to a final decision. The patient should also be involved in rehabilitation, since increasing sensory input can transform distress into eustress. Finally, the patient's individuality should be considered. For example, the nurse could investigate whether the patient is a 'morning' or an 'evening' person, a shift worker, or an unacclimatized traveller, as this could influence assessing, planning, implementing and evaluating care.

Care of unconscious or comatose patients necessitates clinical intervention to maintain physiological equilibrium, so that the endogenous rhythm approximates to its innate time minus the zeitgebers. The nurse

BOX 22.9 Continued

should assume, therefore, that the rhythms are free-running; if the patient is unconscious for a long period of time, or if there is brain injury, then desynchronization must be assumed. In such cases, it is essential that the nurse supports the previous circadian rhythms. In order to do this, the nurse must maintain the patient's physiological equilibrium. The patient should also be helped to reorient the brain to previous temporal and life experiences; this may, for example, involve playing favourite music or a relative talking about the past.

In summary, although not at a rate one would like, research evidence-based practice is being implemented to improve the quality of patient care. Progress in cardiovascular chronobiology research has changed the way in which diagnostic procedures are performed and analysed. For example, 24-hour ambulatory blood pressure (BP) monitoring and Holter monitoring reveal the marked circadian (24-hour) rhythms in BP in hypertensive patients and electrocardiographic events in patients with ischaemic heart disease.

ACTIVITY

Circadian parameters vary in their patterns between people and according to the impact of factors that desynchronize them. Is the individualized care advocated in this section possible on a busy ward? If not, can you suggest any ways to facilitate this, or alternatives?

SUMMARY

1 Human circadian rhythms are bodily processes that are repeated every 24 hours.

2 The genetic (endogenous) component of such rhythms (demonstrated by studies of isolation, older adults, people who are congenitally blind and Inuits) is responsible for producing innate rhythms that are free-running (i.e. outside the 24-hour periodicity).

3 The free-running rhythms are synchronized (entrained) by environmental cues (zeitgebers or synchronizers) to give the 24-hour (circadian) periodicity.

4 Most circadian patterns (e.g. body temperature) show a rise and general peak (or plateau) during the waking hours, and a fall and nadir during the sleeping hours, although some (e.g. the release of growth hormone) display a reversal of this pattern.

5 Individual variation or subjectivity of circadian parameters occurs with relation to the timing of peaks and troughs, the degree of inclines and declines, and the timing of PLDs and dead spots, according to an individual's genotype and their perception of environmental cues.

6 The hypothalamus appears to be the master clock synchronizing the free-running rhythms of the homeostatic control centres, including the pineal gland, since this is responsive to light–dark cues, which are very important zeitgebers.

7 Health is associated with internal synchronization (i.e. all the circadian rhythm parameters being within their homeostatic ranges).

8 Desynchronization occurs when the circadian rhythms are outside their homeostatic range; such a disturbance is known as a phase shift.

9 Phase shifts have been demonstrated in shift workers, people who travel across different time zones, during illness and upon hospitalization. Continued phase shifts lead to illness (psychophysiological homeostatic imbalances), and social problems.

10 Chronobiologists suggest that compensatory changes are necessary to minimize the circadian disturbances. For example, in rotational shift work, shifts should be changed clockwise (i.e. morning to afternoon to evening, etc.). Longer intervals between changes must be introduced so workers have time to 'normalize' their patterns – perhaps this will be reflected by data from longitudinal studies on the 12-hour shift pattern. In the healthcare setting, chronopharmacology removes some adverse drug interactions and decreases the need for hospitalization, and consequently the person's exogenous cues are maintained. This involves dosages and timing of dosages being calculated using the circadian changes that are associated with the illness and the process of hospitalization. Finally, if the health carer is hoping to meet the total needs of the patient, they must take into account the effects of circadian rhythmicity on temporal, physiological and psychological coordination when planning, assessing, implementing and evaluating care, and use this knowledge to aid a more speedy recovery.

REFERENCES

Clancy, J. and McVicar, A.J. (1995) *Physiology and Anatomy. A Homeostatic Approach.* London: Edward Arnold.

Clancy, J. and McVicar, A.J. (2007a) Short-term regulation of acid–base homeostasis. *British Journal of Nursing* **16**(16): 604–7.

Clancy, J. and McVicar, A.J. (2007b) Intermediate and long-term regulation of acid–base homeostasis. *British Journal of Nursing* **16**(17): 1016–19.

Halberg, F. (1959) Chronobiology. *Annual Review of Physiology* **31**: 675–725.

Luce, G.G. (1977) *Body Time.* St Albans: Paladin.

McVicar, A. (2003) Workplace stress in nursing: a literature review. *Journal of Advanced Nursing* **44**(6): 1–10.

Mills, J.N. (1973) *Biological Aspects of Circadian Rhythms.* New York: Plenum Press.

FURTHER READING

Please note: Some of these references are of historical importance in the field of circadian rhythms.

Aschoff, J. (1966) Adaptive cycles. *International Journal of Biometeorology* **10**: 305–24.

Aschoff J. (1981) *Handbook of Behavioural Neurobiology*, vol. 4. *Biological Rhythms.* New York: Plenum.

Baxendale, S., Clancy, J. and McVicar, A.J. (1997) Circadian rhythms: the application to patient care. *British Journal of Nursing* **5**(26): 303–9.

Burgess, H.J., Revell, V.L., and Eastman, C.I. (2008) A three-pulse phase response curve to three milligrams of melatonin in humans. *Journal of Physiology* **586**: 639–47.

Clancy, J. and McVicar, A.J. (1994) Circadian rhythms 1: physiology. *British Journal of Nursing* **3**(13): 657–61.

Clancy, J. and McVicar, A.J. (1994) Circadian rhythms 2: shift work and health. *British Journal of Nursing* **3**(14): 712–17.

Fuller, P.M., Gooley, J.J. and Saper, C.B. (2006) Neurobiology of the sleep–wake cycle: sleep architecture, circadian regulation, and regulatory feedback. *Journal of Biological Rhythms* **21**: 482–93.

Furlan, R., Barbic, F. Piazza, S. Tinelli, M. Seghizzi, P. and Malliani, A. (2000) Modifications of cardiac autonomic profile associated with a shift schedule of work. *Circulation* **102**(16): 1912–16.

Harker, J.E. (1964) *The Physiology of Diurnal Rhythms*. Cambridge: Cambridge University Press.

Klerman, E.B. (2005) Clinical aspects of human circadian rhythms. *Journal of Biological Rhythms* **20**: 375–86.

Klietman, N. (1967) *Sleep and Wakefulness*. Chicago: University of Chicago Press.

Lewy, A.J., Lefler, B.J., Emens, J.S. and Bauer, V.K. (2006) The circadian basis of winter depression. *Proceedings of the National Academy of Sciences, USA* **103**: 7414–19.

Mestel, R. (1994) Mouse gene could help master rhythm. *New Scientist* 7: 15.

Minors, D.S. (1988) *Practical Applications of Circadian Rhythms to Shift Work. The biological clock – Current Approaches*. Southampton: Inprint (litho) Limited.

Minors, D.S. and Waterhouse, J.M. (1985) Circadian rhythms in deep body temperature, urinary excretion and alertness in nurses on night work. *Ergonomics* **28**(11): 523–30.

Moore-Ede, M.C. and Richardson, G.S. (1982) Medical implications of shift work. *Annual Reviews of Medicine* **36**: 607–17.

Petrie, K., Conagelen, J.V., Thompson, L. and Chamberlain, K. (1989) Effects of melatonin on jet lag after long haul flights. *British Medical Journal* **298**: 705–7.

Rutenfranz, E. (1982) Occupational health measures for night and day shift workers. *Journal of Human Ergology* **11**(Suppl.): 17.

Smith L., Folkard S. and Poole, C.J.M. (1994) Increased injuries on night-shift. *Lancet* **344**: 1137–9.

Tureck, F.W. (1981) Are the suprachiasmic nuclei the location of the biological clock in mammals? *Nature* **229**: 289–99.

CASE STUDIES

Healthcare practice: a homeostatic approach

HEALTHCARE PRACTICE: A HOMEOSTATIC APPROACH

INTRODUCTION

This book commenced with an overview of the organization of the human body, and a detailed analysis of the concept of homeostasis as the basis of physiological control and well-being. The intention of this book is to provide the reader with a grasp of homeostatic principles as applied to the maintenance of normal physiology, and to the homeostatic imbalance or failure that is characteristic of ill health. Homeostasis therefore provides a framework for learning that is applicable to all physiological systems, and this is reinforced throughout the book.

While the book is mostly concerned with the application of this concept to physiology in health, with an emphasis as to why processes must occur as they do, it is anticipated that the main readership will be people with an interest in health care. Another aspect therefore is how homeostatic theory relates to the application of care. This is especially evident in Chapters 20–22 which integrate and apply aspects of well-being and healthcare practice that illustrate the interactional and often subjective nature of physiology. For convenience and ease of learning Chapters 2–19 focus on individual physiological constructs of the human body, although the integration between systems should be apparent. It is these latter chapters that provide the basis of this chapter in the context of examples of disorder that are primarily connected to those individual constructs or systems.

This section first revisits the material presented in Chapter 1 to provide the basis of the remainder. This is followed by a series of case studies linked to specific chapters but again identifying how one system integrates with others in health and well-being; these illustrate how healthcare practitioners themselves act as agents of homeostatic control.

The section contents and specific chapter links are:

Case 1: Chapter 1, Introduction to physiology and homeostasis
Case 2: Chapter 2, Cell and tissue functions
Case 3: Chapter 3, The skeleton
Case 4: Chapter 4, Chemical reactions in cells: fundamentals of metabolism
Case 5: Chapter 5, Nutrients and nutrition
Case 6: Chapter 6, Body fluids
Case 7: Chapter 7, The senses

Case 8: Chapter 8, The nervous system
Case 9: Chapter 9, The endocrine system
Case 10: Chapter 10, The digestive system
Case 11: Chapter 11, The cardiovascular system 1: blood
Case 12: Chapter 12, The cardiovascular system 2: heart and circulation
Case 13: Chapter 13, The lymphatic system, immunity and microbiology
Case 14: Chapter 14, The respiratory system
Case 15: Chapter 15, The kidneys and urinary tract
Case 16: Chapter 16, The skin
Case 17: Chapter 17, Skeletal muscle: posture and movement
Case 18: Chapter 18, The reproductive systems
Case 19: Chapter 19, Genes in embryo development and ageing
Case 20: Chapter 20, Pain
Case 21: Chapter 21, Stress
Case 22: Chapter 22, Circadian rhythms

CASE 1. INTRODUCTION: HEALTHCARE PRACTITIONERS AS EXTERNAL AGENTS OF HOMEOSTATIC CONTROL

This case (representing Chapter 1) presents a schema by which healthcare practice can be accommodated within a homeostatic framework, based on the analogy of stages in practice with stages in a homeostatic process. Table 23.1 below summarizes this.

The role of healthcare practitioners in seeking to reverse a homeostatic imbalance essentially makes them external agents of homeostatic control – they are replacing the usual assessment, planning and effector aspects that operate intrinsically in health, but have failed in ill health. This is the focus of the rest of this chapter in which case studies are presented as:

- Scenario
- The condition as a homeostatic imbalance
- Background information
- Presentation
- Healthcare practitioners as external agents of homeostatic control

Table 23.1 Analogy between a homeostatic process and stages in delivery of healthcare practice*

Stages in a homeostatic process	Stages in healthcare practice
Homeostatic set point	Lifestyle, health education practices and well-being (nature–environment interactions).
Parameter change outside the homeostatic range/homeostatic disturbance	Clinical disorder/homeostatic imbalance
Detection of change/magnitude of change/direction/rate	Assessment and diagnosis
Control centre receptors: determination of corrective response	Care planning
Effector response: reversal of homeostatic disturbance/negative feedback	Implementation of care: reversal of homeostatic imbalance/negative feedback
Re-evaluation	Reassessment

*See Chapter 1 for more details and further discussion.

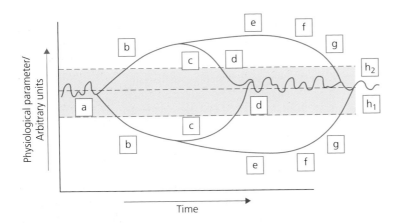

Figure 23.1 Graphical illustration of homeostatic regulation and the role of practitioners as external agents of homeostatic control. See Table 23.1 for comparisons.
a, Parameter within range determined by the homeostatic set point; reflects good health practices based on nature–nurture interactions. **b**, Parameter changing (homeostatic disturbance) owing to impact of lifestyle, etc., or simply random fluctuation. **c**, Initiation of corrective response. **d**, Effector response reversing the disturbance (i.e. negative feedback). **e**, Homeostatic disturbance sustained and increased owing to failure of corrective effector responses (= homeostatic imbalance or illness). **f**, diagnosis and implementation of intervention/care. **g**, Reversal of imbalance (i.e. negative feedback). h_1, h_2, Restoration of parameter to within homeostatic range either by normal homeostatic processes (**b–d**) or by intervention (**e–g**)

– Assessment
– Care planning
– Implementation
– Reassessment/follow-up
• References.

Throughout, the homeostatic graph that was introduced in Chapter 1 and applied at various points in the chapters is presented to illustrate some of the pertinent aspects of intervention in restoring homeostasis, or modulating the imbalance. As an introduction, Figure 23.1 presents the main points in Table 23.1 in this graphical format. In all the graphs in this chapter, box a represents boxes a_1–a_4 in Figure 1.7, p.11, reflecting the individual variability in the homeostatic range. Similarly, the blue areas represent the norm (homeostatic range) 95%.

CASE 2. THE CASE OF A WOMAN WITH BREAST CANCER

This chapter relates specifically to Chapter 2.

SCENARIO

Janet is a 44-year-old married woman who recently discovered a painless lump in her right breast. Her GP referred her to a breast care surgeon, who performed a needle biopsy and subsequently diagnosed an adenocarcinoma ('adeno-' = of glandular tissue, 'carcinoma' = cancerous tumour). Janet was subsequently admitted to hospital for an operation to remove the lump (a lumpectomy) and also for an excision of axillary lymph glands. She was then referred to an oncologist for further treatment, including radiotherapy and cytotoxic chemotherapy.

Breast cancer as a homeostatic imbalance

The main homeostatic imbalance in cancer is a failure of the regulation of cell division. Dividing cells must maintain a rate of tissue growth and replacement conducive to well-being. To this end, the rate of cell division is controlled genetically in response to local tissue conditions, including cell–cell secretions. The genes involved fall into two main categories: proto-oncogenes (which promote cell division) and tumour suppressor genes. It is the complex interactions between these genes and their products that establishes the cell cycle (see Chapter 2, pp.42–6). Cancer arises when the interactions are unbalanced to the extent that the rate of division becomes excessive, and hence the cell cycle is shortened, leading to focal growth (see Figure 2.17b,d,e, p.46). Mutations, some possibly inherited but most acquired, in critical genes are responsible for initiating and promoting the changes, while others produce further unusual characteristics, such as de-differentiation to a simpler form, ectopic production of hormones, independence from normal regulatory controls, 'escape' from the attention of immune cells, and metastasis.

Background

The most common types of breast cancer are infiltrating ductal adenocarcinoma (75%) and infiltrating lobular adenocarcinoma (5–10%). Breast cancer is the most common form of cancer that occurs in women. Currently, the UK has the highest mortality rate in Europe for this disease. The cause of breast cancer is unknown. However, genes (*BRCA1*, *BRCA2*) have recently been identified that are implicated in familial breast cancer. However, only a small percentage of breast cancers show this inherited component and, furthermore, not all women with the gene actually develop the disease. This is because cancer is a polygenic condition (at least 15 genes have been linked to breast cancer) and one or even two genes alone will not necessarily induce its formation (see Box 19.4, p.548).

Hormones, especially excess of oestrogens, play an important role in the development of breast cancer, although their exact role is as yet unclear. Some studies have linked long-term use of high-dose oral contraceptives with an increased incidence, while others suggest that breast-feeding and early age of first pregnancy offer some protection.

Presentation

Cells dividing at an accelerated rate eventually give rise to a palpable mass (tumour). Apart from invading local tissue areas, cancer cells are also capable of migrating (metastasizing) from their sites of origin to develop secondary tumours elsewhere (see Figure 2.17a,e, p.46). The most common sites of metastatic spread from breast cancer are bone and liver, diagnosed by bone and liver scans, respectively. These investigations are not performed routinely, but Janet may undergo them at a later date, or if problems arise. Bone metastases usually present with pain in the affected area. Liver metastases are often asymptomatic until late in the course of the disease, but may present with pain, liver enlargement (hepatomegaly) and/or jaundice.

Healthcare practitioners as external agents of homeostatic control

See Figure 23.2.

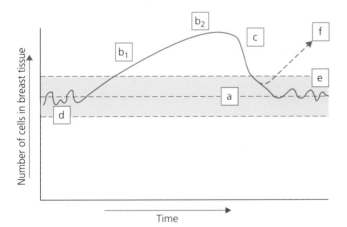

Figure 23.2 Practitioners as external agents of homeostasis in cancer treatment.
a, Cell numbers (breast) appropriate to tissue maintenance and function. **b₁**, Initiator/promoter gene changes remove the 'brakes' on cell division (namely, tumour suppressor gene activity) leading to excessive cell division, and other cell changes characteristic of cancer, and eventually detectable as a primary tumour (**b₂**). **c**, Tumour excision. **d**, Chemotherapy/radiotherapy to remove remnant cancer cells including those that have metastasized away from the breast. **e**, Remission: no evidence of abnormal cell division. **f**, Metastatic growth from cancer cells relocated to other tissues (secondary tumour)

Assessment and planning

Treatment is aimed at surgical removal of the primary tumour, eradication of any remaining abnormal cells that may lead to the development of metastases, and suppression of tumour growth from any remnant cells (see Figure 2.17c, p.46). Care will also involve considerable psychosocial support. The outcome of breast cancer treatment depends largely on the stage of the disease at diagnosis.

Implementation of care

Surgery

Although some tumours are encapsulated, they are not bounded firmly (unlike cysts or nodal tissue) and cells extend out into surrounding tissue. Surgery therefore removes adjoining tissue in an attempt to remove the whole tumour. Cells may also drain from the tumour into lymph, so lymph nodes in the area (i.e. axillary nodes in the case of breast cancer) may also be excised (see Figure 2.17a, p.46). The patient is then at risk of lymphoedema (Figure 2.17d).

Eradication of remaining cells using radiotherapy and chemotherapy

Radiotherapy is a local treatment aimed at destruction of any abnormal cells that may remain in the breast after excision of the tumour. Radiation restores intracellular homeostasis by causing the breakdown of genetic material, thus preventing the accelerated cell division of tumour cells. A number of normal cells in the treatment area will also be affected, but unlike damaged tumour cells, normal cells can repair/reproduce themselves.

Radiotherapy causes extreme fatigue and skin sensitivity; therefore the treatment is given in divided doses and careful observation of the treatment area is required. Although radiotherapy treatment is completely painless, it often produces anxiety. Patients may find the physical environment of the radiotherapy unit overwhelming, particularly the technical equipment. In addition, for the duration of the treatment, the patient has to remain very still on the treatment couch and is alone, although staff will always be visible behind protective lead screens (that do not permit passage of radiation). Ideally, the patient should visit the department before treatment is started to enable them to meet the staff and become familiar with the surroundings.

Chemotherapy is also aimed at the destruction of abnormal cells. Because it is a systemic treatment, given intravenously, side-effects are prevalent. Chemotherapeutic drugs have a variety of actions, but all in some way disrupt cellular growth, either by damaging DNA directly or by interfering with aspects of the cell cycle. Chemotherapy therefore targets normally dividing cells as well as malignant cells. Leucocytes are particularly at risk, so Janet's blood will be monitored at regular intervals for the duration of treatment to enable early diagnosis of leucocyte imbalances.

Chemotherapy is highly toxic and often induces nausea and vomiting. These side-effects can now be controlled effectively with anti-emetic drugs.

Suppression of further tumour growth: anti-hormonal therapy

Hormonal therapy manipulates the hormonal environment of breast tissue cells to suppress cell growth. Oestrogens are important factors in breast cell activity. The drug tamoxifen is an oestrogen antagonist: it binds to oestrogen receptors of cells, thereby inhibiting the growth-stimulating effects of oestrogen and impeding the growth of malignant cells. Not all breast tumours are oestrogen-receptor positive, however. Although early trials suggest that tamoxifen therapy is likely to be beneficial in terms of increased survival, the degree of efficacy and optimal treatment regimens remain unclear, particularly in relation to women who develop breast cancer before the menopause.

Support

Janet will require skilled nursing care to enable her to cope with the demands of her treatment. Patient support and education are an essential part of treatment. Not only will Janet be coming to terms with the diagnosis of a life-threatening disease, but she will also be recovering from surgery and facing several weeks of unpleasant treatment. Janet's family will also require support. Most hospitals now offer the services of specialist breast-care nurses, and there are also a number of charitable organizations and self-help groups that provide care and support for those with breast cancer. The British Association of Cancer United Patients (BACUP) for example, provides booklets and videos, and has a telephone help-line for patients and their relatives.

Case study contributed by Sue Parry and Linda Purdy.

Further reading

Smedira, H.J. (2000) Practical issues in counselling healthy women about their breast cancer risk and use of tamoxifen citrate. *Archives of Internal Medicine* **160**(20): 3034–42.

Zack, E. (2001) Mammography and reduced breast cancer mortality rates. *Medical Surgical Nursing* 10(1): 17–21.

CASE 3. THE CASE OF A WOMAN WITH RHEUMATOID ARTHRITIS

This case study links directly to Chapter 3.

SCENARIO

Mary is a 50-year-old married woman who works as a shop assistant. She visited her general practitioner complaining of extreme tiredness, together with painful, stiff, swollen hands and knees particularly first thing in the morning. She has become limited in her mobility and has difficulty carrying out her routine activities of daily living. Examination confirmed inflammation of the joints of both wrists, the metacarpophalangeal joints (i.e. the joints between the metacarpal bones of the hands and the phalanges of the fingers; see Figure 3.17, p.80), and the proximal interphalangeal joints (i.e. between the finger bones; see Figure 3.17). Joint effusion (excess synovial fluid) restricted Mary's shoulder and knee movements (see Figure 3.16, p.79, and 3.25, p.86).

Routine blood tests revealed that she was anaemic. Her haemoglobin was 9.8 g/dL (normal 12–16 g/dL), but the erythrocytes were of normal size and had normal haemoglobin content (i.e. the anaemia was apparently caused by too few cells rather than any defect of cell structure). Mary also had an elevated erythrocyte sedimentary rate (ESR) at 90 mm/hour (normal 5–15 mm/hour in women) indicative of an inflammatory condition, and a positive rheumatoid factor test. She was referred to the rheumatology department of her local hospital.

On questioning, Mary said she had lost 3 kg in weight, and complained of early-morning joint stiffness that lasted 4–6 hours. A diagnosis of rheumatoid arthritis was made.

Rheumatoid arthritis as a homeostatic imbalance

The cause of rheumatoid arthritis is unknown, but it is an autoimmune problem characterized by the production of autoantibodies to synovial tissue. The condition causes inflammation of the synovial membrane (see Figures 3.23, p.84 and 3.24, p.85) that lines movable joints and tendon sheaths. The inflammation causes pain, stiffness and swelling, which in the long term may result in joint damage and malformation, and hence decreased mobility. It is characterized by periods of remission and flares, and may produce tiredness, anaemia and weight loss. Extra-articular features include nodules of vesicular tissue over bony prominences and possible inflammation of the sclera (scleritis), arteries (arteritis), pericardium (pericarditis) and pleura (pleuritis).

Background

Rheumatoid arthritis is a symmetrical, chronic, debilitating, inflammatory arthritis for which there is no cure, and affects 1% of the UK population (Symmons *et al.,* 2002). The disorder is more common in women than in men (ratio 3:1). It is likely to be caused by a combination of genetic and environmental factors; individuals may have a predisposition to developing rheumatoid arthritis, but it is not inherited directly. As rheumatoid arthritis is much more common in young women than young men under the age of 40 years, this suggests a possible influence of the female sex hormones.

Presentation

Investigations of rheumatoid arthritis demonstrate a number of features:

- Skeletal changes evidenced by X-rays are used in the diagnosis of rheumatoid arthritis, and to monitor the severity and to assess the progression of the disease. Although changes are seen early in the disease, particularly in the hands and feet, approximately 60–70% of patient X-rays will be normal at that stage of the disease.
- Occurrence of anaemia: rheumatoid arthritis is associated with decreased production of erythrocytes. The anaemia results from a poor rate of production, rather than defective cells. Typically, the erythrocytes appear normal and have normal haemoglobin content. This type of anaemia frequently presents in chronic diseases.
- Presence of rheumatoid factor: this is an autoantibody (in fact, a number are involved), usually of the IgM or IgG types,

raised against self-antigens. The presence of rheumatoid factor is helpful to aid diagnosis, and its concentration (titre) appears to relate to the severity of the condition. A new test is for anti-cyclic citrullinated peptide (anti-CCP) autoantibodies, and this is associated with a higher specificity than rheumatoid factor, and has shown to be predictive of joint damage in RA. Kaltenhäuser *et al.* (2007) suggest that it is a better test than measuring rheumatoid factor, particularly early in the disease.

- Elevated erythrocyte sedimentation rate (ESR): a raised ESR is a non-specific measure of inflammation. The ESR is measured simply by allowing a column of blood to separate into cell and plasma components through the effects of gravity. As the cells sediment out, a column of plasma forms; the ESR is a measure of the rate of formation of this column (the higher the ESR, the faster the red cells sediment out; see Box 11.0, p.28). Mary's elevated ESR is typical of autoimmune and inflammatory conditions. What influences the ESR remains unclear but the faster rate of sedimentation in RA possibly relates to changes in plasma protein consistency, but also to the 'stacking' of red cells as rouleaux.
- C-reactive protein (CRP) is an acute-phase protein produced by the liver. It is a marker of inflammation and bacterial infection, and more accurate than an ESR, as this can take a long time to change.

The disease has psychosocial implications and, in particular, can have wide-ranging effects on the family and relationships between loved ones.

The outcome of the disease is variable from a mild self-limiting disease, to those who will continue to have flares with slowly progressing disease, to those with more severe multisystem disease.

Healthcare practitioners as external agents of homeostatic control

Assessment

- Tender joint
- Swollen joint
- Duration of early morning joint stiffness
- Functional measure
- Patient global assessment
- Physician global assessment
- Acute-phase response ESR/CRP
- Pain score on a visual analogue scale (VAS)
- Assessment of joint damage.

Care planning and implementation

See Figure 23.3.

Rheumatoid arthritis requires a multidisciplinary approach from healthcare practitioners. The aims of care are to suppress the inflammatory process, relieve pain and promote optimum function, and to reduce the psychological and social consequences of the condition. The British Society for Rheumatology (2006) guidelines recommend early diagnosis and treatment using disease-modifying anti-rheumatic drugs (DMARDs) or

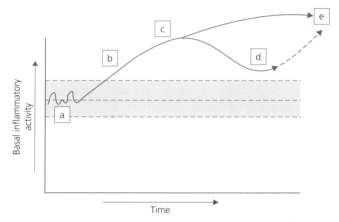

Figure 23.3 Rheumatoid arthritis expressed using the homeostatic graph.
a, Baseline inflammatory responses (note: these will be appropriate to non-rheumatoid occurrences such as infection). **b**, Increased baseline inflammatory activity, indicated by presence of autoantibodies in blood; some early symptoms of rheumatoid arthritis (e.g. joint inflammation). **c**, More active autoantibodies with elevated baseline inflammatory activity, but including other symptoms such as anaemia, raised erythrocyte sedimentation rate (ESR; see text). **d**, Modulation of baseline inflammatory activity by medication with anti-inflammatory drugs; joint function supported by physiotherapy. **e**, Unmodulated inflammatory activity or progression and resistance to anti-inflammatory interventions

biological agents. Patient education is an important aspect of chronic disease management and is usually carried out by specialist nurses. Mary will have to be followed up regularly and many different approaches can be used, from shared care with primary care, to nurse-led follow-up or a combination. Some units encourage patients to contact them when required in between yearly visits.

Promoting optimal function

Mary would have both knees aspirated and injected with a long-acting corticosteroid to counteract the inflammation. Intra-articular steroid injections are very effective for flares, and when only one or two joints are troublesome. They can significantly reduce pain and swelling in a joint for several months.

In line with the British Society for Rheumatology (2006) guidelines, methotrexate, the most commonly used DMARD, will be prescribed 7.5 mg orally once weekly. These drugs are used with the aim of suppressing the inflammatory process, thereby inducing and maintaining remission. They are potentially toxic, so patient needs to be monitored carefully. Regular blood and urine tests, together with direct questioning of the patient, are normally carried out to detect possible side-effects.

Non-steroidal anti-inflammatory drugs (NSAIDs) such as ibuprofen are often prescribed in addition to DMARDs and biological agents as these help relieve the pain, stiffness and inflammation, but they have no effect on the disease progression.

Physiotherapy and occupational therapy are of particular relevance. The physiotherapist aims to maintain physical function and to teach the patient how to exercise their joints. Treatments such as heat, cold and hydrotherapy are administered in the physiotherapy department. The occupational therapist assesses the activities of daily living and teaches joint protection and energy conservation. Aids and appliances can be provided to make carrying out the activities of daily living easier.

Orthotics and prosthetic departments and orthopaedic surgeons may also become involved to enable the patient to remain as independent as possible.

Patient education

- Regarding the disease and its treatments.
- Regular blood test monitoring for methotrexate.

Psychosocial care

Social workers may be involved in community care of people with rheumatoid arthritis, but nurses have a particular role here, both to provide psychosocial support and as a resource in relation to the aspects highlighted above. The role of the nurse is to:

- assess the patient, identify their needs and coordinate their care;
- provide education regarding the disease, and give patients and their family the opportunity to discuss issues with the nurse;
- monitor some of the disease-modifying drugs, and provide access to specialist knowledge and advice through a telephone help-line;
- perform a disease activity score;
- act as a liaison between the community, hospital and patient.

Case study contributed by Janice Mooney.

Further reading

Kaltenhäuser, S.M., Pierer, S., Arnold, M., *et al.* (2007) Antibodies against cyclic citrullinated peptide are associated with the DRB1 shared epitope and predict joint erosion in rheumatoid arthritis. *Rheumatology* **46**: 100–4.

Ramsburg, K.L. (2000) Rheumatoid arthritis. *American Journal of Nursing* **100**(11): 40–3.

Symmons D., Turner G., Webb R. *et al.* (2002) The prevalence of rheumatoid arthritis in the United Kingdom: new estimates for a new century. *Rheumatology* **41**: 793–800.

CASE 4. THE CASE OF A CHILD WITH INSULIN-DEPENDENT DIABETES – TYPE 1

This case study relates specifically to Chapter 4.

SCENARIO

Sara was 8 years old and had recently started drinking large amounts of water, and lots of her favourite squash. She loved karate and was training for her brown belt but had missed two sessions as she said she was 'too tired'. This was so unlike her that her mother was very worried. She discussed it with Sara's grandmother, and was told that similar symp-toms led to the diagnosis of diabetes mellitus in Sara's aunt when she was a very young girl.

The next morning Sara and her mum visited their general practitioner. He listened closely to the story and tested the urine that they had taken with them. The urine contained glucose and ketones. He then tested Sara's blood, by pricking her finger and using a test strip in a glucometer. This revealed a blood glucose level of 11 mmol/L. As this is higher than normal he made an appointment at the diabetes unit at the local hospital.

At the hospital the diabetic nurse practitioner took venous blood to check Sara's blood urea and electrolytes, and a capillary blood gas assessment to ensure Sara was not in diabetic ketoacidosis (DKA); if she had been then she would have been admitted to the children's ward to correct the acidosis. However, as she was not, she was given her first dose of insulin and the nurse arranged to see Sara and her mother at home later that afternoon.

At this meeting the nurse began to educate Sara and her parents about diabetes. Using a flip book of the body she showed them the location of the pancreas and explained that normally the hormone 'insulin' is released by the pancreas to reduce the levels of glucose in the blood. But in Sara's case, not enough insulin was being produced, so insulin would have to be given by injection to supplement the body's supply. This would have to be given before mealtimes so that the insulin was available to help the body process the glucose.

Diabetes as a homeostatic imbalance

In health, fasting blood glucose has a homeostatic range of 3.5–5.5 mmol/L but naturally rises after absorption of a carbohydrate-rich meal. In Sara's case her blood was measured some time after a meal and would be considered higher than it should have been. Insulin is normally secreted from the beta-cells of the islets of Langerhans in the pancreas and utilization of glucose is increased. However, in people who have insulin-dependent diabetes mellitus, now known as Type 1 diabetes, there is little or no production of insulin by the body hence the elevated blood glucose concentration. The excessive presence of glucose in glomerular filtrate interferes with osmosis, and hence water reabsorption, by the kidneys. This is why diabetes (Greek, 'siphon') is characterized by high urine production, and dehydration and thirst.

If the insulin deficiency is profound and continues, the body converts fats and proteins to yield energy (see Figure 4.9, p.101). However the conversion produces ketone bodies and it is these that may induce ketoacidosis.

Background

About 0.25% of all children develop Type 1 diabetes before the age of 15 years. It is more common in developed countries (Hanas, 2007). As noted, Type 1 diabetes is characterized by lack of secretion of insulin. In Sara's case there is suggestion of a familial link.

About 2% of the total UK population have diabetes but the majority have non-insulin-dependent diabetes (Type 2). This form of the disorder is usually found in adulthood and is thought to be an acquired disorder. There is a spectrum of aetiology, ranging from people who are unable to release insulin (not the same as in Type 1 diabetes, in which the production of insulin is deficient) to those who do secrete the hormone but whose target tissues are resistant to its effects. Obesity is a risk factor especially in the latter, but is not the sole cause for Type 2 diabetes.

The symptoms and consequences are much the same as for Type 1 diabetes, so there is a need to control hyperglycaemia. The means of control will include dietary considerations, just as in Sara's condition, but drug intervention is also possible. Tolbutamide might be used to stimulate the pancreas cells to release insulin, or a metabolic drug such as metformin may be used to promote glucose uptake and its utilisation by the tissues. Unfortunately these measures do not replace insulin, so are not appropriate in Sara's case.

Presentation

The main symptoms of insulin-dependent diabetes are:

- hyperglycaemia;
- hyposecretion of insulin;
- glycosuria, as blood glucose rises above the concentration of the renal threshold for glucose appearing in the urine;
- urinary tract infection, arising from the presence of glucose in the urine;
- increased urine production because of the osmotic effects of the glucose in the forming urine;
- thirst and excessive drinking because of the dehydrating effects of the excessive urine production;
- behavioural changes, if the blood glucose reverts rapidly to hypoglycaemia;
- weight loss because of protein metabolism.

There is therefore a need to control the hyperglycaemia, partly because doing so will reverse the other symptoms and partly because persistent hyperglycaemia has long-term consequences for nerve cells and small blood vessels (uncontrolled diabetes raises the risk of peripheral neuropathy and problems arising from poor circulation). Symptoms can include blindness, renal failure, skin ulcers and peripheral necrosis. There is also an elevated risk of intravascular thrombosis events such as coronary heart disease because of the effects of hyperglycaemia and atheroma arising from the release of fatty acids. These long-term changes are irreversible.

In contrast, the brain relies almost exclusively on glucose for energy and so requires a regular supply to maintain its functions. This means that hypoglycaemia must also be avoided during treatment otherwise behavioural disturbances will arise, possibly even coma.

Healthcare practitioners as external agents of homeostatic control

Care planning and implementation

See Figure 23.4.

The presentation of diabetes stems from the hyperglycaemia that arises from lack of insulin secretion after a meal. Restoring blood glucose control will reverse the symptoms if they have not become advanced, for example blindness. Children with diabetes therefore are not 'ill' in the conventional sense and are not neces-

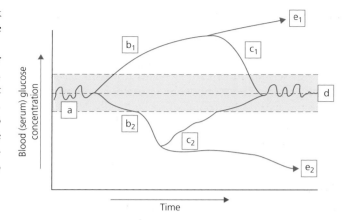

Figure 23.4 Diabetes Type 1 expressed using the homeostatic graph.
a, Normal serum glucose concentration within a child with diabetes as a result of good extrinsic control. **b₁**, Hyperglycaemia caused by excessive intake of carbohydrate. **b₂**, Hypoglycaemia caused by poor carbohydrate intake or increased utilization (e.g. exercise). **c₁**, Effect of administered insulin to restore normal serum glucose concentration. **c₂**, Ingestion of biscuits or dextrosol to increase serum glucose concentration. **d**, Normal serum glucose concentration restored by extrinsic control. **e₁**, Persistent hyperglycaemia resulting from poor control leading to long-term complications. **e₂**, Persistent reduced hypoglycaemia, leading to behavioural disorder or coma

sarily admitted to hospital with suspected diabetes. The aim of care therefore is to replace the missing hormone, but at the same time prevent large fluctuations in blood glucose concentration.

This means injection of insulin at appropriate times, sufficient to prevent hyperglycaemia but not to induce hypoglycaemia. Insulin is given by injection because orally it is broken down. Current paediatric regimes use intermediate-acting insulin such as NovoMix 30, 0.5 units/kg per day in three divided doses before breakfast, lunch and evening tea. This is referred to as a basal bolus regime. The aim is to link insulin more closely to food intake and exercise (Lissauer and Clayden, 2004). A long-acting insulin such as Lantus is administered at night. Insulin injections should be subcutaneous and into a skin fold, but the sites have to be rotated to prevent the formation of lipohypertrophy (fatty lumps), which will delay the absorption of insulin.

Sara and her family will require support in the necessary changes to Sara's lifestyle; the aim is to maintain a 'normal' life style for the child and family. The three main aims for care are:

1 Stabilization of blood glucose concentration, in the range of 4–7 mmol/L, to ensure adequate glucose is available for respiration.
  i This includes the safe administration of insulin.
  ii Monitoring of blood sugar levels.
  iiii Recognizing the signs of hypoglycaemia.
2 For Sara and her parents to be in control of her diabetic condition.
3 For Sara to lead a normal life.
4 To minimize complications of treatment.

The management of diabetes is a balancing act, between meeting energy requirements with a healthy diet and providing enough exogenous insulin so that the body cells can use the glucose provided by the diet.

To assess how Sara is controlling her glucose levels, she and her parents will be taught how to use the glucometer, with the aim of adjusting insulin requirements to match her levels of blood glucose. This is important as insulin acts 'as the key to open the door' for glucose to enter body cells. Normally this blood test will be done about 30 minutes prior to eating one of the three main meals; then the insulin will be given about 10 minutes before eating. It is important that Sara does eat her meal after her injection otherwise the insulin will cause hypoglycaemia. Exercise also reduces blood glucose levels since muscle cells use it to provide energy for activities such as Sara's karate.

Sara and her parents will also receive information from a paediatric dietician regarding her diet, so that the likelihood of episodes of severe hyper/hypoglycaemia can be avoided. A 'diabetic diet' is a normal healthy diet and special foods are not required. However, but a few simple rules have to be followed:

- eat at regular intervals;
- ensure that meals consist of some slowly digested carbohydrate, such as starch in bread and cereals, which maintain glucose levels within the homeostatic range for longer. Short-acting carbohydrates, such as sucrose in sweets, cause a short burst of glucose, and so should be restricted (but not banned!);
- eat extra carbohydrate before taking part in any strenuous exercise.

Another test done regularly (usually 3-monthly) is the measurement of a form of haemoglobin that has glucose attached to it (HbA_1c). This gives an average measurement of the glucose levels over the span of the life of the red blood cell (approximately 120 days) and so indicates how well the diabetes has been controlled.

Sara's diabetic nurse will explain that if Sara needs more glucose, her body will let her know (because of the signs of developing hypoglycaemia). The signs may include feeling dizzy, having trembling or tingling hands or blurred vision; any of these can indicate that hypoglycaemia is developing. It is useful to have a source of glucose available, as hypoglycaemia can develop quickly. Dextrosol tablets maybe kept at hand but sugar lumps or a sweet drink will also work. These foods raise blood glucose quickly and soon reverse the symptoms of hypoglycaemia. Sara's nurse explains that once Sara feels better she should be given something containing long-acting carbohydrate, such as a biscuit or sandwich to stabilize her blood glucose concentration.

Sara's parents will need to be fully informed regarding the condition and on how to use the various equipment, and supported in their new role as parents of a child with a potentially life-threatening condition. To facilitate this appointments are made at the paediatric clinic to meet the diabetic team of consultant, dietitian, specialist nurse, play specialist and often child psychologist. Introductions are arranged to parents of children with diabetes who have offered to support other parents such as Sara's and the excellent charity group Diabetes UK. By knowing about diabetes and who is available to support them, Sara and her parents can gradually regain control of their lives.

For Sara this will include continuing her karate, education, family holidays and special occasions, but also as she moves into her teens the ability to go out with her friends. Eventually, she may want a career, marriage and her own family. These are all possible when she understands, how she can work with her body to maintain control of her diabetes.

Case study contributed by Elaine Domek.

References

Hanas, R. (2007) *Type 1 Diabetes in Children, Adolescents and Young Adults.* 3rd edn. London: Class Publishing.

Lissauer, T., Clayden, G. (2004) *Illustrated Textbook of Paediatrics,* 2nd edn. London: Mosby.

CASE 5. THE CASE OF A BOY WHO IS OBESE

This case study relates specifically to Chapter 5.

> ### SCENARIO
>
> Leo is a 16-year-old boy who has been experiencing recurrent headaches, knee pain and constipation. He has been diagnosed by his general practitioner as being obese, although his mother claims he eats very little. Both his parents and his two siblings are also overweight.
>
> Leo has low self-esteem, spends long periods playing computer games in his bedroom and is socially isolated. He has few friends and is bullied at school.
>
> Nine months later, Leo is reassessed, and his body mass index has risen to within the 98th centile, which warrants further investigations. These tests reveal he has hypertension, elevated serum lipoproteins, elevated insulin and blood glucose levels.

Obesity as a homeostatic imbalance

Overweight and obesity are defined as a high weight-for-height ratio. The body mass index (BMI) is a simple index of weight-for-height that is commonly used in classifying overweight and obesity in adult populations and individuals. It is defined as the weight in kilograms divided by the square of the height in metres (kg/m^2). The World Health Organization (WHO, 2008) defines adults who are 'overweight' as having a BMI equal to or more than 25 kg/m^2, and 'obesity' as a BMI equal to or more than 30 kg/m^2. Obesity can be further classified (Figure 23.5). In children, changes in weight may be confounded by linear growth and puberty related changes in body composition that differ between boys and girls. Therefore, BMI relative to age and sex, in the form of percentiles or standardized z scores, is used to define overweight and obesity in children.

Over time, with no change in behaviour, Leo could progress through each of the BMI categories, at increasing risk to his health and well-being. At any point, adjustments in lifestyle could halt the progression and ideally lower his BMI (Figure 23.5,e).

Overweight and obesity are associated with serious health consequences, especially when combined with poor aerobic fitness (Lee *et al.*, 1999). Raised BMI is a major risk factor for chronic diseases such as cardiovascular disease (mainly heart disease and stroke), diabetes, musculoskeletal disorders (especially back pain and osteoarthritis) and some cancers (e.g. endometrial, breast and colon). The most common sequelae of childhood obesity are hypertension, dyslipidaemia and psychosocial problems (e.g. poor self image, social isolation, suicidal tendencies, eating disorders, drug and alcohol addiction) (Kopelman *et al.*, 2005) Increasing BMI is also associated with an increased risk of mortality (Calle *et al.*, 1999).

Background

Globally, the WHO latest projections (2005) indicated that approximately 1.6 billion adults (age 15+ years) were overweight and at least 400 million adults were obese. In the UK, the prevalence of obesity has increased steadily over recent years. Currently, over 60% of the adult population are overweight. Of these 26.3% of men and 27.9% of women are obese (HSE, 2006).

Obesity is a complex and multifactorial disease. At a simple level, weight is only gained when net energy intake exceeds net energy expenditure over a prolonged period of time (i.e. when the individual is in a state of positive energy balance). However, it is not always possible to find a single explanation as to why this occurs in some individuals and not in others.

Obesity tends to run in families. Children with two obese parents have about a 70% risk of becoming obese compared with less than 20% in children with two lean parents (Association for the Study of Obesity). Perhaps this could be explained by environmental factors since families usually share the same diet, lifestyle and cultural influences. However, studies of adopted children have revealed weight patterns similar to those of their natural rather than their adopted parents (Stunkard *et al.*, 1990). This suggests that obesity does have some genetic basis or is influenced by the intrauterine environment. The degree to which obesity is genetically determined is still under discussion. Detailed studies of genetic transmission, including studies of monozygotic and dizygotic twins, have placed the influence of genetic factors from as low as 5% to more than 50%.

Genes can only exert their effect by increasing energy intake or decreasing energy expenditure, for example through a genetically determined preference for high fat foods or a sedentary lifestyle. The regulation of food intake involves a complex interaction of systems that determine the size, content and frequency of feedings. Presumably, the brain is the final processing centre that translates central and peripheral signals to initiate or stop eating. Neuronal circuits have been identified in the hypothalamus that affect satiation (level of fullness during a meal which regulates the amount of food consumed) and satiety (level of hunger after a meal is consumed which regu-

lates the frequency of eating). Regulatory mechanisms also must be present that integrate determinants of short-term energy intake with long-term energy requirements.

The discovery of leptin, the protein product of the *ob/ob* gene (Zhang *et al.*, 1994) led to a marked increase in understanding the regulation of food intake. Leptin is produced by adipose cells, released into the circulation, and it crosses the blood–brain barrier to bind to its receptor in the hypothalamus, which stimulates the expression of neuropeptides and neurotransmitters that inhibit food intake. Therefore, leptin provides a unique feedback signalling system that transmits information regarding adipose tissue energy stores to the central nervous system. Mutation of the *ob* gene results in profound obesity and type II diabetes.

The rapid increase in the prevalence of obesity over the last 50 years (a very short period of evolution) suggests that obesity is also strongly related to lifestyle rather than genetic factors, although the relationship between lifestyle risk and genetics remains debatable. Global increases in overweight and obesity are attributable to a number of environmental influences including a shift in diet (towards increased intake of readily available energy-dense foods that are high in fat and sugars but low in vitamins, minerals and other micronutrients) and a trend towards decreased physical activity (owing to the increasingly sedentary nature of many forms of work and leisure, changing modes of transportation, and increasing urbanization).

Healthcare practitioners as external agents of homeostatic control

See Figure 23.5.

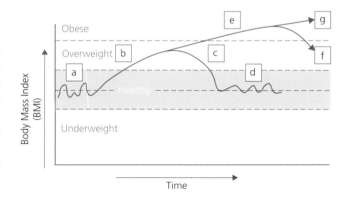

Figure 23.5 Obesity expressed using the homeostatic graph.
a, Weight within the healthy range for age. Body mass index (BMI) is 18–24.9. Energy in = energy expenditure. **b**, 'Overweight' range of BMI (25–29.9). Energy in > energy expenditure. **c**, Effective weight loss programme with return of weight to within healthy range of BMI (**d**). **e**, Sustained weight increase to within the 'obese' range of BMI (class I, 30–34.9; class II. 35–39.9; class III > 40). Increased risk of appearance of comorbid symptoms. In Leo's case, failure to comply with the weight-management programme leads to more weight gain within the 'obese' range of BMI. **f**, An intensive weight-management programme reducing BMI. Comorbidity symptoms may reduce but some may continue as they are irreversible (e.g. diabetes). **g**, Sustained weight within the 'obese' range will further increase the risk of development of comorbid symptoms, with increased risk of death

Assessment

The initial aim of care should focus on assessing lifestyle factors that may influence weight gain. Leo is presenting with a combination of symptoms, which may be exacerbated by his excess weight. However it is excess fat that predisposes an individual to the health risks. The BMI alone cannot distinguish whether a high BMI is the result of high adiposity or elevated levels of lean/muscle tissue (which would occur with sporting activities such as weights/resistance training). Thus it is important to find out how much exercise Leo is doing.

Assess his:

- Height, weight.
- BMI (relate to UK 1990 BMI charts).

Consider intervention (if BMI at 91st centile or above) or further assessment (if BMI at 98th centile or above).

Discuss with him and his parents:

- Energy intake: eating habits (describe a typical meal, portion sizes), types of food and drinks consumed (e.g. how many portions of fruit/vegetables, how many sweetened drinks), pattern of eating (e.g. snacking habits, frequency of eating).
- Energy expenditure: activity habits (how much time spent walking, playing sport, doing exercise, sitting).
- Any worries/concerns, health problems.
- Willingness to modify and/or change energy intake or expenditure.

On initial assessment, Leo's BMI falls within the 91st centile, and according to the assessment it appears that his body is composed of high levels of fat tissue. Leo's lifestyle is cause for concern. His diet consists of mainly fatty fast food (eaten at lunchtime and on the way home from school), crisps, biscuits and fizzy drinks. He never eats any fruit or vegetables and the family does not sit down together for meals at home. He avoids any sport or exercise and admits that the only games he plays are on his computer in his bedroom.

Implementation of care

Following discussion with Leo and his mother, it has been determined that the cause of Leo's obesity is his reliance on high-fat, highly processed foods and consuming more calories than he is burning off. He is therefore in positive energy balance.

With the support of his parents and encouragement from his GP, Leo agrees to change his lifestyle. He promises to exercise on a regular basis instead of spending all his free time in front of the TV and computer. He is also willing to eat more healthily and monitor his caloric intake. He is conscious of the potential health and social benefits and seems determined to succeed in changing his lifestyle.

It is vital to involve the parents from the outset, to build healthy eating and physical activity into daily family routines. During their early years, children's learning about food and eating plays a central role in shaping subsequent food choices, diet quality and weight status. Parents play a powerful role in influencing children's eating habits by purchasing, serving and eating healthy foods and drinks themselves. It is important to teach children how to choose foods that provide all the necessary components for their growth and health. Parents may need guidance on how to make permanent changes in eating habits and avoid over-reliance on the inexpensive, palatable, energy-dense foods that can easily promote overeating and weight gain (Savage et al., 2007).

Untreated, obesity can continue throughout adulthood and increase the risk of chronic health problems.

Evaluation of care

Follow-up evaluations should be offered regularly. Obesity is one of the most difficult and discouraging problems to treat, and long-term success rates remain low. Interventions should be long-term and delivered by appropriately trained personnel. These should be underpinned by relevant information about health risks, goal setting, realistic targets and treatment options. Additional support, advice and guidance can be sought from local/community support groups, voluntary organizations and sports centres. School is an appropriate place for specialized nutritional and exercise programmes, but few such programmes exist.

Reassessment

At Leo's reassessment, no improvements have been made and his BMI has increased. He admits it was really hard to change his behaviour as his parents and siblings were still eating the same foods as before. He was embarrassed going out to do exercise and felt people were laughing at him when he got out of breath. He became really unhappy and ate chocolate to cheer himself up.

As Leo has now moved into the 98th centile for BMI, referral to a specialist multidisciplinary team in secondary care is now advisable. In addition to continued support to modify lifestyle behaviours, this may involve screening for genetic causes of obesity (these are rare, but may be treatable), drug treatment (only if there are physical comorbidities) and, if all other measures fail, bariatric surgery to reduce stomach size. Surgical approaches are reserved for the severely obese.

Case study contributed by Penny Goacher.

References

Association for the Study of Obesity [On-line] http://www.aso.org.uk/portal.aspx (accessed 16/04/2008).

Calle, E.E., Thun, M.J. and Petrelli, J.M. (1999) Body-mass index and mortality in a prospective cohort of US adults. *New England Journal of Medicine* **341**: 1097–105.

Health Survey for England (2006) Latest trends. [On-line] http://www.ic.nhs.uk/webfiles/publications/HSE06/Health%20Survey%20for%20England%202006%20Latest%20Trends.pdf (accessed 16/11/2008).

Kopelman, P.G., Caterson, I.D. and Dietz, W.H. (eds) (2005) *Clinical Obesity in Adults and Children*, 2nd edn. Malden: Blackwell Science.

Lee, C.D., Blair, S.N. and Jackson, A.S. (1999) Cardiorespiratory fitness, body composition, and all-cause and cardiovascular disease mortality in men. *American Journal of Clinical Nutrition* **69**: 373–80.

Savage, J.S., Fisher, J.O. and Birch, L.L. (2007) Parental influence on eating behavior: conception to adolescence. *Journal of Law, Medicine and Ethics* **35**(1): 22–34.

Stunkard, A.J., Harris, J.R., Pedersen, N.L. and McClearn, G.E. (1990) The body-mass index of twins who have been reared apart. *New England Journal of Medicine* **322**(21): 1483–7.

World Health Organisation Global database on body mass index [On-line] http://www.who.int/bmi/index.jsp?introPage=intro_3.html (accessed 16/11/2008).

Zhang Y., Proenca R., Maffei M. *et al.* (1994) Positional cloning of the mouse obese gene and its human homologue *Nature* **372**: 425–32.

Further reading

National Institute of Health and Clinical Excellence. Obesity: the prevention, identification, assessment and management of overweight and obesity in adults and children. [On-line] http://www.nice.org.uk/CG043 (accessed 16/11/2008).

CASE 6. THE CASE OF A 25-YEAR-OLD MAN UNDERGOING EMERGENCY SURGERY

This case links specifically to Chapter 6.

SCENARIO

David Smith is a 25-year-old man brought to the operating theatre after being admitted to the Accident and Emergency Department suffering from extreme blood loss following a stabbing incident. After the initial airway, breathing, circulation (ABC) assessment an intravenous access was secured; he was anaesthetized, his airway intubated and he was placed on a ventilator. A decision was made that David needed urgent surgical intervention to prevent further blood loss. The theatre coordinator was informed and the anaesthetist telephoned the operating department practitioners (ODPs) to alert them to the patient's status and the equipment to be prepared.

Aware that this was a patient suffering massive blood loss and in a compromised state the ODPs prepared an arterial line (an invasive line to monitor blood pressure and to give arterial access for blood gas analysis), central venous pressure monitoring (CVP, to monitor circulating volume and to administer fluids and drugs), a rapid fluid infuser (warms fluids and administers them under pressure), the anaesthetic machine, the operating table and drug infusion pumps.

On arrival the ODP noted that David felt cold and he was very pale. He had an open wound on the lower left of his abdomen through which the bowel was protruding. He had intravenous access in the dorsum of both hands through which Gelofusine (a colloid) was being administered. His electrocardiogram (ECG) monitoring showed an arrhythmia indicative of hyperkalaemia (see Box 12.6, p.319). An arterial blood sample was taken for blood gas analysis.

Hypovolaemia as a homeostatic imbalance

Blood volume in a young adult man is normally around 5–6 L. Small changes can be compensated for as fluid may shift from the tissue fluids into the blood volume. Blood is a composite of plasma and blood cells, and plasma is a component of the extracellular fluid volume. As such it is continuous with the tissue fluids and has similar composition (see pp. 121–2). The cardiovascular system also compensates for any homeostatic disturbances by adjusting cardiac output (through heart rate and stroke volume changes), and by constriction of peripheral blood vessels and so increasing vascular resistance. These two responses help to maintain arterial blood pressure (see Figure 12.26, p.345).

In David's case the loss of blood has been sufficient to produce a significant reduction in blood volume (hypovolaemia) to the extent that these regulatory responses are being overwhelmed.

Background

Shock is a severely compromised circulation of blood (see Figure 12.32, p.355). It has various causes (see Box 12.28, p.354) but in David's case clearly is the result of excessive blood loss from the stab wound. Characteristically, shock presents with a large decrease in blood pressure as a consequence of inadequate circulating blood volume. It is a life-threatening condition because tissues become hypoxic leading to irreversible damage. Thus, if treatment is delayed, David may appear to respond to interventions but if the treatment was too delayed than his circulatory system will gradually decline in function and his blood pressure will fall dangerously (fatally) low. In David's case the hypovolaemia is treated as an emergency, partly because bleeding is continuing and must be arrested, and partly because intervention to restore his circulation must begin as soon as possible.

Presentation and assessment

The following summarizes David's vital signs and blood analyses:

Pulse 120 bpm	(homeostatic range 60–70)
Blood pressure 40/25 mmHg	(homeostatic range 120/80)
Temperature 32.9°C	(homeostatic range 36.9–37.2)
Arterial blood pH 6.96	(homeostatic range 7.35–7.45)
$PaCO_2$ 5.55 kPa	(homeostatic range 4.60–6.40)
PaO_2 41.4 kPa	(homeostatic range 10.6–14.6)
HCO_3 8.9 mmol/L	(homeostatic range 22.0–30.0)
Base excess −22.3 mmol/L	(homeostatic range −2 to +2)
Hb 7.7 g/dL	(homeostatic range 13–18; male)
Na^+ 142 mmol/L	(homeostatic range 134–145)
K^+ 6.1 mmol/L	(homeostatic range 3.6–5.0)
Glucose 11.5 mmol/L	(homeostatic range 3.5–7.0)

David's presentation is typical of a patient who has suffered a large circulating volume loss.

- The tachycardia (fast heart rate) and hypotension (low blood pressure) are indicative of 'adaptive homoeostatic reflexes associated with a low circulating blood volume caused by haemorrhage' (see Figure 12.29a, p.349).
- The fall in blood pressure will set off a sympathetic response; compensatory mechanisms are activated that will increase the rate and force of the heart's contractions in order to maintain an adequate cardiac output. Vasoconstriction also occurs increasing peripheral resistance and therefore venous return. This is why David appears pale and cold (Clancy and McVicar, 1996, 1997).
- Hypothermia is common in trauma patients due to environmental conditions at the scene, inadequate protection, and intravenous fluid administration and on-going blood loss. Hypovolaemic shock leads to decreased cellular perfusion and oxygenation and therefore inadequate heat production (see Figure 2.11, p.36).
- Metabolic acidosis. This can be diagnosed from the blood gas analysis results. pH is a measurement of hydrogen ion concentration. David's pH of 6.96 is indicative of an acidosis (clinical acidosis of the blood is pH < 7.35).
- The PCO_2 is within normal range; therefore the acidosis is not caused by the respiratory component. It is probably caused by excessive production of organic acids (e.g. pyruvic acid and lactic acid) as a result of anaerobic metabolism arising because of his tissue hypoxia. In contrast, the PO_2 is very high as David is being hyperventilated to improve the oxygen perfusion of his tissues and to reduce the acidosis through the respiratory system.
- The bicarbonate ion concentration is low, indicating a metabolic component to the acidosis. The bicarbonate is low because the ions are buffering the excess hydrogen ions (see equation 5, p.130). The base excess also indicates a metabolic acidosis. The base excess is defined as 'the amount of acid (in mmol) required to restore 1 litre of blood to its normal pH, at a normal PCO_2 of 5.3 kPa'. During the calculation any change in pH caused by PCO_2 of the sample is eliminated, therefore it reflects only the metabolic component of any disturbance. The base excess of −22.3 mmol/L indicates that a large amount of bicarbonate has been utilized in the buffering process and will have to be replaced to restore homeostasis.
- The haemoglobin concentration is low because of the loss of blood cells in the haemorrhage, and dilution of remaining blood by tissue fluid moving into the blood volume.
- The potassium (K^+) is high because in an acidosis, potassium excretion is decreased and there is an exchange of intracellular potassium for extracellular hydrogen ions as part of the compensatory response to maintain arterial pH. The potassium is displaced into the blood. The hyperkalaemia may produce cardiac arrhythmias (tall, peaked T-waves) and potentially to cardiac arrest.
- The glucose is raised because of the body's stress response to trauma and surgery. Glucose is mobilised and insulin secretion is inhibited (see Figures 22.6, p.598 and 22.8, p.603).

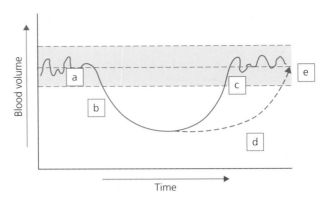

Figure 23.6 Traumatic hypovolaemia and surgical intervention illustrated using the homeostatic graph. **a**, Blood volume, and metabolic parameters associated with good circulation volume (acid–base factors, serum potassium, haemoglobin concentration within homeostatic range for health). **b**, Decreased blood volume as consequence of trauma (in David's case, a stab wound). **c**, Restoration of blood volume by emergency transfusion of colloid and blood cells. However, efficient circulation of blood may remain compromised. **d**, Intervention to restore other symptoms of hypovolaemia (e.g. support for acid–base parameters, serum potassium) while circulating blood volume improves. **e**, Restoration of blood volume, circulating blood volume, and associated metabolic factors to within their homeostatic ranges

Healthcare practitioners as external agents of homeostatic control

Assessment

This is based on the above presentation and a diagnosis of hypovolaemia is made. David's symptoms exist because of a major haemorrhage leading to loss of circulating volume and tissue hypoxia. The aims of care are therefore to prevent further blood loss, repair the cause of the blood loss, restore the circulating volume and correct the acid–base and electrolyte imbalances. David is under a general anaesthetic maintained with a volatile agent (isoflurane), a muscle relaxant and analgesia.

Care planning and implementation

See Figure 23.6.

- *Prevent further blood loss*: immediate surgical intervention. Surgical exploration reveals a wound in the aorta. A surgical clamp is placed on the aorta above the wound in order to prevent further blood loss and to allow a repair to be undertaken. There may also be damage to the spleen leading to blood loss and a splenectomy would be performed if this is the case.
- *Restore circulating volume*: this is achieved through the administration of colloids which are plasma volume expanders (see Chapter 6, p.134) David has suffered major blood loss and his haemoglobin is low, thus affecting oxygen carriage to the tissues (see Figure 14.12. p.416). Red blood cells are transfused to raise the haemoglobin levels and thus oxygen carriage 29 units.
- *Restore acid–base balance*: the treatment of a metabolic acidosis is to treat the cause. In severe cases such as David's the restoration of acid–base homeostasis may be achieved

through the use of an alkali such as sodium bicarbonate. Bicarbonate can generate CO_2 that may enhance the acidosis if there is insufficient respiratory compensation and the extra sodium load can also have metabolic effects. In this case sodium bicarbonate is given, as there is control of David's ventilation.

- *Restore electrolyte balance*: the priority is to correct the elevated potassium levels. David is administered calcium gluconate; this stabilizes cardiac membranes by reversing repolarization abnormalities. At the same time an infusion of insulin and glucose is administered which will transiently move potassium back into the intracellular compartment.
- *Restore normal blood glucose levels*: This is not a priority, but may be facilitated by the insulin/ dextrose infusion (see Chapter 6, p.135).
- *Restore 'physiological' parameters*: raise blood pressure – upon arrival David's blood pressure is dangerously low compromising blood supply to his brain and other major organs. An infusion of noradrenaline (a sympathetic agonist) is administered. Noradrenaline is a catecholamine that increases systemic vascular resistance. The increase in peripheral vascular resistance leads to an increase in systolic and diastolic blood pressure (see Figure 12.29a, p.349). This plus the rapid infusion of fluids will lead to a rise in the blood pressure.
- *Raise temperature*: the fluids are administered through a rapid transfuser that warms the fluids at the same time. A warming blanket that blows warm air is placed over the top of David's body. While the surgical clamp is in place on the aorta there is no point in attempting to warm the lower limbs because there is no circulation.
- *Prevention of coagulopathy*: hypothermia, acidosis and the consequences of a massive blood transfusion can lead to a coagulopathy. Clotting factor therapy involves the transfusion of fresh frozen plasma; platelets and cryoprecipitate.

Evaluation of care

- Repeat blood gas analysis reveals a partial correction of the homeostatic imbalance in that the pH improves to 7.13, bicarbonate to 13.3 mmol/L and the base excess to –14.4 mmol/L. The potassium returns to within normal range to 4.7 mmol/L.
- The blood pressure rises and the tachycardia diminishes. His central venous pressure reading is 10 cmH$_2$O indicating a good circulating volume, but his urine output is minimal.
- The Hb has fallen to 7.5 g/dL indicating a haemodilution which may be caused by the large colloid infusion.
- The temperature has not improved.

The surgical clamp is removed from the aorta after the repair is made. This leads to an enhancement of the acidosis as the circulation is returned to the areas that have had no blood supply during the surgery and have been metabolizing anaerobically.

The surgery has been aimed at damage control (i.e. to control the haemorrhage and to optimize patient survival). Further surgery at this point in such a compromised patient

may not be advisable. The other injuries found are not life threatening and a decision is made to transfer David to the intensive care unit for rewarming and further reversal of the metabolic acidosis. Rewarming will improve tissue perfusion and thus oxygen and nutrient delivery to the cells, thus aiding normal cell metabolism.

David will return to theatre in the next 24 hours when homeostatically stable for further surgery.

Case study contributed by Judy Barker.

Further reading/references

Clancy, J. and McVicar, A.J (1996) Shock: a failure to maintain cardiovascular homeostasis. *British Journal of Theatre Nursing* **6**(6): 19–25.

Clancy, J. and McVicar, A, J. (1997) Hypoxia. A respiratory imbalance. A homeostatic imbalance. *British Journal of Theatre Nursing* **6**(10): 15–20, 1264–70.

Drage, S. and Wilkinson, D. (2001) Acid Base Balance. World Federation of Societies of Anaesthesiologists. http://www.nda.ox.ac.uk/wfsa/html/ul3/u1312_01.htm

McVicar, A.J. and Clancy, J. (1997) The principles of intravenous fluid replacement therapy. *Professional Nurse Supplement* **12**(8): S6–S9.

Montague, S., Watson, R. and Herbert, R. (2005) *Physiology for Nursing Practice*, 3rd edn. London: Elsevier.

Royal College of Surgeons. Arterial blood gases for the surgical trainee. http://www.edu.rcsed.ac.uk/lectures/lt8.htm

Sasada, M. and Smith, S. (2003) *Drugs Used in Anaesthesia and Intensive Care*, 3rd edn. Oxford: OUP.

CASE 7. THE CASE OF A WOMAN WITH CATARACTS

This case links specifically to Chapter 7.

SCENARIO

Averill, aged 64, has been an outgoing community-minded person ever since her two sons moved away from their small town to pursue work, and her husband died suddenly. The boys have their own families and keep regular contact with their mother but have tended not to be concerned for her because of her independent nature, her many interests and her circle of friends. For several years Averill has enjoyed sewing as part of a local craft group, raising funds for a charity. She was a reader at church, played bingo weekly and also wrote poetry with some minor publishing success. The boys are only now beginning to learn through her friends that, over the past year or so, Averill has gradually withdrawn from these pursuits and is becoming a little isolated and depressed, turning down invitations from friends to socialize.

More than a year ago, Averill began to notice that the edges of windows in her house seemed fuzzy, with the light from outside blurring the area around the frame. Over the following months she began to find that her vision seemed to be increasingly cloudy, but initially, when sewing and writing, she could see clearly. This situation gradually deteriorated, though it seemed to improve when she bought some reading glasses. The improvement was only temporary, and eventually, she could no longer distinguish the colours of her materials, and could not see well enough to write or thread a needle. Going out was hazardous, and she began to make excuses to friends and church acquaintances rather than risk falling or looking foolish trying to read in front of a congregation.

Averill felt that she was losing her life and despite a reluctance to make her problems known, she recently visited her general practitioner who diagnosed cataracts and discussed options for treatment.

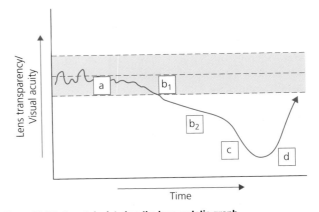

Figure 23.7 Cataract depicted as the homeostatic graph. **a**, Lens transparency/visual acuity within normal range for age. b_1, b_2, Declining visual function as transparency of the lens declines. Visual acuity restricted but compensatable by social awareness, etc. (see text). **c**, Rapidly declining vision as declining lens transparency becomes critical. **d**, Rapid return of visual function almost to normal through surgical replacement of the lens. There may be some remaining deficit requiring further care and support in order to restore normal social activities

Cataracts as a homeostatic imbalance

Cataracts are impaired transparency of the lens in the eye. In most cases the condition is associated with the process of ageing, although less commonly it can be caused by trauma, exposure to X-rays, some poisons, endocrine abnormalities, and can occur before birth as a result of viral infection. The process that maintains transparency in the lens is highly complex and the homeostatic imbalance leading to cataract formation is poorly understood. A range of factors are linked to the disruption to the regulation of proteins, sugars and electrolytes within and around the lens, sometimes interfering with the capacity of membranes to allow diffusion, leading to changes in osmotic gradient. These changes can result in the lens becoming opaque, as can changes to its structure brought about by ultraviolet light or ionizing radiation.

Background

Cataracts may be congenital, traumatic, metabolic (usually related to diabetes or hypoparathyroidism), toxic (often caused by prolonged high dosage of corticosteroids in conditions such as arthritis), secondary to other eye disease, or be caused by over-exposure to ionizing radiation or extreme industrial heat as in occupations such as glass blowing. However, the most common diagnosis is 'senile cataract'. We all begin to lose lens transparency to some degree as we age, though normally sight is not impaired to a problematic level. Some development of cataract can be identified in more than 90% of people over 70 years.

Cataract formation tends to be gradual, but this is very individual and the length of time between noticing the first effects (impaired vision – no other symptoms result from cataracts) and presenting to a general practitioner or optician with the problem varies greatly not only according to speed of cataract development, but equally according to the person's perception of the importance of sight to their way of life.

Senile cataracts fall into three general categories. Seen through an ophthalmoscope, nuclear or 'hard cataracts' have increasing density towards the lens centre and cortical or 'soft cataracts' have 'wedge-shaped' 'spokes'. These two are the most common types, and the third category, posterior subcapsular cataracts, are granular, opaque and 'plaque-like'.

Presentation

Cataracts are not associated with pain or any other symptom, and awareness of their presence occurs to the affected person because of problems with vision. Commonly, vision loss is gradual over months or years, with progression being very individual. Some people have cataracts many years before the condition becomes debilitating. Usually, senile cataracts develop bilaterally as in Averill's case.

In posterior subcapsular cataracts, and to some extent in cortical cataracts, bright light such as sunlight or oncoming car headlights tend to glare. This occurs less frequently in nuclear cataracts. The more serious presentation and the problem that generally leads to a decision to surgically intervene, is the gradual loss of visual acuity.

As cataracts progress there is often a temporary shift towards myopia, with the individual reporting improved near sight. This apparent benefit is soon lost. Sometimes double vision may be reported in one eye.

The impact on an individual's quality of life varies enormously depending on interests, work, level of confidence and general outlook on life as well as environmental factors (living in spacious, well-lit rooms or poorly lit cramped conditions, for example) and social support.

Healthcare practitioners as external agents of homeostatic control

See Figure 23.7.

Assessment

If any condition is able to demonstrate the importance of a good health carer's assessment, then cataract is that condition. The tragedy of this condition is that while it can have such a devastating effect on lives, a simple and inexpensive procedure can dramatically change life for the better.

In the past, eye specialists preferred to wait until the cataract was developed to an extent that vision deteriorated to a very poor level. Advanced technology no longer necessitates this and surgery is considered as soon as soon as sight is impaired enough to begin to negatively impact on activities of living. Therefore a health carer's assessment needs to consider the person as a whole, taking account of social life, including work and hobbies as well as psychological factors and risk to physical health from falls and other incidents such as walking into furniture or sustaining burns or scalds in the kitchen. Assessment therefore must consider potential harm as well as actual, existing problems.

A good observant holistic assessment will aid the decision to undertake surgery at the optimum time, and could well avoid unnecessary suffering. The scenario above provides examples of existing and potential physical, psychological and social factors that require careful assessment.

Care planning and implementation

The care plan in the period prior to admission for the surgical procedure should begin with maintaining a safe environment. Potential hazards in the home environment and in areas where the affected person frequents should be identified and where possible removed. Where this is not possible, the risk of the hazard becoming the cause of injury or harm should be reduced. This will involve not only a physical survey of the areas where the person lives and goes, but also accompanying the person to observe how they carry out chores, travel and socialize.

The plan to eliminate hazards and reduce risks must be sensitive to the individual's dignity and free choice about how they wish to live. It is likely that the person would rather accept some risks and that removing them might have a negative impact on some aspect of life that is important to them. This must be respected and discussions about safety require tact, diplomacy and understanding. As always, working with the affected person to develop the plan rather than attempting to impose it is very important both from the practical point of view of increasing the chance of concordance, and of demonstrating respect.

The plan should address difficulties with social activities. For example, in the scenario above Averill may be avoiding going to her church and reading to the congregation for fear of stumbling and appearing clumsy in full view. It should be possible to work with the church committee to decrease the likelihood of tripping. Sometimes a very inexpensive white or yellow adhesive strip can help to clarify the step up to the altar, for example. There may be large print texts available, or perhaps a small battery light attached to the lectern will help with reading.

A care plan developed in this way, addressing all aspects of living, should help to restore confidence and psychological well-being as well as prevent further physical harm.

A preoperative care plan should allow the patient to express any anxieties about the procedure and should aim to reduce them. In this case, Averill may be concerned about what undergoing the procedure will entail and about the potential for problems after surgery, including a poor outcome with her partial sight being lost or further impaired. The plan should involve taking time to assess these fears by listening and observing verbal and non-verbal cues. Explaining the procedure and the risks and benefits sensitively, responding to cues regarding the level of detail Averill wishes to engage in will help. It is important that the health professional has the skill to assess her level of understanding and whether the interaction has allayed fears satisfactorily for Averill. Attentive listening may suffice, and it is important to know when further information is not required and not helpful.

Implementation

Damage to the lens caused by cataracts cannot be repaired with conservative measures and the homeostatic imbalance regarding regulation of proteins sugars and electrolytes that continues to contribute towards increasing opacity cannot be reversed. Therefore, homeostatic imbalance must be compensated for rather than corrected.

While there may be some truth in claims that a healthy diet can help to slow progression, the only treatment for cataracts is surgical removal of the lens, which can be achieved in several ways. Historically, the intracapsular process involving removal of the capsule intact was generally used, and this is still a useful approach in countries or areas where advanced instruments and irrigation facilities are not available. This approach carries greater risk of complications than the extracapsular procedure that is now much more widely used. Removal may be carried out with surgical instruments, but more often the 'phacoemulsification' procedure involving ultrasound to break down the lens, which is removed by suction, is used.

Evaluation

The postoperative plan must include monitoring for any signs of haemorrhage such as pain in or surrounding the eye especially with sudden onset, or any changes to vision. Eyebrow pain, seeing halos around lights or nausea may indicate raised intraocular pressure. Any of these signs or symptoms (other than pain after perhaps a couple of hours post surgery, which is easily controlled with mild analgesia) must be communicated to the surgeon urgently, while reassuring Averill.

Averill must be taught how to care for her eye at home, by keeping an eye shield on at night and protective glasses on during the day to avoid accidental scratching or knocking. Averill must also be taught to observe for and report any signs of infection such as redness, eyelid oedema, prominent conjunctival vessels, crusting or purulent secretions or a raised local or body temperature. She should be taught to instil eye drops using aseptic technique.

It is important to discuss with Averill how she can begin to re-establish her activities postoperatively. Discussing how she may read, sew and drive; increasing these activities at a pace that is comfortable for her will help to reassure. She should be reminded of restrictions such as lifting heavy items, showering or straining on defecation. She should be helped to understand all medication – what it is for and when and how to take it, and how to carry out eye care. Follow-up appointments must be arranged and the importance of these made clear to Averill.

Case study contributed by Steve Smith.

Further reading

Carpetino-Moyet, L. (2004) *Nursing Care Plans and Documentation*, 4th edn. Philadelphia: Lippincott.

Owsley, C., McGwin, G., Jr, Scilley, K. *et al.* (2007) Impact of cataract surgery on health-related quality of life in nursing home residents *British Journal of Ophthalmology* **91**: 1359–63.

Ross, M., Avery, A. and Foss, A. (2003) Views of older people on cataract surgery options: an assessment of preferences by conjoint analysis, *Quality and Safety in Health Care* **12**: 13–17.

A wealth of information on what cataracts are, signs and symptoms and treatment is available on the Royal National Institute of Blind at: http://www.rnib.org.uk

CASE 8. THE CASE OF A WOMAN WITH DEPRESSION

This chapter links specifically to Chapter 8.

SCENARIO

Nayna Patel is a 43-year-old woman. She is married to Rav and has three sons and one daughter, all of whom are attending university. For her daughter (the youngest child at 18 years) this is her first year away from home. Nayna and her family live with her mother-in-law and her husband's elderly aunt and grandmother. Nayna works part-time in the family shop; there is frequently tension between Nayna and her husband's female relatives. Rav tries to support his wife, but his relatives make it very difficult for him.

Nayna longs to widen her social circle and would (now the children have 'left the nest') like to attend night-school classes. This she is prevented from doing. Over the last few weeks, she has been complaining of pains in her abdomen and legs, she suffers from insomnia, her appetite is reduced and she has been losing weight. When she is not working in the shop or doing housework she lies in bed, complaining of feeling tired, in pain and not being interested in anything.

Depression as a homeostatic imbalance

Depression affects the whole of the person's experience including their physiological self, their thoughts, feelings and behaviour. The term covers a range of mental health problems related to mood. Individuals present with lowered mood and a loss or decrease of interest and pleasure in daily life and experiences. Additionally, there are disorders of thinking, problem-solving and behavioural and physiological symptoms (NICE, 2004; WHO, 1992, 2000). In some cultural groups, depression may present as physical symptoms (this is known as somatization). Often it is not easy initially to identify that the individual with physical symptoms is suffering from depression. Clinical depression is more common in women than in men (indications are that about three times as many women as men suffer from depression; WHO, 2002).

Physiologically, there are many theories that relate to depression, and evidence for an imbalance between excitatory and inhibitory neurotransmitters in neurological pathways (see

Table 23.2 Recognition of severe clinical depression

At least five of the following symptoms are consistently experienced by the client on a daily basis over a 2-week period:

- Constant sad mood
- Loss of interest or pleasure in activities previously enjoyed
- Significant weight loss or gain without dieting, an increased or reduced appetite
- Insomnia or hypersomnia, sleeping problems and early-morning wakening
- Psychomotor agitation or dysfunction
- Fatigue, listlessness or lethargy; loss of energy
- Feelings of worthlessness and guilt
- Lack of concentration, inability to make decisions or think
- Recurrent thoughts of death or suicidal ideas

Adapted from ICD 10 (WHO, 1992).

Figure 8.24, p.192). In particular, the neurotransmitters noradrenaline and serotonin (5-HT) appear to be important in the development of depression. Noradrenaline is involved in the control of mood and emotions, and plays an important role in mood regulation, concentration, attention, memory, sleep and appetite. Serotonin seems to be involved in regulating sleeping–waking cycles and mood control; depression appears to be related to reduced levels of this neurotransmitter (and high levels in mania/hypomania). What remains unclear is how those changes occur.

Background

Many people have normal mood variations, some have long-term low severity low mood (dysthymia) or mood fluctuations (cyclothymic episodes) and distinguishing between these, sadness, and mild to moderate clinical depression can be challenging.

Depressive presentations are the fourth most common cause of disability in the world and are the most common mental disorder in primary care (NICE, 2004). The incidence is rising in the UK; by 2020 it is generally anticipated that depression will become the second highest cause of disability. Depression also has negative effects on comorbid physical illnesses including cardiac disease, myocardial infarction and cancer.

Presentation

Table 23.2 identifies symptoms associated with depression.

Healthcare practitioners as agents of homeostatic control

The healthcare practitioner's role is to establish a therapeutic relationship with the patient and develop a programme of care that offers support and treatment for the symptoms experienced, restores the patient's quality of life and prevents relapse. In the acute phase of a severe (major) clinical depression assessing the risk of suicide (Table 23.3), transporting the patient to a place of safety, managing any medical conditions and physical symptoms associated with the person's depression and selecting and monitoring appropriate antidepressant therapy is crucial. 'Talking treatments', exercise and patient and family education will be useful within the treatment programme as the patient progresses.

Table 23.3 Relevant risk factors for suicide

- Use/misuse of alcohol or drugs
- Hopelessness and helplessness
- Previous suicide attempt
- Recent self-harm; history of violent self-harm (half of those who commit suicide will have self-harmed in the past*)
- Depression – as mood lifts
- Clear plan
- Choice of method
- Young Asian women
- Perception of limited social support and network; social fragmentation
- Relationship problems
- Chronic pain
- Easy access to lethal methods

*NICE (2004).

Assessment

Using rating scales and asking the patient to use self-rating tools is a valuable way to establish an initial benchmark and later to evaluate the patient's progress. An example is an easily accessible self-test, the Patient Health Questionnaire (PHQ-9), that was applied in Nayna's case. It is available at http://www.depression-primarycare.org/clinicians/toolkits/materials/forms/phq9/questionnaire/

Others, such as the Beck Depression Inventory and the Hospital Anxiety and Depression Scale (HADS), should be administered by an appropriately qualified clinician (e.g. a clinical psychologist) and are subject to copyright restrictions.

Use of a person-centred consultation approach asking her open-ended questions helps to communicate the healthcare practitioner's willingness to help Nayna to explore her experience and that she is being listened to.

It is therefore often helpful to support the patient in 'telling their story' (e.g. what a typical day is like; what makes it better or worse) and listening carefully not only to 'what' they say but 'how' they express their narrative. Two simple screening questions may be asked (this can help to screen for depression):

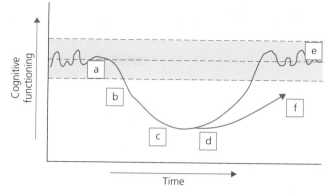

Figure 23.8 Depression depicted as the homeostatic graph.
a, Cognitive functioning within the homeostatic (i.e. equilibrium) range. **b**, Onset of depressive symptoms indicative of neurological/neurotransmitter imbalance between excitatory and inhibitory neural pathways in the central nervous system. **c**, Assessment/diagnosis including evaluation of suicidal tendency (see text). **d**, Implementation of medical intervention for physical symptoms, and cognitive/medical intervention to restore neurological/neurotransmitter homeostasis. **e**, Restoration of an individual's cognitive functioning (homeostasis; equilibrium). **f**, Incomplete return to homeostatic norms in individuals unresponsive to, for example, medication

1 'During the last month, have you often been bothered by feeling down, depressed or hopeless?'
2 'During the last month, have you often been bothered by little interest or pleasure in doing things?'

Questions will be asked of Nayna about her suicidal ideas and whether she has formed a plan. This she denies, saying that she feels 'worthless and as if she is no good as a wife' and is a 'failure not meeting her mother-in-law's requirements for a good daughter'. She also says 'I do not want to let my husband down but I do not want to work in the shop all the time and to feel that my best years are done now that my darling children have left home'. She agrees she feels 'low' and tired all the time and that 'the pains are getting me down'. She also has difficulty in concentrating.

Table 23.4 Flow chart for introducing Nayna's drug therapy

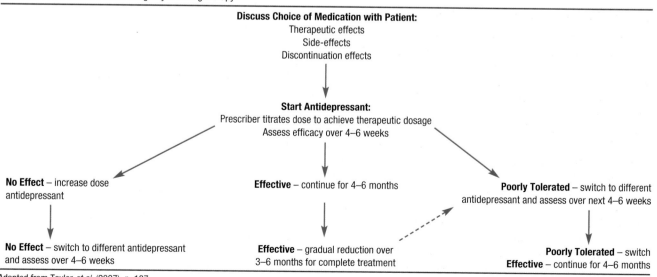

Adapted from Taylor *et al.* (2007), p. 187.

Major depression is diagnosed when other mental health problems physical causes have been excluded. Nayna scores 15 on the PHQ-9 questionnaire, This score indicates that antidepressant therapy and use of psychotherapy would be effective.

Care planning and implementation

See Figure 23.8.

Planning and implementation of care in Nayna's case has two objectives: to control the somatic (physical) symptoms of her depression using drug therapy to redress the imbalance noted earlier, and to provide psychological therapy to help her in the longer term to restore homeostatic balance herself.

Drug therapy

The healthcare practitioner will discuss the therapeutic effects, potential adverse side-effects of the medication and the availability and appropriateness of non-drug approaches. Citalopram is one of the first-line drugs of choice, and this would be prescribed as 20 mg once per day.

Health education is very important. Nayna needs information about how her medication works and possible side-effects, also that she may not see any benefits for 2–3 weeks. The starting dose of 20 mg per day will be reviewed regularly and gradually increased as needed (though evidence for higher doses is not strong; see Taylor *et al.*, 2007, and Table 23.4).

Side-effects include:

- Dyspepsia, nausea and vomiting
- Diarrhoea
- Abdominal pain
- Agitation and anxiety
- Tremor
- Insomnia
- Sexual dysfunction.

Including her husband in the care (which Nayna wants) and explaining to him what depression is, what the treatment plan is and what side-effects to look out for will enable him to support Nayna.

Psychological therapy

Cognitive behavioural therapy (CBT) would help by working on her negative thinking. However, Nayna does not feel able to engage with psychological therapy until she feels less tired and 'stronger', although she (and Rav) agree that it would be a useful goal to work towards in the coming weeks. There is a local women's support group (inter-faith) which runs weekly in the community centre and which Nayna thinks she might try to attend in the coming weeks.

Rav encourages Nayna to tell the children how she is feeling; and, when they do, the children organise a rota to come and spend time with their mother.

Evaluation of care and reassessment

After 4 weeks Nayna returns to the surgery. She is brighter and says that she feels she has more energy and that 'seeing the children has been a real boost'. She is now ready to move on and is referred for CBT; she also plans to go to the local women's group accompanied by her daughter.

Nayna is encouraged not to discontinue the antidepressants. She will need to continue to take them for 4–6 months otherwise she may risk a relapse. Exercise, social activities and spending time with Rav are also activities that are helpful in the prevention of a relapse.

Case study contributed by Derek Shirtliffe and Rosie Day.

References

National Institute of Clinical Excellence (2004) *Depression: Management of Depression in Primary and Secondary Care – NICE guidance.* London: NICE.

Taylor, D., Paton, C. and Kerwin, R. (2007) *The Maudsley Prescribing Guidelines*, 9th edn. London: Informa Healthcare.

World Health Organization (1992) *ICD-10 Classification of Mental and Behavioural Disorders*, Geneva: WHO.

World Health Organization (2000) *WHO Guide to Mental Health in Primary Care*. London: Royal Society of Medicine Ltd.

Further reading

Hamilton, M. (1960) A rating scale for depression. *Journal of Neurology, Neurosurgery and Psychiatry* **23**: 56–62.

Mynors-Wallis, L., Moore, M., Maguire, J. and Hollingbery, T. (2002) *Shared Care in Mental Health*. Oxford: Oxford University Press.

National Institute of Clinical Excellence. The NICE website contains clinical guidelines for both depression and anxiety http://www.nice.org.uk

Zigmond, A.S. and Snaith, R.P. (1983) The Hospital Anxiety and Depression Scale. *Acta Psychiatrica Scandinavica* **67**: 361–70.

CASE 9. THE CASE OF A WOMAN WITH HYPOTHYROIDISM

This case links specifically to Chapter 9.

SCENARIO

Cassandra is 51 years old and has always considered herself as being generally 'fit and well', since she has only ever visited her general practitioner for routine health checks. For the past year Cassandra has experienced persistent fatigue – she frequently falls asleep during the day and in her words 'since menopause I have really slowed down, physically and mentally and I'm no longer interested in making love'. She has noticed she has put on weight, despite a having an extremely modest appetite, her skin has many dry patches, her joints occasionally ache and her fingernails have become brittle and are prone to cracking.

On the advice of her husband and friends Cassandra visited her family doctor recently; her husband and friends were becoming increasingly concerned that she may have diabetes mellitus. The doctor took blood samples, which were analysed for blood glucose, urea and electrolytes and thyroid function tests (TFTs).

The TFTs indicated hypothyroidism:

- thyroid stimulating hormone levels of 4.8 mU/L (homeostatic range: 0.15–3.2 mU/L); and
- free tetra-iodothyronine (T$_4$) of 7 pmol/L (homeostatic range: 10–25 pmol/L).

Cassandra's mum also had hypothyroidism.

Hypothyroidism as a homeostatic imbalance

Thyroid hormone appears to have a critical role in establishing the basal metabolic rate, and it also has 'permissive' effects that facilitate the actions of other hormones, for example catecholamines (see p.206). It is released in response to the presence of a hormone (thyrotropin, or TSH) secreted from the anterior pituitary. This in turn is secreted in the presence of thyrotropin-releasing hormone from the hypothalamus. In other words, this is an example of 'long-loop' feedback control (pp.209, 214) that ensures precise control of the release of thyroid hormone. The release of thyrotropin-releasing hormone, and TSH, is itself inhibited by elevated blood concentrations of thyroid hormone – an example of negative feedback (see Chapter 1, p.13 and Figure 9.8, p.216). In Cassandra's case, the higher than normal TSH concentration suggests a failure of the thyroid gland to respond to it since the lack of thyroid hormone in blood will have a weak negative feedback effect on TSH secretion, hence its elevated concentration. This is an example of primary hypothyroidism.

In secondary and tertiary hypothyroidism (see later) the levels of both thyroid hormone and TSH are low as the problem stems from inadequate production of TSH, and hence poor stimulation of the thyroid gland.

Low secretion of thyroid hormone results in a reduced rate of cellular respiration and therefore low production of ATP, the end product of cellular respiration (see Figure 2.11, p.36 and Equation 4, p.130). Consequently the basal metabolic rate (BMR) is reduced and this reduction is largely responsible for the signs and symptoms experienced in hypothyroidism. The BMR may be only 60% of its homeostatic value, so it is not surprising that cold intolerance is a frequent symptom in patients that are hypothyroidic. A reduction in ATP, a suboptimal body temperature and pH are also responsible (by their link to enzyme function – see p.22) for a slowing down of cognitive processes, bradycardia (hence reduced cardiac output/blood pressure) and respiratory effort, leading to weight gain and fatigue.

Background

Hypothyroidism is more prevalent in women than men and surprisingly common with a reported clinical prevalence of 1 in 20 in postmenopausal women. The condition is rare under the age of 30 years. Approximately 1–2% of the UK population are affected by the condition.

The vast majority of cases of hypothyroidism (including Cassandra's) arise from a destruction or disturbance of the thyroid gland itself (referred to as primary hypothyroidism) by autoimmune mechanisms (a condition called Hashimoto's thyroiditis), or by the over-zealous treatment of hyperthyroidism by anti-thyroid drugs, thyroid ablation (via radiation) and/or surgery (thyroidectomy). A rare cause is failure of the anterior pituitary thyrotropic cells (called secondary hypothyroidism), which fail to produce adequate levels of TSH, or a failure of the hypothalamus cells (called tertiary hypothyroidism), which fail to produce adequate levels of TSH-releasing hormone. When thyroid deficiency is present at birth, the condition has a profound impact on brain development (a condition referred to as cretinism) and is normally caused by a lack of iodine, a constituent of the hormone. In such cases the mother may also suffer from hypothyroidism.

An interesting epidemiological factor is that the Japanese population have a greater prevalence of autoimmune hypothyroidism (Hashimoto's thyroiditis) which suggests strongly that genes play a major part in the development of hypothyroidism. Consequently if these genes have been inherited from parents, or mutations (i.e. changes) to them occur in embryological development, the thyroid will not function properly and congenital hypothyroidism results. Hypothyroidism has an increased incidence in Turner syndrome (i.e. girls born with a missing an X chromosome – see Figure 19.19, p.543) and in people with Down syndrome (people who have been born with an extra chromosome number 21), which indicates that the different genes are on different chromosomes.

Presentation

Early symptoms of hypothyroidism are vague, though extreme fatigue makes it difficult for the patient to complete a full day's work or activities. The patient may become irritable as the condition progresses. Symptoms in addition to those shown by Cassandra include:

- hair thinning and loss;
- numbness and tingling of the fingers;
- the voice occasionally becomes husky. The patient may complain of hoarseness;
- speech is slow;
- the hands and feet increase in size;
- the tongue enlarges;
- constipation;
- a goitre may be present in some patients (i.e. hyperplasia of thyroid nodules; see Figure 9.9a, p.216) this swelling indicates that the thyroid is adapting to produce more thyroxine.

Hypothyroidism in its chronic state also results in the skin becoming thicker and presence of peripheral oedema (a condition known as myxoedema). Myxoedematous coma is the life-threatening end-stage of hypothyroidism, where the patient suffers hypothermia, major cardiovascular imbalances (e.g. hypercholesterolaemia, cardiomyopathy and congestive heart failure), respiratory imbalances (e.g. hypoventilation) and severe metabolic imbalances (e.g. hyponatraemia, hypoglycaemia, hypercapnia, hypoxaemia, lactate acidosis). Hypothyroidism therefore is an illustration of the authors claim in Chapter 1 that illness arises from cellular homeostatic

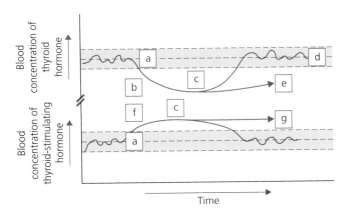

Figure 23.9 Serum concentrations of thyroid hormone and thyroid-stimulating hormone (TSH) concentration in primary hypothyroidism, expressed as the homeostatic graph.
a, Serum thyroid hormone, and TSH, concentration within the homeostatic range appropriate to well-being. b, Reduced thyroid hormone concentration because of inadequate secretion (primary hypothyroidism, e.g. Hashimoto's thyroiditis); onset of symptoms – see text. c, Diagnosis of the condition, and implementation of thyroid hormone replacement therapy; reversal of symptoms if the condition has not been long-standing. d, Effect of replacement therapy to restore serum thyroid hormone concentration to homeostatic range. e, Uncorrected hypothyroidism; exacerbation of symptoms. f, TSH profile in serum; note the increase owing to a loss of negative feedback action from serum thyroid hormone. g, TSH in uncorrected hypothyroidism; the concentration of TSH is usually the means of diagnosis of primary hypothyroidism, for establishing the extent of reversal using thyroid hormone replacement (in a process referred to as titration), and for monitoring if there is progressive loss of thyroid hormone secretion

imbalances, and hence a chemical (in this case thyroid hormone) imbalance, resulting in multiple organ system signs and symptoms, and demonstrates the interdependency of chemical–cell–tissue–organ system functioning.

Healthcare practitioners as external agents of homeostatic control

See Figure 23.9.

Assessment

The majority of patients with hypothyroidism are managed lifelong in primary care and do not require hospital admission; compared with other chronic diseases this condition is well treated and remains reasonably stable all the time. Practice nurses have a key role in education, and empowering patients with hypothyroidism in general practice. At the onset of a patient–nurse interview, the nurse needs to know the signs and symptoms (i.e. homeostatic imbalances) of the condition, since diagnosis relies on the correct assessment of signs and symptoms of the condition; however, diagnosis is only confirmed via thyroid function investigations. These include:

- Serum thyroxine (T_4): this is the total amount of circulating thyroid hormone in the blood.
- Serum tri-iodothyronine (T_3): this is the total amount of circulating T_3, which has actions similar to T_4 in the blood.

- TSH: as noted earlier, this investigation is diagnostic as to whether the problem is with the thyroid or the hypothalamus–pituitary axis.
- Radioactive iodine uptake: a small dose of radioactive iodine is taken orally. The radiation emitted from the thyroid is measured over timed intervals. An underactive thyroid gland will have a low uptake of radioactive iodine.
- Other investigations which identify thyroid dysfunction include fine needle aspiration cytology of the gland, ultrasound, and computed tomography (CT) or magnetic resonance imaging (MRI) scans.

Care planning and implementation

Once the diagnosis is established, the nurse acts as a homeostatic controller in the aggressive management of the condition. The prime objective of care is to re-establish Cassandra's metabolic rate to its homeostatic range by administering dosages of oral thyroxine (levothyroxine), and monitoring its effect (or lack thereof) on the thyroid, so as to remove the signs and symptoms (i.e. homeostatic imbalances) of the condition, but also to avoid symptoms of hyperthyroidism. The nurse should therefore advise Cassandra on the dangers of overdosing on thyroxine.

This hormone replacement therapy is lifelong. Education and support of the patient to adjust to diagnosis is a vital part of nursing care that is carried out by the practice nurse in primary care. The nurse (and husband and friends) should be encouraging Cassandra to be self-caring, where necessary. For example, she should use extra clothing and blankets to protect against cold, avoid use of copious amounts of soap, and use lipid-based creams to treat her dry skin. The nurse (and Cassandra's husband and friends) should be compassionate since other aspects of Cassandra's life will also need reviewing.

If Cassandra is concerned about her weight gain then the nurse could arrange a consultation with a dietitian to recommend an appetizing diet with lower calorie input, and a high protein content, to help her reduce weight.

It may be helpful to some patients to acknowledge that the cause of the condition may be autoimmune; therefore the process of thyroid destruction may be ongoing regardless of replacement of the thyroid extract. Other diseases need to be considered that patients with auto-immune thyroid disease are at increased risk to develop, such as diabetes mellitus (see Box 9.12, p.223), Addison's disease (see Box 9.9, p.220), and pernicious anaemia (see p.243). To rule out the involvement of such diseases a full blood count, fasting glucose, serum vitamin B_{12} and cortisol could be periodically measured.

Evaluation and reassessment of care

It is extremely important that the hormone dosage regime is being calculated for each individual. Thyroxine replacement therapy commences with small doses of 25 or 50 µg in older people or those with coronary heart disease, or higher dose of 100 µg in people under 50 years of age, with the absence of other systemic illnesses. The dose may be increased cautiously until the desired effect is produced; a maintenance dose

100–400 μg once daily is usual. Periodic repeat assessment of blood thyroid hormone and TSH concentrations will be required in case of further reduction of gland activity, and the administered dose should be titrated accordingly.

With good control typically the signs of hypothyroidism disappear quickly (i.e. in a 3- to 12-week period). The patient's vital signs and cognitive level are monitored closely during diagnostic investigations and treatment initiated to detect any deterioration or improvements in symptoms. For example, the nurse must be vigilant for the signs of angina or arrhythmias, especially during the early phases of treatment (see below, 'Further information'). If the patient experiences angina or arrhythmias thyroxine administration must be discontinued immediately, and later resumed when a substitute therapy can be given at lower dosages under the close observation of the clinical team.

The nurse should also be aware that thyroxine interacts with other drugs. For example, thyroxine may cause hyperglycaemia, which for the patient with hypothyroidism and diabetes mellitus will mean that changes in dosages of insulin or oral hypoglycaemic agents will be necessary. Thyroxine also can increase the pharmacological effects of digitalis, anticoagulants, tricyclic antidepressants, etc., therefore careful reassessment of the side-effects of these potential thyroxine–drug interactions is needed.

Further information

If the patient presents with severe hypothyroidism and myxoedema coma, then tri-iodothyronine (T3) may be given intravenously since this has a more immediate effect. Immediately following the life-threatening period, the patient is put back on oral thyroxine.

In advanced myxoedema, the body temperature and heart rate become abnormally low; the skin becomes thickened because the accumulation of mucopolysaccharides in the subcutaneous layer of the skin (see Figure 16.5, p.452). The face becomes expressionless. Patients who have had myxoedema for a long time are at risk of hypercholesterolaemia, atherosclerosis and coronary heart disease. This does not pose much of a problem prior to thyroxine therapy since metabolism is subnormal and the demand for oxygen is consequently low, so the risk of ischaemia is less. However, once thyroxine is administered, the oxygen demand increases, but the supply cannot be met until atherosclerosis improves. This may or may not occur depending upon a whole host of factors associated with nature–nurture interactions. Therefore, signs of ischaemia such as angina or cardiac arrhythmias may occur with thyroxine replacement therapy, since this hormone enhances the cardiovascular effects of adrenaline and noradrenaline.

Case study contributed by John Clancy and Andrew McVicar.

CASE 10. THE CASE OF AN INFANT WITH HYPERTROPHIC PYLORIC STENOSIS

This case study relates specifically to Chapter 10.

SCENARIO

Liam is a 6-week-old infant born at 39 weeks' gestation following a normal pregnancy and delivery. He is breast-fed and was thriving until 5 days ago when he began to vomit after some feeds. Over the past 3 days this has increased and he is now vomiting after every feed. The vomit is projectile, shooting up to a metre away from him. He has been very hungry and, until 24 hours ago, was keen to take another feed immediately after he had vomited. His mother states that he is now not interested in taking feeds and is becoming increasingly listless, his nappies are drier than usual and his stools are more solid and less frequent.

On examination, Liam is lethargic and quiet and does not protest on being handled. His fontanelle is depressed, eyes appear sunken and his skin has lost its elasticity. He looks thin and scrawny and his abdomen is distended.

Hypertrophic pyloric stenosis as a homeostatic imbalance

The pyloric sphincter prevents food from entering the duodenum until gastric digestion has taken place (see Figure 10.9, p.242). It is usually partially open, allowing liquids to pass through. However chyme, the end product of gastric digestion, is semi-liquid and the sphincter needs to be completely open to allow this to pass through.

Hypertrophic pyloric stenosis is caused by the hypertrophy and hyperplasia of the pyloric sphincter occurring during the first weeks of life. The hypertrophy and hyperplasia mainly affects the circular muscles of the pyloric sphincter. The pylorus becomes elongated and thickened causing narrowing of the pyloric canal (Surgical-tutor.org.uk). This results in a gastric outlet obstruction causing compensatory dilation, hypertrophy and hyperperistalsis of the stomach. The obstruction causes vomiting and dehydration (Hockenbury and Wilson, 2007).

As a result of the obstruction to the gastric outlet, food cannot pass into the duodenum and therefore the process of digestion cannot be completed, leading to weight loss and malnutrition. The volume of food in the stomach increases, and vomiting occurs. The loss of fluid in the vomitus causes dehydration and biochemical disturbances (i.e. metabolic alkalosis and hypochloraemia).

Background and presentation

Hypertrophic pyloric stenosis is one of the most common surgical conditions seen in early infancy. It tends to affect male infants, especially first born, more frequently than female infants in the ratio 4:1. There appears to be a definite genetic component because there are an increased number of cases from families where either another sibling or one of the parents has been affected.

The hypertrophy and hyperplasia of the pyloric muscle begins in the early weeks of life causing an obstruction at the pyloric sphincter, partially or completely occluding the gastric outflow from the stomach. Initially, the pyloric sphincter will remain partly open allowing milk to pass through. As the hypertrophy increases less food is able to pass through until eventually the canal is completely occluded.

During the first weeks of life the infant will appear to be thriving, until around 3–5 weeks of age when non-bilious vomiting begins. The frequency of the vomiting gradually increases until it is occurring immediately after every feed. At this point the vomiting will usually be projectile in nature, often being forcefully ejected up to a metre or more away from the infant. In the later stages, vomitus might contain specks of fresh or digested blood, giving it a coffee-ground appearance, owing to inflammation of the gastric mucosa.

Because the obstruction to the gastric outlet prevents the digestive process from being completed, the infant does not receive adequate nutrition resulting in weight loss, malnutrition, failure to thrive and lethargy. The frequent vomiting causes loss of nutrients, dehydration and electrolyte imbalance.

In the early twentieth century pioneering attempts were made to reform the pyloric sphincter (referred to as pyloroplasties) but the majority of cases were unsuccessful, resulting in the death of the infants. In 1912 Conrad Ramstedt described two successful operations for hypertrophic pyloric stenosis. One of the operations involved making an incision in the pyloric muscle and leaving the incision open. The operation performed today is very similar to this and is still known as Ramstedt's pyloroplasty (Surgical-tutor.org.uk).

Hypertrophic pyloric stenosis is seen more frequently in Caucasian infants than in Indian, Asian or African populations. No clear pathophysiological sequence or aetiology has been described to explain why the condition occurs. Several theories have been proposed; these include immature ganglion cells, decreased nitric oxide stimulation of muscle fibres, abnormal circular muscle innervations and abnormal gastrin levels.

Healthcare professionals as external agents of homeostatic control

In 95% of cases the hypertrophied pyloric muscle can be gently palpated through the abdominal wall, whilst the infant is being fed (Thalange *et al.*, 2005). Visible peristaltic waves are often seen moving from left to right across the abdomen. These are caused by the strong peristaltic action taking place in the stomach as the muscles of the stomach wall try to overcome the obstruction. Ultrasound scanning is also frequently used as an aid to diagnosis. Barium swallow can also be used to confirm the diagnosis. This will show delayed gastric emptying, a dilated stomach and a narrowed and attenuated pyloric canal (Glasper *et al.*, 2007).

The role of healthcare professionals in the care of an infant who has hypertrophic pyloric stenosis is to restore homeostasis by surgically correcting the obstruction to the gastric outlet. This will reduce vomiting and provide adequate nutrition for the maintenance of growth and development and to receive an adequate fluid intake to maintain fluid homeostasis.

On admission to hospital, a detailed history will be taken from the parents with particular attention being given to the frequency of vomiting in relation to intake of food and the occurrence of hypertrophic pyloric stenosis in other family members. A detailed physical examination of the infant will

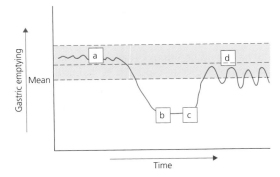

Figure 23.10 Pyloric stenosis depicted as the homeostatic graph.
a, Gastric emptying appropriate for age and feeding pattern of the infant. **b**, Inadequate gastric emptying owing to hypertrophic pyloric stenosis. Liam monitored by preoperative assessment of state of hydration. Preparation for surgery. **c**, Surgical reduction of the hypertrophied sphincter. **d**, Normal gastric emptying largely restored after surgery; postoperative monitoring of hydration, wound healing and analgesia

also take place. The continuous vomiting will cause the infant to display signs of dehydration (sunken fontanelle; sunken eyes; dry skin with loss of elasticity; lethargy; dry mucous membranes; decrease in the volume of urine being passed; and a reduction in the number of stools passed per day). Blood samples will be taken to determine the severity of fluid and electrolyte imbalances. The dehydration and electrolyte imbalance must be corrected before surgery can be performed.

Care planning and implementation

See Figure 23.10.

The focus of preoperative care will be to correct dehydration and electrolyte imbalance, and to prepare the infant and family for surgery. In comparison to older children, infants have a higher percentage of total body water; also, their daily exchange of extracellular fluid is much greater. This can be attributed to the differences in body and organ size and the immaturity of the physiological processes involved in fluid homeostasis. An interruption to fluid intake, as occurs when an infant is vomiting, can soon lead to dehydration. Infants cannot maintain fluid homeostasis if they do not receive an adequate fluid intake. The young infant's ability to concentrate urine is not well developed in the early weeks of life; therefore they produce a larger volume of urine to excrete a given solute load and need a larger fluid intake than older children in order to maintain fluid homeostasis. When fluid intake is decreased, as in the case of Liam because of frequent vomiting, infants can rapidly become dehydrated and solute overloaded (Neill and Knowles, 2004).

Homeostatic mechanisms aimed at water conservation will be activated to compensate for dehydration. The release of aldosterone and antidiuretic hormone promotes renal salt and water retention leading to a decrease in the volume of urine passed (see Chapter 12, p.34, and Chapter 15, p.435). Fluid will also be absorbed from the colon resulting in the stools becoming drier and less frequent.

It is not desirable for Liam to continue to vomit, so he will be nil by mouth and an intravenous infusion of dextrose saline will be commenced to correct dehydration and electrolyte imbalance (see p.135). Liam will be weighed and the volume of fluid to be infused will be calculated depending on the level of dehydration. When dehydration has been corrected, Liam will continue with intravenous maintenance fluids until after surgery has been performed.

During rehydration, frequent assessments of fluid and serum electrolyte levels will be undertaken. Continuous vomiting of gastric content leads to:

- Depletion of sodium, potassium and hydrochloric acid resulting in hypokalaemia, hyponatraemia and metabolic alkalosis. The metabolic alkalosis elevates plasma bicarbonate levels and causes chloride deficiency (Thalange *et al.*, 2006).
- Renal function can be impaired when an infant is dehydrated; therefore the excretion of potassium will also be impaired. Potassium is withdrawn from hyperosmotic cells and may reverse the hypokalaemia (above), now producing a hyperkalaemia. During rehydration, much of the excess extracellular potassium moves back into the intracellular compartment. The complex movements of potassium between the extracellular and intracellular compartments means that any intravenous replacement of potassium will usually be delayed until normal renal function has been restored and the situation is assessed accurately.

The hypertrophied pyloric muscle will cause the stomach to become distended. This will be decompressed by inserting a nasogastric tube, which will be allowed to drain freely into a container and also aspirated 1- to 4-hourly, depending on the amount of gastric fluid being produced. All nasogastric losses will be replaced intravenously, millilitre for millilitre, to prevent further fluid loss and dehydration. A strict record will be maintained of all fluid given intravenously and all fluid lost via the nasogastric tube, the volume of urine passed and any bowel actions.

Observations of vital signs – pulse rate, respiratory rate and temperature – will be recorded 1- to 4-hourly depending on Liam's condition. Blood glucose concentration will be monitored 6-hourly because prolonged vomiting and absence of feeding can deplete glycogen stores. As Liam is not having any fluids by the oral route, his mouth will be kept moist using cooled, boiled water. The integrity of his skin will also be checked regularly because vomiting and dehydration has caused him to lose some of his subcutaneous fat, and for his skin to become dry and less supple.

It is important to correct alkalosis before administering an anaesthetic in order to prevent depression of the respiratory centre because of CO_2 retention, resulting in postoperative apnoea. When Liam's dehydration and electrolyte imbalance has been corrected, he will go to theatre for a laparoscopic pyloroplasty. A small incision is made just above the umbilicus. A laparoscope is inserted and an incision is made in the circular muscle fibres of the pylorus. The incision must not include the submucosa (see Figure 10.9, p.242).

Postoperatively Liam will initially remain nil by mouth and intravenous fluids will be continued. The nasogastric tube will remain *in situ* with free drainage and 2- to 4-hourly aspirations as required. All aspirate will continue to be replaced with normal (isotonic) saline via the intravenous route. Oral feeding will commence 3–6 hours postoperatively, depending on local policy. Feeds will gradually be increased, as tolerated, until the full requirements are being taken and tolerated. The nasogastric tube will be aspirated and spigotted prior to each feed. Vital signs of pulse and respiratory rates will be recorded half-hourly initially, gradually reducing to 4-hourly as Liam's condition dictates. He will also be regularly assessed for pain and appropriate analgesia administered. The wound will be checked frequently for oozing or signs of infection. Liam's malnutrition and dehydration prior to surgery could affect the ability of his body tissues to heal following surgery.

The prognosis following pyloroplasty is very positive. The majority of infants will make a full, uncomplicated recovery and will re-establish their usual feeding regime within a few days. Infants are usually discharged from hospital when they are taking and tolerating their full nutritional requirements. Occasional vomiting might still occur until the pylorus has recovered.

Case study contributed by Theresa Atherton and Wendy Dubbin.

References

Glasper, E., McEwing, G. and Richardson, J. (2007) *Oxford Handbook of Children's and Young People's Nursing*. Oxford: Oxford University Press.

Hockenbury, M. and Wilson, D. (2007) *Wong's Nursing Care of Infants and Children*. St Louis: Elsevier/Mosby.

Neill, S. and Knowles, H. (2004) *The Biology of Child Health*. Basingstoke: Palgrave Macmillan.

Surgical-tutor.org.uk: http://www.surgical-tutor.org.uk (accessed 13 November, 2008).

Thalange, N., Holmes, P., Beach, R., Kinnaid, T. (2005) *Pocket Essentials of Paediatrics*. London: Saunders.

CASE 11. THE CASE OF A WOMAN WITH DEEP VEIN THROMBOSIS (DVT)

This case links specifically with Chapter 11.

SCENARIO

Jane is a 24-year-old woman who was referred to the Deep Vein Thrombosis (DVT) Clinic by her general practitioner. Ten days ago Jane gave birth to a baby girl. Her right leg had now been swollen and painful for 3 days and she was finding it difficult to walk because of the pain in her leg. Examination of Jane's leg revealed pitting oedema, and the leg was warm to touch, with the dorsalis pedis pulse present. The whole leg was swollen; the calf was 40 cm in circumference whereas the left calf was 36 cm, and the left thigh was 46 cm in circumference whereas the left thigh was 44 cm. Her initial observations included:

Blood pressure 116/69 mmHg (normal)
Pulse 80 bpm (normal)
Temperature 36.6°C (normal)
Oxygen saturation on air 98% (normal)
Respiratory rate 14 breaths/minute (normal)

An ultrasound scan of Jane's left leg showed a DVT in the femoral vein. Treatment with oral anticoagulants (warfarin) and subcutaneous low molecular weight heparin was commenced to treat the DVT.

DVT as a homeostatic imbalance

Venous return to the heart is facilitated by muscle movements, breathing movements and the presence of valves within the veins (see Figure 12.18, pp.326–7). Although venous blood still contains significant amounts of oxygen it can become significantly depleted if blood flow becomes severely reduced (referred to as 'stagnant hypoxia'). If this happens the vessel wall is damaged ('roughened') and together with the slow blood flow encourages clot formation by causing platelets to aggregate and stick to the vessel wall. Fibrin strands then trap platelets and red cells to form the clot, or thrombus (see Figure 11.15, p.291). The presence of a clot can precipitate further clotting until the size of the blood clot is such that it begins to occlude the lumen of the vein (Figure 12.13a, p.324). This means that blood leaving a tissue is compromised leading to further hypoxia in that tissue too, hence the feeling of pain.

Thrombus formation usually starts in the valve pockets of calf veins and then extends proximally. Apart from pain, the main danger from a deep vein thrombosis (DVT) is that part of the thrombus can break off, pass around the circulation and lodge in, and obstruct, the pulmonary arteries leading to a potentially fatal pulmonary embolism.

Background

A DVT is a thrombus (blood clot) most commonly seen in the venous system of the leg. Blood flow in the vein can be completely or partially obstructed by the thrombus.

Predisposing factors for the development of DVT were first identified in the nineteenth century. These pathogenic factors are known as Virchow's triad and consist of the following: alterations in blood flow, damage to the vessel wall and hypercoagulability of the blood.

The following are some of the risk factors identified for DVT:

- Recent surgery, especially high-risk procedures such as orthopaedic surgery, can cause damage to the leg veins and alterations in blood flow.
- Previous venous thromboembolism.
- Long-distance travel, and prolonged bed rest, increases the risk of DVT by causing alterations in blood flow and venous stasis.

Jane's case reflects the haemostatic adaptations that occur in pregnancy. The postpartum period is associated with an increase in concentrations of most clotting factors, especially coagulation factors V, VII, VIII, IX, X and von Willebrand fac-

Table 23.5 Clinical model for predicting pre-test probability for deep vein thrombosis (Wells *et al.*, 1997)

Clinical feature	Score
Active cancer (treatment ongoing or within previous 6 months or palliative)	1
Paralysis, paresis, or recent plaster immobilization of the lower extremities	1
Recently bedridden for more than 3 days or major surgery, within 4 weeks	1
Localized tenderness along the distribution of the deep venous system	1
Entire leg swollen	1
Calf swelling by more than 3 cm when compared with the asymptomatic leg (measured 10 cm below tibial tuberosity)	1
Pitting oedema (greater in the symptomatic leg)	1
Collateral superficial veins (non-varicose)	1
Alternative diagnosis as likely as or more likely than that of deep vein thrombosis	−2
In patients with symptoms in both legs the more symptomatic leg is used	

Low probability 0 or less, moderate probability 1–2, high probability 3 or more.

tor. This is accompanied by an increase in fibrinogen levels, while concentrations of the natural anticoagulants protein C and protein S also decrease. These haemostatic changes produce a hypercoagulability state. The changes are thought to result from hormonal changes that help to prevent severe haemorrhage during delivery and in the postpartum period. As noted, however, they do predispose women to complications such as DVT (Brenner, 2004; Franchini, 2006).

Presentation

Someone with a DVT typically complains of unilateral leg swelling, a dull ache and tightness of the calf. Examination of the leg may reveal oedema of the calf and evidence of dilated superficial veins may indicate a collateral circulation that has developed because of disruption to flow in the main vessel. A low-grade fever and tachycardia can also be present, though this was not obvious in Jane's case.

Healthcare practitioners as external agents of homeostatic control

Assessment

A structured assessment of the examination criteria above is combined with a clinical history such as recent surgery, cancer, immobility or pregnancy. The patient is then stratified into low, moderate and high probability for DVT (Wells *et al.*, 1997) (Table 23.5). A pre-test probability score that is low or moderate may then be combined with a D-dimer blood test; the D-dimer is a chemical product of the breakdown of a fibrin clot and its concentrations are raised in the presence of an acute thrombosis. Normal concentrations are expected in the absence of DVT unless other conditions that activate the coagulation system, such as pregnancy and the postpartum period,

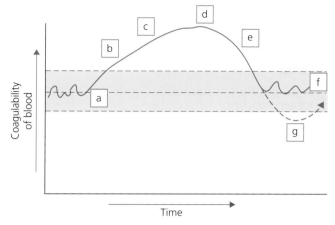

Figure 23.11 Haemostasis, and deep vein thrombosis (DVT), depicted as the homeostatic graph.
a, Coagulability of blood within homeostatic range; balance between intrinsic stimulation of clotting and intrinsic fibrinolysis (thrombolytic) activity. **b**, Localized increase in coagulability of blood within a vein owing to stimulation of the intrinsic clotting mechanism (e.g. because of hypoxaemia, or damage to a blood vessel wall). Risk of DVT. **c**, Diagnosis of DVT and assessment of possible stimulating factors and underlying causes. **d**, Initiation of anticoagulation therapy. **e**, Short-term (e.g. heparin) and medium-term (e.g. warfarin) responses to anticoagulant therapy. **f**, Coagulability returned to homeostatic balance with intrinsic and extrinsic (i.e. pharmacological) thrombolytic activity. Gradual restoration of balance between intrinsic processes as in (**a**); withdrawal of drug therapy. **g**, Thrombolysis is more effective; this imbalance will reduce the clot in the vein (but may increase the risk of its fragmentation, and hence risk of embolism)

recent surgery or cancer, are present. If D-dimer concentration is raised an ultrasound scan will be taken.

All patients with a high probability score are given an ultrasound scan (Fancher *et al.*, 2004). Ultrasound is a non-invasive method for DVT and depends on the non-compressibility of a vein in the presence of a thrombus.

Care planning and implementation

See Figure 23.11.

Following the examination and assessment of Jane the following blood tests were taken: a full blood count, urea and electrolytes, a coagulation screen and liver function tests. It is essential that these bloods are checked before initiating anticoagulant therapy:

- A full blood count is checked for platelet count as platelets are responsible for blood clotting. Because heparins can induce thrombocytopenia it is vital the platelet count is checked; low haemoglobin levels can indicate a bleeding site somewhere.
- Urea and electrolytes are checked as the metabolism of low molecular weight heparin (LMWH) involves renal clearance; in renal failure an accumulation of LMWH may occur, which can result in an increased bleeding risk in patients with renal failure.
- A coagulation screen and liver function test are taken as clotting factors are produced by the liver and liver damage can cause prolonged clotting.

The standard treatment for confirmed DVT is anticoagulation with warfarin tablets and subcutaneous LMWH. This is usually managed on an outpatient basis (Winter *et al.*, 2005). Treatment with anticoagulants will prevent extension of the existing thrombus, embolization of the thrombus and prevent new clots from forming. At the same time the body will act to break down the existing clot through the presence of intrinsic fibrinolysins.

Warfarin is the most commonly used oral anticoagulant in the UK. Warfarin inhibits the synthesis of the vitamin K-dependent clotting factors II, VII, IX and X which are produced by the liver. Warfarin also affects protein C and protein S, which are naturally occurring anticoagulants. Warfarin is absorbed from the gastrointestinal tract and has a half-life of 36–44 hours. The therapeutic effects of warfarin are usually seen after 24–36 hours but can take up to 96 hours to be evident. The effect of warfarin on individuals varies and can be influenced by age, diet, intake of alcohol and medications such as antibiotics. Warfarin therapy is monitored by the prothrombin time, expressed in the measurement of the international normalized ratio (INR); this is done through repeated blood testing. The dose is titrated to achieve a ratio of 2.0–3.0, a ratio thought to provide the lowest combined incidence of bleeding and clotting. Once this is achieved, usually after 5–7 days, LMWH is discontinued. Duration of anticoagulation therapy after a single DVT is usually 3–6 months. Contraindications for the use of warfarin include severe hypertension and active peptic ulcer, as there is an increased risk of haemorrhagic complications. Warfarin is also contraindicated in pregnancy as it is teratogenic and can cause fetal haemorrhage. Cautions for the use of warfarin include recent surgery and hepatic and renal impairment.

Heparin is an anticoagulant that is not active when taken orally as it is digested. It therefore has to be injected. Heparin acts within minutes whereas warfarin acts more slowly and it can take several days to measure the effect. Warfarin and heparin therefore need to be started at the same time. Unfractionated heparin (given intravenously or subcutaneously) is less commonly used because it requires frequent monitoring of the activated partial thromboplastin time (APTT; heparin is especially effective in the final stages of the clotting cascade) to ensure therapeutic and safe anticoagulation.

The dose of LMWH is weight dependent and is given once or twice daily by subcutaneous injection. Laboratory measurements to ensure therapeutic anticoagulation are not generally required. Low molecular weight heparin acts by binding to the intrinsic anticoagulation factor in blood plasma, anti-thrombin. It then accelerates the rate at which anti-thrombin inhibits active factor Xa.

The increased risk of bleeding through use of anticoagulant therapy, and signs of pulmonary embolism that may arise if the clot is mobilized because it has become destabilized and fragmentary (sudden shortness of breath, chest pain and coughing up blood), were explained to Jane and she was advised to seek urgent medical advice should these occur.

Jane's physical activity is limited because of her symptoms. Standing and sitting for long periods should be avoided and short walks taken when able. When sitting, ensure that the legs are elevated on a stool, or rest on a bed or sofa. This will help to reduce leg swelling. Jane is also advised to get measured for a compression stocking once the initial leg swelling has gone down.

Paracetamol for pain relief is safe to take with warfarin. Drugs that inhibit platelet function such as non-steroidal anti-inflammatory drugs (e.g. aspirin) should be avoided, as their anticoagulant properties will increase the risk of bleeding. Jane would also be advised to seek medical advice with future pregnancies as she may require prophylactic anticoagulation.

Patient education is essential to prevent potentially fatal overanticoagulation, which may result in haemorrhage, or under-coagulation, which may result in thrombosis. Education should include the following:

- The anticoagulation record book with target INR, duration and indication for treatment should be explained to the patient.
- The patient should be encouraged to carry an alert card.
- Spontaneous bruising or bleeding that does not stop needs urgent medical attention as this could be a sign of over anticoagulation.
- Patients should also be advised to inform their dentist, doctor or pharmacist that they take warfarin.
- Always check with a GP or pharmacist before taking any medication, including herbal or alternative treatments, to ensure they are safe to take with warfarin.
- Alcohol intake should be limited to one to two units a day.
- Excessive changes in weight should be avoided.
- A healthy balanced diet, with a regular intake of green leafy vegetables (rich in vitamin K), will not cause any disruption to the INR.

In addition, patients should be made aware of post-thrombotic syndrome (PTS), which includes chronic pain, swelling and pigmentation of the leg, and venous ulcers. It can take up to 10 years for it to manifest so all patients should be advised to wear a grade II compression stocking on the previously affected leg to reduce the incidence of developing PTS (Winter et al., 2005).

Case study contributed by Elizabeth Lorie.

References

Brenner, B. (2004) Haemostatic changes in pregnancy. *Thrombosis Research* **114**: 409–14.

Fancher, T., White, R. and Kravitz, R. (2004) Combined use of rapid D-dimer testing and estimation of clinical probability in the diagnosis of deep vein thrombosis: systemic review. *British Medical Journal* **329**: 821–4.

Franchini, M. (2006) Haemostasis and pregnancy. *Journal of Thrombosis and Haemostasis* **95**: 401–13.

Wells, P.S., Anderson, D.R., Bormanis, J. *et al.* (1997) Value of assessment of pre-test probability of deep vein thrombosis in clinical management. *Lancet* **350**: 1795–98.

Winter, M., Keeling, D., Sharpen, F. *et al.* (2005) Procedures for the outpatient management of patients with deep vein thrombosis. *Clinical and Laboratory Haematology* **27**: 61–6.

Further reading

Lip, G. and Blann, A. (2003) *ABC of Antithrombotic therapy.* Oxford: Wiley–Blackwell/BMJ Books.

CASE 12. THE CASE OF A WOMAN WITH MYOCARDIAL INFARCTION

This case links specifically to Chapter 12.

SCENARIO

Jean is 62 years old. She is a slightly overweight retired school teacher who smokes 20 cigarettes a day and takes little recreational exercise. Today, Jean was admitted to the local coronary care unit, having experienced a central crushing chest pain that radiated to her left arm and jaw. The pain occurred at rest, and was accompanied by breathlessness, nausea and vomiting. On examination, Jean was also found to be cold and clammy to the touch; she was also tachycardic and hypotensive.

After a rapid physical examination using the 'ABCDE' approach to sick patient assessment, Jean's electrocardiogram (ECG) was recorded. This demonstrated ST segment elevation over the anterior chest leads (V_1–V_6). As these ECG changes are indicative of an acute anterior myocardial infarction, a blood test for the cardiac specific enzyme troponin I was taken to confirm the diagnosis.

Myocardial infarction as a homeostatic imbalance

Myocardial infarction is a homeostatic imbalance that reflects myocardial oxygen insufficiency, usually arising from a partially or totally occluded coronary artery (generally referred to as myocardial ischaemia; see Figure 12.7, p.313). Blood flow to the tissue beyond the occluded site ceases; if the occlusion is complete, the affected myocardial tissue dies.

Sensory impulses travel from the myocardium via sympathetic nerve fibres to the thoracic sympathetic ganglia and then to nerve roots T1–T5 (see Figure 8.4, p.166). These spinal nerves supply the anterior chest wall but also the inner aspect of the arm and head. For this reason, pain is felt in the region bounded by these nerves, including the left arm.

The poorly functioning myocardium prevents a normal ejection of blood during systole, and so will usually promote a low blood pressure (hypotension). The presence of hypotension can be gauged from the patient's cognitive functions/awareness, and this will form part of the initial assessment. The cardiovascular homeostatic responses to hypotension are to increase heart rate (producing tachycardia) and to promote vasoconstriction in peripheral tissues (and so raise peripheral resistance). These responses were described in Chapter 12. The latter actions explain the pale, cool appearance of Jean's skin.

Vasoconstriction is mediated by sympathetic nerve stimulation, which also causes the skin to sweat, producing clamminess.

Background

Coronary heart disease is caused by atheroma formation. Atherosclerotic plaques form over a period of time in the lumen of arteries (see Figure 12.7c,d, p.313). The plaque consists of soft atheroma – an infiltration of white blood cells (macrophages) engulfs the lipids and forms foam cells and a fibrous cap. Occlusion of the coronary arteries is normally caused by the presence of such atheroma and is usually the result of plaque rupture, resulting in thrombus formation and subsequent artery occlusion. The disorder reinforces the need for cells to receive adequate oxygen. Insufficient oxygen supply to the myocardium inhibits the complete metabolism of glucose for energy; as a result, anaerobic metabolism occurs and lactic acid accumulates. Lactic acid is known to stimulate pain fibres found within the myocardium, so myocardial infarction is commonly associated with severe chest pain. The occurrence of pain at rest is indicative of advanced disease, distinct from more moderate forms that produce pain when the heart is stimulated during activity or excitement.

The risk of suffering a myocardial infarction in a given individual or community reflects the interplay between genetic susceptibility to the disease and environmental factors, such as smoking, elevated cholesterol levels, stress, and lack of physical exercise. In addition, there are gender differences in relation to heart disease, with the incidence being highest in men and postmenopausal women.

Presentation

The diagnosis of acute myocardial infarction (MI) is made in three steps: the patient's history, the electrocardiogram (ECG), and specific cardiac enzyme studies. In many ways, the patient's story of their illness is the prime factor in reaching the diagnosis. However, the history, regardless of how typical it may be, is not diagnostic in its own right, and other steps must be taken to prove that the acute infarction has actually occurred.

The ECG is the single most valuable immediate diagnostic tool. Jean's ECG typically demonstrates that the problem is in the ventricle (primarily the left ventricle). However, additional confirmation of the diagnosis can be made by detecting raised plasma activities of cardiac enzymes (intracellular enzymes that leak from injured myocardial cells into the blood stream). The more extensive the myocardial damage, the greater the release of these enzymes. Particular attention is paid to the enzyme troponin I, which is cardiac specific. Levels of troponin I range from below 0.03 µg/L (negative) to 0.03–0.05 µg/L (medium risk of acute coronary syndrome, or ACS) to 0.05 µg/L upwards, which corroborates the diagnosis of a myocardial infarction. ACS is an umbrella term for the acute cardiac events of unstable angina, non-ST elevation MI and ST elevation MI. A retrospective diagnosis of myocardial infarction can also be made up to 7 days with troponin I. Note that laboratory assays and ranges of biochemical markers for classifying ACS vary between hospital trusts.

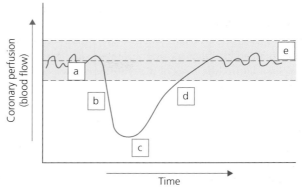

Figure 23.12 Myocardial infarction depicted as the homeostatic graph. a, Coronary perfusion appropriate to well-being. b, Rapid reduction in coronary perfusion caused by blood clot in a coronary artery; myocardium infarcts as it becomes hypoxic. c, Emergency intervention to restore coronary perfusion as much as possible to prevent further infarct (e.g. use of coronary vasodilator drugs). d, Additional improvement in coronary perfusion as thrombolytic therapy becomes effective. e, Restored coronary perfusion. Restoration of cardiac function is dependent on the extent of infarct

Prognosis in myocardial infarction is related principally to the age of the patient and the residual left ventricular function. A major myocardial infarction may result in death from cardiogenic shock, cardiac dysrhythmias or cardiac rupture. If the person recovers, their lifestyle may be restricted by chronic left ventricular failure or by intermittent myocardial ischaemia, particularly when active (angina pectoris).

Healthcare practitioners as external agents of homeostatic control

In the first instance, Jean's treatment will be to ensure survival by improving coronary blood supply and to remove pain. The first 48 hours are the most critical time for Jean. Necrosis can advance for several hours after the infarction (and possibly for a number of days), as does the risk of shock (see Figure 12.32, p.355), so continuous cardiac monitoring is essential in this early phase. Subsequent care will be directed at rehabilitation.

Implementation of care

See Figure 23.12.

Treatment for acute myocardial infarction focuses on recanalization of the occluded artery to limit the size of the infarction (i.e. of the necrotic area). Coronary blood supply is restored either by primary percutaneous coronary intervention or thrombolytic therapy. Immediately following admission, Jean will have an intravenous cannula inserted, and a powerful analgesic such as diamorphine administered for pain relief. Diamorphine acts quickly, and has the added benefits of reducing anxiety, ensuring rest and reducing myocardial preload due to venous pooling. An anti-emetic may be used to counteract consequential nausea.

Other drugs may also be administered:

- Sublingual or intravenous nitrates (e.g. glyceryl trinitrate) will induce dilation of coronary arteries.

- Thrombolytics, such as tenecteplase, may be used to dissolve thrombus clots in coronary arteries. The best results in terms of preserving ventricular function and improving survival are obtained by either starting thrombolytic therapy as soon as possible after the onset of the symptoms or if available primary percutaneous coronary intervention. Thrombolysis reduces mortality in patients with acute myocardial infarction particularly if given soon after the onset of symptoms; many paramedic crews have been trained to assess the patient with chest pain, take an ECG, reach a diagnosis and administer a thrombolytic drug if required all prior to admission to hospital. Aspirin has also been proven to enhance the benefit of either treatment option.
- Beta-blockers such as atenolol following MI may be used to reduce cardiac contractility (and hence the work being done) and to encourage normal cardiac rhythm. If the patient experiences heart failure a beta-blocker such as carvedilol may be the drug of choice as it has the additional action in arteriolar vasodilation therefore reducing the myocardial afterload.

During the acute phase, Jean would be nursed in bed in a semi-recumbent position and attached to continuous cardiac monitoring for constant observation of her heart rate and rhythm. Throughout this time, a nurse would remain with her to monitor her blood pressure and observe for signs of haemodynamic deterioration.

Evaluation of care

Success of treatment and care is measured in three ways: first, that Jean's ECG returns to normal following recanalization of the occluded artery; second, that she experiences no more chest pain; and third that she remains haemodynamically stable.

Rehabilitation

After 48 hours without ischaemic chest pain, Jean will be transferred to a medical ward for mobilization and rehabilitation. During the rehabilitation phase of hospitalization, particular attention is paid to modifying the patient's cardiac risk factors in the hope of preventing recurrent infarction. In Jean's case, she would need advice on stopping smoking, diet and weight loss, and the importance of exercise.

Case study contributed by Julia Hubbard.

Further reading

Department of Health (2000) *National Service Framework for Coronary Heart Disease.* London: Department of Health.

Department of Health (2007) *Progress Report on National Service Framework for Coronary Heart Disease.* London: Department of Health.

Hainsworth, T. (2006) Improving the prevention of cardiovascular disease. *Nursing Times* **102**(7): 23–4.

National Institute for Health and Clinical Excellence (2007) *Guidelines for the Treatment of Acute Coronary Syndromes.* London: NICE.

Opie, S. (2005) *Drugs for the Heart*, 6th edn. Philadelphia: Elsevier Saunders.

Raebuck, A. (2005) Identifying and managing acute coronary syndrome. *Nursing Times* **102**(6): 28–30.

Resuscitation Council (UK) (2006) *The 'ABCDE' Approach to the Sick Patient.* London: Resuscitation Council UK.

CASE 13. THE CASE OF THE YOUNG MAN WITH SYMPTOMATIC HIV/AIDS

This case links specifically to Chapter 13.

SCENARIO

James is 23 years old and was diagnosed as human immunodeficiency virus (HIV) positive 3 years ago. James can recall a period of general malaise and fever-like symptoms approximately 3 months after returning from his travelling abroad. After initially visiting his general practitioner and subsequently being referred to various specialist clinicians James's HIV positive status was confirmed. At the age of 19 years, James decided to take a gap year from university and travelled extensively around Central and Southern Africa and the Far East. During this time James had numerous protected and unprotected sexual contacts. However, for the last 3 years James has been in a loving and stable relationship with his partner Claire, who is aware of James's HIV status.

During the early part of this relationship, James's health status changed from his being HIV positive but asymptomatic, with the development of persistent generalized lymphadenopathy (PGL). Not only were his inguinal, cervical and axillary lymph nodes enlarged, but throughout this time he noticed a recurrence of the initial fever-like symptoms: at times his temperature was elevated, he perspired excessively (particularly at night) and suffered debilitating bouts of persistent diarrhoea and nausea. Oral candidiasis (i.e. thrush) has further diminished James's enjoyment of his food, causing malnutrition and a weight loss (cachexia) from 69 kg to 49.1 kg.

James has suffered from chronic fatigue, lethargy and quite severe mood swings. Within the last 3 weeks he has developed the symptoms of a severe chest infection which has resulted in his re-admission to his local hospital with a diagnosis of *Pneumocystis carinii* pneumonia (PCP). James has been profoundly anxious and depressed at the inexorable progression of his disease and the effect that he sees this as having upon Claire, his family and friends.

James's disease management to date has consisted of antiviral medication (zidovudine/AZT), nutritional supplements and symptomatic treatment for a range of opportunistic infections as these have occurred, with social support, the use of some complementary therapies (Bowen therapy, massage, and relaxation techniques) and counselling, provided through a system of multi-agency cooperation and acquired immune deficiency syndrome (AIDS) charity networks.

AIDS as a homeostatic imbalance

Innate short-lived or natural passive immunity is conferred upon the neonate prenatally and through initial lactation by its mother, but by the time the child is 3 months old it needs to begin to acquire its own immunity which will enable it to produce a specific immune response against invading pathogens. As discussed in Chapter 13 this involves B-lymphocytes responsible for humoral immunity, and T-lymphocytes for cell-mediated immunity.

Acquired immune deficiency syndrome (AIDS) may be seen

predominantly as a dysfunction of cell-mediated immunity, although phagocytic macrophages are also targets of human immunodeficiency virus (HIV). It is a form of secondary immune dysfunction caused by infection with HIV. This is a retrovirus (it contains RNA, not DNA and utilizes reverse transcriptase enzyme to convert the RNA to DNA within an infected cell), with a particular affinity for the helper T-cells which it impairs and destroys. Since helper cells have a central role in immunity (see Figure 13.17, p.383). The virus also impairs the function of cytotoxic and lymphokine-producing T-cells and compromises the efficiency of the B-lymphocytes. The resultant undifferentiated antibody production means that people with symptomatic HIV and AIDS are unable to develop effective and specific humoral immunity to any new antigens. However, the presence of the antibodies is used clinically as the anti-HIV test to determine the HIV status of a person. This, combined with the massive reduction of helper T-cells and the probable impairment of those that survive, produces a terminal immunological deficiency and exposes the individual to repeated opportunistic infections (which may be viral, bacterial or fungal in origin). Collectively, the symptoms produce the characteristic presentation of AIDS.

Background

HIV (see Figure 13.23, p.390) is a blood-borne virus found in body fluids, whose principal mode of transmission is through sexual activity. Globally, unprotected penetrative heterosexual vaginal intercourse with an HIV-infected partner is the most common means by which the vast majority of people become infected with HIV. In Western Europe, North America and Australasia, homosexual or bisexual men, that is, men who have sex with men (MSM), constitute the largest group of individuals who have, so far, become infected with HIV. This is because of the high risk of viral transmission associated with anal sex, the propensity for this sexual practice among MSM, the multiplicity of sexual partners often associated with this group, and the biological factors associated with rectal trauma during penile insertion that allow rectal mucosal cells to be directly infected (Pratt, 2003).

The HIV infection cycle begins as the virus becomes bound to the host cell receptor (adhesion stage). The virus then becomes enclosed in a vesicle which is taken into the cytoplasm of the host cell (penetration stage) where the majority of structure of the virus disintegrates (eclipse stage) freeing both the RNA and the reverse transcriptase enzymes. The enzyme catalyses the copying of RNA to DNA (reverse transcription stage), which then becomes incorporated into the host DNA. The viral DNA now can express its DNA (i.e. genes) to produce viral proteins (i.e. enzymes via transcription and translation stages; see Figure 2.14, p.41) for viral replication. The new viruses are passed out of the host cell into the tissue fluid and blood to infect other host cells.

A long incubation period follows (8–15 years), although some patients will initially experience an acute illness similar in presentation to glandular fever. Antibodies to HIV are generally produced within a 3- to 6-month period (the 'window

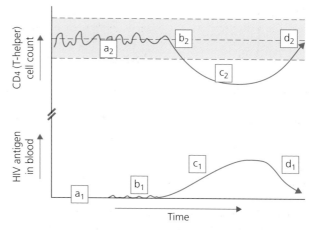

Figure 23.13 Human immunodeficiency virus (HIV)/acquired immune deficiency syndrome (AIDS) depicted as the homeostatic graph.
a_1, Absence of HIV antigen; CD4 cell count normal (a_2). b_1, Sporadic appearance of HIV antigen; CD4 cell count minimally affected (b_2). Generic symptoms of infection (lethargy, general feeling of malaise). This period may last several months or longer. c_1, Progressive increase of HIV antigen in blood indicative of viral infection. Onset of AIDS-like symptoms. CD4 count falling owing to cell destruction by the invading virus (c_2), compromising specific immune responses and allowing opportunistic infections to become problematic. d_1, Reduction of the presence of HIV in blood through the actions of monotherapy or combination drug therapy to prevent CD4 cell infection, and prevention of new viral particles forming within already infected CD4 cells. Some recovery of CD4 cell count as cell infection is reduced (d_2) with restoration of some immunocompetency

period' before which the infected individual undergoes seroconversion, and will then test HIV positive).

The ultimate progression of the disease is determined by a number of factors: the existence of any latent viral infection, other defects or aspects that further compromise the immune system, and what is thought to constitute a genetic predisposition to the development of the various symptoms, which together form the syndrome.

Healthcare practitioners as external agents of homeostatic control

Assessment

The initial diagnosis of James's HIV status probably would be made at a clinic for genitourinary medicine (GUM) clinic, following pre-test counselling from a specialist nurse HIV adviser. This would be followed by post-test counselling and support, with regular attendance the GUM clinic for much of this medical care. Once symptomatic HIV presents, the GP and primary healthcare team will become more fully involved, with community nursing input during acute episodes not requiring hospital admission.

Care planning and implementation

See Figure 23.13.

Ideally, intervention would seek to destroy HIV and restore homeostasis. In reality, intervention has two general aims:

1 To slow the progression of HIV infection.

2 To manage conditions arising from opportunistic infections.

The initial diagnosis of James' HIV positive but asymptomatic status would not be accompanied by any medical intervention, but when the condition known as persistent generalized lymphadenopathy (PGL) was recognized, he would commence continuing treatment with the specific antiviral drug zidovudine (AZT), which inhibits the enzyme (reverse transcriptase). This enzyme is needed to convert RNA to DNA so new viral enzymes can manufacture new HIV. Anti-HIV drugs are most effective when taken in a combination of three or at the same time. This is called combination therapy or HAART (Highly Active Antiretroviral Therapy). All anti-HIV therapies interfere with the way the virus tries to reproduce itself inside a human cell. Although anti-HIV drugs cannot kill the virus completely, they reduce the chance of infected cells producing new HIV particles which could go on to infect even more cells.

The anti-HIV drugs currently available for prescription fall into two main categories: reverse transcriptase inhibitors and protease inhibitors. A single drug from a third class, known as fusion inhibitors, is available to people with limited treatment options (see 'Further information' below).

The success of the human genomics/proteomic projects will no doubt unfold many other potential therapeutic targets against HIV. This combination of drugs has been shown to have some effect in delaying the progression of HIV infection and may even delay the onset of AIDS.

Symptom management is of a prime importance of the healthcare team:

- The persistent diarrhoea is managed through the use of anti-diarrhoea drugs such as loperamide hydrochloride (Imodium), diphenoxylate hydrochloride with atropine sulphate (Lomotil) and codeine phosphate. Replacement fluids such as dioralyte will help to redress fluid and electrolyte loss arising from the diarrhoea.
- Outbreaks of oral candidiasis, as occurred in James, are contained by the topical application of an anti-fungal drug (e.g. nystatin) with the use of proprietary compounds to treat the sores around his mouth and his cracked lips.
- In the early symptomatic stage of the disease, James would be referred to a dietitian for advice, support and access to an appropriate range of nutritional supplements.
- *Pneumocystis carinii* pneumonia (PCP) begins insidiously with a troublesome dry cough and some chest pain, particularly noticeable on inspiration. Upon admission James would be febrile (see Figure 16.13, p.460 and the case study on a febrile toddler, p.664), cyanosed and in acute respiratory distress. His immediate management of pneumonia would require symptom relief and an accurate differential diagnosis to exclude other types of pneumonia. Sputum obtained for culture and sensitivities, with the results of the chest X-ray, will be used to confirm the diagnosis of PCP, hopefully without the need for bronchoscopy and biopsy. There are a variety of drugs now used in the treatment of acute PCP depending on the severity of the illness. High-

dosage intravenous co-trimoxazole (also known as trimethoprim-sulphamethoxazole; TMP-SMX, or Septrin) is the drug of choice for the treatment of PCP. It can be given in low- or high-dose regimes orally or parenterally depending on the severity of the illness.
- The majority of HIV-infected patients develop a drug fever, rash and significant leucopenia (usually granulocytopenia, see p.287) when treated with co-trimoxazole. Antihistamines can be administered to counteract familiar side-effects of rash and itching.
- If the patient develops a significant hypersensitivity to co-trimoxazole, other drugs will be used, including pentamidine isetionate, dapsone and atovaquone. It is fairly common for people with PCP to have other microbial infections in their lungs, such as *Streptococcus* or *Staphylococcus*. This increases the risk that the PCP will become serious. Therefore antibiotic therapy is often given alongside the PCP treatment in order to suppress or eliminate these other infections (Pratt, 2003).

While universal safety precautions are observed by all participating staff, particular care and communication is required to prevent the severity of James's chest infection from compounding his sense of isolation and despair. His partner, Claire, and his family, to whatever extent they are able, should be encouraged to participate in James's care and support. It may be that just by reading to him, that they feel able to contribute to his care, thus helping themselves to come to terms with the situation and providing some pleasure and involvement for James.

The prognosis for James now that PCP has been diagnosed is not good and it is imperative to discuss with him, and those whom he chooses to involve, his future disease management, any respite care which may be afforded (often through the support of an AIDS charity), the continuation of complementary therapies as appropriate, and arrangements for his eventual terminal care.

The homeostatic deficit demonstrated in a person with AIDS is progressive and irrevocable. In the present state of knowledge, there is no way that immunological competence can be restored. Therefore, the need for continued support and counselling of all those who are affected by James's illness cannot be over-estimated.

Further information

It is uncertain when is the best time to begin taking anti-HIV drugs; however the British HIV Association's guidelines on treatment recommend starting treatment if you are ill because of HIV, or if your helper T-cell (called CD4 cell) count is low (below 200 cells/mm^3, a normal count in a healthy HIV-negative adult can vary but is usually between 500 and 1500 cells/mm^3). If you are asymptomatic, and have a higher CD4 count (200–350 cells/mm^3), the decision on whether to start treatment is guided by the speed at which your CD4 is falling and your viral load is increasing.

HAART combinations usually include two drugs from a class of anti-HIV medicines called nucleoside analogues, and one other drug from another class: either non-nucleoside reverse transcriptase inhibitor (NNRTIs) or a protease inhibitor. Some people take four or more drugs, particularly if they are very ill because of HIV, have a very high viral load or have taken several HIV combinations before and have become resistant to some anti-HIV drugs.

- *Reverse transcriptase inhibitors*: there are three classes of anti-HIV drug that target reverse transcriptase:
  - Nucleoside analogues, which include AZT (zidovudine, Retrovir), ddI (didanosine, Videx), 3TC (lamivudine, Epivir), d4T (stavudine, Zerit), abacavir (Ziagen), ddC (zalcitabine, Hivid) and FTC (emtricitabine, Emtriva). AZT and 3TC are also available in a single combined pill called Combivir, AZT, 3TC and abacavir in a single combined pill called Trizivir, and abacavir and 3TC in a combined pill called Kivexa.
  - There are currently two licensed non-nucleoside analogues. These are efavirenz (Sustiva) and nevirapine (Viramune). Delavirdine (Rescriptor) is also available on a named-patient basis.
  - The third class of drugs which attack reverse transcriptase currently available are nucleotide analogues. Tenofovir (Viread) is the only drug in this class currently available for prescription. Tenofovir and FTC are available in a combined pill called Truvada.
- *Protease inhibitors*: protease is a different HIV enzyme which is involved in viral replication once the HIV DNA (see above) has successfully merged with its host's DNA. Protease inhibitor drugs help to prevent an infected cell from producing new infectious virus particles. Currently available licensed protease inhibitors are indinavir (Crixivan), ritonavir (Norvir), nelfinavir (Viracept), saquinavir (which is available in two formulations, Invirase and Fortovase), lopinavir/ritonavir (Kaletra), amprenavir (Agenerase), fos-amprenavir (Telzir) and atazanavir (Reyataz).
- *Fusion inhibitors*: the fusion inhibitor T-20 (Fuzeon) is available to people with limited treatment options.
- *Other drugs*: other drugs from the above classes are in clinical trials to test their effectiveness and safety, as are drugs from other classes of treatment, such as the fusion inhibitors and the immune therapy interleukin-2. The anti-cancer drug hydroxyurea was occasionally (but now rarely) also used in the past as it boosts blood levels of some anti-HIV drugs.
- *Side-effects*: like all medicines, anti-HIV drugs can cause side-effects. Different drugs cause different side-effects. Patients need to ask their doctor or HIV advisors or pharmacist to explain what side-effects can be expected, including mild ones which disappear, and serious ones which should be reported to the doctor straight away.
- *Resistance*: resistance can develop whenever HIV continues to reproduce whilst anti-HIV drugs are being taken. However, resistance can be delayed, perhaps indefinitely, by taking drugs in powerful combinations which suppress viral load to very low levels. HIV that is resistant to one anti-HIV drug is likely to still be susceptible to some other anti-HIV drugs. However, if the patient become resistant to one drug in a class, they may be resistant to other similar drugs and this could limit their future treatment options.

Case study contributed by Judith Tyler and Iain Shuttleworth.

References

Pratt, R.J. (2003) *AIDS: a Strategy for Nursing Care*, 5th edn. London: Edward Arnold.

Further reading

HIV-AIDSMAP: http://www.aidsmap.com (accessed 20 November, 2008).

Joint United Nations Programme on Aids (UNAIDS) and World Health Organization (WHO) (2000) *Report on the Global HIV/AIDS Epidemic*, UNAIDS/00, 13E. Geneva: UNAIDS/WHO (cited in Pratt, 2003).

Vernumd, S.F., Tabereaux, P.B. and Kaslow, R.A. Epidemiology of HIV sexual transmission. In: Merigan, T.C., Bartless, J.G. and Bolognesi, D. (eds) (1999) *Textbook of AIDS Medicine*, 2nd edn. Baltimore: Williams & Wilkins, 101–9 (cited in Pratt, 2003).

CASE 14. THE CASE OF A BOY WITH ASTHMA

This case links directly to Chapter 14.

SCENARIO

Adam is a 13-year-old boy. He has been diagnosed with asthma since he was 5 years old following a history of recurrent chest infections and a nocturnal cough. Adam's mother and sister also have asthma.

He has been using regular inhaled corticosteroids as a 'preventer' and a short-acting beta-2 adrenoceptor agonist when required as a 'reliever' to control his asthma symptoms. Recently, Adam began to experience an increase in his symptoms and was needing to use his reliever inhaler daily, suggesting that his asthma was not very well controlled. Adam's mother made an appointment for him to see a nurse with training in asthma management at his doctor's surgery.

Asthma as a homeostatic imbalance

Asthma is an obstructive lung disease, the obstruction is reversible either spontaneously or as a result of treatment. Its cause is not completely understood but for certain individuals many triggers cause bronchoconstriction. The airways become hyper-responsive and inflamed resulting in oedema, epithelial damage and increased mucus secretion; this results in a narrowing of the airways.

The main mechanisms involve an abnormal response initiating a specific allergen hypersensitivity response following previous exposure. This results in antigen–antibody reactions, which induce the release of large quantities of chemicals, enzymes and cell stimulators. The consequence is chronic inflammation with infiltration of lymphocytes, eosinophils and mast cells (basophils).

Background

Inhaled allergens are the most common route for precipitating allergic (or atopic) asthma, especially in children. Inhaled allergens include pollens from grass, trees and weeds, fungi, the house-dust mite and animal dander. Pollens and fungal allergens tend to cause seasonal symptoms of allergic rhinitis and/or conjunctivitis. Allergy to house-dust mites is extremely common, causing IgE-mediated hypersensitivity reactions in asthma (Figure 13.24, p.391). Specific IgE antibody to the common inhalant allergens can be found in serum samples of atopic individuals, who may have raised concentrations.

Asthma is defined by its intermittent and variable nature and can present at various stages in life. Symptoms can appear and disappear rapidly within 24 hours or may disappear for longer periods, months or even years. It is not uncommon for some children to cease experiencing symptoms with increasing age, but symptoms may recur later in life. This may be explained by the possible dynamic nature of homeostasis (see Chapter 1, p.42).

Although the mechanisms underlying the inflammatory response in the airways are still not fully understood, it has become clear that both genetic predisposition and subsequent environmental exposure to an allergen are inextricably linked to the development of the disease. A number of genes have been identified that contribute to a person's susceptibility to developing the disease: chromosomes 5, 6, 11, 12 and 14 have been implicated to date. Chromosome 5 is showing particular promise, as it is known to be a region rich in genes coding for key molecules involved in the inflammatory response presented in asthma. Alongside these, interest in a gene known as *ADAM33* on chromosome 20, which is expressed in muscle and lung cells, is believed to be related to asthma as it may cause the airways to over-respond initiating constriction.

Many studies have revealed the strong correlation between asthma and genetic inheritance. However studies involving identical twins (who share the same genes) reveal that although they have the same chance of developing the disease, often only one twin might present the signs and symptoms of the disease. It is suggested that we inherit a tendency to develop asthma, which will only come to fruition if the individual is exposed to the environmental stimuli that triggers the gene expression. Therefore, asthma is thought to result from nature–nurture interactions.

Presentation

Such pathology presents as variable airflow obstruction associated with the inflammation of the airways, and symptoms of cough, wheeze, tightness in the chest and paroxysms of dyspnoea. The excessive airway narrowing occurs in response to a variety of provoking stimuli, such as the allergens mentioned, environmental pollutants, exercise, infections, drugs and psychological factors, including stress or anxiety.

The narrowing of the airway is detectable by an investigation in which Adam exhaled forcibly through a peak flow meter. Increased airway resistance will impede the maximal

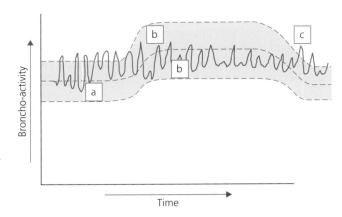

Figure 23.14 Asthma depicted as the homeostatic graph.
a, Bronchohyperactivity fluctuating with time, at times outside of homeodynamic parameters (= imbalance, signs and symptoms of disease; inflammatory response). **b**, Parameters raised through environment/genetic triggers. Bronchohyperactivity now inside the homeodynamic parameters (see text). Signs and symptoms of disease cease. **c**, Parameters may drop again later in life resulting in return of signs and symptoms

flow rate that he should be capable of achieving or the best he achieved when asymptomatic. This is a quick, relatively easy to perform and inexpensive tool used in the asthma management for individuals other than young children (who cannot perform the task effectively) to aid clinical decisions.

Healthcare practitioners as external agents of homeostatic control

Assessment

See Figure 23.14.

At the doctor's surgery the nurse took a recent history from Adam and his mother, it was clear his asthma had increased in severity; notably, Adam had developed a persistent cough and was showing signs of allergic rhinitis (hay fever). Adam also had a history of mild eczema and episodes of allergic conjunctivitis, demonstrating signs of an atopic immune system. Adam's school work was being affected by his symptoms and both him and his mother were becoming increasingly anxious.

The nurse performed the following examinations:

- peak expiratory flow rate (PEFR);
- chest auscultation.

Adam's chest was clear of any abnormal breath sounds such as wheeze but his PEFR was reduced from his previous best value for his age and height, providing signs of increased airway resistance. This confirmed that Adams asthma was not being controlled effectively by his current inhaled medication.

Care planning and implementation

Once asthma is diagnosed the aim of care is to control symptoms and restore normal or best possible airway function. It comprises effective management by both the patient and healthcare worker. Regular 6-monthly reviews should be maintained to monitor response and adjust treatment accordingly, reaffirming patient education and updating self-management plans. Appropriate pharmacological therapies may be stepped up or down according to asthma guidelines (BTS/SIGN, 2004).

The means of treating asthma are to control the airways either by preventing the onset of a severe attack, or by maintaining the airway should an attack occur. The drugs are usually administered via an inhaler device or a spacer. Spacers, either large-volume spacers or smaller aero-spacers, are devices that assist the patient (particularly children or the elderly) to administer their inhaled drugs effectively, as the synchronization involving the intake of a breath with the operation of an inhaler device is not required. The lung deposition of the drug is increased and side-effects such as oral thrush from inhaled corticosteroids reduced. Patients commenced on inhalers would be expected to show some response within 5–7 days.

Preventing inflammation and bronchoconstriction

Drug therapy includes:

- A short-acting beta-2 adrenoceptor agonist, such as salbutamol, to be used as required. These drugs act to promote the bronchodilator actions of the sympathetic nervous system on airways.
- Regular (daily) inhaled corticosteroids, which stabilize eosinophils, reduce bronchial inflammation and mucus hypersecretion, can reverse epithelial damage.

Adam now required an add-on therapy as his asthma symptoms were inadequately controlled by the inhaled corticosteroids and short-acting beta-2 agonist he had been using. Adam had moved up to Step 3 of the Asthma Guidelines (BTS/ SIGN, 2004), from mild to moderate persistent asthma, which recommends adding in further medication – either a long-acting beta-2 adrenoceptor agonist or leukotriene receptor antagonist.

With Adam's history of atopy, the nurse chose to trial a leukotriene receptor antagonist (an oral medication) as trials have shown this drug works well in allergic asthma.

Cysteinyl leukotrienes are released from mast cells and are involved in the complex inflammatory process. Antileukotriene medications block the leukotriene receptor sites, inhibiting their action. There are many other chemicals released by mast cells in this response and leukotriene receptor antagonists are only effective in blocking some of these pathways; because of this it is not an effective asthma treatment for all individuals. Adam would trial the drug for 1 month and return for review.

Indicators of assessing the outcome of asthma treatment include:

- frequency of relief medication;
- limitation of activity;
- amount of daytime and night-time cough and/or wheeze;
- peak flow reading.

Health education and support

Health education will provide Adam and his mother with information about the disease process, allergen avoidance,

treatment and action plans. Continuing support for the family will be provided via the nurse-led asthma clinic or GP. The family will be encouraged to monitor Adam's peak flow readings and symptoms to see if the drug added in to his current inhaler regime offers any benefits in controlling his asthma.

Successful management in children involves participation from all family members in partnership with the health professional. Education is the foundation for long-term control with fewer exacerbations, less use of reliever medication and less time off school.

Case contributed by Helen Bell and Val Gerrard.

Reference

British Thoracic Society (BTS)/Scottish Intercollegiate Guidelines Network (SIGN) (2004) *British Guidelines on the Management of Asthma*. Edinburgh: BTS/SIGN.

Further reading

Cross, S. and Burns, D. (2005) *Vital Asthma*. London: Class Publishing.

Townsend, H., Hails, S. and McKean, M. (2007) Management of asthma in children. *British Medical Journal* **335**: 253–7.

CASE 15. THE CASE OF A MAN PRESENTING FOR HAEMODIALYSIS

This case links specifically to Chapter 15.

SCENARIO

Daniel is a 27-year-old single man who is unemployed. He lives with his mother. He has one young child who he sees intermittently. He has a history of poor attendance at health consultations and has done so since a child. He is well known to the GP. He attends complaining of increasing nausea and lethargy. He is low in mood and has difficulty in carrying out his activities of daily living. He is known to the renal services to be at chronic kidney disease stages 4/5. After several days of severe lethargy and increasing nausea, his mother persuades him to attend his GP. Daniel's GP orders urgent urea and electrolytes (U&Es). On the basis of these and presenting symptoms he liaises with the renal team who suggest Daniel attends. Daniel did not report any renal problems in his family. His mother and father are still alive. His renal dysfunction is confirmed mechanical, not familial.

A tunnelled permanent central cannula has been placed and haemodialysis subsequently booked.

Renal failure as a homeostatic imbalance

Renal failure particularly presents as an imbalance in blood biochemistry, since a major role of the kidneys is to maintain homeostasis of body fluid composition. 'Uraemia' is a generic term used to cover a multitude of signs and symptoms. In Daniel's case, urea and creatinine levels were elevated outside homeostatic range:

- Urea: 17.7 mmol/L (homeostatic range: 2.5–6.7 mmol/L).

- Creatinine: 1301 µmol/L (homeostatic range: 70–150 µmol/L).

There are differences between first dialysis for chronic kidney disease (CKD) patients and first dialysis for acute renal failure (ARF) patients. A CKD first dialysis is considered less complicated because of the chronic nature of the presenting patient. The patient's uraemic status would typically have developed over months/years in comparison to that of ARF, which is often developed over a few hours. As a consequence of this, patients often respond differently depending on their presenting status of either CKD or ARF.

Specifically, a patient's urea level is of concern and gives the practitioner an indication of what dialysis prescription might be required. In general, it is now recognized that a patient's pre-(first) dialysis serum urea level should be reduced by 30% and no more. This is in order to guard against dialysis disequilibrium syndrome (DDS). This can be a problem in both CKD and ARF patients although primarily ARF where patients typically present with extremely high urea levels. The syndrome is characterized by the following symptoms: headache, nausea, disorientation, restlessness, blurred vision, fits, coma and occasionally death occurring during or after haemodialysis. Milder and somewhat more common symptoms include cramps, nausea and dizziness. Levy *et al.* (2004) suggest this is caused by cerebral oedema owing to an osmotic influx of water into the brain following removal of urea before equilibrium across cell membranes occurs. However, Porth (2005) describes urea as an 'ineffective osmole' suggesting that although osmotically active it is lipid soluble and therefore distributes evenly across either side of the cell membrane. However, it is the initial shift (prior to redistribution) that causes cerebral oedema and the above-mentioned potential medical problems.

Anaemia in CKD is linked to the reduced production of the hormone erythropoietin. This hormone is involved in red blood cell production between the committed erythroid precursor stage and the release of reticulocytes into the blood. Daniel was clearly suffering iron-deficiency anaemia:

- Haemoglobin (Hb) measured at 7.3 g/dL (normal 13–18 g/dL).
- Serum iron was suboptimal at 9.1 µmol/L.
- Haematocrit levels measured 0.219 (normal value 0.4–0.52).
- Serum ferritin levels were 55 µg/L. Note: in haemodialysis current target levels differ between renal units although Steddon *et al.* (2006) recommend 150–500 µg/L.

Presentation

Presenting signs and symptoms are uraemia, nausea, pallor, lethargy and hypertension (blood pressure upon admission: 189/107 mmHg). Peripheral oedema may be present, secondary to fluid and electrolyte retention (though not in Daniel's case). His jugular venous pressure (JVP), an indicator of fluid overload, was also normal. He appeared to have arrived at CKD stage 5.

Uraemia often manifests itself with nausea and vomiting if changes are great enough. Lethargy is also not unusual, and is multifactorial. It is often linked to the general toxic state of a patient (along with nausea) but is also strongly linked with anaemia (Stein *et al.*, 2004). Daniel complained of lethargy and malaise but notably he had pallor, suggestive of anaemia.

Healthcare practitioners as external agents of homeostatic control

Daniel was attending for haemodialysis. The nurse using good assessment skills can act as an agent of homeostatic control. In assessing the patients fluid status using peripheral oedema, JVP and blood pressure, the nurse can judge if there is any excess fluid which will then be removed during haemodialysis.

His pre (first) dialysis blood samples showed the following (with reference to normal/Renal Association 2007 Guidelines):

- Urea: 17.7 mmol/L (elevated)
- Creatinine: 1301 µmol/L (elevated)
- Phosphate: 2.05 mmol/L (normal)
- Potassium: 5.0 mmol/L (normal)
- Sodium: 139 mmol/L (normal)
- Corrected calcium: 2.33 mmol/L (normal)
- Haemoglobin: 7.3 g/dL (low)
- Haematocrit: 0.219 (low)
- Ferritin: 55 µg/L (low)
- Serum iron: 9.1 µmol/L (low).

Assessment

Fluid assessment

Upon questioning, Daniel denied dyspnoea at rest or upon exertion. His ankles were examined for any signs of oedema but they appeared normal. In younger adults skin turgor is not always evident because of well-maintained elasticity of the skin; it is more evident in the elderly where this elasticity has lessened. Epstein *et al.* (2003) suggests that the skin between the medial maleolus and Achilles tendon would usually be concave in appearance. With fluid accumulation this becomes flat and then convex. This was not noted but in order to confirm examination, the patient's sacral area/lower back were checked for oedema.

His JVP was noted. Examination of this is most certainly not definitive as a measure of fluid status but adds to other evidence. The internal jugular vein is joined directly with the superior vena cava and right atrium without intervening valves. The JVP is indicative of the amount of 'input' into the aforementioned atrium. Normal pressure in the right atrium is equivalent to that exerted by a 10–12 cm column of blood. By reclining the patient to a 45° angle a 'normal' jugular venous pulsation should be visible just above the clavicle. Every increment above this level indicates fluid overload or possible cardiac dysfunction, most commonly tricuspid regurgitation (Epstein *et al.*, 2003). Daniel's JVP was just visible above the clavicle. Considering the absence of dyspnoea, lack of peripheral oedema and normal JVP, Daniel was not obviously fluid overloaded.

Blood pressure assessment

Countering the lack of signs of significant fluid overload was

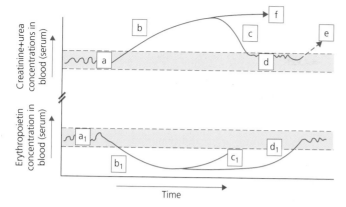

Figure 23.15 Renal failure depicted as the homeostatic graph.
a, Serum creatinine/urea concentration in health. Glomerular filtration conducive to efficient excretion of these, matching the rate of their production through metabolism. **b**, Increasing serum creatinine/urea concentrations as reduction in glomerular filtration compromises their excretion; production by metabolism now greater than excretion. **c**, Rapid decrease in serum creatinine/urea concentrations through efficient haemodialysis (i.e. replacing renal function), restoring near-normality (**d**). **e**, Gradual reversal of the effects of the haemodialysis session as impaired renal function again causes serum creatinine/urea concentrations to rise. Analogous to situation in (**b**). **f**, Chronic failure: continued increase in serum creatinine/urea concentrations (between haemodialysis sessions) as glomerular filtration continues to decrease over time. a_1, Erythropoietin serum concentration appropriate to maintain erythrocyte numbers in blood. b_1, Erythropoietin concentration too low to replace normal erythrocyte destruction rate; packed cell volume/haematocrit falls producing anaemia. c_1, Erythrocyte concentration increasing again following administration of synthetic erythropoietin (epoetin; see text). d_1, Normalization of erythrocyte concentration but now dependent on repeat hormone replacement with epoetin

his presenting hypertension. Blood pressure management is very important when caring for CKD patients. Steddon *et al.* (2006) suggest that diastolic blood pressure is the best indicator of cardiovascular risk in those under the age of 50 years. A simple reduction in diastolic pressure of 10 mmHg is associated with reductions in death from stroke and ischaemic heart disease of 50%. The Renal Association (2007) suggests a normotensive state should be aimed for with pre- and post-dialysis. It is also of note that Parfrey and Foley (1999), while investigating cardiovascular disease in patients on haemodialysis, found that a 35-year-old on haemodialysis had the same risk of death from cardiovascular disease as an 80-year-old in the general population.

Upon arrival Daniel's blood pressure measured 189/107 mmHg. Excessive fluid load is known to contribute to hypertension because of the increased cardiac output, unless of course this fluid is stored interstitially, but as previously mentioned there were no obvious signs of oedema. Daniel's hypertension might therefore be classed as 'essential' (i.e. no known cause) rather than secondary to his renal failure. Steddon *et al.* (2006) describe essential hypertension as a heterogeneous genetic and environmental condition. However, there is also the possibility that the release of renin from the kidneys is increased in response to the low perfusion in renal failure, and

this would trigger the renin–angiotensin system (see Chapter 9), and so there remains the possibility that Daniel's hypertension is secondary to the failure.

Urea and electrolytes assessment

See Figure 23.15.

Urea and creatinine remain the standard blood serum measurements of kidney function as their excretion is predominantly dependent on the rate of glomerular filtration (see Chapter 15, pp.425–9). They therefore allow for a relatively quick exploration of kidney filtering ability. They also enable one to act as an external agent of homeostatic control by prescribing the amount of haemodialysis to be administered (hours on machine), potassium content of dialysate fluid (normally 0–3 mmol/L) and size of dialyser to be used (depending on solute clearance required). They allow one to consider/exclude dehydration as a contributor to the blood analysis profile. This is typically true of an elderly patient who attends via a GP referral having suffered marked deterioration in kidney function, having previously endured a slow loss in function. Such a patient becomes increasingly uraemic, suffers a loss of appetite, marked weight loss and dehydration. However, with rehydration one might sometimes see an improvement in U&Es and subsequent discharge although of course the threat of further decline is a very real possibility. Daniel attended with lower results, although still alarmingly high. Young males tend to have a healthy protein intake, accounting for a higher urea level, while they also carry a larger muscle mass, accounting for a higher creatinine. However, a loss of appetite was not considered in Daniel's case.

Corrected calcium and phosphate levels would be requested. Phosphate is reabsorbed from the filtrate into the epithelial cells of the proximal tubule. In CKD, such homeostatic action is usually lost and resultant hyperphosphataemia occurs. Good control of phosphate is essential in protecting against vascular calcification (Goldsmith *et al.*, 1997; see also Chapter 6). It also reduces the incidence of renal bone disease.

The kidneys generally excrete calcium normally despite the renal failure by changes to the (passive) reabsorption in the renal tubule (Porth, 2005). Any mismatch is readily compensated for by changes in absorption of the ion from the bowel, and/or uptake/release from bone (see p.128 and Figure 9.10, p.217).

A normal serum calcium concentration and hyperphosphataemia were confirmed by Daniel's blood profile. This would help in determining the calcium level of the dialysate used. It also led to the prescribing of a phosphate-binding agent as a high phosphate and normal calcium level were noted; the risk is that this combination may promote the deposition of calcium phosphates in blood vessels producing arteriosclerosis (Figure 12.13a,b, p.324) and hence increased risk of ischaemic heart disease and cardiac failure (Foley *et al.*, 1996). The agent was therefore a calcium-containing medication called Adcal. If the patient had attended with both raised calcium and phosphate one might have prescribed sevelamer or Fosrenol, containing no calcium yet able to bind phosphate.

A raised phosphate level had been expected, this being common in CKD. It is difficult to control phosphate through diet alone.

Daniel was informed of the need to take these tablets with food. He was informed that if he did not do this, the tablets would have no effect and his phosphate level would continue to be a problem. We suggested that gastrointestinal disturbances were the main side-effect although uncommon. 'Safety netting' is a relatively easy practice to undertake in the haemodialysis setting. Daniel would be attending thrice weekly for long-term haemodialysis. Therefore, any medical problems caused by medication would be noted on subsequent visits. The nurse (prescriber) again acts as an external agent for homeostatic control by prescribing phosphate-binding agents after reviewing blood results.

Haematological assessment

A full blood count (FBC) was requested in order to ascertain Daniel's basic haematological status. The role of erythropoietin has been discussed in maintaining an adequate Hb. It was previously noted that Daniel had pallor and claimed lethargy and malaise.

Daniel's anaemia would be a problem. Once started on haemodialysis, the target level for patients is still subject to great debate. British guidelines suggest 10.5–12.5 g/dL (Renal Association, 2007). European Best Practice Guidelines (2000) suggest a level of 11 g/dL. The counterargument to higher Hb levels is an increasing incremental risk of access thrombosis (Besarab et al., 1998). Such concerns have yet to be confirmed using large cohort studies. In my multi-unit experience, a level of 11–12 g/dL is usually accepted.

Either way, Daniel was anaemic; therefore he was prescribed epoetin alfa (Eprex), 4000 IU, thrice weekly on haemodialysis. This was per BNF (2007) instructions of 50 IU/kg thrice weekly. Daniel was 71 kg, so 50 × 71 = 3550, rounded up to the nearest prefilled syringe amount of 4000 IU. Epoetin alfa usually takes a few weeks to have a perceivable effect. Owing to his young age, renal transplant would be the ultimate aim and so blood transfusion to correct anaemia is normally avoided, unless medically necessary, since the administration of blood products increases antibodies against future transplanted organs and hence increases rejection risk.

Again, the nurse can act as an external agent of homeostatic control. The nurse prescriber is able to review blood results noting anaemia and iron deficiency, then prescribing erythropoietin. The non-prescriber acts as an agent in the act of administering this intravenous medication.

Linked to FBC is ferritin, a carrier of iron. It is important for the patient to have good iron stores in order to optimize Hb in each erythrocyte. The Renal Association standard (2007) suggests a serum ferritin < 100 ng/mL and no higher than 800 ng/mL. This was subsequently found to be suboptimal at 55 µg/mL leading to prescription of Venofer (iron sucrose), 100 mg, once weekly on haemodialysis. Daniel was informed that the first dose is given by a doctor in order to test for allergic reaction.

Evaluation and reassessment of care

Once commenced, haemodialysis is normally a life-long treatment until a transplant is available or the death of the patient. Reassessment entails monthly (or very regular) blood analysis observing U&Es, bone (calcium/phosphate) and haematological composition. The nurse acts as an external agent of homeostatic control by manipulating elements of the patient's haemodialysis in order to increase or suppress specific blood levels and to control signs and symptoms such as dyspnoea and peripheral oedema.

Case study contributed by Carolyn Galpin and Mark Prentice.

References

Besarab, A., Bolton, W.K., Browne, J.K. et al. (1998) The effects of normal as compared with low hematocrit values in patients with cardiac disease who are receiving hemodialysis and epoetin. *New England Journal of Medicine* **339**(9): 584–90.

Epstein, O., Perkin, G.D., Cookson, J. and de Bono, D.P. (2003) *Clinical Examination*, 3rd edn. Edinburgh: Mosby.

Foley, R.N., Parfrey, P.S., Harnett, J.D. et al. (1996) Hypocalcaemia, morbidity, and mortality in end-stage renal disease. *American Journal of Nephrology* **16**(5): 386–93.

Goldsmith, D.J., Covic, A., Sambrook, P.A. and Ackrill, P. (1997) Vascular calcification in long-term haemodialysis patients in a single unit: a retrospective analysis. *Nephron.* **77**: 37–43.

Levy, J., Morgan, J. and Brown, E. (2004) *Oxford Handbook of Dialysis*, 2nd edn. Oxford: Oxford University Press.

London BMJ Publishing Group Ltd and Royal Pharmaceutical Society of Great Britain (2007) *British National Formulary – 52*. London: BMJ Publishing Group Ltd and Royal Pharmaceutical Society of Great Britain.

Parfrey, P.S. and Foley, R.N. (1999) The clinical epidemiology of cardiac disease in chronic renal failure. *Journal of the American Society of Nephrology* **10**: 1606–15.

Porth, C.M. (2005) *Pathophysiology – Concepts of Altered Health States*, 7th edn. Philadelphia: Lippincott Williams & Wilkins.

Renal Association (2007) *Clinical Practice Guidelines*, 4th edn. Accessed on-line: http://www.renal.org/guidelines

Steddon, S., Ashman, N., Chesser, A. and Cunningham, J. (2006) *Oxford Handbook of Nephrology and Hypertension*. Oxford: Oxford University Press.

Stein, A. Wild, J. and Cook, P. (2004) *Vital Nephrology*. London: Class Publishing.

Working Party for European Best Practice Guidelines (2000) European Best Practice Guidelines for the management of anaemia in patients with chronic renal failure. *Nephrology Dialysis Transplantation* **15**(Suppl. 4).

CASE 16. THE CASE OF CASSIUS, A FEBRILE TODDLER

This case links specifically to Chapter 16.

Cassius has had a febrile seizure and has been brought to the hospital by ambulance. Cassius is 18 months old, fully immunized and has been, to date, a healthy baby and toddler, reaching all his normal milestones of development. Over the last 24 hours, he has been miserable, hot, irritable, pulling at his ear and disinterested in food. Alison, his mother was concerned and took Cassius to see their GP who diagnosed otitis media (i.e. a middle ear infection; see p.155) and prescribed antibiotics. It was while Alison was at the chemist waiting for the prescription that Cassius had what she described as a fit.

An ambulance was called and according to their records, Cassius had stopped fitting by the time they arrived. Alison thought it had lasted about 3 minutes and she described his arms and legs shaking with some stiffening of his limbs, during this time he appeared to her, to be unresponsive.

On admission to the Accident and Emergency Department (A&E) of the local hospital, Cassius had had no further fits and had not required oxygen during the transfer. The crew recorded his O_2 saturation, at 94–97% in air. The A&E staff rapidly assessed his level of consciousness, airway, breathing and circulation (ABC) as he was still sleepy. Some secretions were suctioned gently from his nose and mouth; then a set of baseline observations was recorded by the staff. These included temperature, pulse and respiration and blood glucose monitoring. The nurse would have liked to check his blood pressure, but Cassius became so distressed when she applied the sphygmomanometer cuff that the attempt was abandoned. A child who is distressed will have a raised blood pressure and in these circumstances the measurement does not provide any useful clinical information.

Cassius's temperature is taken with a tympanic membrane sensor and a value of 40°C recorded; this is higher than normal. The tympanic method is a very accurate way of recording a child's temperature in seconds, rather than other methods that take between 4 and 6 minutes and require a great deal of cooperation from the child (see Box 16.14, p.455). Cassius's pulse and respiration are both elevated.

With Alison's help, Cassius is stripped to his nappy and a thin T-shirt. The doctor examines him and prescribes some rectal paracetamol and, concurring with the GP on the diagnosis of otitis media, an antibiotic. These are administered in A&E department and Alison is encouraged to give Cassius some of his favourite squash while waiting to be transferred to the ward for a period of observation. The nurse explains to Alison about febrile seizures, then gives Alison a handout that reinforces the main points made. As this is his first febrile seizure, he will be admitted to the ward until he is fully recovered.

Fever as a homeostatic imbalance

The normal set point for core temperature in a toddler is 36.7–37.7° C, but with infection, pyrogens produced by bacteria and some of Cassius's white blood cells (WBCs) can cause an increase in the set point (see Figure 16.13, p.460). Cassius's temperature of 40°C results from this resetting. So fever (pyrexia) is actually an adaptive response, achieved with resetting of homeostatic parameters. The elevated (aerobic) metabolism that generates the extra heat in pyrexia will also generate more carbon dioxide, so this will trigger a response in the peripheral chemoreceptors (see Figure 14.14, p.418). This explains Cassius's increased respiratory rate, while his increased pulse rate is also associated with his increased metabolic rate. The tissues have an increased oxygen demand and the circulation increases to respond accordingly.

Background

Febrile convulsions affect 3–5% of all children and tend to occur between the ages of 6 months and 3 years. They usually accompany intercurrent infections, typically viral illness, tonsillitis, pharyngitis, otitis media and urinary tract infections (UTIs). They are unusual after the age of 5 years. Otitis media is very common in early childhood because of the shortness of the auditory tube that links the back of the nasopharynx, with the middle ear providing a route for infective agents to access the middle ear. The distance becomes greater as the tube grows with the child and middle ear infections become less frequent.

A young child's hypothalamus is immature, which means that the new set point is likely to be higher than might be anticipated from the extent of the infection, thus making the child more susceptible to extreme temperature changes. Neural tissue is especially susceptible to changes in core temperature and a high core temperature excites a group of cells known as the 'epileptogenic' focus. This explains Cassius's fit at the onset of fever. Febrile seizures or fits are generalized, being of a tonic/clonic nature with the tonic phase lasting for 10–20 seconds and the clonic phase for about 30 seconds; however, this does depend on the individual and can last from a few seconds to 30 minutes.

Healthcare practitioners as external agents of homeostatic control

The aims of care are:

- safety of child;
- establishing a diagnosis;
- prevention of further fitting;
- supporting parents;
- education of parents around child's illness so facilitating safe discharge.

Assessment

Initially in A&E, the aim was to establish the nature of Cassius's problem. So he was rapidly assessed using the 'ABC' process in order to check for respiratory or circulatory distress. His mouth and nose were suctioned to remove any collection of secretions. Infants and toddlers tend to nose breath, so secretions will raise airway resistance and increase respiratory effort.

Baseline observations of temperature, pulse and respiration (TPR) were recorded to facilitate continued monitoring for changes that might indicate he is likely to fit again (temperature 40°C, pulse 170 beats per minute, respiration 42 per minute). His blood glucose level was checked and was 4.2 mmol/L (within normal limits, 3–7 mmol/L). Hypoglycaemia may cause fits. A full physical examination and history was taken to rule out other causes for the fit and establish a diagnosis.

Care planning and implementation

See Figure 23.16.

Cassius would be encouraged to drink; squash is usually more palatable than water. His increased metabolic rate can

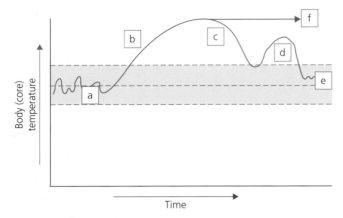

Figure 23.16 Pyrexia depicted using the homeostatic graph.
a, Body temperature before febrile episode within homeostatic range for age group (36.7–37.7°C): balance between heat loss and heat gain. **b**, Rising temperature as the rate of heat gain now exceeds the rate of heat loss. In pyrexia this occurs partly because of an increased metabolic rate as a consequence of infection, but also because of a resetting of the homeostatic set point by pyrogens produced by the bacteria and by cells of Cassius' immune system. If the set point is too high for normal neural function then a fit may ensue, as in Cassius' case. **c**, Effect of antipyretic drug to reverse the actions of pyrogens, and other interventions to promote heat loss (e.g. removal of clothing). **d**, Unstable temperature as antipyretic medication needs replenishing – tendency for temperature to increase again as the bacterial infection persists. Following antibiotic therapy and activity from Cassius' own immune mechanisms, the body temperature returns to normal range. **e**, Over the next 24 hours the set point will return to normal. **f**, Worst case scenario: no intervention takes place. Temperature remains at the new set point with the risk of prolonged or frequent fits, and a potential to cause neural damage

easily lead to dehydration. This problem may be exacerbated in toddlers by their large surface area relative to their body size (roughly twice that of an adult) from which perspiration can take place.

Cassius may suffer from physical fatigue following the fit making him reluctant to drink. An antipyretic drug, such as paracetamol would be administered either orally or rectally. The rectal mucosa is thin, so rectal administration is a very efficient way to administer drugs as they are absorbed relatively quickly, if the rectum is empty. In addition Cassius's distress makes it likely he would resist attempts to make him swallow a strange liquid in an unknown environment, so rectal administration can be less distressing and he is likely to receive the full dose.

As a focus for the infection has been identified Cassius would be commenced on oral antibiotics, to assist his immune system in removing the bacteria.

A persistently raised temperature following administration of an antipyretic means that further fits may occur if other steps are not taken to cool the child. Reducing Cassius's clothes to the minimum will reduce trapped air and lessen any insulating effect that the clothes produce. In this way, conductive heat loss to the environment is enhanced.

Regular monitoring of his vital signs will take place on the ward, usually 2- to 3-hourly when paracetamol is used, as it reaches its maximum effect in 2.5 hours. The nurses will also

observe closely for changes in his behaviour and the general condition of his skin.

His parents have undergone a very frightening experience; most parents are convinced their child will die when it happens the first time. These feelings need to be addressed and support with reassurance offered. The reassurance is based on the fact that for many families their child will only have one febrile seizure. The likely occurrence of a second fit is only 30% of children over 1 year of age, with no family history of febrile seizures and pyrexia in excess of 40°C.

Education is centred round giving the parents the skills to recognize when the child is becoming pyrexial and the appropriate steps to take to reduce pyrexia, as well as the confidence to cope with a further seizure if it occurs. For example:

- If the child appears hot when a hand is places on the nape of neck or abdomen it is advisable to remove outer layers of clothes to enable cooling to take place.
- Administer an antipyretic such as oral soluble paracetamol in the recommended dose and strength for the child's age if the child's temperature appears to be increasing.
- Encourage high fluid intake, seek medical advice if fever persists.
- A further aspect is the safe positioning of the child and how to maintain a clear airway, if this becomes compromised.

FURTHER READING

Barnes, K. (ed.) (2003) *Paediatrics – a Clinical Guide for Nurse Practitioners.* London: Elsevier Science Limited.

Dunlop, S. and Taitz, J. (2005) Retrospective review of the management of simple febrile convulsions at a tertiary paediatric institution. *Journal of Paediatric Child Health* **41**(12): 647–51.

Hawksworth, D.L. (2000) Simple febrile convulsions: evidence for best practice. *Journal of Child Health Care* **4**(4): 149–53.

MacDonald, B.K., Johnson, A.L., Sander, J.W. and Shorvon, S.D. (1999) Febrile convulsions in 220 children – neurological sequelae at 12 years follow-up. *European Neurology* **41**(4): 179–86.

NICE (2007) *Feverish Illness in Children: Assessment/Initial No. 47 Management in Children Younger than 5 Years* (Quick Reference Guide). London: National Institute for Health and Clinical Excellence.

Case study contributed by Elaine Domek.

CASE 17. THE CASE OF A PERSON WITH IMPAIRED MOBILITY FOLLOWING A STROKE

This chapter links specifically to Chapter 17.

SCENARIO

It had been a good day for Philip and Mary, at last getting to spend some time in the garden after almost a week of sitting indoors avoiding the rain. Mary was pleased to see Philip active, as she often worried about his lifestyle, which she believed to be unhealthy. Philip had protested that he eats healthy foods, and gets into the garden whenever the weather is fine. But Mary had often pointed out that he smokes, sits for long periods in front of the TV, and while its true he likes the garden, she'd like to see him walk at a good pace regularly, as she has to when she walks the dog and walks to the shops. Mary has managed to keep fairly trim since they reached their sixties a few years ago, while Philip has put on 3 stones, or about 20 kg.

Soon after supper, Mary went up to bed, leaving Philip watching the highlights of the day's football on TV. At 3 a.m. she woke and realized Philip had not come up to bed. It was not unusual to find that he had fallen asleep downstairs, so she went to wake him. Philip wasn't difficult to wake, and as he started making a move to get up, Mary headed for the door. Before she got there, Philip fell back into his chair and Mary turned to see him slumped over to his left side. His speech was slurred as he tried to explain that he felt light-headed, and the left side of his face felt strange and tingly. He couldn't move his left arm. Mary saw that his mouth was drooping towards the left. She called an ambulance and the crew arrived within minutes. The paramedic carried out a 'FAST' test, checking for signs of stroke: facial weakness (seeing if the patient can smile, and whether the mouth and /or eye has drooped); arm weakness (checking if the patient is able to raise both arms); speech problems (listening to whether the patient speaks clearly). Philip was found to have impairment in all these areas and was admitted to a specialist stroke unit in the nearby hospital.

Within several hours, following a computed tomography scan, Philip had been diagnosed with an ischaemic cerebral vascular accident (a stroke; see Box 8.13, p.183) caused by a blood clot rather than a haemorrhage. He was treated early with an intravenous tissue plasminogen activator (clot-busting medication; see Box 11.23, pp.297–8) and aspirin (anti-platelet medication).

In the specialist stroke unit, a rehabilitation programme involving an interdisciplinary team began early and continued when Philip returned home with occupational therapy and outpatient attendance at physiotherapy and speech and language clinics. Mary and Philip were both considered important members of the therapeutic team, and appreciated feeling included in discussions and decision-making and in evaluating Philip's progress.

Stroke as a homeostatic imbalance

Ischemic stroke may be caused by a thrombus, an embolus, or systemic hypoperfusion as in shock (see Figures 12.32, p.355). Many types of embolus originating elsewhere in the body could lead to a stroke including thrombotic (most commonly), gas, fat (from damaged bone), cancer cells or clumps of bacteria, typically from endocarditis. Blockage of circulation to a small or large area can arise from any of these causes, leaving affected tissue starved of oxygen. Nervous tissue cannot survive more than a few minutes without an oxygen supply. Similarly, bleeding within the brain (haemorrhagic stroke) leaves an area without blood and therefore oxygen supply. As there are multiple possible causes of stroke, there are many ways that stroke might be considered in terms of homeostatic imbalance.

Background

Stroke is the third most common cause of death in the Western world, after coronary disease and cancer. There are one or two cases of stroke in 1000 Western people each year. In England alone, each year 110 000 people suffer a stroke. As indicated above there are various possible causes for a cerebral vascular accident (CVA) leading to a stroke (the terms CVA and stroke tend to be used synonymously as they will be here, but when necessary to distinguish, CVA refers to the event within the brain and stroke refers to the resulting effects in the body).

Around 80–85% of strokes are ischaemic and 15–20% are primarily haemorrhagic. Some 20% of ischaemic strokes are the result of atherosclerotic cerebrovascular disease, 25% are caused by small penetrating arterial disease (lacunar strokes), and 20% are caused by cardiogenic emboli, most commonly resulting from atrial fibrillation, but may also result from valvular or ventricular disease or other cardiac causes. In approximately 30% cases of ischaemic stroke, no cause is identified (cryptogenic) and about 5% are identified as having 'unusual causes' which include prothrombotic states, arteritis, migraine vasospasm and drug misuse (Lip *et al.*, 2002). A transient ischaemic attack (TIA) is often described as a 'mini' stroke, and is diagnosed when the effects of a stroke last 24 hours or less. It must be regarded as a serious medical condition requiring investigation because the risk of stroke following a TIA is high.

The importance of distinguishing early between haemorrhagic and ischaemic strokes is widely recognized and a computed tomography (CT) scan should be available immediately on admission so that those confirmed with a diagnosis of ischaemic stroke can commence on 'clot-busting' medication (e.g. a TPA, or tissue plasminogen activator, within 3 hours, along with anti-platelet medication such as aspirin). However, there remains controversy over some of the published evidence for the use of TPA with allegations that some authors promoting its use have a conflict of interest.

Nevertheless, early CT scanning, diagnosis and treatment is generally accepted as very important for a good outcome. The UK government acknowledges that while the attention Philip received in the above scenario is desirable, at the time of writing he would be in a minority. Not all paramedics have the training to identify stroke and the knowledge to locate a specialized stroke unit when appropriate. Not all hospitals can provide a CT scan within 24 hours, let alone 3 hours, and problems with accessing diagnosis and early treatment can be particularly insurmountable at weekends in some areas. A need to improve stroke facilities was identified in the government's National Service Framework for older people in 2001, and the 'National Stroke Strategy' (Department of Health, 2007) following from this is aimed at meeting specific goals that would make Philip's experience of service provision the norm.

Presentation

A diagnosis of stroke should be considered if a patient presented with any acute neurological deficit or altered level of consciousness. The symptoms will vary with each individual, depending on which area of the brain is affected and to what extent. Facial paresis, arm weakness and speech impairment are important indicators. There is no reliable way to distinguish haemorrhagic from ischaemic stroke without a CT scan,

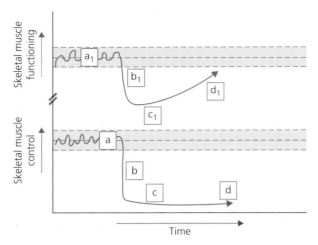

Figure 23.17 Cerebrovascular accident (CVA; stroke) expressed as the homeostatic graph.
a, Skeletal muscle control appropriate to function; sensory input and neurological output operating within tight homeostatic range to maintain normal posture/movement control (**a₁**, see below). **b**, Rapid decline in skeletal muscle control, depending upon the degree of brain infarction following CVA.
c,d, Sustained loss of control (hemiparesis; see Chapter 17) due to irreversible brain infarct. **a₁**, Skeletal muscle functioning appropriate for maintenance of posture/movement. **b₁**, Rapid decline in skeletal muscle functioning due to CVA (**b**, above). **c₁**, Sustained poor functioning owing to hemiparesis, complicated by psychological factors (e.g. fear of falling) and sociocultural factors. See text.
d₁, Some improvement in skeletal muscle functioning as remaining neurological control is used more efficiently following intervention of healthcare practitioners to improve psychological and sociocultural outcomes

but raised intracranial pressure indicated by nausea, vomiting and headache occur more often in haemorrhagic stroke.

When a stroke is associated with the anterior cerebral artery, frontal lobe function is affected, tending to result in contralateral lower limb weakness, awkward gait and personality change linked to altered mental status. If the middle cerebral artery is affected there tends to be a contralateral hemiparesis with ipsilateral hemianopia. There may be loss of ability to recognize people and objects.

When the lesion occurs in the dominant (for most people the left) hemisphere, there may be receptive or expressive aphasia, and if the parietal cortex is damaged, there may be neglect of the contralateral side. The person may not be able to acknowledge the existence of the opposite side of the body, or even the corresponding side of environment or objects. Classically, when asked to draw a clock face, only half of the clock will be drawn, including say, numbers 12–6, and the affected person is unable to acknowledge that some of the drawing is missing

If the damage is to the posterior cerebral artery vision is affected. There also tends to be altered mental status and memory impairment. A lesion affecting the vertebrobasilar artery may cause a wide variety of deficits linked to cranial nerve, cerebellum and brainstem functions. There may be vertigo, visual field deficit, dysphagia and dysarthria, syncope and ataxia. A loss of pain and temperature sensation may occur on the face (ipsilateral) and body (contralateral).

Healthcare practitioners as external agents of homeostatic control

Interventions aimed at restoring homeostasis depend on the variety of associated and causal factors. Anti-platelet and anti-coagulant medication for example are aimed at bringing the blood clotting mechanism within safe limits, where this has been indicated (e.g. in ischaemic stroke). Hypertension may have been a factor in haemorrhagic stroke, requiring efforts to bring blood pressure back to within a normal, healthy range. It may be necessary to work to return oxygen saturation to satisfactory levels, or the stroke may have resulted in problems with swallowing, requiring healthcare professionals to assist in achieving homeostasis with regard to hydration and nutrition.

The impact of stroke can be so global that there may be many other areas where homeostasis is adversely affected, and so healthcare practitioners must carefully consider the whole person.

Assessment

See Figure 23.17.

The many aspects of the impact of stroke have been identified above, and a health carer's assessment must consider all of these, taking a holistic approach so that the psychological and social factors are considered along with physiological problems. Here, the focus is on the impact on movement.

The assessment should be systematic and a conceptual framework such as the Roper, Logan and Tierney model (see Box 1.2, p.8) can help to structure it. The problem for the individual is a reduction in the previous level of independence. Factors that will influence ability to increase independence and must be considered are:

- *Physical/biological*: problems are individual, but typically, for example where there is a hemiparesis (weakness on the side of the body opposite to the affected part of the brain), there is some degree of paralysis. The paralysis can be flaccid or spastic, or often may begin flaccid and become spastic over time. In flaccid paralysis, the limb lacks muscle tone, for example an arm may hang heavily from the shoulder. This is because no nerve impulse is transmitted to the muscles. A shoulder in this case might easily become dislocated through poor handling by care workers and there is a serious risk of damage to muscles, ligaments and tendons if the limbs are not well protected and supported. In a spastic paralysis, there is too much muscle tone, there being a lack of control over the impulse to contract. Resulting contractions can be extremely painful and with limbs pulled into awkward postures, quite disabling.

- *Psychological*: the experience of a stroke can be understandably frightening, and may result in a loss of confidence in ever being able to walk again. Fear of falling may be based on a logical conclusion that further injury would set back recovery enormously. However, the fear may become more disabling than the physical problem if allowed to prevent efforts to practise mobilizing and regaining independence in movement. There is often depression associated with stroke and the low mood may reduce motivation to work to achieve independent mobility.

- *Sociocultural*: depending on the individual's social and cultural background there may be expectations that, for example, a person who has suffered an illness such as a stroke should rest in bed a great deal and allow others to tend to their needs, or that it is important to shrug off the experience and 'get on with it'. Factors like this, and religious beliefs, family values, and so on, are likely to influence the level of dependence or independence greatly, and it is important for a health carer to get to know the person well enough to understand these influences and take them into account in making an assessment.

- *Environmental*: there are many factors concerning home environments that can help or hinder a person's ability to mobilize independently following a stroke. It is useful to imagine having the same impairments as the patient – this may be a weak arm, or both limbs on one side of the body, an unsteady gait, poor balance, or choreic movements or tremor, depending on the part of the brain damaged by the stroke. Walk around the house and garden imagining how you would or would not be able to negotiate stairs for example, doorways, a small room such as a toilet, and how you would step into the bath. If you fell in a small room, behind the door, could someone get in and have enough room to help you stand?

Care planning and implementation

The care plan aimed at improving independence in mobilizing should be led by the assessment. It should involve and draw on the expertise of an interdisciplinary team. The physical assessment should inform a plan for medication, and appropriate physiotherapy, and training for the main caregiver in how to assist with mobilizing safely, avoiding injury to the patient or to themselves. The psychological assessment should inform a plan for increasing motivation to mobilize and lifting the mood. Clinical depression should be treated. Allowing time for venting frustration and expressing fears about mobilizing is important. An environmental plan should take account of recommendations by the occupational therapist and other healthcare workers involved, and must respect the individuality and wishes of the patient and main caregiver. Handrails, for example, that seem appropriate to professionals may not be acceptable changes in the house for those that have to live there.

It can be tempting for some health carers to over-prioritize their concerns about litigation, and make sure that if the patient does have a fall, they will be seen to have put as many preventative measures in place as possible, even if these are not appreciated by the patient or caregiver. This approach can lead to the avoidance of taking even necessary risks that are important in restoring independence. Work with the patient and caregiver instead, and prioritize what they need to mobilize safely as far as is reasonable, but comfortably and as independently as is manageable to the patient. If you document your reasons for taking any clearly calculated risks that are outweighed by the benefits of being independent, you will be able to address concerns about litigation confidently without being over-zealous.

Case study contributed by Steve Smith.

References

Department of Health (2007) *National Stroke Strategy*. London: Department of Health.

Lip, G., Kamath, S. and Hart, R. (2002) ABC of antithrombic therapy: antithrombic therapy for cardiovascular disorders. *British Medical Journal* **325**: 1161–3.

Further reading

Alarcón, F., Zijlmans, J., Dueñas, G. and Cevallos, N. (2004) Post-stroke movement disorders: report of 56 patients. *Journal of Neurology Neurosurgery and Psychiatry* **75**: 1568–74.

Boyle, R. (2006) *Mending Hearts and Brains – Clinical Case for Change*. London: Department of Health.

Hansard (2007) House of Commons Debates, 11th July. http://www.publications.parliament.uk/pa/cm/cmhansrd.htm

Roper, N. and Logan, A. (2000) *Model of Nursing Based on Activities of Living*. Edinburgh: Churchill Livingstone.

CASE 18. THE CASE OF A MAN WITH BENIGN PROSTATIC HYPERPLASIA (BPH)

This case links specifically to Chapter 18.

SCENARIO

Bill was 72, and retired from the civil service 7 years previously. He had enjoyed good health, but in latter years had suffered from nocturia (passing urine two to three times each night), hesitancy and decreasing flow without consulting his GP believing it to be a normal phenomenon males suffer as ageing occurs.

However 8 months ago, Bill suffered an acute bout of urinary retention. He had a hot bath, which resolved it. The next morning, he consulted his GP. On physical examination nothing abnormal was detected. His urinalysis was clear, and nothing abnormal was found on palpation of his kidneys and abdomen. There was no evidence of bladder distension, but the GP found a large soft prostate gland on digital rectal examination. An International Prostate Symptom Score was also performed. As Bill had suffered an episode of resolved retention, the GP decided to refer him to a consultant urologist. In the meantime, a blood specimen was obtained to check urea, electrolytes and prostatic acid phosphatase (PAP) concentrations. Urea and electrolytes were normal, but the PAP level was elevated. This enzyme is produced by the prostate and can be a marker for a prostate tumour; in addition its elevated blood concentration is indicative of hyperplasia. It is noted that the reliability of PAP in screening and diagnostic accuracy for prostate cancer has been questioned (Department of Health, 2004) and can give false positives and negatives.

The British Urological Foundation (2007) asserts that the main function of the prostate gland is during ejaculation. Sperm is stored in a jelly-like matrix and at the time of ejaculation sperm are mixed with fluid from the prostate gland. Prostatic acid phosphatase liquidises the ejaculate in order to improve the chances of fertilization (British Urological Foundation, 2007).

A biopsy under general anaesthetic found no evidence of malignancy, and Bill was diagnosed with benign nodular hyperplasia of the prostate. Because of his symptoms, he was placed on the waiting list for a transurethral resection of prostate (TURP). However, while awaiting his surgery, Bill suffered a series of lower urinary tract infections, common in BPH (British Urological Foundation, 2007), which were treated with the appropriate antibiotics by his GP.

However, at one stage, Bill was admitted to the local hospital in acute retention of urine and had to be urethrally catheterized to relieve the urinary obstruction. Bill eventually had his TURP. However he experienced postoperative complications and further episodes of lower urinary tract infections, with frequency of micturition and nocturia. A rectal examination by the GP confirmed a still-sizeable prostate remnant. He was therefore referred back to the consultant. In the meantime, Bill lost weight and generally felt unwell. A cystoscopy carried out under general anaesthesia showed a grossly trabeculated bladder, and a residual volume of urine of 950 mL. A further TURP was then carried out. This was successful; Bill has had no problems since and subsequently gained weight.

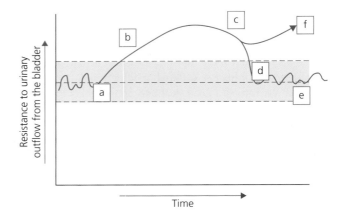

Figure 23.18 Prostate hyperplasia depicted as the homeostatic graph.
a, Urinary outflow resistance appropriate to age. **b**, Increased resistance (and hence decreased rate of outflow) owing to urethral compression by the enlarged prostate gland (note: the urethra passes through this gland; see Figure 18.2, p.486). **c**, Reduced resistance (hence improved urinary outflow) through pharmacological intervention to dilate the urethra. **d**, Surgical reduction of the prostate gland, restoring resistance and outflow to within the normal range for age (**e**). **f**, Resistance remains elevated as a consequence of urethral damage sustained during the surgical procedure

Benign prostatic hyperplasia as a homeostatic imbalance

The reason for the hyperplasia is unclear. Isaacs and Coffey (1989) assert that one major theory includes the hypothesis that pathological benign prostate hyperplasia (BPH) is caused by a shift in prostatic androgen metabolism that occurs with ageing, which leads to an abnormal accumulation of dihydrotestosterone. They suggest that the presence of prostate-specific antigen (PSA) in the patient's blood is an enzyme associated with the prostate and is indicative of hyperplasia of the gland (Department of Health, 2000).

Background

The prostate gland has three zones, the peripheral, transitional and central (British Urological Foundation, 2007). However with BPH it is the central part, the transitional zone, where the hyperplasia of the cells takes place (British Urological Foundation 2007). Further, the main difficulty with the central overgrowth is the physiological decrease in the lumen of the urethra that can lead to the symptoms and the potential for lower urinary tract symptoms, urinary obstruction, potentially resulting in acute retention of urine, referred to as bladder outflow obstruction (BOO). Prostate cancer and prostatitis are usually confined to the peripheral zone (British Urological Foundation, 2007).

Presentation

Because of its anatomical position surrounding the urethra, benign enlargement of the prostate is likely to obstruct urine flow (British Urological Foundation, 2007) resulting in homeostatic imbalance of bladder function. The resulting symptoms from urethral obstruction can vary, depending on whether the obstruction is chronic or acute. In chronic obstruction, frequency, dribbling, urgency, nocturia, incontinence, hesitancy, and stream and intensity decrease can be experienced. In acute obstruction, anuria, pain and a distended palpable bladder usually present as an emergency episode, and the patient needs to be urethrally catheterized. It is important to realize that BPH can be managed surgically or medically (NICE, 2005).

Urethral obstruction may also lead to problems with the urethra, ureters and kidneys (see Figure 15.2, p.423):

- The urethra may become distorted and displaced, so urine flow is impeded further.
- If urine is not excreted sufficiently, dilation of the renal pelvis and calyces, and the collecting ducts, will occur, leading to renal failure if left untreated. The excretion of waste products is essential for the homeostatic maintenance of all systems in the body.
- If renal failure occurs, a gross disturbance of body fluid composition arises (see p.661), which would eventually be fatal if uncorrected.
- If the bladder wall is affected, there is incomplete emptying with urinary stasis. This predisposes to the formation of stones (calculi) and infection, as stagnant urine serves as a culture for bacterial growth.

The presence of urinary retention is detectable by palpation, and by the symptoms described by the patient. While renal failure or depressed renal function could be expected to produce a change in blood chemistry, routine electrolyte checks are performed to assess renal function by measuring urea and creatinine regularly. The clinical conclusion was that his problem was prostate enlargement, rather than secondary to other systems.

Healthcare practitioners as external agents of homeostatic control

Care planning and implementation

Bill's treatment would be aimed at restoring the normal flow of urine to improve symptoms. This in turn will restore normal fluid and electrolyte balance, which may have been disrupted by the obstructive process. In the case described the prostate enlargement had not been malignant, but surgery was still indicated. Had malignancy been present, then he would also, with his consent, received oncology treatment for the tumour.

The National Institute of Clinical Excellence (2005) advocates medical and/or surgical approaches to care. See Figure 23.18.

Medical

Medical interventions, with the use of pharmacodynamics, aim to work in two ways, first with alpha-1 blockers, such as doxazosin (British Urological Foundation, 2007). They add that they are administered once a day and produce a rapid and sustainable improvement of lower urinary tract symptoms and flow. The British Urological Foundation (2007) purport that they do prevent the eventual need for surgical treatment. They act by blocking alpha-1 adrenoceptors in prostatic smooth muscle and in the bladder neck. This reduces the outflow obstruction. Symptoms usually improve within 2–3 weeks and they can be use as a long-term option. The second medical approach is the use 5α-reductase inhibitors such as finasteride. The British Urological Foundation (2007) proposes that they improve both symptom scores and urine flow rates. Unlike alpha-1 blockers, 5α-reductase inhibitors are capable of reversing the natural history of BPH (British Urological Foundation, 2007), but can take up to 6 months to observe the benefits. Patients who respond best tend to be those with large prostates and elevated PSA levels (British Urological Foundation, 2007). A combined approach of both is also advocated (Department of Health, 2000).

New advances and medical techniques are being used in BPH. Examples of this are potassium-titanyl-phosphate (KTP) laser vaporization of the prostate for benign prostatic obstruction (NICE, 2005) and transurethral needle ablation (British Urological Foundation, 2007).

Before the prostate hyperplasia was advanced, Bill's first bout of urinary retention was reversed by a hot bath. The bath probably caused muscle relaxation.

Sex steroid activities that may have contributed to the hyperplasia may also be modified pharmacologically. For example, the 5α-reductase inhibitor, finasteride, blocks the formation of dihydrotestosterone and induces shrinkage of hyperplastic tissue in the prostate.

Surgical

Eventually, surgical resection of the prostate (i.e. prostatectomy) will be necessary. While it is a commonly applied surgical procedure, the position of the prostate in relation to the urethra and bladder can make it difficult to sufficiently reduce the gland without causing extensive damage to the urethra. A risk of this method is that the ejaculatory ducts may be damaged where they exit into the urethra (see Figure 18.2, p.486), thus making ejaculation impossible.

Case study contributed by Linda Purdy and Louise Fuller.

References

British Urological Foundation (2007) http://www.britishurologicalfoundation.org.uk

Department of Health (2000) *The NHS Prostate Cancer Programme.* London: DH.

Department of Health (2004) *Making Progress on Prostate Cancer.* London: DH.

Isaacs, J.T. and Coffey, D.S. (1989) Etiology and disease process of benign prostatic hyperplasia. *Prostate Supplement* **2**: 33–50.

National Institute of Health and Clinical Excellence (2005) *Prostate Cancer: Diagnosis and Treatment.* London: NICE.

Useful websites

http://www.britishurologicalfoundation.org.uk/index.html

http://www.dh.gov.uk/en/index.htm

http://www.nice.org.uk/

http://www.prostate-cancer.org.uk/

http://www.cancerscreening.nhs.uk/prostate/index.html

CASE 19. THE CASE OF A FAMILY WITH HUNTINGTON'S DISEASE

This case relates specifically to Chapter 19.

SCENARIO

Tracey and John have lived together for 3 years and now Tracey is pregnant. She is anxious because John's family have a history of misfortune and illness that she fears may have genetic implications for her child. John's father, Mike, died in a car accident a year ago. His temperament had been increasingly erratic in the 2 years Tracey had known him. John's grandmother had died in a care home before Tracey met John. Apparently she had a mental illness, but Tracey had found that the family did not like talking about it. John's uncle Jim, aunt Amy and two cousins, Sophie and James, live nearby, but John and his family do not have much contact with them. John says that uncle Jim has a drink problem and is an embarrassment. He can be seen frequently walking in town with an awkward, clumsy gait, and on the few occasions they have met, Tracey has noticed that his speech is slurred, and that his hands are fidgeting constantly, his limbs jerk and his face grimaces. Tracey has always thought there was more to uncle Jim's problem than can be explained by alcohol consumption.

Her fears were confirmed recently when, with John, she met Sophie who asked if they were going to have the baby tested. John had quickly changed the subject, and later, would not discuss what Sophie might have meant. Tracey went to her GP to ask if he knew of anything in the family that might have implications for her baby. The GP felt that he could not discuss or disclose anything that might be confidential to other patients of his, including John's relatives. His guarded response led Tracey to demand answers from John, who eventually told her that his uncle Jim has been diagnosed with Huntington's disease (HD). John explained that this illness tends to develop in mid-life, and that Jim's diagnosis means that he has a copy of the (dominant) gene that causes Huntington's disease and so his children Sophie and James are both at 50% risk of inheriting the gene and hence of HD. John says that the family now believe his grandmother probably had HD but was never diagnosed, and that his father might have had it, but having died in the car crash, this cannot be established. If his father did have a copy of the gene this may or may not have been inherited by John and so he too would have a 50/50 chance that he has the faulty HD gene. If he does have it then he will one day develop HD. (Note though that his risk of having inherited the HD gene depends upon the genotype of his parents; see Figure 19.20, p.545.)

Tracey says she will have her unborn baby tested for the gene, and if the result is positive she will have a termination. John says he will not allow this: if the baby were positive, it would mean that John is positive also, and John has opted not to know his status. The couple agree to an appointment with a genetic counsellor, to see if they can be helped to work through their dilemma.

Huntington's disease as a homeostatic imbalance

Huntington's disease (HD) is caused by a mutation – a trinucleotide expansion – on a single gene on the short arm of chromosome 4. This was discovered in 1993, and genetic testing for HD has been possible since then. The non-mutated gene is necessary for life and is involved in the production of a protein (huntingtin) that has a poorly understood function related to the development of the central nervous system. The trinucleotide sequence is CAG CAG CAG, etc., repeated in the healthy gene some 8–36 times (see Figure 2.14, p.41). In the faulty or mutated gene, the sequence repeats beyond the homeostatic range, and occurs more than 40, often 60+ or even 100 times. There is a tendency for an association between higher numbers of CAG repeats, and earlier onset with more rapid disease progression. This association is not strong enough to make it possible to determine from the numbers of CAG repeats shown in a HD test result how early or late in life symptoms may manifest in an individual.

As a result of this mutation, cellular death occurs in the basal ganglia, in particular the putamen and caudate nuclei, areas deep in the brain involved in the coordination of movement (see Figure 8.9, p.173). Neural pathways affected lead to disrupted function in the cortex, and particularly the prefrontal motor cortex (see Figure 8.8, p.173), associated with higher functioning such as thinking flexibly, containing impulses and the ability to consider alternative views.

Background

HD is named after George Huntington, a GP whose grandfather and father, also doctors, had monitored a family affected by movement disorder and cognitive decline. In his 1871 publication, George Huntington succinctly described the nature of the disease and its dominant hereditary pattern, distinguish-

ing it from other conditions associated with chorea. It is estimated that between 1 in 10 000 and 1 in 14 000 people of Western origin have HD, with pockets of higher prevalence within the UK in Grampian, East Anglia and South Wales. Globally, Maracaibo in Venezuela and Tasmania are areas of higher than average occurrence of HD.

Presentation

Specifically, in time (40+ years in age), people with HD have trouble with 'flexible' thinking, required for planning and organising. Faces tend to be recognized but facial expressions become difficult to distinguish, particularly an expression of 'disgust'. People with HD are often 'fixed' into a line of thought (referred to as 'perseveration') and may discuss a topic intelligently, but will be unable to cope with attempts to change their view or switch topic. The control of movement becomes disordered, with characteristic 'dance-like' movements appearing (see below).

Healthcare practitioners acting as external agents of homeostatic control

The reason for the expanded trinucleotide (CAG) repetition beyond the homeostatic range as described above is currently poorly understood, as is the way in which the excess protein (huntingtin) production damages specific neuronal pathways particularly in the caudate nucleus and putamen in the basal ganglia, leaving other pathways intact despite wide distribution of the protein.

Ongoing research projects include those that centre on explaining the genetic mutation, interfering with protein production (by inhibiting mutant receptor activation; blocking the mutant gene; competitively inhibiting the enzyme, a product of the mutant gene) and cellular transplantation at the damaged sites within the brain – though this is not without its dangers of damage to surrounding tissues.

Currently, healthcare practitioners are unable to restore homeostasis and must focus on assessing the impact of disease on individuals and the family (HD provides a clear example of the way in which genetic conditions impact on whole families, including those at risk and those providing care as well as those physiologically affected), with a view to planning and implementing input aimed at relieving the effects of HD.

Assessment

A dominant genetic neurodegenerative condition such as HD affects the whole family in a very much more literal sense than most other illnesses. Family and individual assessments are necessary.

Family assessment

The family in the above scenario are struggling to function effectively with particular regard to carrying out the activity of living (see Figure 1.1, p.8) of communicating. Secrets about the family history, and the diagnosis and consequent misunderstandings about the reasons for the behaviour of relatives, have led to potential mistrust, anger and resentment. Tracey

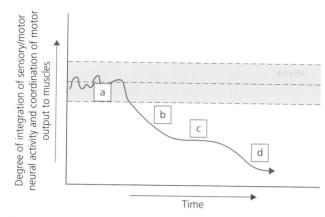

Figure 23.19 Progression of Huntington's disease depicted as the homeostatic graph.

a, Integration of sensory inputs to and motor outputs from the brain, producing posture/movement control appropriate to activity. **b**, Failing control through gene activation and onset of Huntington's disease that prevents modulation of motor outputs from the brain. Integration and coordination impaired, primarily because of inappropriate activity of the basal ganglia (see Box 17.13, p.482). Behavioural changes are also apparent. **c**, Apparent interruption of rate of declining function through effective physiotherapy and occupational therapy that improves posture control despite declining function of the basal ganglia. **d**, Progression of Huntington's disease as basal ganglia function declines further. Exacerbation of poor posture/movement control. Changes are irreversible

does not have the knowledge she feels she needs about her unborn child's health status and future prospects, and may feel that she has unwittingly become responsible for caring for John possibly in the near future and perhaps for many years, and then for her child, if and when he or she becomes ill with HD. She believes this is knowledge to which she was entitled, but John feels he has a right to keep his own risk status confidential.

Individual assessment

John may or may not have the faulty HD gene. If he does, he will certainly develop HD at some time, probably in mid-life, provided that he lives long enough. There are three aspects of HD to consider regarding the direct impact on an individual: movement disorder, cognitive decline and psychiatric problems.

Regarding movement disorder, if John does develop HD, his fingers and hands may initially fidget, and gradually awkward upper and lower limb involuntary movements will become noticeable. Over time his whole torso will begin to writhe and eventually the involvement of intercostal and accessory muscles will interfere with breathing, and consequently with speech and swallowing. In later stages muscular control of the epiglottis and the throat and face add further to swallowing problems and common causes of death include aspiration pneumonia and choking.

Cognitive decline in HD develops insidiously. Because of difficulties in thinking flexibly, ability to change a line of thinking and consider alternative perspectives, if John were to develop HD, he would be likely to be considered as unreasonable and selfish, and the limited ability to control impulses

may result in apparently aggressive behaviour, especially if he cannot get what he wants as soon as he wants it, or if a view he expresses is confronted.

Psychiatric disturbance varies individually, and may range from mild to severe depression, and in some cases there are episodes of florid psychosis.

Care planning and implementation

See Figure 23.19.

A care plan might be organized around the three aspects of HD described above. Care should be taken to avoid resorting to medical solutions where more conservative approaches may be effective. There is currently no cure for HD; hence the healthcare practitioner would not be able to restore the homeostatic status for the patient but good care approaches and some medication for specific symptoms can be effective in relieving signs and symptoms of the condition without restoring the homeostatic status.

The plan should aim at facilitating independence to the extent that is possible safely and should consider all the factors that can interfere with independence. It should be noted that while HD is known for chorea (dance-like involuntary movement), this movement tends to be more socially than physically disabling, while dystonia, spasticity and rigidity are among movement problems that do tend to cause falls and interfere with mobilizing. These can be aggravated if chorea is treated without due consideration, with medication such as tetrabenazine. Good physiotherapy and occupational therapy can aid posture and maximize control of movement, especially if sessions are reinforced by nurses or others involved in promoting independence in carrying out activities of living.

The plan should involve frequently reviewing cognitive ability, and should anticipate increasing difficulty with adapting to change and inconsistencies. A predictable day becomes important in reducing frustration and consequent anger.

Psychiatric problems are unique to individuals if and when they occur, and can be planned for under guidance of a psychiatric team.

Implementation of the care plan requires a flexible approach, based on a good long-term rapport between the care team and the patient and family. Ideally, this rapport should be established early, for example, admission to a long-term care facility may be less traumatic if preceded by some respite stays, and visits at home by staff.

Evaluation of care

Evaluation requires honesty, and objectivity. This can be problematic, because staff members at long-term facilities are very involved with the people they care for and can easily feel demoralized if their efforts are criticized. They have to be taught how to work as a team to try approaches and to objectively consider what has been successful and what was less so. Team leaders need to be sensitive and encouraging towards staff.

Case study contributed by Steve Smith.

CASE STUDIES

Further reading

Pollard, J. (2003) *Caregivers Handbook for Advanced–stage Huntington's Disease*, London: Huntington's Disease Association.

Quarrel, O. (1999) *Huntington's Disease: The Facts*. Oxford: Oxford University Press.

Rosenblatt, A., Ranen, N., Nance, M. and Paulsen, J. (1999) *A Physician's Guide to the Management of Huntington's Disease*. London: Huntington's Disease Association.

Smith, S. (2005) *Huntington's Disease: A Nursing Guide*. Ely: Fern House.

Trejo, A., Tarrats, R.M., Alonso, M.E. *et al.* (2004) Assessment of the nutrition status of patients with Huntington's disease. *Nutrition* **20**(2): 192–6.

Wexler, A. (1995) *Mapping Fate*. New York: Times Books.

CASE 20. THE CASE OF A 53-YEAR-OLD MAN UNDERGOING LAPAROSCOPIC CHOLECYSTECTOMY

This chapter links specifically with Chapter 20.

SCENARIO

Roger Browne is a 53-year-old married man who has been admitted to hospital for a laparoscopic cholecystectomy (surgical removal of the gall bladder using a minimally invasive approach) following an 8-month history of symptomatic cholecystitis. Initial attempts to remove the gall bladder using the laparoscopic method had proved difficult, as there were many adhesions, causing the surgeon to proceed to an open approach to remove the gall bladder.

Background and presentation

Acute postoperative pain is not uncommon and usually has a has a clear cause. With effective management acute pain can be either minimized or totally removed.

Pain following surgery is described as nociceptive, caused by noxious or damaging stimuli (i.e. surgical incision and removal of tissue; see Figure 20.1, p.562). This type of pain can be further divided into visceral (arises from internal organs) or somatic (localized pain). Roger was initially having a laparoscopic approach to surgery but owing to unforeseen complications, a more invasive, open method had to be employed. Roger is suffering from pain caused by surgical intervention and specific laparoscopic pain causing conditions.

Pain arises as a response to injury and inflammatory response of the body (see Figure 11.16, p.293) initiated by the surgical incision (see Figures 11.13b, p.290, 11.14a, p.291 and 21.1, p.562); all combine to cause pain for the patient. Postoperative pain (i.e. a cellular imbalance whereby pain-producing disturbances are greater than inhibiting neurotransmitters/neuromodulators) affects the patient in many ways (i.e.

has a knock-on effect, producing disturbances to organ system function, thus demonstrating the interdependency of body components, as discussed in Chapter 1, pp.8–10), for example:

- The respiratory system is affected by the patient not breathing optimally or coughing which in turn leads can lead to respiratory complications such as hypoxia.
- An increase sympathetic activity (see Figures 12.11, p.321, 12.22b, p.340 and 12.28b, p.347) can result in raised blood pressure and tachycardia resulting in increased oxygen demand potentiating the possibility of myocardial ischaemia (see Figures 12.13a,b, p.324 and 12.7c, p.313). If the patient is reluctant to move due to pain, this can lead to risk of deep vein thrombosis and pulmonary embolism (see Figures.12.18e, p.328.
- Pain can cause the patient further anxiety and lead to increased tiredness as well as a fear that those who are charged with their care are not discharging their duties to the highest level.
- Patients having laparoscopic surgery suffer from pain not only caused by surgery but by residual pneumoperitoneum (caused by gas used to insufflate the abdominal cavity) or specific complications such as biliary leak or gall stone disease (see Box 10.15, p.247).

Healthcare practitioners as external agents of homeostatic control

Assessment

Prior to surgery Roger was seen by the surgical team and the anaesthetist. He was given information regarding the procedure and its risk. Postoperative pain management was also discussed, allowing Roger to ask questions and clarify options. This process also gave the anaesthetist the opportunity to identify Rogers's suitability for pain reliving methods such as patient-controlled anaesthesia (PCA). By having all necessary information preoperatively, Roger was able to give informed consent.

On transfer to the postoperative recovery room, the patient was initially assessed using the ABC approach which established that he was breathing, tachycardic, had raised blood pressure and was able to respond to simple instructions:

- Pulse: 98 bpm (normal 60–70 bpm).
- Blood pressure: 150/95 mmHg (normal 120/80 mmHg).
- Temperature: 37.7°C (normal 36.9–37.2°C).
- Respiratory rate: 20 (normal 12–16).

As Roger is in pain he is becoming anxious. This is causing an increase in cardiovascular activity resulting in tachycardia and hypertension, thus increasing the risk of myocardial damage (see Figure 12.13b, p.324).

Roger's anxiety is also causing an increasing his respiratory rate; however due to the surgical approach his depth of breathing is reduced (Figures 14.13, p.417 and 14.14, p.418). His ineffective breathing owing to pain is affecting his respiratory effort potentially leading to respiratory complications. The response by the body to the surgery and the effects of using insufflatory gas is raising his pain level.

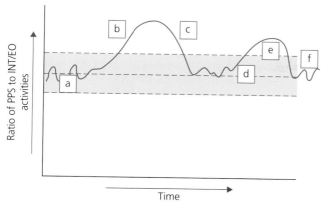

Figure 23.20 Surgical pain and management expressed as the homeostatic graph.

a, Ratio of pain-producing substances (PPS) to inhibitory neurotransmitters (INT)/endogenous opiates (EO) within normal range. **b**, PPS are greater than INT/EO (i.e. the ratio increases). This is caused by the effect of surgical intervention and administration of insufflatory gas to inflate the abdomen. If this situation continues into the postoperative period then the patient will experience considerable pain. **c**, Administration of morphine during surgery as a preventative method supplements the activity of endogenous opiates (i.e. ratio of PPS to INT/EO now restored, or even reduced beyond normal; not shown in the diagram). Further intervention (e.g. intravenous paracetamol) may also be used as a non-opiate intervention if the patient is in pain during recovery. **d**, Failure to manage the PPS to INT/EO ratio effectively during the postoperative period, leading to perception of pain and associated respiratory and cardiovascular complications. **e**, Intervention of opiate delivery via a patient-controlled analgesia device allowing the patient to self-manage the PPS to INT/EO ratio, leading to reduced pain, and (**f**) normalization of respiratory and cardiovascular parameters, as well as reduced anxiety levels

Care planning and implementation

See Figure 23.20.

Because of effective patient preparation, Roger was not given any premedication. By giving him appropriate information and undertaking good preoperative preparation his anxiety levels were reduced. On arrival in the postoperative care unit Roger would be assessed for breathing and circulation. Appropriate procedures would be undertaken to ensure that he had a secure airway, stable blood pressure and that all other body system parameters were within recognized acceptable parameters (e.g. respiration, oxygen saturation and temperature). Pain assessment would also be undertaken and the correct treatment procedures implemented, incorporating pharmacological and non-pharmacological methods. The aim of effective pain assessment would be to establish levels of pain that Roger had and to ensure that his pain was relieved to allow him to return to the ward in a comfortable condition. Other factors such as fluid therapy, relieving anxiety and ensuring a safe environment would also be implemented.

Postoperative recovery practitioners have a duty to deliver effective postoperative pain relief, their main objectives being the control of discomfort and side-effects of treatment of pain caused by surgery by using the most effective method(s) possible. This will lead to the minimizing of patient morbidity and mortality.

Primary pharmacological management of postoperative pain

Roger was able to respond to simple questions and pain assessment indicated that he was in pain. Reassurance was given and advice sought from the anaesthetist, who suggested initially that intravenous paracetamol be prescribed. Initial pharmacological approaches to the management of postoperative pain focus on the use of paracetamol and/or non-steroidal anti-inflammatory drugs (NSAIDs). With any of these drugs, the practitioner must be aware of their mode of action (see Figure 21.6, p.562) and side-effects as well as patient allergy and condition. There are minimal side-effects (but avoid in patients with liver/renal impairment) and paracetamol does not have any anti-inflammatory effect.

NSAIDs, such as diclofenac, have various properties including anti-inflammatory, analgesic and antipyretic effects. The NSAID group of drugs work by reducing the production of the enzyme cyclo-oxygenase and therefore reducing the production of prostaglandin.

Common side-effects are related to the increase in gastric toxicity and NSAIDs should be avoided in patients with asthma, reduced liver function and when other drugs such as aspirin are being used as part of an anticoagulation therapy programme.

Patient-controlled analgesia

After a short period, further pain assessment indicated that paracetamol was not sufficient to relieve Roger's pain and further advice was sought. The anaesthetist requested that Roger was given morphine using PCA. This involves the patient self-administering opioid (e.g. morphine) pain relief using an infusion-pump device. It is vital that any patient being considered for PCA has suitable comprehension of what the method involves and how to use the equipment. The technique allows the patient to self-administer pain relief on a 'when needed' basis, thus avoiding breaks in administration of pain relief and the requirement of staff to administer a drug. The most common drug used is morphine, which is given usually in a 5 mg bolus that provides analgesia yet avoids potential overdose complications such as respiratory depression. The PCA device has a lockout time which prevents subsequent doses of opiate being delivered no matter how many times the patient attempts to do so. Staff should also be aware of problems such as siphoning or faulty equipment. The PCA was duly commenced and gradually Roger's pain levels diminished. Roger had good comprehension of how the PCA device worked and was able to self-administer pain relief effectively

Complementary approaches

Although traditional approaches to pain such as pharmacological methods are still the most common way of relieving a patient's pain following surgery, the use of an eclectic approach to pain management considering all alternatives can be beneficial. Alternative methods include altering patient position (if safe to do so), and simply offering reassurance. Effective preoperative patient assessments by anaesthetists or specialist pain practitioners, including discussion of methods of postoperative pain relief can also help to reduce patient anxiety following surgery. Other therapies to consider where appropriate include, heat and cold, transcutaneous electrical nerve stimulation (TENS), music therapy and acupuncture (although some of these methods may not be appropriate in the postoperative care setting). Roger will be positioned to allow him to get as comfortable as possible and throughout his postoperative care, reassurance and effective communication will be given.

Evaluation of care (reassessment)

Although the main treatment pathway for postoperative pain is the use of pharmacological methods, it is worthwhile that the practitioner considers all alternative methods of managing pain to allow the development of an integrated approach to treat the patients' distress and discomfort. The effective management of Roger's pain will reduce anxiety, re establish normal respiratory and cardiovascular parameters and allow Roger to return to the ward.

Case study contributed by David Huggins.

Further reading

MacLellan, K. (2006) *Expanding Nursing and Health Care Practice*. Cheltenham: Nelson Thornes.

Pudner, R. (2005) *Nursing the Surgical Patient*, 2nd edn. London: Elsevier.

Woodhead, K. and Wicker, P. (2005) *A Textbook of Perioperative Care*. London: Churchill Livingstone.

CASE 21. THE CASES OF (A) A WOMAN WITH OCCUPATIONAL HYPERSTRESS, AND (B) A MAN WITH OCCUPATIONAL HYPOSTRESS

These cases link specifically to Chapter 21.

SCENARIO

Case (a)
Polly is a 23-year-old paediatric nurse. Previously enthusiastic, sensitive and compassionate, during the past 6 months Polly has become cool and detached towards her patients, uncommunicative with them, and aloof and distant from her colleagues. Her delivery of care has remained competent, but she feels beset by doubts as to her own ability, constantly checking and rechecking procedures and equipment with which she has been involved. There never seems time to complete everything expected of her, and the increasing difficulty that she finds in expressing herself in the nursing care plans means that this aspect of her work is left to the last possible moment. She has begun to dread returning to work following her time off duty, and has missed several days suffering from migraine.

Polly lives with her boyfriend, Tom, who has little patience with her current moods and feels that if she no longer likes children then she should change her job.

Case (b)
Gordon is 43 years old and has recently lost his job as manager of a farm when the owner sold it to a large cooperative with its own management structure. He has been applying for similar positions without success, a factor he attributes to his age and to his reluctance to move out of the area and disrupt his children's secondary schooling. He has had to leave the tied house that went with his post and has moved into rented council accommodation. To continue to support his family, Gordon has reluctantly accepted a position as a tractor driver on a neighbouring farm.

The reality of the situation is that he has moved from a position of considerable responsibility and great variety (managing a team of men and a substantial budget on a large farm with mixed arable enterprises and a pedigree breeding stock of pigs, sheep and cattle). His current role is subordinate; his salary, status and standard of living are reduced, and he finds the work repetitive, boring and lacking in any stimulation or challenge.

Gordon visits his general practitioner and complains of tiredness, poor sleep and indigestion.

Hyperstress and hypostress as homeostatic imbalances

Although the concept of stress is relatively modern, its study has attracted an immense amount of interest, and a variety of definitions and models have emerged (see Chapter 21). Stress has been identified as constituting a response to potentially damaging demands upon the person. This focus produced a preoccupation with the causative components of stress that has dominated research in this field. Subsequent work has developed the concept of negative stressors, and sought to identify these in relation to significant life events (see Figure 21.3, p.592). The results of negative stress have been seen in terms of occupational dissatisfaction, disengagement and 'burnout' (see Box 21.5, p.599, and Table 21.2, p.589).

While the traditional approach has concentrated on the negative effects of stress, the contemporary stance, in defining stress in terms of homeostatic balance, admits to the concept of deleterious and beneficial stress, respectively, 'distress' and 'eustress'. Furthermore, a normal individual range is established, beyond the bounds of which that person can be said to be experiencing hyperstress or hypostress (i.e. of the stress threshold) (Figures 21.2, p.590 and 21.5, p.597). To date, research has concentrated on hyperstress, with only a comparatively recent recognition of the potentially, equally injurious situation in which sustained hypostress occurs. Occupational areas that make low demands on the workers but provide little support (or actual constraint) in fulfilling those demands are potentially more stressful than highly demanding areas that give a good level of support.

Background and presentation

Given the situations as they are presented, it seems probable that Polly is suffering from occupational hyperstress (see Figure 21.4a, p.596). It seems likely that the principal cause of her hyperstress is occupationally based, as she is showing the characteristic symptoms of 'burnout' (an extreme reaction to unrelieved stress that has long been associated with those engaged in the 'caring professions'). These can be summarized as disaffection and withdrawal of involvement with those for whom they care. However, Tom's recent lack of sympathy,

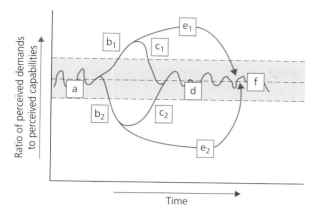

Figure 23.21 Occupational hyper- and hypo-stress depicted as the homeostatic graph.

a, Stress level maintained within homeostatic norms: perceived capabilities, perceived demands. **b₁**,**b₂**, Distress. In **b₁**, perceived capabilities are less than perceived demands (= hyperstress); in **b₂**, perceived capabilities are greater than perceived demands (= hypostress). In each case, stress-related symptoms may be observed. **c₁**,**c₂**, Reduction in capability–demand mismatches by identification of stressors and stress management (**c₁**), or use of alternative stimuli to promote eustress (**c₂**). **d**, Return of stress levels to normal (eustress). **e₁**,**e₂**, Failure to restore capability–demand mismatch, with exacerbation of signs and symptoms, and possibly stress-related disorders. **f**, Intervention to control symptoms, and facilitate return to norms

while it may be purely a response to the change he sees in Polly, could be indicative of deeper problems within the relationship that may have affected Polly's ability to cope with the demands of her job.

Gordon's description of boredom and frustration in his work, and the feeling of 'being tired doing nothing', support his hypostress (see Figure 21.4a, p.596). He demonstrates increased psychological and physiological morbidity, including boredom, lethargy and chronic tiredness. He is disaffected, and shows lack of motivation and a range of psychosomatic disorders, leading to increased incidence of sickness and absenteeism. He is showing signs of depression. Severe depression may arise, with the risk of suicide. However, Gordon has recently experienced significant trauma in losing a responsible job and an established home, and these events cause distress. This emphasizes the difficulty in determining a rigid 'diagnosis' of hyperstress or hypostress, and endorses the concept of constantly fluctuating levels of stress.

Healthcare practitioners as external agents of homeostatic control

See Figure 23.21.

These cases relate to people who are currently experiencing distress thought to be principally occupational in origin. Current thinking favours an eclectic approach that recognizes the complex interrelationship between mind and body, and cause and effect. Stress may be viewed, therefore, as a homeostatic disturbance/imbalance (see Figure 21.2, p.590, and Tables 21.1, p.587, and 21.2, p.589) that arises when there is actual or perceived demand–capability mismatch between the person and their environment (see Figure 21.4, p.596).

In the context of assisting the person to return to a level of stress within the normal homeostatic range defined by their stress thresholds, the model of clinical supervision that is advocated is one of support and development, rather than the more narrow regulation and standard setting.

Care planning and implementation of care

Hyperstress

Appropriate support for Polly will be identified only once the predominant source of her distress is recognized. It may be that Polly's stress is not isolated but indicative of job dissatisfaction among her colleagues. Any recent changes in practice (e.g. altered shift patterns) and any undue pressures should be identified and, where possible, measures taken to address these. As Polly's stress appears to be occupationally founded, support must be provided in the workplace. This will operate at two levels: individual support for Polly through involvement of the occupational health department and awareness of her manager, and an assessment of the current environment within the paediatric unit where she works.

Support will entail the following:

- Those caring for her, and Polly herself, must recognize that the level of stress she is experiencing is outside the usual limits within which her previous homeostatic norm has naturally fluctuated. During this time, the demands made upon her were within her individual capability.
- Care for Polly will need to restore the homeostasis by reducing stress levels to below the upper homeostatic parameter (see Figure 21.2, p.590). Specialist psychological intervention may be indicated, with the appropriate medical treatment for her presenting 'physiological' problems, such as her migraine.
- An individual programme of stress reduction should be instituted, incorporating techniques whereby Polly will be able to recognize and use the beneficial effects of everyday beneficial stressors (eustressors) to counteract the adverse effects of her current hyperstress.
- Medical, nursing and/or specialist counselling intervention will need to address the occupational focus of her distress, probably by providing career guidance. Has her original ambition in joining the paediatric unit been realized? If so, does she still feel that this is appropriate, or can she be developed in the role, and what will facilitate her career development? If not, what alternatives are there, and how can she access them? (Note that in either eventuality, it is important to concentrate on Polly's strengths and aspects about which she feels positive and less distressed.)

The importance of a non-judgemental approach is paramount. Hyperstress and 'burnout' are known to affect those who are caring and conscientious. Above all, a level of care should be instituted that effectively restores the state of equilibrium between demands and capabilities, irrespective of Polly's ultimate decisions about her work and her relationships.

Hypostress

Although Gordon's problems seem to be related to hypostress, there is a possibility that some of his symptoms arise from other causes. Gordon will therefore require medical investigation in case there is a non-occupational cause for his symptoms. His GP will wish to exclude other 'biochemico-physiological' causes for his tiredness (e.g. possible anaemia, diabetes, hypothyroidism, etc.) and establish the reason for his indigestion (e.g. ulcer, hiatus hernia, etc.). The sleep problem will need to be investigated thoroughly, as a history of disturbed rest and early-morning waking may indicate a level of clinical depression that will require immediate intervention to prevent suicidal behaviour.

While these investigations are being conducted, and treatment and, where necessary, specialist referral, is being undertaken, Gordon will need help in restoring his presenting homeostatic imbalance:

- Gordon needs to be able to utilize everyday eustressors that will help to restore homeostasis. Measures to promote the beneficial effects of eustressors that will provide an alternative source of stimulation and a necessary 'healthy' stress response might include working with Gordon to get him to recognize remaining areas of challenge in his life.

- Gordon has suffered an inevitable loss of self-esteem, and the lack of challenge and respect in his current work endorse this. He may be experiencing a sense of shame where his family and wider circle of friends are concerned, tension in his relationships and feelings of profound isolation.

- The fact that Gordon has sought medical opinion is encouraging, since it shows recognition on his part of the need for action to restore equilibrium in his life. Support for Gordon will need to capitalize and develop this self-awareness, to promote alternative strategies for him to adopt in relation to his work. It may be that he can be encouraged to find some unrealized potential in the job, or he may be able to find this fulfilment in other interests, family, hobbies or organizations. Given his former level of responsibility and involvement, the challenges he needs to develop to establish a pattern of healthy stressors in his life are more likely to be found in social/community activities, where he can use his former expertise and regain his self-respect.

Case study contributed by Judith Tyler.

Further reading

Dickinson, T. and Wright, K.M. (2008) Stress and burnout in forensic mental health nursing: a literature review. *British Journal of Nursing* **17**(2): 82–7.

Edwards, D., Burnard, P., Coyle, D., Fothergill, A. and Hannigan, B. (2000) Stress and burnout in community mental health nursing: a review of the literature. *Journal of Psychiatric and Mental Health Nursing* **7**(1): 7–14.

Sauter, S., Murphy, L., Colligan, M. *et al.* (2008) *Stress at Work. Publication No. 99-101*. Washington, DC: National Institute of Occupational Safety and Health (this publication highlights knowledge about the causes of stress at work and outlines steps that can be taken to prevent job stress).

Useful websites

http://www.helpguide.org/mental/work_stress_management.htm

http://www.cdc.gov/niosh/stresswk.html

Post-traumatic stress disorder:
http://www.rcpsych.ac.uk/mentalhealthinfoproblems/posttraumaticstressdisorder/posttraumaticstressdisorder.aspx

Coping with stress:
http://www.rcpsych.ac.uk/mentalhealthinfo/mentalhealthandgrowingup/32copingwithstress.aspx

Stress:
http://www.rcpsych.ac.uk/mentalhealthinformation/mentalhealthproblems/stress.aspx

CASE 22. THE CASE OF A MAN WITH LEARNING DISABILITIES LEAVING A LONG-STAY HOSPITAL

This case links specifically to Chapter 22.

> **SCENARIO**
>
> Simon is a 50-year-old man with mild learning disabilities, as established by assessment using Wechsler Adult Intelligence Scales (WAIS-III). He has lived in a hospital for people with learning disabilities for the last 40 years. During his stay in the hospital, he has lived in a variety of settings. For the past 5 years, he has shared accommodation with 14 other men who have various learning disabilities. In the last 2 weeks, Simon has left the hospital in order to live in an ordinary dwelling with four other people who have learning disabilities.
>
> With the goal of Simon's complete independence in mind, staff have been working with him to determine what his wants and needs are associated with his future life. Following discussion, Simon has revealed that he is experiencing a number of problems following his move from the hospital environment. The problems are principally connected with disturbed sleep, lack of appetite and general tiredness.

Leaving a long-stay institution as a homeostatic imbalance

A substantial number of people with learning disabilities have spent the majority of their lives in hospital wards. It has been recognized for some time, however, that many people with learning disabilities do not require care that necessitates their stay in a hospital setting, since they are not subject to an ongoing acute illness of any kind.

For many people, resettlement means giving up routines and a way of life that has been theirs for most of their childhood and adult life. In many cases, this traditional regime of care will have involved practices that have perpetuated the dependence of clients upon carers, and led to the erosion of their ability to indulge in decision making. Simon's symptoms are indicative of this and probably result from a desynchronization of his circadian rhythms (e.g. body temperature, serum constituents; see Figure 22.1, p.610 and 22.4, p.612).

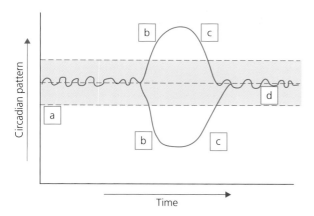

Figure 23.22 Circadian desynchronization.
a, Parameters fluctuating within range established by circadian entrainment within the hospital. **b**, Circadian pattern desynchronized by loss of institutionally imposed cues and incorporation of new cues (from the community). **c**, Nursing intervention to re-establish resynchronization (i.e. short term to encourage sleep–wake and mealtime patterns as they were in hospital, and long term to encourage the establishment of rhythms based on new cues). **d**, Parameters fluctuating within range now established by cues provided by the community environment

Circadian rhythms refer to events that are repeated in the body every 24 hours. When rhythms follow the expected patterns, the body is said to be in a state of internal synchronization.

Background and presentation

The potential for desynchronization is greater in people such as Simon, because he has been subjected to institutional practices and so has experienced regular exogenous cues that will have helped him to maintain the synchronization of his circadian rhythms. This helps to explain the tiredness and lack of appetite he demonstrates in his new lifestyle and environment. The situation is probably exacerbated by his learning disability, since this reduces his capacity to interpret and react to the changes in his lifestyle.

Healthcare practitioners as external agents of homeostatic control

Care planning and implementation of care

The main thrust of the care is aimed at transferring the locus of power away from its traditional location in the hands of carers to the prerogative of clients. Much of the creation of power is associated with the possession of information and the subsequent decision making that takes place. Institutions have reinforced tendencies in which clients are acted upon by carers, rather than with carers, leading to institutionalized practices. Community care emphasizes the client's rights as having the same human value as other members of the community. The small scale of the home in which Simon now lives makes privacy and dignity more possible, and avoids the distress and dehumanization that may accompany overcrowding.

The two main aims of care for someone in Simon's position will therefore be to reduce the impact of the changes associated with his move from hospital to community and to facilitate the resynchronization of his circadian rhythms once the move has occurred.

Reducing the impact of Simon's move

The move should be gradual. With this in mind, a number of occasions on which Simon can stay in the new home might be arranged for a number of months, with the duration of the stay being increased gradually. Thus, in the first instance Simon might attend the home in order to have a meal with some of the clients who already live there. Following this, he might stay overnight in the home. With time, he might extend his stay to a whole weekend.

Facilitating resynchronization of Simon's circadian rhythms

In accordance with a person-centred approach, Simon's symptoms should be discussed with him to clarify that his problems are associated with the difference between his present lifestyle and his previous residence in the hospital environment. For example, it might be identified that previously he was woken in the morning by carers at an early hour because of the necessity to eat breakfast and leave the home area to attend day care. He now has responsibility for this activity himself and is free to remain in bed longer if he so wishes. However, it is likely that Simon will find that he is unable to sleep beyond the time dictated by his previous routine. Similarly, if he ate meals according to a schedule devised for the convenience of the hospital kitchen, then he would be free in his new environment to have meals when he wants or in cooperation with other residents in the home.

In order to compensate for the desynchronizing effect of the shift between the long-established routines and those that are new, staff would agree with Simon to affect a number of changes to enable him to achieve circadian homeostasis once more. For example, Simon's sleep pattern should adapt over a longer exposure time, but short-term strategies might involve him having a short nap around lunchtime in the day-care service that he attends. This would enable him to avoid the fatigue caused by lack of sleep that he had been experiencing.

Another strategy that might be used is to encourage Simon to adopt an activity programme that involves cycling to improve his level of overall fitness. The benefits of this are an increased resistance to fatigue, and a raising of Simon's feeling of well-being.

Evaluation and reassessment

- Simon should have access to advocacy services that can ensure he is able to develop self-assertive skills in order that he can participate fully in decision making.
- Simon should be given further information so that he can consider seeking attendance on further educational courses and employment. This may further widen his range of friends and acquaintances and give him increased economic independence.
- The care team working in the home should encourage

Simon to talk about his previous experiences in the hospital environment as he may have unresolved feelings of anger about his earlier restricted lifestyle. The team could help Simon to record his thoughts and feelings in an anthology that both celebrates and criticizes his lived experiences.

- The care team should ensure that Simon has healthcare facilitation as many of his health needs may have been overlooked during his previous residence in hospital.

Case study contributed by Derek Shirtliffe.

Further reading

Department of Health (2007) *Valuing People Now: From Progress to Transformation – a Consultation on the Next Three Years of Learning Disability Policy.* London: Department of Health.

APPENDICES

UNITS OF MEASUREMENTS

INTERNATIONAL SYSTEM OF UNITS

The International System of Units (Syst me Internationale, or SI units) is a system of standard units used by the scientific, medical, and technical fraternity throughout most of the world. Most units used in this country are now SI units (e.g. grams, litres) but some imperial units (e.g. pounds, stones, pints, and gallons) are still in everyday usage.

The following are SI units for various parameters. Note that the basic SI unit for temperature is the Kelvin but the use of a Celsius scale is more practical for most measurements, since 0 Kelvin is −273 °C!

MEASUREMENT SI UNIT AND SYMBOL	
Mass	gram (g)
Length	metre (m)
Volume	litre (l)
Temperature	degrees Kelvin (K) (or Celsius, °C)
Time second (s)	
Amount of substance	mole (mol)
Pressure	pascal (Pa)
Frequency	hertz (Hz)
Energy/heat	joule (J)
Radioactivity	becquerel (Bq)
Forcenewton (N)	
Electrical potential	volt (V)
Electric current	ampere (A)
Power	watt (W)

The following are some useful conversions from Imperial to SI units.

Lengths

LENGTH	METRIC EQUIVALENT
1 yard (yd)	0.9144 metre (m)
1 foot (ft)	0.31 metre (m)
1 inch (in)	2.54 centimetres (cm)
25.4 millimetres (mm)	

METRIC LENGTH	EQUIVALENT
1 metre (m)	100 centimetres (cm)
1000 millimetres (mm)	
39.37 inches (in)	
1 centimetre (cm)	10 millimetres (mm)
0.39 inches (in)	
1 millimetre (mm)	0.1 centimetre (cm)
1000 micrometres (μm)	
1 micrometre (μm)	1000 nanometres (nm)

Weights

WEIGHTS	METRIC EQUIVALENT
1 pound (lb)	373 grams (g)
	373 000 milligrams (mg)
1 ounce (oz)	31.1 grams (g)
	31 000 milligrams (mg)

METRIC WEIGHT	EQUIVALENT
1 kilogram (kg)	1000 grams (g)
	1000 000 milligrams (mg)
	1000 000 000 micrograms (μg)
	32 ounces (oz)
	2.7 pounds (lb)
1 gram (g)	1000 milligrams (mg)
	1000 000 micrograms (μg)
1 milligram (mg)	1000 micrograms (μg)

Volumes

VOLUME	METRIC EQUIVALENT
1 fluid ounce (fl oz)	29.6 millilitres (ml)
	29.6 cubic centimetres (cm^3)
1 pint (pt)	473 millilitres (ml)
	473 cubic centimetres (cm^3)

METRIC VOLUME	EQUIVALENT
1 litre (l)	1000 millilitres (ml)
	1000 cubic centimetres (cm^3)
	2.1 pints (pt)
1 millilitre (ml)	1 cubic centimetre (cm^3)

FACTORS, PREFIXES AND SYMBOLS FOR DECIMAL MULTIPLES

FACTOR	PREFIX	SYMBOL
10^6	mega	M
10^3	kilo	k
10^2	hecto	h
10^1	deca	da
10^{-1}	deci	d
10^{-2}	centi	c
10^{-3}	milli	m
10^{-6}	micro	μ
10^{-9}	nano	n
10^{-12}	pico	p

UNITS OF CONCENTRATION, PRESSURE AND OSMOTIC PRESSURE

Substance concentration, the pressure of a gas or fluid, and the osmotic pressure of a fluid, are important measurements in physiology and it is worthwhile considering the units used in more detail.

Units of concentration

The concentrations of substances in body fluids and urine may be expressed as grams or milligrams per unit volume, for example grams per litre (written as g/l). Although widely used, such units are of limited use in considering chemical activities because they give no indication of the concentration of atoms or molecules present. Atoms of different elements are of different size and mass and so the number of atoms in, say, a milligram will vary between substances. The SI unit of concentration is called the mole, and 1 mole of an element will contain 6.02×10^{23} atoms (called Avogadro's number); if the substance consists of molecules then a mole of the substance will contain that number of molecules. A mole of atoms or molecules is also equal to the atomic, or molecular, weight of the substance.

Consider glucose (chemical formula $C_6H_{12}O_6$):

$$\begin{array}{ccc} 1 \text{ mole} & & 180 \text{ g} \\ \text{of} & = & \text{of} & (= \text{its molecular weight}) \\ \text{glucose} & & \text{glucose} \end{array}$$

made up of 6 moles of carbon atoms

6 × atomic weight of carbon	= (6 × 12 = 72 g)
12 moles of hydrogen atoms	(12 × 1 = 12 g)
and 6 moles of oxygen atoms	(6 × 16 = 96 g)
	180 g

(Note that hydrogen is the atomic 'standard', i.e. 1 mole weighs 1 g.)

A molar solution of a substance contains 1 mole of it per litre of solution (usually dissolved in water). A molar solution of glucose, therefore, will contain 180 g of glucose per litre. This is actually a very high concentration, far higher than is found in body fluids. The concentrations of substances in physiological fluids are usually given in millimoles (1 mmol = 1 mole $\times$ 10^{-3}) or micromole (1 μmol = 1 mole $\times$ 10^{-6}). Some biochemicals are of even lower concentrations and are measured in nanomoles (1 nmol = 1 mole $\times$ 10^{-9}) or even picomoles (1 pmol = 1 mole $\times$ 10^{-12}).

Sometimes the concentration of a hormone or an enzyme is recorded in Units or milliUnits per millilitre. In this case, the unit relates to the biological activity of the substance, with 1 milliUnit producing a known, quantified physiological response.

Units of pressure

Fluids are non-compressible. Gases, however, can be compressed into a smaller volume or expanded into a larger one. Such compressions and expansions alter the concentration of gas molecules as the same number of molecules are now contained in different volumes. Pressure is a measure of the interactions made between gas molecules and the surface of its container or chamber – the greater the concentration of a gas, the more interactions there will be per unit time. Traditionally, pressure was measured by observing how high mercury would rise up a thin tube as a consequence of collisions between gas molecules and the surface of the pool of mercury in which the tube stood. At sea level, standard air pressure is 760 mm of mercury (written as 760 mmHg; the symbol for mercury is Hg).

The SI unit for pressure is the pascal (Pa) although mmHg (or even mmH_2O for low pressure; water has a lower density than mercury) is still used for many parameters, such as blood pressure (note that pressure also applies to fluids within enclosed chambers, such as blood vessels). The pressures of respiratory gases are usually given in kilopascals (kPa) and 1 kPa approximates to 7.6 mmHg. For example, the pressure of oxygen in the alveoli after inspiration is 13.3 Pa (equivalent to about 100 mmHg).

Units of osmotic pressure (osmolarity)

The direct measurement of osmotic pressure of a solution is difficult when dealing with small samples of body fluid. However, osmotic pressure is directly related to the concentration of solute in the solution. A convenient means of measuring the total concentration of solute, and therefore its osmotic potential, is to measure how much the freezing point of the solvent (i.e. water) has been depressed by the solute. Body fluids contain a variety of substances and the unit of concentration of solute used is the osmole, to distinguish it from the mole unit for the concentrations of individual substances present. Physiological fluids are normally in the milliosmole range, for example plasma has an osmolarity of about 285 mosmol per litre. The higher the osmolar concentration, the greater the osmotic potential of the fluid.

BLOOD VALUES AND URINALYSIS

BLOOD, PLASMA OR SERUM VALUES

TEST	NORMAL VALUES*	SIGNIFICANCE OF CHANGE
Bicarbonate	22–26 mmol/l	↑in metabolic alkalosis ↑in respiratory alkalosis ↓in metabolic acidosis
Blood urea nitrogen (BUN)	5–25 mg/dl	↑with increased protein intake ↓in kidney failure
Blood volume	*Women*: 65 ml/kg body weight *Men*: 69 ml/kg body weight	↓during a haemorrhage
Calcium	8.4–10.5 mg/dl	↑in hypervitaminosis D ↑in hyperparathyroidism ↑in bone cancer and other bone diseases ↓in severe diarrhoea ↓in hypoparathyroidism ↓in avitaminosis D (rickets and osteomatacia)
Chloride	96–107 mmol/l	↑in hyperventilation ↑in kidney disease ↑in Cushing's syndrome ↓in diabetic acidosis ↓in severe diarrhoea ↓in severe burns ↓in Addison's disease
Clotting time	5–10 minutes	↓in haemophilia ↓(occasionally) in other clotting disorders
Creatine phosphokinase (CPK)	*Women*: 0–14 IU/l *Men*: 0–20 IU/l	↑in Duchenne muscular dystrophy ↑during myocardial infarction ↑in muscle trauma
Glucose	70–110 mg/dl (fasting) (4–6 mmol/l approx.)	↑in diabetes mellitus ↑in liver disease ↑during pregnancy ↑in hyperthyroidism ↓in hypothyroidism ↓in Addison's disease ↓in hyperinsulinism
Haematocrit (packed cell volume)	*Women*: 38–47% *Men*: 40–54%	↑in polycythaemia ↑in severe dehydration ↓in anaemia ↓in leukaemia ↓in hyperthyroidism ↓in cirrhosis of liver

TEST	NORMAL VALUES*	SIGNIFICANCE OF CHANGE
Haemoglobin	*Women*: 12–16 g/dl *Men*: 13–18 g/dl *Newborn*: 14–20 g/dl	↑in polycythaemia ↑in chronic obstructive pulmonary disease ↑in congestive heart failure ↓in anaemia ↓in hyperthyroidism ↓in cirrhosis of liver
Iron	50–150 µg/dl (can be higher in male)	↑in liver disease ↑in anaemia (some forms) ↓in iron-deficiency anaemia
Lactate dehydrogenase isoenzymes (LDH_{1-5})	60–120 u/ml	↑during myocardial infarction ↑in anaemia (several forms) ↑in liver disease ↑in acute leukaemia and other cancers

Lipids – total
  Cholesterol – total
    High-density lipoprotein (HDL)
 	
    Low-density lipoprotein (LDL)
	450–1000 mg/dl
	120–220 mg/dl
	>40 mg/dl
	
	<180 mg/dl
		↑(total) in diabetes mellitus
		↑(total) in kidney disease
		↑(total) in hypothyroidism
		↓(total) in hyperthyroidism
		↑in inherited hypercholesterolaernia
		↑(cholesterol) in chronic hepatitis
		↓(cholesterol) in acute hepatitis
		↑(HDL) with regular exercise

Mean corpuscular volume	82–98 µl	↑or↓in various forms of anaemia
Osmolality	285–295 mosmol/l	↑or↓in fluid and electroyte imbalances
PCO_2	35–43 mmHg (4.6–5.7 kPa)	↑in severe vomiting ↑in respiratory disorders ↑in obstruction of intestines ↓in acidosis ↓in severe diarrhoea ↓in kidney disease
pH	7.35–7.45	↑during hyperventilation ↑in Cushing's syndrome ↓during hypoventilation ↓in acidosis ↓in Addison's disease
Plasma volume	*Women*: 40 ml/kg body weight *Men*: 39 ml/kg body weight	↑or ↓in fluid and electrolyte imbalances ↓during haemorrhage
Platelet count	150 000–400 000/mm^3	↑in heart disease ↑in cancer ↑in cirrhosis of liver ↑after trauma ↓in anaemia (some forms) ↓during chemotherapy ↓in some allergies
PO_2	75–100 mmHg (10–13.3 kPa)	↑in polycythaemia (breathing standard air) ↓in anaemia ↓in chronic obstructive pulmonary disease
Potassium	3.8–5.1 mmol/l	↑in hypoaldosteronism ↑in acute kidney failure ↓in vomiting or diarrhoea ↓in starvation

Protein – total
  Albumin
  Globulin
	6–8.4 g/dl
	3.5–5 g/dl
	2.3–3.5 g/dl
		↑(total) in severe dehydration
		↓(total) during haemorrhage
		↓(total) in starvation

TEST	NORMAL VALUES*	SIGNIFICANCE OF CHANGE
Red blood cell count	*Women*: 4.2–5.4 million/mm^3 *Men*: 4.5–6.2 million/mm^3	↑in polycythaemia ↑in dehydration ↓in anaemia (several forms) ↓in Addison's disease ↓in systemic lupus erythematosus
Reticulocyte count	25 000–75 000/mm^3 (0.5–1.5% of RBC count)	↑in haemolytic anaemia ↑in leukaemia and metastatic carcinoma ↓in pernicious anaemia ↓in iron-deficiency anaemia ↓during radiation therapy
Sodium	136–145 mmol/l	↑in dehydration ↑in trauma or disease of the central nervous system ↑or↓in kidney disorders ↓in excessive sweating, vomiting, diarrhoea ↓in burns (sodium shift into cells)
Transaminase	10–40 u/ml	↑during myocardial infarction ↑in liver disease
Viscosity	1.4–1.8 times the viscosity of water	↑in polycythaemia ↑in dehydration

White blood cell count
  Total
  Neutrophils
  Eosinophils
  Basophils
  Lymphocytes
  Monocytes
	
	4500–11 000/mm^3
	60–70% of total
	2–4% of total
	0.5–1% of total
	20–25% of total
	3–8% of total
		↑(total) in acute infections
		↑(total) in trauma
		↑(total) some cancers
		↓(total) in anaemia (some forms)
		↓(total) during chemotherapy
		↑(neutrophils) in acute infection
		↑(eosinophils) in allergies
		↓(basophil) in severe allergies
		↑(lymphocyte) during antibody reactions
		↑(monocyte) in chronic infections

* Values vary with the analysis method used and between individuals.

1 dl = 100 ml.

URINE COMPONENTS

TEST	NORMAL VALUES*	SIGNIFICANCE OF CHANGE
Routine urinalysis Acetone and acetoacetate	 None	↑during fasting ↑in diabetic acidosis
Albumin	None to trace	↑in hypertension ↑in kidney disease ↑after strenuous exercise (temporary)
Calcium	<150 mg/day	↑in hyperparathyroidism ↓in hypoparathyroidism
Colour	Transparent yellow, straw-coloured, or amber	Abnormal colour or cloudiness may indicate: blood in urine, bile, bacteria, drugs, food pigments, or high solute concentration
Odour	Characteristics slight odour	Acetone odour in diabetes mellitus (diabetic ketosis)
Osmolality	500–800 mosmol/l	↑in dehydration ↑in heart failure ↓in diabetes insipidus ↓in aldosteronism

TEST	NORMAL VALUES*	SIGNIFICANCE OF CHANGE
pH	4.6–8.0	↑in alkalosis ↑during urinary infections ↓in dehydration ↓in emphysema
Potassium	25–100 mmol/l	↑dehydration ↑in chronic kidney failure ↓in diarrhoea or vomiting ↓in adrenal insufficiency
Sodium	75–200 mg/day	↑in starvation ↑in dehydration ↓acute kidney failure ↓in Cushing's syndrome
Creatinine clearance Glucose	100–140 ml/min 0	↑in kidney disease ↑in diabetes mellitus ↑in hyperthyroidism ↑in hypersecretion of adrenal cortex
Urea clearance	>40 ml blood cleared per min	↑in some kidney diseases
Urea	25–35 g/day	↑in some liver diseases ↑in haemolytic anaemia ↓during obstruction of bile ducts ↓in severe diarrhoea
Microscopic examination Bacteria	<10 000/ml	↑during urinary infections
Blood cells (RBC)	0-trace	↑in pyelonephritis ↑from damage by calculi ↑in infection ↑in cancer
Blood cells (WBC)	0-trace	↑in infections

COMMON PREFIXES, SUFFIXES AND ROOTS

WORD PARTS COMMONLY USED AS PREFIXES

Word part	Meaning	Example	Meaning of example
a-	Without, not	Apnoea	Cessation of breathing
af-	Toward	Afferent	Carrying toward
an-	Without, not	Anuria	Absence of urination
ante-	Before	Antenatal	Before birth
anti-	Against, resisting	Antibody	Unit that resists foreign substances
auto-	Self	Autoimmunity	Self-immunity
bi-	Two; double	Bicuspid	Two-pointed
circum-	Around	Circumcision	Cutting around
co-, con-	With; together	Congenital	Born with
contra-	Against	Contraceptive	Against conception
de-	Down from, undoing	Defibrillation	Stop fibrillation
dia-	Across, through	Diarrhoea	Flow through (intestine)
dipl-	Twofold, double	Diploid	Two sets of chromosomes
dys-	Bad; disordered; difficult	Dysplasia	Disordered growth
ectop-	Displaced	Ectopic pregnancy	Displaced pregnancy
ef-	Away from	Efferent	Carrying away from
endo-	Within	Endocarditis	Inflammation of heart lining
epi-	Upon	Epimysium	Covering of a muscle
ex-, exo-	Out of, out from	Exophthalmos	Protruding eyes
extra-	Outside of	Extraperitoneal	Outside of peritoneum
eu-	Good	Eupnoea	Good (normal) breathing
hapl-	Single	Haploid	Single set of chromosomes
Haem-, haemat-	Blood	Haematuria	Bloody urine
hemi-	Half	Hemiplegia	Paralysis in half the body
Hom(e)o-	Same; equal	Homeostasis	Standing the same
hyper-	Over; above	Hyperplasia	Excessive growth
hypo-	Under; below	Hypodermic	Below the skin
infra-	Below, beneath	Infraorbital	Below the (eye) orbit
inter-	Between	Intervertebral	between vertebrae
intra-	Within	Intracranial	Within the skull
iso-	Same, equal	Isometric	Same length
macro-	Large	Macrophage	Large eater (phagocyte)
mes-	Middle	Mesentery	Middle of intestine
micro-	Small; millionth	Microcytic	Small-celled
milli-	Thousandth	Millilitre	Thousandth of a litre
mono-	One (single)	Monosomy	Single chromosome
non-	Not	Non-dysjunction	Not disjoined
para-	By the side of; near	Parathyroid	Near the thyroid
per-	Through	Permeable	Able to go through
peri-	Around; surrounding	Pericardium	Covering of the heart
poly-	Many	Polycythaemia	Condition of many blood cells
post-	After	Postmortem	After death
pre-	Before	Premenstrual	Before menstruation
pro-	First; promoting	Progesterone	Hormone that promotes pregnancy
quadr-	Four	Quadriplegia	Paralysis in four limbs
re-	Back again	Reflux	Backflow
retro-	Behind	Retroperitoneal	Behind the peritoneum
semi-	Half	Semilunar	Half-moon
sub-	Under	Subcutaneous	Under the skin
super-, supra-	Over, above, excessive	Superior	Above
trans-	Across; through	Transcutaneous	Through the skin
tri-	Three; triple	Triplegia	Paralysis of three limbs

WORD PARTS COMMONLY USED AS SUFFIXES

Word part	Meaning	Example	Meaning of example
-aemia	Refers to blood condition	Hypercholesterolaemia	High blood cholesterol level
-al, -ac	Pertaining to	Intestinal	Pertaining to the intestines
-algia	Pain	Neuralgia	Nerve pain
-aps, -apt	Fit; fasten	Synapse	Fasten together
-arche	Beginning; origin	Menarche	First menstruation
-ase	Signifies an enzyme	Lipase	Enzyme that acts on lipids
-blast	Sprout; make	Osteoblast	Bone maker
-centesis	A piercing	Amniocentesis	Piercing the amniotic sac
-cide	To kill	Fungicide	Fungus killer
-clast	Break; destroy	Osteoclast	Bone breaker
-crine	Release; secrete	Endocrine	Secrete within
-ectomy	A cutting out	Appendectomy	Removal of the appendix
-emesis	Vomiting	Haematemesis	Vomiting blood
-gen	Creates; forms	Lactogen	Milk producer
-genesis	Creation, production	Oogenesis	Egg production
-graph(y)	To write, draw	Electrocardiograph	Apparatus that records heart's electrical activity
-hydrate	Containing H_2O (water)	Dehydration	Loss of water
-ia, -sia	Condition; process	Arthralgia	Condition of joint pain
-iasis	Abnormal condition	Giardiasis	*Giardia* infestation
-ic, -ac	Pertaining to	Cardiac	Pertaining to the heart
-in	Signifies a protein	Renin	Kidney protein
-ism	Signifies 'condition of'	Gigantism	Condition of gigantic size
-itis	Signifies 'inflammation of'	Gastritis	Stomach inflammation
-lepsy	Seizure	Epilepsy	Seizure upon seizure
-logy	Study of	Cardiology	Study of the heart
-lunar	Moon; moon-like	Semilunar	Half-moon
-malacia	Softening	Osteomalacia	Bone softening
-megaly	Enlargement	Splenomegaly	Spleen enlargement
-metric, -metry	Measurement, length	Isometric	Same length
-oma	Tumour	Lipoma	Fatty tumour
-opia	Vision, vision condition	Myopia	Nearsightedness
-ose	Signifies a carbohydrate (especially sugar)	Lactose	Milk sugar
-osis	Condition, process	Dermatosis	Skin condition
-oscopy	Viewing	Laparoscopy	Viewing the abdominal cavity
-ostomy	Formation of an opening	Tracheostomy	Forming an opening in the trachea
-otomy	Cut	Lobotomy	Cut of a lobe
-philic	Loving	Hydrophilic	Water-loving
-penia	Lack	Leucopenia	Lack of white (cells)
-phobic	Fearing	Hydrophobic	Water-fearing
-plasia	Growth, formation	Hyperplasia	Excessive growth
-plasm	Substance, matter	Neoplasm	New matter
-plegia	Paralysis	Triplegia	Paralysis in three limbs
-pnoea	Breath, breathing	Apnoea	Cessation of breathing
-(r)rhage, -(r)rhagia	Breaking out, discharge	Haemorrhage	Blood discharge
-(r)rhoea	Flow	Diarrhoea	Flow through (intestines)
-some	Body	Chromosome	Stained body
-tensin, -tension	Pressure	Hypertension	High pressure
-tonic	Pressure, tension	Isotonic	Same pressure
-uria	Refers to urine condition	Proteinuria	Protein in the urine

WORD PARTS COMMONLY USED AS ROOTS

Word part	Meaning	Example	Meaning of example
acro-	Extremity	Acromegaly	Enlargement of extremities
aden-	Gland	Adenoma	Tumour of glandular tissue
aesthe-	Sensation	Anaesthesia	Condition of no sensation
alveol-	Small, hollow, cavity	Alveolus	Small air sac in the lung
angi-	Vessel	Angioplasty	Reshaping a vessel
arthr-	Joint	Arthritis	Joint inflammation
bar-	Pressure	Baroreceptor	Pressure receptor
bili-	Bile	Bilirubin	Orange-yellow bile pigment
brachi-	Arm	Brachial	Pertaining to the arm
brady-	Slow	Bradycardia	Slow heart rate
bronch-	Air passage	Bronchitis	Inflammation of pulmonary passages
(bronchi)			
calc-	Calcium; limestone	Hypocalcaemia	Low blood calcium level
carcin-	Cancer	Carcinogen	Cancer-producer
card-	Heart	Cardiology	Study of the heart
cephal-	Head, brain	Encephalitis	Brain inflammation
cerv-	Neck	Cervicitis	Inflammation of (uterine) cervix
chem-	Chemical	Chemotherapy	Chemical treatment
chol-	Bile	Chotecystectomy	Removal of bile (gall) bladder
chondr-	Cartilage	Chondroma	Tumour of cartilage tissue
chrom-	Colour	Chromosome	Stained body
corp-	Body	Corpus luteum	Yellow body
cortico-	Pertaining to cortex	Corticosteroid	Steroid secreted by (adrenal) cortex
crani-	Skull	Intracranial	Within the skull
crypt-	Hidden	Cryptorchidism	Undescended testis
cusp-	Point	Tricuspid	Three-pointed
cut(an)-	Skin	Transcutaneous	Through the skin
cyan-	Blue	Cyanosis	Condition of blueness
cyst-	Bladder	Cystitis	Bladder inflammation
cyt-	Cell	Cytotoxin	Cell poison
dactyl-	Fingers, toes (digits)	Syndactyly	Joined digits
dendr-	Tree; branched	Oligodendrocyte	Branched nervous tissue cell
derm-	Skin	Dermatitis	Skin inflammation
diastol-	Relax; stand apart	Diastole	Relaxation phase of heart beat
ejacul-	To throw out	Ejaculation	Expulsion (of semen)
electr-	Electrical	Electrocardiogram	Record of electrical activity of heart
enter-	Intestine	Enteritis	Intestinal inflammation
eryth(r)-	Red	Erythrocyte	Red (blood) cell
gastr-	Stomach	Gastritis	Stomach inflammation
gest-	To bear, carry	Gestation	Pregnancy
gingiv-	Gums	Gingivitis	Gum inflammation
glomer-	Wound into a ball	Glomerulus	Rounded tuft of vessels
gloss-	Tongue	Hypoglossal	Under the tongue
gluc-	Glucose, sugar	Glucosuria	Glucose in urine
glyc-	Sugar (carbohydrate); glucose	Glycolipid	Carbohydrate–lipid combination
hepat-	Liver	Hepatitis	Liver inflammation
hist-	Tissue	Histology	Study of tissues
hydro-	Water	Hydrocephalus	Water on the brain
hyster-	Uterus	Hysterectomy	Removal of the uterus
kal-	Potassium	Hyperkalaemia	Elevated blood potassium level
kary-	Nucleus	Karyotype	Array of chromosomes from nucleus
lact-	Milk; milk production	Lactose	Milk sugar
leuc-	White	Leucorrhoea	White flow (discharge)
lig-	To tie, bind	Ligament	Tissue that binds bones
lip-	Lipid (fat)	Lipoma	Fatty tumour
lys-	Break apart	Haemolysis	Breaking of blood cells
mal-	Bad	Malabsorption	Improper absorption
melan-	Black	Melanin	Black protein
men-, mens-, (menstru-)	Month (monthly)	Amenorrhoea	Absence of monthly flow
metr-	Uterus	Endometrium	Uterine lining
muta-	Change	Mutagen	Change-maker
my-, myo-	Muscle	Myopathy	Muscle disease
myel-	Marrow	Myeloma	(Bone) marrow tumour

myx-	Mucus	Myxoedema	Mucous oedema
nat-	Birth	Neonatal	Pertaining to newborns (infants)
natr-	Sodium	Natriuresis	Elevated sodium in urine
nephr-	Nephron, kidney	Nephritis	Kidney inflammation
neur-	Nerve	Neuralgia	Nerve pain
noct-, nyct-	Night	Nocturia	Urination at night
ocul-	Eye	Binocular	Two-eyed
odont-	Tooth	Periodontitis	Inflammation (of tissue) around the teeth
onco-	Cancer	Oncogene	Cancer gene
ophthalm-	Eye	Ophthalmology	Study of the eye
osteo-	Bone	Osteoma	Bone tumour
oto-	Ear	Otosclerosis	Hardening of ear tissue
ov-, oo-	Egg	Oogenesis	Egg production
oxy-	Oxygen	Oxyhaemoglobin	Oxygen–haemoglobin combination
path-	Disease	Neuropathy	Nerve disease
phag-	Eat	Phagocytosis	cell eating
pharm-	drug	Pharmacology	Study of drugs
photo-	Light	Photopigment	Light-sensitive pigment
physio-	Nature (function) of	Physiology	Study of biological function
pino-	Drink	Pinocytosis	Cell drinking
plex-	Twisted; woven	Nerve plexus	Complex of interwoven nerve fibres
pneumo-	Air, breath	Pneumothorax	Air in the thorax
pneumon-	Lung	Pneumonia	Lung condition
pod-	Foot	Podocyte	Cell with feet
poie-	Make; produce	Haemopoiesis	Blood cell production
presby-	Old	Presbyopia	Old vision
proct-	Rectum	Proctoscope	Instrument for viewing the rectum
pseud-	False	Pseudopodia	False feet
psych-	Mind	Psychiatry	Treatment of the mind
pyel-	Pelvis	Pyelogram	Image of the kidney pelvis
pyro-	Heat; fever	Pyrogen	Fever producer
ren-	Kidney	Renocortical	Referring to the cortex of the kidney
sarco-	Flesh; muscle	Sarcolemma	Muscle fibre membrane
semen-, semin-	Seed; sperm	Seminiferous tubule	Sperm-bearing tubule
sept-	Contamination	Septicaemia	Contamination of the blood
sigm-	Greek Σ or Roman S	Sigmoid colon	S-shaped colon
son-	Sound	Sonography	Imaging using sound
spiro-, -spire	Breathe	Spirometry	Measurement of breathing
stat-, stas-	A standing, stopping	Homeostasis	Staying the same
syn-	Together	Syndrome	Sings appearing together
systol-	Contract; stand together	Systole	Contraction phase of the heart beat
tachy-	Fast	Tachycardia	Rapid heart rate
therm-	Heat	Thermoreceptor	Heat receptor
thromb-	Clot	Thrombosis	Condition of abnormal blood clotting
tox-	Poison	Cytotoxin	Cell poison
troph-	Grow; nourish	Hypertrophy	Excessive growth
tympan-	Drum	Tympanum	Eardrum
varic-	Enlarged vessel	Varicose vein	Enlarged vein
vas-	Vessel, duct	Vasoconstriction	Vessel narrowing
vol-	Volume	Hypovolaemic	Characterized by low volume

* Tables in Appendix C are reproduced, with permission from Thibeaudeau, G.A. and Patton, K.T. (1992). *The human body in health and disease*. St Louis: Mosby.

* A term ending in -*graph* refers to apparatus that results in a visual and/or recorded representation of biological phenomena, whereas a term ending in -*graphy* is the technique or process of using the apparatus. A term ending in -*gram* is the record itself. Example: In electrocardio*graphy*, an electrocardio*graph* is used in producing an electrocardio*gram*.

SYMBOLS AND COMMON CLINICAL ABBREVIATIONS

Many medical terms are commonly expressed in abbreviated form. The following list is designed to familiarize you with some of these abbreviations. Most of the terms have been used in the book, however, some are included because they are frequently used.

SYMBOLS

♀, 0	female
♂,	male
∞	infinity
α	alpha
β	beta
γ	gamma

ABBREVIATIONS

Ab	antibody; abortion
ACTH	adrenocorticotropic hormone
ADH	antidiuretic hormone
Ag	antigen
AIDS	acquired immune deficiency syndrome
ANS	autonomic nervous system
ARD	acute respiratory system
ARF	acute renal failure
ATP	adenosine triphosphate
AV	atrioventricular
BBB	bloodÑbrain barrier; bundle branch block
BBT	basal body temperature
BMR	basal metabolic rate
BP	blood pressure
BPM	beats per minute
BS	blood sugar
C	Celsius
CABG	coronary artery bypass grafting
CAD	coronary artery disease
CCU	cardiac care unit; coronary care unit
CF	cystic fibrosis; cardiac failure
CH	cholesterol
CHF	congestive heart failure
CNS	central nervous system
CO	cardiac output; carbon monoxide
COAD	chronic obstructive airways disease
CSF	cerebrospinal fluid
CVA	cerebrovascular accident
CVD	cardiovascular disease
CVS	chorionic villus sampling
DBP	diastolic blood pressure
DNA	deoxyribonucleic acid
DVT	deep venous thrombosis
ECF	extracellular fluid
ECG	electrocardiogram
EEG	electroencephalogram
EM	electron micrograph
EMG	electromyogram
EPSP	excitatory post-synaptic potential
ER	endoplasmic reticulum
ESR	erythrocyte sedimentation rate
ESV	end-systolic volume
F	Fahrenheit
FAS	fetal alcohol syndrome
FSH	follicle-stimulating hormone
GAS	general adaptation syndrome
GFR	glomerular filtration rate
GI	gastrointestinal
GIFT	gamete intrafallopian transfer
Hb	haemoglobin
hCG	human chorionic gonadotropin
Hct	haematocrit
HDL	high-density lipoprotein
HDN	haemolytic disease of newborn
HF	heart failure
hGH	human growth hormone
HR	heart rate
HSV	herpes simplex virus
ICF	intracellular fluid
Ig	immunoglobin
IPSP	inhibitory post-synaptic potential
IUD	intrauterine device
i.v.	intravenous
IVC	inferior vena cava
IVF	in vitro fertilization
KS	Kaposl's sarcoma
kPa	kilopascal
LDL	low-density lipoprotein
LH	luteinizing hormone
mEq/l	milliequivalents per litre
MI	myocardial infarction
mm³	cubic millimetre
mmHg	millimetres of mercury
MS	multiple sclerosis
MSH	melanocyte-stimulating hormone
NSAID	non-steroidal anti-inflammatory drug

NTP	normal temperature and pressure		SA	sinoatrial
OD	overdose		SBP	systolic blood pressure
OT	oxytocin		SCA	sickle cell anaemia
P	pressure		SCD	sudden cardiac death
PCP	*Pneumocystis carinii* pneumonia		SCID	severe combined immunodeficiency syndrome
PCV	packed cell volume		SIDS	sudden infant death syndrome
PG	prostaglandin		SNS	somatic nervous system
pH	hydrogen ion concentration		STD	sexually transmitted disease
PKU	phenylketonuria		SV	stroke volume
PMS	premenstrual syndrome		SVC	superior vena cava
PNS	peripheral nervous system		T	temperature
PRL	prolactin		TB	tuberculosis
PROG	progesterone		TIA	transient ischaemic attack
PTH	parathyroid hormone		TPR	temperature, pulse, and respiration
RBC	red blood cell; red blood count		TSH	thyroid-stimulating hormone
RDS	respiratory distress syndrome		URI	upper respiratory infection
REM	rapid eye movement		UTI	urinary tract infection
Rh	rhesus		UV	ultraviolet
RNA	ribonucleic acid		VF	ventricular fibrillation
RR	respiratory rate		VS	vital signs
RRR	regular rate and rhythm (heart)		WBC	white blood cell; white blood count

Index

Figures and tables are comprehensively referred to from the text. Therefore, significant material in figures and tables have only been given a page reference in the absence of text referring to that figure or table on that page.